Veterinary Pathophysiology

Veterinary Pathophysiology

Edited by

Robert H. Dunlop

Charles-Henri Malbert

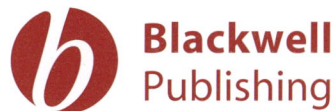

Blackwell Publishing Professional
2121 State Avenue, Ames, Iowa 50014, USA

Orders: 1-800-862-6657
Office: 1-515-292-0140
Fax: 1-515-292-3348
Web site: www.blackwellprofessional.com

Blackwell Publishing Ltd
9600 Garsington Road, Oxford OX4 2DQ, UK
Tel.: +44 (0)1865 776868

Blackwell Publishing Asia
550 Swanston Street, Carlton, Victoria 3053, Australia
Tel.: +61 (0)3 8359 1011

First edition, 2004

Veterinary pathophysiology/[edited by] Robert H. Dunlop, Charles H. Malbert.—1st ed.
        p. ; cm.
Includes bibliographical references and index.
    ISBN-13: 978-0-8138-2826-8 (alk. paper)
    ISBN-10: 0-8138-2826-0 (alk. paper)
  1. Veterinary pathophysiology.
    [DNLM: 1. Animal Diseases—physiopathology. 2. Veterinary Medicine—methods. SF 745 V5876 2003]
I. Dunlop, Robert H. II. Malbert, Charles H. (Charles-Henri)
    SF769.4.V48 2004
    636.089'607—dc21

                                                                        2003013530

The last digit is the print number: 9 8 7 6 5 4 3 2

DEDICATION TO YVES RUCKEBUSCH

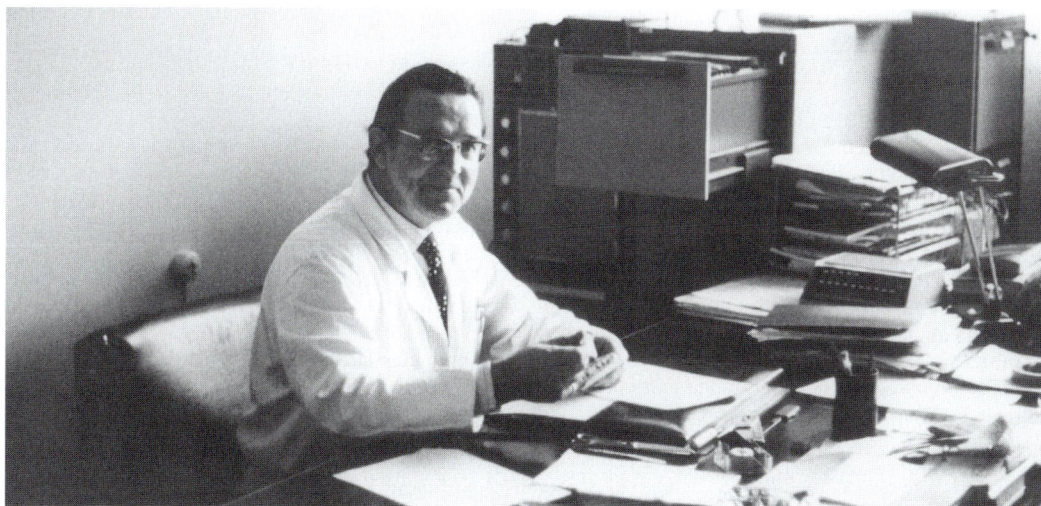

THIS BOOK IS A DEDICATION TO THE ACADEMIC PASSION OF DR. YVES RUCKEBUSCH who was influential for the genesis of the theme of veterinary pathophsyiology and therapeutics.

Yves Ruckebusch (1931–1989): A Memoir by L.P. Phaneuf, Montreal.

On Saturday, December 16, 1989, a cerebral hemorrhage quietly ended the life of Yves Ruckebusch. Ten months earlier, he had survived cardiac arrest and had been granted a reprieve without cerebral anoxia. He credited his so-called second life to the rapid and persistent cardiorespiratory re-animation performed by his research collaborator, Dr. Charles-H. Malbert, who had mastered this emergency technique in the military service. After prolonged hospitalization, much of it in the intensive care unit, he was recuperating and learning to use his indomitable energy with some restraint. A week before his death, he participated actively in a meeting on a subject he was closely associated with—substances acting therapeutically or helpful for animal production (SATHAP; *SITAPA or substances d'intervention therapeutique et d'aide aux productions animales*).

An only child, he was born on December 1, 1931, and raised on a farm in northern France, on the Flemish-Belgium border. The war years of his youth had imprinted him with a deep humanitarian trait and a firm belief in international cooperation. Benevolent, with a keen sense of humor and without affectation, he always responded to the quest for knowledge and enjoyed the company of colleagues. Eventually, most foreign visitors would sign his guest book and come to his home to share a hospitable dinner prepared by his gracious scientist-wife, Michele Ruckebusch-Cordier. In contrast, his agrarian upbringing had endowed him with a capacity for practical and efficient work, which was fed by a phenomenal and dedicated energy. For instance, convinced that English was essential for publication of his research outside France, he would arrange for Anglophone colleagues to review one or several of his manuscripts during the course of a visit in Toulouse. The drafts, dutifully prepared before their arrival, also served to update them on the current research of the laboratory. Besides provoking relevant questions, the exercise led to a friendly exchange of ideas in his open-door office over a cup of coffee obtained from an ever-present coffee pot.

Although modest, in spite of his scientific fame and influence, Yves Ruckebusch was grateful for the recognition granted by colleagues from all parts of the world. On the walls of his office were honorary degrees from the University of Ghent, the University of Liege, and the University of Montreal, and the certificate of honorary membership of the European association for Veterinary Pharmacology and Toxicology, as well as a memento photograph from a group of American veterinary pharmacologists—some of the marks of esteem shown by the scientific community.

These lines aim at remembering Yves Ruckebusch, a man who will be missed by his colleagues and friends all over the world. The work of Professor Ruckebusch, his important contribution to fundamental research in gastrointestinal physiology and pharmacology, is in itself a memorial. Knowledge in the field of gastrointestinal science will continue to progress and undoubtedly will undergo evolution, but we are confident that his scientific legacy will not be lost to posterity.

Extracts from professors P.L. Toutain (Toulouse) and A.S.J.P.A.M. van Miert (Utrecht).

DR. YVES RUCKEBUSCH, honorary member of EAVPT and active member of the editorial board of the *Journal of Veterinary Pharmacology and Therapeutics.*

Dr. Ruckebusch's contributions to our profession were both considerable and distinctive (see also *J.vet. Pharmacol. Therap., 9, 350-351).* He was a real personality, prototype of a gifted teacher and research worker and an active editor and author, who published several textbooks including *Physiologie, Pharmacologie et Therapeutique Animales* (second edition, 1981). With L. P. Phaneuf (Saint-Hyacinthe, Canada) and R.H. Dunlop (St. Paul, USA) he prepared *Small and Large Animal Physiolo*gy. His lectures reflected the breadth of his knowledge, including a lively interest in the history of veterinary medicine, the depth of his scientific thinking, and the charm and humor of his personality. He carefully guided students, co-workers and guest workers from abroad through the complex field of comparative veterinary physiology and pharmacology. Yves Ruckebusch's major scientific interests were in the area of sleep patterns and regulation in the horse and ruminants, the function of the forestomach system, and the pattern of intestinal motility in several animal species, including dogs, cats, and rats. His influence can be seen from the large number and high quality of papers he published and, perhaps even more importantly, from the many scientists who trained under his guidance, including Laplace, Bueno, Fioramonti, Malbert, Toutain; Latour and of many other scholars who worked in his laboratory at Toulouse; Bell (UK) Dallaire, Phaneuf (Canada), Hara (Japan), Hornicke (Germany), Koritz, Merritt, Dunlop (USA), Soldani (Italy), Tomov (Bulgaria), and many others. Yves Ruckebusch was an active participant in the international congresses devoted to ruminant physiology. During the first EAVPT congress (Zeist, 1979) he invited all participants to come to Toulouse to attend a second meeting (1982). The widely acknowledged success of this congress can be largely attributed to the tireless efforts of Yves Ruckebusch (see also *J.vet. Pharmacol. Therap. 5, 295-296).* Another successful congress organized by Ruckebusch was the 5th International Symposium on Ruminant Physiology held at Clermont-Ferrand in September 1979. Recognition of his stature among professional physiologists was indicated by his selection to author the section on the digestive physiology of ruminants in the prestigious *Handbook of Physiology.* Similar recognition resulted in his outstanding paper in the book, *The Ruminant.* For further details of Ruckebusch's see the following references: Toutain, P.L."Yves Ruckebusch 1931-1989" in *Revue Medecine Veterinaire,* 1990, 141, 2: 83-86: Toutain, P.L. and Van Miert, A.S.J.P.A.M

Editorial: "In appreciation of Professor Yves Ruckebusch",
J.vet Pharmacol, Therap. 1990. Vol. 13. Page 112

DR. CHARLES-HENRI MALBERT adds the following personal comments about his debt to his mentor, Yves Ruckebusch

During the numerous evenings spent in the experimental lab trying to understand the intricacies of gastrointestinal smooth muscle physiology and waiting for a migrating motor complex to occur, Yves Ruckebusch was eloquent on his own conception of physiology within the veterinary schools. Yves Ruckebusch's vision was two sided. On the one hand, he was strongly convinced of the need for excellence, hence a necessity for high standards in fundamental physiology. On the other hand, he believed the end product of teaching must supply a better understanding of the mechanisms involved in diseases to ultimately provide cures. One of the greatest merits of Yves Ruckebusch was to understand that these goals were not antagonistic but rather that they need each other's advances in the sciences. That's why during his academic career he was strongly supportive of joined meetings between physiologists and practitioners following the position exemplified by his intellectual guide Claude Bernard in his classic work *Principes de Medecine Experimentale.* In this book, we tried to follow Yves Ruckebusch's conception and most chapters will supply the latest fundamental physiological principals with some examples of their alterations occurring during pathophysiological processes.

DR. ROBERT H. DUNLOP adds the following.

The career paths of Yves Ruckebusch and Bob Dunlop crossed over the years at various ruminant research meetings involving digestive physiology and neuroscience. In 1978 Yves invited me to join him in Toulouse for a study leave endowing me with the remarkable privilege of sharing his office. We developed a close intellectual relationship in the very dynamic research group of his Service de Physiologie. We concurred in the view that there was a primary defect in the established curricula of most veterinary schools, namely the lack of a focus on the nature of dysfunctions occurring during the early stages of diseases and during subsequent changes over their time course. We recognized that this process of "pathophysiology" involved complex changes in homeostatic regulatory interactions and adaptive behaviors. We concluded that pathophysiology was the true basis of clinical veterinary internal medicine and vowed to collaborate in producing a trail-blazing text on this subject to promote its adoption as part of core curricula.. Tragically, Yves did not survive to see our vision realized. Fortunately, in 1998, Charles Malbert agreed to join me in fulfilling the objective. This book, involving 27 authors, is the result.

CONTENTS

CONTRIBUTORS

David John Argyle (Chapter 2)
Associate Professor of Oncology
Department of Medical Sciences
School of Veterinary Medicine
University of Wisconsin
Madison, WI 53706-1102, USA
E-mail: argyled@svm.vetmed.wisc.edu

Tatiana Art (Chapter 5)
Faculty of Veterinary Medicine
Department of Functional Sciences
University of Liege
B-4000 Liege, Belgium
E-mail: tatiana.art@ulg.ac.be

Cleta Sue Bailey (Chapter 9)
Professor Emeritus
Department of Surgical and Radiological Sciences
School of Veterinary Medicine
University of California
Davis, CA 95616, USA
E-mail: csbailey@ucdavis.edu

Anthony T. Blikslager (Chapter 4)
Department of Clinical Sciences
College of Veterinary Medicine
North Carolina State University
Raleigh, NC 27606, USA
E-mail: Anthony_Blikslager@ncsu.edu

Donald M. Broom (Chapter 10)
Department of Clinical Veterinary Medicine
University of Cambridge
Cambridge CB3 0ES, England
E-mail: ljr27@cam.ac.uk

Charles C. Capen (Chapter 12)
Distinguished University Professor and Chairman
Department of Veterinary Biosciences
Ohio State University
Columbus, OH 43210, USA
E-mail: capen.2@osu.edu

Robert H. Dunlop (Chapters 9 and 13)
Professor Emeritus, University of Minnesota
Bandon, OR 97411, USA
E-mail: rhdunlop@aol.com

Marie-Louise Grondahl (Chapter 4)
Laboratorieleder
Fertilitets Klinikken
Hvidovre Hospital
DK-2650 Hvidovre, Denmark
E-mail: marie.groendahl@hh.hosp.dk

Pascal Gustin (Chapter 5)
Faculty of Veterinary Medicine
Department of Functional Sciences
University of Liege
B-4000 Liege, Belgium
E-mail: pascal.gustin@ulg.ac.be

Robert L. Hamlin (Chapter 6)
Department of Veterinary Biosciences
Ohio State University
Columbus, OH 43210, USA
E-mail: hamlin.1@osu.edu

Julien Hamoir (Chapter 5)
Faculty of Veterinary Medicine
Department of Functional Sciences
University of Liege
B-4000 Liege, Belgium
E-mail: julien.hamoir@ulg.ac.be

M. Anthony Hayes (Chapter 11)
Department of Pathobiology
University of Guelph
Guelph, Ontario, Canada N1G 2W1
E-mail: ahayes@uoguelph.ca

Samuel L. Jones (Chapter 4)
Assistant Professor of Equine Medicine
Department of Clinical Sciences
College of Veterinary Medicine
North Carolina State University
Raleigh, NC 27606, USA
E-mail: sam_jones@ncsu.edu

Richard D. Kirkden (Chapter 10)
Department of Clinical Veterinary Medicine
University of Cambridge
Cambridge CB3 0ES, England
E-mail: rdkirkd@purdue.edu

Pierre Lekeux (Chapter 5)
Faculty of Veterinary Medicine
Department of Functional Sciences
University of Liege
B-4000 Liege, Belgium
E-mail: pierre.lekeux@ulg.ac.be

Scott Madill (Chapter 7)
College of Veterinary Medicine
University of Minnesota
St. Paul, MN 55108, USA
E-mail: madil001@tc.umn.edu

Charles-Henri Malbert (Chapter 4)
Director of Research
DVM, Dr es Sci
UMRVP, INRA
F-35590 Saint-Gilles, France
E-mail: malbert@st-gilles.rennes.inra.fr

Alfred M. Merritt (Chapter 4)
Department of Large Animal Clinical Sciences
College of Veterinary Medicine
University of Florida
Gainesville, FL 32610-0136, USA
E-mail: MerrittA@mail.vetmed.ufl.edu

Alastair R. Michell (Chapter 1)
Mill Barn, Mill Lane
Exning, Nr. Newmarket
Suffolk CB8 7JW, England
E-mail: bobmichell@hotmail.com

Lubna Nasir (Chapter 2)
Faculty of Veterinary Medicine
Division of Small Animal Clinical Studies
University of Glasgow
Glasgow G61 1QH, Scotland
E-mail: L.Nasir@vet.gla.ac.uk

Timothy D. O'Brien (Chapter 12)
Veterinary Diagnostic Medicine Department
College of Veterinary Medicine
University of Minnesota
St. Paul, MN 55105, USA
E-mail: obrie004@umn.edu

Richard A. Squires (Chapter 3)
Veterinary Clinic
Massey University
Palmerston North, New Zealand
E-mail: R.A.Squires@massey.ac.nz

Arnold A. Stokhof (Chapter 6)
Faculteit der Diergeneeskunde
Vakgroep Geneeskunde van Gezelschapsdieren
Utrecht University
3584 CM Utrecht, The Netherlands
E-mail: A.A.Stokhof@vet.uu.nl

Mats H.T. Troedsson (Chapter 7)
Professor of Theriogenology
Department of Veterinary Science
University of Florida
Gainesville, FL 32610, USA
E-mail: troedssonm@mai.vetmed.ufl.edu

Stephanie J. Valberg (Chapter 8)
Associate Professor
CAPS Department
College of Veterinary Medicine
University of Minnesota
St. Paul, MN 55108, USA
E-mail: valbe001@umn.edu

Marc Vandevelde (Chapter 9)
Institute of Animal Neurology
University of Bern
CH-3012 Bern, Switzerland
E-mail: marc.vandevelde@itn.unibe.ch

Andreas Zurbriggen (Chapter 9)
Institute of Animal Neurology
University of Bern
CH-3012 Bern, Switzerland
E-mail: contact Vandevelde

PREFACE

The central goals of both human and veterinary medicine are similar: to prevent or cure diseases, to palliate what cannot be cured (yet), and to prevent a life's potential fulfillment from being suppressed by the processes and pressures of disease. The reductionist approach in biomedical research has achieved remarkable advances in identifying molecular events contributing to dysfunction. However, leading thinkers believe that there is a need for greater investment aimed at better understanding the changing complex of functional interactions involved in the pathophysiology of specific clinical diseases ("Physician-researchers needed to move cures out of the rat's cage," by Sharon Begley, *Wall Street J*, 22 April).

Toward this aim, a quotation from Greger and Windhorst identifies the challenge of the physiological sciences very succinctly and clearly:

> The challenge is to cope with the rising flood of outcomes of reductionism research and, at the same time deal with the fundamental question of how the parts and pieces interact. How cells are coordinated to function as an organ, how the organs are coordinated and cooperate in systems, and how the systems' functions are integrated in the somatomotor and neurovegetative behavior of the whole organism when adapting to internal and external needs—a highly dynamic science based on functional thinking and embedded in the fascinating ever-continuing process of learning more about life. [To which R.H.D. would add, "including its resilience and its frailty."] A hierarchy of biological rhythms superimposed on homeostatic autoregulatory feedback circuits plays an important role in coordination of various body functions. This requires crossing borders to new ways of thinking and other disciplines and concepts—the mathematics of rhythmic self-organizing systems. Note the PNI paradigm: Psychoneuroimmunology. [Greger R, Windhorst U. 1996. *Comprehensive Human Physiology*, 2 vols. New York: Springer]

They quote W.B. Cannon: "Indeed, regulation in the organism is the central problem in physiology."

The veterinary profession provides health-related needs for all kinds of animals. Many of its members are also engaged in the quest for solutions to human suffering. Today, its specialists maintain and treat a fascinating range of mammals, birds, and less sentient creatures in their diverse functions through comparative medicine. These roles encompass physical deployment of energy, food and fiber production, companionship, disease modeling as laboratory species, and even tissue and organ replacement and overcoming genetic deficiencies or traumatic injuries. Historically, the profession has made enormous contributions to advancing understanding of infectious and nutritional diseases and of host resistance to infections and infestations, including the vector-borne epidemics. Now it needs to focus on the challenge of understanding the failures of homeostatic and regulatory processes in diseases that lead to impairment through pathophysiology or escape from controls of cellular proliferation as in neoplasia.

Whereas our understanding of physiology is becoming more and more accurate, going from the whole body to organ, then to cell, and ultimately to gene, the intricate mechanisms linking all of these are not yet fully understood even for normal animals and much less in sick animals or people. This failure has been somewhat hidden from the public by the benefits of the remarkable achievements attributable to antibiotic therapy. Nevertheless, the increasing outbreaks of functional disorders leave practitioners (of human or animal medicine) without the desired standard of efficacy and safety. For instance, in human medicine, irritable bowel syndrome, which represents in Europe more than 60% of the diseases in gastroenterology, is still without a real cure. Similarly, cancer therapy is still using, albeit somewhat more efficiently, drugs designed in the late 1960s! The big challenge facing us in the early years of this new *century21* is that, by increasing understanding of the processes by which diseases are occurring, we expect to gain insights toward new therapeutic approaches, especially for the so-called functional diseases.

A prerequisite for achieving such progress is to develop appropriate animal models for the diseases, be they human or animal. In fact, today the majority of physiologically oriented researchers work on a *pathophysiological* rather than a normal animal model. As physiologists, to reach our aim we will need (a) appropriate animal models to portray key features of the functional disorder and (b) effective tools to evaluate the adequacy of the models to define the nature of the problem. At present, these goals are far from being reached for the majority of diseases. Whereas the last decade has been dominated by gene physiology, it is likely that the next one will demand a more clever selection and deployment of new animal models based on advancing knowledge of evolutionary mechanisms and pathophysiology. This might be the first step toward gaining a better understanding of disease at all levels from the gene to the whole body. If successful, this step will help us to design new therapies ranging from gene modification to the development of strategies that promote reversal of the destructive changes in failing homeostatic regulatory systems.

Veterinary support staff must perform a wide range of duties, including many relating to restraint. Human medicine has a massive supporting arm of professional nurses and technological assistants. Most textbooks on human pathophysiology have been written by nurses who have advanced training. Also, there is a wide range of specialized technical services conducted by technologists. Only within the last decade have physician-researchers begun to address the field of pathophysiology in texts. Jack Lange, who developed the series of widely used state-of-the-art medical texts covering a wide range of medical disciplines with frequent revisions, noted the importance of the omission of pathophysiology from his list of texts. His first edition of *Pathophysiology of Disease: An Introduction to Clinical Medicine* appeared in 1995. Its evolution was rapid; by 2003, this title was already in its 4th edition (edited by Stephen J. McPhee, V.R. Lingappa, and W.F. Ganong), a clear indication that it was meeting a long-overdue need. Our text is aimed at meeting a similar need in veterinary medicine.

The study of pathophysiology is the logical basis for the study of clinical veterinary medicine. It is the prerequisite for pharmacotherapy and, where appropriate, surgical intervention. L. Meyer Jones developed his trailblazing *Veterinary Pharmacology and Therapeutics* that illustrates the differences in scope between the pharmacotherapy of domestic animals and humans in 1954 (current edition edited by Richard Adams). Goodman and Gilman's *The Pharmacological Basis of Therapeutics* first appeared in 1941, and its latest edition continues to lead the field for the human species. This 2001 edition reveals the staggering diversity of medications available for human patients. This illustrates the urgency of the need for a much greater focus on the understanding of the interactions among the multitude of functional components that make up the mammalian body and mind and participate in resistance to infections. Also, it must be noted that every therapeutic manipulation needs to be evaluated for its potential to further imbalance the situation in disease. The remarkable capacity of the body for self-healing through its homeostatic and immunologic responses once the initial insults have been ameliorated must be exploited and not impaired by side effects of medication.

The paths of Yves Ruckebusch and Bob Dunlop

crossed in 1978 when an opportunity arose to join Yves for a short sabbatical in his Service de Physiologie in Toulouse. That visit had an enormous impact on our thinking and research focus. It led to our identifying the urgent need to apply the principles of homeostasis and behavioral adaptation to advance understanding of pathophysiology in clinical disease. More significantly, we jointly concurred that there was a lack of recognition of the importance of pathophysiology in the veterinary medicine curriculum. Consequently, we made a mutual vow to develop a trailblazing text on the subject to meet this need.

Tragically, Yves died before this vision could be fulfilled. Fortunately, Yves's protégé, Charles-Henri Malbert, agreed to join Dunlop in 1998 to plan a veterinary pathophysiology textbook. Our goal was to create a comprehensible innovative way of looking at how dysfunctions arise and distort homeostatic regulatory systems and behavioral adaptations within the whole mammalian organism as a function of time. We were greatly encouraged by the enthusiastic response of the outstanding international veterinary scholars we invited to join us in this challenging endeavor. We were delighted that Iowa State Press agreed to take it on, perceiving it to be an important initiative.

Our aim was to focus on getting veterinary students and scholars to establish a new framework of thinking about the nature of disease—to avoid being overwhelmed by detail so that they can be motivated to think critically about the interactions among factors that contribute to the discernable dysfunctions. Then, they can develop the confidence to participate in the process of challenging existing ideas and advancing understanding. This should help in encouraging the participants to seek opportunities to engage in relevant research on animal diseases. The conceptual approach should prove valuable in problem-based learning.

The goal is to stimulate biomedical motivation to strive to gain understanding of the subtleties of disease processes and their consequences that defy knowing. These must be pursued with tenacity so that they may gradually yield their secrets. The path to advancing understanding of veterinary pathophysiology is rooted in our curiosity, be it innate or aroused by mentors or experience, our creative ideas, and intuitions that can be tested and lead us toward the goals. The aim of this work is to be both scholarly and practical. Although the text includes some coverage of categories of diseases, often focusing somewhat on body systems and touching on some topics relevant to various domesticated species, it was not our goal to be encyclopedic or comprehensive. There are some splendid clinical texts that do that. Biomedical knowledge is a very dynamic process—a demanding quest for unlimited exploration of the compass of comparative aspects of the dysfunctions to which the mortal body is prone.

ROBERT H. DUNLOP
CHARLES-HENRI MALBERT

ACKNOWLEDGMENTS

This book, as any, is the result of many people working toward a common goal. Assembling the 27 contributors was but the first step. Several established veterinary scholars gave the editors invaluable advice on candidates for chapter authorship. Particular mention must be made of N. Ole Nielsen, formerly Veterinary Dean of the University of Sasketchewan and then of the University of Guelph, Ontario, who gave significant advice on how to address the very difficult chapter on host-pathogen interactions.

The task of honing the chapters into final form proved to be far more heroic than anticipated. Charles Malbert did the initial formatting of the text and played an essential role in ensuring that all illustrations met publication standards. Josephine Dunlop rigorously managed the many drafts of each chapter. Without her ability and dedication there simply would be no book! In addition, several family members were recruited to lend various skills to the effort: R. Hugo Dunlop of Bendigo, Victoria, Australia; Lachlan S. Dunlop of Saint Paul, Minnesota; Tasha White of Walnut Creek, California; Karma Dunlop of Fulham, London, UK; and Boadie and Anne Dunlop, of Atlanta, Georgia. Thanks are also due to Willa Landino, an Oregon neighbor, for volunteering her artistic talent with several illustrations.

A number of Iowa State Press (Blackwell Publishing) staff participated in developing and producing the book. David Rosenbaum, senior acquisitions editor, recognized from the very beginning the trail-blazing significance of the proposal to produce a book in this field and gave it his unstinting support. Cheryl Garton, publishing assistant, kept the pressure on, ensuring no necessary steps were left unfulfilled and helped numerous authors meet administrative requirements. Judi Brown, project manager/editor, guided the production process through copy editing, composition, proofreading, and indexing. John Flukas, the copy editor, had the formidable task of checking every detail of the manuscript, including text, references, tables, legends, and captions. His remarkable ability to do this rapidly was impressive. Jamie Johnson, editorial computer specialist, inventoried and organized the materials before they went into production. Justin Eccles, designer, played a major role in helping to create an attractive and meaningful cover design. He also checked the suitability and quality of illustrations, fine-tuned the book design and lent recommendations on the best use of color within the book. Helen Flockhart proofread the entire book, adding yet another level of checking details as well as the words. And indexer Don Glassman, combed the text for the most important elements and developed a listing that is inclusive and user-friendly.

ROBERT H. DUNLOP

Veterinary
Pathophysiology

PHYSIOLOGY AND PATHOPHYSIOLOGY OF THE INTERNAL ENVIRONMENT

Alastair R. Michell

PHYSIOLOGY AND PATHOPHYSIOLOGY: IS THERE A REAL DIFFERENCE? In the 19th century, much of the study of animals centered on confining them, provoking them, and seeing what they did; increasingly, we appreciate the greater value obtained from understanding how they respond to the natural disturbances of everyday existence. The grand tradition of physiological research has been to isolate a system, subject it to stimulation, even extreme, and observe the consequences in comparison with those expected from current hypotheses. Pathophysiology observes the behavior of systems responding to the stimuli imposed by disease. Frequently, by comparing outcomes with current concepts, it provides the stimulus to modify or create new hypotheses concerning regulatory mechanisms. These outcomes usually reflect a balance between adaptive and maladaptive responses, rather than total failure of the system. Sometimes, notably in shock, the outcome is a caricature of the adaptive response—recognizable but exaggerated to an absurd and damaging degree. Pathophysiology is the bedrock of internal medicine, and many conditions misconceived primarily as infections (e.g., diarrhea or fever) are better understood in terms of the dysregulatory mechanisms involved.

There is a conceit among traditional physiologists that pathophysiology can be deduced from existing concepts of the normal regulatory system. But it is frequently the case that accurate observation of responses to disease necessitates modification of existing concepts of regulation or, at least, the recognition that they are unable to explain consistent aberrations observed in patients. The situation is exemplified by sodium; at face value, the regulation of body sodium is amply explained in physiology textbooks. So it should be—it is the most important ion in the extracellular fluid, the internal environment. It is readily measured and has been exhaustively studied. Yet, in the case of one of its most common clinical disturbances, certainly the most obvious and historically one of the oldest recognized, our explanations fail: we are unable to provide a convincing explanation for any of the common clinical forms of generalized edema without invoking abstractions to hide the gaps between the data and the theory.

The 1960s saw the physiology of aldosterone and renal function as a sufficient basis to explain clinical disturbances of body sodium. It was the pathophysiologists who showed the inadequacy of such a concept, for example, because the clinical outcome of excessive aldosterone secretion is not edema but hypokalemia. Indeed, even now, it requires insights from herbivores to realize that the key role of aldosterone is probably in the regulation of body potassium rather than sodium. Certainly, the 1980s showed the importance of an array of other hormones in regulating or modulating body sodium, not least those responsible for the excretion of excess. The 1990s, through the applications of molecular biology, revealed a bewildering variety of other effects of these hormones (e.g., angiotensin) and a remarkable range of tissues, which they may affect. But there is a difference between description of complexity and understanding; unless we have reproducible observations, which yield consistent predictions or explanations, we do not truly understand the system.

Regulation and Dysregulation. The most familiar concept of physiological regulation is based on the maintenance of a *set-point* or target value of a variable by detecting any divergence (*error signal*) and initiating a response that corrects the disturbance (and eliminates the error signal)—this is *negative feedback*, exemplified in thermostats, cruise control systems, and textbook accounts of the regulation of body temperature, plasma sodium concentration, arterial pressure, etc. In pathophysiology, such responses are frequently superseded by *positive feedback* in which the response amplifies the disturbance—as exemplified by power steering or by physiological systems requiring a rapid, self-accelerating response (e.g., the uterus during parturition, the bladder during micturition, the neural membrane during depolarization, or the clotting system following injury). Thus, the vasoconstrictor response to hypovolemia defends arterial pressure against the consequences of hemorrhage and, by dropping the downstream capillary pressure, assists the return of fluid from the interstitial space to the intravascular compartment, reducing the extent of both hypovolemia and hypotension. But vasoconstriction that is too intense or too protracted leads to capillary leakage, and any further vasoconstriction intensifies the problem rather than corrects it. Shock involves a number of systems—vascular, cytokine, coagulatory—in the distortion of responses that are fundamentally defensive, but if triggered too intensely, too protractedly, or in response to inappropriate stimuli, reinforce the breakdown of normal regulation; ultimately, the animal is killed by the misapplication of its regulatory mechanisms.

Physiology embraces the mechanisms that enable animals to maintain the integrity of the internal environment (not necessarily its constancy), according to the changing demands of the external environment or of reproduction. *Pathophysiology* is the study of normal regulatory mechanisms responding to the abnormal circumstances associated with disease; it is the physiology of survival in an abnormal internal environment. They are inseparable and truly symbiotic.

COMPLEXITY OF PATHOPHYSIOLOGY. In the physiology of disease, as in life, truth is rarely pure and never simple. Those who recall Apollo 13, the events or the film, saw perhaps the outstanding example of improvisation of engineering systems to circumvent the results of dysfunction and ensure survival. As ever with such improvisations, there were *trade-offs*; the spacecraft's systems did not function optimally or even adequately, but survival was achieved.

Compensation and Trade-offs. Such trade-offs are also typical of the adaptive responses seen in pathophysiology, most famously in the intact nephron hypothesis of chronic renal failure. The overall decline in renal function, expressed as the decline in glomerular filtration rate (GFR) reflects a permanently reduced nephron population, but the residual renal function reflects the heightened activity of the surviving nephrons, working individually with their own GFRs at supranormal levels and increased flows within their tubules. Not surprisingly, they can not achieve the extremes of composition required for maximal renal function, and the patient, therefore, is stable in a stable environment with a stable diet, but the capacity to respond to challenges such as a sudden dietary change or dehydration is reduced. The kidney is "inflexible," like an aircraft flying with two engines shut down. Similarly, the increased heart rate that compensates for anemia or early cardiac failure, to maintain adequate resting perfusion, encroaches on the functional reserve available for exertion. Moreover, since high heart rates encroach on the duration of diastole, which is also the period of optimal coronary perfusion, they ultimately impede myocardial oxygen supply. The mobilization of bone mineral in chronic renal failure stabilizes plasma calcium concentration, but the trade-off is soft-tissue calcification and skeletal damage. The colon can reduce or conceal the effects of inadequate salt and water reabsorption in the small intestine by engaging its functional reserve capacity and increasing its absorption of both, but the trade-off is increased fecal loss of potassium. Thirst normally serves to stabilize plasma sodium concentration, which is increased when the body loses water and corrected by drinking. During hypovolemia, however, the set-point for thirst (and for the release of antidiuretic hormone, ADH) becomes the restoration of circulating volume, and the trade-off for the resulting improvement is the dilution of plasma sodium concentration by the additional water. During diarrhea, the kidneys, by responding to ADH, can reduce urine output to a degree that may virtually balance the increased fecal water loss; the trade-off is the associated distortion of the segmental balance of renal function (see the section *Renal Interactions*) and the resulting impairment of the regulation of plasma composition.

Set-points: Movable Targets. While physiology has traditionally emphasized the constancy of set-points, any effective regulatory system is capable of adjustment of set-point according to changing demands; cruise controls, thermostats, and auto pilots are all routinely reset in response to changed circumstances. Total body water is reasonably constant, but it is not the same in the young as in the elderly, nor during the reproductive cycle, particularly during pregnancy, and it often changes with season or climate. Nocturnal arterial pressure and diurnal arterial pressure are different and so is body temperature, to a heightened extent in animals such as camels, which by radiation save on their water requirement for evaporative cooling by allowing their daytime temperature to rise and shedding the excess heat to the cool night environment. Fever is a regulated rise in temperature to a new set-point, which is then defended—cooling thus provokes further heat conservation or generation. Heatstroke involves overwhelming of the capacity of the system; hence, cooling is essential. Nonsteroidal anti-inflammatory drugs correct an elevated set-point; hence, they are effective in fever but not in heatstroke. That does not mean they are appropriate in fever, since its effects, during infections, are more likely to be beneficial than harmful unless the rise in temperature is extreme (Michell 1982; Kluger 1993; Blumenthal 1997). An idiosyncratic reaction to halothane triggers a rare, dangerous rise in body temperature (malignant hyperthermia), combining accelerated heat production with restriction of heat loss; it can occur in people or in pigs and occasionally in cats (Michell 1994a). There is a growing appreciation of the fact that the effectiveness of a given dose of a drug (e.g., a diuretic) may vary with the time of day; moreover, if the effects are not sustained, the kidney is likely to "correct" for these effects during the interval until the next dose.

Renal Interactions. The understanding of physiological regulation is easiest in the context of single regulatory loops, but in reality interactions between systems is commonplace and underlies many aspects of pathophysiology. Thus, the kidney can stabilize plasma pH not only by altering excretion of hydrogen ions, but also by altering plasma bicarbonate, for example, increasing it to offset the rise in plasma carbon dioxide (CO_2). As a result, animals with chronic respiratory problems are more vulnerable when they have coexisting renal disease. Animals with metabolic acidosis can reduce their plasma CO_2 through hyperventilation, but less readily with coexisting respiratory disease, and the ability to compensate for the metabolic acidosis of diarrhea or the potential metabolic alkalosis of vomiting are both undermined by chronic renal failure, which may precipitate both forms of alimentary dysfunction. The kidney and liver both catabolize hormones, so failure of either may disturb endocrine function. The liver also generates albumin, essential for the maintenance of intravascular volume as against extravascular (interstitial) fluid volume, and, through the production of glutamine and removal of ammonia,

the liver plays a subsidiary role in the regulation of acid-base balance (Michell et al. 1989); thus, the ability of the kidney to defend plasma volume and composition may be undermined by hepatic dysfunction.

Within the kidney, the function of the different nephron segments is usually portrayed in sequential isolation, whereas the balance between the segments themselves is vital for normal regulatory function. Thus, sodium is mostly reabsorbed in the proximal tubules, according to the demands of plasma volume; proximal tubular fluid, being essentially similar to plasma in sodium concentration and being rapidly produced from plasma by the glomeruli, is an ideal fluid to restore plasma volume during hypovolemia. But if the proportion of glomerular filtrate absorbed proximally is increased, sodium delivery to more distal segments of the nephron is reduced, and their function, which is to regulate plasma composition, is impaired. Thus, inadequate delivery to the loop of Henle diminishes its ability to produce maximally dilute urine (and thus excrete water to correct hyponatremia) or to generate maximally concentrated interstitial fluid within the renal medulla (thus diminishing the ability to conserve water from the collecting duct in response to ADH and correct hypernatremia).

Severe hypovolemia also diminishes the supply of sodium to the aldosterone-sensitive segments of the distal nephron and impedes the excretion of hydrogen ions or potassium in exchange for the conservation of sodium, thus predisposing an animal to hyperkalemia. On the other hand, milder hypovolemia may allow sufficient distal delivery for the increased reabsorption of sodium to cause potassium depletion, especially during anorexia, when potassium intake is also reduced. The reason why correction of plasma volume is the paramount objective of fluid therapy is not simply that this is the prerequisite for the avoidance or treatment of shock, but because it normalizes the balance of segmental function within the nephrons, restoring their ability to correct abnormalities of plasma composition.

DISTURBANCES OF INTRACELLULAR ELECTROLYTES. Extracellular fluid provides the internal environment of the cells; the majority is the interstitial fluid in the tissue spaces (about 15% of body weight), whereas plasma, the intravascular portion, is merely 5% of body weight; its importance derives from its function, not its size. Intracellular fluid is about twice as large as extracellular fluid (about 40% of body weight), so total body water is about 60% of the weight of a mature animal, or less if it is fat and more if it is young and lean, and especially if it is newly born.

Plasma (X^+): Not the Whole Story. While the emphasis of homeostasis is always on the maintenance of the extracellular environment, particularly on the composition of plasma (and therefore interstitial fluid), this is an incomplete view of regulation. Plasma potassium concentration and magnesium concentration both matter, but these are predominantly intracellular ions, and cellular depletion may be even more important. Moreover, the latter can coexist with normal or even elevated concentrations in plasma; a calf dying of acute diarrhea concurrently suffers massive loss of intracellular potassium (due both to external losses and intracellular movement of hydrogen ions) and lethal hyperkalemia due to loss of intracellular potassium and to impaired excretion. Intracellular potassium is about 25 times as concentrated as extracellular fluid, and intracellular fluid is about twice its volume, so small changes in the transmembrane distribution of potassium have a huge impact on its plasma concentration (Michell 1995a, Antes et al. 1998).

The regulation and abnormalities of individual ions can not be viewed in isolation: when proximal reabsorption of glomerular filtrate is reduced in order to correct expanded extracellular fluid volume, not only is the excretion of sodium and water appropriately increased, so is that of divalent ions, inappropriately. Aldosterone is routinely portrayed as a sodium-conserving hormone that happens to raise potassium excretion—probably because the latter poses little problem in people on mixed diets with low potassium intakes, often below 10 mmol/day (Mandal 1997; Morris et al. 1999). But herbivores such as sheep face the conundrum of a high obligatory potassium intake (often above 500 mmol/day) combined with the problem of excreting it even when the intakes of sodium and water are low; the cardiac effects of doubling the plasma potassium concentration are potentially fatal. The role of aldosterone in promoting distal excretion of potassium is then vital, as is the restoration of sodium intake to levels enabling sufficient delivery of sodium to the distal nephron, since the enhanced potassium excretion is indirectly dependent on enhanced reabsorption of sodium. The kidney responds to several hormones, including angiotensin II, atrial natriuretic peptide (ANP), and active sodium transport inhibitor/endogenous digitalis-like inhibitor (ASTI/EDLI), in adjusting sodium excretion, whereas only aldosterone fulfills the criteria for a homeostatic loop to promote potassium excretion: hyperkalemia promotes aldosterone secretion, and this promotes renal and colonic excretion of potassium and sequestration of potassium, via saliva, into the rumen. It also promotes uptake from extracellular fluid into cells, as does insulin, which is also stimulated by hyperkalemia and which can be given to treat hyperkalemia (Michell et al. 1989; Greenberg 1998). In severe hypervolemia, the kidney escapes from the sodium-retaining effects of aldosterone (by decreasing proximal sodium reabsorption and overwhelming the distal nephron with unabsorbable quantities of sodium). Conversely, in diuretic-induced sodium depletion, the subsequent compensatory sodium retention is not aldosterone dependent (Ellison 1999). The kidney never escapes from the potassium-related effects of aldosterone, unlike the sodium-related effects. Thus the hallmark of pathological excess secretion of aldosterone is not edema but potassium depletion. The rumen provides a large reservoir of sodium or potassium, according to the salivary Na/K ratio, which is dictated by aldosterone. Small changes in food intake, such as those at estrus, can have substantial effects on electrolyte excretion (Michell 1981; Michell and Noakes 1985).

Cows recumbent with hypocalcemia or raving with hypomagnesemia both contain abundant calcium (in bone) or magnesium (in bone and cells) but are unable to mobilize it. Worse, the low plasma magnesium reduces both the responsiveness of the parathyroid gland to hypocalcemia and the effect of parathyroid hormone (PTH) on bone (Kelepouris and Agus 1998). Deficits of the two major intracellular cations—potassium and magnesium—are interlinked by the fact that delivery of potassium to the intracellular fluid depends on the sodium pump, the magnesium-dependent enzyme Na-K ATPase.

MULTIPLE CONTROL SYSTEMS. Just as vital systems on spacecraft have redundancy—that is, backup systems that can compensate for failure of primary systems—it may take a double insult to overcome physiological regulatory mechanisms. Thus, plasma sodium concentration is regulated by the adjustment of water balance, mainly through changes in thirst (except in species drinking for habit or flavor), and secondarily through changes in urine concentration modulated by the release of ADH and the renal response to it. Pure water loss (which is clinically unusual compared with dehydration, which is usually applied to mixed loss of water and electrolytes) raises plasma sodium concentration and thereby triggers increased drinking and decreased urinary excretion of water, thus correcting the disturbance. The biggest potential water losses are those of diabetes insipidus—failure of the secretion of ADH or the renal response to it. Although this massively increases urine output, there is no hypernatremia because thirst compensates and drinking increases in parallel; a wasteful increase in water turnover prevents a dangerous increase in plasma sodium concentration. The clinical lesson is obvious but widely disregarded: detection of hypernatremia indicates not only loss of water but interference with compensatory drinking because the animal is too weak, can not retain what it drinks, finds drinking painful, or is inadvertently water deprived (e.g., by a frozen water supply).

Regulatory Responses Also Oppose Therapeutic Interventions. We realize increasingly that therapeutic intervention against one physiological system may be undermined by the response of other systems; a diuretic acting in the distal nephron has its effects blunted by the counterregulatory response in the proximal tubule and the loop. Therapeutic interventions may also undermine these backups (e.g., the kidney is defended against excessive vasoconstriction by a prostaglandin-mediated response); hence, hypovolemic animals on steroidal anti-inflammatories may be more vulnerable to shutdown of renal function. Equally, some animals may maintain a normal GFR through elevated concentrations of angiotensin (which preferentially constricts the efferent arteriole), and they experience a decline in renal function in response to angiotensin-converting enzyme (ACE) inhibitors (despite their normally beneficial effects in chronic renal failure). Specific transport functions in the nephron and elsewhere may be accomplished by several different pumps sharing similar characteristics, enabling redundancy to protect vital systems from failure of a single mechanism (Caviston et al. 1999).

Attempts to intervene against cytokine systems involved in shock, especially septic shock, increasingly reveal the existence of counterregulatory cytokine systems that undermine or eliminate the intended beneficial effect. Increasingly, our concepts of single regulatory loops, perhaps with reinforcing backup loops, as the elegantly simple basis for physiological regulation have to be replaced by the complexity of multiple interacting networks. Accordingly, we realize that therapeutic interventions may thereby become blunted or transient in their effects.

These considerations are not intended to be discouraging but to encourage a sense of realism. In internal medicine, we frequently seek to replace, temporarily or permanently, the role of the natural regulatory system. Unless we understand its complexity, and its adaptability, we are likely to be disappointed by the effectiveness of seemingly rational strategies. In particular, when we recall that so many mechanisms on which we intervene have a normal role, but abnormal characteristics, in disease, we readily understand the balance between the beneficial and detrimental effects of many appropriate drugs. Add to that the growing realization of the component of genetic individuality in governing patterns of response, or of diet in influencing many mediators (e.g., omega fatty acids, which influence eicosanoids), and we realize that within the general characteristics of their disease, each patient is ultimately unique. Thereby hangs the importance of the art, alongside the science, in clinical judgment.

DISTURBANCES IN BODY SODIUM. *Sodium* is the osmotic skeleton of the extracellular fluid (ECF); it dictates its volume. *Plasma sodium concentration* is the marker for total body water, since water moves freely across most cell membranes. When it does, cells shrink or swell, which matters most when they are as vital as brain cells and are constrained within the rigid cranium; this, rather than effects on membrane potentials, explains the predominance of neurological signs with abnormalities in plasma sodium concentration, both hyponatremia and hypernatremia. Since the brain, given time, can alter the concentration of intracellular solutes to alleviate changes in cell volume, it is not just the extent of the abnormality, but the speed of onset, that dictates its clinical impact; remarkable abnormali-

ties are tolerable if they develop slowly enough. Clearly, overrapid correction can precipitate further dangerous changes in cell volume, since the brain cells also need time to correct the compensatory changes in their solute content (Michell 1995a). Thus, duration of the disturbance, as well as its severity, is an important element of therapeutic decisions regarding plasma sodium concentration, especially hypernatremia, which, if sustained, can inflict lasting brain damage.

Total Sodium = ECF Volume: Plasma (Na⁺) = Total Water. Disturbances in body sodium, whether retention or depletion, manifest primarily as changes in extracellular volume, not in plasma sodium concentration, though these may occur secondarily. Thus, sodium depletion leads to hypovolemia, whereas sodium retention is associated with edema. The physiology textbooks suggest that we understand the regulation of body sodium, but the pathogenesis of edema suggests otherwise. Sodium is also involved in the regulation of arterial pressure; the kidney is the long-term regulator of arterial pressure (unlike the baroreceptors, which are mainly involved in responses to short-term disturbances, e.g., due to hemorrhage or postural change). The renal regulation or arterial pressure depends on *pressure natriuresis*, the rapid increase in sodium excretion in response to sustained rises in arterial pressure. There are many publications on the relationship between the control of renal sodium excretion and the regulation of blood pressure or extracellular volume, but few attempt to reconcile the demands of these two separate regulatory requirements; clinically, hypertension and edema do not tend to coexist and, if they do, the reasons are separate.

Medical textbooks generally present the regulation of body sodium as synonymous with the regulation of renal sodium excretion. This is certainly important, but once again multiple systems are involved, and those who have the fortune to work with a range of species are readily aware of the importance of salt appetite in determining sodium intake, and of the importance of enteric regulation of fecal sodium excretion, especially in herbivores. Indeed, the gut has some of the attributes of a giant nephron, and diarrhea shares important characteristics with diuresis (Michell 2000a). The main clinical impact of sustained consumption of excess sodium, apart from increased water turnover, is on arterial pressure (by predisposing an animal to hypertension), and the main clinical cause of fluid and electrolyte disturbances is diarrhea rather than renal failure: the renocentric view of sodium regulation is incomplete once we consider the realities of pathophysiology. Delays in the progress of understanding the pathophysiology of sodium have risen precisely from the fact that its physiology has been parceled out between organ-focused physiologists who are blind to the complexity of the interactions. Other than acute diarrhea, the greatest natural challenges to body sodium regulation are those associated with pregnancy and lactation, and, certainly in herbivores, the reproductive cycle provides a fascinating demonstration of the interactions between the several mechanisms—enteric, behavioral, and renal—responsible for the maintenance of body sodium.

If we accept that the main impact of sodium on ECF is to dictate its volume, the first question a mechanic would ask is "Where is volume measured?" The second might be "Are there reserves of sodium and, if so, where are they measured?" There are reserves, in bone and certainly, in herbivores, within the gut, but we do not know how they are measured or regulated. The most important "pool" of extracellular fluid is in the interstitial space, expanded in edema and reduced to boost plasma volume through the vasoconstrictor response to hypovolemia. We have no idea how, or whether, interstitial volume is monitored, yet an engineer would find it hard to design an adequate control system without information about this vital statistic. No city could function on data about pump speeds, pipe pressures, and outflows with no knowledge of the whereabouts or fullness of the reservoirs. We measure what is most accessible, including renal function, and we neglect problems that are too intractable to be fashionable and too slow to generate the rapid "hits" needed to keep grant income flowing. That is why today we know a lot about renal function and about hormones, and other factors that regulate it or affect it, but we can not truthfully, rigorously, explain the causation of any common form of generalized edema to an intelligent school graduate.

RENAL AND ENTERIC SODIUM REGULATION. Both in the nephron and the gut, fluids and electrolytes vital to the integrity of the extracellular fluid are transferred to a separate compartment at hazardous rates that would be unsustainable if there were not mechanisms to ensure reabsorption and restoration to plasma. With the nephron, there is a wealth of research concerning this *glomerulotubular balance*, ensuring that if GFR changes, there is usually a matching change in reabsorption. This ensures internal sodium balance; that is, increased delivery of sodium to the tubules is matched by increased salvage, safeguarding extracellular volume. The demands of external balance are the opposite: that if excess sodium is consumed, it is successfully excreted. Some of the renal mechanisms ensuring this are now understood, but the enteric mechanisms reconciling the conflicting requirements of both internal and external sodium balance have scarcely been studied (Michell 2000a).

The small intestine, like the proximal tubule, essentially reabsorbs large volumes of salt and water without major changes in their concentration, whereas in the distal nephron, as in the colon, the quantities absorbed are smaller but decisive in reducing external losses, where necessary, virtually to zero, and in facilitating the aldosterone-mediated excretion of potassium when sodium is conserved. In both the gut and the nephron, the distal effects are capable of being overwhelmed by changes in proximal reabsorption because earlier segments deal with far greater total fluxes. Thus, during excessive aldosterone secretion, the resulting expansion in ECF volume reduces proximal reabsorption and allows excretion of excess sodium before edema develops, and despite the continuing aldosterone-driven distal conservation of sodium; the distal pumps are overwhelmed. Similarly, in diarrhea, the enormous compensatory capacity of the colon, which allows substantial increases in fluid content of material leaving the small intestine to be concealed by continued production of normal feces, is finally overwhelmed, and fecal fluid losses become obvious and dangerous. Fecal potassium losses will also be increased by aldosterone-driven sodium conservation in the colon.

From a human perspective, it seems obvious that the regulation of sodium and water balance is renally driven, and involvement of the intestine is simply to balance secretory and reabsorptive fluxes. When we look at herbivores, however, a more complex and interesting picture emerges, with sodium balance also powerfully influenced by salt appetite and by enteric regulation of sodium excretion: in many normal herbivores, this is the main excretory route on diets adequate in sodium but free of excess; excess sodium is mainly excreted renally (Michell 1995a). It would be interesting to know whether, in those few remaining human communities that remain essentially herbivorous and where excess sodium intake has been avoided, the intestine also plays a greater role in the regulation of sodium and water balance. Certainly, once it is realized that diarrhea is fundamentally a failure of net sodium and water absorption, which overwhelms the compensatory capacity of the colon, it becomes less surprising that diarrhea remains the main cause of serious fluid, electrolyte, and acid-base disturbances in most species and that a key component of therapy is to reverse this failure with an oral rehydration solution designed to restore net uptake of sodium and water (and to correct metabolic acidosis). Thus, oral rehydration is not merely symptomatic but attacks a fundamental therapeutic target; moreover, the most modern solutions can support recovery of villus architecture and renal function, which is surprisingly sensitive even to modest hypovolemia in diarrheic calves (Brooks et al. 1997; Michell 1998a).

Segmental Function in the Nephron. Many veterinary and medical graduates will recall renal function as a series of fiendishly complex contraflows on a series of separate motorways, with the glomerulus, proximal tubule, loop, and distal nephron as the major highways, but each capable of subdivision into regions of scenic or functional diversity. As with motorways, the preoccupation appears to be with flows within each segment rather than the overall traffic flow. The latter, like overall renal function, is crucially dependent on the balance of events between segments. For example, it has sometimes been naively remarked that, in diarrheic patients, the total fluid losses may not be dramatically increased, because the increased fecal output can be offset by reduced urine output, in effect equating the pathological loss of a liter of fecal fluid with the normal excretion in urine. Equally, the traffic flow on most of the southbound freeway is normal whether the traffic arrives in London or is all diverted around it, but the functional consequences are very different. The ability of the kidney to minimize fluid loss, and therefore contraction of extracellular volume, is crucially dependent on adaptations that undermine the defense of plasma composition; moreover, renal function as a whole is compromised by the reduction in GFR. The very definition of GFR as a clearance—that is, the plasma concentration at which a particular solute output can be maintained—implies unacceptable increases in plasma solute concentrations unless they are subject to adaptive changes in secretion, reabsorption, or extrarenal excretion.

clearance of Z
= U/P concentration of Z × urine flow per time
= urinary excretion of Z, per plasma
  concentration of Z

GFR is thus a key expression of the efficiency of renal function, as well as its magnitude. It is, not surprisingly, subject to highly efficient regulation because the smallest mismatch between GFR and net tubular reabsorption can convert a tiny percentage error into fluid losses equivalent to or far exceeding those of a major hemorrhage. In ourselves, failure to absorb 1% of glomerular filtrate would cause 2 L of loss in a day. Thus, GFR is protected from reduction of arterial pressure through a range; renal perfusion, per se, is protected (*autoregulation*) and, even at a reduced perfusion rate, GFR can be stabilized by increased intraglomerular pressure (raised efferent arteriolar resistance or reduced afferent arteriolar tone) allowing increased filtration fraction. This also favors a balancing increase in proximal tubular reabsorption, because the relevant capillaries are downstream of the efferent arterioles, and their perfusion pressure is therefore reduced, allowing the increased albumin concentration in the plasma arriving from the hyperfiltrating glomeruli to attract fluid back into circulation. Thus, when a given GFR is sustained through increased filtration fraction, more retention of sodium and water is likely than when filtration fraction is normal. The beneficial effect of glomerulotubular balance is that, if GFR does change, the tubule is likely to minimize any consequential change in net excretion. GFR increases after the digestion of meat meals in response to the associated amino acids.

Inconstancy of Glomerular Filtration Rate. Sustained, rather than temporary, hyperfiltration (together with compensatory nephron growth) also features in the response of the kidney to chronic renal failure (i.e., progressive nephron loss). The surviving intact nephrons increase their size and workload (i.e., their

GFR). But the increased filtration fraction underlying hyperfiltration may also reduce the perfusion of the downstream tubular capillaries sufficient to damage the tissues dependent on them, and this may contribute to the relentlessly progressive nature of the condition (Maschio and Oldrizzi 2000). It is not the increased GFR but the associated increase in intraglomerular pressure that predisposes to progression, as does systemic hypertension, proteinuria, numerous growth factors, cytokines, and a number of other factors, some of which (phosphate, omega-3 lipids and, in diabetics, dietary protein) are amenable to dietary manipulation (Michell 1999; El Nahas 2000; Maschio and Oldrizzi 2000). If the dietary sodium and potassium are to be excreted by a reduced nephron population, there need to be adaptive increases in the single nephron excretion of both ions, involving increased levels of ANP and increased Na-K ATPase activity in the distal nephron (to facilitate potassium secretion) (Michell 1995a; Franz et al. 2001). Indeed, in some cats with chronic renal failure, the efficiency of potassium excretion is maintained so well, in the face of reduced dietary intake, that potassium depletion may occur, inflicting muscle damage and further renal damage (Michell 1994a).

There are also mechanisms to adjust GFR in response to changes in fluid delivery to the distal nephron (tubuloglomerular balance). Nitric oxide is an important mediator of tubuloglomerular balance, but it also affects tubular reabsorption of sodium and protects renal perfusion against excessive vasoconstriction (Gabbai 1999). Adaptive increases in GFR also occur in salt loading (in response to the resulting increase in extracellular volume) and during pregnancy. GFR is adaptively reduced during even modest exercise in horses: this contrasts with the picture seen in people where GFR is "protected" unless the exercise is extreme compared with the level of fitness. Why should it be protected? Granted that coronary and cerebral perfusion are sacrosanct, and that blood volume is far smaller than the total volume of vessels capable of being perfused, any unnecessary renal perfusion will restrict muscle perfusion in animals attempting to escape predators. Seen from the standpoint of survival rather than the supreme importance of renal function, it seems obvious that this redistribution of blood flow is beneficial (Gleadhill et al. 2000). Renal function can be severely compromised by anesthesia, especially through hypotension or impeded autoregulation (depending on the agent), and by the effects of surgery (which can be neural as well as cardiovascular) and is much more vulnerable if there is also hypovolemia (Michell et al. 1989).

Tubular Reabsorption. Glomerular filtrate differs from plasma only in the absence of proteins similar to or larger than albumin in size (though charge also affects the likelihood of filtration) and the fact that ion concentrations, for divalent ions such as Ca or Mg which are partly bound in plasma, correspond approximately to the free, not the total, plasma concentration. For all ions, slight differences in concentrations between plasma and glomerular filtrate reflect the influence of the negative charge on albumin, for which there is an unavoidable concentration gradient between the two. Since ECF is essentially a saline solution and, in particular, since its volume is dictated by sodium which therefore acts as its "osmotic skeleton," resisting the osmotic pull of the intracellular solutes, glomerular filtrate is an ideal fluid for rapidly altering plasma volume and, hence, extracellular volume. Thus, the reabsorption of proximal tubular fluid is primarily adjusted to the need to defend plasma volume, increasing during hypovolemia and decreasing when plasma volume is expanded. Moreover, these adjustments do not affect the concentration of sodium in plasma, allowing independent regulation of ECF volume (via total body sodium) and plasma sodium concentration (via total body water).

The regulation of plasma composition is mainly (but not totally) dependent on subsequent segments of the nephron and, apart form the importance of restoration of plasma volume in avoiding hypovolemic shock, restoration of plasma volume is the key to successful fluid therapy, because, by removing the need for supranormal reabsorption of fluid from the proximal tubule, it promotes restoration of normal distal delivery of tubular fluid. It thus allows the loop and distal nephron (distal tubules and collecting duct) to resume their normal functions, which contribute to the regulation of plasma concentrations of sodium, potassium, and hydrogen ions, rather than regulation of ECF volume. The kidney of a healthy normovolemic animal is extremely accurate in regulating normal plasma composition, whereas the changes in segmental balance of reabsorption in hypovolemic animals mean that, in protecting plasma volume, the kidneys create or permit abnormalities in plasma composition.

Water Excretion and Plasma (Na$^+$). Plasma sodium concentration is primarily regulated by thirst and ADH: both are stimulated extremely sensitively by small increments in plasma sodium concentration that signal pure water loss. Hyponatremia, signaling dilution by excess body water, suppresses both the intake and renal retention of water (suppression of ADH). The exception is during hypovolemia that is sufficiently severe to promote thirst and ADH secretion in defense of plasma volume, at the expense of plasma sodium concentration. Again, correction of hypovolemia serves to correct plasma composition. In the majority of species for which drinking equates with intake of pure water, thirst, rather then the renal-ADH mechanism, is the primary hour-by-hour regulatory mechanism, with the kidney as a backup. This is the opposite of the picture conveyed in textbooks on human physiology for the understandable reason that most human drinking is of flavored fluids drunk for pleasure, social, or habitual reasons, thus giving the kidney the task of excreting the obligatory excess of fluid. It can do this because the

loop creates a maximally dilute tubular fluid that, if unaltered in the collecting duct, enables excretion of watery, low-sodium urine. On the other hand, the loop also creates an interstitial fluid rich in sodium and urea, which surrounds the collecting ducts so that, when their permeability is increased by ADH, the osmotic gradient pulls water out of tubular fluid into interstitial fluid and thence into plasma. The loop is therefore essential for the generation of both maximally concentrated and maximally dilute urine, the two prerequisites for the regulation of water balance and plasma sodium concentration.

Maximally concentrated urine also requires a normally sensitive system governing the synthesis and release of ADH, a normal response to it (increased permeability) in the collecting duct, and a normal degree of impermeability in its absence. Maximum concentrating capacity also requires the ability to sustain high concentrations of urea, as well as sodium in the medullary interstitial fluid surrounding the collecting ducts. The extremely low perfusion rate of the medulla avoids the "washout" of concentrated interstitial fluid that would otherwise undermine water conservation. Nevertheless, even without the concentrated medullary interstitial fluid, the cortical collecting duct is surrounded by interstitial fluid that resembles the rest of extracellular fluid, so it is much more concentrated than fully dilute urine: it is therefore an important site for water reabsorption from tubular fluid. When ADH increases water reabsorption, there is also increased resorption of urea, via different sites; this causes the preferential increase in plasma urea, compared with creatinine, seen in dehydration with prerenal failure.

Water movement at different nephron sites depends on specific protein channels known as *aquaporins*, of which at least six have been characterized and others are known (Kwon et al. 2001). Those in the proximal tubule and thin descending limb of the loop differ from those in the collecting duct, and abnormalities of the latter occur in diabetes insipidus (inadequate production) and overproduction in conditions such as heart failure and inappropriate secretion of ADH, which are associated with pathological water retention. Aquaporins provide an excellent example of the power of molecular biology to open up new avenues of research by identifying a specific molecule in an *unexpected* site; they were originally identified in red cells during research on Rhesus factor, but subsequently got their identification in the nephron, which revealed their functional importance (Laski and Pressley 1999). Aquaporins are also found in the small intestine and colon, notably the type also found in the proximal tubule; this type is also present in the peritoneal membranes and may have a key effect on the efficiency of peritoneal dialysis. The specific type found in the collecting duct responds to ADH with increased synthesis and altered intracellular distribution. Biologically, water movement is such a fundamental process that we should not perhaps be surprised that plants also have aquaporins (Zeidel 1998). Before long, further understanding of these channels may allow the design of drugs appropriate to certain disturbances in water balance. ADH also activates receptors in the thick ascending limb of the loop, thereby promoting the sodium transport into medullary interstitial fluid, which is vital for the subsequent conservation of water in the collecting ducts. Synthetic antagonists (V_2 receptor antagonists) are already in use to treat some conditions where nonosmotic stimulation of ADH (such as that seen in hypovolemia but also in pregnancy and cardiac or hepatic failure) leads to excessive water retention and, hence, to hyponatremia (Cardenas and Gines 2001).

Clinically, then, how should we view hyponatremia (Michell 1995a; Palevsky 1998; Verbalis 1998)?

• The usual cause of hyponatremia is hypovolemia, rather than overhydration.
• Hyponatremia requires not only a predominant water loss (correctly called *hypertonic dehydration*, to reflect the effect on ECF) but an inability to correct via thirst (water access restricted or the animal is too weak to drink, inhibited by pain, or unable to retain what it drinks).
• Because water crosses most cell membranes freely, hyponatremia or hypernatremia respectively imply that water flows into or out of intracellular fluid, causing cells to swell or shrink. This matters most in brain because it is surrounded by the rigid cranium. Given time, brain cells are particularly adept at adjusting their intracellular concentration of organic solutes to offset these potentially damaging osmotic gradients. It also takes time to adjust these intracellular solutes back to normal after plasma sodium concentration recovers (Michell 1995a; Ayus and Arieff 1996). Thus, the risk of an abnormal plasma sodium concentration causing its most obvious and dangerous effects on brain depends not only on the extent of the rise or fall but the speed at which it occurred. Insidious hyponatremia may be well tolerated even when severe, but the instantaneous correction of any severe hypernatremia or hyponatremia is potentially dangerous even if correction does not overshoot normal plasma concentration.

Hyponatremia is readily caused by injudicious use of low-sodium parenteral solutions in hypovolemic patients. Apart from being inappropriate, because only a solution with a sodium concentration similar to plasma is efficient in boosting extracellular volume, such solutions are potentially hazardous, especially in surgical patients in whom, apart from stimuli arising from actual fluid deficits, there is often disproportionate retention of water compared with sodium, during recovery. Low-sodium solutions are also mistakenly advised for cardiac patients, to "avoid salt loading." But, even in cardiac patients, the reason for giving the parenteral solution is to repair extracellular volume, and every liter of extracellular fluid inescapably requires around 145 mmol of sodium to act as its osmotic skeleton and maintain its volume (Michell 1994b, 1995a).

Other Aspects of Renal Tubular Function. The importance of the distal nephron in regulating sodium and potassium excretion has already been described, but it is also an important site of calcium reabsorption, independent of sodium, under the influence of PTH, whereas magnesium is predominantly reabsorbed in the loop and potassium in the proximal tubule, virtually completely—hence the dependence on distal excretion. PTH also enables the proximal tubule to promote phosphate excretion by suppression of reabsorption. Thus, when bone mineral is mobilized by PTH in response to inadequate calcium intake or inadequate intake of vitamin D or inadequate activation to calcitriol, PTH appropriately promotes the necessary retention of the calcium and the excretion of the unnecessary phosphate. Since the latter depends on suppression of reabsorption from glomerular filtrate, it is made impotent by gross reductions in GFR, since reduction of reabsorption scarcely matters if little is filtered in the first place. That is the particular problem of patients with chronic renal failure and, together with adverse effects of the associated changes in PTH secretion (which increases in response to hyperphosphatemia, as well as hypocalcemia), it is the reason why it is essential to control their phosphate intake (Michell 1995a, b).

As well as phosphate, a number of specific carriers in the proximal tubule enable the excretion of organic compounds, many of them weak acids, and among these are important hepatic metabolites and many drugs. The latter, such as diuretics and some antibiotics, are expected to act within the urinary system. Thus, the efficiency of secretion into urine, or elimination form the body, can be vitally affected by overall renal function (reflected by GFR) but especially by competition for the same secretory route or by the effects of urine pH. The latter will depend on the pK of the organic acid (hence, its tendency to associate or dissociate in response to pH) and on membrane solubility of the undissociated form. The effect of pH should also depend on the predominant site of reabsorption, because urine pH gradients are essentially attained in the distal, rather than the proximal, nephron. The significance of low urine pH is that it indicates that loading of the urinary buffers is complete: it is the hydrogen ions carried on the buffers that represent significant excretion of hydrogen ions, whereas the free concentration, even in maximally acidified urine, is minuscule—the hydrogen ions in 0.5 mL of gastric acid would require a gallon of urine to be excreted at pH 4.5, were it not for the urinary buffers.

The proximal tubule contributes to regulation of acid-base balance by reabsorbing bicarbonate (both directly, and indirectly by recycling with some secreted hydrogen ions as carbonate acid, i.e., dissolved CO_2) and by loading the urinary buffers with secreted hydrogen ions, whereas hydrogen-ion secretion in the distal nephron, which is also facilitated by aldosterone, serves to acidify urine in the sense of lowering its pH to the levels characteristic of carnivores and omnivores. In contrast, mature herbivores produce more alkaline urine. Interestingly, in preruminant calves, urine is acidic and contains significant phosphate buffer, but, in mature ruminants, the main route from plasma for phosphate is into saliva rather than urine; nevertheless, as in the kidney, the hormone involved is still PTH. As well as phosphate, ammonia secreted from the proximal tubule is a vital urinary buffer and is dependent on an adequate supply of glutamine. The liver, through its role in urea synthesis and glutamine supply, plays an important subsidiary role in the regulation of plasma pH.

Apart from the hormones that control renal function, many affect it in ways not yet understood; for example, calcitonin affects renal sodium excretion, but we are unaware of any functional significance, whereas catecholamines and prostaglandins have multiple effects that await functional clarification (Michell 1995a). Among them is a very important renoprotective effect of prostaglandins during widespread vasoconstriction; this protection is undermined by nonsteroid antiinflammatory drugs (NSAIDs), thus predisposing patients to acute renal failure. As well as hormones already mentioned, those with an important regulatory role for sodium excretion include angiotensin, which not only promotes aldosterone secretion but also sodium reabsorption [and is also an extremely potent vasoconstrictor (Ultendahl and Aurell 1998)], and also two types of hormone promoting the excretion of the excess sodium present in most diets, including even those of most herbivores. ASTI/EDLI is an active sodium-transport inhibitor produced, probably from the brain, in response to sodium loading, whereas ANP is a hormone produced by the heart and serves to reduce circulating volume and thereby offloads the left ventricle. ANP not only accelerates urinary sodium excretion but promotes transfer of fluid from plasma into interstitial fluid. The pressure (downstream of constricted arterioles) enables it to serve as a reservoir via capillary uptake of fluid. EDLI, as an endogenous digitalis-like inhibitor of sodium transport, probably represents the evolutionary reason for the existence of cardiac glycoside receptors, in a manner analogous to endogenous opiates and morphine. Although the most familiar effects of angiotensin are renal, it also increases thirst and has widespread cellular effects; hence, the effects of ACE inhibitors (which prevent its activation to angiotensin II) are not restricted to those on renal function or arterial pressure (Michell 1999).

How Does the Kidney Reconcile Its Multiple Functions? Renal regulation of sodium balance and the control of GFR are not only essential to the stabilization of ECF volume but also to the long-term stability of arterial pressure. Sustained increases in pressure provide a strong stimulus for a compensatory pressure natriuresis, and defects in this are probably important in the involvement of dietary sodium in the pathogenesis of hypertension, alongside changes in the production of ASTI/EDLI leading to alterations in the ionic content of arteriolar cells (Michell 1995a). How these two aspects of the regulation of renal sodium excretion are reconciled is scarcely considered in the literature because of the specialized fragmentation of research "fields". From a whole-animal standpoint, this is only one glaring deficiency in the general assumption that sodium regulation is well understood. We know many of the instruments and some of the instrumental themes, but few have considered the shape of the symphony. We will return to this in the later parts of this chapter when we consider edema and hypertension, which, alongside renal failure, hypovolemia, and shock, are among the most important clinical disturbances of the systems supporting the fluid environment of the cells.

SHOCK. No clinical condition more decisively illustrates the balance between adaptive and maladaptive responses that characterizes so much of pathophysiology and that imposes on therapy such a fine line between triumph and disaster.

Clinically, the main forms of shock are hypovolemic (including hemorrhagic and traumatic), endotoxic, septic (which has bacteria in circulation and includes the effect of exotoxins), neurogenic (e.g., following spinal trauma—but includes some effects of endotoxin), anaphylactic (triggered by a hypersensitivity reaction and includes histamine among its mediators), and cardiogenic (caused by acute heart failure, seldom recognized in veterinary practice and physiologically very different from other forms). Functionally, and therefore in the targets for the therapy, there is substantial overlap, especially between hypovolemic shock and endotoxic or septic shock.

Hypovolemia and Defense of Arterial Pressure: Effects on Capillary Perfusion. Hypovolemic shock is a caricature of the physiological response to hemorrhage (Michell 1989). Thus, peripheral vasoconstriction protects arterial pressure and facilitates capillary uptake of fluid from the interstitial space, but, if sustained for too long, if too widespread, or if triggered by inappropriate stimuli, the adverse effects predominate. Among these are tissue hypoxia and cell damage, leading to acidosis and hyperkalemia, and increased capillary permeability, leading to further leakage of plasma and a rising packed-cell volume. The additional oxygen capacity of the higher red cell concentration is almost immaterial in a shocked recumbent animal, whereas the associated increase in viscosity is disastrous for capillary perfusion. Peripheral circulatory failure with inadequate capillary flow is the central feature of hypovolemic shock, whether or not cardiac performance is also impaired. The key to therapy, therefore, is restoration of circulating volume and avoidance of increased blood viscosity or further vasoconstriction. Hypotension per se is not an issue until shock is profound, and a slightly subnormal arterial pressure may help to avoid secondary bleeding due to clot displacement. Abnormal clotting is another feature of shock, initially excessive and then impeded by consumption of precursors for fibrin production (Michell 1989; Vervloet et al. 1998): while sensitization of coagulation seems an appropriate response to hemorrhage, it is inappropriate in other causes of hypovolemic shock (e.g., diarrhea or burns) and may further prejudice capillary perfusion.

Endotoxic and Septic Shock. The other main form of shock is endotoxic, but there is considerable overlap in the final common pathways, because splanchnic vasoconstriction, through its effect on intestinal membranes and on the liver, increases the risk of access of microorganisms or toxins to the systemic circulation (Michell 1989, 1995a; Rowlands et al. 1999). The hemodynamic effects of endotoxin produce regional hyperperfusion, necessitating excessive constriction in other capillary beds, and this, together with increased capillary permeability, results in elements of hypovolemic shock in endotoxemia. A key element of endotoxin shock (or of septic shock, which is very similar) is the abnormal presence in circulation of a variety of inflammatory mediators, together with the effects of these and others in the peripheral circulation—for example, endothelins, eicosanoids, free radicals, nitric oxide, interleukins, tumor-necrosis factor, and platelet-activating factor (Michell 1995a, 1997a, b; Bellingan 1999; Wheeler and Bernard 1999; Wort and Evans 1999). The hope is that, in due course, specific antibodies or receptor antagonists will provide effective remedies according to the type of shock and its duration. In both forms of shock, the combination of defective circulation and abnormal cell metabolism makes tissue hypoxia a serious problem—hence the continuing importance of circulatory and ventilatory support. In septic shock, cardiac output can be supranormal, but tissue perfusion is still compromised by excessive perfusion of inappropriate regions.

Although shock generally causes tachycardia, it can also present with bradycardia and inadequate arteriolar tone; both are reversible by repair of circulating volume (Jacobson et al. 1994). This important clinical observation is absent from most textbooks because of the difficulty in explaining it (Jacobson and Secker 1994). Shock can occur in the context of a more protracted metabolic response to trauma, characterized by exaggerated catabolism that is not easily corrected by even high levels of calorie supplementation (Griffiths et al. 1999). As we understand more of the detailed pathophysiology of the different forms of shock, we will increasingly find that as well as the similarities of approach, based on shared final common pathways, we will acquire far more specific treatments appropriate to the type of shock and the time since its onset. One leading medical expert recently suggested that septic shock was still so prevalent, so expensive to treat, and so lethal that if an effective vaccine appeared, it could be cost effective.

Constraints on Progress. In assessing new therapies, the lessons of the last 30 years will remain valid:

- Agents that work well as pretreatments in models may be less effective (e.g., corticosteroids) or dangerous (β-blockers) once shock is established.
- Agents that prolong survival do not necessarily reduce mortality.
- Since many of the pathophysiological responses underlying the therapeutic targets combine adaptive and potentially adverse effects, new therapies frequently generate conflicting data.
- The ethical and technical problems of designing clinical trials in such a lethal condition, where each patient, their injuries, and their responses are in a sense unique, and where the duty to save life may override the duty to obey a protocol (e.g., with regard to ancillary therapies).
- Sadly there is a pattern for new drugs to emerge from sound theory and encouraging results in experimental animals, only to founder on dubious efficacy in patients or on unanticipated hazards.

No therapy illustrates this better than high-dose intravenous corticosteroids, still widely used in veterinary patients, but with the identical product now contraindicated in human patients. Few if any drugs offer a wider spectrum of pharmacological properties that should benefit patients with shock, especially if administered early. Yet there is very little satisfactory peer-reviewed clinical trial evidence to substantiate their effectiveness, and what there is has been open to serious criticism. In human patients, their use became contraindicated when a tiny minority of patients with unsuspected renal failure had increased mortality following corticosteroid therapy for shock. In veterinary patients, they have mainly been used for companion animals with hypovolemic shock, because the cost of providing the obligatory high dose rate in larger animals like horses is prohibitive. Most of the evidence for their efficacy, of which a significant amount is in experimental dog models (some of them horrific and inappropriate), relates to endotoxic, not hypovolemic, shock. Would I use them in my own dog? Definitely, because the theoretical and anecdotal evidence is persuasive, and the level of therapeutic risk that paralyzes human medicine in a climate imposed by fear of litigation is, mercifully, well within what we regard as highly acceptable, faced with an inherently lethal clinical emergency. I would accept a 1 in a 1000 adverse event—but no doctor could any longer afford to, because, in court, the newly expert barrister would ask coldly, "Doctor, were you unaware of the published evidence regarding the risks of...?" It will be interesting to see how events turn out for low-volume hypertonic saline, used not as fluid replacement (which remains essential) but as an adjunctive stimulus to cardiovascular function. Currently, the hazards seem minimal (except perhaps in horses and poorly interpreted rat experiments), the mode of action is only partly explained, and the majority of the clinical evidence so far seems encouraging (Michell 1995a, 1997a, b).

ACID-BASE DISTURBANCES. The predominant buffer system of blood is the bicarbonate system with hemoglobin taking a subsidiary but important role. Within cells, various proteins are important, and intracellular transfer of excess hydrogen ions is an important adaptation to chronic acidosis. Phosphate also provides intracellular buffering alongside its vital role as a urinary buffer; in plasma, it is a relatively unimportant buffer. Chemically, buffers are effective only for a pH range within about 1.0 of their pK, and this means that at a physiological pH (7.40), bicarbonate with its pK of 6.1 is not the optimal in vitro buffer. But acid-base regulation goes beyond the in vitro properties of buffers: the bicarbonate buffer system derives its power from the fact that its two major components, bicarbonate and carbonic acid (dissolved CO_2), are capable of being independently controlled, the former by the kidneys and the latter through the regulation of respiration:

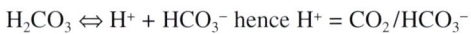

$$H_2CO_3 \Leftrightarrow H^+ + HCO_3^- \text{ hence } H^+ = CO_2/HCO_3^-$$

The latter, unlike the logarithmic Henderson-Hasselbalch equation, is not mathematically correct, but it is the key to understanding the pathophysiology of acid-base disturbances (Michell et al. 1989; Michell 1994a; Palazzo 1997).

Defenses Against Acidosis and Alkalosis. When hydrogen ions accumulate, they titrate bicarbonate, and its concentration falls; this, rather than the change in pH, defines the acidosis as metabolic. If pH falls because of retained CO_2, the acidosis is defined as respiratory, and alkalosis is similarly metabolic or respiratory, depending whether the primary change is a rise in bicarbonate or a fall in CO_2. Abnormal pH, if it is sufficiently severe or sustained, threatens survival through a multitude of effects, not least on the charge on proteins, the distribution of solutes (including potassium) across membranes, the activity of enzymes, and the release of oxygen from hemoglobin or calcium from albumin. On the other hand, even if the concentration of CO_2 and bicarbonate are both abnormal, pH is defended provided the *ratio* remains constant. Thus, the physiological response to a respiratory disturbance is renal alteration of bicarbonate in the same direction as the change of CO_2, restoring the ratio toward normal. Hence, a chronic respiratory acidosis is frequently accompanied by a compensatory, secondary, bicarbonate retention (not a metabolic alkalosis). Similarly, metabolic acidosis is sensitively compensated for by the hyperventilation to match the fall in bicarbonate with an appropriate fall in CO_2. In contrast, metabolic alkalosis (caused by loss or sequestration of gastric or abomasal acid) is poorly served by respiratory compensation, because the price of the requisite CO_2 retention would be inadequate pulmonary oxygenation of arterial blood. Fortunately, metabolic alkalosis is well served by the fact that the kidney is very resistant to excess bicarbonate reabsorption unless a patient is hypovolemic; hence, correction of hypovolemia with a bicarbonate-free solution (i.e., saline) is the appropriate remedy—there is no need to replace lost acid. Because hypovolemic animals, under the influence of aldosterone, secrete hydrogen ions or potassium as they retrieve sodium in the distal nephron, cell deficits of potassium encourage unwanted excretion of hydrogen ions in animals with metabolic alkalosis. Although saline will help, by correcting hypovolemia, the provision of additional potassium may facilitate recovery.

The kidney is the only significant excretion route for hydrogen ions, and animals with metabolic acidosis, the most common and life-threatening acid-base disturbance, depend on respiratory compensation but ultimately enhanced renal excretion of hydrogen ions to survive. The latter may be facilitated by increased generation of ammonia buffer from glutamine during sustained acidosis.

The clinician can accelerate survival by providing additional bicarbonate either directly or in the form of precursors such as lactate or citrate that yield bicarbonate once they are metabolized. Excessively fast administration of bicarbonate may impede release of oxygen from hemoglobin in the tissue capillaries and can suppress ionized calcium concentration (by increasing binding to albumin) as well as allow hyperkalemia to give way rapidly to hypokalemia as plasma pH rises. While much is made of paradoxical hyperventilation in humans [because CO_2 rises rapidly after treatment in both plasma and cerebrospinal fluid (CSF), whereas CSF bicarbonate lags behind, leaving CSF with a relative excess of CO_2], our experience in diarrheic calves is that excess bicarbonate in some individuals suppresses ventilation, perhaps because endotoxemia allows increased blood-brain barrier permeability and overspill of bicarbonate into CSF. The acidosis of diarrhea is not simply due to a bicarbonate loss but to compromised renal function caused by hypovolemia (prerenal failure) and by fermentation causing abnormal production of organic acids within the intestine. In severe hypovolemia, underperfused hypoxic tissues generate additional acid, including lactic acid. Healthy, normally perfused liver has a huge capacity to metabolize lactic acid, replacing it in plasma with bicarbonate; hence, the rapid recovery of healthy athletes and the ability to use lactate, e.g., in Hartmann's solution, as a source of bicarbonate.

Treatment. Metabolic acidosis or alkalosis, as already indicated, can be corrected by appropriate fluid therapy (oral or parenteral), but respiratory disturbance can not (except with certain solutions not in routine clinical use); the requirement for respiratory disturbances is to restore normal gas exchange. The risk of excess bicarbonate has already been discussed, and excessive inappropriate use of bicarbonate-free solutions causes dilutional acidosis (by reducing bicarbonate concentration). Quantitative evaluation of acid-base disturbances is therefore vital: in the case of canine gastric torsion, for example, metabolic acidosis or alkalosis may result, whereas in diarrheic calves it is a reasonable prediction that they are acidotic, but, without a measurement, the clinician lacks a safe basis for daring to provide the huge amounts of bicarbonate that they may actually require. The necessary measurement is plasma bicarbonate, either from a blood-gas machine or, much faster and cheaper, a measure of total CO_2, e.g., from the Harleco micro apparatus (Michell et al 1989). This simply liberates CO_2 from bicarbonate by addition of acid, as in the classic *Van Slyke*, technique. The measured CO_2 is compared with that from a standard bicarbonate solution in a small custom-built machine that does not even require electricity. Although called total CO_2, this is a measure of bicarbonate and thus a sound guide for correction of metabolic acidosis or alkalosis. CO_2 originally in the sample is also liberated, but its concentration, expressed in micromoles per liter, is so minute, compared with bicarbonate, that it has no significant impact on the evaluation of the metabolic disturbance.

Clinical Acid-Base Assessment: SID, a Sadly Inappropriate Distraction. Unfortunately, and unlike human medicine, no veterinary account of acid-base balance is complete without reference to SID, strong ion difference, which has a cult-following among some North American veterinarians. It does have some interesting applications, especially in respiratory or exercise physiology, or in attempting to predict the effect of diet on acid-base balance, but as a basis for the routine management of clinical disturbances, it is terrifyingly complicated, demands multiple measurements with their cumulative uncertainties, and can lead to lethal decisions, at least in diarrheic calves; it is also logically flawed (Michell 1994b; Grove-White and Michell 2001).

SID is similar to but far more complicated than *anion gap*, the concentration sum of $(Na + K) - (HCO_3 + Cl)$. This reflects the contribution to acid-base disturbances of routinely unmeasured anions, notably of organic acids such as lactate. It therefore helps to distinguish (apart from clinical considerations) between acidosis due to bicarbonate loss and those due to accumulation of acid (in which anion gap is increased) (Ishihara and Szerlip 1998).

Any consistently reproducible measurement has a legitimate sphere of interpretation. The problem with SID is its practicality and its safety in the management of clinical cases of metabolic acidosis or alkalosis, regardless of its proclaimed theoretical interest. The latter seems to rest on the recurrent trap of regarding physiological regulation of acid-base balance in terms of in vitro buffering rather than in terms of the dynamically responsive systems of intact animals. It also includes assertions that are measurably incorrect, for example, that "as lactate and chloride are strong ions, they can not affect acid-base balance," whereas they are both instrumental in improving metabolic acidosis or alkalosis, respectively. Even more extraordinary, hydrogen-ion concentration per se is regarded as an unimportant outcome rather than a primary consideration for both phys-

iological regulation and clinical management. Were this so, it seems remarkable that proton pumps should be so important or that, across a range of vertebrates, the usual pH, which varies with temperature, maintains a relatively fixed distance from the neutral pH, which also varies with temperature. Exactly the same is seen in mammals, thanks to the effect of the imidazole residues of hemoglobin, and this casts serious doubt on the circumstances in which "correction" of blood-gas data for abnormalities of body temperature is actually valid (Michell et al. 1989; Michell 1994a; Danzi and Pozos 1994). The reason for this parallel movement of "normal" pH and neutral pH as temperature changes is that the separation between them determines the balance between associated and dissociated forms of a vital range of organic molecules, including many proteins, not just buffers, and this has profound functional implications. It therefore seems beyond credibility that plasma pH, the pH of the internal environment, should have evolved as a happenstance of "strong ion difference," not least when Na, K, and bicarbonate are subject to independent regulatory mechanisms.

RENAL FAILURE. Not all renal dysfunction results in renal failure that has the specific meaning that GFR is reduced below normal (Narins 1994; Michell 1995b, 1999; Gleadhill and Michell 1996; Barber and Elliott 1996; Brady et al. 1996; Thadhani et al. 1996). Thus, defective urinary acidification (renal acidosis), glomerulonephritis leading to proteinuria (failure to restrain macromolecules), and defective proximal tubular reabsorption (Fanconi syndrome) do not inherently involve renal failure, though it may appear subsequently. Essentially there are five forms of renal failure:

- Chronic: An insidious reduction of the nephron population, compensated for by the surviving intact nephrons, but usually relentlessly progressive and invariably irreversible.
- Acute-on-chronic: As above but presenting suddenly due to decompensation, for example, as a result of acute hypovolemia.
- Acute, prerenal: Sudden decline in renal function provoked by inadequate perfusion, for example, cardiac failure or hypovolemia. The nephron population is normal and remains so unless the condition is protracted.
- Acute, postrenal: As above but provoked by urinary obstruction or by bladder rupture so that urinary solutes accumulate through failure of elimination.
- Acute, intrarenal—the usual context in which acute renal failure (ARF) is considered: A sudden collapse of renal function caused, for example, by toxins or by internal maldistribution of blood flow (as in hepatorenal syndrome (Michell 1995a; Epstein 1997) with underperfusion of the cortex and relative overperfusion of the medulla. Unlike in chronic renal failure, all nephrons are probably dysfunctional, and there is no scope for compensatory responses.

Acute Renal Failure. The renal cortex and the renal medulla are at the extremes of perfusion, with the latter being close to hypoxia even in normality, while the kidneys receive 25% of cardiac output. In ARF, there is severe reduction of renal perfusion with a disproportionately greater fall in GFR, suggesting redistribution of blood toward the medulla. Cortical underperfusion impedes tubular reabsorption and reduces GFR, while medullary overperfusion washes out the concentrated interstitial fluid needed for urinary concentration. Nevertheless, the outer medulla may experience sufficient fall in perfusion to impede its functions through hypoxia. The atypical (but not invariable) result therefore is the paradoxical production of small volumes of urine that, instead of being concentrated and low in sodium, as in response to dehydration, is dilute but contains substantial amounts of sodium. Sometimes, if the impairment of tubular reabsorption is even more severe than the fall in GFR, an atypical form of ARF can occur with increased urine output. In recovery, urine output is high because of prior retention of water and electrolytes and continuing tubular dysfunction. Key components of the development of ARF are afferent arteriolar constriction (leading to reduced GFR), abnormal backleak of urinary solutes from tubular fluid, and ultimately blockage by tubular debris. Additional problems may arise from redistribution of Na-K ATPase in proximal tubular cells (Michell 1995a; Paller 1998; Sutton and Molitoris 1998). Endothelins appear to be important as causes of the excessive vasoconstriction (Kelly and Molitoris 2000). As with most aspects of renal function, the role of nitric oxide in ARF appears to be complex, potentially important, but, as yet, very incompletely defined (Gabbai 1999).

Recovery from ARF depends on the cause and in particular whether tubular basement membranes are damaged, which limits the capacity for repair; the balance between cell death and repair depends on the relative activation of extracellular regulated—or stress-activated—protein kinases, while apoptosis (regulated cell death) can contribute both to loss of tubular function and to remodeling and recovery (Lieberthal 1998; Safirstein et al. 1998). The fundamental defects are functional, rather than structural: hence, unlike in chronic renal failure, recovery is possible (despite high initial mortality) and can be complete, given time (Liano and Pascual 1998). ARF does not characteristically predispose patients to subsequent development of chronic renal failure.

Chronic Renal Failure. In chronic renal failure, the symptoms reflect failure of the regulatory, endocrine, and excretory functions of the kidney. The endocrine functions include not only the production of renin, erythropoietin, prostaglandins, and the final activation of calcitriol (1,25-dihydroxycholecalciferol, the active hormonal form of vitamin D) but the proximal tubular reabsorption and catabolism of proteins smaller than albumin, several of which, like insulin, are hormones. A wide range of endocrine disturbances are therefore possible and also include reduced target-organ responsiveness resulting from the uremic environment. The latter refers to the complex deterioration of plasma composition, not the results of increased urea concentrations, since it is a relatively harmless excretory product (as is creatinine). Increased plasma concentration of nitrogenous end products (urea and creatinine) constitutes azotemia; uremia means that the increases are associated with sufficient decline in renal function to be symptomatic. Because these changes progress so insidiously and are so advanced by the time they become obvious, one of the key problems in renal medicine is the availability of simple, affordable, precise methods to measure GFR or other indices of normal renal function (Michell 1995b; Gleadhill and Michell 1996).

In dogs and cats, a frequent sign of chronic renal failure is polyuria, together with compensatory polydipsia. This probably reflects medullary damage and, perhaps, reduced sensitivity to ADH. Generation of maximally concentrated medullary interstitial fluid, and therefore maximal capacity to concentrate the urine, probably requires an intact population of loops, not a mixture of intact and nonfunctional nephrons. This sign may be more obvious in dogs and cats than in people because animals drink in a regulatory fashion and normally produce concentrated urine whereas people, in a sense, are "normally" polyuric in order to eliminate excess fluid drunk for nonregulatory reasons. In people, where glomerulonephritis is common, albuminuria is almost the hallmark of renal disease, but renal failure can occur without it. On the other hand, tests for *microalbuminuria* (detection of a trace concentration of albumin by using specific antibodies) enable detection of increased intraglomerular pressure. This may well be one of the critical aspects of progression of chronic renal failure—sustaining GFR at supranormal levels in surviving intact nephrons but inducing damage that hastens their demise. The value of ACE inhibitors or angiotensin receptor antagonists in renal disease lies not only in lowering arterial blood pressure, but also, among other properties, the ability to preferentially relax the efferent arteriole and reduce intraglomerular pressure. Conversely, diabetics risk renal damage even with arterial pressures in the high-normal range, because their afferent arterioles are relaxed, so a greater proportion of the arterial pressure is transmitted to the glomeruli (Michell 1999; Mogensen 2000).

EDEMA, HYPERTENSION, AND DIURETICS. Most people with chronic renal failure become hypertensive, as do many cats; interestingly dogs, though susceptible to hypertension, and classic experimental models for its study, are relatively resistant to it when they have renal insufficiency (Michell et al. 1997). In dialysis patients, hypertension is frequently exacerbated by hypervolemia (Zucchelli and Santoro 2000), but more generally hypertension and edema do not inherently tend to coexist. Fundamentally, that is not surprising—hypertension generally involves excessive peripheral resistance that, by reducing the perfusion pressure of downstream capillaries, tends to promote uptake of interstitial fluid, as in the natural response to hypovolemia including hemorrhage (see the section *Shock*). Edema, conversely, involves the expansion of the interstitial fluid from plasma. Since this involves the expansion of a large compartment from a small one, it could not continue unless the latter were continuously replenished (i.e., the kidney retained additional sodium and water). Thus, although the kidneys are seldom regarded as the primary cause of edema (except, for example, through excessive leakage of albumin), they are always the enabling cause because they continue to replenish plasma volume. Diuretics are mainly used in veterinary medicine to treat edema by impeding renal sodium retention: the definition of a clinically useful diuretic is not simply that it promotes urine output (as would water or alcohol) but that it promotes sodium excretion.

The main use of diuretics in people is to treat hypertension, although they are being overtaken by newer agents, especially calcium channel blockers, ACE inhibitors, and angiotensin receptor antagonists. The causes of hypertension are multifactorial and include genetic and endocrine factors (including prostaglandins, endothelins, and nitric oxide) and reduced renal perfusion, which liberates excess renin and angiotensin; renal artery stenosis is, in fact, one of the few entirely reversible causes of hypertension. It is an example of secondary hypertension, which is probably the predominant form in animals. Most human hypertension, however, is *essential* or primary; that is, as yet the cause is unknown. A number of interesting breeds of dog routinely run "normal" pressure well into the human hypertensive range (Michell 2000b), but the defining feature of hypertension is not statistical; it is the range of pressures above which the probability of cardiovascular and hence coronary, myocardial, ocular, renal, or cerebral damage is increased. We do not yet know whether the high-pressure breeds are showing an adaptive increase in pressure, in which case the factors sustaining it and preventing damage are of great interest, or whether they are models of essential hypertension. Nor do we know which pressures are damaging: systolic, diastolic, or pulse pressure, daytime or nocturnal pressure. We do know that in people the rapid morning rise is a period of cardiovascular hazard (Michell 1997c).

The most obvious role for diuretics is to reduce extracellular volume, which inevitably must eventually reduce arterial (and venous) pressure. That does not underlie their sustained efficacy in hypertension, which seems more related to their effects on the intracellular electrolytes of the arterioles and thereby on their responsiveness to constrictor or dilator stimuli. The oldest accurate, clinical insight is probably that derived from Chinese medicine, identifying the link between renal disease, salt intake, and increased pressure in the pulse. Over 2000 years later, one of the keystones of antihypertensive therapy, and thereby one of the most profitable classes of drug, remains those which promote increased excretion of sodium: the diuretics.

Sodium and Hypertension, What, then, is the role of sodium, or salt (since some see importance in the anion), in the pathogenesis of hypertension? There are two sorts of answer—mechanistic and observational— and both continue to cause controversy. The most coherent causal hypothesis remains that of De Wardener and Haddy (see Michell 1995a), which is essentially as follows: Excess salt, by provoking chronic expansion of extracellular volume, causes increased secretion of natriuretic hormones; (a) those that inhibit sodium transport do so in the kidneys, where the response is appropriate, but also (b) in the arterioles, where the consequences are a secondary increase in intracellular calcium (in exchange for the surplus intracellular sodium accumulated through inhibition of the sodium pumps) and, therefore, supranormal responsiveness to constrictor stimuli.

The most persuasive observational data are that, almost without exception, civilizations with high salt intake are more prone to hypertension, and those with the highest intakes are extremely susceptible, whereas, at the other extreme, those with intakes close to or only slightly above the likely nutritional requirement are almost without hypertension. There appears to be no exception to the rule that, in civilizations on such "low" (i.e., nonexorbitant) salt intakes, primary hypertension is virtually unknown and blood pressure scarcely rises with age. The age-related rise in arterial pressure, tolerated as normal in Western medicine, appears to be a hallmark of chronic ingestion of excess sodium, compared with nutritional need: it is also seen in dogs and cats, which also routinely consume far more sodium than their daily requirement, though in these species, since they seldom (if ever) suffer from primary hypertension, it is a moot point whether it does them any harm.

Hypertension is not the only adverse effect of chronic ingestion of excess sodium; among those which have received most attention is that, in postmenopausal women, the excretion of excess calcium alongside sodium (as a result of suppression of proximal tubular reabsorption) predisposes those women to osteoporosis. The fact that excretion of excess sodium can predispose to "unintended" renal loss of divalent ions is worth remembering in any species, for example, in considering the pathogenesis of ruminant hypocalcemia or hypomagnesemia.

There is, however, a more fundamental link between sodium and hypertension, which is encompassed in Guyton's hypothesis that the kidneys are the long-term regulators of arterial pressure, through pressure natriuresis: increased pressure sensitively increases sodium excretion until normal pressure is regained. The slope of this relationship is steep; that is, hypertension powerfully increases corrective excretion of sodium, and conditions that predispose to hypertension, such as chronic renal failure, do so by flattening the slope so that a greater rise in pressure is needed to achieve the same acceleration of sodium excretion. It must be said that this very satisfying concept is substantially based on computer models using data from experimental dogs subjected to extremely high sodium intakes. It also poses a question to which we will return: What is normal pressure: daytime, nocturnal, the pressure that I had two minutes ago or 10 minutes ago?

Arterial Pressure: Stable Yet Inconstant. It remains extremely difficult to reconcile the demands placed on long-term regulation of arterial pressure with the fact of its extreme short-term lability. It is not unusual, in normal individuals, to have daytime diastolic pressures above their nocturnal systolics. How would you decide to fill your car if the gas gauge constantly and largely inexplicably fluctuated between levels close to full and not far above empty? The preoccupation with baroreceptors, protecting arterial pressure against postural change or hemorrhage, together with the difficulty until recently of chronic noninvasive (*ambulatory*) monitoring of arterial pressure have left generations of clinical students with a deceptive impression of arterial pressure as one of the physiological set-points, like body temperature, which is most rigorously and effectively defended, despite the fact that the inconstancy of arterial pressure was obvious 270 years ago. Minute-to-minute, year-to-year, regulation of arterial pressure is, in fact, nothing like the regulation of temperature in a thermostatically controlled room. Perhaps the most remarkable observation, taken for granted, is that despite this striking short-term variability, and the carelessness with which blood pressure is usually measured in people, individuals tend to have characteristic, reasonably repeatable, pressures in long-term studies; this has been repeatedly shown in humans (*tracking*) and is also seen in dogs (Swales 1996; Bodey and Michell 1997).

CAUSES OF EDEMA. The textbook causes of edema are entirely obvious and logical in terms of fluid exchange between capillaries and interstitial fluid. Fluid leaves the capillaries to replenish interstitial fluid, the environment of the cells, thanks to the pressure gradient at the arterial end. At the venous end, capillaries retrieve interstitial fluid because their perfusion pressure has fallen, but, with the increased concentration of albumin resulting from the preceding fluid loss, there is a favorable oncotic (colloid osmotic) gradient for fluid uptake. Clearly, this depends on the oncotic gradient remaining intact, and it is normally protected by the acceleration of lymphatic drainage whenever interstitial protein increases (through capillary leakage or cell turnover or damage).

The oncotic gradient is undermined by lymphatic obstruction or by capillary leakage, which is why these are powerful causes of edema, alongside increased capillary pressure resulting from arteriolar dilatation or impaired venous drainage (obstruction or cardiac failure). The oncotic gradient is also undermined by reduced plasma albumin (hepatic disease, enteric or renal protein loss), but this has to be severe before edema becomes obvious because of the "safety factor" provided by acceleration of lymphatic drainage when excess interstitial fluid starts to accumulate. It is the unique route for removal of excess interstitial protein provided by the lymphatics that makes them so important in edema; it is a smaller route for fluid removal than the venous end of the capillaries, but the only one available to proteins. Similarly, the significance of increased capillary permeability is not primarily leakage of water (to which capillaries are mostly freely permeable) but of albumin, undermining the oncotic gradient for fluid removal from tissue spaces: when the mesh of a trawler net is made larger, it is the small fish that fall out faster, not the water. To these factors, which have been familiar for decades, more recent research has added the role of adsorption of fluid onto the structural components of the interstitial spaces and of drastic reductions in interstitial pressure as factors in the rapid formation of edema, together with the ability of β integrins to increase tension on the fibrous networks that oppose swelling of the hyaluron gel (Michell 1995a; Reed at al. 2001).

So, with the exception of pregnancy, the causes of edema seem obvious: impeded venous return in heart failure, protein leakage in glomerulonephritis, and inadequate production of albumin in hepatic disease, perhaps together with the effect of abnormally accumulating toxins on capillary permeability (which is also altered during pregnancy). The kidney restores plasma volume, enabling the continuing expansion of interstitial volume. Of course, if the kidney were to chronically retain excess sodium, that would also cause edema because the expanded extracellular volume would overfill the interstitial compartment; reduced arteriolar tone, to maintain arterial pressure, would raise downstream capillary pressure and favor outward flow of fluid from capillaries into the tissue spaces, the reverse of the response to hemorrhage. More interestingly, ANP prevents excessive plasma volume (and potential cardiac overload) not only by increasing sodium excretion, but also by promoting transfer from plasma to interstitial fluid. It may seem anomalous that a salt-shedding hormone should thereby favor edema, but it illustrates the reservoir function of interstitial fluid—that is, to facilitate the maintenance of appropriate plasma volume by providing protection against both depletion and excess. Bone may serve a similar function for sodium, since, like calcium, its active extrusion from cells precludes significant intracellular reserves, but we know little about this. Although ANP is the best understood of the natriuretic peptides, others may also be important, including those from the brain and the kidneys (Michell 1995a; Drummer 2001).

Cardiac edema occurs amid continuing controversy regarding *forward* versus *backward* failure and growing understanding of the balance between adaptive and harmful aspects of the neuroendocrine responses, notably those affecting sodium balance and vascular tone, which are triggered by inadequate cardiac function—that is, inability to sustain an acceptable cardiac output without an unacceptable rise in filling pressure (Michell 1995a; Pacher 2001; Schrier et al. 2001). There is also the potential for new understanding of the adverse effects of endothelins on myocardial perfusion and ventricular remodeling in chronic failure to lead to therapeutic use of endothelin antagonists (Pacher 2001). Endothelial abnormalities may also exacerbate exercise intolerance. ANP levels increase but insufficiently to prevent edema; natriuretic peptide assays in plasma may help the clinical investigation of cardiac dysfunction (Haggstrom et al. 2000; Sisson 2000). Hepatic failure poses multiple factors affecting vascular permeability, distribution of blood volume (not least, the huge volume of portal capillaries), hepatic metabolism of hormones, neuroendocrine responses, renal function, and perhaps receptor sites involved in regulation of sodium balance, apart from the oncotic effects of defective albumin synthesis (Michell 1995b, 1996; Moller and Henriksen 1997; Cardenas and Gines 2001; Magri et al. 2001). As a result, not only edema but hyponatremia are common; as with cardiac edema, ANP increases, but not sufficiently to prevent edema (Levy 1997). Biliary stasis adds the effect of bile acids to cause both oxidative damage to tubular cells and to inhibit tubular reabsorption of sodium (Bomzon et al. 1997).

The Shortcomings of the Obvious. The basic principles underlying accumulation of excess interstitial fluid are, therefore, well understood, as are predisposing factors arising from specific failures of organ function. Why then does controversy continue to rage concerning the causes of edema, and why do they remain so uncertain that we could not confidently explain any of the common clinical causes of generalized edema to a truly inquisitive student? The nub of the problem is twofold:

• Does the kidney truly participate merely by replenishing plasma volume, or does it fuel the development of edema through primary overretention of sodium and water? Is edema, therefore, a condition associated with an "underfilled" or an "overfilled" intravascular compartment?
• Where, physiologically, are "underfill" or "overfill" detected, and what measurements will resolve our uncertainty?

The problems surrounding this controversy relate to technical, observational, and conceptual problems (Michell 1995b, 1996). At the dawn of the century of postgenomic medicine, 2000 years after the Sabbath on which Jesus saw fit to cure it (St Luke 14:2), "the dropsy" continues to defy us. The prerequisite for clarification was identified over 50 years ago by Peters (1948):

> The most crucial problem related to the formation of edema is the discovery of the criteria by which the kidneys determine whether to accelerate or retard the reabsorption of sodium.

Not the mechanisms (ANP, aldosterone, or GFR) but the criteria: How does the body measure total body sodium, and how does it relate that to sodium excretion in the context of regulating both arterial pressure and extracellular volume? Thirty years beyond my PhD, the answers are as elusive as when I began it, and the questions attract far less attention amid the delights of defining an ever-expanding and surprising range of mediators, receptors, and their genetic regulators.

Both of the key questions are obscured by a convenient device for tidying up the intelligibility of textbooks by reconciling with the theory almost any measurement that conflicts with it: effective arterial blood volume (EABV). This has evolved through several subtly different meanings, but essentially it says that even when measurements suggest that plasma volume is increased, it may actually be reduced in some unknown site where a hypothetical subcompartment (EABV) is monitored. The fact that the site is unknown, the compartment hypothetical, in a sense does not matter: we simply do not know how or where the body monitors total sodium or its crucial derivative, extracellular volume, whether interstitial or in plasma. There could be other important derivatives, for example, rate of lymphatic drainage in key sites, or, since the sodium pump is a major determinant of energy use, the rate of sodium transport, in response to natriuretic hormones. The question, with regard to EABV, is does it help, or is it simply a satisfying fiction (Michell 1996, 1998b)? Before returning finally to this issue, there are aspects of the use of diuretics that deserve further comment.

USE AND LIMITATIONS OF DIURETICS. Diuretics remain the frontline treatment for edema in animals. Moreover, edema may seem merely cosmetic with the exceptions of pulmonary or cerebral edema [which both have very different pathophysiology (Michell 1995b; Kempski 2001)], but it can be very uncomfortable, and the increased interstitial fluid may increase diffusion distances between cells and capillaries, so treatment matters. Like other antihypertensive drugs, the reason for the available plethora is not so much shortcomings of efficacy but the importance of side-effects and associated noncompliance in drugs used for extended periods, often lifelong.

Side Effects. The dose-response curve of diuretics tends to be steep, so that once there is a clear response, there is little likelihood of a useful increase in response from increased dosage, nor is there much likelihood of a further response from additional diuretics primarily affecting the same segment of the nephron. Increased dosage is much more likely to generate side effects than additional therapeutic benefit (Michell 1995b; Ellison 1999; Kaplan 1999). Among the many potential side effects, which range from irritating or inconvenient to potentially serious, hypovolemia, hypomagnesemia, and hypokalemia are important. Diuretic-induced potassium depletion results from increased delivery of fluid to the distal nephron and the effects of aldosterone. One approach to prevention, therefore, is the use of *potassium-sparing diuretics*, which act on the distal nephron to reduce sodium reabsorption, producing a modest natriuresis but an important reduction in potassium excretion (Michell 1995b; Hebert 1999). Although not conventionally included in this group, ACE inhibitors have an additive effect to restrict potassium excretion by reducing angiotensin-driven secretion of aldosterone. Hyperkalemia, should it occur, provides an independent drive to restore aldosterone secretion. Potassium-sparing diuretics are especially useful in hepatic disease where aldosterone levels are pathologically elevated (Brater 1999). Apart from other interactions between hypokalemia and hypomagnesemia already considered, diuretics often induce unwanted urinary loss of magnesium and calcium as well as potassium particularly in the case of loop diuretics, since this is the main site of magnesium and calcium reabsorption (Michell 1995b; Kelepouris and Agus 1998; Friedman and Bushinsky 1999; Wilcox 1999), whereas thiazides promote calcium reabsorption from the distal nephron. The efficacy of loop diuretics in nephrotic edema is restricted by binding to albumin in tubular fluid (Brater 1999).

Hypovolemia is the most dangerous potential effect of excessive diuresis, and it will result from a rate of urinary fluid loss that exceeds the maximum speed of mobilization of edema fluid. A more intense diuresis is both pointless and dangerous. This calls into question the habitual use of potent short-acting diuretics, notably loop diuretics; at worst, they produce a brief period of excessive diuresis followed by an extended period in which the kidney can compensate for the period of diuresis—that is, negate the purpose of giving the drug. It is essential to be aware that whenever diuretics are used, any nephron segment that is unaffected will be compensating for (i.e., opposing) their effects, and any time free of effective concentrations will allow even the target segments to compensate. Most diuretics only have major effects in one segment, whether or not they have minor effects in others. The exception is osmotic diuretics, but these are inappropriate in generalized edema, because they promote expansion of extracellular fluid (from intracellular fluid) and a watery diuresis; hence, unlike other diuretics, they tend to cause hypernatremia rather than hyponatremia.

CONCLUSION: EDEMA AND UNDERSTANDING OF THE REGULATION OF TOTAL BODY SODIUM. We do not understand how the body measures its total sodium (which includes the large amount in bone), but, more important, we do not understand how it measures the volume of the main functional compartment for sodium: the extracellular fluid. It is, therefore, scarcely surprising that the causes of edema, the pathological expansion of the larger component of extracellular fluid in the tissue spaces (interstitial fluid), still eludes rigorous explanation. It is also obvious that any research addressing changes in the volume of interstitial fluid faces daunting technical difficulties since, in normality, most of the fluid is associated with structural components as a gel and accumulation of free fluid is seen only in edema; if some specific pool of interstitial fluid, perhaps in the special permeability areas of the brain (Michell 1995a), serves as an index of total interstitial volume, its location remains unknown, although with newer noninvasive techniques, such as functional magnetic resonance imaging, investigation of the function of even the most inaccessible regions becomes potentially feasible. Once such areas are examined and characterized, it will seem remarkable that, at least at the start of the 21st century, we could claim to understand so much about the pathophysiology of edema when we know so little about the regulation of total extracellular sodium, as opposed to plasma volume. It is as if we had to manage a car in which we knew the pressure and flow rate of the gas supplied to the cylinders but had no means of guessing the level in the tank. In pregnancy, when both plasma and interstitial volume are definitely expanded, we neither understand the basis for excessive sodium retention (Michell 1996, 1998b) nor, indeed, in what sense it is excessive, granted that it is virtually a physiological feature of normal pregnancy (Michell 1995a; Lindheimer et al. 1999). We can not explain the most natural and recurrent challenge to salt and water regulation.

The Gap Between What Is Said and What Is Known. The problem is that because we do not know the crucial monitoring site or what it measures, we infer what it concludes about total extracellular sodium from our own interpretation of responses seen in the known mechanisms associated with the cardiovascular system, including the relevant hormones. Thus, even if measured ECF volume is supranormal, elevation of peripheral resistance, aldosterone, angiotensin, and ADH and suppression of ANP would all suggest that "the system" still perceived that the extracellular space was underfilled and sought to remedy the perceived deficit. But these observed changes could, in fact, form part of the primary disturbance, in which case extracellular fluid would inevitably become overfilled (Michell 1996). Moreover, a system that is underfilled by day could be overfilled by night when recumbency and inactivity allow redistribution of fluid. Moreover, in theory, it seems plausible that baselines defining the error signals that determine regulatory changes in sodium excretion are more likely to be those occurring during the stable nocturnal period—that is, those least likely to be measured (Michell 1997c; Moller and Henriksen 1997).

Unfortunately, the uncertainties surrounding the techniques for the measurement of extracellular volume, already substantial, are maximized by abnormalities of tissue perfusion or capillary permeability (Michell 1996); if we could only measure plasma sodium concentration with an accuracy of 5% to 10%, I doubt whether we would yet understand the regulation of water balance; we would probably relate it simply to the defense against hypovolemia or, heaven forbid, to "effective plasma sodium concentration"—that is, the concentration in a hypothetical compartment that, unlike measured concentration, changed in accordance with our theories.

If any blood volume were to serve as a proxy for extracellular volume, it would seem more likely to be some aspect of venous capacitance, since, like interstitial fluid, this serves a "reservoir" function and during hypovolemia provides a "reserve" of blood available to the high-pressure arterial delivery side of the circulation. This makes it even more remarkable that a concept that began in 1958 as effective *extracellular* volume should have evolved decisively into effective *arterial* blood volume. Arterial physiology is primarily focused on pressure, whereas volume is more important in the venous system. In other words, EABV becomes an astigmatic way of viewing arterial pressure; indeed, one of the most enthusiastic exponents presents evidence for "a decrease in EABV, due either to a fall in cardiac output or a decrease in peripheral resistance" (Michell 1996). The outcome of a change in cardiac output and peripheral resistance, whatever it does to conceptual EABV, alters arterial pressure. In fact, underfilling of EABV seems to have great difficulty in being distinguished from something far more familiar and readily measurable: hypotension. Unfortunately, much that we do understand about hypotension would not conform to the expectations of EABV protagonists. Despite this, EABV is alive and well and still regarded as an "explanation" for edema (Kurtzman 2001; Schrier 2001).

Does it matter? Unfortunately it does: Santa Claus is a wonderful story but does not explain the packages that fill the stockings on Christmas morning. The understanding of the physiology of corticosteroids would have been hampered, not advanced, had we clung unflinchingly to a quest to relate any unexpected aspect of their regulation to "virtual stress." We, especially we clinicians, faced with students or by clients informed by access to the internet, must distinguish between explanations that stem from repeatable observations and those that stem from concepts which, though attractive and perhaps capable of ultimately being substantiated, derive their strength from their logic rather than from specific data. We may be aware,

uncomfortably often, that our advice rests on the latter category, but the growing appetite for evidence-based medicine will not long allow such approaches to go unchallenged (Michell 2000c). As veterinary clinicians, we have the advantage of instinctive insight into species diversity, and the lessons that may be drawn from it, for example, regarding the regulation of sodium and water balance. In sheep, for example, that most physiological but most demanding and recurrent challenge, the reproductive cycle (including pregnancy and lactation) demonstrates the interplay between the various mechanisms, not just renal, that interact to regulate sodium balance (Michell 1995a). The gap between what is said and what is known should help to clarify the research that needs to be done.

If we truly understood how body sodium was regulated, reconciling the demands of both arterial pressure and extracellular volume, and their natural variability, on renal sodium excretion, we might understand how "the system" was so comprehensively defeated in the pathogenesis of edema. To gain that knowledge, we need to admit our bewilderment, not cling to security blankets such as effective arterial blood volume, myths that reassure but do not inform. *That is the fundamental importance of pathophysiology—to refine what we understand about physiology and, by identifying consistent anomalies, to define what we need to discover.*

REFERENCES

Michell AR. 1995a. The Clinical Biology of Sodium. Oxford: Pergamon (Elsevier Science). This reference serves as a general source of primary publications for this chapter.

Antes LM, Kujubu DA, Fernandez PC. 1998. Hypokalemia and the pathology of ion transport. Semin Nephrol 18:31–45.

Ayus JC, Arieff AI. 1996. Abnormalities of water metabolism in the elderly. Semin Nephrol 16:277–288.

Barber BJ, Elliott J. 1996. Assessment of parathyroid function in renal failure. In: Bainbridge J, Elliott J, eds. Manual of Canine and Feline Nephrology and Urology. Cheltenham, UK: British Small Animal Veterinary Association, pp 117–123.

Bellingan G. 1999. Inflammatory cell activation in sepsis. Br Med Bull 55:12–29.

Blumenthal I. 1997. Fever: Concepts old and new. J R Soc Med 90:391–393.

Bodey AR, Michell AR. 1997. Longitudinal studies of reproducibility and variability of indirect (oscillometric) blood pressure measurements in dogs: Evidence for tracking. Res Vet Sci 63:15–21.

Bomzon A, Holt S, Moore K. 1997. Bile acids, oxidative stress, and renal function in biliary obstruction. Semin Nephrol 17:549–562.

Brady HR, Brenner BM, Lieberthal W. 1996. Acute renal failure. In: Brenner BM, ed. Brenner and Rector's The Kidney, 5th ed. Philadelphia: WB Saunders, 2:1200–1252.

Brater DC. 1999. Use of diuretics in cirrhosis and nephrotic syndrome. Semin Nephrol 19:575–580.

Brooks HW, Gleadhill A, Wagstaff AJ, Michell AR. 1997. Fallibility of plasma urea and creatinine as indices of renal function in diarrheic calves treated with conventional or nutritional oral rehydration solutions. Br Vet J 154:35–39.

Cardenas A, Gines O. 2001. Pathogenesis and treatment of fluid and electrolyte imbalances in cirrhosis. Semin Nephrol 21:308–316.

Caviston TL, Campbell WG, Wingo CS, Cain BD. 1999. Molecular identification of the renal H+, K+-ATPases. Semin Nephrol 19:431–437.

Danzi DF, Pozos RS. 1994. Accidental hypothermia. N Engl J Med 331:1756–1760.

Drummer C. 2001. Involvement of the renal natriuretic peptide urodilatin in body fluid regulation. Semin Nephrol 21:239–243.

Ellison DH. 1999. Diuretic resistance: Physiology and therapeutics. Semin Nephrol 19:581–597.

El Nahas AM. 2000. Mechanisms and Management of Chronic Renal Failure. Oxford: Oxford University Press, pp 20–103 and 146–210.

Epstein M. 1997. Hepatorenal syndrome, emerging perspectives. Semin Nephrol 17:563–575.

Franz M, Woloszczuk W, Horl WH. 2001. Plasma concentration and urinary excretion of N-terminal proatrial natriuretic peptides in patients with kidney diseases. Kidney Int 59:1929–1934.

Friedman PA, Bushinsky DA. 1999. Diuretic effects on calcium metabolism. Semin Nephrol 19:551–556.

Gabbai FB. 1999. Nitric oxide and its relationship to nephrology. Semin Nephrol 19:251–263.

Gleadhill A, Michell AR. 1996. Clinical measurement of renal function. In: Bainbridge J, Elliott J, eds. Manual of Canine and Feline Nephrology and Urology. Cheltenham, UK: British Small Annual Veterinary Association, pp 107–116.

Gleadhill A, Marlin D, Harris PA, Michell AR. 2000. Reduction of renal function in exercising horses. Equine Vet J 32:509–514.

Greenberg A. 1998. Hyperkalemia: Treatment options. Semin Nephrol 18:46–57.

Griffiths RD, Hinds CJ, Little RA. 1999. Manipulating the metabolic response to injury. Br Med Bull 55:181–195.

Grove-White DH, Michell AR. 2001. Comparison of the measurement of total carbon dioxide and strong ion difference for the evaluation of metabolic acidosis in diarrheic calves. Vet Rec 148:365–370.

Haggstrom J, Hansson K, Kvart C, et al. 2000. Relationship between different natriuretic peptides and severity of naturally acquired mitral regurgitation in dogs with chronic myxomatous valve disease. J Vet Cardiol 2:7–16.

Hebert SC. 1999. Molecular mechanisms of diuretics. Semin Nephrol 19:504–523.

Ishihara K, Szerlip HM. 1998. Anion gap acidosis. Semin Nephrol 18:83–97.

Jacobsen J, Secker N. 1994. Changing concepts of hypovolemic shock. In: Secker NH, Pawelczyk JA, Ludbrook J, eds. Blood Loss and Shock. London: Edward Arnold, pp 3–9.

Jacobsen TN, Jost CMT, Converse RI, Victor RG. 1994. In: Secker NH, Pawelczyk JA, Ludbrook J, eds. Blood Loss and Shock. London: Edward Arnold, pp 47–59.

Kaplan NM. 1999. Diuretics: Correct use in hypertension. Semin Nephrol 19:569–574.

Kelepouris E, Agus ZS. 1998. Hypomagnesemia: Renal magnesium handling. Semin Nephrol 18:58–73.

Kelly KJ, Molitoris BA. 2000. Acute renal failure in the new millennium. Semin Nephrol 20:4–19.

Kempski O. 2001. Cerebral edema. Semin Nephrol 21:303–307.

Kluger MJ. 1993. Attitudes to fever. In: Michell AR, ed. History of the Healing Professions: The Advancement of Veterinary Science. Oxford: CAB International, 3:65–72.

Kurtzman NA. 2001. Nephritic edema. Semin Nephrol 21:257–261.

Kwon TH, Hager H, Nejsum LN, et al. 2001. Physiology and pathophysiology of renal aquaporins. Semin Nephrol 21:231–238.

Laski ME, Pressley TA. 1999. Aquaporin mediated water flux as a target for diuretic development. Semin Nephrol 19:533–550.

Levy M. 1997. Atrial natriuretic peptide: Renal effects in cirrhosis of the liver. Semin Nephrol 17:520–529.

Liano F, Pascual J. 1998. Outcomes in acute renal failure. Semin Nephrol 18:541–550.

Lieberthal W, Koh JS, Levine JS. 1998. Necrosis and apoptosis in acute renal failure. Semin Nephrol 19:505–518.

Lindheimer MD, Roberts JM, Cunningham FG. 1999. Chesley's Hypertensive Disorders of Pregnancy. Stamford, CT: Appleton and Lange, pp 3–42.

Magri P, Auletta M, Andreucci M, et al. 2001. Sodium retention in the preascitic stage of cirrhosis. Semin Nephrol 21:317–322.

Mandal AK. 1997. Hypokalemia and hyperkalemia. Med Clin North Am 81:611–639.

Maschio G, Oldrizzi L. 2000. Progression of renal disease. Kidney Int 57(Suppl 75):S1–S76.

Michell AR. 1981. Fluid and electrolyte excretion in sheep: Comparison of reduced food and water with oestrus. Q J Exp Physiol 66:515–521.

Michell AR. 1982. Current concepts of fever. J Small Anim Pract 23:185–193.

Michell AR. 1989. Shock in companion animals. Vet Annu 29:48–58.

Michell AR. 1994a. Physiology. In: Hall LW, Taylor PM, eds. Anaesthesia of the Cat. London: Bailliere Tindall, pp 12–39.

Michell AR. 1994b. Small animal fluid therapy. J Small Anim Pract 35:559–565 and 613–619.

Michell AR. 1995a. The Clinical Biology of Sodium. Oxford: Pergamon (Elsevier Science).

Michell AR. 1995b. Progression of renal failure: Have we progressed? Vet Annu 35:159–176.

Michell AR 1996. Effective blood volume: An effective concept or a modern myth? Perspect Biol Med 39:471–490.

Michell AR. 1997a. Circulatory shock: Pathophysiology and management. Proc Assoc Vet Pharmacol Ther 15:48–53.

Michell AR. 1997b. Circulatory shock: New developments in therapy. Proc Assoc Vet Pharmacol Ther 15:78–83.

Michell AR. 1997c. Long term control of blood pressure and sodium balance: Is the baseline nocturnal? Perspect Biol Med 40:516–528.

Michell AR. 1998a. Oral rehydration for diarrhea: Symptomatic treatment or fundamental therapy. J Comp Pathol 118:175–193.

Michell AR. 1998b. Sodium retention and edema. Perspect Biol Med 41:461–462.

Michell AR. 1999. Diet and chronic renal failure: Is 'self-sustaining progression' in terminal decline? J Nutr Environ Med 9:63–76.

Michell AR. 2000a. Diuresis and diarrhea: Is the gut a misunderstood nephron? Perspect Biol Med 43:399–405.

Michell AR. 2000b. Hypertension in dogs: The value of comparative medicine. J R Soc Med 93:451–452.

Michell AR. 2000c. Only one medicine: The future of comparative medicine and clinical research. Res Vet Sci 69:101–106.

Michell AR, Noakes DE. 1985. The effect of estrogen and progesterone on sodium, potassium and water balance in sheep. Res Vet Sci 38:46–53.

Michell AR, Bywater R, Clarke KW, et al. 1989. Veterinary Fluid Therapy. Oxford: Blackwell Scientific.

Michell AR, Bodey AR, Gleadhill AG. 1997. Absence of hypertension in dogs with chronic renal insufficiency. Renal Fail 19:61–69.

Mogensen CE. 2000. Diabetic nephropathy: Natural history and management. In: El Nahas AM, ed. Mechanisms and Clinical Management of Chronic Renal Failure. Oxford: Oxford University Press, pp 211–240.

Moller S, Henriksen JH. 1997. Circulatory abnormalities in cirrhosis with focus on neurohumoral aspects. Semin Nephrol 17:505–519.

Morris RC, Schmidlin O, Tanaka M, et al. 1999. Differing effects of supplemental potassium chloride and potassium bicarbonate: Pathophysiological and clinical implications. Semin Nephrol 19:487–493.

Narins RG. 1994. In: Maxwell & Kleeman's Clinical Disorders of Fluid & Electrolyte Metabolism, 5th ed. New York: McGraw-Hill, pp 1153–1212.

Pacher R. 2001. Pathogenesis of heart failure. Semin Nephrol 21:273–277.

Palazzo M. 1997. Disturbances of acid-base and electrolyte balance. In: Garrard C, Foex P, Westaby S, eds. Principles and Practice of Critical Care. Oxford: Blackwell Scientific, pp 225–275.

Palevsky PM. 1998. Hypernatremia. Semin Nephrol 18:20–30.

Paller MS. 1998. Acute renal failure, controversies, clinical trials and future directions. Semin Nephrol 18:482–489.

Peters JP. 1948. The role sodium in the production of edema. N Engl J Med 239:353–362.

Reed RK, Berg A, Gjerde EB, Rubin K. 2001. Control of interstitial fluid pressure: Role of β-integrins. Semin Nephrol 21:222–230.

Rowlands BJ, Soong CV, Gardiner KR. 1999. The gastrointestinal tract as a barrier in sepsis. Br Med Bull 55:196–211.

Safirstein R, Di Mari J, Megyesi J, Price P. 1998. Mechanisms of renal repair and survival following acute injury. Semin Nephrol 18:519–522.

Schrier RW, Cadnapaphornchai MA, Ohara M. 2001. Water retention and aquaporins in heart failure, liver disease and pregnancy. J R Soc Med 94:265–269.

Schwartz D, Blantz RC. 1999 Schwartz. Nitric oxide, sepsis and the kidney. Semin Nephrol 19:272–276.

Sisson D. 2000. The diagnostic potential of natriuretic peptides in heart failure. J Vet Cardiol 2:5–6.

Sutton TA, Molitoris BA. 1998. Mechanisms of cellular injury in ischemic acute renal failure. Semin Nephrol 18:490–497.

Swales JD. 1996. Textbook of Hypertension. Oxford: Blackwell Scientific, pp 14–15.

Thadhani R, Pascual M, Bonventre JV. 1996. Acute renal failure. N Engl J Med 334:1448–1460.

Ultendahl HR, Aurell KM. 1998. Renin-Angiotensin. London: Portland Press, pp 115–168.

Verbalis JG. 1998. Adaptation to chronic hyponatremia: Implications for symptomatology, diagnosis and therapy. Semin Nephrol 18:3–19.

Vervloet MG, Thijs LG, Hack CE. 1998. Derangements of coagulation and fibrinolysis in critically ill patients with sepsis and septic shock. Semin Thromb Hemost 24:13–44.

Wheeler AP, Bernard GR. 1999. Treating patients with severe sepsis. N Engl J Med 340:207–214.

Wilcox CS. 1999. Metabolic and adverse effects of diuretics. Semin Nephrol 19:557–568.

Wort SJ, Evans TW. 1999. The role of endothelium in modulating vascular control in sepsis and related conditions. Br Med Bull 55:30–48.

Zeidel M. 1998. Recent advances in water transport. Semin Nephrol 18:167–177.

Zucchelli P, Santoro A. 2000. Dry weight in hemodialysis: Volemic control. Semin Nephrol 21:286–290.

2

PATHOPHYSIOLOGY OF CELLULAR REGULATION, CELL DEATH, AND CANCER

David John Argyle and Lubna Nasir

Throughout this textbook, reference has been made to the importance of homeostasis and how disruption of homeostasis can lead to, or be a consequence of, disease states. Cells are the fundamental building blocks of any organism, and an understanding of cell biology is a prerequisite for an understanding of disease. There has been an overwhelming increase in our understanding of how cells behave both as individual units and also within multicellular organisms. Central to cellular homeostasis is the ability of cells to proliferate, control proliferation, and communicate. Intercellular signals enable each cell to take on its position and specialized role in the body, and intracellular signaling is vital to control cell function. These communication networks orchestrate the process of cellular homeostasis, the failure of which leads to injury or disease.

Of major significance to the health of animals is the development of malignant tumors following a breakdown in the normal homeostatic processes that control cell division, proliferation, and differentiation. To understand the mechanisms by which a normal cell becomes a cancer cell, one must first have a working understanding of normal mechanisms of cellular behavior, growth, and proliferation control and the complex issues of cell signaling. These complex mechanisms of control form the basis of Part 1 of this chapter and describe normal cellular physiology with special reference to the control of the cell cycle. In Part 2, we describe the central role of the cell cycle in the development of the malignant phenotype and attempt to simplify recent advances in cancer research by defining cancer in terms of the acquisition of six fundamental traits. Part 3 reviews the etiology of cancers in domestic animals. Part 4 describes the molecular pathology and the new technologies that are enabling us to define the genetic basis of cancer and improve diagnosis. In Part 5, the interaction of the malignant phenotype with the host immune system along with the role of the immune system are described. In Part 6, we discuss the clinical manifestations of cancer, the biological basis of conventional therapies, and some of the new genetic approaches to treatment.

PART 1: THE NORMAL CELL AND ITS HOMEOSTATIC MECHANISMS: CELLULAR HOMEOSTASIS AND PROLIFERATION TOWARD MALIGNANCY

CELLS ARE THE BASIC BUILDING BLOCKS OF ALL ORGANISMS. Mammalian cells are termed *eukaryotic* and have three main components: the plasma membrane, a fluid filling called the cytoplasm, and the organelles within the cell (Figure 2.1). The plasma membranes of the cell enclose the cytoplasm and functions in cellular mobility and the maintenance of cellular shape. They are composed of phospholipid and protein in a motile, asymmetrical structure. They form the outer structures of the intracellular organelles, including the nucleus, and are highly specialized structures inextricably linked to normal cell function and homeostasis. The membranes control the composition of the space that they enclose, having the ability to move molecules from one side to the other via transport mechanisms. Consequently, they can profoundly affect metabolic pathways and play a vital role in cell-to-cell communication via the expression of specialized receptors for hormones, chemicals, and other proteins.

THE NUCLEUS HOUSES THE CELL'S GENETIC BLUEPRINT. The nucleus is the largest of the cell organelles and is surrounded by a double membrane termed the *nuclear envelope*. The outer membrane is continuous with the endoplasmic reticulum, and the entire envelope structure contains pores to allow the passage of proteins and RNA between the cytoplasm and the nuclear contents.

The nucleus is composed of the nucleolus, DNA, DNA-binding proteins, and histones. To protect the DNA, the histone proteins enable the DNA to be folded into chromosomes. The primary function of the nucleus is cell division and the control of the genetic material. Within the nucleus, genetic material is transcribed into RNA, which can be processed onto messenger, transport, or ribosomal RNA and introduced to the cytoplasm, where it directs cellular activities. RNA is processed mostly in the nucleolus.

OTHER CELLULAR ORGANELLES RESIDE IN THE CYTOPLASMIC SPACE. The cytoplasm is an aqueous solution or cytosol that contains many enzymes involved in metabolism and ribosomes involved in protein production. The other organelles are suspended in the cytoplasm surrounded by a plasma

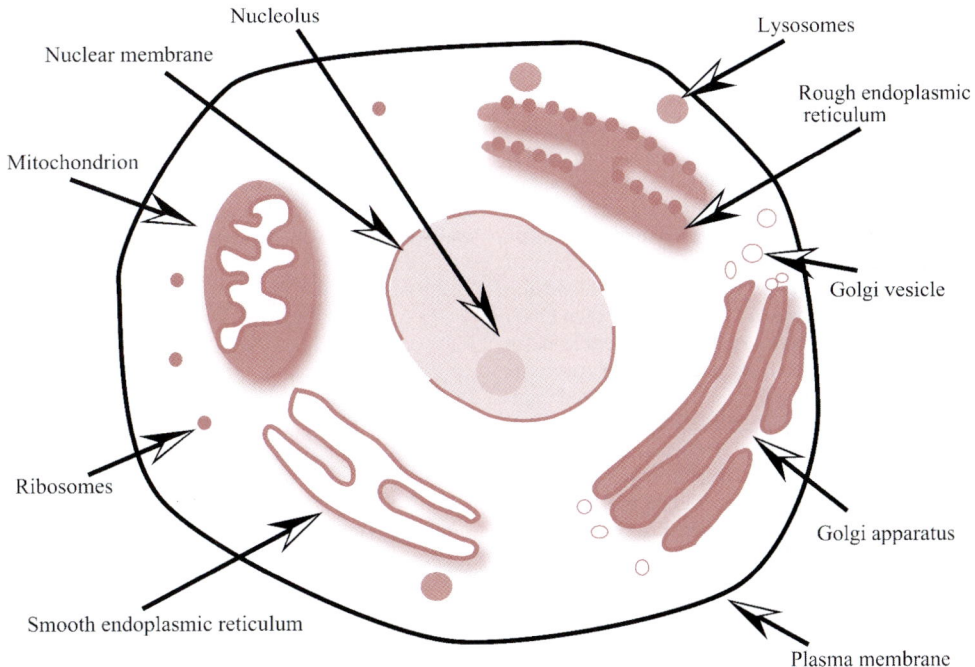

FIG. 2.1—The structure of eukaryotic cells. The cell is a dynamic three-dimensional structure that interacts closely with its environment and other cells to retain homeostasis.

membrane. Ribosomes are RNA-protein complexes that are synthesized in the nucleolus and transported to the cytoplasm via the nuclear pores, where they attach to the endoplasmic reticulum to provide sites for protein synthesis.

The endoplasmic reticulum is continuous with the nuclear membrane and specializes in the synthesis and transport of protein and lipid. It is composed of a network of cisternae that extend throughout the cytoplasm and may be granular (rough endoplasmic reticulum) or agranular (smooth endoplasmic reticulum). The granular nature of rough endoplasmic reticulum is formed by the attachment of ribosomes involved in protein production. The smooth endoplasmic reticulum contains many enzymes involved in the production of steroid hormones and involved in a number of reactions required to remove toxic substances from the cell.

The Golgi complex is continuous with the endoplasmic reticulum and often located close to the nucleus. Here, proteins from the endoplasmic reticulum are processed and packaged into small vesicles that bud from the complex for distribution to intracellular or extracellular locations. Lysosomes are specialized vesicles that arise from the Golgi apparatus and contain a cocktail of hydrolases. Lysosomes can digest cellular contents, but their membranes create a protective shield for the cell. They are necessary for normal digestion of cellular nutrients, intracellular debris, and potentially harmful extracellular substances that must be removed from the body. Lysosomal abnormalities are involved in a number of conditions that involve cellular injury or death.

The mitochondria are intimately involved with cellular energy metabolism. They are rod-shaped organelles bound by a double plasma membrane. The inner membrane is folded to form partitions called cristae. The inner membrane also contains the enzymes of the respiratory chain and is responsible for the production of most of a cell's energy in the form of adenosine triphosphate. The mitochondria contain their own DNA in the form of a supercoiled circular double-helix strand of about 16 kb. The majority of proteins involved in oxidative phosphorylation are derived from nuclear DNA, with mitochondria DNA providing only a fraction of protein required. However, there is currently a great deal of interest in mitochondrial DNA because it is subject to a much higher mutation rate than is nuclear DNA because of its exposure to reactive oxygen species during oxidative phosphorylation. This may have implications for cellular aging mechanisms and the generation of malignant cells.

CELL DIVISION IS A TIGHTLY REGULATED PROCESS. Within an animal, all cells are subject to wear and tear, making cellular reproduction a necessity for maintenance of the individual. Gametes are reproduced by the process of meiosis, whereas somatic cell reproduction involves two sequential phases known as mitosis and cytokinesis. *Mitosis* is nuclear division, and *cytokinesis* involves the division of the cytoplasm, the two occurring in close succession. Nuclear division is preceded by a doubling of the genetic material of the cell during a period known as *interphase*. As well as a copying of the chromosomes, this period is characterized by marked cellular activity in terms of RNA, protein, and lipid production. The alternation between mitosis and interphase in all tissues is often referred to as the *cell cycle*. The phases of the cell cycle are shown in Figure 2.2.

Interphase (G_1, G_2, and S phases) is the longest phase of the cell cycle. During interphase, the chromatin is very long and slender, but progressively shortens and thickens as interphase progresses. The first phase of mitosis is the *prophase*, during which the chromosomes first appear. As the phase progresses, the chromosomes appear as two identical sister chromatids joined at the centromere. As the nuclear membrane disappears, spindle fibers form and radiate from the two centrioles, each located at opposite poles of the cell. The spindle fibers serve to pull the chromosomes to opposite sides of the cell.

During *metaphase*, the spindle fibers pull the centromeres of the chromosomes, which become aligned to the middle of the spindle often referred to as the *equatorial plate*. During *anaphase*, the centromeres split, and the sister chromatids are pulled apart by the contraction of the spindle fibers. The final stage of cell division is *telophase*, which is characterized by the formation of a nuclear membrane around each group of chromosomes, followed by cytokinesis or separation of the cytoplasm to produce two identical diploid cells.

Although the four stages of mitosis and cytokinesis last only about 1 hour, the whole cell cycle lasts for about 12 to 24 hours. In adult life, rates of cell division vary depending on cell type. For example, nerve cells

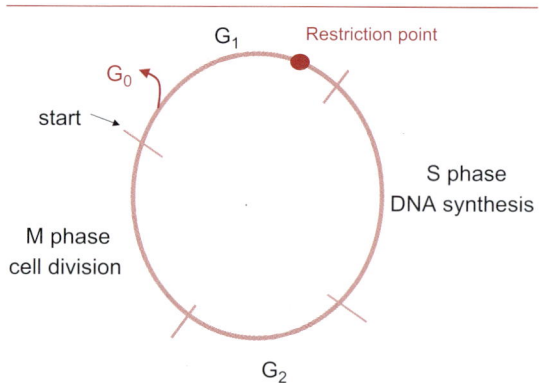

FIG. 2.2—The cell cycle. Cells are stimulated to divide in G_1. Once the cell has passed the restriction point, the cell is committed to cycle. The cycle is tightly regulated by both intracellular and extracellular signals. S phase represents a period of DNA synthesis, which progresses to G_2 and finally cell division (M phase).

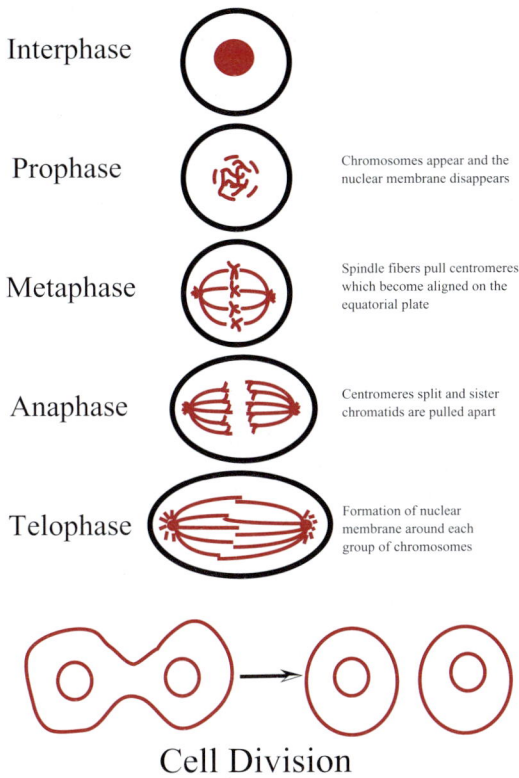

Interphase

Prophase

Chromosomes appear and the nuclear membrane disappears

Metaphase

Spindle fibers pull centromeres which become aligned on the equatorial plate

Anaphase

Centromeres split and sister chromatids are pulled apart

Telophase

Formation of nuclear membrane around each group of chromosomes

Cell Division

FIG. 2.3—The stages of mitosis. *Interphase* represents the longest phase and is a period of DNA synthesis and replication. *Prophase* sees the first appearance of the chromosomes and dissolution of the nuclear membrane During *metaphase* and *anaphase*, the spindles pull the centromeres, which initially align on the equatorial plate. Centromeres ultimately split, and sister chromatids are pulled apart. During *telophase*, a nuclear membrane forms around each group of chromosomes and the cell ultimately divides.

divide very slowly or lose their ability to replicate. In comparison, cells of epithelial origin often divide continuously and rapidly. The difference between cells that divide slowly compared with those that divide rapidly is the time spent in G_1 of the cell cycle. Cells that divide slowly may spend days in G_1, but, once the S phase begins, progression through mitosis takes a fairly constant amount of time.

GROWTH FACTORS STIMULATE CELL DIVISION. Growth factors are highly specialized proteins that stimulate cell division. Specific subsets of cells require specific growth factors for cell division and are characterized by having specific cell surface receptors. It is clear from seminal experiments in growth-factor biology that these compounds are also involved in cellular differentiation. In contrast, autocrine messengers exist that can downregulate growth stimulation (Table 2.1).

CELLULAR PROLIFERATION IS CONTROLLED THROUGH THE CYCLINS, CYCLIN-DEPENDENT KINASES, AND THEIR INHIBITORS. Cells are stimulated to enter the cell cycle in response to external factors, including growth factors and cell adhesion. During the G_1 phase of the cell cycle, cells respond to mitogenic signals. Once the cell cycle has traversed the restriction (R) point in the G_1 phase, cell-cycle transitions become autonomous (Figure 2.4).

Progression through the cell cycle is mediated by the sequential activation and inactivation of a class of proteins called *cyclin-dependent kinases* (CDKs), which consist of an inactive conserved catalytic core and are regulated at three levels:

1. CDK activity requires the association with regulatory subunits known as *cyclins*. The level of CDKs remains constant throughout the cell cycle, but the concentration of cyclins varies in a phase-specific manner.

TABLE 2.1—Growth factors

Growth factor	Physiological action
Platelet-derived growth factor (PDGF)	Proliferation of connective tissue cells and neuroglia
Epidermal growth factor (EGF)	Proliferation of epidermal cells
Insulin-like growth factor I (IGF-I)	Collaborates with EGF and PDGF and stimulates proliferation of fat and connective tissue cells
Insulin-like growth factor II (IGF-II)	As for IGF-I
Vascular endothelial growth factor (VEGF)	Involved in stimulating angiogenesis
Transforming growth factor β (TGF-β)	Stimulates or inhibits the response of cells to other growth factors
Fibroblast growth factor (FGF)	Stimulates the proliferation of fibroblasts and myoblasts
Interleukin 2 (IL-2)	Stimulates the proliferation of T lymphocytes
Nerve growth factor (NGF)	Promotes axon growth
Hemopoietic growth factors: G-CSF, GM-CSF, M-CSF, IL-3, SCF, and erythropoietin)	Stimulate blood precursor cells
SCF, stem cell factor.	

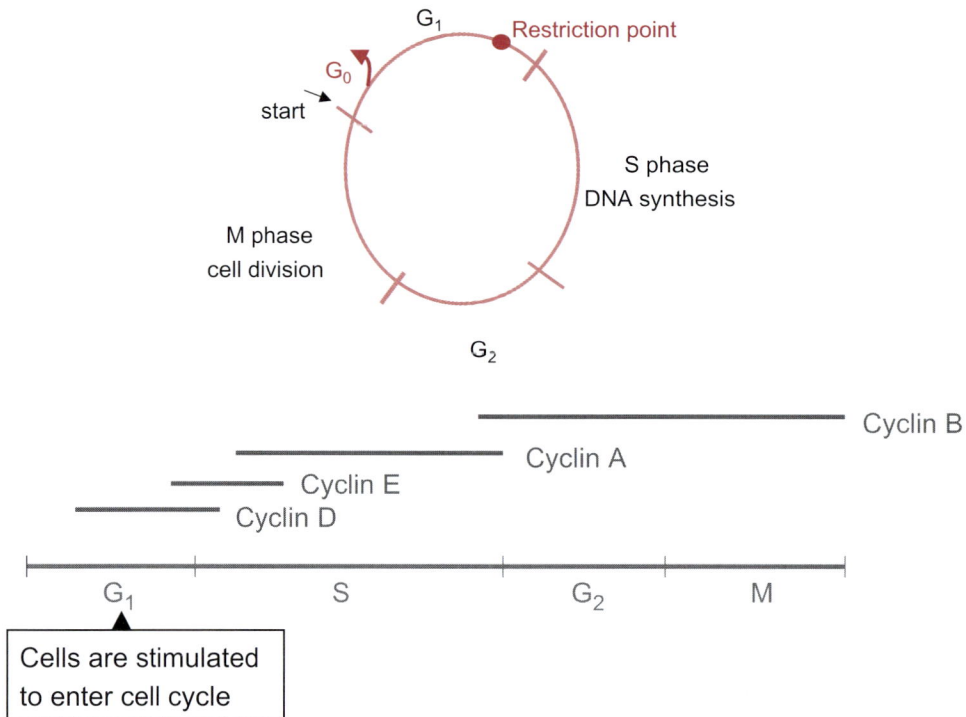

FIG. 2.4—Cells are stimulated to enter the cell cycle in response to external factors, including growth factors and cell adhesion. During the G_1 phase of the cell cycle, cells are responsive to mitogenic signals. Once the cell cycle has traversed the restriction point (R) in the G_1 phase, the cell-cycle transitions become autonomous. Progression through the cell cycle is mediated by the sequential activation and inactivation of a class of proteins called cyclin-dependent kinases (CDKs). CDK activity requires the association with regulatory subunits known as cyclins (D, E, A, and B).

Thus, the periodic synthesis and destruction of cyclins provides the primary level of cell-cycle control (Figure 2.4).

2. The activity of cyclin-CDK complexes is also regulated by phosphorylation. Activation of cyclin-CDK complexes requires phosphorylation by CDK-activating kinases (CAKs), and the phosphorylation at threonine and serine residues suppresses activity.

3. CDKs are also tightly regulated by a class of inhibitory proteins known as *cyclin-dependent kinase inhibitors* (CDKIs), which can block G_1/S progression by binding cyclin-CDK complexes and can be classified into two groups: (a) The INK4A family (p15^{INK4b}, p16^{INK4a}, p18^{INK4c}, and p19^{INK4d}). These act primarily on cdk4 and cdk6 complexes and prevent the association with cyclin D. (b) CIP/KIP family (p21^{Cip1}, p27^{Kip1}, and p57^{Kip2}). These are less specific and can act to inactivate various cyclin/CDK complexes.

PROGRESSION THROUGH THE CELL CYCLE INVOLVES THE RETINOBLASTOMA PROTEIN. The first class of proteins induced in G_1 following mitogenic stimulation of the cell cycle is the class D cyclins, which in turn activate CDK4 and CDK6. CDK-cycling complexes cause phosphorylation of the substrate retinoblastoma protein (Rb), which results in dissociation of the transcription factor E_2F from the Rb protein (Figure 2.5). The phosphorylation status of Rb plays a critical role in regulating G_1 progression, and Rb is the molecular device that serves as the R-point switch; phosphorylated Rb releases E_2F, enabling transcription of numerous E_2-responsive genes involved in DNA synthesis, whereas unphosphorylated protein Rb (pRb) remains associated with E_2F, thereby inhibiting cell-cycle progression. During G_1 progression, E_2F activation also leads to induction of cyclin E, which associates with CDK2, and the CDK2-cyclin E complex maintains Rb in the phosphorylated state and is essential for cells to enter the S phase of the cell cycle. At the G_1/S phase transition, E_2F induces cyclin A. During early S phase, cyclins D and E are degraded, and cyclin A associates with CDK2 and CDK1, and this kinase activity is essential for entry into S phase, completion of S phase, and entry into M phase. Mitosis is regulated by CDK1 in association with cyclins A and B, causing phosphorylation of cytoskeletal proteins, including histones and lamins.

CELLULAR RESPONSES TO DNA DAMAGE. When normal cells are subjected to stress signals,

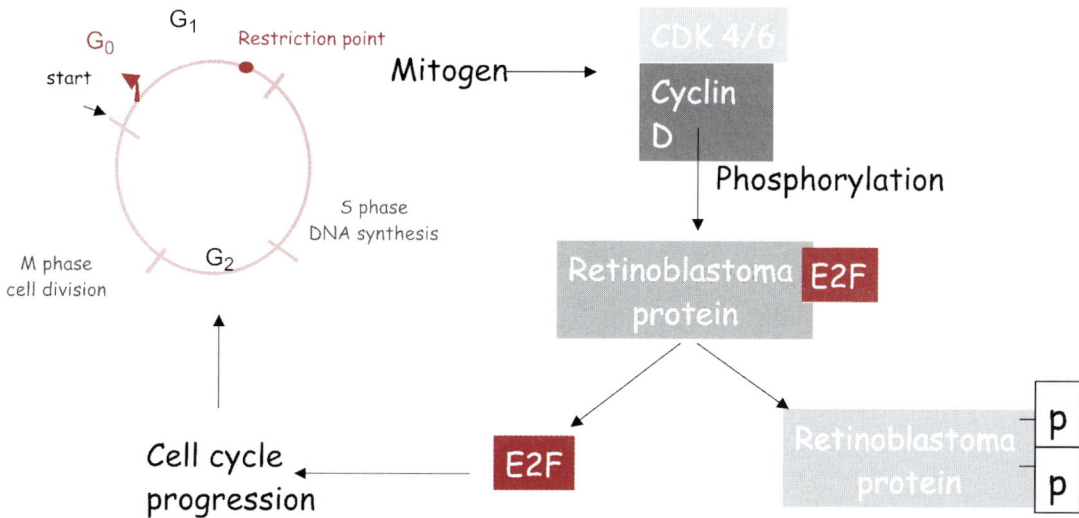

FIG. 2.5—The first class of proteins induced in G_1 following mitogenic stimulation of the cell cycle are the class D cyclins, which in turn activate cyclin-dependent kinase 4 (CDK4) and CDK6. Cyclin D-CDK complexes cause phosphorylation of the substrate retinoblastoma (Rb) protein, which results in dissociation of the transcription factor E2F from the Rb protein. Phosphorylated Rb releases E2F, enabling transcription of numerous E_2-responsive genes involved in DNA synthesis. Unphosphorylated protein Rb (pRb) remains associated with E2F and thereby inhibits cell-cycle progression. During G_1 progression, activation of E2F also leads to induction of cyclin E. Cyclin E associates with CDK2, and the cyclin E-CDK2 complex maintains Rb in the phosphorylated state and is essential for cells to enter the S phase of cell cycle. At the G_1/S-phase transition, E2F induces cyclin A.

radiation, DNA damage, or oxygen depletion, the majority have the ability to cause cell-cycle arrest in G_1, S, and G_2 phases or enter programmed cell death (*apoptosis*) or both. Within cells, surveillance systems called *checkpoints* operate to recognize and respond to DNA damage. Cell-cycle checkpoints occur in the G_1 phase in response to DNA damage, during S phase to monitor the quality of DNA replication and the occurrence of DNA damage, and during the G_2/M phase to examine the status of the spindle. Of these, the DNA damage-induced checkpoint mediated by the tumor-suppressor protein P53 is the most well studied.

The P53 protein plays an important role in maintaining genomic stability and forms part of a stress-response pathway to various exogenous and endogenous DNA-damage signals, including γ-irradiation, ultraviolet (UV) irradiation, chemicals, and oxidative stress.

P53 FUNCTIONS AS A GENOMIC POLICE OFFICER. The P53 response to stress may be mediated by DNA-dependent protein kinase (DNA-PK) or by the ataxia-telangiectasia mutated kinase and leads to phosphorylation of the N terminus of P53 protein. In normal cells, P53 is short lived, but phosphorylated P53 is stabilized and can thus function as a transcriptional regulator binding to sequences and transactivating a number of genes, including *p21*. P21 protein has

a high affinity for G_1 CDK-cyclin complexes and acts as a CDK inhibitor inhibiting kinase activity, thereby arresting cells in the G_1 phase. By holding cells in G_1, the replication of damaged DNA is prevented, and the cells own DNA-repair machinery has the opportunity to repair damage prior to reentering the active growth cycle (Figure 2.6).

The cellular levels of P53 are regulated by the product of another gene: *mdm2*(mouse double minute 2 oncogene) (Figure 2.7). The principle role of MDM2 is to act as a negative regulator of P53 function. One mechanism by which MDM2 may downregulate P53 is to target P53 for degradation. The P53 protein is maintained in normal cells as an unstable protein, and its interaction with MDM2 can target P53 for degradation via a ubiquitin proteosome pathway. MDM2 can also control P53 function by suppressing P53 transcriptional activity. MDM2 is a transcriptional target of P53, and expression is induced by the binding of P53 to an internal promoter within the *mdm2* gene. MDM2 can in turn bind to a domain within the amino terminus of P53, thereby inhibiting the transcriptional activity and G_1 arrest function of P53 by masking access to the transcriptional machinery.

CELL-CYCLE ARREST OR APOPTOSIS?. Apoptosis is the mechanism by which cells commit suicide and occurs during normal development and cellular turnover. In contrast to necrosis, apoptosis is a distinct

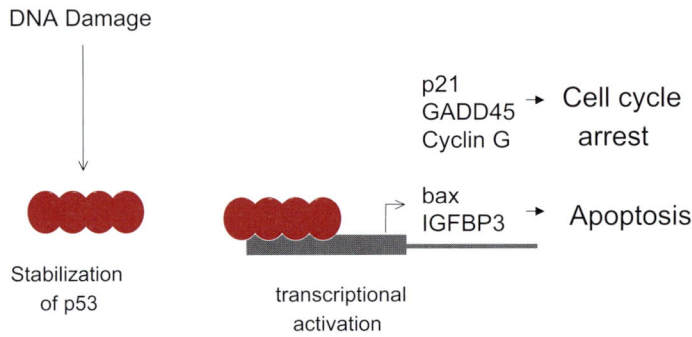

FIG. 2.6—Cell-cycle checkpoint: role of the p53 tumor-suppressor protein. In normal cells, p53 is short lived. When a cell is exposed to a DNA-damaging agent, however, p53 can become phosphorylated. Phosphorylated p53 is stable and can then function as a transcriptional regulator binding to sequences and transactivating a number of genes, including p21. p21 has a high affinity for G_1 cyclin-dependent kinase (CDK)-cyclin complexes and acts as a CDK inhibitor of kinase activity, thereby arresting cells in G_1. By holding cells in G_1, the replication of damaged DNA is prevented, and the cell's own DNA repair machinery has the opportunity to repair damage prior to reentering the active growth cycle. Alternatively, p53 stabilization may lead to apoptosis via the bax pathway.

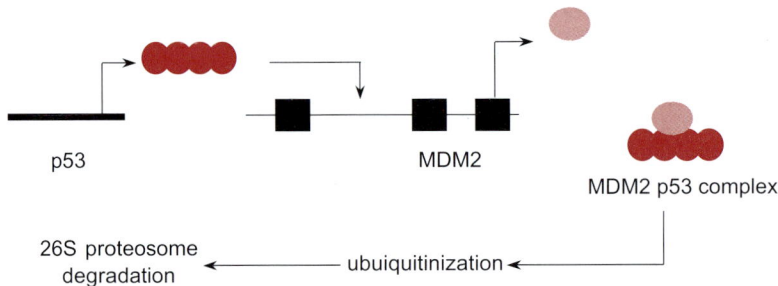

FIG. 2.7—Relationship between p53 and MDM2. The cellular levels of p53 are regulated by the product of another gene *mdm2* (mouse double minute 2 oncogene). The principle role of *mdm2* is to act as a negative regulator of p53 function.

type of cell death characterized by programmed self-destruction of cells that occurs in disease states as well as part of normal physiological cell turnover. Whereas necrosis is characterized by swelling of the cell and lysis, in apoptosis there is cellular and nuclear shrinkage followed by fragmentation and subsequent phagocytosis. The molecular mechanisms involved in apoptosis are shown in Figure 2.8.

A wide variety of signals can initiate an apoptotic response, including Fas ligand, tumor-necrosis factor, and oncogenes. Where cells are damaged and are unable to repair DNA, *p53* expression aids in pushing the cells into programmed death or apoptosis. In one such mechanism, the expression of *p53* can downregulate expression of the *bcl2* gene. This has the effect of allowing the expression of the Myc transcription factor, which promotes apoptosis.

SUMMARY. The cell cycle ensures a regulated process so that each cell can complete DNA replication before cell division occurs. The cell responds to growth and environmental signals through the cell cycle. Components of the cell cycle that have a stimulatory effect include the cyclins and the cyclin-dependent kinases. The negative influences come from a series of checkpoints that respond to external stimuli. These include tumor-suppressor genes such as *p53* and *Rb*, and genes involved in DNA repair (Figure 2.9).

DNA replication is also subject to the introduction of errors, and these are closely monitored by a class of enzymes call *DNA-repair enzymes*. Consequently, there are a number of safeguards within the cell cycle to ensure that normal cells are produced during division and that the DNA is accurately replicated. In Part 2, we describe how these systems are overcome to produce a malignant cancer cell.

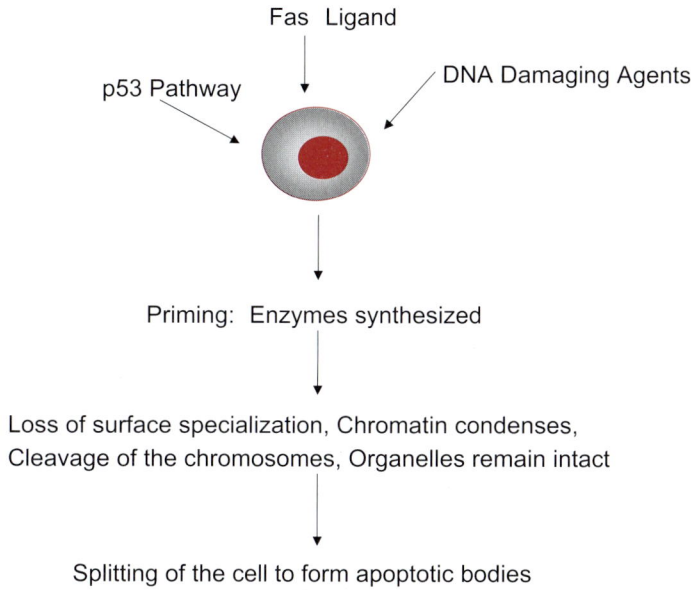

FIG. 2.8—Processes in apoptosis. Fas ligand, tumor-necrosis factor, the p53 pathway, and certain oncogenes can initiate apoptosis. Where cells are damaged and are unable to repair DNA, p53 expression aids in pushing the cell into programmed death or apoptosis. In one such mechanism, the expression of p53 can downregulate expression of the *Bcl2* gene. This has the effect of allowing the expression of the myc transcription factor, which promotes apoptosis.

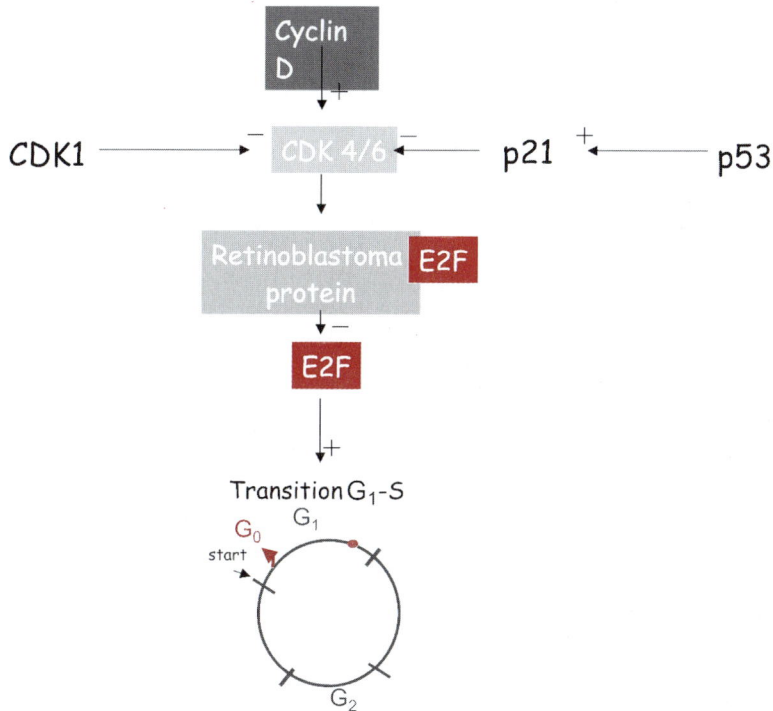

FIG. 2.9—The cell responds to growth and environmental signals through the cell cycle. Components of the cell cycle that have a stimulatory effect include the cyclins and the cyclin dependent kinases. The negative influences come from a series of checkpoints that respond to external stimuli. These include tumor-suppressor genes such as p53 and Rb (retinoblastoma), as well as genes involved in DNA repair.

KEY REFERENCES AND FURTHER READING
Alberts B, Bray D, Johnson A, et al. 1997. Essential Cell Biology. New York: Garland.
McCance KL, Roberts LK. 1997. Tumour invasion and metastasis. In: McCance KL, Huether SE, eds. Pathophysiology, the Biological Basis of Disease in Adults and Children, 3rd ed. St Louis: CV Mosby, pp 350–372.
Peckham M, Pinedo H, Veronesi U, eds. 1995. Oxford Textbook of Oncology. New York: Oxford University Press.
Watson JD, Gilman M, Witkowski J, Zoller M. 1992. Recombinant DNA. New York: Freeman.

PART 2: MOLECULAR MECHANISMS IN CANCER, A DISEASE OF GROWTH, DIVISION, AND CELLULAR DIFFERENTIATION

From our discussion of normal cell biology, it is apparent that cells of multicellular organisms form part of a specialized society that cooperates to promote survival of the organism. In this, cell division, proliferation, and differentiation are strictly controlled, and a balance exists between normal cell birth and the natural cell death rate. Derangement of these normal homeostatic mechanisms can lead to uncontrolled proliferation leading to a malignant phenotype.

Cancer in humans has been known since society learned to record its activities. However, it is interesting to note that its importance as one of the civilized world's biggest killers is a relatively recent entity. This is because improvements in public health and vaccination have led to a massive reduction in the classical causes of death (i.e., infectious diseases), and more people now survive to an age where cancer becomes important.

Cancer in animals is also well documented throughout history but has taken on significance over the past 100 years for a number of reasons. Studies on chicken, feline, and bovine retroviruses have made significant contributions to our overall understanding of carcinogenesis and the discovery of oncogenes and tumor-suppressor genes. Further contributions to our understanding of viral oncogenesis have come from studies of the DNA papillomaviruses in cattle and horses, which have complemented research into cervical cancer in women. More recently, cancer in animals has taken on more of a significant role in clinical veterinary medicine. The increase in companion-animal practice and advances in human medicine have led to treatment of cancer in pet animals as accepted and expected clinical practice. Dogs have the highest rate of malignant tumors of the domestic species and are second only to horses for benign tumor rate. This has implications in terms of health and welfare of this species but also suggests that dogs may represent a further natural outbred model of cancer for parallel studies in humans. This complementary cancer research has paved the way for the development of programs of research in comparative medicine that has benefits for both people and the veterinary species.

CAN WE DEFINE CANCER? It is difficult to define a cancer cell in absolute terms. Tumors are usually phenotypically recognized by the fact the their cells show abnormal growth patterns and are no longer under the control of the cell's normal homeostatic growth-controlling mechanisms. Although the range of mechanisms involved in the development of tumors and the spectrum of tissues from which tumors are derived is diverse, they can be classified into three broad types.

Benign Tumors. Broadly speaking, these arise in any of the tissues of the body and grow locally. Their clinical significance is there ability to cause local pressure, cause obstruction, or form a space-occupying lesion, such as a benign brain tumor. Benign tumors do not metastasize (Table 2.2).

In situ Tumors. These are often small tumors that arise in the epithelium. Histologically, the lesion appears to contain cancer cells, but the tumor remains in the epithelial layer and does not invade the basement membrane or the supporting mesenchyme. A typical example of this is preinvasive squamous cell carcinoma affecting the nasal planum of cats and is often referred to as Bowen's disease.

Cancer. This refers to a malignant tumor that has the capacity for both local invasion and distant spread by the process of metastasis.

CARCINOGENESIS IS A MULTISTEP PROCESS. Cancer is a disorder of cells and, although it usually appears as a tumor made up of a mass of cells, this

TABLE 2.2—Characteristics of benign and malignant tumors

Characteristic	Malignant	Benign
Differentiation	Broad range of degrees of differentiation giving rise to an atypical structure	Tumor tissue closely resembles the structure of the parent tissue
Rate of growth	Range of growth rates but may be rapid with abnormal mitoses	Usually slow or intermittent growth; mitoses are rare
Mode of growth	Growth by expansion, and then by infiltration, giving poorly defined borders	Growth by expansion
Metastasis	Can occur	Never occurs

is the phenotypic end result of a whole series of changes that may have taken a long time to develop. The application of a cancer-producing agent (*carcinogen*) to tissues does not lead to the immediate production of a cancer cell. Following the initiating step produced by the agent, there follows a period of tumor promotion. This promotion may be caused by the same initiating agent or by other substances such as normal growth promoters or hormones. The initiating step is rapid and affects the genetic material of the cell. If the cell does not repair this damage, then promoting factors may progress the cell toward a malignant phenotype (Figure 2.10).

In contrast to initiation, progression may be very slow and may not even become manifest in the lifetime of the animal. Each stage of multistep carcinogenesis reflects genetic changes in the cell, with a selection advantage that drives the progression toward a highly malignant cell. The age-dependent incidence of cancer suggests a requirement for between four and seven rate-limiting, stochastic events to produce the malignant phenotype (Figure 2.11).

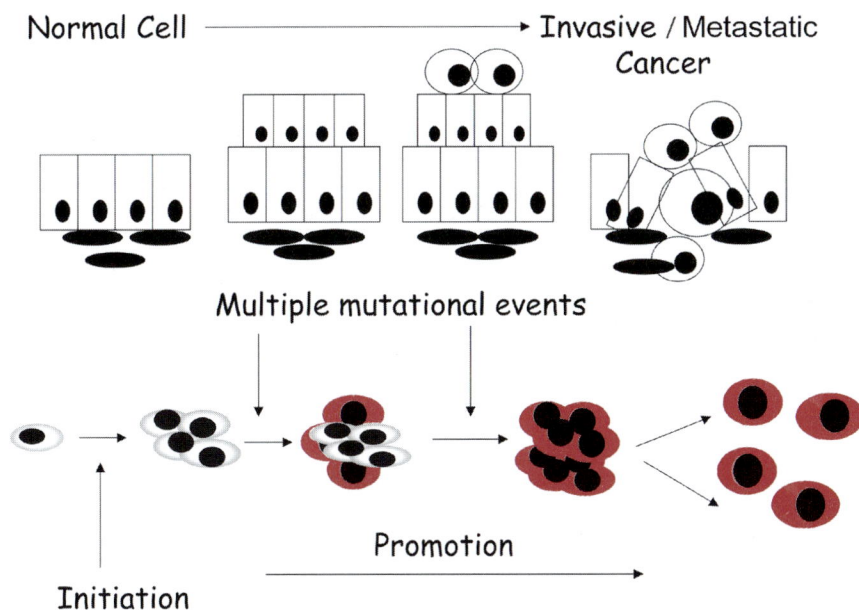

FIG. 2.10—Cancer is the phenotypic end result of a whole series of changes that may have taken a long time to develop. The application of a cancer-producing agent (carcinogen) to tissues does not lead to the immediate production of a cancer cell. Following the initiation step produced by the agent, there follows a period of tumor promotion. The initiating step is rapid and affects the genetic material of the cell. If the cell does not repair this damage, then promoting factors may progress the cell toward a malignant phenotype. Each step in the progression may represent a selective growth advantage over the previous one.

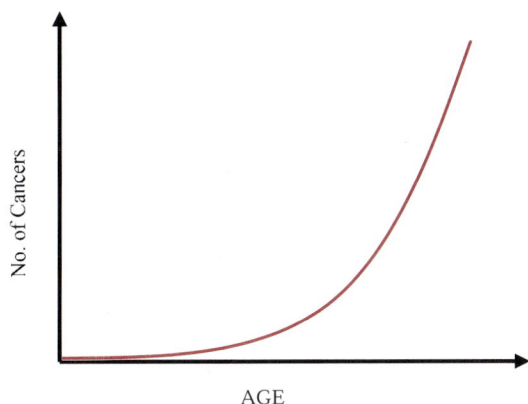

FIG. 2.11—This graph shows the age-dependent incidence of cancer, which suggests a requirement of a number of stochastic events to produce a malignant phenotype.

The whole sequence of events in the process of tumor formation is a consequence of changes at the genetic level. Over the past 25 years, cancer research has generated a rich and complex body of information revealing that cancer is a disease involving dynamic changes in the genome. This foundation has been set in the discovery of the so-called cancer genes or *oncogenes* and *tumor-suppressor genes*. Mutations that produce oncogenes with dominant gain of function and tumor-suppressor genes with recessive loss of function have been identified through their alteration in human and animal cancer cells and by their elicitation of cancer phenotypes in experimental models. Central to the discovery of oncogenes and tumor-suppressor genes were seminal experiments performed in virally induced tumors.

ONCOGENES. The RNA tumor viruses (*retroviruses*) provided the first evidence that genetic factors play a role in the development of cancer. The initial observation came in 1910, when Rous demonstrated that a filterable agent (later termed avian leukosis virus) could produce lymphoid tumors in chickens. As cancer in chickens was not considered important, it was not for several years that the significance of this discovery was realized.

Retroviruses have three core genes (*gag*, *pol*, and *env*) and an additional gene that gives the virus the ability to transform cells (see Part 3 of this chapter). Retroviral sequences that are responsible for transforming properties are called viral oncogenes (v-*onc*). The names of these genes are derived from the tumors in which they were first described (e.g., v-*ras* from rat sarcoma virus).

Viral oncogenes were subsequently shown to have cellular homologues called *cellular oncogenes* (c-*onc*). Later the term *proto-oncogene* was used to describe cellular oncogenes that do not have transforming potential to form tumors in their native state but can be altered to lead to malignancy. Most proto-oncogenes are key genes involved in the control of cell growth and proliferation, and their roles are complex. For simplicity, their sites and modes of action in the normal cell can be separated as follows (Figure 2.12):

- Growth factors
- Growth-factor receptors
- Protein kinases
- Signal transducers
- Nuclear proteins and transcription factors

Growth Factors. These are molecules that act on the cell via cell surface receptors. Their contribution to carcinogenesis may be through excessive production of the growth factor or where a growth factor is expressed in a cell but does not normally function in that cell.

Growth-factor Receptors. Several proto-oncogene-derived proteins form part of cell surface receptors for growth factors. The binding of ligand to receptor is the initial stage of delivery of mitogenic signals to cells. The role of these signals in carcinogenesis may be through structural alterations in these proteins.

Protein Kinases. These are associated with the inner surface of the plasma membrane and are involved in signal transduction following ligand receptor binding. Structural changes in these genes and proteins lead to

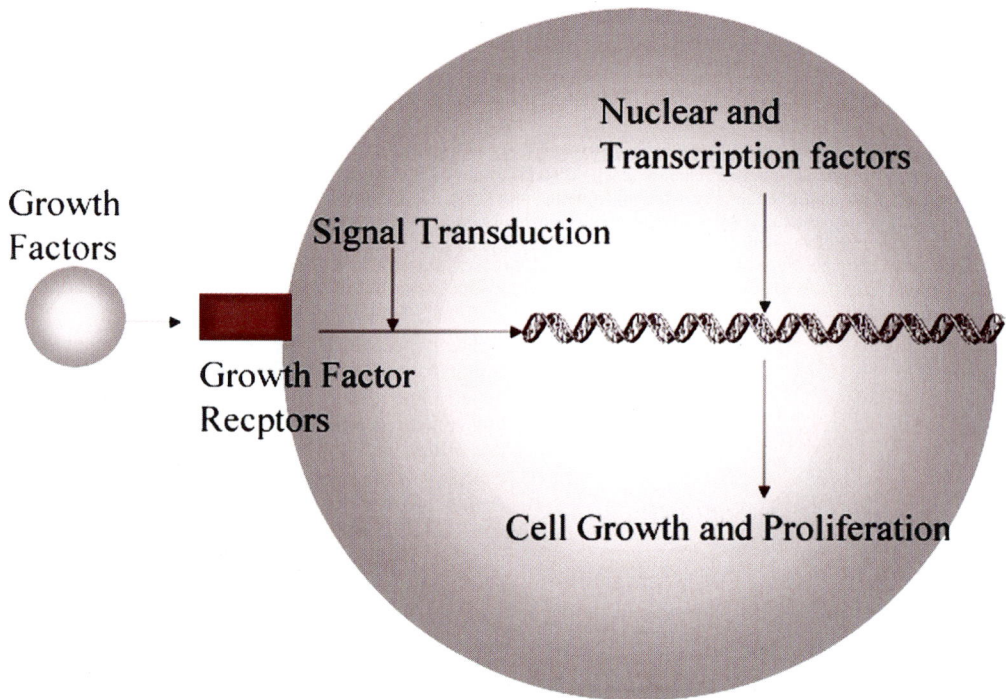

FIG. 2.12— Oncogenes: dominant gain in function. Oncogenes are normal cellular genes involved in cell division and differentiation. Oncogenes may be growth factors, growth-factor receptors, signal transducers, protein kinases, nuclear proteins, or transcription factors.

increased kinase activity that can have profound effects on signal transduction pathways.

Signal Transduction. The binding of an extracellular growth factor to the membrane receptor leads to a series of events by which the mitogenic signal is transduced to the nucleus of the cell. Intimate to this signaling are the second messengers such as GTP (guanosine triphosphate) and proteins that bind GTP (G proteins). During signal transduction, GTP is converted to GDP (guanosine diphosphate) by the GTPase activity of G proteins. A group of proto-oncogenes called *Ras* encode proteins with GTPase and GTP-binding activity and, in the normal cell, help to modulate cellular proliferation. Mutations in the *ras* proto-oncogene can contribute to uncontrolled cellular proliferation.

Nuclear Proteins and Transcription Factors. These proto-oncogenes encode proteins that control gene expression. Where these genes may have a role in cellular proliferation, changes in transcription-factor activity may contribute to the development of the malignant genotype.

MECHANISMS BY WHICH ONCOGENES BECOME ACTIVATED. The advent of recombinant DNA technology has enabled scientists to unravel a number of mechanisms by which the normal products of proto-oncogenes can be disrupted to produce uncontrolled cell division (Figure 2.13).

Chromosomal Translocation. Where proto-oncogenes are translocated within the genome—that is, from one chromosome to another—their function can be greatly altered. The classical example in human medicine is the chromosomal breakpoint that produces the Philadelphia chromosome found in chronic granulocytic leukemia. This involves the translocation of the c-*abl* oncogene on chromosome 9 to a gene (*bcr*) on chromosome 22. The *abl-bcr* hybrid gene produces a novel transcript whose protein product has tyrosine kinase activity and can contribute to uncontrolled cellular proliferation. Transgenic mice for this chimeric gene develop lymphoblastic leukemia and lymphoma.

Gene Amplification. Quantitation of gene copy number is possible by Southern hybridization and subsequent densimetric analysis comparing the expression of *housekeeping* genes. Amplification of oncogenes can occur in a number of tumor types and has been demonstrated in childhood neuroblastoma, where the myc proto-oncogene (nuclear transcription factor) is amplified up to 300 times. A further example is the *mdm2* proto-oncogene, which has been identified in dogs and horses and has recently been shown to be amplified in a proportion of canine soft-tissue sarcomas.

Point Mutations. These are single base changes in the DNA sequence of proto-oncogenes leading to the production of abnormal proteins. A classical example is the *ras* proto-oncogene, where point mutations are a consistent finding in a number of tumors.

Viral Insertions. The discovery of oncogenes was through studies of the tumor-causing viruses. In some circumstances, proto-oncogene function can be damaged by the insertion of viral elements. A more detailed

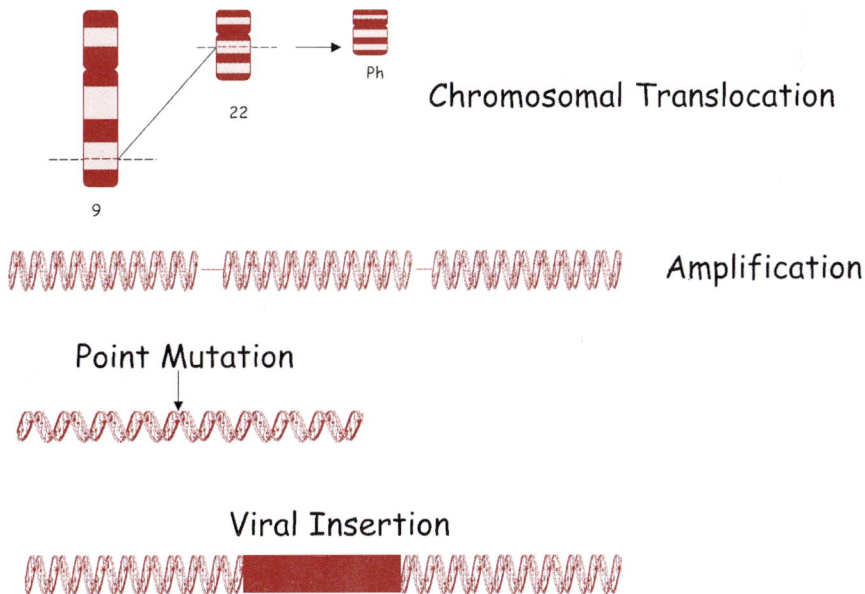

FIG. 2.13—Methods of oncogene activation.

account of viral oncogenesis is presented in the following chapter.

TUMOR-SUPPRESSOR GENES. Changes in genes can lead to either a stimulatory or an inhibitory effect on cell growth and proliferation. The stimulatory effects are provided by the proto-oncogenes already described. Mutations or translocations of these genes produce positive signals leading to uncontrolled growth. In contrast, tumor formation can result from a loss of inhibitory functions associated with another class of cellular genes called the tumor-suppressor genes. The discovery of these genes began by observations of inherited cancer syndromes in children, in particular studies of *retinoblastoma*. In the early 1970s, epidemiological studies of both retinoblastoma and Wilms' tumor led Knundson to propose his "two hit" theory of tumorigenesis.

RETINOBLASTOMA FORMS THE FIRST CLUES TO THE EXISTENCE OF TUMOR-SUP-PRESSOR GENES. Retinoblastoma occurs in two forms: sporadic and inherited (accounting for 40% of cases). In the inherited form, the mode of inheritance is autosomal dominant, and about half the children are affected by the condition. Knudson's model required the retinoblastoma tumor cells (in either sporadic or inherited form) to acquire two separate genetic changes in the DNA before tumor development. The first or pre-

disposing event could be inherited through the germline (familial retinoblastoma) or arise de novo in somatic cells (sporadic form). The second event occurred in somatic cells. Thus, in sporadic retinoblastoma, both events arose in the retinal cells. However, in familial retinoblastoma, the individual had already inherited one mutant gene and only required a second hit in the remaining normal gene in somatic cells.

The mode of inheritance of retinoblastoma is dominant with incomplete penetrance. At the cellular level, however, loss or inactivation of both alleles is required to change the cell's phenotype. The retinoblastoma gene codes for *Rb*, which has been already described as a normal cellular gene involved in control of the cell cycle. The *Rb* is described as a tumor suppressor and, in a cell with only one normal allele, that allele usually produces enough tumor-suppressor product to remain normal. Genetically, mutations in tumor-suppressor genes behave very differently from oncogene mutations. Whereas activating oncogene mutations are dominant to wild type (they emit their proliferating signals regardless of the wild-type gene product), suppressor mutations are recessive. Mutation in one gene copy usually has no effect, as long as a reasonable amount of wild-type protein remains (Figure 2.14). Consequently, some texts refer to tumor-suppressor genes as recessive oncogenes.

More recently, Knundson's hypothesis was confirmed when the *Rb* gene was cloned and characterized. The retinoblastoma tumor-suppressor Rb is the principle member of a family of proteins that also encompass

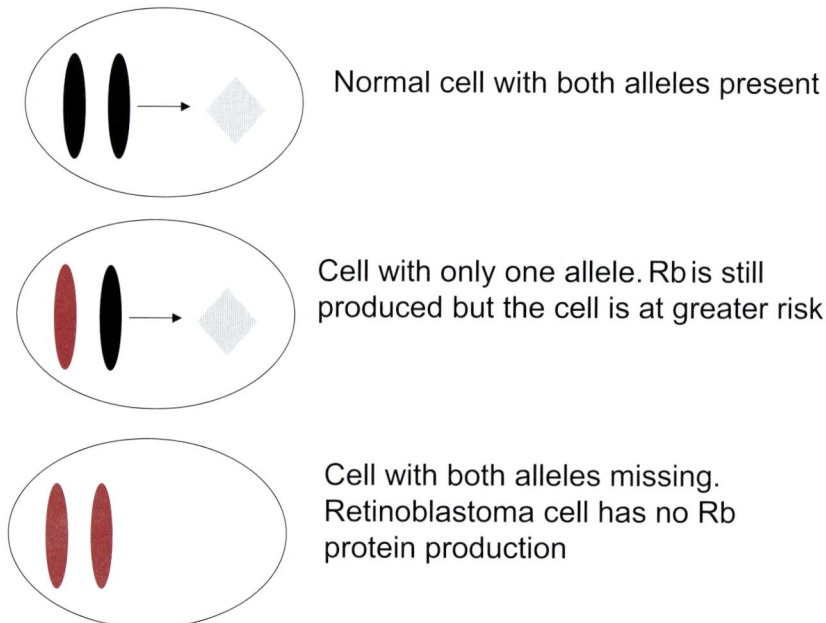

Normal cell with both alleles present

Cell with only one allele. Rb is still produced but the cell is at greater risk

Cell with both alleles missing. Retinoblastoma cell has no Rb protein production

FIG. 2.14—In contrast to oncogene mutations, suppressor gene mutations are recessive. Mutation in one copy usually has no effect on the individual, as long as a sufficient amount of protein is provided by the normal allele. Rb, retinoblastoma.

pRb2/p130 and p107. Rb plays a central role in regulating cell-cycle progression in G_1, and disruption of Rb function has been found to be a common feature of many human cancers as well as the classical retinoblastoma tumor. Rb function can be abrogated by point mutations, by deletions, or by complex formation with viral oncoproteins such as simian vacuolating virus 40 (SV 40) large-T-antigen, adenoviral E_{1A} protein. The function of additional proteins associated with the Rb pathway is also subjected to deregulation in human cancers, including overexpression of D-type cyclins, overexpression of CDK4, and downregulation of the CDKI cell-cycle inhibitor p16.

Whereas cell-cycle control via the Rb pathway is lost commonly in many human tumors, little is known about the role of Rb, cyclin D, CDK4, and p16 in domesticated animal tumors.

THE *P53* TUMOR-SUPPRESSOR GENE. *p53* is a gene whose product is intimately involved in cell-cycle control. Its discovery by Sir David Lane marked a major milestone in cancer research and has enabled greater understanding of molecular mechanisms of cancer and identified potential targets for therapeutic intervention.

In the preceding section, we described *p53* as the guardian of the genome, by virtue of its ability to push cells into arrest or apoptosis depending on the degree of DNA damage. Thus, the *p53* tumor-suppressor gene plays an important role in cell-cycle progression, in regulation of gene expression, and in the cellular response mechanisms to DNA damage. Under normal physiological conditions, wild-type *p53* can bind specific DNA sequences and regulate transcription of a number of genes involved in cell-cycle progression and apoptotic pathways, including *p21^wafl/cip1* and *bax*. The *p53*-mediated mechanisms are responsible for tumor suppression and prevent accumulation of potentially oncogenic mutations and genomic instability. Failure by *p53* to activate such cellular functions may ultimately result in abnormal uncontrolled cell growth leading to tumorigenic transformation.

p53 is the most frequently inactivated gene in human neoplasia, with functional loss commonly occurring through gene mutational events, including nonsense, missense, and splice-site mutations, allelic loss, rearrangements, and deletions. However, *p53* function can also be abrogated by several nonmutational mechanisms, including nuclear exclusion, complex formation with a number of viral proteins, and through overexpression of the cellular oncogene *mdm2*.

The homologues of *p53* and *mdm2* have both been identified in domestic animal species, and a number of studies indicate that this gene also has a central role in the progression of veterinary cancers. A summary of these studies and the role of *p53* in carcinogenesis is presented in Figure 2.15 and Table 2.3.

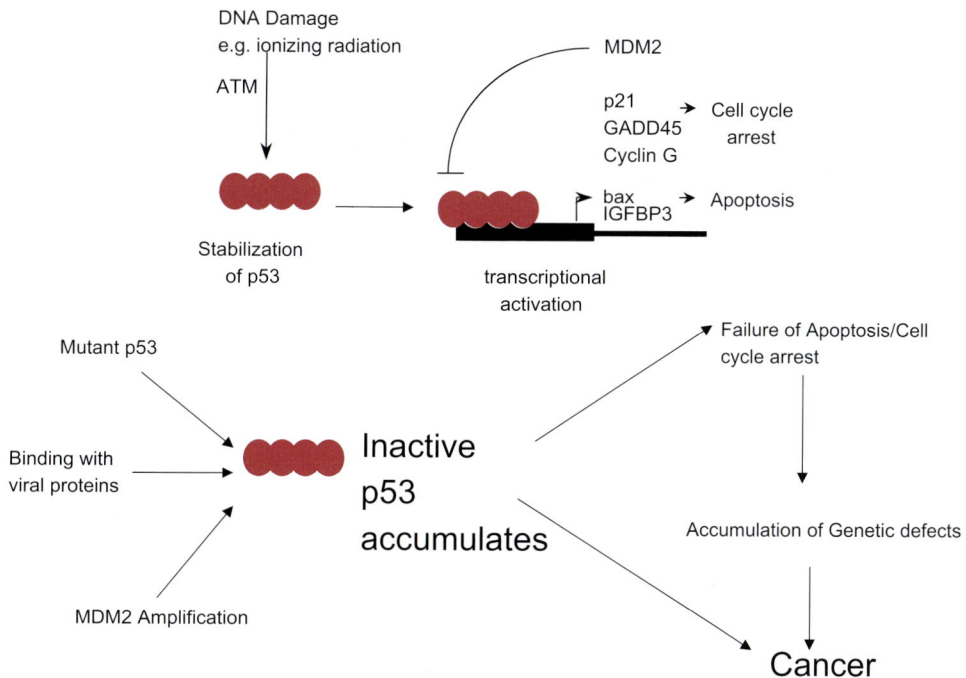

FIG. 2.15—The role of p53 in protecting the cell against DNA damage is seen by its ability to cause cell-cycle arrest or apoptosis. Failure of these mechanisms by P53 inactivation or mutation can lead to the accumulation of DNA damage and development of the malignant phenotype.

TABLE 2.3—Oncogene and tumor-suppressor gene abnormalities detected in animal cancers

Gene	Tumor type	Species
Myc oncogene	Lymphoma	Cat (FeLV)
		Chicken (ALV)
	Plasma cell tumor	Dog
Ras oncogene	Lung carcinoma	Dog
	Acute myeloid leukemia	Dog
MDM2 oncogene	Soft-tissue sarcoma	Dog
p53 tumor-suppressor gene	Mammary carcinoma	Cat
	Squamous cell carcinoma	Cat
	Osteosarcoma	Cat
	Soft-tissue sarcoma	Cat
	Osteosarcoma	Dog
	Lymphoma	Dog
	Mammary Carcinoma	Dog
	Nasal Carcinoma	Dog
	Sarcoid	Horse

ALV, avian leukosis virus; and FeLV, feline leukemia virus.

CANCER ARISES THROUGH MULTIPLE MOLECULAR MECHANISMS. As discussed, the advances in our understanding of normal cell biology and the processes that lead to malignancy have increased dramatically over the past 30 years. It is a daunting prospect that, if cancer research continues at the same pace, then levels of complexity will be added to make it more difficult to "see the forest for the trees." However, it may be worth considering a far more optimistic approach. Research during the last decade has shown us that transformation of a normal cell into a malignant cell requires very few molecular, biochemical, and cellular changes that can be considered as acquired capabilities. Further, despite the wide diversity of cancer types, these acquired capabilities appear to be common to all types of cancer. The optimistic view of increasing simplicity is further endorsed by the fact that all normal cells, irrespective of origin and phenotype, carry similar molecular mechanisms that regulate cell proliferation, differentiation, aging, and cell death.

We have discussed that tumorigenesis is a multistep process and that these steps reflect genetic alterations that drive the progression of a normal cell into a highly malignant cancer cell. This is supported by the finding that genomes of tumor cells are invariably altered at multiple sites. The spectrum of changes ranges from subtle point mutations in growth-regulatory genes to obvious changes in chromosomal complement.

Cancer cells have defects in regulatory circuits that govern cellular proliferation and homeostasis. It has been suggested that the vast array of cancer genotypes is a manifestation of only six alterations in cellular physiology that collectively dictate malignant growth. These acquired characteristics can be summarized under the following headings (Figure 2.16):

- Self-sufficient growth
- Insensitivity to antigrowth signals
- Evasion of programmed cell death (apoptosis)
- Limitless replicative potential
- Sustained angiogenesis
- Tissue invasion and metastasis

In one sense, cancer is a very common disease in animals and people, but the development of cancer is actually a rare event. When one considers the number of cells in the body, the proliferation of these cells, and the potential for malignant transformation, then the development of a single cancer is rare. This is because of the cell's own natural defenses against progression toward the malignant phenotype. Each of the acquired capabilities previously described represents a breach in the cell's own homeostatic mechanisms that are in place to prevent the development of cancer. Next is an overview of these traits and the strategies by which they are acquired in cancer cells.

SELF-SUFFICIENCY IN GROWTH SIGNALS. Normal cells require mitogenic stimuli for growth and proliferation. These signals are transmitted to the nucleus by the binding of signaling molecules to specific receptors, the diffusion of growth factors into the cell, extracellular matrix components, or cell-to-cell adhesions or interactions. As previously discussed, many oncogenes act by mimicking normal growth signals. Tumor cells do not depend on external mitogenic stimuli for proliferation and sustained growth but are self-sufficient. The liberation from dependency on exogenous signals severely disrupts normal cellular homeostasis. The mechanisms by which this occurs are summarized in Figure 2.17.

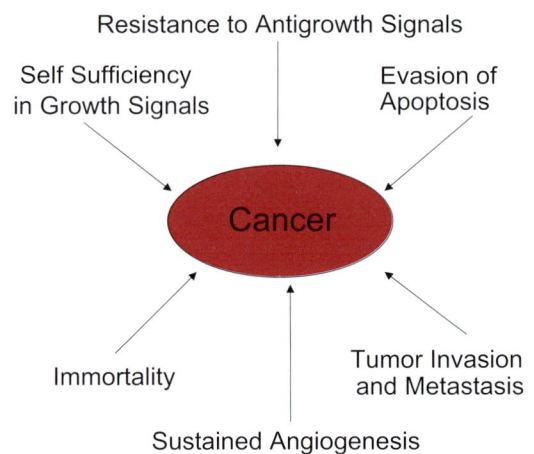

FIG. 2.16—The acquired capabilities of cancer.

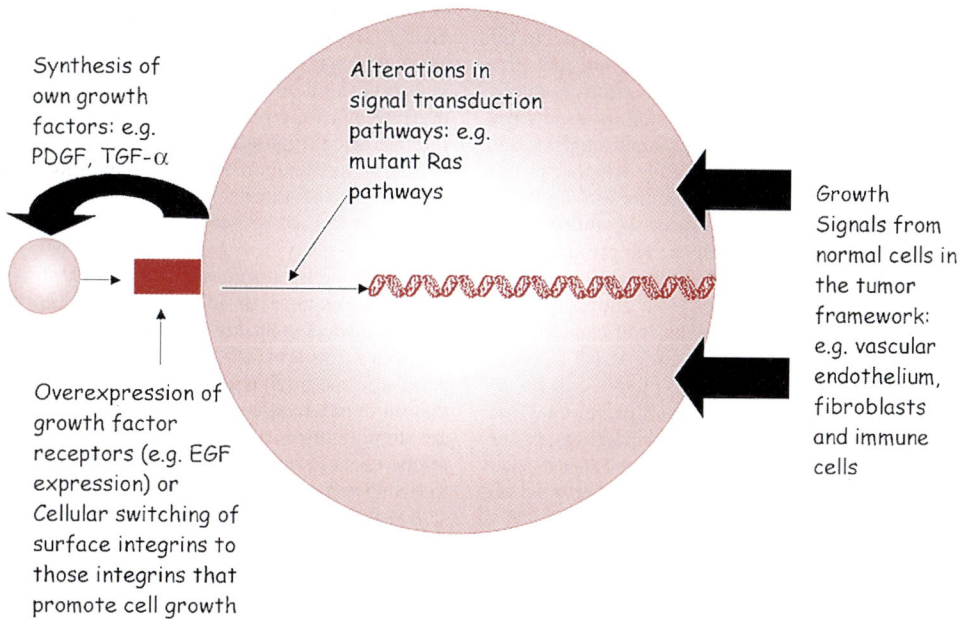

FIG. 2.17—The acquisition of self-sufficiency in growth signals. EGF, epidermal growth factor; PDGF, platelet-derived growth factor; and TGF-α, transforming growth factor β.

Although the acquisition of growth-signaling autonomy by cancer cells is conceptually satisfying, it is too simplistic. One of the major problems in cancer research is to focus on the cancer cell in isolation. It is now apparent that we must also consider the contribution of the tumor microenvironment to the survival of cancer cells. Within normal tissues, paracrine and endocrine signals contribute greatly to growth and proliferation. Cell-to-cell growth signaling is also likely to operate in cancer cells and may be as important as some of the autonomous mechanisms of tumor growth. It has recently been suggested that growth signals for the proliferation of carcinoma cells are derived from the tumor stromal elements. It is therefore possible that the survival of tumor cells not only relies on the acquisition of growth-signal autonomy but may also require the recruitment of local cells to provide them with growth signals (Figure 2.18).

INSENSITIVITY TO ANTIGROWTH SIGNALS.
Within the normal cell, multiple antiproliferative signals operate to maintain cellular quiescence and homeostasis. These signals include soluble growth inhibitors that act via cell surface receptors and immobilized inhibitors that are embedded in the extracellular matrix and on the surface of nearby cells. The signals operate

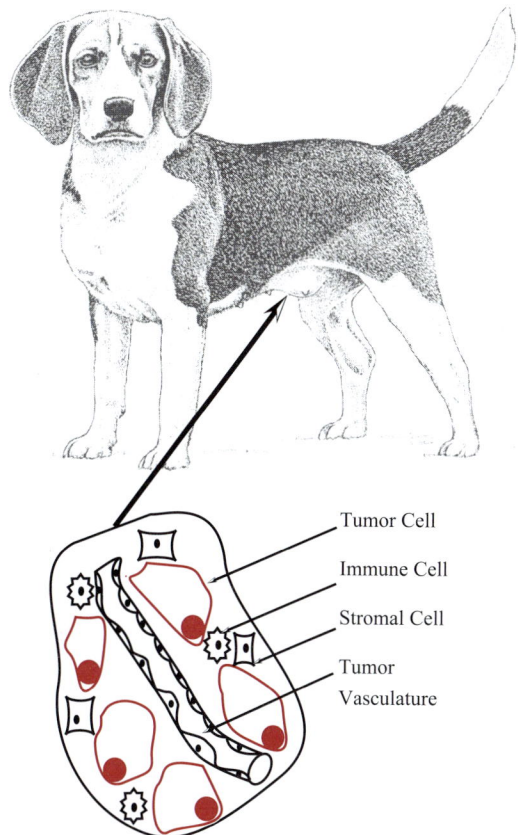

FIG. 2.18—The tumor microenvironment may play a major contributing role in the promotion of malignancy. This includes the local vasculature and stromal elements.

to push the cell either into G_0 or into a postmitotic state (usually associated with the acquisition of specific differentiation–associated characteristics) and are thus intimately associated with cell-cycle control mechanisms. As discussed in Part 1, cells monitor their external environment during the progression through G_1 and, on the basis of external stimuli, decide whether to proliferate, to become quiescent, or to enter into a postmitotic state. At the basic level, most of the antiproliferative signals are funneled through the Rb protein and its close relatives. Disruption of Rb allows cell proliferation and renders the cell insensitive to antiproliferative signals such as that provided by the well-characterized transforming growth factor (TGF-β). The Rb signaling circuit and the associated extrinsic factors can be disrupted in a number of ways, as shown in Figure 2.19.

However, the development of the malignant phenotype depends on more than the avoidance of cytostatic mechanisms. The cell also needs to avoid terminal differentiation and the postmitotic state. One example of how tumor cells manage this is provided by studies on the myc oncogene product, which is a nuclear transcription factor that has growth-stimulating effects in association with another protein called Max. During normal development, the growth-inducing effect of MYC-MAX complexes can be supplanted by alternative complexes of max with a group of transcription factors known as Mad. Mad-Max complexes elicit signals for terminal differentiation. However, where the myc oncogene is amplified (as occurs in many tumor types), the balance of complexes is shifted in favor of myc-max, thereby impairing differentiation and promoting proliferation.

EVADING APOPTOSIS OR PROGRAMMED CELL DEATH. An overview of the mechanisms of apoptosis and its role in normal cellular homeostasis was presented in Part 1. The growth of any tumor depends not only on the rate of cell division, but also the rate of cellular attrition (that is mainly provided by apoptotic mechanisms). Basic molecular and pathological studies of tumors have confirmed that acquired resistance toward apoptosis is a hallmark of all types of cancer.

Cancer cells, through a variety of strategies, can acquire resistance to apoptosis, and one of the most common ways is through loss of function of the tumor-suppressor protein P53. Loss of P53 protein function is most often through mutation but can also be via sequestration or inactivation of the protein by viral proteins or by amplification of other oncogenes such as *mdm2*. Removal of normal P53 function leads to failure of the cell's sensor mechanism for DNA damage. When the cell suffers an insult such as UV radiation, hypoxia, or exposure to DNA-damaging agents, signals are funneled through P53 to either cause cell-cycle arrest or apoptosis. Failure of this mechanism can contribute to the progression of a cell toward malignancy and promote the accumulation of genetic defects.

LIMITLESS REPLICATIVE CAPACITY. Much of our understanding of cellular aging is derived from observations of cultured cells in vitro. From these studies, it is clear that normal somatic cells have a finite replicative potential when cultured in vitro. After an estimated 50 cell divisions, cells enter an irre-

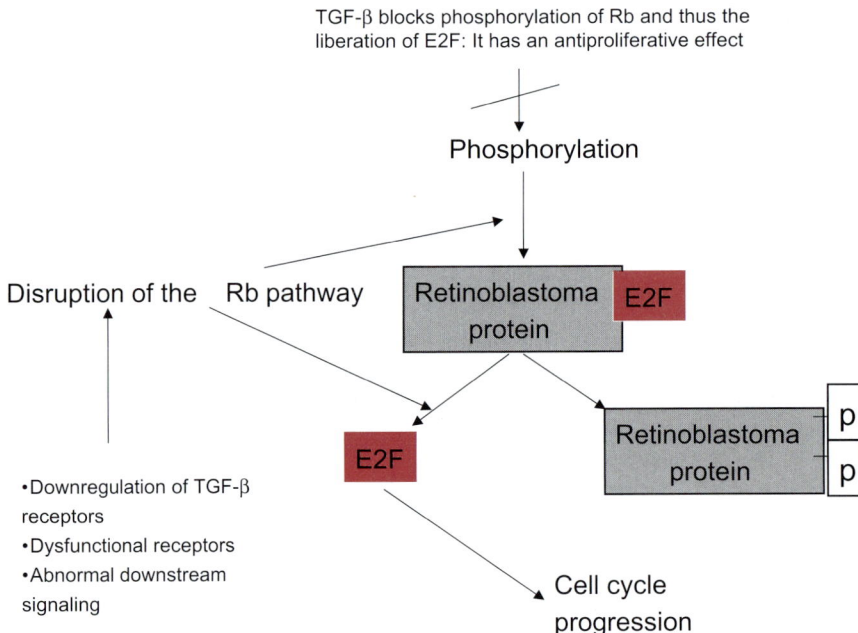

FIG. 2.19—Disruption of the retinoblastoma protein (Rb) signaling pathway in cancer.

versible (and prolonged) state of cellular senescence (sometimes referred to as *mortality stage 1* or M1). This period is characterized by arrest of proliferation without loss of biochemical function or viability. At the end of this period, cells exhibit altered morphology and chromosomal instability, a state often referred to as *crisis* (*mortality stage 2* or M2) (see Figure 2.20).

This phenomenon has been explained by studies on the ends of linear chromosomes, which contain specialized nucleoprotein structures where noncoding DNA sequences are arranged in tandemly repeated units of the hexanucleotide TTAGGG (referred to as telomeres).

During cell division, replication of linear chromosomes leads to a net loss of around 50 to 200 nucleotides from the chromosomal ends, mainly due to the unidirectional polarity of synthesis of the growing DNA strand in a 5′ to 3′ direction (the end-replication problem) (Figure 2.21). Thus, during each cell division, there is telomeric attrition. Both Watson and Oblivnokov, who also originally suggested that telomeric shortening gave rise to the signal for cellular senescence, described this observation. In fact, some 30 years later, and through the power of molecular biology, it is clear that the telomeric attrition is intimately linked to progression of the cell to senescence and crisis. We shall return to telomeres later in the chapter during discussions on cancer progression.

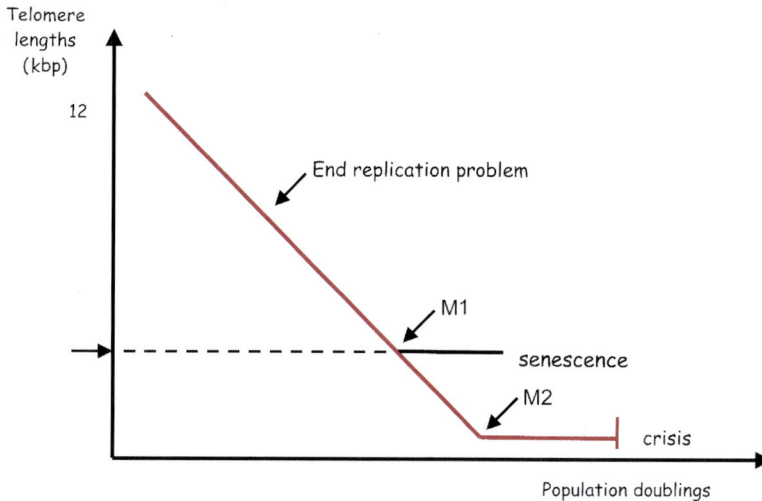

FIG. 2.20—Telomere length dynamics in normal cellular aging. M1 and M2, mortality stages 1 and 2.

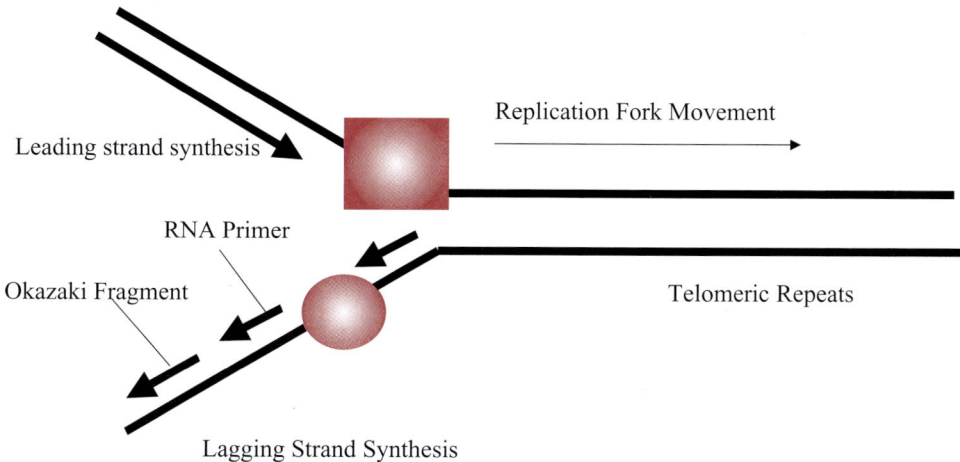

FIG. 2.21—The inability of chromosomes to completely replicate their extreme 5′ ends (the end-replication problem) leads to attrition of telomeres at each cell division.

The aforementioned three acquired capabilities are not sufficient to ensure the survival of a tumor. The cell must also overcome replicative senescence and crisis. It has now been demonstrated in human tumors and, more recently, dog tumors, that telomere maintenance is a feature of virtually all cancer types. Tumor cells succeed in telomeric maintenance by the expression of the enzyme telomerase. From studies on cellular senescence, expression of the enzyme telomerase has emerged as a central unifying mechanism underlying the immortal phenotype of cancer cells and has thus become the most common marker of malignant cells. *Telomerase* is a ribonucleoprotein enzyme that maintains the protective structures at the ends of eukaryotic chromosomes, called *telomeres*. In humans, telomerase expression is repressed in most somatic tissues, and telomeres shorten with each progressive cell division. In contrast, telomerase activity is a common finding in many malignancies resulting in stabilized telomere length. It is now well documented that the level of telomerase in malignant tissue compared with that in normal tissue is much higher, and this differential is greater than that for classical enzymatic targets such as thymidylate synthase, dihydrofolate reductase, or topoisomerase II (Figure 2.22).

Telomerase biology is complex, and the mechanisms by which telomerase becomes reactivated in tumor cells is the subject of intense research. However, this represents an exciting opportunity for further understanding the complex biology of cancer and also the identification of completely novel targets for therapy.

SUSTAINED ANGIOGENESIS. For any normal or tumor cell to survive, then, it must be supplied with adequate oxygen and nutrient supplies by the vasculature. During normal organogenesis, the development of the parenchyma is carefully coordinated with the growth of new blood vessels or angiogenesis. Once a tissue has been formed, angiogenesis becomes carefully regulated and part of the normal homeostatic processes of the body. During the development of cancerous lesions, one would suspect that the proliferating cells within the tumor would have intrinsic capability to encourage angiogenesis. In fact, the experimental evidence suggests that cells within a developing tumor initially lack any angiogenic capabilities. Consequently, for a tumor mass to survive and grow, it must acquire this capability of sustained angiogenesis.

The whole process of angiogenesis is governed by positive and negative signals provided by soluble factors and their receptors, integrins, and adhesion molecules that mediate cell-matrix and cell-cell associations. The classical examples of positive angiogenic factors are vascular endothelial growth factor (VEGF) and basic fibroblast growth factor (BFGF). Each of these molecules binds to specific receptors on the surface of endothelial cells to elicit their effects.

The ability of a tumor to induce and sustain angiogenesis seems to be acquired in a stepwise fashion during carcinogenesis and via an *angiogenic switch* from vascular quiescence. It has been postulated that this acquired capability is an early event in tumorigenesis and that the *switch* is provided by a change in balance of angiogenic inducers and inhibitors via upregulation of expression of VEGF/BFGF compared with normal tissue. In other tumors, there may be downregulation of angiogenic inhibitors such as thrombospondin 1. The mechanisms by which gene expression profiles are altered are poorly understood. However, in one classi-

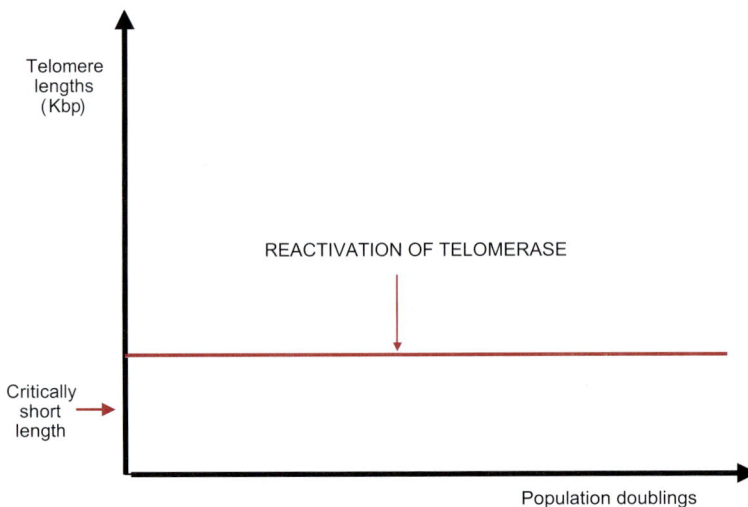

FIG. 2.22—Reactivation of the enzyme telomerase maintains telomere lengths and offers the cancer cell a mechanism of immortality.

cal example, P53 positively regulates thrombospondin 1 levels and so loss of normal P53 function will reduce antiangiogenic signals. In a similar way, activation of the *ras* oncogene in certain tumors can upregulate VEGF expression and promote angiogenesis.

Another level of angiogenic regulation is provided by the extracellular matrix. Proteases within the matrix may control the availability of angiogenic factors stored in the extracellular matrix, the system representing a complex homeostatic regulatory circuit. The matrix metalloproteinases (see the next section) have also been implicated in the angiogenic switch and are upregulated in certain tumor types promoting both angiogenesis and invasion.

The angiogenesis story is yet another clear example of the danger of considering a cancer as just a mass of tumor cells in isolation. It should be becoming clearer that the tumor microenvironment plays a critical role in sustained tumor growth and represents an exciting target for therapeutic intervention.

TISSUE INVASION AND METASTASIS. We have discussed that one of the major differentiating factors between benign and malignant tumors is the capability of malignant tumors to spread via the blood or lymphatics and form colonies or metastases in distant parts of the body. It is well recognized that the cause of death in 90% of both human and domestic animal cancers is through metastatic disease.

The capability of tumors to invade local tissues and spread to distant sites enables cancer cells to escape the primary tumor mass and colonize areas of the body where space and nutrients are not limiting. As with the establishment of the primary tumor, the successful establishment of metastatic lesions is dependent on the previous five capabilities already discussed.

The mechanisms by which a tumor is able to invade and metastasize are complex and not completely understood. However, they involve the physical coupling of cells to the microenvironment and the parallel activation of extracellular proteases. A three-step theory has been proposed to describe the sequence of events during local invasion of a tumor of the extracellular matrix (Figure 2.23). These steps include attachment of tumor cells to the matrix, degradation of the matrix, and locomotion into the matrix. The attachment of tumor cells is provided by alterations in molecules such as the CAMs (cell-associating molecules) (e.g., members of the calcium-dependent cadherin families). In particular, many epithelial tumors lose the ability to express E cadherin, which promotes the capability of cancer cells to invade. Once anchored, the tumor cell secretes (or induces host cells to produce) proteases to degrade the matrix. In particular, type IV collagenase (a matrix metalloproteinase) is a powerful proteolytic enzyme intimately involved with the process of invasion. In the third stage of invasion, the tumor cells produce pseudopodia that facilitate movement by the attachment to blood vessels that cross the basement membrane. The tumor cells then continue this process of invasive growth.

Invasion is a prerequisite for ultimate metastatic spread. Metastasis occurs by three basic mechanisms: direct or continuous extension, lymphatic spread, or dissemination by the bloodstream. Continuous extension is a direct result of local invasion and enables tumors to break into other tissue spaces. A classical example is transserosal spread of abdominal tumors such as that seen with splenic hemagiosarcoma in dogs.

True metastasis via the blood and lymphatics involves a sequential series of steps involving local invasion, penetration into blood vessels or lymphatics, release of tumor cells into these circulatory pathways,

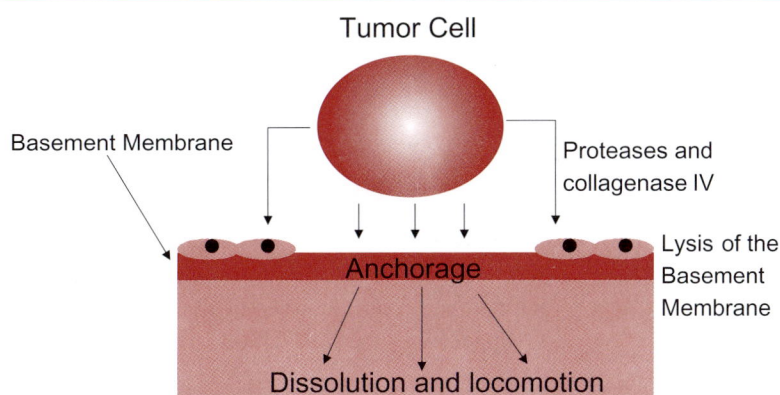

FIG. 2.23—Invasion is a prerequisite to metastatic spread. The attachment of tumor cells is provided by alterations in molecules such as the CAMs (cell-associating molecules, e.g., members of the calcium-dependent cadherin families). In particular, many epithelial tumors lose the ability to express E cadherin, which promotes the ability of cancer cells to invade. Once anchored, the tumor cell secretes (or induces host cells to produce) proteases to degrade the matrix. In particular, type IV collagenase (a matrix metalloproteinase) is a powerful proteolytic enzyme intimately involved with the process of invasion. In the third stage of invasion, the tumor cells produce pseudopodia, which facilitate movement by the attachment to blood vessels that cross the basement membrane. The tumor cells then continue this process of invasive growth.

extravasation into secondary sites, and finally adherence and proliferation at distant sites. The mechanisms of metastasis are summarized in Figure 2.24.

The distribution of metastatic lesions is often predicted by patterns of blood and lymphatic flow. There are, however, circumstances where certain tumor deposits show tropism for organs that are difficult to explain just by the dynamics of fluid flow. In these circumstances, it is suggested that this organ tropism is through growth-factor expression or receptor expression in the target tissue.

THE ROLE OF GENOME INSTABILITY. In the foregoing section, we placed decades of fundamental cancer research into six neatly defined boxes, each representing the capabilities that a normal cell needs to acquire to show the hallmarks of malignancy. Most of these capabilities require changes in the genome through mutation or amplification of chromosomal translocation. However, the process of mutation is actually inefficient because of the complex and fastidious maintenance mechanisms of the normal cell that monitor DNA damage and regulate repair enzymes. Because of this, it is difficult to explain why cancers arise in animals at all, as the acquisition of all traits would seem an impossible task. It may be argued that genomes must attain increased mutability in order to develop into a cancer cell. Alternatively to explain increased mutability, it is the caretaker mechanisms that are affected first. In particular, loss of P53 function leads to failure of the cell to arrest or apoptose in response to DNA damage. We have not included genomic instability in the aforementioned six categories because we consider that it represents the means that enable evolving premalignant cells to reach these six biological end points.

THE PATHWAYS TO CANCER. In the foregoing section, we outlined the six acquired capabilities of cancer cells. It is important to stress that the pathways for cells becoming malignant are highly variable. Mutations in certain oncogenes can occur early in the progression of some tumors and late in others. As a consequence, the acquisition of the essential cancer characteristics may appear at different times in the progression of different cancers. Furthermore, in certain tumors, a specific genetic event may, on its own, contribute only partially to the acquisition of a single capability, whereas, in others, it may contribute to the simultaneous acquisition of multiple capabilities. However, irrespective of the path taken, the hallmark capabilities of cancer will remain common for multiple cancer types and will help clarify mechanisms, prognosis, and the development of new treatments (Figure 2.25).

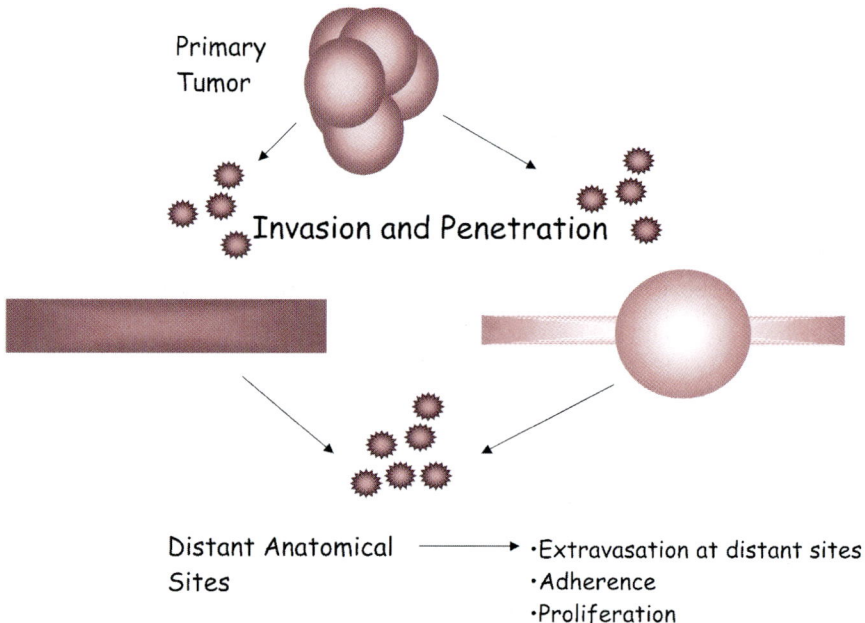

FIG. 2.24—Cancer cells metastasize via the bloodstream or via the lymphatics. In addition, they can extend along tissue planes, especially across the body cavities (transcoelomic spread).

1 Self-Sufficiency in Growth Signals
2 Resistance to Antigrowth Signals
3 Evasion of Apoptosis
4 Immortality
5 Sustained Angiogenesis
6 Tumor Invasion and Metastasis

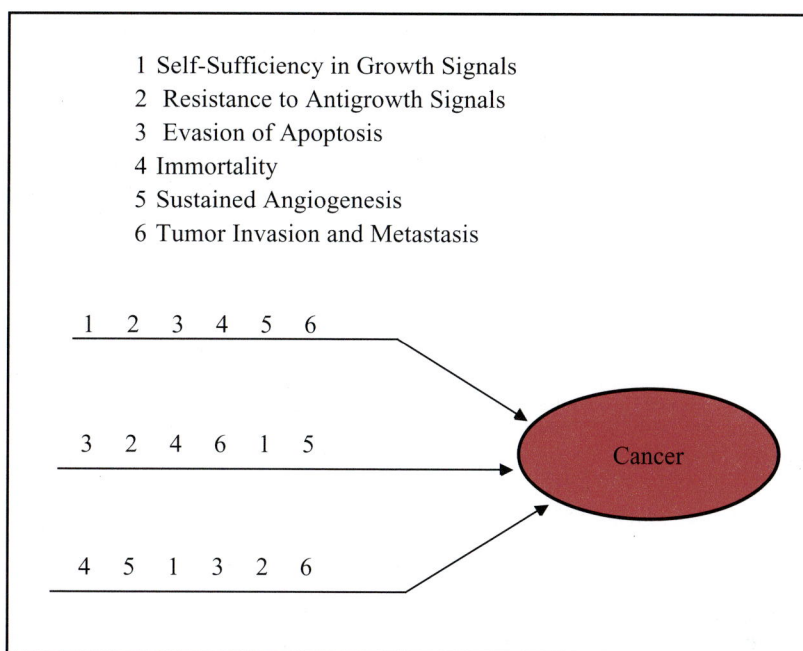

FIG. 2.25—It is important to stress that the pathways for cells becoming malignant are highly variable. Mutations in certain oncogenes can occur early in the progression of some tumors and late in others. As a consequence, the acquisition of the essential cancer characteristics may appear at different times in the progression of different cancers. In this diagram, we can see the different sequence of acquisitions that may occur for a cell to become malignant.

KEY REFERENCES AND FURTHER READING

Bergers G, Hanahan D, Coussens LM. 1998. Angiogenesis and apoptosis are cellular parameters of neoplastic progression in transgenic mouse models of tumorigenesis. Int J Dev Biol 42:995–1002.

Bergers G, Javaherian K, Lo K-M, et al. 1999. Effects of angiogenesis inhibitors on multistage carcinogenesis in mice. Science 284:808–812.

Biller BJ, Kitchel B, Casey D, Cadile DA. 1998. Evaluation of an assay for detecting telomerase activity in neoplastic tissues of dogs. Am J Vet Res 59:1526–1528.

Blasco MA, Funk W, Villeponteau B, Greider CW. 1995. Functional characterization and developmental regulation of mouse telomerase RNA. Science 269:1267–1270.

Blasco MA, Lee H-W, Hande MP, et al. 1997. Telomere shortening and tumour formation by mouse cells lacking telomerase RNA. Cell 91:25–34.

Bouck N, Stellmach V, Hsu SC. 1996. How tumors become angiogenic. Adv Cancer Res 69:135–174.

Chambers AF, Matrisian LM. 1997. Changing views of the role of matrix metalloproteinases in metastasis. J Natl Cancer Inst 89:1260–1270.

Datto MB, Hu PP, Kowalik TF, et al. 1997. The viral oncoprotein E1A blocks transforming growth factor mediated induction of p21/WAF1/Cip1 and p15/INK4B. Mol Cell Biol 17:2030–2037.

Evan G, Littlewood T. 1998. A matter of life and cell death. Science 281:1317–1322.

Hanahan D, Folkman J. 1996. Patterns and emerging mechanisms of the angiogenic switch during tumorigenesis. Cell 86:353–364.

Hanahan D, Weinberg RA. 2000. The hallmarks of cancer. Cell 100:57–70.

Harris CC. 1996. p53 tumor suppressor gene: From the basic research laboratory to the clinic—an abridged historical perspective. Carcinogenesis 17:1187–1198.

Haupt Y, Maya R, Kazaz A, Oren M. 1997. Mdm2 promotes the rapid degradation of p53. Nature 387:296–299.

Hayflick L. 1997. Mortality and immortality at the cellular level: A review. Biochemistry 62:1180–1190.

Lane DP. 1992. Guardian of the genome. Nature 358:15–16.

Levine AJ. 1997. p53, the cellular gatekeeper for growth and division. Cell 88:323–331.

McCance KL, Roberts LK. 1997. The biology of cancer. In: McCance KL, Huether SE, eds. Pathophysiology, the Biological Basis of Disease in Adults and Children, 3rd ed. St Louis: CV Mosby, pp 304–349.

McCance KL, Roberts LK. 1997. Tumour invasion and metastasis. In: McCance KL, Huether SE, eds. Pathophysiology, the Biological Basis of Disease in Adults and Children, 3rd ed. St Louis: CV Mosby, pp 350–372.

McKenzie K, Umbricht CB, Sukumar S. 1999. Applications of telomerase research in the fight against cancer. Mol Med Today 5:114–122.

Nasir L, Argyle DJ. 1999. Mutational analysis of p53 in two cases of bull mastiff lymphosarcoma. Vet Rec 145:23–24.

Nasir L, Argyle DJ, McFarlane ST, Reid SWJ. 1998. Nucleotide sequence of a highly conserved region of the canine p53 tumour suppressor gene. DNA Sequence 8:83–86.

Nasir L, Krasner H, Argyle DJ, Williams A. 2000. A study of p53 tumour suppressor gene immunoreactivity in feline neoplasia. Cancer Lett 155:1–7.

Nasir L, Burr P, McFarlane S, et al. 2000. Cloning, sequence analysis and expression of the cDNA's encoding the canine and equine homologues of the mouse double minute two proto-oncogene. Cancer Lett 152:9–13.

Nasir L, Devlin P, McKevitt T, et al. 2001. Telomere lengths and telomerase activity in dog tissues: A potential model system to study human telomere and telomerase biology. Neoplasia 3:351–359.

Nasir L, Rutteman GR, Reid SW, et al. 2001. Analysis of *p53* mutational events and MDM2 amplification in canine soft-tissue sarcomas. Cancer Lett 174:83–89.

Oliner JD, Kinzler KW, Meltzer PS, et al. 1992. Amplification of a gene encoding a p53 associated protein in human sarcomas. Nature 358:80–83.

Shay JW, Wright WE. 1996. Telomerase activity in human cancer. Curr Opin Oncol 8:66–71.

Stetler-Stevenson WG. 1999. Matrix metalloproteinases in angiogenesis: A moving target for therapeutic intervention. J Clin Invest 103:1237–1241.

Teich NM. 1997. Oncogenes and cancer. In: Franks LM, Teich NM, eds. The Molecular and Cellular Biology of Cancer, 3rd ed. New York: Oxford University Press, pp 169–201.

Vogelstein B, Kinzler KW. 1992. P53 function and dysfunction. Cell 70:525–526.

Weinberg RA. 1995. The retinoblastoma protein and cell cycle control. Cell 81:323–330.

Wu X, Bayle JH, Olson D, Levine AJ. 1993. The *p53-mdm2* autoregulatory loop. Genes Dev 7:1126–1132.

Wyllie AH, Kerr JF, Currie AR. 1980. Cell death: The significance of apoptosis. Int Rev Cytol 68:251–306.

Yazawa M, Okuda M, Setoguchi A, et al. 1999. Measurement of telomerase activity in dog tumours. J Vet Med Sci 61:1125–1129.

Zhu J, Wang H, Bishop JM, Blackburn EH. 1999. Telomerase extends the life-span of virus-transformed human cells without net telomere lengthening. Proc Natl Acad Sci USA 96:3723–3728.

PART 3: THE ETIOLOGY OF CANCERS IN DOMESTIC ANIMALS

Throughout this chapter, we have reinforced the concept that carcinogenesis is multistep rather than a reflection of a single event. In many circumstances, exposure to one tumor-inducing agent or carcinogen only provides one step toward the development of the malignant phenotype. The nature of tumor-inducing agents has been crucial to our understanding of cancer formation because they all have the common property of being able to affect host DNA via genetic or epigenetic means. In particular, seminal experiments in animal retroviruses led to the discovery of oncogenes, which was a turning point in our understanding of cancer biology. The following is a short synopsis of our understanding of the etiologic agents involved in the production of cancers in animals. These agents can be broadly divided into the oncogenic viruses, chemical carcinogens, and physical agents such as radiation.

ONCOGENIC VIRUSES. The oncogenic viruses are a diverse group of pathogens that include all the major families of the DNA viruses and a class of RNA viruses known as *retroviruses*. Although diverse, one almost universal feature is the importance of a DNA stage in the replication of the viral genome.

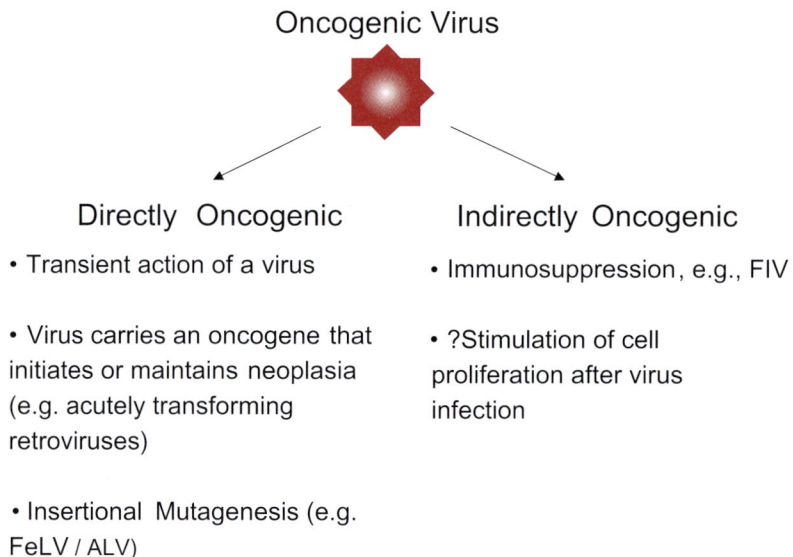

Oncogenic Virus

Directly Oncogenic

• Transient action of a virus

• Virus carries an oncogene that initiates or maintains neoplasia (e.g. acutely transforming retroviruses)

• Insertional Mutagenesis (e.g. FeLV / ALV)

Indirectly Oncogenic

• Immunosuppression, e.g., FIV

• ?Stimulation of cell proliferation after virus infection

FIG. 2.26—The major mechanisms of viral oncogenesis. ALV, avian leukosis virus; FeLV, feline leukemia virus; and FIV, feline immunodeficiency virus.

RNA Viruses

RETROVIRUSES ARE IMPORTANT ONCOGENIC VIRUSES OF CATS, CATTLE, AND CHICKENS. Studies on animal retroviruses have been seminal to our understanding of viral and nonviral oncogenesis. The mechanisms by which these viruses cause neoplastic transformation can be broadly divided into indirect and direct mechanisms (summarized in Figure 2.26 and Table 2.4).

The important oncogenic viruses in veterinary medicine include those of cats, chickens, and cattle, the latter two profoundly affecting agricultural economics. The replication cycle of a typical retrovirus is shown in Figure 2.27. The provirus of a typical oncogenic retrovirus contains three gene blocks. The *gag* gene encodes the core viral proteins, the *pol* gene encodes the reverse transcriptase, and the *env* gene encodes the envelope glycoproteins (Figure 2.28).

RETROVIRUSES CAN BE ACUTELY TRANSFORMING. Very occasionally, novel retroviruses are isolated from leukemias or sarcomas in animals that have been viremic with a leukemia virus for some time. These viruses induce tumors very rapidly when inoculated into members of the species of origin and are referred to as *acutely transforming oncoviruses*. The prototype of the acutely transforming virus is the *Rous sarcoma*

TABLE 2.4—Major oncogenic viruses of domestic animals

Virus classification	Virus	Associated tumors
Retroviruses		
Oncoviruses (type C)	Avian leukosis virus (ALV)	Lymphomas and leukemias
	Feline leukemia virus (FeLV)	Lymphomas and leukemias (usually T cell)
	Bovine leukemia virus (BLV)	Lymphomas and leukemias (B cell)
Oncoviruses (type D)	Sheep pulmonary adenomatosis (SPA)	Lung tumors
Lentiviruses	Feline immunodeficiency virus (FIV)	B-cell lymphomas
Papovirus	Papilloma of various species	Warts in various species
		Alimentary tract/bladder cancer in cattle associated with bracken fern
		Skin carcinoma (esp. cattle) associated with sunlight exposure
		?Sarcoids in horses
Adenovirus	Types 2, 5, and 12	Sarcomas in hamsters
Herpes viruses	Marek's disease of fowl	T-cell neurolymphomatosis

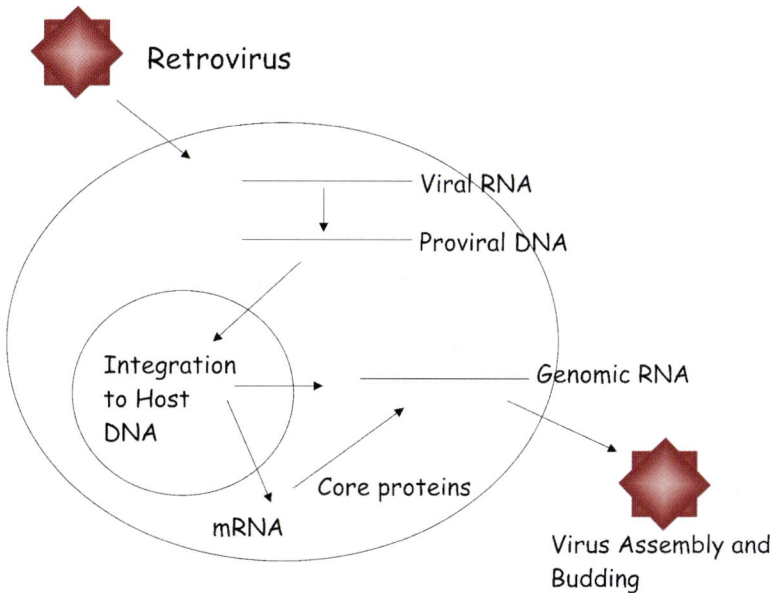

FIG. 2.27—The life cycle of a retrovirus. The retrovirus is a double-stranded RNA virus, which, on entry into the cell, reverse transcribes into proviral DNA. This DNA can integrate into the host cell genome. Expression of viral proteins then enables assembly and budding of the virus.

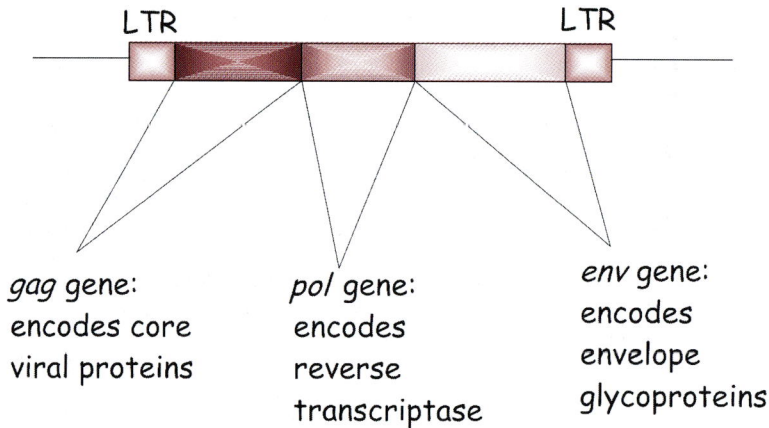

FIG. 2.28—Structure of a typical retroviral provirus. LTR, long terminal repeats: enhancer/promoter sequences.

virus (RSV), which was isolated from a chicken in 1911. Subsequently, many more have been isolated from animals infected with avian, feline, murine, or simian oncoviruses. The mechanism by which these viruses are generated is shown in Figure 2.29. They are generated by a rare recombinational event between the leukemia virus with which the animal was originally infected and a cellular proto-oncogene. In this, part of the viral genome is deleted and replaced with the cellular oncogene. The virus then becomes acutely transforming because this oncogene is now under the tran-scriptional control of the very efficient viral promoters and so infection of a cell and insertion of this continuously expressed oncogene into the cellular genome allows rapid progression toward malignancy. Evidence suggests that these acutely transforming viruses are not transmitted naturally, but all events occur in the individual animal. Because the virus has itself lost some of its own genetic material, it is defective for replication. However, it is spread throughout an animal by the provision of help from the normal leukemia virus, which provides the missing proteins in coinfected cells.

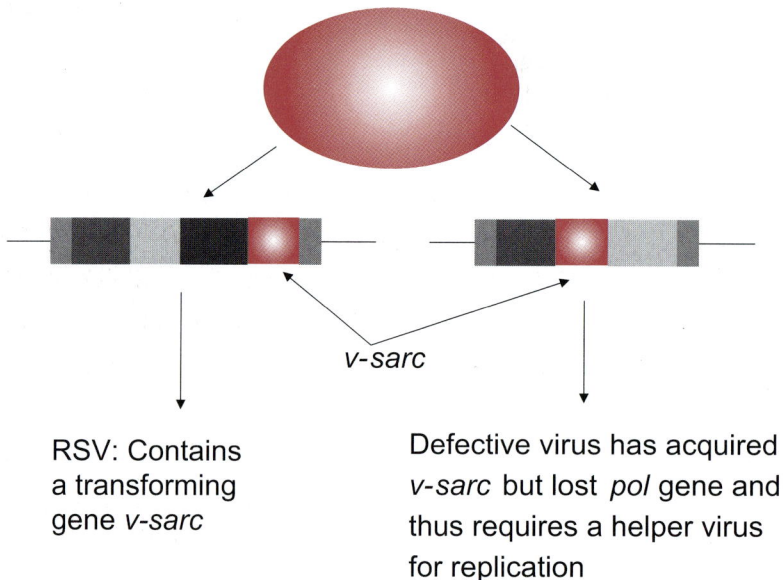

FIG. 2.29— Transduction of cellular oncogenes to create acutely transforming retroviruses. Acutely transforming viruses are generated by a rare recombinational event between the leukemia virus with which the animal was originally infected and a cellular proto-oncogene. In this, part of the viral genome is deleted and replaced with the cellular oncogene. The virus then becomes acutely transforming because this oncogene is now under the transcriptional control of the very efficient viral promoters, and so infection of a cell and insertion of this continuously expressed oncogene into the cellular genome enables rapid progression toward malignancy. RSV, Rous sarcoma virus.

RETROVIRUSES CAN ACTIVATE ONCOGENES BY INSERTIONAL MUTAGENESIS. In addition to the previously described mechanism of the virus being able to capture or transduce cellular oncogenes, retroviruses can activate cellular oncogenes by integrating adjacent to them. A good example of this is the *myc* gene, which is frequently activated in feline T-cell lymphomas. In one mode, the virus integrates adjacent to the oncogene and transcription initiation in the viral LTR (long terminal repeat) proceeds into the adjacent oncogene, producing a hybrid messenger RNA (mRNA). In a second form, the enhancer of the virus overrides the regulation of the *c-onc* transcription from its normal promoter (Figure 2.30).

AVIAN LEUKOSIS VIRUS. The retroviruses of chickens were the first tumor viruses to be discovered and have played a crucial role in understanding tumor virology and oncogenesis. Avian leukosis virus (ALV) causes a variety of hemopoietic tumors in domestic poultry, the most common of which is lymphoid leukosis characterized by the malignant infiltration of malignant B cells into the liver, spleen, and bursa of Fabricius.

Although all birds in commercial poultry flocks are exposed to the virus, and many birds become persistently infected, relatively few develop clinical disease. The major route of transmission is via eggs of carrier hens, virus being shed into the albumin by cells of the oviduct. Chickens hatched from these eggs are persistently infected.

The formation of tumors by ALV is through immunosuppression by the virus combined with insertion of proviral DNA into the host cell genome. In over 80% of B-cell tumors induced by experimental inoculation of ALV, the provirus integrates within or close to the c-*myc* locus. As discussed previously, *myc* is an oncogene intimately associated with cell-cycle pro-

gression and proliferation. Where there is integration close to the Myc locus, the gene becomes controlled by the powerful viral promoters, leading to upregulated *myc* expression and prevention of cells entering G_0 of the cell cycle (Figure 2.30).

FELINE LEUKEMIA VIRUS. Hemopoietic tumors are the most commonly diagnosed neoplasms in cats, accounting for around 30% to 40% of all tumors, and this is directly related to feline leukemia virus (FeLV). FeLV isolates are classified into three distinct subgroups (A, B, and C) on the basis of viral interference with superinfection. These subgroups most likely define envelope subtypes that use different cellular receptor molecules for viral entry. FeLV A is ecotropic (can only infect feline cells) and represents the dominant form of FeLV. FeLV B is polytropic (can also infect human cells) and is overrepresented in cases of virally induced lymphoma in cats. FeLV B isolates are thought to arise de novo from recombination events between FeLV A and feline endogenous sequences present in the feline genome. FeLV C is also thought to arise de novo by mutation of the *env* gene in FeLV A and is not transmitted in nature. It is uniquely associated with the development of pure red cell aplasia (PRCA) in cats.

Persistently viremic cats are the main source of infection. The virus is secreted continuously in the saliva and spread by intimate social contact. The virus can also be spread congenitally from an infected queen to her kittens. In the first few weeks after viral exposure, interactions between the virus and the host's immune system determine the outcome of infection. The potential outcomes of infection include persistent viral infection, latent infection, and the establishment of complete immunity and viral clearance. It is the persistently viremic cats that go on to develop FeLV-associated diseases (Figure 2.31).

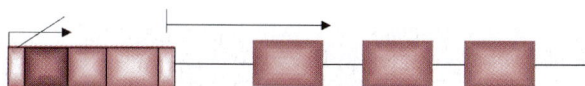

1) Integration of virus adjacent to *myc* locus in ALV. *Myc* comes under the control of viral promoters

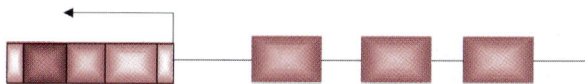

2) Enhancer of the virus overrides the regulation of the cellular oncogene: e.g. enhancer insertion at *C-myc* in FeLV.

FIG. 2.30—Mechanisms of insertional mutagenesis by retroviruses. ALV, avian leukosis virus; and FeLV, feline leukemia virus.

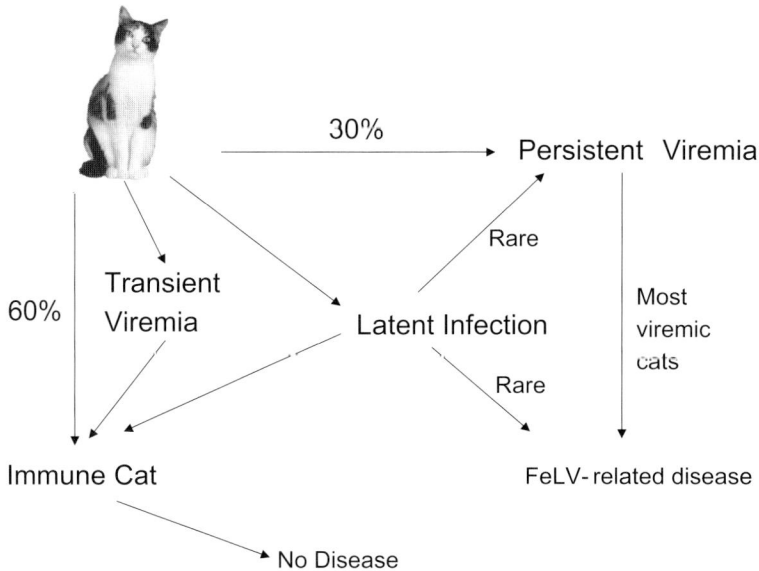

FIG. 2.31—The potential outcomes of feline leukemia virus (FeLV) infection in cats.

Malignant diseases associated with FeLV include lymphomas and leukemias. Lymphoma is the most common tumor of cats and can present most commonly in thymic, multicentric, and alimentary forms. Essentially, the mechanisms of tumorigenesis are very similar for ALV, in that there is both immunosuppression of the host and insertional effects of proviral DNA on cellular oncogenes such as *myc*. However, it is important to note that FeLV is not isolated from all cats with lymphoma. Only 80% of cats with thymic lymphoma are viremic, whereas only 60% and 30% are viremic in the multicentric and alimentary forms, respectively. There is some evidence to suggest, however, that these viruses may be involved as an initiating event before being cleared by the animal's immune system.

FeLV is also associated with nonmalignant diseases such as bone marrow failure, immunosuppression, and reproductive failure. The pathogenesis of these conditions is poorly understood.

FELINE IMMUNODEFICIENCY VIRUS AND TUMORIGENESIS. In contrast to the oncogenic retroviruses, feline immunodeficiency virus (FIV) is a lentivirus. Lentiviruses are retroviruses that classically cause diseases with a slow incubation period and include FIV, human immunodeficiency virus (HIV), maedi-visna, and equine infectious anemia. FIV has also been associated with neoplastic disease in cats, especially lymphomas. These can largely be explained by the immunosuppression caused by the virus; however, a direct effect associated with viral insertional mutagenesis has been postulated.

BOVINE LEUKEMIA VIRUS. Leukemia and/or lymphoma complex occurs in both a sporadic form and an enzootic form. The enzootic form is associated with bovine leukemia virus (BLV), which shares many similarities to human T-cell leukemia/lymphoma virus I (HTLV-I) infection.

Enzootic bovine leukosis occurs as clusters in multiple-case herds as compared with the sporadic form, which occurs in low-incidence herds. Differences in the clinicopathological form of the disease and age distribution between these epidemiological types are recognized. The three main clinicopathological types of lymphoma in cattle are multicentric, thymic, and cutaneous. In the sporadic form, thymic and multicentric forms occur at roughly the same frequency, but the skin form is rare. In the enzootic form, all cases are of the multicentric variety. Further, the sporadic form is a disease of young cattle, but the enzootic form usually occurs in cattle over 4 years of age.

In contrast FeLV and ALV, BLV has a remarkable cell association and is found only in the latent form in B cells. Although all three viruses are considered type C retroviruses (based on electron microscopy), BLV cases have no free virus in the blood. Further, all EBL tumors are clonal, since the proviral DNA is found in the same site in all of the tumor cells from an individual animal. However, there is no preferred integration site in chromosomal DNA, since BLV proviruses are found in different sites in tumors from different cattle.

In further contrast to the feline virus, BLV also contains an additional *tax* gene to *gag*, *pol*, and *env*. This gene regulates the transcription of the provirus, which is often transcriptionally silent. When it is activated, the first mRNA produced encodes the *tax* gene. The product of this gene activates other cellular proteins that bind the LTR and upregulate transcription. Consequently, the expression of the TAX protein acts as a positive-feedback loop in the replication cycle (Figure 2.32). The TAX protein can also transactivate

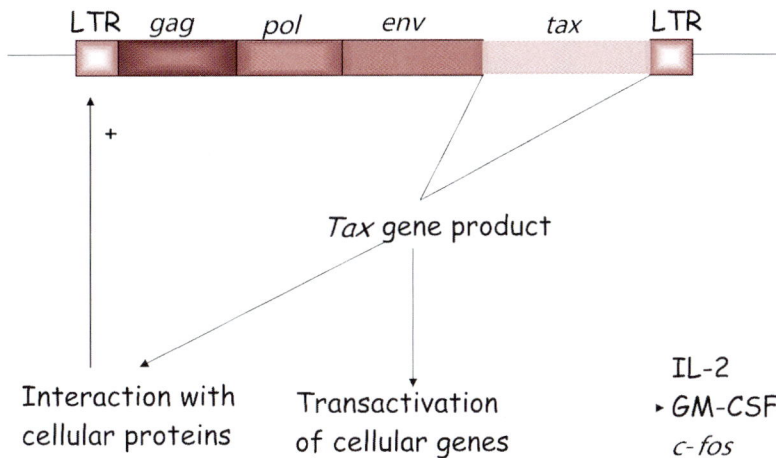

FIG. 2.32—The role of the gene *tax* in bovine leukemia virus (BLV) infection. This gene regulates the transcription of the provirus, which is often transcriptionally silent. When it is activated, the first mRNA produced encodes the *tax* gene. The product of this gene activates other cellular proteins that bind the long terminal repeat (LTR) and upregulate transcription. Consequently, the expression of the tax protein acts as a positive-feedback loop in the replication cycle. The tax protein can also transactivate certain cellular genes that may be involved in tumor production. GM-CSF, granulocyte-macrophage colony-stimulating factor; and IL-2, interleukin 2.

certain cellular genes that may be involved in tumor production.

SHEEP PULMONARY ADENOMATOSIS. This is a relatively common tumor of sheep caused by a type D ovine retrovirus. Up to 20% of Scottish sheep are infected by the virus, and the tumor it causes is considered the most common neoplasm of sheep. The condition is often referred to by its South African name: *Jaagsiekte*.

DNA Viruses. Many of the DNA viruses have been associated with the development of cancer in animals and people. In particular, the papillomaviruses (which are small DNA viruses) have long been known to cause tumors in many animals. In general, papillomaviruses give rise to warts, but these lesions can become malignant, depending on a number of several other predisposing factors. In contrast, herpesviruses are large DNA viruses and are known to cause Marek's disease in chickens. From the aspect of comparative medicine, the herpesviruses are extensively studied in humans through their involvement in Epstein-Barr virus (EBV)-associated lymphomas and Kaposi's sarcoma.

PAPILLOMAVIRUSES ARE IMPORTANT ANIMAL PATHOGENS. Papillomaviruses are important pathogens of animals and can give rise to warts in many species, including cattle, horses, and dogs. They are oncogenic viruses and infect cutaneous and mucous epithelia to induce the production of wart lesions. Most often, these wart lesions are overcome by the immune system and disappear from the animal over a 6-month period. In horses, warts often appear when the animals are stressed, such as at the start of the horse-racing season in early spring. In dogs, warts appear most commonly in young dogs and disappear after around 6 months. The life cycle of the virus is tightly coupled with the differentiation process of the epithelial cell. In certain circumstances, the benign wart will persist and transform into a squamous cell carcinoma.

The most extensively studied of the papillomaviruses are the bovine papillomaviruses (BPVs), which have also been used as model systems to study the role of cocarcinogens in the development of cancer. BPVs fall into two groups: subgroup A, comprising the fibropapillomaviruses BPV-1, 2, and 5; and subgroup B, comprising the epitheliotropic papillomaviruses BPV-3, 4, and 6. BPV-2 is the virus of common cutaneous warts in cattle. The high-risk viruses have early gene products known as E6 and E7, which can immortalize cells and thus contribute to the development of malignancy. However, as we have discussed, the progression to produce a malignant cell requires a number of genetic insults in addition to the effects of E6 and E7 proteins. These proteins can bind to both P53 and Rb proteins, thereby conferring a further growth advantage of the infected cell (Figure 2.33).

In healthy cattle, papillomas normally regress, but in cattle exposed to cocarcinogens, there is a positive correlation between warts and the development of cancer. BPV-2 has been associated with bladder cancer in cattle, and BPV-4 is associated with a syndrome of upper alimentary tract cancer in bracken-fed cattle.

BRACKEN FERN: A COCARCINOGEN (BOVINE). Bracken fern is a cocarcinogen where cattle are infected with papillomavirus.

VIRUS ──────→ E6 ──────────────→ Inactivation of p53

VIRUS ──────→ E7 ──────────────→ Inactivation of Rb

Bracken / UV ──────────────→ Co-carcinogens

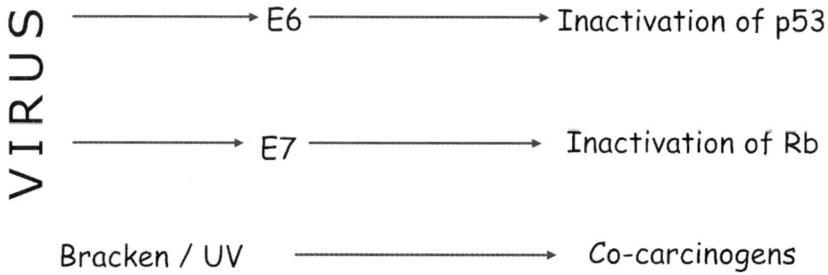

FIG. 2.33—The role of bovine papilloma viruses (BPVs) in the development of cancer. BPVs fall into two groups. Subgroup A comprises the fibropapillomaviruses BPV-1, 2, and 5, Subgroup B comprises the epitheliotropic papillomaviruses BPV-3, 4, and 6. BPV-2 is the virus of common cutaneous warts in cattle. The high-risk viruses have early gene products known as E6 and E7, which can immortalize cells and thus contribute to the development of malignancy. These proteins can bind to both p53 and retinoblastoma (Rb) proteins, thereby conferring a further growth advantage of the infected cell. UV, ultraviolet.

Field cases of alimentary tract cancer were found to occur at high frequency in areas such as the Nasampolai Valley of Kenya and the Western Highlands of Scotland where the cattle were grazing on bracken (*Pteridium aquilinum*)-infected land. Bracken-fed cattle become chronically immunosuppressed and develop chronic enzootic hematuria and bladder tumors, as well as a high incidence of alimentary tract cancers. Papillomas develop and concurrently transform into cancer in this site through the immunosuppressive and carcinogenic effects of the sesquiterpene pterosins and pterosides present in bracken. Additional agents, such as ptaquiloside and α-ecdysone, are also found in bracken and are associated with producing changes, such as chromosomal aberrations, in cells. More recently, it has been demonstrated experimentally that the components of bracken fern may activate viral oncogenes such as E7 to drive the cells toward malignancy. Further, activation of the *ras* proto-oncogene and inactivation of the *p53* tumor-suppressor gene may also play a role in the pathogenesis of this disease.

The papilloma-carcinoma syndrome of cattle was one of the first examples of papillomavirus-induced cancer and has benefited both human and veterinary studies. Further, the role of papillomaviruses in these lesions has led to extensive research in developing papillomavirus vaccines, the benefits of which will be felt by both people and animals alike.

SARCOIDS IN HORSES ARE ASSOCIATED WITH PAPILLOMAVIRUSES. The equine sarcoid is a fibropapillomatous disease of horses, donkeys, and mules that presents in four different clinical forms: verrucose, fibroblastic, mixed, and occult. The disease is the most common equine neoplasm and affects equids worldwide. It is not metastatic, but lesions rarely regress, and currently there is no ubiquitously effective therapy. The great majority of reports in the peer-reviewed literature support the hypothesis that the pathogenesis of this tumor is associated with papillomaviral infection. Papillomaviruses are ubiquitous viruses infecting people and animals. They are strictly species specific with

the exception of BPV types 1 and 2, which can infect horses. Although an equine papillomavirus (EqPV) has been identified, equine sarcoids are associated with BPV in the only documented case of natural cross-species infection. Despite infection by the same agent, there are numerous differences between infection in cattle and in horses. Infection by BPV-½ in cattle results in formation of cutaneous fibropapillomas: benign tumors with a fibroblastic component and an epithelial component, productive for infectious progeny virus, and spontaneously regressing. Infection by BPV-½ in horses results in sarcoids, which have a number of clinical manifestations, all of which appear to be nonproductive for virus, locally aggressive and nonregressing. In both types of lesions, the viral genome is maintained as an episome. There are variations, however, in nucleotide sequence between BPV in cattle and BPV in horses, although it is unknown whether these variations play a part in the different pathogenesis in the two species and in the four different clinical types of equine sarcoid. It is also unknown why fibropapillomas regress following a cell-mediated immune response by the host, whereas naturally occurring sarcoids do not, while experimentally induced sarcoids do regress. Even though BPV-½ has been shown by a number of workers to be associated with the lesions, the viral genomes isolated from different clinical manifestations of the disease have not been exhaustively analyzed. Similarly, localization of the BPV genome within tumors has been reported by one group, but this was performed on a limited number of tumors and did not differentiate the viral types at the genomic level. In consideration of the population aspects of the disease, epidemics have been described, but it is not clear whether an epidemic curve in large populations could be explained by direct animal-to-animal transmission or by vector-borne transmission, or indeed whether the viral types isolated from affected animals are related at all; consideration of attack rate and transmission of the virus has hitherto been clouded by lack of definition of viral type and the true proportion of susceptible animals.

Few studies have addressed the molecular mechanisms at play in such tumors, but it is quite possible that a combination of immunosuppression and the association between viral oncoproteins and the loss of the normal tumor-suppressive properties within cells play a part.

HERPESVIRUS CAUSES MAREK'S DISEASE IN CHICKENS. Marek's disease is a commercially important lymphoproliferative disease of domestic chickens that is caused by an oncogenic herpesvirus. Two main forms of the disease are recognized: the classical and the acute forms. In classical Marek's disease, paralysis is the predominant clinical feature through the infiltration of peripheral nerves with neoplastic lymphoid cells. In the more common acute form of the disease, lymphoid infiltration of the visceral organs predominates, leading to death through multiorgan failure. The pathogenesis of Marek's disease is complex. Natural infection involves the inhalation of infected dander, followed by infection of the lymphoid tissue (predominantly the B cells). The infection of these cells is nonproductive in that viral antigen is expressed on the surface of cells, but no free virus is released. The majority of virus is carried in a lymphocyte-associated viremia to the feather-follicle epithelium, which is the only cell type that supports productive replication. Cell-free virus is released from the dying keratinized cells in the feather follicle, thus maintaining the cycle of virus transmission.

CHEMICAL CARCINOGENS. In 1775, Sir Percival Potts perceived the relationship between the high incidence of scrotal cancer in chimney sweeps and their chronic exposure to soot. He also noted that skin cancer in the general population was a disease of middle to late age, whereas the chimney-sweep boys, who often started at the age of 4 years, developed cancer in their teens. These observations demonstrated the link between chemicals such as hydrocarbons and the development of cancer. Since that time, the role of chemical carcinogens has been extensively studied in human medicine and, to a lesser extent, in veterinary medicine. The role of tobacco smoke and asbestos are well documented from epidemiological studies in human cancer patients, but their role in veterinary cancer medicine is still unclear. However, there are clear examples of chemical-induced carcinogenesis playing a role in veterinary cancers. In the foregoing section, we described the role of papillomaviruses in cattle tumors and that chemical carcinogens supplied by bracken fern provide a cofactor for malignant transformation. Further, epidemiological studies have linked the use of herbicides with the development of canine lymphoma. However, the data presented for the latter have been questioned, and the role of herbicides and pesticides in domestic animal cancers still remains unclear. Food substances can also be carcinogenic, and notable is aflatoxin, an alkaloid produced by *Aspergillus* species that grows on badly stored peanuts. A classical veterinary case was an epizootic of liver cancer in trout reaching up to 60% incidence in Denmark and Kenya, which had been fed on a batch of moldy peanuts in hatcheries in Denmark.

Of major importance is the use of chemicals that induce chronic inflammation. The use of cyclophosphamide for treatment of cancer patients can lead to chronic inflammation of the bladder due to the filtration of a product of drug breakdown called acrolein. Although not common, there are case reports of transitional carcinoma in dogs developing after treatment with cyclophosphamide.

CHRONIC INFLAMMATION, BACTERIA, AND CANCER. Over the past 100 years, a focus on the role of viruses in cancer has led to huge strides in our understanding of carcinogenesis. However, a number of neglected areas of study are currently becoming more fashionable. These include the role of chronic inflammation and/or the role of bacterial agents in the promotion of the malignant phenotype.

There is still very little known about the role of inflammation, chronic irritation, or traumas in the development of cancer, and many reports have largely been anecdotal. However, there are a number of important observations that have been made that warrant further investigation:

• There is epidemiological evidence to suggest that primary bone neoplasia may occur at the site of a previous fracture or repair. In most documented cases, however, there has been a complication of surgery, such as low-grade osteomyelitis, that may have contributed to the development of cancer. In addition, the presence of microfractures through increased mechanical stress in the growing long bones of the giant breeds may contribute to the higher incidence of bone cancer in these dogs. Although very few molecular studies have been performed, one may suggest that this may be through increased cell-cycle activity in these sites and therefore an increased likelihood of a mutational event occurring.

• Case reports have described the development of squamous cell carcinomas at the sites of both burns and scar tissue in horses. The development of tumors at the site of previous burns in people is well recognized.

• It has been suggested that epitheliotropic lymphoma in dogs may develop through persistent antigenic stimulation in the skin. Although C-type retroviral particles have been isolated from canine lymphoma cells in culture, there has been no definitive isolation of a canine retrovirus, and its presence is still speculative. However, persistent stimulation of lymphoid cells in the skin may allow the selection of malignant cells and the establishment of the tumor. A similar situation occurs in human gastric lymphoma associated with *Helicobacter pylori* infection.

• We are still uncertain of the trigger in injection-site-associated sarcomas in cats. As described, numerous theories have been suggested, including the roles of the adjuvant and of the vaccine itself. However, there is good epidemiological evidence that these lesions are solely due to vaccine administration. In essence, this may not be a reflection of what is injected or applied but may just reflect local irritation that is adding another step toward malignancy. A more extreme manifestation of this is trauma-associated neoplasia. This is far more anecdotal in veterinary practice but is well recognized in people. D.J.A. has treated at least two dogs that developed highly aggressive sarcomas at the site of extensive trauma, one of which followed a dogfight. One can only speculate at the pathogenesis, but it may be associated with excessive cell division, inflammatory responses, and inflammatory mediators in the site, contributing to progression to malignancy. Further, there are reports in the literature of the development of intraocular neoplasia associated with eye trauma. It has been suggested that this may involve the release of lens epithelia into the aqueous environment.

• Although not well studied in animals, *Helicobacter pylori* has emerged as a highly important human pathogen, especially in its association with gastric ulcer disease and gastric carcinoma. The role of this bacteria in this disease is now undisputed, and it is regarded as a causal agent of human cancer. Further, it is also associated with the development of human gastric lymphoma through chronic inflammation.

PARASITIC INFECTIONS. Very little is documented with regard to the role of parasites in carcinogenesis. The most-quoted example is that of the helminth infection *Spirocerca lupi*. This parasite, which is endemic to Africa and the Southeastern United States, causes esophageal tumors (fibrosarcomas or osteosarcomas in dogs and foxes). Worm eggs develop into larvae in an intermediate host. In dogs, ingested larvae migrate to the esophagus via the aorta and form highly vascular fibroblastic nodules that can undergo malignant transformation to form either fibrosarcomas or osteosarcomas.

PHYSICAL AGENTS. Radiation is a well-known carcinogen in animals and people. Either the mutagenic effects of radiation cause errors in DNA replication, or the indirect effect of radiation causes the production of oxygen free radicals. For this reason, exposure to either diagnostic or therapeutic radiation should be kept to an absolute minimum.

In terms of UV radiation, the association between sunlight and the development of malignancies has been recognized for over 100 years and has been one of the most extensively studied physical causes of cancer. In people, the association between the frequency and severity of sunburns during childhood and the eventual development of malignant melanoma has been proven in epidemiological studies.

In domestic animals, the best-documented examples of this kind are in the development of squamous cell carcinomas in white cats, in whiteface cattle, and possibly in gray horses. In white cats, the ear tips and the nasal planum are susceptible to chronic inflammatory dermatitis that may be initiated by excessive exposure to direct sunlight containing UV radiation (especially UVB). A photon of UVB can be directly transforming by its subcellular effects on DNA. However, it has also been suggested that a contributing mechanism may be immunosuppression as a consequence of UV exposure. In this, UVB photons can convert transurocyanic acid in the skin to cisurocyanic acid that can have profound effects on antigen-presenting cell function and T-cell activity.

THE ROLE OF HORMONES IN CANCER. The relationship between hormones and cancer has been studied extensively in human medicine. In particular, cancer of the breast, endometrium, ovary, and prostate occur in hormone-responsive tissues, and these tumors may require hormones for their continued growth. Hormones can influence cancer development by enhancing cellular replication in cells that may have already acquired a number of genetic hits toward malignancy. Estrogen is known to influence the development of benign vaginal fibromas in bitches that regress after an ovariohysterectomy. In addition, it is well documented that early ovariohysterectomy in bitches is protective against mammary carcinoma. The hormonal influences on breast cancer are far better defined for women than dogs. The complete role of estrogens and progesterones, and the significance of receptor expression on canine mammary tumors, are still under investigation. Other examples of hormonal influences on neoplasia are presented in Table 2.5.

GENETIC PREDISPOSITION TO CANCER. In people, a number of inherited syndromes give rise to familial cancer syndromes. The best characterized are Li-Fraumeni syndrome (inheritance of an abnormal copy of the *p53* allele) and retinoblastoma (inheritance of an abnormal copy of the *Rb* allele). In both of these, the defect is in a tumor-suppressor gene and therefore requires that both alleles are lost for abnormal function. However, affected individuals are more likely to develop cancers at a younger age. Other inherited cancers include Wilms' tumor (*WT-1*), familial adenomatous polyposis (FAP), and breast cancer (*BRCA-1* and *BRCA-1&2*).

TABLE 2.5—Hormone associations and neoplasia

Hormone	Associated neoplasm
Estrogen	Mammary tumors
	Vaginal fibroma (dogs)
Progestrogen	Fibromatous hyperplasia in cats
	?Mammary tumors in dogs
Testosterone	Perianal adenoma in dogs
	?Prostatic tumors

No specific hereditary genes have been identified in domestic animals. However, it is well recognized that certain dog breeds have a predisposition to certain cancers (Table 2.6). In addition, a germline mutation in *p53* has been identified in a bullmastiff with lymphoma. This breed has a particular predisposition to lymphoid neoplasia.

TABLE 2.6—Dog breed predispositions to cancer

Breed	Tumor
Bullmastiff	Lymphoma
Boxer	Mast cell tumor
	Brain tumor
Flat-coated retriever	Soft-tissue sarcoma
German shepherd	Hemangiosarcoma
Bernese mountain dog	Histiocytosis
Belgian shepherd	Gastric carcinoma
Irish wolfhound/Great Dane	Osteosarcoma
Labrador retriever	Fibrosarcoma

KEY REFERENCES AND FURTHER READING

Adams GE, Cox R. 1997. Radiation carcinogenesis. In: Franks LM, Teich NM, eds. The Molecular and Cellular Biology of Cancer, 3rd ed. New York: Oxford University Press, pp 130–150.

Balmain A, Brown K. 1988. Oncogene activation in chemical carcinogenesis. Adv Cancer Res 51:147–182.

Campo MS, Jarrett WF, Barron R, et al. 1992. Association of bovine papillomavirus type 2 and bracken fern with bladder cancer in cattle. Cancer Res 52:6898–6904.

Campo MS, O'Neil BW, Barron RJ, Jarrett WF. 1994. Experimental reproduction of the papilloma-carcinoma complex of the alimentary canal in cattle. Carcinogenesis 15:1597–1601.

Doddy FD, Glickman LT, Glickman NW, Janovitz FB. 1996. Feline fibrosarcomas at vaccination sites and non-vaccination sites. J Comp Pathol 114:165–174.

Donner P, Greiser-Wilkie I, Moelling K. 1982. Nuclear localization and DNA binding of the transforming gene product of avian myelocyomatosis virus. Nature 296:262–266.

Ferrer JF. 1980. Bovine lymphosarcoma. Adv Vet Sci Comp Med 24:1–67.

Gaukroger JM, Bradley A, Chandrachud L, et al. 1993. Interaction between bovine papillomavirus type 4 and cocarcinogens in the production of malignant tumours. J Gen Virol 74(Pt 10):2275–2280.

Jarrett WF. 1985. Bovine papillomaviruses. Clin Dermatol 3:8–19.

Jarrett O. 1991. Overview of feline leukemia virus research. J Am Vet Med Assoc 199:1279–1281.

Jarrett O. 1999. Strategies of retrovirus survival in the cat. Vet Microbiol 69:99–107.

Jarrett O, Onions D. 1992. Leukaemogenic viruses. In: Whittaker JA, ed. Leukaemia, 2nd ed. Oxford: Blackwell Scientific, pp 34–63.

Lancaster WD, Olson C, Meinke W. 1977. Bovine papillomavirus: Presence of virus-specific DNA sequences in naturally occurring equine tumors. Proc Natl Acad Sci USA 74:524–528.

McEntee MC, Page RL. 2001. Feline vaccine-associated sarcomas. J Vet Intern Med 15:176–182.

McNiel EA. 2001. Vaccine-associated sarcomas in cats: A unique cancer model. Clin Orthop 382:21–27.

Neil JC, Hughs D, McFarlane R, et al. 1984. Transduction and rearrangement of the *myc* gene by feline leukaemia virus in naturally occurring T cell leukaemias. Nature 308:814–820.

O'Byrne KJ, Dalgleish AG. 2001. Chronic immune activation and inflammation as the cause of malignancy. Br J Cancer 85:473–483.

Onions DE. 1984. A prospective study of familial canine lymphosarcoma. J Natl Cancer Inst 72:909–912.

Onions DE, Jarrett O. 1987. Naturally occurring tumours in animals as a model for human disease. Cancer Surv 6:1–181.

Onions DE, Lees G, Forrest D, et al. 1987. Recombinant feline viruses containing the *myc* gene rapidly produce clonal tumours expressing T-cell antigen receptor gene transcripts. Int J Cancer 40:40–45.

Powell PC. 1984. Marek's disease and its causative virus. In: Goldman JM, Jarrett O, eds. Mechanisms of Viral Leukaemogenesis. Edinburgh: Churchill Livingstone, pp 155–183.

Reid SW, Smith KT, Jarrett WF. 1994. Detection, cloning and characterisation of papillomaviral DNA present in sarcoid tumours of *Equus asinus*. Vet Rec 135:430–432.

Schat KA. 1987. Marek's disease: A model for protection against herpesvirus-induced tumours. Cancer Surv 6:1–38.

Tennent R, Wigley C, Balmain A. 1997. Chemical carcinogenesis. In: Franks LM, Teich NM, eds. The Molecular and Cellular Biology of Cancer, 3rd ed. New York: Oxford University Press, pp 106–129.

Veldhoen N, Stewart J, Brown R, Milner J. 1998. Mutations of the *p53* gene in canine lymphoma and evidence for germ line *p53* mutations in the dog. Oncogene 16:249–255.

Vousden KH. 1994. Cell transformation by human papillomaviruses. In: Minsen B, ed. Viruses and Cancer. Cambridge: Cambridge University Press, pp 27–46.

Weiss RA, Teich N, Varmus H, Coffin J. 1984. The Molecular Biology of Tumour Viruses: RNA Tumour Viruses, 2nd ed. Cold Spring Harbor, NY: Cold Spring Harbor Laboratory.

Wyke J. 1997. Viruses and cancer. In: Franks LM, Teich NM, eds. The Molecular and Cellular Biology of Cancer, 3rd ed. New York: Oxford University Press, pp 151–168.

PART 4: MOLECULAR PATHOLOGY OF CANCER

TUMOR NOMENCLATURE AND THE PHENOTYPIC DIAGNOSIS OF CANCER. Classically, the histological and thus phenotypic naming of tumors is performed to benefit clinicians in designing the most appropriate treatment strategy based on a knowledge of the natural history of that particular tumor type. Tumors are described to specify their tissue of origin, which may either be mesenchymal, epithelial, or hematogenous.

The diagnosis of a tumor has classically relied on traditional anatomic pathology and light microscopy using one or two staining techniques. The diagnosis of a tumor is based on the cellular morphology and the staining characteristics of the cells. In some circumstances, the decision on whether a tumor is benign or malignant can often depend on the behavior of the cells at the interface between normal and abnormal tissue. A classical example of this is the differentiation of benign and malignant lesions of the colon in dogs. The decision to call a tumor malignant is based on demonstrating the invasive nature of the malignant form into the underlying tissues.

As well as classifying tumors, a histopathologist can somewhat predict the behavior of a tumor based on the organization and appearance of the neoplastic cells. This grading of tumors is often of great value to the clinician in introducing the most appropriate therapy. Grading systems are well worked out in human medicine but are still crude in veterinary medicine, producing a fairly course subdivision of tumors often based on the number of mitoses observed expressed as the mitotic index.

Although the microscopic examination of tissue sections is the basis for cancer diagnosis, in recent years specific staining techniques have been developed that allow for identification of various cell and tissue components. The application of techniques such as immunocytochemistry, in situ hybridization, and flow cytometry has resulted in radical changes in diagnostic criteria and in the identification of many previously unrecognized tumor-specific proteins by, for example, staining techniques to highlight mucin production, interstitial collagen, muscle fibers, glycogen, and melanin pigment.

IMMUNOCYTOCHEMISTRY. Immunocytochemistry is commonly used in the diagnosis and monitoring of malignant disease. Specific antibodies are used to bind cellular or tissue components, and the bound antibody is subjected to a detection system that enables clear visualization of the bound antibody. It enables the identification of both nuclear and cytoplasmic proteins and is used in tumor diagnosis to detect the origin of malignancy and tumor stage. Such information enables clinicians and researchers to pinpoint the treatment that is likely to have the best rate of success. For example, immunohistochemistry is used to detect membrane expression of the c-*erbB-2* oncogene in human breast cancers. Expression of c-*erbB-2* is significantly related to positive lymph nodes, poor nuclear grade, lack of steroid receptors and high proliferative activity. Patients expressing this antigen have a poor prognosis. As discussed in Part 2, P53 is an important tumor-suppressor protein that is abnormally expressed in human cancers and in cancers in domesticated animals. Mutation in the *p53* gene leads to accumulating or mutant protein (usually in the nucleus), which may be detected by using immunohistochemistry. Figure 2.34 shows the immunohistochemical expression of abnormal P53 protein in canine osteosarcoma cells.

IN SITU HYBRIDIZATION. ISH is a technique that enables detection of a target DNA or RNA sequence in a tissue section by use of a labeled nucleic acid probe. This technique offers a direct approach for cellular localization and quantitation of nucleic acid sequences of relatively low copy number. ISH is commonly used by cancer researchers to identify sites of cellular mRNA expression and viral genomes. It was originally

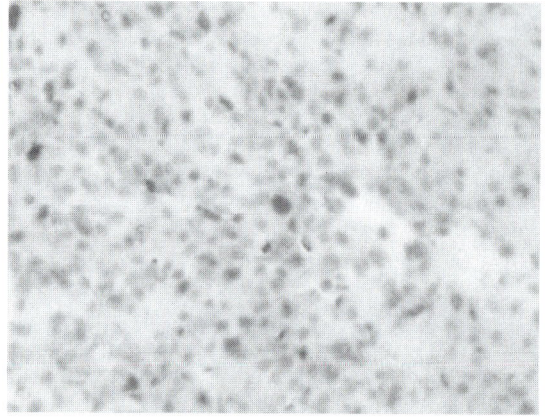

FIG. 2.34—Abnormal p53 protein expression detected by immunohistochemistry in canine osteosarcoma cells (cells stained brown overexpress p53).

developed to visualize nucleic acids in tissue sections, but more recently the technology has been improved such that the nucleic acids can also be detected on chromosomes and interphase nuclei. Complementary probes are commonly linked to fluorescent molecules for visualization of the target and referred to as FISH (fluorescent in situ hybridization).

FLOW CYTOMETRY. Flow cytometry is a technique that utilizes a laser to count or measure large numbers of cells. A suspension of single cells or nuclei is stained with a fluorescent dye that binds to the DNA; the amount of dye bound is proportional to the amount of DNA. The stained cells or nuclei are then introduced into the flow cytometer, and the fluorescent light emitted generates an electronic pulse that is proportional to the total fluorescence emission from the cell. Flow cytometry is commonly used to identify subpopulations of lymphocytes by use of monoclonal antibodies to various cell surface antigens. Different cell populations of the hematopoietic system express different cell surface antigens at various stages of maturation. By detecting and measuring these expressed antigens, flow cytometry can aid in the classification of the cell lineage of leukemias and lymphomas. Flow cytometry can be used to calculate the percentage of a cell population in each phase of the cell cycle. The percentage of cells in the S phase gives an indication of proliferative activity. Similarly, flow cytometry can be used to establish the nuclear DNA content. Normal cells have a diploid DNA content, whereas cancer cells from different species are often associated with an abnormal DNA content, known as aneuploidy (Figure 2.35).

DETECTION OF GENETIC ABNORMALITIES. Over the past two decades, a number of molecular techniques have been developed that have greatly aided the identification of genetic abnormalities in cancer tissues

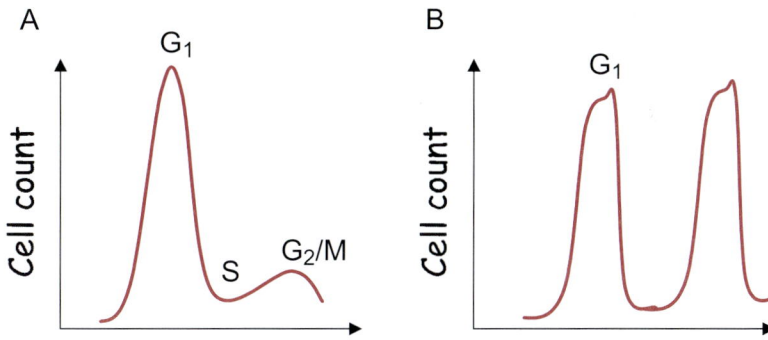

FIG. 2.35—Flow-cytometric data are usually presented as histograms, and variations in the histogram pattern can reveal the presence of cells with abnormal DNA contents. **A:** Most normal cells are in the G_0/G_1 phase of the cell cycle, with a DNA content of 2 N. **B:** Aneuploid cells with an abnormal DNA content are detected by the presence of additional peaks.

not only in human tumors but in domesticated animal cancers. These techniques are rapidly joining the clinical tools used in veterinary and human cancer diagnosis and treatment.

Polymerase Chain Reaction. The development of the polymerase chain reaction (PCR) by Kary Mullis in the 1980s has revolutionized the ways in which DNA molecules can be studied. Using this technique, a given nucleotide sequence can be selectively and rapidly amplified in large amounts from any DNA that contains it.

There are essentially three basic steps in PCR, as shown in Figure 2.36.

First, the double-stranded DNA is heat denatured to separate the two DNA strands. In the second step, short synthetic oligonucleotides complementary to a specific gene sequence of interest are then allowed to anneal to complementary regions within the single-stranded DNA. Specific enzymes that can add nucleotide bases to DNA (known as polymerases) are used to add complementary nucleotides to the DNA from the end of the primer along the rest of the single-stranded DNA templates, thereby making multiple copies of the DNA segment between the two primers. The process is repeated for multiple cycles to yield a large amount of the desired DNA region. Additionally, such techniques may be used to detect very low levels of disease, so-called minimal residual disease (MRD) studies.

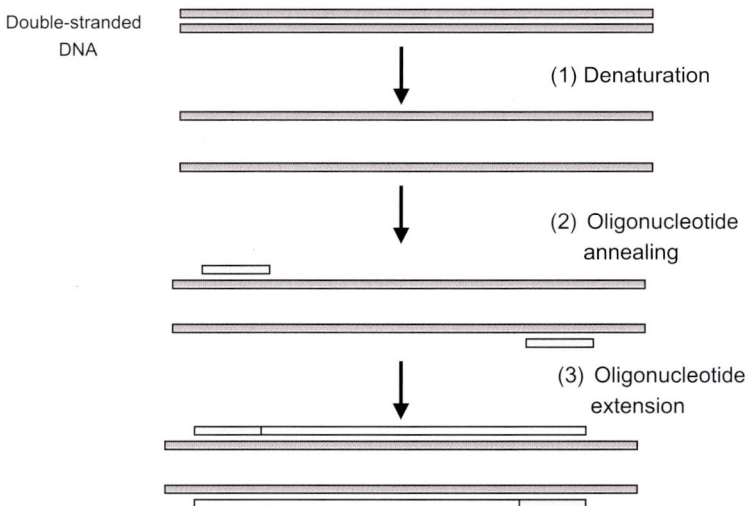

FIG. 2.36—The steps in the polymerase chain reaction. Firstly, the double-stranded DNA is heat denatured to separate the two DNA strands. In the second step, short synthetic oligonucleotides complementary to a specific gene sequence of interest are then allowed to anneal to complementary regions within the single-stranded DNA strands. Specific enzymes that can add nucleotide bases to DNA (known as polymerases) are used to add complementary nucleotides to the DNA from the end of the primer along the rest of the single-stranded DNA templates, thereby making multiple copies of the DNA segment between the two primers. The process is repeated for multiple cycles to yield a large amount of the desired DNA region.

Applications of the Polymerase Chain Reaction.
PCR is commonly used for the diagnosis of many
human genetic disorders, and its potential in veterinary
oncology is currently being investigated. The technology allows for the detection of mutations within specific genes in tumor tissues and can also be used to
screen for polymorphisms. In diseases of viral origin,
samples may be screened by PCR to detect the viral
pathogens, and microorganisms can readily be detected
in specimens by PCR.

Mutational Analysis. Gene mutations are common
events in cancers, and their identification plays an
important role in aiding prognosis and determining the
most appropriate therapeutic strategy. Mutation analyses of specific tumor-suppressor genes have been an
important area of research over the past decade and
have not only demonstrated the role of mutations in
cancer progression but have identified potential targets
for therapy.

SINGLE-STRANDED CONFORMATIONAL POLYMOR-
PHISM ANALYSIS. SSCP, which is one of the most
common techniques used to screen for unknown gene
mutations, is based on the mobility of single-stranded
molecules, as shown in Figure 2.37.

The sequence of interest is amplified by PCR, and
the products of amplification subjected to electrophoresis using conditions that separate the double-stranded
DNA into single-stranded molecules (denaturing gel
electrophoresis). Single-stranded molecules containing
gene mutations show altered mobility under denaturing
conditions and can readily be detected as abnormal
bands following electrophoresis.

DENATURING GRADIENT GEL ELECTROPHORESIS.
This is also based on the mobility of single-stranded
molecules. PCR products or small genomic fragments
are hybridized to a DNA probe. If the template contains
a mutation, then a region of mismatch is formed on
hybridization; such molecules are known as heteroduplexes. Hybridized products are electrophoresed
through an increasingly linear denaturant gradient. As
the DNA migrates into higher denaturing conditions, it
reaches a point where it begins to melt, which is determined by the sequence composition. The partial melting severely retards the progress of the molecule in the
gel, which can be identified as a mobility shift (Figure
2.38).

Further, a number of additional techniques that are
often used include heteroduplex analysis and the chemical cleavage of mismatch (CCM) method. Homodu-
plex molecules form when two complementary DNA
strands from identical alleles are base paired, whereas
heteroduplex molecules contain regions of mismatch
due to sequence variation. The latter show altered
migration patterns compared with the former, and this
can be used as a simple technique to screen for mutations. Alternatively, the mismatched base pairs can be
treated with specific chemicals causing cleavage of
mismatches, which results in products of different
sizes.

The techniques just described provide no information on the nature of the mutation but do provide rapid
screening strategies. The nature of the mutation must
be established by DNA sequencing, which is regarded
as the gold standard for mutation detection. The
methodology for DNA sequencing was first described
in the 1970s by Sanger, Maxim, and Gilbert using man-

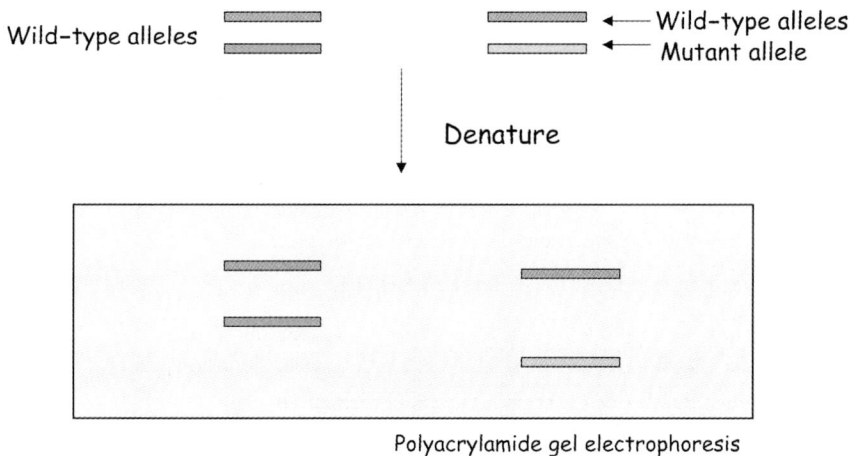

FIG. 2.37—In single-stranded conformational polymorphism analysis, the sequence of interest is amplified by polymerase
chain reaction, and the products of amplification are subjected to electrophoresis using conditions that separate the double-
stranded DNA into single-stranded molecules (denaturing gel electrophoresis). Single-stranded molecules containing gene
mutations show altered mobility under denaturing conditions and can readily be detected as abnormal bands following
electrophoresis.

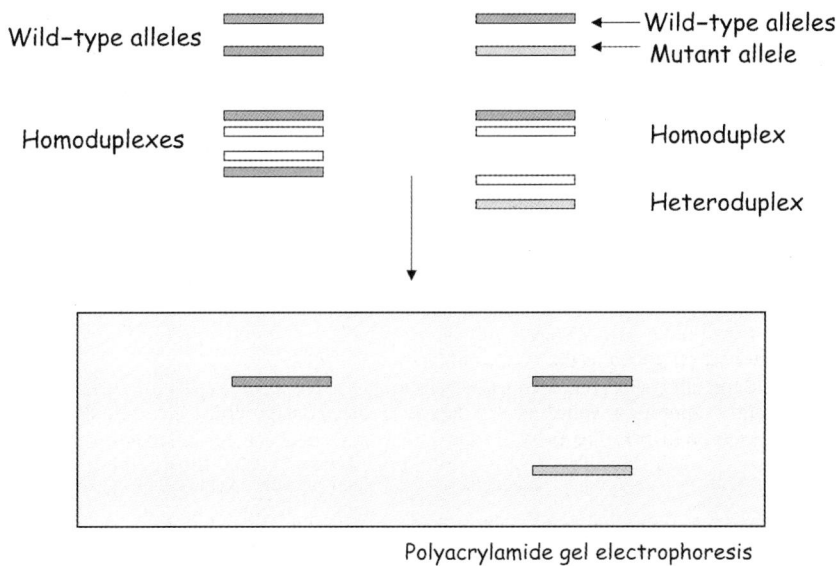

FIG. 2.38—In denaturing gradient gel electrophoresis, polymerase chain reaction products or small genomic fragments are hybridized to a DNA probe. If the template contains a mutation, a region of mismatch is formed on hybridization; such molecules are known as heteroduplexes. Hybridized products are electrophoresed through an increasingly linear denaturant gradient. As the DNA migrates into higher denaturing conditions, DNA reaches a point where it begins to melt, which is determined by the sequence composition. The partial melting severely retards the progress of the molecule in the gel, which can be identified as a mobility shift.

ual chemical cleavage or dideoxy-chain termination. The manual techniques have now been largely superseded by automated DNA sequencers using fluorescent labels, enabling larger DNA fragments to be sequenced more quickly.

Chromosomal Analysis. As discussed previously, gene mutations are a common genetic event associated with cancers not only in humans but also in domesticated species. Changes at the chromosomal level— for example, changes in chromosome number or chromosome structure—also represent a common feature of many tumor cells. Such mutations can be detected by chromosomal analysis by studying the karyotype, which represents the chromosomal makeup of a particular subject. To prepare a karyotype, metaphase cells are required, and peripheral blood lymphocytes are commonly used. However, any growing tissue, including bone marrow, skin fibroblasts, or tumor cells, can also be used. Mononuclear cells are isolated from heparinized blood samples and incubated with a mitogen (phytohemagglutinin) to stimulate the proliferation. Following 24 to 72 hours of incubation, the cells are arrested in the metaphase of cell division by the addition of colchicine (which disrupts mitotic spindle and prevents mitosis). The chromosomes are then swollen by the addition of a hypotonic solution and dropped onto microscope slides and allowed to air-dry. The chromosomes must be stained for visualization and for routine karotyping. Giemsa (G) staining is used. G banding produces characteristic banding patterns for each chromosome pair, and the banding pattern is related to the density of the chromatin within the chromosomes. Stained chromosomes are photographed and the chromosome pairs arranged in order of decreasing size. Examination of the karyotype allows any abnormalities in the number of chromosomes or the structure of chromosomes to be readily identified.

While karyotypic analysis of metaphase chromosomes is commonly used to analyze tumor cell chromosomes for cancer diagnosis and research, in some instances the identification of subtle abnormalities or complex chromosomal rearrangements is very difficult. This has led to the development of a number of new techniques.

CHROMOSOME PAINTING. This is the hybridization of fluorescently labeled chromosome-specific sequences (probes) to chromosome preparations. Chromosome painting allows individual chromosomes to be detected and enables the accurate identification of both numerical and structural chromosomal aberrations. This technique has become an important tool in veterinary cancer diagnosis, since it can be applied to cross-species comparisons. For example, the simultaneous hybridization of multiple chromosome-painting probes, each tagged with a specific fluorochrome combination, has resulted in the differential color display of human and canine chromosomes.

MICROARRAY TECHNOLOGY. Microarray or chip technology, which is a recent development in molecular biology, enables the simultaneous analysis of hundreds of genes. To use chip technology, DNA fragments corresponding to specific genes are loaded onto a glass microscope slide in a high-density grid known as an array. The array is then exposed to fluorescently labeled DNA, or a complementary DNA (cDNA) copy of mRNA from a sample of interest, which hybridizes with the DNA on the array. The levels of hybridization are then analyzed by quantifying fluorescence, and the results are color coded (Figure 2.39). The genes that are the most active (i.e., have the highest level of hybridization) appear as red, whereas the genes that are repressed (hybridize the least) are green. This powerful technology is currently being used in research to learn which genes are turned on or off in cancers.

SUMMARY. Classical pathological and histological techniques for the diagnosis of cancer are now being supported by more sophisticated techniques that enable the identification of specific abnormalities at the gene level. One may speculate that the phenotypic diagnosis of cancer is decreasing in significance as we identify specific molecular abnormalities that are associated with specific prognoses or outcomes of specific therapies. It may be that the future will enable the genotypic diagnosis of cancer based on technologies such as microarray, which will allow a more precise treatment modality to be employed.

KEY REFERENCES AND FURTHER READING

Bertucci F, Houlgatte R, Nguyen C, et al. 2001. Gene expression profiling of cancer by use of DNA arrays: How far from the clinic? Lancet Oncol 2:674–682.

Dunn KA, Thomas R, Binns MM, Breen M. 2000. Comparative genomic hybridization (CGH) in dogs: Application to the study of a canine glial tumour cell line. Vet J 160:77–82.

Khan J, Wei JS, Ringner M, et al. 2001. Classification and diagnostic prediction of cancers using gene expression profiling and artificial neural networks. Nat Med 7:673–679.

Lemoine NR, Stamp G. 1997. The molecular pathology of cancer. In: Franks LM, Teich NM, eds. The Molecular and Cellular Biology of Cancer, 3rd ed. New York: Oxford University Press, pp 264–272.

Naito N, Kawai A, Ouchida M, et al. 2000. A reverse transcriptase-polymerase chain reaction assay in the diagnosis of soft tissue sarcomas. Cancer 89:1992–1998.

Ramaswamy S, Tamayo P, Rifkin R, et al. 2001. Multiclass cancer diagnosis using tumor gene expression signatures. Proc Natl Acad Sci USA 98:15,149–15,154.

Thomas R, Smith KC, Gould R, et al. 2001. Molecular cytogenetic analysis of a novel high-grade canine T-lymphoblastic lymphoma demonstrating co-expression of CD3 and CD79a cell markers. Chromosome Res 9:649–657.

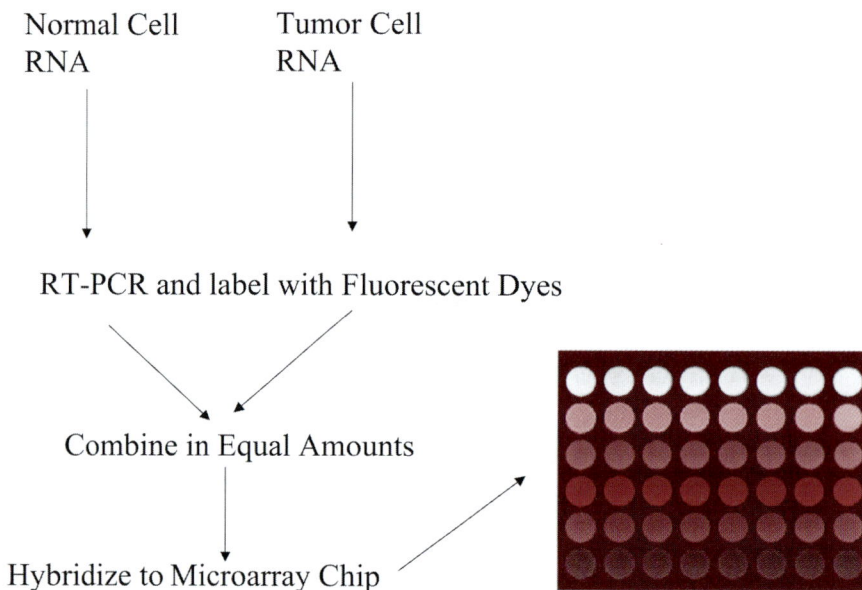

FIG. 2.39—An example of a microarray chip readout. Initially, tumor and normal tissue RNA is isolated. This is reverse transcribed to form cDNA libraries, which are labeled with fluorescent dyes and mixed in equal amounts. The mixture is then hybridized to a chip containing a number of genes from that species. The fluorescence indicates whether a gene is upregulated or downregulated in a sample. ■ represents low hybridization, and red represents increased hybridization. This system enables rapid genetic profiling of tumors. RT-PCR, reverse transcriptase-polymerase chain reaction.

PART 5: TUMOR IMMUNOLOGY

The immune system of the domestic species has evolved to recognize antigens that are considered to be nonself or foreign. For cancer cells to be recognized by the immune system, they must express nonself-antigens or altered self-antigens. The role of the immune system in controlling cancer has followed a continuous sine wave of optimism and pessimism among researchers in the field. As far back as 1908, Paul Erlich proposed that the transformation of normal cells into cancer cells was a common event in the body but did not give rise to cancers by virtue of immunosurveillance and the expression of foreign antigens by the tumor cells. The general concept of tumor cells expressing antigens recognizable as nonself by the immune system and the role of the immune system in cancer have since been supported by experimental evidence:

- Histologically, tumor masses are surrounded and often infiltrated by immune effector cells such as T lymphocytes, natural killer (NK) cells, and macrophages.
- Lymphocyte proliferation is often present in lymph nodes that drain tumor sites.
- Increased expression of major histocompatibility complex (MHC) class II molecules in tumors is an indicator of cytokine effector functions within the tumor microenvironment.
- Tumor antigens have been recognized.
- Cancer occurs at a higher frequency in immunocompromised animals (e.g., cats with FIV infection).

- Patients with lymphocytic infiltrates within tumors often correlate with a better prognosis than those patients whose tumors demonstrate little immune cell infiltration.
- There is abundant experimental evidence that tumors can stimulate specific T-cell responses.

Tumor cells are able to express molecules that act as antigens for recognition by the immune system. However, it is clear that the concept of immunosurveillance (as originally proposed by Erlich) is ineffective, as aggressive cancers can arise in normal as well as in immunocompromised animals. It is fair to assume, then, that the natural immune response to tumors is generally weak, and/or tumors have developed mechanisms by which they can escape immune recognition.

TUMOR ANTIGENS HAVE BEEN DEFINED IN ANIMALS AND PEOPLE. The term tumor-specific antigen (TSA) is used to describe molecules that allow tumors to be recognized by the immune system (Figure 2.40). An overview of the categories of tumor antigens and their association is presented.

It is important to recognize that the antigens expressed by these tumors do not necessarily induce protective immunity and that tumors have evolved complex mechanisms to overcome immune recognition. However, despite tumor immunology having sat on the fringe of mainstream cancer therapy research for many years, it is now clear that tumors can express antigens that are recognized by the immune system, manipulation of the immune system can aid regression

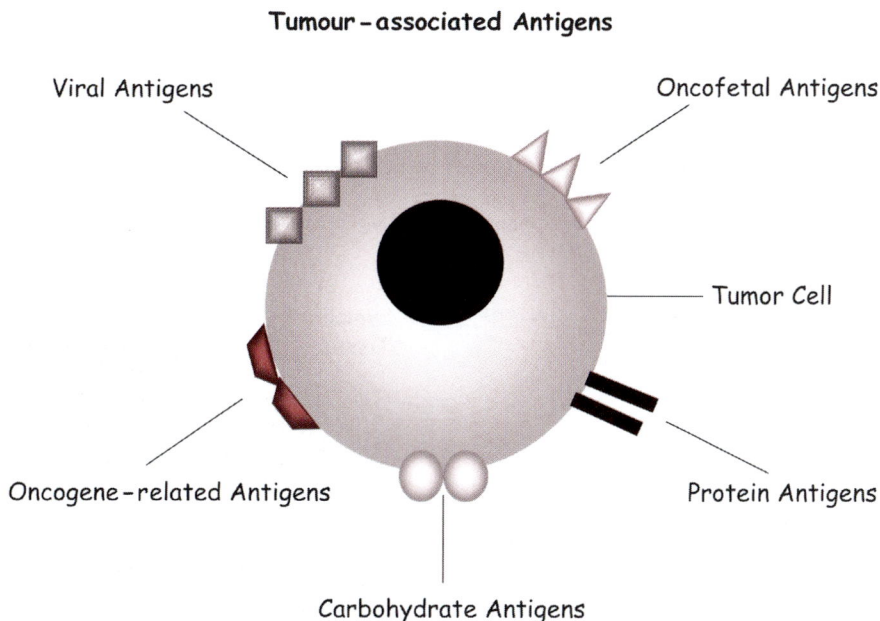

FIG. 2.40—Tumor-associated antigens.

of certain cancers, and antitumor T cells can be generated by cancer patients, but the cancer operates various mechanisms that can limit the effects of immune effector cells.

Viral Antigens. These are products expressed in virally transduced cells and common to all tumors induced by the same virus. A classical example of this is FeLV-induced lymphoid malignancies where virus-infected cells express the viral protein gp70 on their surface. In addition, feline oncornavirus-associated cell membrane antigen (FOCMA) has been defined on lymphomas from cats that are either virus positive or virus negative for FcLV. Interestingly, in cats that develop high levels of anti-FOCMA antibodies after FeLV infection, there appears to be a lower incidence of lymphoid-related malignancies. The fact that some virus-negative tumors also express FOCMA may be associated with endogenous retroviral elements in the feline genome.

Another example of virus-associated tumor antigens are those defined in Marek's disease (Figure 2.41).

Cell lines derived from Marek's disease lymphomas express a membrane antigen that is considered to be specific for transformed cells. This antigen [Marek's disease tumor-associated surface antigen (MATSA)] is distinct from antigens induced in infected cells. In contrast to FOCMA in cats, there is no evidence of a host humoral response to MATSA in chickens.

Oncofetal Antigens. These represent molecules that are expressed by cells during certain stages of embry-onic development but are usually absent on normal adult cells. Homologues of these antigens occur in domestic animals, but they are best characterized in people. The two most studied antigens in human medicine are α-fetoprotein and carcinoembryonic antigens.

α-Fetoprotein, which is an α-globulin that is secreted by embryonic liver cells, constitutes around 90% of the total globulin in the blood of human embryos. This level rapidly declines after birth, but high levels of this protein have been detected in patients suffering from hepatic and pancreatic carcinomas. In addition, high levels at the time of diagnosis correlate with poor prognosis. Although detection of this protein in adults is indicative of neoplastic disease, it should also be noted that increased levels have also been associated with acute viral hepatitis.

Carcinoembryonic antigen (CEA) is a glycoprotein that is associated with the mucous coating of the fetal gut, pancreas, and liver during embryonic development. High levels of this antigen have been found in patients with cancers of the colon and breast.

Oncogene-related Antigens. Numerous oncogene-encoded proteins (or tumor-suppressor gene-encoded proteins) can act as antigens and are associated with certain malignancies. For example, *Rb* and *p53* products can be expressed as tumor antigens. Some tumors of our domestic species such as canine osteosarcoma, feline vaccine-induced sarcomas, and equine sarcoids are associated with accumulation of *p53* products.

Carbohydrate Antigens. These are carbohydrate antigens that arise through alterations in the normal glyco-

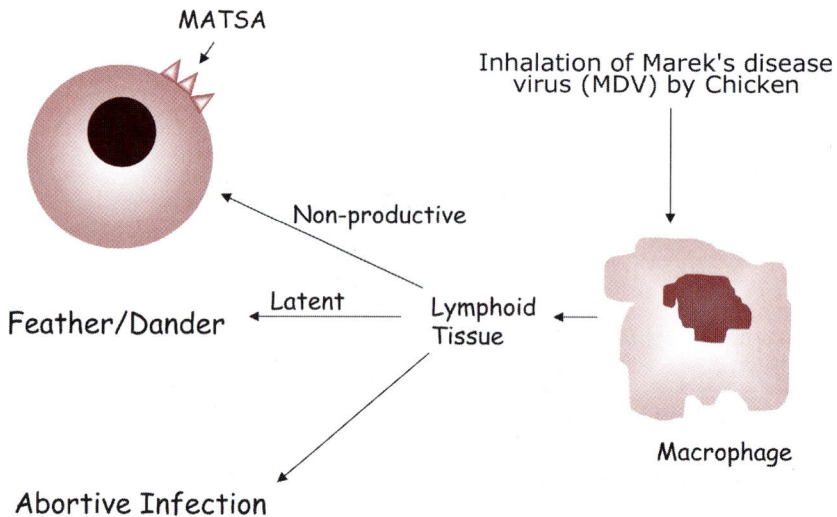

FIG. 2.41—Cell lines derived from Marek's disease lymphomas express a membrane antigen that is considered to be specific for transformed cells. This antigen (Marek's disease tumor-associated surface antigen or MATSA) is distinct from antigens induced in infected cells. There is no evidence of a host humoral response to MATSA in chickens.

sylation of proteins or lipids. Expression of these antigens has been correlated in human medicine with increased tumor invasiveness and decreased patient survival.

Protein Antigens. These are abnormally expressed proteins, which often have a normal (e.g., enzyme) function. They may be located in the nucleus, in the cytoplasm, or on the surface of the cell. In humans, prostate-specific antigen (PSA) is an enzyme that is frequently expressed by prostate tumors. Serum levels of PSA are often high in patients with prostatic carcinoma. PSA is also expressed in canine prostatic cancer and can be detected in biopsy samples by immunohistochemistry. It is also worthy of note that PSA is also expressed in benign prostatic hyperplasia in dogs, but the distribution of the expression within the prostate appears different from carcinoma when immunohistochemistry is used.

IMMUNE MECHANISMS FOR DEFENSE AGAINST TUMORS. As with other antigens, TSAs can elicit both protective and suppressive immune responses. The main defense mechanisms are summarized in Figure 2.42.

B cells serve the host by the production of TSA-reactive antibodies. These antibodies may help to define TSAs and aid in diagnosis but tend not to be protective for the host. Where they have been shown to have a protective function is through their ability to activate complement pathways to induce complement-mediated lysis or cause antibody-dependent cell-mediated cytotoxicity (ADCC). In the latter method, cells of the immune system are able to recognize tumors by the coating of tumor cells with tumor-specific antibodies. Binding to these antibodies occurs through the Fc receptor, and the ADCC cell causes death of the tumor cell by a lytic event. Macrophages, neutrophils, NK cells, and some lymphocytes can function as ADCC cells.

In some circumstances, antibodies directed at TSAs can be cross-reactive with self-epitopes present on normal tissues. When this occurs, one of many paraneoplastic syndromes that can occur is a corresponding immune-mediated disease associated with the malignant condition. Examples of this include immune-

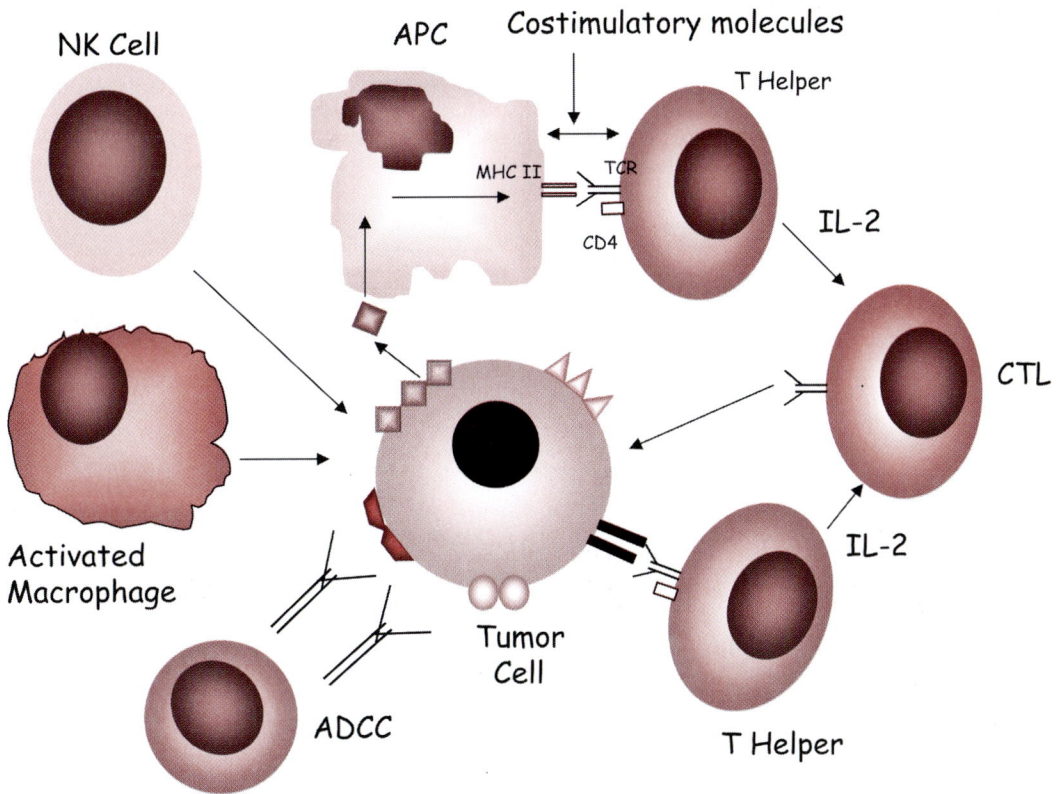

FIG. 2.42—The main immunologic mechanisms involved in tumor immunology. These include both MHC-restricted and non-MHC-restricted mechanisms. It is recognized that cell-mediated immunity plays a greater role in antitumor immunity than do humoral responses. APC, antigen-presenting cell; CTL, cytotoxic T lymphocyte; IL, interleukin; MHC, major histocompatibility complex; NK, natural killer; and TCR, T-cell receptor.

mediated arthritis, hemolytic anemia, and myasthenia gravis associated with thymoma in dogs.

Intense research has defined that the most protective form of immunity against cancer is provided by the cell-mediated arm of the immune system. Macrophages and NK cells can effect tumor cell killing via non-antibody-dependent means and in a non-MHC-restricted fashion. In these situations, local stimulation for macrophage and NK activity may be provided by cytokines such as interleukin 12 (IL-12) and interferon-γ. However, cytotoxic T lymphocytes (CTLs) are the most effective mediators of tumor rejection. CTLs are TSA specific and become activated following antigen presentation by antigen-presenting cells (in association with MHC class II molecules) and are subsequently further activated via helper T cells. CTLs or tumor-infiltrating lymphocytes (TILs) are then able to recognize tumor cells expressing TSAs in association with MHC class I molecules. Some tumor cells also express MHC class II molecules and can themselves act as antigen-presenting cells. The TILs cause death by direct lysis of tumor cells. The role of the CD4+ T helper cells is to provide the correct cytokine environment (mainly through the expression of Th1-type cytokines (i.e., cytokines that promote cell-mediated immunity) such as IL-12, IL-18, interferon-γ, and IL-2) to drive cell-mediated responses and activation of the CD8+ TILs.

TUMOR CELLS CAN EVADE IMMUNE RECOGNITION. From the processes of tumor immunology just described, it is clear that some cancer cells can evade immune recognition. A detailed description of these mechanisms is not within the scope of this text, but they are summarized below and in Figure 2.43.

• Class I MHC molecules may be down regulated on tumor cells so that they cannot form complexes of processed tumor antigen peptides and MHC molecules required for CTL recognition. A classic example of this is found in transmissible venereal tumor of dogs. Transplantation of tumor cells from an affected dog to its mate during coitus leads to successful growth of the tumor in the recipient because the tumor fails to express MHC class I molecules.
• Very few tumor cells express MHC class II molecules and so activation of CTLs relies on successful penetration of the tumor by professional antigen-presenting cells. If this does not occur, there will be suboptimal activation of CTL responses.
• Even in tumors that express MHC molecules, activation of CTLs requires a second signal provided by costimulatory molecules CD28 and B7. Some tumors fail to express B7 and therefore fail to elicit CTL activation and lead to a situation regarded as T-cell anergy.

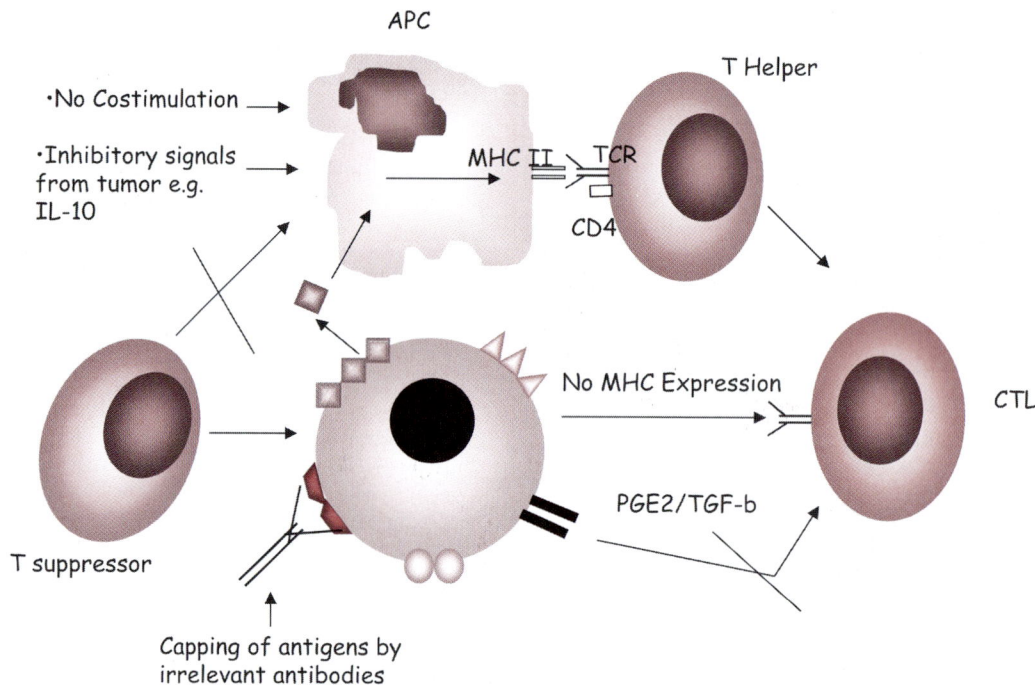

FIG. 2.43—Mechanisms by which tumors evade the immune system. APC, antigen-presenting cell; IL, interleukin; MHC, major histocompatibility complex; PGE, prostaglandin E; TGF, transforming growth factor; and TCR, T-cell receptor.

• Some tumors produce cytokine molecules, such as TGF-β, that downregulate the immune system.

• Antitumor immunity may result in the selection of tumor cells within a mass that no longer expresses immunogenic peptide-MHC molecules. This may arise through mutations or deletions in genes encoding the tumor antigens. Alternatively, immunoselection may favor the growth of tumor cells with deletions or mutations in MHC genes whose products are required to present antigenic peptides. These mutations are more likely in cancer cells because of the high mitotic rate of the cells and also the inherent genomic instability.

PROSPECTS FOR THE FUTURE. Because of the potential of the immune system as a natural defense mechanism, the augmentation of this response has been a subject of intense research in the fight to find effective cancer therapeutics or an effective cancer vaccine. Strategies have ranged from very crude cancer vaccines to more sophisticated methods of cytokine gene transfer and dendritic cell vaccines. The prospect of developing a protective vaccine for cancer (rather than an immunotherapy) is also the subject of intense research. However, the development of such an agent will rely on the comprehensive characterization of tumor-associated antigens and a clearer understanding of the mechanisms involved in generating effective antitumor immune responses.

KEY REFERENCES AND FURTHER READING
Abbas AK. 2000. Tumour immunology. In: Abbas AK, Lichtman AH, Pober JS, eds. Cellular and Molecular Immunology. Philadelphia: WB Saunders, pp 356–375.
Balkwill F. 1997. Cytokines and cancer. In: Franks LM, Teich NM, eds. The Molecular and Cellular Biology of Cancer, 3rd ed. New York: Oxford University Press, pp 380–390.
Beverley P. 1997. Immunology of cancer. In: Franks LM, Teich NM, eds. The Molecular and Cellular Biology of Cancer, 3rd ed. New York: Oxford University Press, pp 311–329.
Hoag GS, MacEwen G. 2001. Immunology and biological therapy of cancer. In: Withrow SJ, MacEwen EG, eds. Small Animal Clinical Oncology, 3rd ed. Philadelphia: WB Saunders, pp 138–168.
Jager D, Jager E, Knuth A. 2001. Immune responses to tumour antigens: Implications for antigen specific immunotherapy of cancer. J Clin Pathol 54:669–674.
Rosenberg SA. 2001. Progress in human tumour immunology and immunotherapy. Nature 411:380–384.

PART 6: CLINICAL MANIFESTATIONS OF CANCER AND THERAPEUTIC INTERVENTION

CLINICAL PRESENTATION, DIAGNOSIS, AND STAGING OF CANCER IN ANIMALS. Animals are brought to veterinarians because of either the effects of a solid mass or the systemic effects of a tumor. For instance, cattle with thymic lymphosarcoma usually present with marked head and brisket edema (i.e., a manifestation of the physical effects of the tumor). Further examples of this include the noticing of lumps or bumps on the skin or perhaps signs such as vomiting because of mechanical obstruction of the bowel from a luminal tumor. The systemic effects of a tumor can be more subtle and complex. In leukemias, animals may present with general lethargy because of progressive anemia. Animals with insulin-secreting tumors of the pancreas may present with syncopal episodes because of episodes of hypoglycemia. Many of these systemic effects are referred to as paraneoplastic syndromes.

A detailed discussion of the clinical approaches to cancer is not within the scope of this text. However, the major objective for any clinician is to define the nature and the extent of the disease. This involves clinical and clinicopathological assessment of the primary tumor, the draining lymph nodes, and compartments of the body in the search for distant metastases. This may involve a combination of biopsy, diagnostic imaging, and clinical pathology. When all the information has been gathered, the patient can be staged. This is a predictive assignment that enables the clinician to provide an accurate prognosis and deliver the most appropriate treatment.

Systemic Manifestations of Cancer Are Often Referred to as Paraneoplastic Syndromes. Paraneoplastic syndromes are remote and often insidious effects of cancer, not mediated directly by local infiltration or metastatic spread. These syndromes are of extreme importance because

1. They may be the only presenting feature of a treatable tumor.
2. They can be life-threatening, and their early detection is central to case management.
3. They run parallel to the course of the cancer and can act as markers of disease activity.

The causes of paraneoplastic syndromes are not fully understood, but in general two mechanisms have been identified: (a) the inappropriate secretion of hormones or growth factors and (b) the cross-reaction of antitumor antibodies with normal tissue (Figures 2.44 and 2.45).

Inappropriate hormone secretion occurs through excessive or unregulated secretion by the normal source of the hormone or synthesis by an organ or tissue not normally associated with that hormone (*Ectopic secretion*). In addition to the endocrine syndromes, abnormal hormone or growth-factor production may contribute to other paraneoplastic syndromes such as fever, hematologic abnormalities, and cachexia.

The second group of paraneoplastic syndromes are those caused by antitumor antibodies that may cross-react with normal tissue, which has been suggested as the probable cause of paraneoplastic syndromes affecting the nervous system (e.g., myasthenia gravis) and the hematologic system. In addition, circulating immune complexes may be associated with tumor-

Paraneoplastic Hypercalcemia

Production of PTH-rP

Direct Bone Resorption

Tumor Induced Production of Calcitriol

Osteoclastic Activating Factors

Tumor Induced Production of Prostaglandins

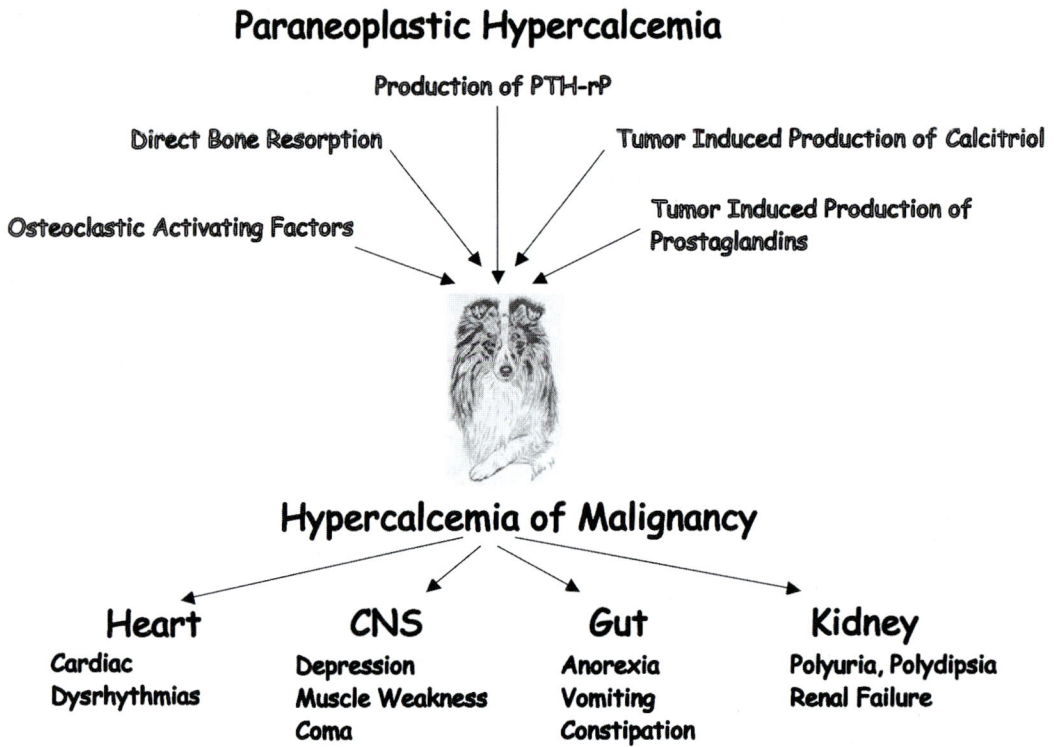

Hypercalcemia of Malignancy

Heart
Cardiac
Dysrhythmias

CNS
Depression
Muscle Weakness
Coma

Gut
Anorexia
Vomiting
Constipation

Kidney
Polyuria, Polydipsia
Renal Failure

FIG. 2.44—The pathogenesis and clinical consequences of paraneoplastic hypercalcemia. PTH-rP, parathyroid hormone-related peptide.

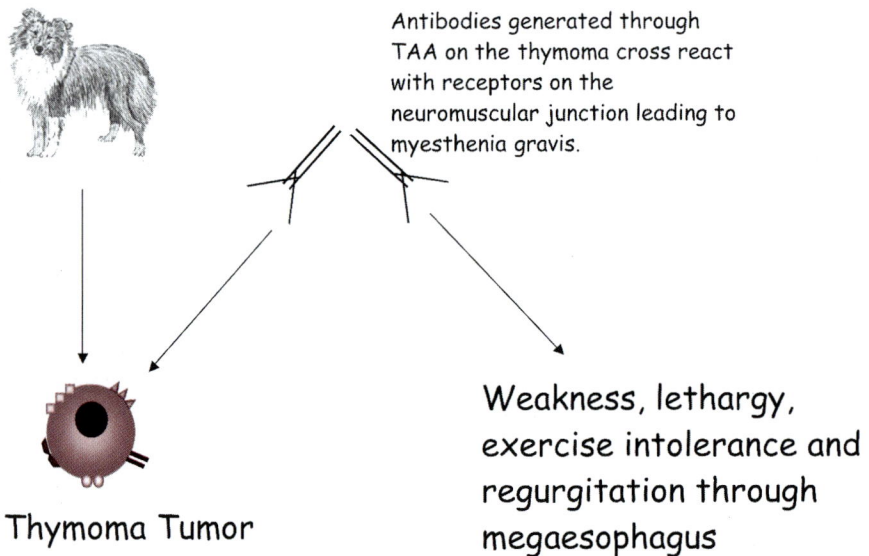

Antibodies generated through TAA on the thymoma cross react with receptors on the neuromuscular junction leading to myesthenia gravis.

Thymoma Tumor

Weakness, lethargy, exercise intolerance and regurgitation through megaesophagus

FIG. 2.45—The pathogenesis of paraneoplastic myasthenia gravis associated with lymphoma in the dog. TAA, tumor-associated antigen.

associated arthropathies and glomerulonephropathies (e.g., amyloidosis).

The following list is a short synopsis of syndromes that can be associated with malignancy (see Tables 2.7, 2.8, and 2.9).

HYPERCALCEMIA OF MALIGNANCY. Hypercalcemia, which is the most common topical paraneoplastic syndrome in dogs and cats, is frequently associated with malignant disease. It is due to an increase in bone resorption and calcium absorption, but the pathogenesis of these processes remains unknown in many cases. Five major groups of patients with hypercalcemia can be identified, depending on the type of malignancy:

1. Lymphosarcoma and other hematogenous malignancies
2. Adenocarcinoma of apocrine glands of the anal sac
3. Solid tumors that occasionally cause hypercalcemia (e.g., testicular interstitial cell tumor, seminoma, fibrosarcoma, and thymoma)
4. Solid tumors with primary or metastatic bone invasion (e.g., carcinoma of mammary gland, prostate, exocrine pancreas, and lung)
5. Primary adenoma/adenocarcinoma of the parathyroid

The potential causes of hypercalcemia of malignancy include (a) direct resorption of bone by tumor cells, (b) tumor-associated production of osteoclastic activating factors (cytokines), (c) tumor-induced production of calcitriol, (d) tumor-induced production of prostaglandins, and (e) tumor-induced production of parathyroid hormone-related peptide (PTH-rP). Dogs with lymphoma and anal sac adenocarcinoma most commonly develop cancer-associated hypercalcemia

from production of PTH-rP. Tumors that are associated with local osteolytic hypercalcemia include lymphoma, multiple myeloma, and mammary gland neoplasia.

The clinical manifestations of hypercalcemia reflect the important role of calcium in maintaining the stability and excitability of cellular membranes. The effects of hypercalcemia become particularly evident in the gastrointestinal, neuromuscular, renal, and cardiovas-

TABLE 2.7—Hematologic complications of cancer

Condition	Cause
Anemia	Infiltration of the marrow with tumor cells
	Anemia of chronic disease
	Estrogen-producing tumor (e.g., Sertoli cell tumor)
	Immune-mediated anemia associated with malignancy
	Microangiopathic hemolytic anemia (e.g., splenic hemangiosarcoma)
	Disseminated intravascular coagulation (DIC)
	Hemorrhage
Bleeding	Thrombocytopenia (tumor infiltration of the marrow, DIC, immune mediated, and sequestration of platelets)
	Bleeding from a tumor
	Gastrointestinal bleeding as part of hypergastrinemia or hyperhistaminemia
	DIC
Hyperviscosity syndrome	Polycythemia associated with primary erythrocytosis or renal tumors causing localized hypoxia
	Excessive production of γ-globulins from myeloma
	High numbers of white cells in leukemia
Other cytopenias	Marrow infiltration by tumor cells
	Leukemic process overcrowding normal cell production

TABLE 2.8—Metabolic and endocrine disorders associated with neoplasia

Syndrome	Tumor	Clinical manifestations
Hypercalcemia	Lymphoid tumors	Polyuria/polydipsia
	Anal sac carcinoma	Anorexia/vomiting
	Parathyroid adenoma	Constipation
		Cardiac dysrhythmias
		Tremors/weakness
Hypoglycemia	Insulinoma	Weakness/episodic collapse
	Hepatic tumors	
	Leukemias	
Hyperhistaminemia	Mast cell tumors	Localized swelling of the tumor
		Gastrointestinal ulceration leading to vomiting, anorexia, melena, and anemia
Hypergastrinemia	Gastrin-producing pancreatic tumor	Gastrointestinal ulceration
Hyperthyroidism	Thyroid adenoma (cats)	Polyuria/polydipsia
	Thyroid carcinoma (dogs)	Weight loss
		Tachycardia
		Hyperexcitability
Hyperadrenocorticism	Adrenal adenoma/ carcinoma	Polyuria/polydipsia
		Muscle weakness
	Pituitary tumor	Hair loss
		Polyphagia

TABLE 2.9—Other paraneoplastic syndromes

Tumor types	Syndrome	Suggested mechanism
Thymoma	Myasthenia gravis	Autoantibodies directed at thymoma antigens are cross-reactive with nicotinic acetylcholine receptors
Insulinoma (plus a variety of other tumors, including hemangiosarcoma)	Peripheral Neuropathy	Demyelination and axonal degeneration, which is possibly immune mediated
Tumors in the thoracic cavity mainly; however, have been associated with nonneoplastic lesions of the thorax and a few abdominal tumors	Hypertrophic osteopathy (Marie's disease)	Palisading periosteal new bone formation on the distal limbs; etiology unknown
Glucagon-producing pancreatic carcinoma (also noted in liver disease and often accompanied by diabetes mellitus)	Hepatocutaneous syndrome (necrolytic migratory erythema)	Etiology unknown; may be hormonally mediated
Nodular dermatofibrosis	Renal cystadenocarcinoma in German shepherds	Cutaneous nodules associated with bilateral renal tumors; autosomal recessive mode of inheritance
Thymoma in cats	Exfoliative dermatitis	Immune mediated

cular systems, causing anorexia, vomiting, and constipation; pancreatitis and peptic ulcers; depression; lethargy; muscle weakness; and finally coma. Hypercalcemia may be associated with cardiac arrhythmias, and the most common cause of death in hypercalcemic patients is cardiac arrest. A poorly understood but important adverse effect of hypercalcemia occurs in the kidneys, resulting in polyuria with secondary polydipsia. This vicious cycle leads to further renal impairment with subsequent azotemia, acidosis, and eventual renal failure. Hypercalcemia, even with accompanying mild renal failure, can be reversed, but if it is not treated, it will cause fatal complications. The management of hypercalcemia requires restoration of the circulating volume, promotion of calciuresis, and treatment of the primary cause.

HYPERGASTRINEMIA. The secretion of gastrin by pancreatic tumors, known as *Zollinger-Ellison syndrome*, and the release of histamine by mast cell tumor degranulation promote gastric acid secretion and can lead to gastroduodenal ulcers. Vomiting, acute intraluminal bleeding, and gastric perforations can all ensue. In addition, mast cell degranulation may precipitate an anaphylactoid reaction and shock that require treatment with fluids, corticosteroids, and antihistamines.

HYPERHISTAMINEMIA. Hyperhistaminemia associated with mast cell tumors is more common than is generally appreciated. Mast cells are intimately involved with inflammation and type I hypersensitivity reactions. Mast cell tumors that have a reasonable degree of differentiation will also contain active granules containing heparin and histamine. Histamine release from tumors can lead to localized edema and swelling. In addition, the effect of degranulation and release of histamine on the gastrointestinal tract is to promote ulcer formation. Consequently, animals with active mast cell tumors may have vomiting and melena through ulceration and gastrointestinal bleeding. Also, the tumor may be red and swollen or fluctuate in size. Degranulation and heparin release may cause bleeding tendencies especially at surgery, when the mass is being manipulated.

HYOGLYCEMIA. The opposing effects of insulin and glucagon tightly regulate blood glucose levels. Hypoglycemia is a dangerous metabolic abnormality because glucose is the major energy substrate of the brain. Neurological signs of hypoglycemia include confusion, weakness, hindlimb paresis, grand mal seizures, and coma. Catecholamine release in response to hypoglycemia can cause tachycardia, dilated pupils, and nervousness. The severity of the clinical signs depends on the degree, duration, and rate of development of the hypoglycemia and the degree of susceptibility of the individual patient.

The most common malignancy that is associated with hypoglycemia is *insulinoma*. However, large hepatic tumors, lymphosarcoma, and hemangiosarcoma have all been associated with hypoglycemia. Insulinomas are functional, insulin-secreting beta-cell tumors of the pancreas. The clinical features of insulinomas are related to the *hypoglycemia*. However, in some cases, there can be an associated *peripheral polyneuropathy*. These polyneuropathies may be associated with defective metabolism in the peripheral nerves or may be associated with the development of cross-reactive tumor-associated antibodies. Diagnosis is based on the demonstration of hypoglycemia and concurrent hyperinsulinemia.

DISSEMINATED INTRAVASCULAR COAGULATION. DIC is a common acquired coagulopathy seen in a number of disease states such as trauma, neoplasia, and certain hemolytic diseases. DIC occurs when there is diffuse activation of the hemostatic mechanism in vivo and can be initiated by several mechanisms, the most common of which are the escape of tissue substances into the circulation, endothelial damage with exposure of components of vessel walls, and vascular stasis with acidosis and electrolyte imbalance. The findings in most cases reflect the generation of thrombin in the circulation.

CANCER CACHEXIA. Cancer cachexia is a complicated paraneoplastic condition that manifests as weight loss in the face of adequate calorific intake. Even in anorexic patients, the degree of weight loss is still disproportionate. Research has demonstrated that there are dramatic alterations in carbohydrate, lipid, and protein metabolism in cancer patients, and this may be, in part, mediated by cytokines such as IL-1, tumor-necrosis factor, and IL-6. It has been suggested that tumors prefer to handle glucose anaerobically rather than aerobically, leading to the excessive production of lactate that has to be converted to glucose by the liver. This leads to a net energy deficit and the theoretical risk of lactic acidosis. In any treatment regime, it must be ensured that the patient consumes an adequate quantity of highly bioavailable nutrients present in a palatable form.

FEVER. Tumor-associated fever is usually defined as unexplained elevated body temperature that coincides with the growth or the elimination of a tumor. Tumor-associated fevers can be caused by

1. Rapid turnover/metabolism of cells (e.g., in leukemia)
2. Leukopenia and subsequent infection
3. Release of tumor pyrogens, which have direct action on the hypothalamus

HYPERTROPHIC OSTEOPATHY, This is a relatively common condition that occurs in the bones of the extremities with a periosteal proliferation and subsequent osteophyte development that palisades from the cortical bone at 90°. The exact pathogenesis is uncertain, but there is often an association with thoracic neoplasia. Lameness resolves on removal of the tumor, but radiological changes may take several months or years to resolve.

CANCER THERAPIES

Choice of Treatment in Cancer Depends on a Number of Factors. The option to treat cancer in veterinary patients is limited to companion animals. The main treatment modalities include surgery, radiotherapy, and chemotherapy, the choice of which depends on the following criteria:

- Tumor type
- Disease stage
- Veterinarians skills and facilities
- Owner compliance
- Cost

Radiotherapy Can Be Used to Treat Cancer. Radiation causes ionization within DNA molecules of the cell. Although the most important target for damage is nuclear DNA, damage to the lipids and proteins of the cell membrane may also be involved. Radiation may damage DNA directly, or indirectly by the production of free radicals and highly reactive ions that damage the DNA. The mechanism depends on the type of radiation used. In the clinic, the responses of tissue to radiation are also affected by the characteristics of the tissue or tumor itself.

1. Rate of cell division: The damage to cellular DNA in response to ionizing radiation occurs very rapidly. However, the dose of radiation required to kill a cell outright, by completely destroying its ability to function, is very high. Within the therapeutic range, the DNA damage is subtler, allowing normal function until the cell tries to divide, when it cannot and dies. Thus, the damage done to the cells by radiation is not apparent until they try to divide, resulting in a variable delay in the response of tissues and tumors. Rapidly dividing tissues will express their responses to radiation within days or weeks, whereas slowly dividing tissue such as bone may not show the full effects of radiation for months or years. This principle is important in understanding the side effects of radiation.

2. Tumor volume: Smaller tumors are generally more sensitive to radiation because they are dividing more rapidly, with a higher growth fraction and a greater proportion of cells in the sensitive M phase of the cell cycle. In addition, these tumors are less likely to contain a large number of hypoxic cells and are easier to dose accurately and uniformly. The converse is true of very large tumors.

3. Inherent cell sensitivity: Unfortunately, neoplastic cells are not inherently more radiosensitive than normal cells. Generally, rapidly dividing normal or neoplastic cells are more radiosensitive than slowly dividing cells. It is wrong to imagine that the growth fraction of tumors is greater than that of normal tissues, because this is often not the case. In addition, some rapidly dividing tumors with high growth fractions appear to be fairly radioresistant: this may reflect tremendous ability to repair and repopulate between treatments, and/or tumor cell hypoxia.

Tumors of different histological types show different radiosensitivity. In general, carcinomas are more radiosensitive than sarcomas. However, the same type of tumor may show different radiosensitivity (and other characteristics of biological behavior) in different sites and in different species.

Chemotherapy Can Be Used to Treat Primary Cancer and Metastatic Disease. At the turn of the 20th century, cancer was regarded as a disease that began locally and, only at a very late stage, spread to distant sites. Thus, initial attempts at disease control were confined to radical local excision or radiotherapy. Over time, it became clear that many tumors metastasize early, and patients may still die despite the primary tumor site remaining clear. It was therefore necessary to develop some form of systemic therapy. Many of the cancer chemotherapy drugs used today stem from seminal experiments conducted during the 1940s onward. Alkylating agents originated from research into chemical warfare, and the antimetabolite class of drugs was born from research into nutrition and nucleic acid metabolism.

THE CENTRAL TARGET FOR CHEMOTHERAPY DRUGS IS DNA. In many branches of pharmacology, the aim is to treat a disease with a drug that is specific for the disease or the diseased tissue. In cancer patients, this specificity is, in part, provided by the rapidly dividing cells of the tumor as compared with the rest of the animal's normal tissues. This is because most chemotherapeutic or cytotoxic drugs act upon the process of *cell growth and division*. However, normal cells of the bone marrow and the gut are also rapidly dividing and can be affected by cytotoxic drugs. The cytotoxic drugs used in cancer chemotherapy can be broadly divided into the following six classes on the basis of their mode of action: alkylating agents, antimetabolites, antitumor

antibiotics, vinca alkaloids, hormones, and some miscellaneous agents (Figure 2.46).

THE KINETICS OF TUMOR GROWTH ARE IMPORTANT IN THE BIOLOGY OF CHEMOTHERAPY. To understand the concept behind the success of chemotherapy, one must first consider the principles of tumor development and growth. Cancer is a genetic disease arising as a result in changes in the cellular DNA. Following malignant transformation of one cell, there will be a certain period (which may be months or years) before which the tumor becomes *clinically detectable* (i.e., by palpation or by diagnostic imaging). Tumor growth kinetics is such that there is an initial rapid growth curve that then flattens as the growth rate slows. This is known as *Gompertzian* growth and is depicted in Figure 2.47. The slowing of growth may be for several reasons, including outgrowth of its major nutrient supply. Chemotherapy is most effective when tumors are rapidly growing, but unfortunately most tumors become clinically detectable during the slower plateau phase of growth.

In addition to changes in growth rate, a naturally occurring tumor will evolve in other ways. Although classically a tumor is considered to be clonal in origin, tumor cells within a population can accumulate other mutations, which can alter their biological properties. These may include biochemical changes to improve their ability to expel cytotoxic drugs or their ability to metastasize. This is known as *tumor cell heterogeneity* and can be a determining factor in the success or fail-

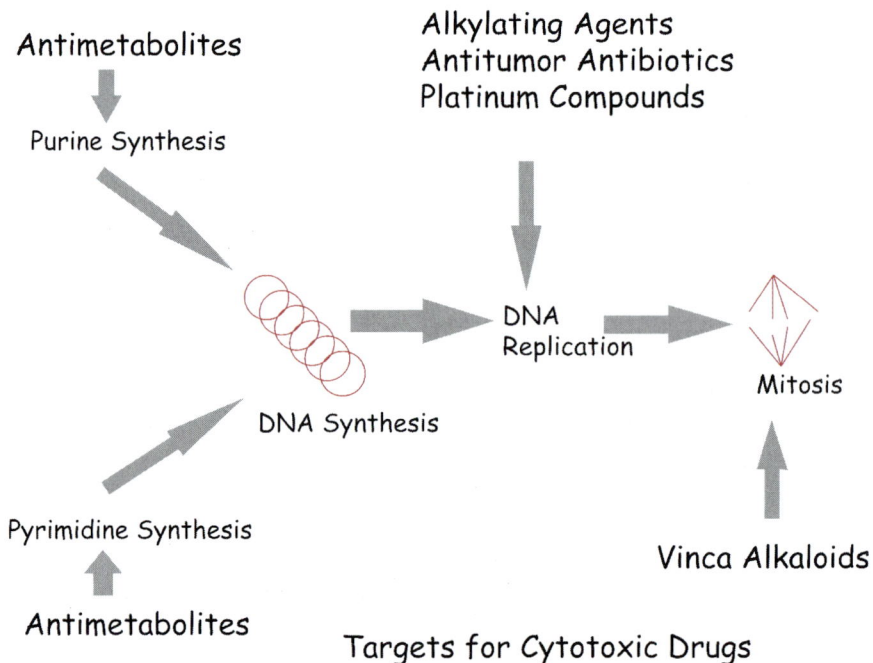

FIG. 2.46—The major targets of cytotoxic chemotherapeutic drugs. The major target is DNA replication.

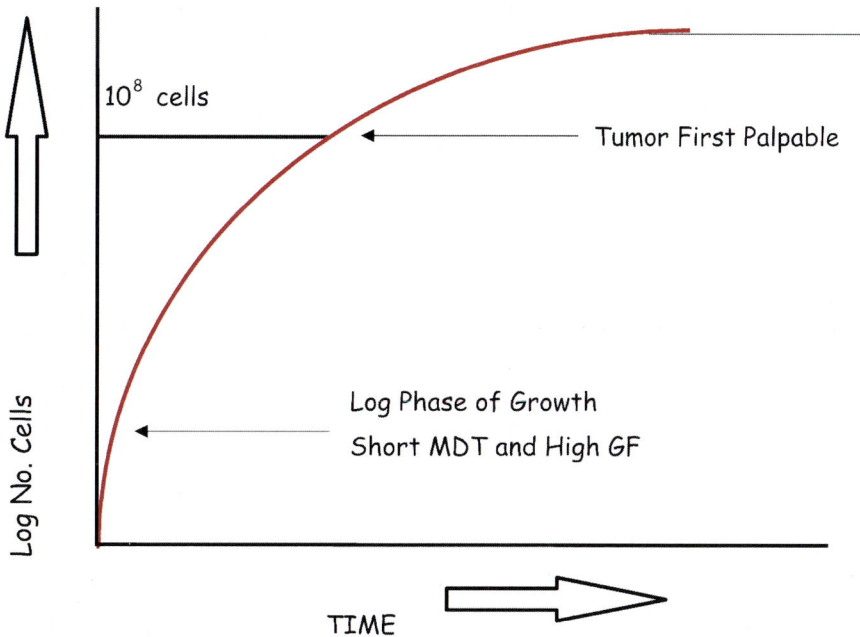

FIG. 2.47—The Gompertzian growth curve of tumors. In the early stages of growth, there is a low mass-doubling time (MDT) and a high growth fraction (GF). Later, there is a high MDT and a low GF. This may limit the success of anticancer chemotherapy for large, bulky tumors.

ure of chemotherapy. Among a general population of cancer cells, if there is a small population of cells that are resistant to a particular cytotoxic drug, continued use of that drug can lead to selection for the resistant cells, eventually leading to treatment failure.

EFFECT OF GROWTH KINETICS ON CHEMOTHERAPY. Cell division is a cyclical process whereby a cell programmed to divide will progress through several stages involving growth and DNA replication, ultimately leading to mitotic division. Cells that are not dividing are said to be in G_0 or the *resting phase* but can be recruited into the cell cycle in response to stimuli. Some cytotoxic drugs are termed *cell-cycle specific*, in that they are only active on cells at a certain stage of cell division (e.g., vincristine during the M phase). Other drugs such as cyclophosphamide are not cell cycle specific and act on all dividing cells. Cells in G_0 are relatively resistant to the action of cytotoxic drugs, so it can be said that a deciding factor in the success of chemotherapy is the number of tumor cells within a population that are in G_0.

The actual growth rate of a tumor is described in terms of *mass-doubling time* (MDT), or the time taken for a tumor to double in size. As described earlier, tumor growth is considered to be Gompertzian, which means that MDTs are much shorter during the early stages of tumor growth. It follows that MDT is a function of the number of cells that are actively dividing, or the *growth fraction* (GF), the cell *cycle time*, and the *number* of cells being lost by cell death.

Thus, tumors with a high growth fraction have a short MDT. Because most chemotherapeutic agents act upon the process of cell division, it follows that chemotherapy is likely to be more successful where tumors have a high GF and a low MDT. A number of important points can be drawn from these observations:

1. Small tumors with a high growth fraction and short MDT will be more susceptible to the action of cytotoxic drugs.
2. Initially, metastatic lesions have a higher GF and shorter MDT than the primary tumor from which they arose.
3. When tumor cells are left behind at the site of surgery, they tend to move into a phase of cell division and adopt a higher GF and shorter MDT than the removed mass. This is known as *recruitment*.

Considering the above, it can be appreciated that chemotherapy may be of greatest use in small, rapidly dividing tumors or metastatic disease or where there has been incomplete removal of the primary tumor at surgery.

BOTH TUMOR CELL TYPE AND DRUG RESISTANCE CAN AFFECT THE SUCCESS OF CHEMOTHERAPY. Although the GF and MDT are important in determining the success of chemotherapy, even some tumor types that are rapidly growing will not respond well to cytotoxic drugs, by virtue of their inherent resistance to antineoplastic agents.

Drug resistance is the ability of a tumor cell to survive the actions of an anticancer agent. Drug resistance can be an *inherent* feature of the particular tumor or can be *acquired resistance*, arising through genetic mutations within the tumor. Several mechanisms exist that may confer resistance to anticancer agents. Drugs that share similar chemistry often share resistance mechanisms, which allows us to choose sensible rescue drugs. However, relapsing tumors can acquire resistance to drugs that have not been used to treat the tumor initially. This phenomenon is known as *multidrug resistance* (MDR). In practice, drug resistance is the most common form of treatment failure.

Understanding the Pathophysiology of Cancer Is Helping to Develop Novel Drugs. Despite advances in radiotherapy and chemotherapy, cancer remains a disease of high mortality, largely through metastatic disease. In the previous sections, we have tried to make clear that cancer biology is developing into a far more logical science where one can define the six fundamental characteristics of a cancer cell. Radiotherapy and chemotherapy are crude treatments relying on the fact that tumors contain rapidly dividing cells. However, by having a clearer understanding of the basic mechanisms of cancer development, one can develop drugs that are far more specific for the cancer phenotype. These drugs include angiogenesis inhibitors to cut off the nutrient supply to tumors, inhibitors of metastasis, kinase inhibitors, and molecules that may enhance the

antitumor immune response. As described in Part 2, telomerase has emerged as a near universal molecular marker of cancer, and research is under way to look at mechanisms by which telomerase can be inhibited to cause cell death (Figure 2.48).

Harnessing the Immune System May Complement Existing Therapies. Immunotherapy is treatment by immunologic means and can be divided into active and passive forms. In active immunotherapy, the patient's own immune system is stimulated to respond to tumor, whereas, in passive immunotherapy, there is adoptive transfer of immune cells. We have previously discussed the role of the immune system in cancer and how tumors have evolved mechanisms to overcome host immunity. Consequently, many protocols involving immunotherapy or the development of cancer vaccines have largely failed. There have been clear examples in the veterinary literature of adopting immunotherapy approaches to cancer in animals. These have been largely based on nonspecific immunostimulation using substances such as injectable bacillus Calmette-Guérin (BCG) vaccine to cause regression of sarcoids in horses and also muramyl tripeptides as an adjuvant to more classical approaches.

Although many previous strategies have failed to consistently improve the outlook of cancer patients, there is now a greater understanding of the presentation of antigens to the immune system and the orchestration of host responses by cytokines. During the last two

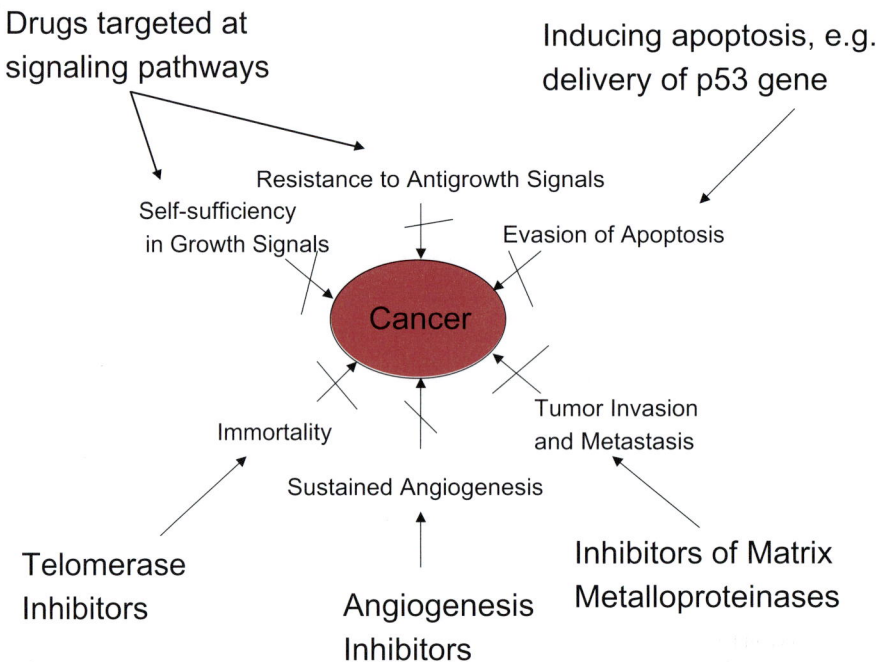

FIG. 2.48—A greater understanding of the molecular biology of cancer is enabling the identification of new targets for therapeutic intervention.

decades of the 20th century, there was great excitement about antibody therapy and the production of monoclonal antibodies to tumor tissues. However, it is now clear that the most important mechanisms in cancer immunology are cell-mediated responses. Harnessing cell-mediated responses is far more difficult, even now that reagents such as IL-2 and other cytokines are available. Recombinant IL-2 has been used to help treat malignancies in both people and dogs. One of the problems with using recombinant cytokines is that they are essentially autocrine or paracrine molecules that are being asked to act as endocrine molecules when given systemically. Consequently, it is difficult to achieve doses that have biological effect without causing toxicity to the host. It does seem, however, that recombinant molecules are tolerated well by dogs and cats compared with people.

In alternative strategies, there have been attempts to isolate TILs from biopsy material. TILs are CD8+ cells that are tumor specific and can be expanded ex vivo by incubation with a cocktail of cytokines, including IL-2. Once expanded, these TILs are delivered back to the patient in an attempt to target micrometastatic disease. This has proved useful in some circumstances but is cumbersome and time consuming. Workers have tried to establish similar effects by expanding patient dendritic cells by addition of cytokines and priming with (or pulsing) with tumor antigens. This again is a cumbersome process that is unlikely to reach its way into the veterinary clinic in the immediate future.

It seems likely that effective cancer immunotherapy will require a combination of approaches that may include delivery of cytokine molecules and/or costimulatory molecules and/or tumor-specific antigens (Figure 2.49). The advent of technologies such as phage display for identifying tumor-specific antigens may hold exciting keys for the development of novel therapeutics. Further, instead of delivery of cytokines in the form of recombinant proteins, a more likely avenue is to use the genes for cytokines and gene-transfer technology for delivery (see below).

Gene Therapy Offers a Completely New Pharmacological Approach. Gene therapy is the introduction of genetic material into a cell in vivo to ameliorate a disease process. This is one of the newest areas of pharmacology and could potentially play a major role in the development of new cancer therapeutic agents. However, results from many of the clinical trials have been disappointing, and major technical hurdles need to be overcome before gene therapy can become accepted clinical practice.

There Are Essentially Three Broad Approaches to Gene Therapeutics for Cancer (Figure 2.50).

1. *Rescue* of the cancer cell through gene-replacement, antisense, or related therapies that overcome the genetic abnormalities associated with the cancer phenotype
2. Destruction of the cancer cell through introduction of *suicide* genes or prodrug activating genes, which result in the death of the transduced cell
3. The introduction of genes such as cytokine genes that enhance the immune response against the tumor

Delivery of Genes to Cancer Cells Requires a Vector. The delivery of genes to cancer cells requires a vehicle

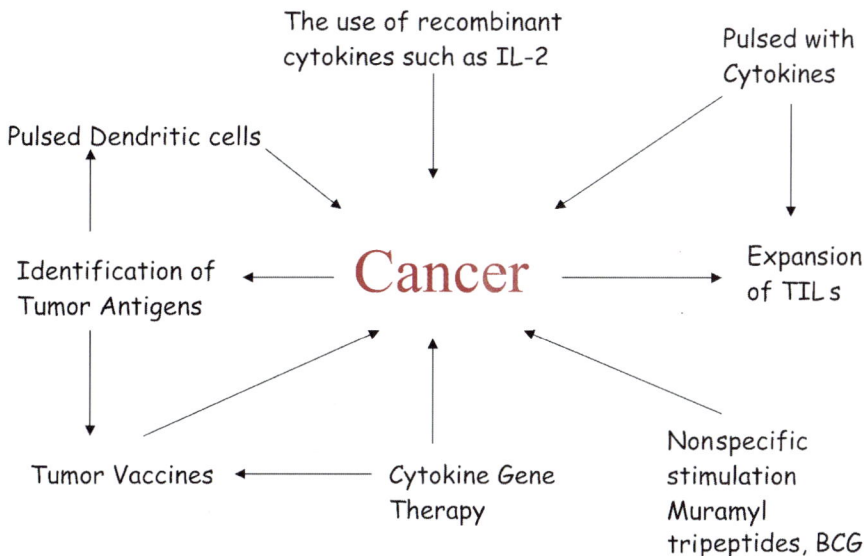

FIG. 2.49—Methods by which immunotherapy is being employed to treat cancer. BCG, bacillus Calmette-Guérin; IL-2, interleukin 2; and TILs, tumor-infiltrating lymphocytes.

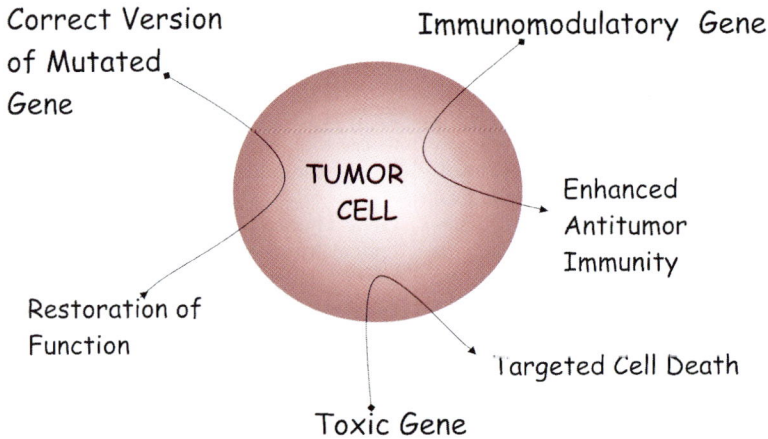

FIG. 2.50—Potential gene-therapy strategies to treat cancer.

or vector. The ability of viruses to enter cells and the ability of some (mainly retroviruses) to integrate genetic material into the host genome make them seem ideal vectors for gene delivery. Further, the use of recombinant DNA technology allows us to unravel the genetic machinery of the virus and insert our own gene of interest so that it can be delivered to cells consistently. Many of the early gene-transfer studies were performed using retroviruses or adenoviruses, which had been modified to prevent replication and virus-associated disease. Although still used, the concerns over safety using viruses have led many workers to investigate nonviral delivery systems such as naked DNA or liposome complexes.

Delivery of Therapeutic Genes. Genes can be delivered to patients directly (in vivo delivery) or via ex vivo delivery. The latter is a more cumbersome method that involves the removal of target cells (in this case, tumor cells) from the patient, transduction with the therapeutic genes, and then delivery of the cells back to the patient after they have been irradiated. However, this method has been largely superseded by direct in vivo delivery (Figure 2.51).

The efficient targeted transduction of genes to tumor cells still remains one of the major obstacles in the way of developing cancer gene therapy. The development of vectors that restrict gene expression to specific cell populations is therefore of great importance not only in terms of developing systemic gene therapy for metastatic disease but also in local gene therapy, where the efficacy and safety of gene transfer can be maximized by keeping the expression of the transgene in normal tissue to a minimum. Targeting studies have included surface targeting of the vector (e.g., receptor-based approaches) and transcriptional targeting using transcriptional mechanisms that are unique to cancer cells. In this system, the promoter for a gene that is expressed only in cancer cells is used in the gene-therapy vector to drive expression of the therapeutic gene. In this way, the novel gene will be expressed only in cancer cells and not in any normal cells that the vector enters. The success of transcriptional targeting depends on differential expression of genes in cancer cells compared with normal cells, and several studies have focused on using tissue-specific promoters such as tyrosinase (melanoma), osteocalcin (osteosarcoma), and *MUC1* (breast cancer). As many of these promoters are specific to cancer types, the possibility of developing a transcriptionally targeted promoter with a broader spectrum of activity is an attractive one. The development of such a system relies on the identification of a gene/protein that is unique to a broad range of cancer types. As we have previously discussed, telomerase has emerged as the most common tumor marker and currently this system is under investigation as a mechanism for targeting toxic genes to cancer cells.

One of the most common approaches to cancer gene therapy is gene-directed enzyme prodrug therapy (GDEPT). In GDEPT, a gene is delivered to cancer cells, which has little effect on the cell. However, this gene is capable of converting an exogenously delivered prodrug to a much more active compound. If the activation of this prodrug occurs only in the cancer cell, then GDEPT has achieved a form of localized chemotherapy that has spared any normal tissues.

Alternative approaches include the delivery of normal oncogenes or tumor-suppressor genes to cancer cells that are known to have defective homologues. One example of this is the delivery of a normal copy of the *p53* gene to cancer cells that are defective for this gene. Cells that are defective for *p53* fail to undergo cell-cycle arrest or apoptosis when damaged. Delivery of the *p53* gene may help the tumor cell to achieve apoptosis via either the *p21* or the *bcl2* pathway. Unfor-

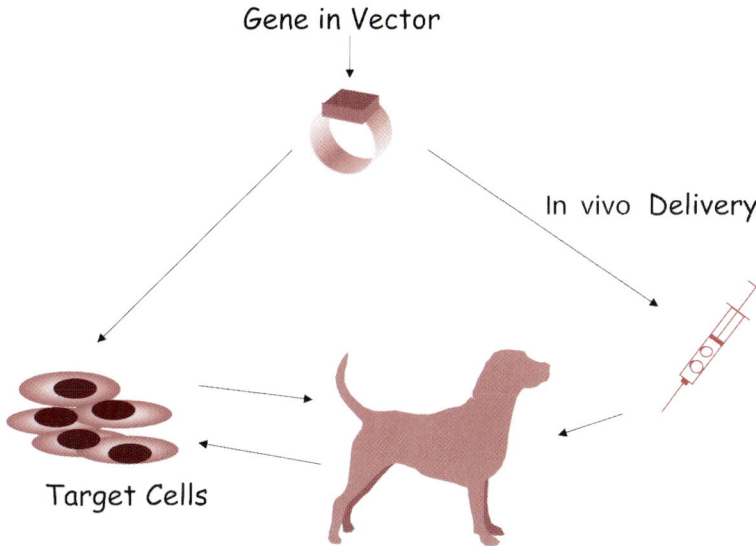

FIG. 2.51—Gene delivery to veterinary patients is the key to the success of this form of therapy in the clinic. The gene needs to be delivered in a vector either directly (in vivo) or indirectly (ex vivo). In the latter, target cells (tumor cells) are removed from the patient and then returned carrying a therapeutic gene(s). This is a laborious method, and most gene-delivery systems are now based on a direct method.

tunately, the success of this approach relies on the delivery of the normal gene to the majority of cancer cells, a technology that is not achievable at present. In contrast, cell killing using the GDEPT system relies only on a small proportion of the cells receiving the therapeutic gene. This is because the toxic metabolites generated during activation can leak across gap junctions for a bystander effect.

Gene Therapy Offers a Further Mechanism for Enhancing Antitumor Immunity. There is increasing evidence that in situ cell destruction through prodrug activation can result in an immune response. Consequently, efforts have focused on the coexpression of immunostimulatory molecules (in particular, cytokines) to further enhance the antitumor immune response. Numerous cytokine genes from domestic animal species have been cloned, sequenced, and expressed. Evidence derived from animal model systems suggests that the local production of cytokines within or around a tumor mass may enhance the antitumor immune response or reverse T-cell anergy. It is anticipated that a combined prodrug-activating and cytokine approach may enhance both primary tumor cell destruction and the development of an antitumor immune response that is directed at established or micrometastatic disease (Figure 2.52).

As discussed, cell-mediated responses are important in the antitumor immune response, and this is reflected in the choice of cytokines used for such studies, includ-

ing IL-12 and IL-18. These cytokines enhances T-cell proliferation, augment natural killer cell activity, and are inducers of interferon-γ. Recent work suggests that a combination of IL-12 and IL-18 may be synergistic in abrogating tumor development and that IL-12 has a role in inhibition of angiogenesis through activation of NK cytotoxicity.

CONCLUSIONS. In this chapter, we have summarized the normal physiology of the cell and the mechanisms by which cancers arise. The cell clearly has many regulatory pathways that try to prevent cancer. The transformation to malignancy requires the acquisition of six fundamental capabilities involving changes to the host DNA. The immune system plays a role in surveillance of cancer, but cancer cells have evolved many mechanisms to overcome the immune response. Despite our increased understanding of cancer biology, the classical treatments of radiotherapy and chemotherapy have changed little over the past 100 years. The next two decades however, will further unravel the complex mechanisms of tumorigenesis and help us to define the fundamental mechanisms more clearly. Coupled with this is an exponential growth curve in our ability to manipulate DNA and host immunity such that we are entering a new dawn of therapy where molecular medicine will sit comfortably alongside conventional treatments to develop more effective strategies to diagnose, prevent, and treat cancer in domestic animals.

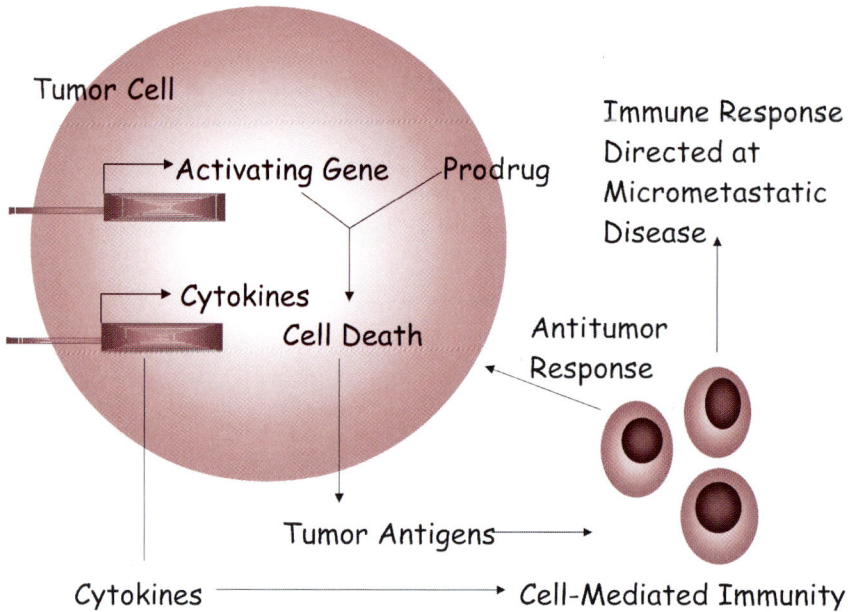

FIG. 2.52—Combining strategies for gene therapy of cancer. In this, a toxic gene is delivered to cancer cells, which causes cell death in situ. To spare normal tissue, this gene is exquisitely targeted to cancer cells. The environment created by the dying cancer cells promotes the exposure of tumor-associated antigens to the immune system. The subsequent antitumor immune response may be augmented by the coexpression of cytokines that promote cell-mediated immune responses. This has the potential to lead antitumor responses in sites of micrometastases.

KEY REFERENCES AND FURTHER READING

Argyle DJ. 1999. Gene therapy in veterinary medicine. Vet Rec 144:369–376.

Argyle DJ, Nicolson L, McGillivery C, Onions DE. 1999. Cloning, sequencing and characterisation of canine IL-18. Immunogenetics 49:541–543.

Blackwood L, Argyle DJ. 2002. Feline hyperthyroidism: Advances towards novel molecular therapeutics. J Small Anim Pract 43:58–66.

Blackwood L, Onions DE, Argyle DJ. 2001a. The feline thyroglobulin promoter: Towards targeted gene therapy of hyperthyroidism. Domest Anim Endocrinol 20:185–201.

Blackwood L, O'Shaughnessy PJ, Reid SJ, Argyle DJ. 2001. *E. coli* nitroreductase/CB1954: In vitro studies into a potential system for feline cancer gene therapy. Vet J 161:269–279.

Dachs GU, Dougherty GJ, Stratford IJ, Chaplin DJ. 1997. Targeting gene therapy to cancer. Oncol Res 9:313–325.

Dobson JM, Gorman NT. 1994. Cancer Chemotherapy in Small Animal Practice. Oxford: Blackwell Scientific.

Harris J, Sikora K. 1993. Gene therapy in the clinic. Mol Aspects Med 14:251–546.

Keller ET, Burkholder JK, Shi F, et al. 1996. In vivo particle mediated cytokine gene transfer into canine oral mucosa and epidermis. Cancer Gene Ther 3:186–191.

Vile RG, Hart IR. 1993. In-vitro and in-vivo targeting of gene expression to melanoma cells. Cancer Res 53:962–967.

Withrow S, MacEwen G, eds. 1996. Small Animal Clinical Oncology, 2nd ed. Philadelphia: WB Saunders.

Withrow S, MacEwen G. 2001. Tumour immunology and immunotherapy. In: Withrow S, MacEwen G, eds. Small Animal Clinical Oncology, 3rd ed. Philadelphia: WB Saunders pp 138–168.

Yang N, Sun WH. 1995. Gene and non-viral approaches to cancer gene therapy. Nat Med 1:481–483.

HOST-PATHOGEN INTERACTIONS

Richard A. Squires

AGENTS OF INFECTIOUS DISEASE

Introduction. Veterinarians take care of an extraordinary variety of species of vertebrates; in some countries, they care for invertebrates—such as tarantulas and shrimp—too. As if this bewildering variety of patients was not interesting and challenging enough, consider for a moment that each individual animal under a veterinarian's care is not—in fact—a single individual, but a multitudinous throng of coexisting organisms. Viruses, bacteria, protozoa, helminths, and insects are just some of the kinds of organisms that might be along for a ride with the average veterinary patient. Even with modern parasiticides, the average vertebrate harbors billions of microorganisms on its skin and particularly within its gastrointestinal tract. Yet, despite the profusion of potentially harmful inhabitants upon and inside them, most veterinary patients manage to remain healthy. This chapter examines some of the many mechanisms by which this at-first-glance precarious *détente* is able to persist. Given that this is a *patho*physiology book, we naturally concentrate on what happens when the balance is upset and things go wrong, particularly from the host's point of view. Along the way, we examine some situations where the microbial passengers are far more than mere freeloaders—situations in which their presence is essential to the survival of their host. We'll see that some host-microbe relationships are extremely ancient and mutually beneficial; so much so that the distinction between host and microbe has, in some cases, become quite blurred.

This first section of this host-pathogen chapter describes the bewildering variety of organisms that have adopted an infectious or parasitic way of life. Some of means by which they gain entry to hosts' bodies, persist there, and cause disease are described. A few examples of desirable infections are also mentioned. In the second section, host and environmental factors relevant to infectious diseases are considered separately, for simplicity's sake. Along the way, numerous exemplar infectious diseases of veterinary importance are described in order to illuminate the interplay between host, infectious agents, and environment.

This book is not large enough to serve adequately as a textbook of veterinary microbiology or immunology. Readers are encouraged to seek further information elsewhere to build strength in these important and ever-growing disciplines (Greene 1998; Tizard 2000).

Simple to extremely complex organisms can host infectious agents. For example, bacteria can be infected by a range of viruses that have evolved to parasitize them; these viruses are called *bacteriophages* or *phages* for short (literally, bacteria eaters). In some parts of the world, bacteriophages are used—instead of or in addition to—antibiotics, to treat serious bacterial infections of people and animals. Molecular biologists also make extensive use of bacteriophages as tools to manipulate DNA.

Even the simplest of eukaryotes (e.g., yeasts) can themselves become infected. In the southeastern United States and the Ohio-Mississippi river valleys, the dimorphic fungus *Blastomyces dermatitidis* can cause life-threatening pneumonia in dogs and people (Krohne 2000). *Blastomyces dermatitidis* is also known to be endemic in Africa, where it seems to be somewhat less pathogenic. A Ugandan strain of *B. dermatitidis* was found to be infected by a novel double-stranded RNA virus (Kohno et al. 1994). Virus-infected yeast cells had an unusual shape, being oblong or dumbbell-like. They did not seem to be budding properly. It is tempting to consider that the virus infection might be responsible for making some strains of African *B. dermatitidis* less pathogenic, but this has not been proven.

It seems that colonization by infectious agents is a general feature of all but the very simplest of life-forms. Infections can reach down, right to the genomic level. Well-studied yeasts, like *Candida albicans* and *Cryptococcus neoformans*, host a wide array of mobile DNA elements in their genomes. These intragenomic "inhabitants" are closely related to the DNA forms of retroviruses [the family of viruses that includes human immunodeficiency virus (HIV) and feline leukemia virus (FeLV)]. These DNA elements can move around in the host genome. As they do so, they may disrupt host genes and cause disease. Such simple disease-causing genomic elements span the boundary between what is *living* and *nonliving* (Holton et al. 2001). They inhabit (or infest, depending on your viewpoint) the genomes of all eukaryotes studied to date.

Not only do hosts vary in complexity, but the infectious agents themselves do, too. Organisms that infect or infest animals range in complexity from prions (infectious proteins devoid of nucleic acid) right up to insects (e.g., *Cuterebra* larvae that develop under the skin of companion animals). Why is it so attractive for a microbe or larger parasite—like a worm or insect—to set up home inside or upon a larger organism? Some of the answers to this question are quite straightforward. The outside world is generally drier, colder, and less well protected from other adverse elements—such as ultraviolet light—than is the inside of an animal's body. To a microbe or larger parasite, parts of the host's body and/or the substances transiting through it represent a rich supply of nutrients. Organisms that adopt a parasitic lifestyle are generally less prone to predation than are their free-living relatives. Infectious agents can travel and become widely dispersed if their host animal ranges over a large geographic area—always assuming there is a way for the microbe to leave one host animal's body and enter another.

This begs the question of how and when infectious agents gain entry to their host's body. Some have evolved structures and/or life stages that are specifically designed to be able to penetrate a host's body. For example, the third larval stage of most species of hookworm (e.g., *Ancylostoma caninum* of dogs and *Bunostomum phlebotomum* of cattle) can actively penetrate the skin or mucous membranes of their hosts and thence travel hematogenously (i.e., via the bloodstream) to the small intestine. Other infectious agents depend on being carried into their host's body by various substances or objects. Substances that adhere to, and transmit, infectious agents are sometimes termed *fomites*. Living organisms that transmit infectious agents are more usually termed *vectors*. Many substances enter or come very close to animals' bodies. Almost all of these can carry microbes and larger parasites into the host's body. Air, dust, food, drinking water, teeth, claws, biting insects' mouthparts, projectiles, surgical instruments, and sexual organs all penetrate or come into direct contact with animal bodies. All can carry infectious agents into an animal's body and can thus be termed fomites or vectors. Some microbes enter animal bodies even before birth or hatching. Many more enter shortly after hatching or birth (e.g., as a consequence of maternal grooming or in colostrum or milk). Some infectious agents—those that blur the distinction between microbe and host—are passed genomically from parent to offspring in a Mendelian fashion and are thus present from conception.

Up to this point, the impression may have been given that life is a bed of roses for the invaders and that host animals are easy prey. Nothing could be further from the truth. Animals have evolved robust barrier defenses and sophisticated, multilayered immune systems to help them avoid becoming overwhelmed by invading organisms. Nevertheless, microbes and even larger parasites such as worms and insects evolve more quickly than veterinary patients and have developed multifarious strategies to penetrate external barriers, circumvent host immunity, and establish persistent infections and infestations. We deal with some of these strategies later.

Only a minority of infectious agents cause disease and are thus termed *pathogens*. The *virulence* of a pathogen (i.e., the extent to which it causes disease compared with its close relatives) is determined by a variety of host and pathogen factors. Some examples of pathogenic mechanisms are

• Some bacterial organisms secrete *toxins* that directly damage host tissues. The more virulent organisms produce more toxin, or perhaps a more potent toxin.

• Other infectious agents provoke an intense inflammatory and immune response by the host, which is, itself, damaging to the host. This process is sometimes termed *immunopathogenesis*. The more virulent organisms provoke more damaging, excessive, inflammation and immune response.

• Some pathogens cause *direct injury* to cells and tissues. For example, some viruses that take over cellular machinery for the purpose of making more virus particles eventually cause cell lysis. Some intestinal nematodes invade mucosal surfaces and cause ulceration and hemorrhage.

• In some infections, a mixture of two or more of the foregoing mechanisms applies.

Figure 3.1 summarizes the pathogenesis of infectious diseases. Table 3.1 provides a list of useful definitions.

TABLE 3.1—Useful definitions

Colonization: Similar to infection. However, this word is used by some authors to connote the overgrowth of normal flora by potentially pathogenic organisms.
Commensalism: A relationship between host and infecting organism that causes detrimental effects to neither.
Congenital infection: Infection present at birth.
Fomite: An inanimate object or substance that transmits infectious organisms from one individual to another.
Flora: Those organisms that usually occupy ecological niches within the host body and do no harm. Indeed, they may prevent colonization by potential pathogens.
Host: An organism capable of supporting the growth and nutrition of another organism upon or inside itself.
Infection: The presence and (usually) multiplication of a living organism upon or inside a host.
Infectious disease: An illness sustained by the host as a consequence of an infection or infestation. By no means do all infections cause disease.
Infestation: Similar to infection, but usually connotes the presence of one or more reasonably large parasitic organisms rather than microbes.
Microflora: Those organisms that usually occupy ecological niches within the host body and do no harm. Indeed, they may prevent colonization by potential pathogens (synonymous with *flora*).
Mutualism: A relationship between host and infecting organism from which both derive benefit. An example would be the production of vitamins by intestinal microflora.
Obligate pathogen: Some authors use this term to describe organisms that almost invariably cause disease when they are present in a host.

continued

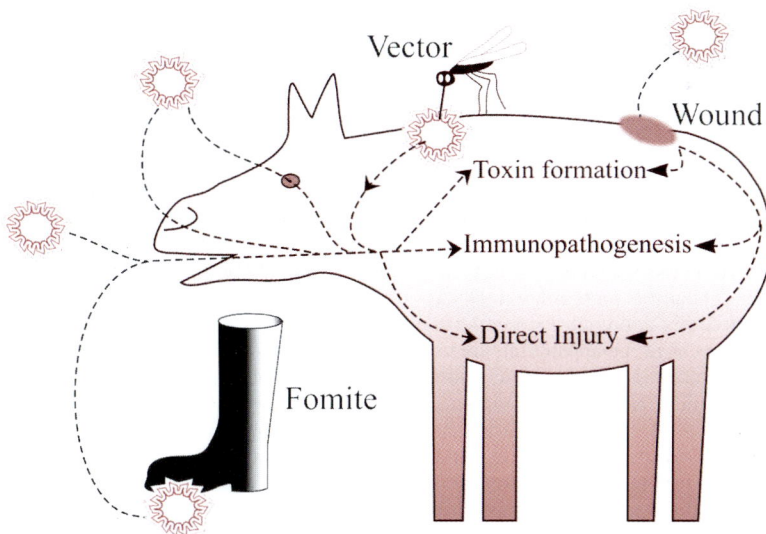

FIG. 3.1—Pathogenesis of infectious disease. Organisms gain entry to the host's body by a variety of routes, including ingestion, inhalation, injection by biting vectors, and direct entry through wounds and abrasions. The host may be exposed to organisms present on fomites. Within the host's body, disease arises as a consequence of direct injury, the effects of toxins and, importantly, as a consequence of the interaction between the pathogen and the host's immune system (immunopathogenesis).

TABLE 3.1—(continued)

Opportunistic pathogen: An organism that usually causes no harm to members of the host species (it may be part of normal flora), but may cause disease if the host is immunosuppressed, or if the organism inadvertently gains entry to host tissues via a puncture wound. Examples include *Pneumocystis carini* pneumonia in canine renal transplant recipients, cryptococcosis in feline immunodeficiency virus-infected cats, and cutaneous sportrichosis in dogs, cats, and people.

Parasitism: A relationship between host and infecting organism from which only the infecting organism derives benefit.

Pathogen (pathogenic organism): An infecting organism that can cause disease. When pathogens are present in a host, they usually cause disease.

Saprophyte: A harmless, free-living organism that usually derives its nutritional needs from decaying matter in the environment. Rarely, saprophytes may gain entry to a host body and cause disease.

Vector: An organism—such as a mosquito or a tick—that can carry disease-causing microorganisms from one host to another.

Virulence: The degree to which an organism is pathogenic, compared with its relatives. The more virulent an organism is, the more severe is the disease it can cause.

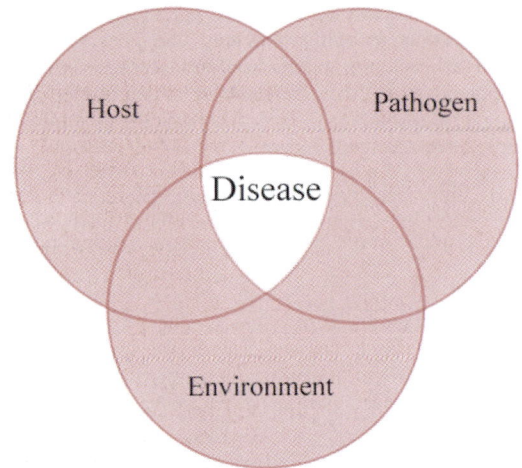

FIG. 3.2—A Venn diagram representing the interrelationship between host, pathogen, and environmental factors in the causation of infectious diseases. Disease occurs only when and where the three sets of predisposing factors converge.

From the foregoing points, it will be clear that an interplay between host and pathogen factors is essential for disease to develop. A third factor, important in many infectious diseases, is the *environment*. Some infectious agents will cause disease only in susceptible hosts under particular environmental conditions. For example, some infectious respiratory diseases of pigs can be avoided if stocking rate (i.e., population density) and air quality (particularly ammonia concentration) are managed correctly. The Venn diagram in Figure 3.2 is a simplified representation of the relationship between host, pathogen, and environmental factors. Disease occurs only when and where the three sets of predisposing factors converge.

Major Categories of Infectious Agent. In the past, all living organisms were categorized as being either plants or animals. Modern methods for analysis of phylogenetic relationships (including recombinant DNA technology) have revealed this approach to be overly simplistic. Debate continues as to the appropriate number and boundaries of fundamental taxonomic categories (domains) into which all living organisms should be designated. Many authorities believe that there are three domains—Archaea, Bacteria, and Eukarya—but this classification scheme does not deal adequately with the prions, viroids, and viruses that span the boundary between living and nonliving. Another recently formulated scheme divides all living things into Viroids, Viruses, Archaea (formerly Archaebacteria), Bacteria (formerly Eubacteria), Eukarya, and Unclassified. Thus, in both schemes, all organisms with distinct cell nuclei—whether unicellular or multicellular—fall into one major group (the Eukarya). Eukarya are further divided into plants, animals, fungi, and pro-

tista. This last group, protista, is the most heterogeneous and least cohesive, including every eukaryote that does not fit properly into one of the other three categories. It is likely that the number and arrangement of fundamental categories of life will change as our understanding of phylogeny improves still further. Nevertheless, using either of the foregoing classification schemes, it is evident that infectious organisms are extremely widespread and diverse in nature. All of these taxonomic groups, except for Viroids, Archaea, and Plantae, contain members known to be pathogenic to animals. In addition, many archaeal species inhabit the gastrointestinal tracts of animals—particularly herbivores—where they are thought to be harmless or beneficial. Prions, viruses, bacteria, fungi, protozoa, and larger parasitic organisms such as helminths and arthropods all infect animals under the care of veterinarians. Infectious organisms have evolved an enormously elaborate and diverse range of capabilities to assist them to overcome the barriers and other defense mechanisms of their prospective hosts. We next examine some of these groups of infectious organisms and their capabilities in more detail.

PRIONS. Prions are infectious agents that do not contain a nucleic acid (Collinge 2001). Simpler than viruses, they consist only of an abnormal protein (PrP, prion protein). The archetypal prion disease is scrapie of sheep. More recently, bovine spongiform encephalopathy (mad cow disease), and variant Creutzfeldt-Jakob disease of people, other prion diseases, have been very much in the news. Cats have also been reported to develop a spongiform encephalopathy is some countries. The abnormal PrP usually gains entry to the host animal when the host ingests infected material from another animal. Upon gaining entry to the host's brain, the infecting PrP is thought to act rather like an enzyme and convert a counterpart or progenitor normal protein (produced in the normal brain) into more abnormal PrP. Thus, a chain reaction or vicious circle of abnormal protein production begins: the more PrP that is produced, the more is available to catalyze conversion of the normal counterpart or "progenitor PrP" to PrP. A large amount of PrP accumulates in the brain, and although it causes no inflammation or immune response, it leads to progressive disruption of normal brain function.

Infection is not the only way that animals can acquire prion diseases. Spontaneous mutation of the gene encoding the aforementioned normal progenitor PrP can lead to the production of PrP in what is essentially a genetic disease. Members of some families are prone to develop prion diseases because they inherit a mutated PrP progenitor gene. Interestingly, brain tissue taken from such spontaneous or familial cases of prion disease is infectious when given to normal animals. Thus, prion diseases blur the boundary between genetic and infectious diseases in an interesting and rather chilling way.

VIROIDS. These tiny relatives of RNA viruses lack a viral capsid. They infect plants and cause disease but are not known to cause animal diseases. They have been well reviewed and are not considered further here (Diener 1999).

VIRUSES. Other than prions and viroids, these obligate intracellular organisms are the smallest infectious agents. They consist chemically of protein, nucleic acid (DNA or RNA; not both) and, in some cases, carbohydrate and lipid. Protein predominates and is arranged as a coat (capsid) around the virus particle. The capsid is made up of numerous identical capsomere building blocks arranged to produce a variety of capsid shapes, including icosahedral and helical forms. Viruses are classified into families according to their nucleic acid content (mostly double-stranded DNA or single-stranded RNA), their capsid shape, and the presence or absence of a lipid envelope around the capsid (usually derived from the host nuclear or cytoplasmic membrane). The classification of viruses is continually being updated as our knowledge grows.

Viruses are incapable of replicating outside of a living cell; thus, they must gain entry to cells. They usually achieve this as a consequence of a specific interaction between a host cell surface receptor and a viral surface molecule. Viral capsid or envelope proteins may be involved in the interaction. Having gained entry to the cell, viruses must uncoat to reveal their nucleic acid and then subvert cellular machinery to make copies of themselves. This usually happens in the cytoplasm for RNA viruses and in the cell nucleus for DNA viruses, but there are exceptions. Copies of some viruses bud from the surfaces of infected cells without damaging the host cell. Other viruses typically cause cell lysis and are released when the cell dies.

Viruses cause a huge variety of acute and chronic diseases in the species under the care of veterinarians. For example, herpesviruses and influenzaviruses can cause acute respiratory disease in horses. Equine herpesviruses can also establish latent infection in the trigeminal ganglia and lymphoid tissues. Subsequent viral reactivation can cause clinical disease and viral shedding during periods of stress. In contrast, feline immunodeficiency virus (FIV) infection typically does not cause noticeable acute disease. Long after the initial infection, it may cause immunodeficiency (associated with opportunistic infections), neurological impairment and, eventually, death. Occasionally this virus, like FeLV, is associated with the development of lymphoid neoplasia.

BACTERIA. Bacteria are unicellular organisms, most of which are capable of living and replicating outside of host cells. They are termed *prokaryotes* because they lack a distinct cell nucleus. Compared with eukaryotic cells (those with a cell nucleus and, usually, other organized cellular organelles), bacterial cells are small and structurally simple. However, they do contain DNA, RNA, ribosomes, and everything else necessary for their own growth and reproduction. Most bacteria are similar in size to the mitochondria of eukaryotic cells; indeed, many biologists believe that mitochondria evolved from prokaryotic organisms that were living as commensals inside larger cells.

Bacteria do not contain mitochondria or other organized structures such as a Golgi apparatus or endoplasmic reticulum. Their genome consists of a single, circular, double-stranded DNA chromosome. There may also be several smaller circular double-stranded DNA molecules called plasmids inside a bacterial cell. Plasmids can be exchanged between bacterial cells in a process reminiscent of sex. Most of the time, plasmids exist in a supercoiled state in the bacterial cell. However, they can uncoil and serve as a template for production of mRNA and protein. Plasmids generally encode specialist phenotypic traits such as resistance to toxins and antibiotics. Mainstream housekeeping traits are encoded on the main chromosome.

Bacteria are surrounded by a cytoplasmic membrane, beyond which most have a *peptidoglycan polymeric cell wall*. Synthesis of this polymer is not carried out by animals, so interference with this process is a suitable target for the development of antibacterial drugs. The cell wall is rigid and dictates the shape of the bacterium (e.g., coccoid, helical, or elongated). Beyond their cell walls, some bacteria have a protective *capsule* and/or slime. Most capsules and slimes are composed of polysaccharides, some of polypeptides, and some of both. Capsules and slime can help to protect bacteria from uptake and ingestion by host immune cells.

Some bacteria have one or more whiplike appendages—termed *flagellae*—that enable them to move around within their aqueous environment. At the base of each flagellum is a "motor" that causes a rotary motion of the entire extracellular part of the flagellum. Each flagellum thus functions rather like a mixture between a gondola's oar and a propeller.

Pili or *fimbriae* are hairlike protuberances that some bacteria possess. They are shorter and thinner than flagellae. Some pili enable bacteria to adhere to host cell surfaces. Others, termed *sex pili*, enable the transfer of plasmids between bacterial cells.

Most bacteria reproduce by simple cell division. Under suitable conditions, a single bacterial cell can replicate to produce millions in several hours. Bacteria with strict growth requirements are termed *fastidious*. Those that require oxygen for growth are termed *aerobes*, whereas those that cannot survive in an oxygen-containing environment are called *anaerobes*. Those that can survive in the presence of oxygen or in anaerobic conditions are called *facultative anaerobes*.

A few groups of potentially pathogenic bacteria deserve special mention. *Mycoplasmas*, known since 1898, are less than one-third the size of most bacteria, and their genome is about half the size of the average bacterial chromosome. They are the smallest and simplest prokaryotes capable of replicating themselves by using their own enzymatic machinery. Mycoplasmas lack rigid cell walls and hence vary markedly in shape. They are resistant to antibacterial drugs that target cell wall synthesis. Some reproduce sexually rather than by binary fission. Many live as commensals on the mucous membranes of the respiratory, urogenital, and gastrointestinal tracts of their hosts. Others can cause pneumonia, arthritis, mastitis, and genital infections.

Rickettsiae, Chlamydiae, Ehrlichiae, and Coxiella are all obligate intracellular bacterial organisms. In this respect, they sit at the boundary between bacteria and viruses. However, in other respects, they are far more like bacteria than viruses. They form rigid peptidoglycan cell walls, are susceptible to various antibiotics, and reproduce by binary fission. They can carry out many of the metabolic activities of free-living, extracellular bacteria, but some require energy in the form of adenosine triphosphate (ATP) from the host cell, and others require various other nutrients and vitamins. Chlamydiae are transmitted directly between host animals, whereas rickettsiae and ehrlichiae are usually transmitted via arthropod vectors (e.g., ticks). Rickettsiae can cause potentially lethal diseases like Rocky Mountain spotted fever. *Coxiella burnetti* is the causative agent of Q fever in people. It can infect animals important to veterinarians, including cattle, sheep, and goats. People may become infected at abattoirs during meat processing, if the organism becomes aerosolized. In people, *C. burnetti* causes a nonspecific febrile illness with headache, painful joints, and mild pneumonia.

FUNGI. Fungi include some of the simplest of eukaryotes. Most are free-living saprophytic organisms, but a minority live as parasites or commensal organisms in and upon plants and animals. Fungi cause many economically important plant diseases but fewer parasitic diseases in the animal species under the care of veterinarians. Ingestion of certain fungus-infected plant materials can cause a range of economically important diseases in herbivores, but these are really intoxications rather than true infectious diseases.

Fungal diseases of animals are often relatively mild and involve only the skin, but there are some more serious *systemic mycoses* that involve deeper tissues. Although sexual reproduction is possible, most fungi arise from spores—termed *conidia*—that are produced asexually. From conidia grow *hyphae*, elongated filamentous structures that may branch and develop cross walls (*septae*). A mass of hyphae forms a mat termed a *mycelium*. For example, the hyphae of the potentially pathogenic fungus *Aspergillus fumigatus* are characteristically branching and septate and may form visible mycelia in the respiratory structures of animals. In dogs, *A. fumigatus* can cause destructive rhinitis (inflammation inside the nasal cavities). In horses, *A. fumigatus* can erode arterial walls in the guttural pouches, leading to massive, life-threatening epistaxis (nosebleeding). In numerous bird species *A. fumigatus* infects the air sacs and lungs, often leading to death.

Some parasitic fungi are found as simple, round-to-oval yeast forms. An example is *Malassezia pachydermatis*, which is a common commensal organism in canine ears but can multiply to massively elevated numbers and contribute to extremely uncomfortable disease under suitable environmental conditions (e.g., wax accumulation, excessive moisture, or compromised skin barrier due to inflammation).

Some fungi (e.g., *Blastomyces dermatitidis* and *Candida albicans*) grow as yeasts at one temperature and as molds (or mycelia) at another and are hence termed *dimorphic*. It is the yeast form of dimorphic fungi that usually grows in mammalian and avian tissues and the mycelial form that grows in the usually much cooler external environment. Dimorphic growth facilitates the dispersal of the organism: yeasts are relatively fragile and replicate only by simple budding, whereas massive numbers of hardy conidia are released into the atmosphere from specialized hyphal reproductive structures. *Blastomyces dermatitidis*, which has already been mentioned as a cause of pneumonia in a wide range of mammalian species, can also cause ulcerated skin lesions, osteomyelitis, and genitourinary and ocular lesions. *Candida albicans* can cause dermatitis and mucous membrane infections in debilitated animals, especially if immunosuppressant drugs or broad-spectrum antibiotics have been used long term.

PROTOZOA. Protozoa are unicellular eukaryotes with many features reminiscent of simple animals. Like fungi, most are free-living. Amoebas are archetypal. In the five-kingdom classification scheme outlined earlier, all protozoans belong in the kingdom Protista or Protoctista. In addition to amoebas (among the very simplest of all eukaryotes), there are flagellated and ciliated protozoa, sporozoans, and microsporidians of veterinary and medical importance.

Some of the ciliated protozoa are among the most complex of unicellular organisms. Apart from cilia for motility, they also have weapons for capturing food and defending themselves and structures for expelling excess water and other waste substances. Parasitic protozoa cause a wide variety of diseases in their hosts. Many protozoal infections cause gastrointestinal signs (e.g., anorexia, vomiting, diarrhea, and weight loss), enlarged lymph nodes (termed *lymphadenopathy*), and/or anemia in their hosts, though all manner of other disease manifestations are possible.

LARGER PARASITES. Helminths and arthropods are the most important of the larger parasites. Helminths, in decreasing order of veterinary importance, include nematodes (roundworms), platyhelminths (flukes and tapeworms), acanthocephalids (thorny-headed worms, pathogenic to aquatic birds and, occasionally, to pigs), and annelids (segmented worms, including leeches). Helminth infestations of farmed animals are of huge economic importance in many parts of the world.

Ticks, mites, and insects are the most important of the arthropod parasites. Ticks and mites are by far the most numerous and diverse of the arachnids, and, by virtue of their parasitic lifestyle and their potential to cause and transmit diseases, they are the best studied, too. A diverse range of insects pursues a parasitic way of life. Fleas, lice, biting flies (including mosquitoes and midges), and true bugs (Hemiptera) all parasitize animals of veterinary importance.

The bites of some of these larger parasites are uncomfortable (e.g., tabanid flies) and may reduce farm animal productivity, but it is the potential of some of these parasites to transmit life-threatening microbial infectious diseases that makes them particularly important.

Virulence Factors. From the foregoing, it is apparent that a horde of diverse organisms infects and infests animals of veterinary importance. Every successful parasite or infectious organism has evolved a repertoire of mechanisms to gain entry to its host and, once there, to evade eviction and to flourish. Given the diversity of infectious organisms, it is not surprising that innumerable subtly different approaches have evolved. However, the fundamental obstacles that must be overcome to gain entry and to persist depend more on the host than on the infectious organism. Hence, some intriguing examples of convergent evolution can be found when one studies the attributes and mechanisms employed by organisms in the process of establishing and maintaining infections.

ADHESION. Although some infectious agents can infect a wide variety of hosts (e.g., the rabies virus), most show a high degree of *host specificity*. Hosts of a particular species are favored. Sometimes, the specificity extends below the species level to certain breeds, races, or strains of host animal. Often, infection is restricted to particular organs, tissues, and/or cells within the host's body. Some of this specificity can be explained in terms of an inability of infectious agents to adhere to cells or tissues other than the ones to which they are adapted. Adhesion of microbes generally involves a rather specific interaction between molecules on the surface of the infectious agent (termed *ligands* or *adhesins*) and *receptors* in the host's cell surface membranes. For example, FIV—like other retroviruses—has multiple copies of a surface glycoprotein (termed SU, for surface) decorating its outer envelope. Retroviral SU molecules bind host cell surface receptors in an adhesion process that can lead to cell-cell fusion as well as entry of viruses into cells. Some strains of FIV—particularly some that are adapted to grow in vitro—are known to bind a host cell surface molecule called CXCR4 as their primary receptor (Willett and Hosie 1999). CXCR4 is an α–chemokine receptor and is present on cells of a wide range of animals, including people and cats. Actually, CXCR4 is an important coreceptor for some strains of HIV-1, needed for cell entry along with the better-known CD4 receptor. Each host species has a slightly different form of CXCR4; that of cats has an amino acid sequence 94.9% similar to that of humans. CXCR4 is expressed only on certain host cells, for example, astrocytes and lymphocytes; and these are the kinds of cell that can therefore be infected by CXCR4-dependent strains of FIV. Studying such strains of FIV is beginning to yield insights, not only into feline immunodeficiency, but also into human AIDS-associated dementia and immunodeficiency.

Bacteria, fungi, and protozoa similarly express adhesion molecules on their surfaces; in the case of bacteria, often on their pili or fimbriae. Bacterial, fungal, and protozoal adhesion molecules are usually termed adhesins or colonization factors. Chemically, most adhesins are glycoproteins or lipoproteins. They often bind to sugar moieties on the surfaces of host cells. Expression or lack of expression of adhesins can be a defining feature of bacterial virulence. For example, in a recent study, 56% of *Escherichia coli* isolates obtained from canine fecal samples gathered in a public park were described as pathogenic because they were *papG* allele III positive. *papG* allele III is a gene that encodes variant III of the P-fimbrial adhesin molecule PapG. A later study showed many canine urinary *E. coli* strains also to be *papG* allele III positive. Interestingly, *papG* allele III positive strains of *E. coli* are pathogenic to people, so canine urine and feces may act as an important and worrying reservoir of human pathogens (Johnson et al. 2001). In Figure 3.3, a bacterium with surface pili is shown. As an inset, the location of adhesin molecules (such as PapG) at the tip of a pilus is shown.

Further evidence that bacterial, fungal, and protozoal adhesins are bona fide virulence factors comes from the fact that novel vaccines made from adhesins seem to protect against disease. An *E. coli* pilus vaccine pro-

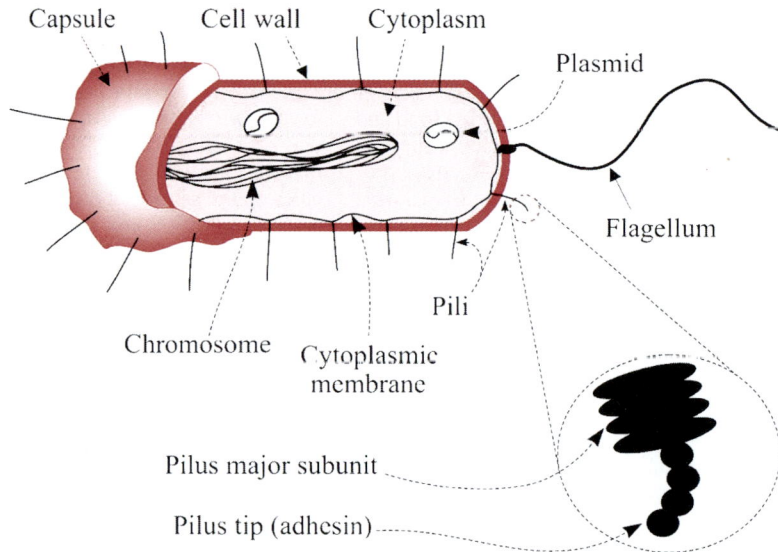

Capsule   Cell wall   Cytoplasm

Plasmid

Chromosome   Cytoplasmic membrane

Pili

Flagellum

Pilus major subunit

Pilus tip (adhesin)

FIG. 3.3—Many species of bacteria bear long, flexible, proteinaceous appendages on their surfaces, termed fimbriae or pili. These structures are important in adhesion to host cells. Formerly, pili were thought to be homopolymeric, composed of about 1000 identical copies of a single structural subunit. More recently, it has been shown that minor proteins are located at the distal end of the organelle. These adhesin molecules bind to host cell surface molecules, usually carbohydrates.

tects swine against diarrhea (scours). A peptide vaccine made from the *Entamoeba histolytica* galactose-binding adhesin protected gerbils against amebic liver abscesses (Lotter et al. 2000). A novel vaccine being developed from the *B. dermatitidis* adhesin WI-1 shows promise (Klein 2000).

When microbes grow in clusters, or colonies, not all of them need to adhere directly to host cells or other solid surfaces. Staphylococci can attach to indwelling intravenous plastic catheters and eventually form a confluent biofilm over the plastic surface. Some of the bacteria are undoubtedly attached to the plastic by nonspecific electrostatic, hydrophobic, and other forces, but many more are held together by bacterially produced slime. Because catheters so easily become infected, aseptic technique is essential during catheter placement. If a catheter-associated bacterial infection becomes established, antibiotics are usually ineffective, in part because of the slime. Removal of the catheter is the best course of action.

Larger infectious agents and parasites attach or "adhere" to their hosts by various anatomical structures including mouthparts and legs. Hooks and suckers often provide a tenacious grip, for example, that achieved by feeding ticks.

In many cases, the receptors and mechanisms used by infectious agents of veterinary importance to attach to host cells have not yet been properly identified. The specific pathophysiological consequences of receptor occupation by microbial ligands have, likewise, not been studied in depth. In the future, when receptor-ligand interactions are understood in more detail, exciting new opportunities to understand disease mechanisms and therefore to develop more effective therapeutic interventions will be presented.

INVASION. Invasive factors enable infectious agents to penetrate host barriers. Many bacterial, fungal, and protozoal invasive factors are secreted enzymes capable of breaching cell membranes (e.g., phospholipases) or digesting connective tissues (e.g., elastase, collagenase, hyaluronidase, and protease). Such bludgeoning tactics can cause much tissue damage and are not without risk to the invader. As our understanding of microbial pathogenesis improves, it is becoming clear that many infectious agents use much more subtle and sophisticated methods to invade their hosts' cells and tissues.

Nearly all host cells have *integrin* receptors on their surfaces. Integrins consist of α and β chains, and there are many variant forms. They enable cells to recognize one another and to recognize elements of the extracellular matrix. Integrins interact with the cell's actin cytoskeleton, providing a mechanism for the plasma membrane to interact with the cell's interior and initiate changes in the cell's shape. Integrins are able to mediate cellular activation, adhesion, migration, and phagocytosis by interacting with various ligands in their environment. Importantly, integrins found on leukocyte cell surfaces are activated by many cellular stimuli, such as bacterial components, chemokines, cytokines, and immunoglobulin G (IgG)-containing immune complexes.

Since integrins are almost ubiquitous on host cell surfaces and their ligation can initiate phagocytosis (i.e., ingestion by the host cell), it is not surprising that microbial invaders have evolved to take advantage of them as a means of gaining entry to cells. Some viruses and bacteria mimic host proteins and thereby subvert integrins to invade cells. For example, enteropathogenic *Yersinia* bacterial organisms express a protein termed *invasin* on their surfaces. Invasin is a ligand for β_1 integrins present on the surfaces of intestinal epithelial cells. The invasin-integrin interaction induces uptake of the bacterium by the intestinal epithelial cell (Isberg et al. 2000).

More impressively, several groups of bacteria engineer their own phagocytosis by macrophages, one of the larger cells of the immune system. They achieve this apparently dangerous feat by attaching complement—in the form of C3bi—to themselves. Macrophages ingest organisms that are coated with C3bi complement by using an integrin called CR3. Normally, bacteria would be killed and digested after ingestion by a macrophage, but CR3-mediated phagocytosis of C3bi-opsonized bacteria does not activate microbicidal responses inside the macrophage, so the bacteria can survive. Some of these macrophage invaders have further mechanisms that enable them to interfere with intracellular signaling pathways to prevent further microbicidal responses. By invading phagocytes, these pathogens find a safe haven inside the very cells that should be attacking them.

Larger infectious agents and parasites may burrow or puncture their way through host barrier defenses to gain entry. Biting mouthparts of insects, ticks, and leeches are all too familiar to us. Less well known are the ancylostomatoid hookworms that parasitize all higher mammals except members of the Equidae. L_3 larvae of some of these worms are quite effective at penetrating the skin of their hosts, in addition to using the more conventional fecal-oral transmission route. Not surprisingly, some microbes have evolved to take advantage of the very convenient activities of these larger parasites and use them as *vectors*. For example, Babesiae, Ehrlichiae, Rickettsiae, and the spirochete *Borrelia burgdorferi* are transmitted to their mammalian hosts by various species of ticks. Bloodsucking sand flies transmit leishmaniasis, and reduviid bugs transmit trypanosomiasis. Many more examples could be cited.

One particularly intriguing example of a microbe that uses a vector to invade its host concerns so-called salmon poisoning disease of dogs (Gorham and Foreyt 1998). This is a rickettsial infection caused by *Neorickettsia helminthoeca*. The vector of the causal organism in this case is a trematode (fluke) that infests salmon. The fluke *Nanophyetus salmincola* harbors the rickettsiae throughout its life cycle, from egg to adult. Dogs become infested and infected when they eat dead salmon. The trematode infests the dog successfully, but, more importantly, the rickettsial organism gains entry to the dog's body and causes a rapidly fatal illness characterized by fever, anorexia, weight loss, and enlarged lymph nodes (termed *lymphadenopathy*). This is an intriguing expression of the saying, "Little fleas have lesser fleas upon their backs to bite them, and lesser fleas have smaller fleas and so ad infinitum."

EVASION. Once infectious agents have invaded the host's body, they must evade various host immune defenses (as covered in detail in the next section). They must successfully spread throughout the host tissues to which they are adapted and, usually, they must reproduce. A wide variety of evasive tactics are employed; one we have already encountered is invasion of cells. Under some circumstances, the intracellular environment is a safe haven, well away from immune surveillance. Evasive tactics may be very simple: for example, motile bacteria like *Helicobacter felis* can move away from danger; alternatively the tactics may be highly sophisticated: some protozoa express a sequence of different antigens on their cell surfaces during the course of infection, so as to evade detection by the immune system—an example of a protozoal "leopard changing its spots" with alarming frequency.

Sturdy cell walls, bacterially produced slime, and polysaccharide capsules can help pathogens to avoid immune destruction. Yet, bacterial cell walls are more than a resilient barrier to the outside world. Pathogenic strains of *Staphylococcus aureus* have substantial amounts of a protein, termed *protein A*, as part of their cell walls. Protein A can bind to one end—called the F_c (short for *fragment crystallizable*) end—of antibody molecules of the IgG class. F_c is needed to bind to receptors on immune cells in order for antibody-mediated phagocytosis (i.e., ingestion of antibody-coated pathogens) to take place. By binding to the F_c portions of many IgG molecules, protein A "mops up" many antibody molecules that would otherwise be available to attack *S. aureus*. Other cell wall constituents of both Gram-positive and Gram-negative bacteria have been shown to block antibody- and complement-mediated bacterial cell lysis by a variety of other mechanisms (Wilks and Sissons 1997).

Trypanosoma brucei is the protozoal causative agent of African trypanosomiasis, an important disease of animals and people (it causes sleeping sickness in people). Dogs are particularly susceptible to the subspecies *T. brucei brucei*. Trypanosomiasis is transmitted by tsetse flies of the genus *Glossina*. *Trypanosoma brucei* is covered by a confluent glycoprotein layer that limits activation of one immune component—complement—on its surface but can also serve as a target for antibody attack. This glycoprotein layer undergoes continual, rapid, and spontaneous variation in composition; hence, it is called the variable surface glycoprotein (VSG). By constantly varying the composition of its VSG coat, *T. brucei* can remain one step ahead of the host immune system. There are estimated to be more than 1000 different VSG-encoding genes in the trypanosomal genome, so the potential for variation, and hence immune evasion, is huge.

Furthermore, infectious agents have an impressive array of offensive and defensive mechanisms that come into play only once they have engaged the immune system in combat. We have already learned that some microbes can survive or even encourage phagocytosis by macrophages and evade being killed once inside the immune cells. We say more about the interplay between microbes and the immune system in the next section.

TOXIGENICITY. Adhesion, invasion, and evasion are undoubtedly crucial capabilities of infectious agents. Toxin production is not always crucial to the pathogen. In contemplating toxin production, we are for the first time examining a characteristic of infectious agents very much from the viewpoint of the host, not the pathogen. Not surprisingly, a hugely diverse range of toxins is produced by infectious agents; after all, anything toxic to the host animal qualifies. In many cases, the toxicity of a microbial product does, indeed, contribute to the evolutionary success of the pathogen. In other cases, however, the toxicity of a particular microbial product is unfortunate for the host but largely irrelevant to the pathogen.

Many bacteria produce toxins. These can be divided into cell-associated *endotoxins*, produced by Gram-negative bacteria, and proteinaceous *exotoxins*, which are usually secreted by the organisms that produce them.

Exotoxins are potent and often responsible for the clinical features of bacterial infectious disease, including death. Both Gram-positive and Gram-negative bacteria produce exotoxins. Some of the more familiar exotoxins are those produced by clostridial organisms. For example, tetanospasmin, produced by *C. tetani*, and various neurotoxins produced by *C. botulinum* are responsible for most of the clinical features of tetanus and botulism, respectively.

Bacillus anthracis, the causative agent of anthrax, produces two distinct A-B binary exotoxins from three precursors named protective antigen (PA), edema factor (EF), and lethal factor (LF). Individually, these components cause no harm, but when either EF or LF is given with PA, disease or death ensues. PA is a receptor-binding protein, named for its protective effect when included in anthrax vaccines. Once PA has bound to its high-affinity cell surface receptor, it is proteolytically cleaved, exposing a binding site to which EF or LF can bind. EF and LF combine with PA molecules to form the A-B binary toxins *Edema toxin* and *Lethal toxin*, respectively. These toxins enter cells by endocytosis and PA subsequently assists LF and EF to enter the cytosol where they exert their pathogenic effects (Ascenzi et al. 2002) (see Figure 3.4).

Other exotoxins work by disrupting cell membranes. Some have phospholipase activity (e.g., the α-toxin of *Clostridium perfringens*), whereas others insert themselves into the lipid bilayer, forming a protein pore that disrupts the cell's ability to conserve its internal environment (e.g., the α-toxin and the δ-toxin of *S. aureus*).

Still other exotoxins act like peptide hormones, signaling across intact cell membranes. Heat-stable enterotoxins of strains of *E. coli*, related to those that cause diarrhea in piglets, bind to cell-membrane guanylate cyclase and cause an increase in intracellular cyclic guanosine monophosphate. In turn, this causes changes in sodium and chloride transmembrane transport and leads to a voluminous secretory diarrhea.

Toxin production benefits bacteria in a wide variety of ways. By causing diarrhea, organisms increase the volume and dispersion of infected material that may be encountered by potential, new hosts. Antimicrobial substances may be diluted. Nutrients, particularly iron, may be made more available by toxins that lyse host cells. Some clostridial toxins damage tissues in a way that promotes an anaerobic environment, essential for these organisms to grow optimally. Many exotoxins are antiphagocytic.

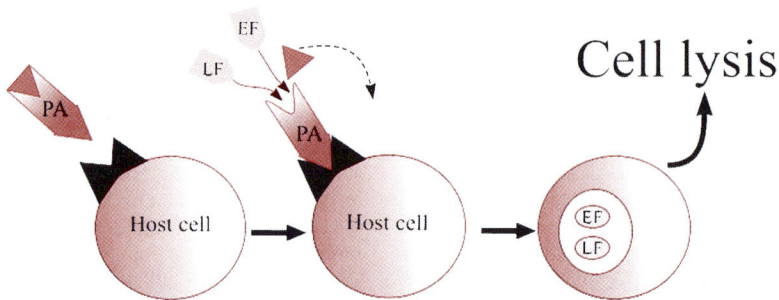

FIG. 3.4—Toxigenicity of *Bacillus anthracis*. *Bacillus anthracis*, the causative agent of anthrax, produces two distinct A-B binary exotoxins from three precursors: protective antigen (PA), edema factor (EF), and lethal factor (LF). Individually, each component causes no harm, but when either EF or LF is given with PA, disease or death ensues. PA is a receptor-binding protein, named for its protective effect when included in anthrax vaccines. Once PA has bound to its high-affinity cell surface receptor, it is proteolytically cleaved, exposing a binding site to which EF or LF can bind. EF and LF combine with PA molecules to form the A-B binary toxins edema toxin and lethal toxin, respectively. These toxins enter cells by endocytosis, and PA subsequently assists LF and EF to enter the cytosol, where they exert their pathogenic effects. (Adapted from Ascenzi et al. 2002.)

Endotoxins differ substantially from exotoxins. Produced by Gram-negative organisms, endotoxins are not secreted; rather, they are passively released during cell growth and at the time of bacterial cell lysis. Chemically, they are heat-stable lipopolysaccharides (LPS); in fact, the terms LPS and endotoxin are often used synonymously. The toxic activity resides in the lipid portion of the endotoxin molecule, while repeating sugar moieties on a long side chain may engender an immune response in some hosts. Endotoxins form a substantial portion of the cell walls of Gram-negative bacteria.

Endotoxins have numerous, incompletely understood, adverse effects upon the host. Much of the damage inflicted is indirect, being caused by overzealous release of inflammatory mediators and other substances by the host's immune system. Endotoxins contribute substantially to the pathogenesis of often-fatal septic shock, although, again, this clinical entity is incompletely understood. Endotoxemia (i.e., endotoxin in the blood) has been associated with fever, hypoglycemia, hypotension (low blood pressure), shock, disseminated intravascular coagulation, multiple-organ failure, and death.

LPS molecules in the cell walls of Gram-negative bacteria form a physical barrier to attack by the immune system. The long, externally exposed carbohydrate side chains help keep components of the host's immune system (e.g., complement membrane-attack complex; see the section *Complement*) at arm's length. The toxicity of LPS/endotoxin is largely a consequence of the host's immune response; it is not clear that this toxicity is of primary importance to the pathogen.

Bacterial toxins have been well studied, but, of course, bacteria are not the only infectious agents that produce toxins. A few viral components are directly toxic; for instance, the transmembrane protein of some strains of FeLV has been reported to be immunosuppressive. Invasive fungi, protozoa, and even arthropod parasites produce toxins (e.g., the one causing tick paralysis in dogs). Some of the fungal toxins of greatest veterinary importance are not produced by infectious organisms per se. Rather, they are ingested preformed in contaminated food, as is also typical for the clostridial botulinum toxin. Herbivores that ingest ergot alkaloids or sporidesmin develop ergotism and facial eczema, respectively. Ingestion of penitrem A, a toxin produced by *Penicillium crustosum* when grown on moldy walnuts, can lead to a severe tremoring illness in California dogs.

CYTOPATHICITY. Viruses do not generally produce toxins but may damage cells by a variety of mechanisms, including subversion of cellular machinery for production of more viral particles. One of the most obvious cytopathic effects is virally mediated cell lysis. From the virus's viewpoint, lytic infection releases a large number of viral particles quickly. Conversely, viruses that bud from cell membranes without destroying their host cell (e.g., retroviruses) can persist and replicate within an infected cell over a long period. Some viruses use both strategies; for example, some herpesviruses (like the one that causes feline rhinotracheitis) lytically infect epithelial cells but can persist for extremely long periods in trigeminal ganglion sensory neurons without killing them. How they manage to behave so differently in these two separate cellular environments is uncertain but may have something to do with the relatively long distance between the sensory nerve endings where herpesviruses gain entry to sensory neurons and the cell bodies where they replicate.

Cell lysis is not the only cytopathic effect caused by viruses. For example, there are quite a number of theories about how lentiviral immunodeficiency viruses like bovine immunodeficiency virus (BIV), FIV, and HIV may kill cells. High-level budding of virus particles from cell surfaces may adversely increase cell-membrane permeability, leading to cell death. Interaction of viral surface glycoprotein (SU) on infected cells with receptors on uninfected cells may lead to cell-cell fusion and, eventually, the formation of large, nonviable, multinucleate syncytia. Buildup of viral proteins and circular proviral DNA molecules inside host cells may be directly toxic. There is growing evidence that induction of apoptosis (programmed cell death) by viruses may be an important cytopathic effect. Conversely, some viruses produce antiapoptotic signals to extend the life of the infected cell so that it can continue to produce virus particles for longer.

It is important to realize that the recognition of a striking cytopathic effect caused by a virus in cells grown outside the body (i.e., in tissue culture) does not guarantee that the virus will be a highly pathogenic one. For example, foamy viruses like feline syncytium-forming virus produce a startling cytopathic effect in vitro but are uniformly nonpathogenic in vivo (Linial 2000). This may be a consequence of an effective host immune response in vivo or may be due to altered expression of gene products by the virus in the two different environments (in vivo versus in vitro).

MUTAGENESIS AND ONCOGENESIS. Infectious agents can cause mutations in host cells either indirectly or directly. Such mutations sometimes lead to the development of cancer (i.e., oncogenesis; see Chapter 13). A wide variety of infectious agents can cause mutations indirectly; for example, by inducing inflammation and/or dramatically increasing the replication rate of some host cells and therefore increasing the raw material upon which natural mutagenic agents (like cosmic rays) can act. Direct mutagenesis is most likely to be caused by certain DNA viruses and retroviruses because they have the most intimate association with host cell DNA. Of the viruses implicated in the causation of cancer, the retroviruses have been most thoroughly studied. FeLV, discovered by a veterinarian in Scotland in 1964, was the first retrovirus proved to cause a naturally occurring cancer in an outbred mammalian species.

Integration of retroviral proviral DNA into a host cell chromosome represents, by definition, a mutational event. Many such insertional mutations will cause no deleterious effects to the cell and produce no phenotypic change in the host. Integration at other genomic sites may produce a lethal effect. If integration confers a selective advantage upon the infected cell, then its progeny cells will increase in number. An extreme example of this is retroviral oncogenesis, in which infected cells continue to grow and replicate beyond control.

Certain cellular genes, termed *proto-oncogenes* or *cellular oncogenes*, can be activated by retroviral provirus integration to increase the probability of neoplastic transformation of the infected cell. Tumors caused in this way often develop only after a long latent period. This is, at least in part, because proviral insertion in the necessary position relative to a proto-oncogene is a chance event that takes time to occur. Because of the long latent period, retroviruses acting via this oncogenic mechanism are sometimes termed *weakly oncogenic*. Less frequently, retroviruses capture or *transduce* proto-oncogenes. The transduced oncogene usually replaces one of the recipient virus's essential genes, so a defective virus results. However, with the assistance of a normal helper virus, such defective oncogene-carrying viruses can infect new cells and rapidly cause neoplastic transformation (see Figure 3.5). Such oncogene-carrying retroviruses are termed *strongly oncogenic*. Actually, oncogenes were first dis-

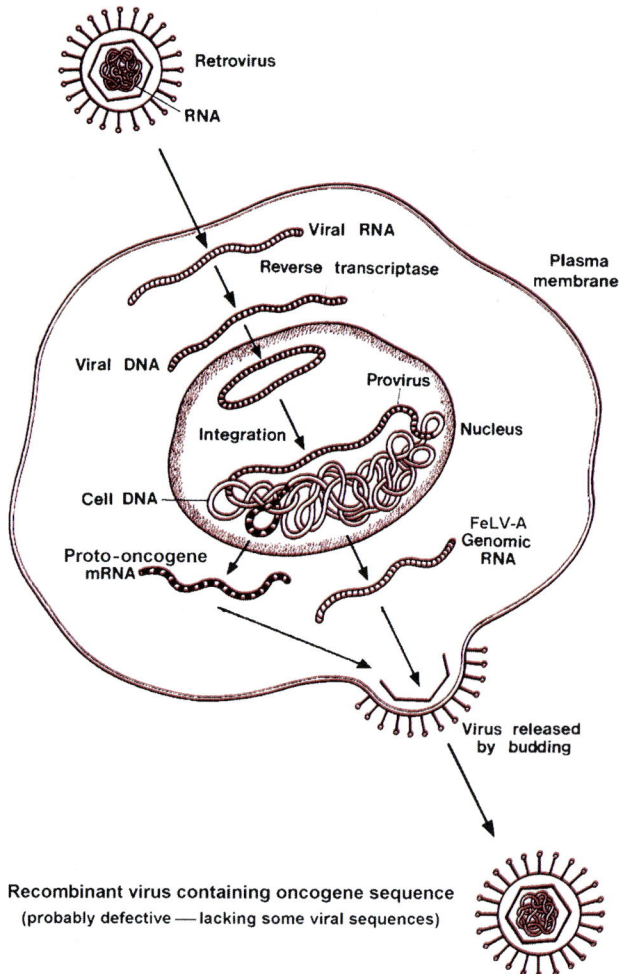

FIG. 3.5—Viruses can cause neoplasia by a variety of means. One method used by some retroviruses involves the capture or transduction of cellular proto-oncogenes. The transduced oncogene usually replaces one of the recipient virus's essential genes so that a defective virus results. However, with the assistance of a normal helper virus, such defective oncogene-carrying viruses can infect new cells and rapidly cause neoplastic transformation. FeLV-A, feline leukemia virus A.

covered in such strongly oncogenic, recombinant retroviruses. It was only later realized that retroviral oncogenes (v-*onc*s) are derived from cellular progenitor genes (c-*onc*s).

Turning our attention away from viruses, a much more complex parasitic organism that is frequently associated with oncogenesis is the nematode of canids and wild felids: *Spirocerca lupi*. A recent review of South African cases of *S. lupi* infestation in dogs suggests that almost half of all diagnosed cases are associated with development of esophageal cancer, usually osteosarcoma or fibrosarcoma. Other studies suggest that a much smaller proportion of infested dogs develop neoplasia. Eggs of this large, coiled reddish worm are present in the feces of infested dogs. Eggs are ingested inadvertently by a coprophagous beetle, in whose body cavity they hatch, develop to L_3, and encyst. The beetle is either ingested directly by a dog or else eaten by a paratenic host (e.g., a lizard or bird), which is subsequently eaten by a dog. L_3 larvae are released in the dog's stomach and migrate into and along the wall of the gastroepiploic artery to reach the thoracic aorta. After several months, parasites emerge from the aortic wall and invade the adjacent esophagus, where they provoke chronic inflammation and formation of a large fibrous nodule, in which they live, reproduce, and from which the females release eggs into the esophageal lumen. It is clearly to the advantage of the parasite that it can provoke chronic inflammation and consequent formation of the large fibrous nodule in which it lives. Some of these nodules go on to become neoplastic. This is very unfortunate for the host but probably largely irrelevant to the parasite. The processes by which chronic inflammation sometimes leads to neoplasia are highly important—for example, in terms of the role of *Helicobacter pylori*-associated gastritis in the genesis of gastric carcinoma. Unfortunately, these processes are, as yet, incompletely understood.

Desirable Infections. Some of the relationships between infectious agents and their hosts are truly ancient. It is certainly not in any infectious agent's best interest to annihilate its host species outright, so, not surprisingly, many examples of a mature *détente* between host and infectious agent can be found in nature. Indeed, one could reasonably argue that, over millennia, a pathogen might be expected to become progressively less pathogenic to its chosen host as their relationship matures. Conversely, when a pathogen jumps species, i.e., manages to establish a productive infection in a species other than its usual one, it may at first be exceedingly pathogenic to members of the new host species. Another less teleological way of expressing this notion is to argue that nature may select against host-pathogen relationships in which the pathogen is exceedingly pathogenic in favor of those in which the pathogen is less pathogenic to its host. Of course, this will depend on many factors, including whether the

pathogen significantly affects the overall reproductive success of its host. However, I am unaware of any research proving that infections evolve to become milder over time.

Perhaps the most extreme example of the maturing of a relationship between host and infectious agent is one in which the infectious agent becomes useful, or even essential, to its host. We have already mentioned that mitochondria are thought to represent the descendants of commensal bacteria living within eukaryotic cells. Perhaps the next most obvious example of a vital infection concerns the billions of archaea, bacteria, protozoa, and fungi that inhabit the gastrointestinal tracts of ruminants and many other herbivores. These organisms are essential for their hosts to digest the structural plant materials, such as cellulose, that they depend upon. Without them, their hosts would suffer starvation and death.

Endogenous retroviruses, or their close relatives, infest all animals studied to date at a genomic level. Arguably, these are the most fundamental of all parasites. Recently, it has become apparent that the proportion of mammalian DNA contributed by endogenous retroviruses and their relatives has been grossly underestimated. Although 8% of the human genome is comprised of endogenous retroviruses and their close relatives, a staggering 45% of the human genome consists of retrovirus-like elements and their more distant relatives, such as nonviral retroposons and transposons. We know from comparing the genomes of diverse animals that many endogenous retroviral elements are indeed ancient. Most are mutating gradually, or eroding; they can be considered clinically irrelevant "genomic fossils." However, a few ancient ones have an almost pristine structure; it has been persuasively argued that they are being conserved because they serve a useful (or, stated another way, evolutionarily adaptive) purpose. Usually, their presumed function is obscure; however, in a few cases, a purpose is becoming evident. For example, endogenous retroviruses may play a role in human salivary amylase expression (Ting et al. 1992; Samuelson et al. 1996) and mammalian placental morphogenesis (Mi et al. 2000)

HOST RESPONSES TO INFECTION

Overview. As stated in the last section, despite their panoply of highly evolved defensive and offensive mechanisms, infectious agents do not get it all their own way. Their hosts have necessarily evolved sophisticated immune defenses to avoid becoming overwhelmed by invaders. In many situations, hosts have forged stalwart alliances with some organisms, tolerating or even encouraging their presence, in order to thwart the colonizing efforts of more pathogenic organisms. Barriers such as skin and mucous membranes are challenging for invaders to penetrate, not only because of their robust physicochemical properties appreciable from examination of a histological snapshot, but also because of impressive dynamic properties. Skin is continually exfoliating, casting off would-be invaders. Some mucous membranes are equipped with beating cilia and special mucus, actively carrying away organisms that alight on their surfaces on a so-called *mucociliary escalator* or *blanket*. Those organisms that manage to get past these primary barriers encounter a battery of immune defenses of startling range and complexity. The host may raise its body temperature to a level at which the invader finds it difficult to function. Vital nutrients may be actively sequestered by the host, in places where the invader cannot gain access. Various antimicrobial cells and substances already present in the host's body prior to the arrival of the invader are immediately available to defend. Most impressive of all, though, is that a tailored immune response, exquisitely appropriate to the particular type of infection, is rapidly mounted by the host. Moreover, the specificity and intensity of this response improve over the course of infection. After an infection, the host's immune system can often "remember" the infectious agent for years so that it is all the more ready to deal with subsequent infections by the same type of organism.

Immune defenses are commonly divided into two fundamental categories, often termed *innate* and *adaptive*. More recently, the words *constitutive* and *nonspecific* have been used by some authors in place of the word innate and the word *responsive* in place of adaptive. Innate immunity is the first line of defense; this term describes those elements of the immune system that are already present before an infection begins for the first time. The adaptive immune system consists of those elements that mount a specific response after an infection begins or when a repeat infection occurs. In my view, none of the terms currently used to describe these two major categories of immunity ideally capture the distinction. However, this should not be a cause for concern to readers, since the difference is not of overwhelming importance, and, in any case, the boundary between the two categories is becoming increasingly blurred, with some overlap.

In this section, we first consider nonspecific, innate components of the immune system and later deal with the more specific, adaptive responses. Wherever possible, I mention relevant examples of situations in which the interaction between pathogen and host immune system does not lead to rapid extinction of the infection but rather leads to disease. Readers are reminded that this chapter cannot hope to provide an exhaustive description of vertebrate immunology. The intention is to deal with aspects of the *patho*physiology of the immune system—particularly those caused by interaction with pathogens—not to provide a detailed description of the immune system. Readers are encouraged to read other texts in combination with this one if they need to deepen their understanding of essential immunology in order to properly understand the examples provided (e.g., see Tizard 2000)

Innate or Nonspecific Immune Defenses

NORMAL FLORA. In most healthy animals, internal tissues are devoid of microorganisms. The skin and mucosae, on the other hand, are continually exposed to organisms in the environment and are readily colonized by certain microbial species. The mixture of organisms usually present at any particular healthy anatomic location is termed the *normal flora*. It has been estimated that a normal human being has about 10^{12} bacteria on his or her skin, 10^{10} in the mouth, and 10^{14} in the gastrointestinal tract. By extrapolation, this means that the number of bacterial cells living inside and upon a typical mammalian body far exceeds the number of mammalian cells making up that body (Henderson and Wilson 1998).

The normal flora of the various animals of veterinary importance has not been studied exhaustively but is undoubtedly extremely complex. In most monogastric animals, normal flora includes a few eukaryotic fungi and protists, and some methanogenic archaeal organisms that colonize the large intestine. In ruminants and some other herbivores, far more archaea are present in the gastrointestinal tract. More than 200 species of bacteria contribute to the normal flora of humans; the figure is likely to be similar for other monogastric omnivores and carnivores like dogs and cats. The composition of the normal flora depends to a large extent upon the species, breed, age, and sex of the host. Food being eaten (i.e., quantity and type), stress being experienced, drug therapy, and the presence or absence of intercurrent illnesses also have an influence.

Hosts and their normal flora are thought to interact dynamically rather than displaying mutual indifference, although the details of the profusion of interrelationships are far from being completely understood. Usually, both host and bacteria derive benefit from each other, their relationship thus being mutualistic. The normal flora obtains a supply of nutrients, shelter and protection, and a means of dissemination. The host gains certain nutrients from its flora, "priming" stimulation of its immune system, and exclusion of some potential pathogens.

Just as pathogens must adhere to host cells in order to initiate infection, so members of the normal flora are likely to interact with host cells via receptor–ligand interactions. However, less is known about how members of the normal flora interact with host cells than is known about pathogens. Members of normal flora exhibit *tissue tropism*; that is, they tend to occupy rather restricted ecological niches within or upon their host's body. Perhaps essential nutrients or other environmental conditions (e.g., pH or oxygen concentration) required by a particular species of bacterium are available in only one location, or receptors needed for bacterial adhesion are only found there. The degree of tissue tropism can be extreme. Some organisms are found on the tongue but not on the gums. In the gut, different organisms predominate at different distances from mouth to anus, but also cross-sectionally some organisms favor the deep glandular crypts, whereas others are more numerous at the villous apices or in the luminal fluid.

The normal flora provides a number of important advantages to the host, some of which have been inferred from studies of *germ-free animals*. Such animals must be obtained by cesarean operation, since bacterial colonization of the skin occurs as the newborn animal passes through the birth canal, and colonization of the gastrointestinal tract begins with the very first feed. Such animals must obviously be raised with strict barrier nursing and scrupulous attention to detail, since "germs" are ubiquitous.

By competing for adhesion sites or for essential nutrients, members of the normal flora help prevent colonization of host tissues by pathogens. This is thought by many investigators to be their most important beneficial effect. Normal flora also produce inhibitory substances that kill or slow the growth of potential pathogens. Some of these substances are relatively nonselective (e.g., lactic acid, fatty acids, and hydrogen peroxide). Others are potent and highly specific: *Bacteriocins* are proteins or protein complexes produced by bacteria with bactericidal activity directed against species that are usually closely related to the producer (Mishra and Lambert 1996).

Another important beneficial effect of the normal flora is the production of so-called cross-reactive antibodies. Although normal flora is indigenous, it can still provoke an immunologic response. Low levels of antibodies are produced against members of the normal flora. Some of these antibodies cross-react with related pathogens and can therefore decrease the likelihood of infection or invasion.

Normal flora is essential for proper development of parts of the gastrointestinal tract (e.g., cecum and Peyer's patches). Germ-free animals have enlarged, thin-walled cecums, compared with those of conventional animals. Intestinal lymphatic tissues of germ-free animals are poorly responsive to stimuli compared with those of conventional animals.

Finally, some members of the normal flora synthesize essential vitamins that are absorbed as nutrients by the host (e.g., vitamins K and B_{12}). Germ-free animals sometimes need vitamin K supplementation in their diets, because they lack the assistance of normal flora to make it.

BARRIERS. The external body surfaces represent the first line of defense against microbial invaders. These barriers consist of the skin; the mucosae of the gastrointestinal, genitourinary, and respiratory tracts; and the ocular mucosae. In addition to their normal flora, these surfaces present other obstacles to potential invaders.

The importance of intact skin as a barrier against the entry of microbial invaders becomes abundantly clear when one is required to take care of burn victims. Burnt skin, or denuded subcutaneous tissue, is a much less effective barrier than is healthy skin to the entry of microbes. Patients with skin burns are particularly prone to develop bacterial infections. Keratinized skin provides a confluent cover over most of the body. It is usually relatively dry and contains antimicrobial fatty acids in sebum. Continual desquamation of superficial layers helps to limit microbial colonization.

The oral cavity normally harbors a huge, diverse, and finely balanced population of normal flora. Chronic antibiotic therapy can disrupt this ecosystem and lead to overgrowth by pathogenic bacteria or fungi (e.g., *C. albicans*). Saliva and other secretions normally wash away food debris, excess bacteria, and exfoliated cells. Saliva also contains *lysozyme*, a cationic antibacterial enzyme. Some diseases and drugs cause a failure of saliva secretion, leading to a chronically dry mouth (*xerostomia*) and predisposing to bacterial overgrowth. Similarly, diseases that cause dry eyes (termed *keratoconjunctivitis sicca*) predispose to conjunctival and corneal infections. This can happen, for example, when a disease targets and damages the tear-producing lacrimal apparatus.

The extremely low pH and protective layer of mucus in the stomach represent another, highly effective barrier to microbial colonization. Most bacteria entering the stomach are killed and digested. However, a few species of bacteria have evolved to survive passage through the stomach, and some can even live in there. For example, *Helicobacter felis* (in dogs and cats) and *H. pylori* (in people) can cause gastric inflammation. In people, *H. pylori* has been shown to cause gastric ulcers and to predispose toward development of gastric neoplasia. *Helicobacter* organisms are motile, perhaps enabling them to swim away from areas of extremely low pH. They also synthesize large amounts of the enzyme urease. By hydrolyzing urea to carbon dioxide and ammonia, urease may create a more neutral pH microenvironment around the producer organisms. However, urease production is not essential for the survival of *H. pylori* once colonization has established, so other bacterial defensive mechanisms or resistance factors must exist. If the stomach pH is chronically raised by antacid drugs such as histamine type 2 receptor antagonists (e.g., ranitidine or famotidine), then bacterial colonization by a wide range of pathogenic organisms is facilitated.

In the intestines, normal flora, mucus, and rapid epithelial cell turnover provide important barriers to colonization. Enzymes and bile will digest many potential pathogens. Peristalsis flushes away replicating organisms. If a pathogen replicates to high numbers and is detected, the rate of peristalsis can be dramatically increased to hasten the expurgation of the pathogen. Secretory diarrhea can help to dilute microbial toxins, but, if it is too severe, it can rapidly cause life-threatening dehydration.

In the genitourinary tract, many of the same barriers are present. Lactic acid-producing bacteria, which are part of the normal vaginal flora of some species, are protective. Mucopolysaccharide secretions make it more difficult for bacteria to access adhesion receptors on host cell membranes. The high osmolality of urine impedes microbial growth. The flow of urine is said to prevent some ascending urinary tract infections, although strong evidence for this hypothesis is lacking. However, it is true that some diseases that cause urinary stasis predispose to bacterial urinary tract infections.

The respiratory tract has a well-developed set of defensive barriers, including the mucociliary escalator. Larger infectious particles (>5 to 10 μm) in the airstream usually collide with the mucosa of the highly convoluted nasal turbinates, or hit the wall of the pharynx, and get sneezed out or swallowed. Smaller particles (<3 μm) more readily pass through the laryngeal opening. Those that reach the alveoli are usually phagocytosed by macrophages and removed. More commonly, particles alight on the thin blanket of mucus that covers the walls of the trachea, bronchi, and bronchioles. From there, they are carried back up toward the larynx on a moving layer of mucous. Rhythmic, coordinated beating of cilia on the respiratory epithelial cells is what continuously propels the mucus layer toward the mouth. Some animals have an inherited disorder of ciliary motility termed *ciliary dyskinesia* or *Kartagener's syndrome*. Their mucociliary escalator does not work properly. Such animals are prone to chronic coughing and progressive bronchial disease because they fail to clear mucus, irritants, and pathogens effectively from their airways. Interestingly, some pathogens have evolved the capacity to paralyze or destroy respiratory cilia, thus improving their chances of colonizing the respiratory tract. Canine parainfluenzavirus tends to denude respiratory epithelial cells of their cilia, and *Bordetella bronchiseptica* produces toxins that paralyze cilia (i.e., cause ciliostasis) as well as impede phagocytosis. Both of these infectious agents facilitate the colonization of the respiratory tract by other, opportunistic, organisms.

Beyond these physicochemical defenses, there is emerging evidence that epithelial barrier cells synthesize a range of potent and vitally important antimicrobial peptides (Zasloff 2002). About 500 such peptides have so far been reported, and many more are being identified each year. These evolutionarily ancient defensive weapons are found in plants and animals—indeed, in all multicellular organisms studied to date. Most of these peptides target microbial cell membranes and take advantage of fundamental differences between the membranes of microbes and multicellular organisms. Because of the fundamental basis of their action, microbes evolve resistance to these peptides only with great difficulty. Although they share essential structural features, the diversity of antimicrobial peptides is staggering; it has been argued that each species has evolved its own particular repertoire of unique peptides ideally suited to deal with the microbes in their environment. As an example, investigators have recently isolated a 5-kilodalton (kD) antimicrobial peptide from human psoriasis lesions and cloned the encoding gene from keratinocytes. This molecule, termed β-defensin 3, is particularly effective against the potential skin pathogen *S. aureus*. It is highly likely that the species under the care of veterinarians synthesize their own antimicrobial peptides. Some of these may eventually be cloned and used to treat infections resistant to more conventional antimicrobial agents.

FEVER. Fever, which should be distinguished from hyperthermia (Dunn and Greene 1998) is an ancient, effective, but incompletely understood antimicrobial defense mechanism. Interestingly, it is not restricted to warm-blooded animals (i.e., endotherms or homeotherms). Cold-blooded animals (e.g., some fish, lizards, and toads) exhibit behavioral "fever" in response to pyrogenic stimuli. Given a choice, infected cold-blooded animals move to locations that raise their body temperature above what they would normally find most comfortable. Mammals and birds, on the other hand, increase the *set-point* of their *thermoregulatory center* to induce fever. The thermoregulatory center, which is located in the preoptic region of the rostral hypothalamus, consists of two subcenters: a rostral heat-loss center (influenced by the parasympathetic limb of the autonomic nervous system) and a caudal heat-production center (influenced mainly by the sympathetic nervous system). Increased thermogenesis (e.g., by shivering) and decreased heat loss (e.g., by cutaneous vasoconstriction) lead to an elevated body temperature.

The fact that fever is so widespread in nature has been viewed as strong evidence that it is an important, adaptive host response. It is argued that this metabolically expensive defense mechanism would not have evolved and been conserved so widely within the animal kingdom unless fever provided some net benefit to the host (Mackowiak 1994).

The benefits of fever are clearer for some infections than for others. Mice that had their body temperatures artificially raised slightly were more resistant to a wide range of viral infections and to *Cryptococcus neoformans* infection, but were less resistant to infection with a streptococcus. Of course, artificial elevation of body temperature is not the same as fever induction.

Cytokines are soluble molecules (often peptides) released by cells that help mediate immune responses. They are discussed in more detail a little later. For now, we need to know that fever is associated with five major pyrogenic cytokines [these are interleukin 1β (IL-1β), tumor-necrosis factor α (TNF-α), IL-6, interferon, and IL-2]. These cytokines have immune-potentiating capabilities that enhance resistance to a range of infections.

Until recently, it was thought that cytokines circulated to the brain (specifically, the circumventricular organs, where there is no blood-brain barrier) and acted directly on the rostral hypothalamus to cause fever. More recently, substantial evidence has been accumulated to suggest that vagal afferent nerve fibers play an active role in conveying peripheral immune signals to the brain. For example, many of the central nervous system effects caused by intraperitoneal administration of bacterial LPS or IL-1β—including fever—are markedly attenuated or suppressed following subdi-aphragmatic transection of the vagus nerve. How cytokines released peripherally in response to infection transfer their signals to the brain remains something of a mystery (Konsman and Cartmell 1997).

IRON SEQUESTRATION. Iron is a component or cofac-tor of many bacterial enzyme systems, but the amount of free iron in host tissues is extremely low (of the order of 10^{-18} M). Most of the iron in host tissues that might otherwise be available to bacteria is bound to high-affinity binding proteins such as transferrin and lactoferrin. Of necessity, bacteria have evolved highly efficient mechanisms to scavenge iron from these bind-ing proteins. Some bacteria, such as *E. coli* and *Kleb-siella* species, secrete high-affinity extracellular iron-chelating molecules, termed *siderophores* or *siderochromes*. Other species of bacteria express recep-tors for transferrin and/or lactoferrin on their surfaces and internalize iron this way. Still others remove iron from host binding proteins by proteolytic cleavage.

An ancient antimicrobial defense mechanism involves sequestration of iron away from the bacterial invaders that need it. Most recirculating iron in the host body is released from senescent erythrocytes as hemo-globin and converted to ferritin and hemosiderin inside mononuclear phagocytes. From these cells, it is usually transferred to serum transferrin for delivery to red blood cell precursors in the bone marrow. Infection can cause sustained release by leukocytes of a cytokine (IL-1) that prevents mononuclear phagocytes from releasing their load of iron. This induced mild iron-deficiency state, if long-standing enough, can be associated with a mild to moderate nonregenerative anemia. Nonregenerative anemia associated with infection or inflammation can be distinguished from blood-loss anemia by examining a bone marrow sample with a Prussian blue stain: in anemia of inflammation, iron-replete mononuclear cells are present in the marrow.

NATURAL ANTIBODIES. *Antibodies*, or *immunoglobu-lin* molecules, are glycoproteins made by cells of the immune system that selectively bind and neutralize for-eign molecules, or parts of molecules, termed *antigens*. Binding of antigens by antibodies is often an important early step in an effective immune response to a patho-genic invader. Antigen-specific antibodies are "made [or, more correctly, selected] to order" when the immune system encounters a foreign molecule that is part of an invader. Antibodies and antigens are there-fore discussed further in the section *Adaptive Immune Defenses*. For the time being, it is sufficient to know that some types of potentially pathogenic infectious agents are neutralized by preexisting antibodies the *very first time* they enter the host body. This fortunate event (from the host's viewpoint) happens even though the immune system has never before been exposed to that particular antigen. These preexisting antibodies (termed *natural* antibodies)—part of the innate or non-specific immune system—can be found in umbilical cord blood (at least in humans) and thus can arise spon-taneously without need of prior exposure to pathogens or normal flora (Boes 2000).

There are various classes, or isotypes, of immunoglobulin (IgA, IgD, IgG, and IgM). Natural antibodies mostly belong to the pentameric IgM class. Compared with the enormous number of different kinds of antibodies that are "made to order," a relatively lim-ited repertoire of natural antibodies is produced. Fortu-nately, natural antibodies have broad specificities, mak-ing up for the limited repertoire. Affinities for antigens are relatively low but compensated for by the pen-tameric structure of IgM (10 antigen-binding sites per molecule versus 2 for IgG). Natural antibodies tend to be polyreactive to a broad range of phylogenetically conserved structures, such as nucleic acids, carbohy-drates, and phospholipids (Boes 2000). Despite their rather low specificity, natural antibodies can neutralize some important potential pathogens (e.g., *Listeria monocytogenes*, influenzavirus, vesicular stomatitis virus, and invading intestinal bacteria; Boes 2000) and thus play a significant role in innate immunity.

PHAGOCYTOSIS. *Phagocytes* are immune cells that engulf bacteria and other harmful cells or particles and kill and digest them (their name is derived from the Greek, *phagein*, "to eat"). *Neutrophils* and *macrophages* are the most important of the phagocytes, but *eosinophils*, *basophils*, and *monocytes* play a sig-nificant role in defense against some invaders.

Migration of phagocytes to a site of tissue infection represents an early and fundamental defensive response to infection. The processes by which phago-cytes are "called to arms" are intricately orchestrated. Chemical signals are released by bacterial cells, dam-aged host tissues, or immune cells that have already been recruited. These signal molecules (including bac-terial endotoxin, IL-1, and TNF-α) cause vascular endothelial cells promptly to begin to express adhesion molecules that can "capture" circulating phagocytes. There are two main categories of endothelial adhesion molecules: *selectins* and members of the *immunoglob-ulin gene superfamily*; both categories comprise of gly-coproteins. Members of the immunoglobulin gene superfamily relevant here include vascular cell adhe-sion molecule 1 (VCAM-1), intercellular cell adhesion molecule 1 (ICAM-1, or CD54) and ICAM-2. After endothelial cells express selectins, phagocytes begin to attach and roll along the inside of the vascular endothe-lium. Next, they flatten against the endothelial lining, and *integrins* on their cell membranes (e.g., CD11b/CD18) attach to ICAM/VCAM firmly. Next, pseudopods project from the phagocyte and probe between endothelial cells, enabling the phagocyte to emigrate from the blood vessel and gain entry to the infected tissue.

Phagocytes are able to recognize and attach to bac-teria in part because they express receptors that can bind the carbohydrate molecules present on many bac-terial cell surfaces. Bacteria in an infected site may also become coated with host molecules such as antibodies of the IgG class and the C3b component of complement (discussed in more detail later). Phagocytes have receptors for both of these host molecules. Indeed, bacteria coated with IgG antibodies and the C3b component of complement are very much more likely to be phagocytosed. They are said to be *opsonized* by these host molecules (*opsonization* literally means prepared for eating; from the Greek *opsonein*, a "relish").

Phagocytosis requires adhesion of the invading organism to the phagocyte cell membrane, followed by engulfment by coalescing pseudopods. The invading organism is locked within a membrane-bound vesicle, or *phagosome*, which almost immediately fuses with lysosomal granules (to become what is sometimes called a *phagolysosome*), and a number of microbicidal mechanisms swing into action.

OXIDATIVE KILLING. Binding of an invading microorganism to the phagosome-lining membrane initiates a rapid increase in oxidative activity, termed the *respiratory burst*, within the phagocyte. In essence, this involves a stepwise reduction of molecular oxygen to hydrogen peroxide, which is toxic to engulfed microorganisms. Much glucose and oxygen are consumed in the process; indeed, oxygen consumption by the phagocyte increases two- to 20-fold during the respiratory burst. Reduction of molecular oxygen is catalyzed by a nonheme oxidase located on the phagocyte plasma membrane. This oxidase acts on reduced nicotinamide adenine dinucleotide phosphate (NADPH). NADPH, the hydrogen donor (and electron donor) for the process, is continuously regenerated by a sudden increase in anaerobic glucose metabolism via the hexose monophosphate shunt. A unique *phagosome cytochrome*, termed *b558*, is the terminal electron donor to molecular oxygen, producing reactive oxygen intermediates; 90% of the molecular oxygen gains one electron and is converted to an *oxygen free radical*, the *superoxide anion* ($O_2^-\bullet$). Other oxygen free radicals that are produced include the hydroxyl radical ($\bullet OH$) and singlet oxygen ($O\bullet$). Two superoxide anions can combine with two hydrogen ions to form hydrogen peroxide (H_2O_2) and oxygen. This reaction is catalyzed by the enzyme *superoxide dismutase*. Hydrogen peroxide is, itself, toxic to ingested microorganisms, but when it combines with halides in the phagolysosome, the toxic effect is amplified about 50-fold. The reaction of hydrogen peroxide with halide is catalyzed by the enzyme *myeloperoxidase*. The most likely chemical product of the hydrogen peroxide-myeloperoxidase-halide interaction is hypochlorous acid (essentially, bleach).

OTHER KILLING MECHANISMS. The pH inside of the phagolysosome declines to 3.5–4.0, in part as a consequence of active proton pumps in the membrane, and partly because protons are released during the respiratory burst. This relatively low pH can itself damage or prevent the replication of some microorganisms. However, it is probably more important that a low pH promotes the production of hydrogen peroxide and is optimal for the majority of lysosomal enzymes that help to break down invading microorganisms inside the phagolysosome. Lysozyme (muramidase) is a well-known cationic enzyme found in phagolysosomes that degrades some bacterial peptidoglycans by cleaving glycosidic linkages between N-acetylmuramic acid and N-acetylglucosamine.

Lactoferrin is an iron-binding protein, sometimes present in phagolysosomes, that acts to deprive microorganisms of the essential nutrient, iron.

The phagolysosome contains various other cationic proteins with antibacterial activities. These tend to be active at a slightly higher, neutral pH. Examples include *bactericidal/permeability-increasing protein* (BPI) and *defensins*, a family of cysteine-rich, small, bactericidal peptides. BPI and defensins destabilize bacterial cell membranes and render them more permeable (Wilks and Sissons 1997). Lysosomal hydrolases finish off the job of digesting bacteria but usually act after the microbes have been killed.

HOW PATHOGENS AVOID OR SURVIVE PHAGOCYTOSIS. Some bacteria and fungi, such as *Cryptococcus neoformans*, klebsiellae, and streptococci surround themselves with polysaccharide capsules that are antiphagocytic. Capsules may be relatively permeable to large proteins like antibodies: deposition of antibodies and complement in an intracapsular or subcapsular location means that these opsonizing molecules are sequestered away from the receptors on phagocytic cells, so effective opsonization may not be able to take place.

As mentioned in the previous section, some pathogens that infect macrophages intracellularly (e.g., *Leishmania donovani*) enter cells by interacting with complement receptors (specifically, CR3 integrin receptors that bind complement component C3bi) rather than antibody (F_c) receptors. This is advantageous to the invader because, unlike F_c receptors, CR3 integrin receptors are not linked to activation of NADPH oxidase, and so the respiratory burst is not triggered by their "backdoor" ligation.

Most intracellular pathogens can produce enzymes that destroy hydrogen peroxide and superoxide. Catalase and superoxide dismutase are well-studied examples. Some organisms also produce substances that may hinder the respiratory burst. The membrane lipophosphoglycan (LPG) of *L. donovani* is reported to inhibit protein kinase C, a key component in the signal transduction pathway leading to activation of NADPH oxidase and thence to superoxide production. LPG, like many of the larger microbial polysaccharides (e.g., mannitol), can also act as a nonspecific scavenger of toxic oxygen free radicals. However, the role of LPG as a common virulence factor in *Leishmania* species is cast into question by recent studies that show it to be an essential virulence factor in *L. major*, but not in *L. mexicana*. Other glycoconjugates [e.g., proteophosphoglycans (PPGs)] may act as virulence factors in those species for which LPG is not essential (Späth et al. 2000).

Three further approaches worthy of note have evolved to enable intracellular pathogens to evade nonoxidative killing:

• Some pathogens, such as *Toxoplasma gondii*, can impede fusion of the phagosome with lysosomes.
• Other organisms (e.g., mycobacteria) can withstand the hostile phagolysosomal environment and even replicate there. How they resist annihilation within a structure specifically designed to kill bacteria is incompletely understood, but somehow the bacteria are able to control and alter the phagosome internal environment. Thus, the interior of phagosomes infected by mycobacteria do not become acidified and show a specific lack of the proton pumps essential for normal, complete acidification.
• Other organisms escape from the phagolysosome into the cytoplasm by rupturing their way out. The cytosol is a much less hostile environment in which to grow and replicate. *Listeria monocytogenes* is a bacterial cause of disease in many species of veterinary importance, particularly in ruminants. The ability of *L. monocytogenes* to escape from the phagosome has been shown by deletion mutagenesis to depend on the bacterial product *listeriolysin*.

INHERITED AND ACQUIRED DEFECTS OF PHAGOCYTES. Numerous qualitative and quantitative inherited disorders of phagocytes exist in the species of veterinary interest. Some functional defects can lead to dramatically increased cell numbers because those cells that are present do not function properly; that is, a qualitative abnormality can lead to a quantitative one. In general, inherited disorders of phagocytes lead to an increased susceptibility of the host to infections, particularly bacterial infections. Inherited disorders can affect any of the stages of phagocyte function—that is, adherence to endothelial cells, migration/chemotaxis, phagocytosis, fusion of lysosomes to phagosomes, generation of the respiratory burst, nonoxidative killing, and digestion of the engulfed organisms once they have been killed.

An example of an inherited disorder of neutrophil function exists in Holstein cattle. This disorder is termed *bovine leukocyte adhesion deficiency* (BLAD) and has a simple autosomal recessive inheritance. Neutrophils of homozygous calves lack effective adhesion glycoproteins (β_2 integrins) on their surfaces because of a mutation in the common β chain that the β_2 integrins share. Recurrent nonsuppurative bacterial infections, persistent neutrophilia (often extreme, exceeding 100,000 cells/μL), and lymphocytosis are observed. Affected calves are usually stunted and suffer from recurrent pneumonia, ulcerative stomatitis, and enteritis. Death usually supervenes between 2 weeks and 8 months of age.

A very similar leukocyte adhesion deficiency affects Irish setters. It is sometimes still called *Irish setter granulocytopathy*, although *canine leukocyte adhesion deficiency* (CLAD) would nowadays be a more precise

term. In one study, 12 Irish setter puppies from six litters were investigated. They had severe recurrent infections, neutrophilia, and low body weights. Investigations revealed a leukocyte adhesion deficiency with a total lack of CD11b/CD18. Neutrophils from these dogs were functionally impaired, with a total lack of ability to ingest C3b-opsonized particles. There was also a decreased ability to ingest IgG-opsonized particles and less adherence to nylon wool compared with neutrophils from healthy control dogs. Not surprisingly, given what is now understood about this disorder, the respiratory burst was normal in these patients.

A wide range of qualitative and quantitative *acquired* disorders also affects phagocytes. One of the simplest and most common is an insufficient number of phagocytic cells. For example, insufficient neutrophils (*neutropenia*) can be caused by drugs (e.g., antineoplastic chemotherapeutic agents or excessive estrogen), viruses (e.g., canine parvovirus type 2, FeLV, or FIV), other infectious agents (e.g., Ehrlichiae), invasion of bone marrow by cancer cells (e.g., lymphoma), and—rarely—immune destruction of neutrophils.

Diabetes mellitus reversibly impairs locomotion of neutrophils. Corticosteroids impair neutrophil chemotaxis and cause failure of lysosomal fusion with phagosomes. Morphine and various hyperosmolar states (such as some forms of diabetes mellitus, again) cause difficulties with phagocytic engulfment of particles.

COMPLEMENT. The complement system consists of about 20 different proteins that function together to play an important role in acute inflammation, hemostasis, phagocytosis, and other aspects of immune defense. The numbered complement proteins are sequentially cleaved and/or activated in an amplifying cascade to carry out the following functions:

• Lysis of bacteria by generation of the *membrane-attack complex* of complement
• Enhancement of phagocytosis by coating of invading microorganisms (i.e., opsonization)
• Release of chemotactic signals to "recruit" phagocytes and other immune cells
• Assistance with binding of antigen to antigen-presenting cells (APCs) and B lymphocytes
• Prevention of precipitation and promotion of removal of immune complexes

Other *complement-control proteins* exert a moderating influence on the amplification process and prevent excessive activation by targeting key activated-complement intermediaries.

Complement can be activated in two main ways: via the *classical pathway* or via the *alternate pathway*.

THE CLASSICAL PATHWAY. With few exceptions, membrane-bound antigen-antibody complexes are required to activate the classical complement pathway. Each of the nine complement components that contribute to the classical pathway is given a number preceded by the letter C. C1 is a trimolecular complex made up of C1q, C1r, and C1s. C1q has an interesting structure, with a collagen-like stem and six heads. Complement activation begins when at least two of the C1q heads bind to F_c portions of one or more bound antibody molecules. Antibodies of the IgG class are monomeric; i.e., they have only one F_c per molecule, so at the very least two IgG molecules would need to be bound in close proximity to activate C1q. By contrast, IgM antibodies are pentameric, with five F_c portions per molecule. Clearly, IgM antibodies are much more effective at activating complement via the classical pathway than are IgG antibodies, since a single membrane-bound IgM molecule is more than sufficient to activate C1q. Upon activation, C1q forms a complex with C1r and C1s. The complex has esterase activity: it first binds and cleaves C4 to produce C4a and C4b. Then, activated C1 binds C2 to produce C2a and C2b. Next, C4b and C2a combine to form a complex (C4b,2a) that has enzymatic activity. C4b,2a is the main convertase for cleavage of C3, a pivotal step in complement activation. Cleavage of C3 releases C3a (which is chemotactic for phagocytes and a potent stimulator of mast cell degranulation) and C3b, which adheres to the surface of the same cell to which the initiating antibody/antibodies were bound.

As previously mentioned, some phagocytes have receptors for C3b, so this activated-complement component exhibits *immune adherence* properties. In other words, it serves as an *opsonin*.

The last stage of complement activation involves the formation of the membrane-attack complex. The ultimate effect of this multimolecular complex is to create a pore in the membrane, leading eventually to cell lysis. C5 binds nonenzymatically to C3b. C5 is next cleaved by the complex C4b,2a,3b. The smaller cleavage product (C5a) is strongly chemotactic for phagocytes. The larger fragment (C5b) combines with C6 and C7 to form a stable trimolecular complex that is also chemotactic for phagocytes. A molecule of C8 interacts to form C5b,6,7,8. Finally, this complex binds to and induces the polymerization of six molecules of C9 to produce the membrane-attack complex that perforates the membrane of the antibody-coated cell, causing it to become disrupted.

THE ALTERNATIVE PATHWAY. The most important difference between the classical and alternative pathways is that the latter does not require the presence of antigen-antibody complexes for activation to begin. In this sense, the alternative pathway might rather simplistically be viewed as being a component of natural or innate immunity, and the classical pathway as being a component of acquired immunity. However, there are a few exceptions to the rule that the classical pathway must be activated by membrane-bound antibodies. For example, some retroviruses, mycoplasmata, and Gram-positive and Gram-negative bacteria can directly bind C1q to initiate complement activation via the classical pathway.

Complement activation via the alternative pathway can be initiated by several stimuli:

- The presence of cells infected by certain viruses
- The presence of one or more of many species of Gram-positive and Gram-negative bacteria
- The presence of trypanosomes or fungi
- The presence of certain carbohydrates or endotoxins; for example, those that might be found in bacterial cell walls

Activation via the alternative pathway begins with the C3 molecule, which has an internal thiol ester that undergoes continual, spontaneous, low-grade hydrolysis under normal conditions. Hydrolyzed C3 [termed $C3(H_2O)$] can bind to another, nonnumbered complement component called factor B. Once combined with $C3(H_2O)$, factor B becomes susceptible to cleavage by complement factor D. Cleavage of factor B releases a small fragment (Ba). The larger fragment (Bb) remains associated with $C3(H_2O)$ in a complex termed the *priming C3 convertase* [$C3(H_2O)$,Bb]. This priming convertase is a weak C3-cleaving enzyme. It causes continuous, low-grade cleavage of C3 to produce C3b. If some of the newly formed C3b binds to a suitable cell surface, it can combine reversibly with native factor B to form a complex (C3b,B). Factor D then cleaves the factor B portion of C3b,B to form C3b,Bb—a highly efficient *amplification C3 convertase* that is stabilized by factor P (properdin). If the C3b,Bb complex forms or is deposited on the surface of a foreign invader, a positive-feedback loop of activation of the alternative pathway ensues. This response is normally kept from getting out of hand by modulatory C3b-inactivator molecules.

C3b,Bb combines with a second molecule of C3b to produce the C5 convertase C3b,Bb,3b. From the point of C5 cleavage onward, the alternative pathway merges with the classical pathway; in other words, from C5 cleavage onward is a common pathway (Woolf 2000).

INHERITED AND ACQUIRED HYPOCOMPLEMENTEMIAS. Numerous inherited and acquired complement deficiencies have been described in people (Winkelstein 1998), but less is known about the species of veterinary importance. In people, inherited deficiencies are known to exist for all of the numbered complement components, as well as for some of the complement-control proteins, like factor H. Most of these conditions are inherited as autosomal recessive traits, some are X-linked.

Complete C3 deficiency has been described as an autosomal recessive condition in a colony of Brittany spaniels with spinal muscular atrophy (Blum et al. 1985, cited in Giger and Greene 1998). Affected dogs had defective chemotaxis and phagocytosis, and were more prone to infections, particularly bacterial infections, than normal. The immunodeficiency was relatively mild, but some life-threatening infections such as pneumonia did develop. Other recognized primary complement deficiencies of animals include C6 deficiency in Angora rabbits and rats, C5 deficiency in inbred mice, and multiple complement component deficiencies in guinea pigs (C4, C2, and partial C3 deficiency). Yorkshire pigs suffer from a deficiency of the complement-control protein, factor H.

Various acquired or secondary complement-deficiency states are known to exist in humans. It is likely that most of these also affect the species of direct veterinary interest. *Newborn infants* are hypocomplementemic compared with adults; *premature babies* more so. Nearly all of the numbered complement components are low compared with adults. *Nephrotic patients* with heavy proteinuria have low levels of factor B, which compromises complement activation via the alternative pathway and means they have poor serum-opsonizing activity. Presumably factor B is lost, along with albumin, in the urine.

In one veterinary study, almost all *FeLV-infected cats with lymphoma* were found to be hypocomplementemic as a consequence of factor depletion. Complement was shown to have been activated via the classical pathway. About 50% of FeLV-infected cats without lymphoma and 50% of lymphoma-bearing FeLV-negative cats were also found to be hypocomplementemic.

UNUSUAL INTERACTIONS OF PATHOGENS WITH COMPLEMENT. We have already encountered a way in which pathogens "take advantage of" the complement system rather than being damaged or destroyed by it. This involved use by some organisms of complement receptors on phagocyte cell surfaces as a portal to gain entry to cells. You will recall that ligation of complement receptors does not necessarily activate quiescent phagocytes, such as macrophages. Some *mycobacteria* actually coat themselves with C3b in order to gain entry to the interior of phagocytes by this means.

Adaptive Immune Defenses. For some people, *adaptive immunity* (also called *acquired specific immunity*) is what the immune system is really all about—they view innate immunity as a bit of a bore—more to do with inflammation than *real* immunity. This seems a little unfair, given what we have already learned about the sophistication of some innate immune responses and their crucial role in defense against some invading pathogens. However, it is perfectly true that adaptive immunity is one of the crowning achievements of vertebrate evolution and a highly impressive example of "genomic parsimony"—that is, how relatively short lengths of DNA coding sequence can be used to achieve immunity against a very broad range of potential pathogens.

If it works properly, the adaptive immune system is able to

- Recognize foreign invaders
- Mount a targeted, specific attack upon each invader

- "Remember" previous infections and mount a more rapid, effective response if the same infectious agent attacks on subsequent occasions

ANTIGENS. Invading organisms have molecules in or upon themselves that can be recognized as foreign by the immune system; these molecules are called *antigens* (or *immunogens* if they are sufficient to provoke an effective immune response). Most antigens are proteins, polypeptides, or polysaccharides. Molecules that are too small (less than about 2.5 kD) cannot act as antigens; most antigens are, in fact, larger than 10 kD. Despite this minimum-size restriction, the specific determinants on the surfaces of antigens that are recognized by the immune system are very much smaller, consisting of just a few amino acids or sugar residues. These so-called *epitopes* are the fundamental targets of the immune system; each evokes a specific immune response. There are usually multiple epitopes on a single antigen.

Some molecules that are too small to act as antigens in their own rights can bind to larger carrier molecules (generally proteins) and be recognized that way. The small molecule in this situation is termed a *hapten*. After an immune response has been evoked by the hapten-carrier combination, the free hapten may be able to be recognized independently, for example, in plasma. Some drugs (e.g., trimethoprim-sulfa) can act as haptens, leading to immune-complex formation and adverse drug reactions.

Since antigens are recognized by the immune system, it would clearly be to the advantage of invading pathogens if they could "cloak" or hide their antigens, or perhaps regularly change them, staying one step ahead of the host's immune system. We have already learned that some groups of bacteria surround themselves with relatively permeable capsules that help to prevent opsonization by sequestering antibodies within the substance of the capsule. Most such capsules are made of relatively nonimmunogenic substances, so they effectively cloak the bacterium's cell wall antigens and yet do not provoke much of an immune response themselves.

There is an example of a tight-knit group of infectious agents that have evolved to change their surface antigens to evade the immune system. *African trypanosomiasis* is a term used to describe a group of closely related protozoal diseases of huge economic and social impact. Different forms of disease affect several species of veterinary importance, as well as afflicting humans. African trypanosomiasis of humans is *sleeping sickness*, a desperately serious disease.

The genus *Trypanosoma* (family: Trypanosomatidae; order: Kinetoplastida) comprises unicellular flagellates that parasitize members of all vertebrate classes. Species of veterinary importance include *Trypanosoma equiperdum* (horses), *T. brucei brucei* (dogs), *T. congolense* (also dogs), and *T. simiae* (pigs). The characteristic forms of trypanosomes are the epimastigotes found in the invertebrate vectors and the trypomastigotes found in the blood and tissues of vertebrate hosts. Bloodsucking arthropods (insects or arachnids) can serve as vectors for mammalian, avian, and some amphibian and reptilian trypanosomes. Trypanosomes of fish and certain other amphibians and reptiles are transmitted by leeches. The mammalian trypanosomes are divided into the *Salivaria* and the *Stercoraria* according to their mode of transmission, which is predominantly inoculative (by tsetse flies) for the Salivaria and contaminative (by a variety of bloodsucking insects) for the Stercoraria (Haag et al. 1998). They note that chronic infections with trypanosomes dwelling extracellularly in the blood and tissues of their hosts are observed in all vertebrate classes. They present a molecular phylogenetic reconstruction of trypanosome evolution based on nucleotide sequences of small subunit rRNA genes. The evolutionary tree suggests an ancient split into one branch containing all Salivarian trypanosomes and a branch containing all non-Salivarian lineages. The latter branch splits into a clade containing bird, reptilian, and Stercorarian trypanosomes infecting mammals and a clade with a branch of fish trypanosomes and a branch of reptilian/amphibian lineages. The branching order of the non-Salivarian trypanosomes supports host-parasite cospeciation scenarios, but also suggests host switches, e.g., between bird and reptilian trypanosomes. The tree is discussed in relation to the modes of adaptation that allow trypanosomes to infect immunocompetent vertebrates. Most importantly, the early divergence of the Salivarian lineages suggests that the presence of a dense proteinaceous surface coat that is subject to antigenic variation is a unique invention of this group of parasites.

All members of Salivaria are thought to evade the humoral immune responses of their hosts by the sequential expression of VSGs, which cover the parasites in a confluent protective coat. At a given time, a particular trypanosomal cell or clone expresses only one of over 1000 VSG genes that it has. As mentioned in the last section, when sufficient antibody accumulates in the host's plasma to bring about large-scale complement-mediated lysis of organisms, the trypanosomes simply express the next VSG gene in sequence. Their surface coat is changed—a case of a "protozoal leopard changing its spots"! This is achieved by a DNA rearrangement involving duplication of the latest VSG gene at a genomic expression site. In due course, when antibody to the latest VSG has had time to form, the process is repeated. During the course of infection of an individual host, the extent of parasitemia rises and falls cyclically every few days. Each new wave of parasites expresses a new variant form of VSG, which is not (yet) recognized by the host's immune system. Given that the process can be repeated many times over, this adaptation clearly has a

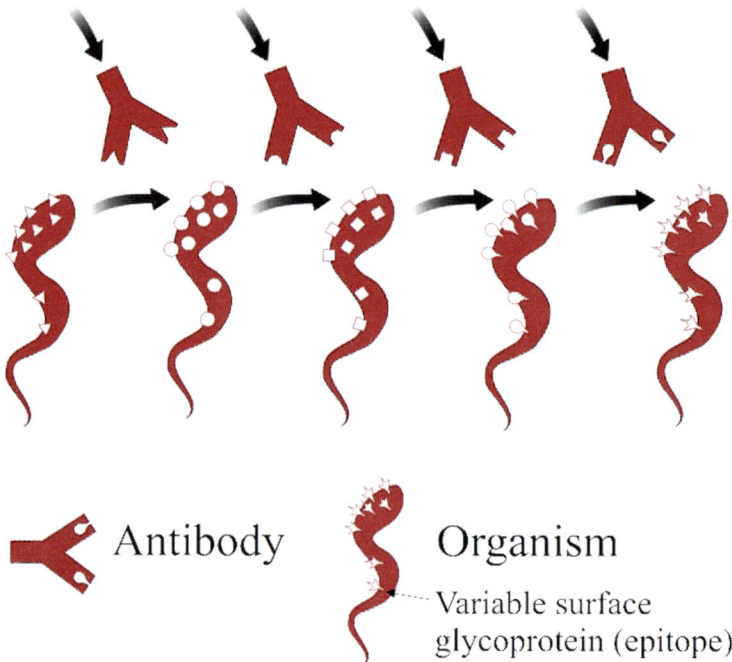

FIG. 3.6—Some pathogens, including African salivarid trypanosomes and influenzaviruses, evade the host immune system by varying their surface antigens. All members of Salivaria are thought to evade humoral immune responses by the sequential expression of variable surface glycoproteins (VSGs), which cover the parasites in a confluent protective coat. At any given time, a particular trypanosomal cell or clone expresses only one of over 1000 VSG genes that it has. When sufficient specific antibody accumulates in the host's plasma to bring about large-scale complement-mediated lysis of organisms, the trypanosomes express the next VSG gene in sequence. They thus remain one step ahead of the humoral immune response.

huge impact on the success of the pathogen, as it can stay consistently one step ahead of the host's immune system. This particular method of changing surface antigen expression seems to be a unique adaptation of African salivarid trypanosomes. Figure 3.6 illustrates how African trypanosomes alter their surface antigen expression over time to evade immune detection.

Antigenic variation is also important for the survival of some viral pathogens. Influenzaviruses (members of the family *Orthomyxoviridae*) are categorized serologically into types A, B, and C. The antigens that are used to differentiate the three serotypes are *internal* nucleoproteins; hence, those of intact virus particles are not accessible to host antibodies. However, the virus also bears two variable major surface antigens: hemagglutinin (H) and neuraminidase (N); these are important targets for host antibodies. All three serotypes of influenzavirus may alter both H and N gradually by mutation, a process known as *antigenic drift*. Additionally, type A viruses (but not types B or C) can express one of at least 15 different subtypes of H and at least nine subtypes of N. The emergence of strains expressing different combinations of these H and N surface antigens is called *antigenic shift*. So far, only H1–3 and N1–2 have been found in the vast majority of human influenzaviruses. However, mice, ferrets, pigs, horses, and sea mammals express many other, different combinations; for example, an equine influenza A virus that arrived in South Africa in 1986 from the United States of America expressed H_3N_8.

Antigenic shift and drift enable influenzaviruses to escape host immune responses. It is thought that animal orthomyxoviruses serve as a reservoir for generation of novel antigenic variants that eventually may infect people. There is ample evidence to suggest that all mammalian influenza A viruses were originally derived from those of wild waterfowl. In addition to those influenzaviruses that are already well established in mammals, new viruses have been transmitted to both mammals and to poultry from wild waterfowl in recent years, causing significant outbreaks of disease. Influenzaviruses have an eight-segmented RNA genome and may acquire alternative RNA segments from other animal species, thus undergoing antigenic shift by a reassortment process that can occur when cells are infected by two or more viruses of different strains. The transmission of avian influenzaviruses (or, at least, of avian viral genes) to people is postulated to occur indirectly through pigs, which serve as the intermediate host (Webster 1997).

ANTIBODIES AND THE HUMORAL IMMUNE RESPONSE. Before we consider antibodies themselves, we need to spend a few moments thinking about the cells involved in making them. *Small lymphocytes* are arguably the most important cells involved in adaptive immunity. There are two major categories: *B cells* and *T cells*. B cells mature to become the *plasma cells* that are responsible for making antibodies. T cells cannot do this, but they have a broad range of other, crucial responsibilities, including attacking pathogens inside and outside of infected host cells, regulating immune responses, and helping B cells to make antibodies. Various APCs (including monocytes, macrophages, and dendritic cells) play an important role by ingesting, processing, and then appropriately presenting antigen fragments in a way that allows them to be recognized by T cells. Soluble "communication molecules" called *cytokines* are made by cells of the immune system and exert powerful effects on close and (less often) distant cells. The term cytokine is a general one; it includes a huge and growing number of *lymphokines*, *chemokines*, *interleukins*, and many other classes of molecule. Cytokines, APCs, and T cells will be discussed after we consider antibodies and the cells that make them.

ANTIBODY STRUCTURE AND FUNCTION. Functionally, antibodies are molecules that bind specifically to particular antigens. Structurally, they are glycoprotein molecules made by plasma cells, the mature, differentiated form of B cells. Antibodies form part of the globulin fraction of plasma and are also known as *immunoglobulins*. Because antibodies are dissolved in plasma and other body fluids, and their effects are exerted by these cell-free solutions, the old-fashioned term *humoral immunity* is still used sometimes to refer to antibody-mediated immunity.

Several classes and subclasses of immunoglobulin with substantially differing structures exist (e.g., IgA, IgD, IgE, IgG1, IgG2a, IgG2b, and IgM1). For example, IgM antibodies are pentamers, whereas IgA molecules usually exist as dimers. Members of the other three antibody classes are monomers. Each antibody monomer actually consists of four polypeptide chains: two identical light chains and two identical heavy ones linked together by disulfide bonds to form a Y shape. Each heavy and light chain has a downstream constant part and an upstream variable part. The constant part has an amino acid sequence that is identical for all antibodies of a given class or subclass. The variable part has an amino acid sequence that differs widely among members of the same class or subclass. It is the variable parts of the heavy and light chains that, together, make up the antigen-binding site. Each antibody monomer has two identical *antigen-binding sites* or *fragments* (2 x F_{ab} at the tops of the limbs of the Y). Each plasma cell clone makes antibodies with almost unique antigen-binding sites. It is the great diversity of antigen-binding sites made by different plasma cell clones that enables the humoral immune system to respond effectively to so many diverse antigens. The potential diversity in antigen-binding site specificities is simply enormous, because both heavy and light chains are formed from genes that have previously undergone a gene-rearrangement process. Germline DNA contains a large number of "choices" of gene segments for possible inclusion in antigen-binding sites (this is true for both heavy and light chains). During B-cell ontogeny, one of hundreds of variable (V) segments, one of several joining (J) segments, and (in heavy chains) one of several diversity (D) segments are selected, essentially at random, and spliced to a constant (C) segment. The enormous diversity of antibody specificity thus results from a huge number of possible V(D)J permutations.

The differences between the subclasses of antibody do not relate to antibody specificity, but rather to various housekeeping aspects of antibody function. Subclasses differ in the number of disulfide bonds between heavy and light chains and the number and kinds of carbohydrate residues attached to the polypeptide chains. These differences are found toward the bottoms of the limbs of the Y and on its stalk, in a part of the antibody molecule called F_c. F_c gets its name because papain digests antibody molecules by cleaving them near the top of the stalk of the Y. The F_c stalk fragments readily crystallize if purified. These downstream carboxy-terminal F_c structures confer upon the different antibody classes and subclasses their differing abilities to bind to immune cells (e.g., phagocytes and mast cells), to activate complement, etc.

The binding of antibody to antigen can have important immunologic benefits:

- Agglutination and lysis of bacteria (IgM antibodies)
- Opsonization of bacteria, protozoa, and fungi
- Initiation of the classical complement pathway by binding the Clq complement component (IgM1 antibodies)
- Protecting the tissues underneath epithelial barriers in the respiratory tract, gut, eyes, and urinary tract from being invaded by microorganisms (secretory IgA)
- Killing infected cells by antibody-dependent cell-mediated cytotoxicity (ADCC); in this process, antibody bound to antigen on the surface of an infected cell (e.g., viral antigen) subsequently binds to F_c receptors on natural killer (NK) cells
- Neutralizing toxins and some other bacterial products that would otherwise enable the bacteria to avoid detection and removal by the immune system (Woolf 2000).

ACTIVATION OF B CELLS. Antigens are recognized and bound by B cells via *surface immunoglobulin* molecules. In other words, immunoglobulins serve both as the secreted effector molecules of plasma cells and also as B-cell receptors. The variable domains of these surface immunoglobulins bind precisely to their cognate epitopes (i.e., the particular ones they recognize). As previously discussed, each B-cell clone is programmed to bind to a particular epitope. It is the specificity of their surface immunoglobulins' variable regions that determines which clones of B cells will proliferate and differentiate in response to a particular infection.

All unstimulated B cells express IgM on their surfaces, and about 70% of them also express IgD. Relatively few express IgM along with one of the other immunoglobulin classes. When stimulated by interaction with their cognate epitope and activated, B cells bearing IgM or IgM/IgD on their surfaces give rise to clones of plasma cells that produce only IgM. B cells bearing IgM and immunoglobulin of one of the other classes (e.g., IgA, IgE, or IgG) go on to produce clones of plasma cells that switch over from producing IgM to produce whatever other class of immunoglobulin was originally on their surface. This *class switching* (also called *isotype switching*) is a routine part of the humoral immune response and involves a sophisticated process of immunoglobulin gene rearrangement in the activated B cell.

To be activated by most antigens, B cells need assistance from T helper cells. This is how it works: First of all, specific antigen binds to surface immunoglobulin on a B cell. The antigen-antibody complex is internalized by pinocytosis. The antigen is processed inside the B cell, and relevant fragments of the antigen are delivered back to the cell surface to be presented in the cleft of polymorphic cell surface molecules, called *major histocompatibility (MHC) class II molecules*, that are present on B-cell surfaces. It is important that B cells express MHC class II molecules on their surfaces (as, indeed, do other "professional" APCs) because the antigen fragment *must* be presented to the T helper cell in association with an MHC class II molecule; otherwise, it will not be recognized. If the "right" (i.e., cognate) T cell interacts with the B cell, it will promptly recognize and respond to correctly presented antigen by directly delivering signals to that B-cell membrane that cause proliferation and differentiation of the B cell into antibody-secreting plasma cells. As usual, the direct-signaling system involves a receptor-ligand interaction. *CD40* is an important activating molecule on the surface of the APC (in this case, the B cell). It interacts with *CD40 ligand* on the surface of the T helper cell. In addition to this direct signaling, activated T helper cells release a range of cytokines that stimulate B cells to proliferate (IL-2 and IL-4) and differentiate (IL-4, IL-6, IL-10, interferon-γ). Some activated B cells differentiate into antibody-producing plasma cells and a smaller number into long-lived *memory cells*.

As stated, activation of B cells usually requires the assistance of T cells. However, some antigens (so-called *T-independent antigens*) can trigger B cells to respond without the assistance of T helper cells. T-independent antigens are polymers; they include such molecules as bacterial lipopolysaccharides, pneumococcal polysaccharides, and dextran, among others. The antibody response to these antigens is extraordinary, consisting almost exclusively of IgM. In response to T-independent antigens, very few memory cells are produced, and tolerance to these antigens is easily induced.

INHERITED IMMUNOGLOBULIN DEFICIENCIES. Animals suffer for a number of inherited (or primary), selective, and nonselective immunoglobulin deficiencies. Often, the genetic basis for these disorders is incompletely understood. One such disorder is *selec-*

tive IgA deficiency. This disorder, the mode of inheritance of which is unknown, affects German shepherd dogs, Chinese shar-peis, and beagles. Serum IgA levels are normally low in healthy young dogs, so serum IgA levels of suspected patients must be compared with those of age-matched controls. Affected dogs are usually presented as youngsters with recurrent otitis, pyoderma, gastroenteritis, and chronic respiratory infections.

Another, seemingly distinct immunodeficiency of Chinese shar-peis involved both humoral and cellular immune responses. Levels of IgM, IgA and, in some cases, IgG were decreased, as were T-cell responses. Affected dogs developed recurrent infections and malignancies.

Another incompletely understood immunodeficiency syndrome affects juvenile llamas. Failure of passive transfer of maternal antibodies has been ruled out as the cause. Affected animals suffer from a wasting illness with recurrent infections. All llamas affected with the immunodeficiency syndrome had low serum IgG concentrations (e.g., prevaccination titers against *Clostridium perfringens* C and D toxoids, ≤1:100), and no increase in titer following vaccination. A retroviral cause was suspected but has not been confirmed. A primary immunodeficiency affecting B-cell development seems more likely at this stage.

Hypogammaglobulinemia may be seen as a component of a more generalized inherited immunodeficiency, such as X-linked severe combined immunodeficiency. This will be discussed under the heading of inherited disorders of cellular immunity.

ACQUIRED IMMUNOGLOBULIN ABNORMALITIES. Failure of passive transfer (FPT) of immunoglobulin is a common form of acquired immunodeficiency in horses and farm animals. Kittens and puppies seem to be relatively resistant to the adverse effects of colostrum deprivation. FPT is by no means a death sentence, but it does predispose foals and young farm animals to bacterial infections and septicemia. It can be prevented if farmers pursue optimal perinatal management practices.

Hypergammaglobulinemia may be associated with various infections (e.g., feline infectious peritonitis virus, FIV, and ehrlichiosis), neoplasms (e.g., multiple myeloma, lymphoma, and lymphoid leukemia), and other chronic inflammatory diseases. There is also a benign hypergammaglobulinemia seen in extreme old age. If it is sufficiently severe, hypergammaglobulinemia can cause *hyperviscosity syndrome*, characterized by seizures, epistaxis, renal failure, and retinopathy.

IMMUNE-COMPLEX DISEASE. Unfortunately, antibodies produced as part of an immune response to some pathogens are sometimes a major cause of the resulting disease.

Feline infectious peritonitis (FIP), caused by feline coronavirus (FCoV), is an *immune complex-mediated disease* involving viral antigen, antiviral antibodies, and complement. Not only is the host's immune response ineffective, it is central to the pathogenesis of this disease. Notably, cats that lack anti-FCoV antibodies do not develop FIP, nor do FCoV-seropositive cats whose complement has been artificially removed using cobra venom factor (Addie and Jarrett 1998).

FIP may occur as a result of circulating immune complexes coming out of circulation and lodging in blood vessel walls (Addie and Jarrett 1998). Alternatively, complexes may form locally within the blood vessel walls. Either way, they fix complement and can lead to dramatically increased vascular permeability with resulting leakage and/or the formation of pyogranulomata. The pathological consequences of in vivo immune-complex formation depend on the size of the complexes and their particular antibody-antigen content. Immune-complex deposition is more likely to happen where blood flow is turbulent or blood pressures are high. Such conditions are found at forks and tight U bends in blood vessels. FIP lesions are most common in the kidney, peritoneum, and uveal tract of the eye, sites of high blood pressure and turbulent flow. Effusive (wet) FIP is characterized by accumulation of proteinaceous fluid in the pleural, pericardial, and peritoneal cavities. It is usually a more acute form of the disease than is dry (noneffusive) FIP. Cats that develop effusive FIP may have a very large quantity of circulating virus, leading to massive formation of circulating immune complexes and damage to many blood vessels. Noneffusive FIP may result if fewer circulating immune complexes are formed, if circulating immune complexes fail to lodge in blood vessel walls, or if they do not fix much complement (Addie and Jarrett 1998).

Preexisting antibodies against a particular infectious agent usually protect animals against subsequent challenge with that same invader. However, in some experimental studies of FCoV infection, an enhanced form of disease occurred in seropositive cats compared with seronegative ones. One proposed mechanism for this antibody-dependent enhancement of disease was that antibody facilitated the uptake of FCoV into macrophages. However, subsequent field trials have not confirmed antibody-dependent enhancement of disease for FIP (Addie and Jarrett 1998). Nevertheless, it is clear that anti-FCoV antibodies contribute centrally to the pathogenesis of this disease.

MOLECULAR MIMICRY. Another situation in which antibodies can cause disease involves something termed *molecular mimicry* (Rose 2001). This term is not ideal because the word *mimicry* suggests *active* imitation, and this gives the wrong impression. Molecular mimicry is merely unfortunate happenstance. An epitope on an invading pathogen provokes an immune response. Unfortunately, this epitope resembles a host *self*-epitope, so that antibodies raised against the pathogen cross-react with self-antigens, leading to an *autoimmune disease*. One rather poorly characterized example concerns *Lyme borreliosis.* Antimyelin basic protein antibodies are frequently detected in the cerebrospinal fluid of patients with Lyme disease, and molecular mimicry between host antigens and *Borrelia burgdorferi* antigens is believed to contribute to the neuropathogenesis.

A better example of strongly suspected molecular mimicry concerns so-called *Reiter's syndrome*, which is a form of reactive arthritis/conjunctivitis/urethritis of people that follows various bacterial infections (most notably chlamydial urethritis). Tissues of 75% of affected individuals bear a particular histocompatibility antigen (i.e., tissue type): HLA-B27. Cross-reacting antibodies are strongly suspected to be involved in the pathogenesis, although this has not been confirmed definitively, and cytotoxic T lymphocytes may be involved. Another example from human medicine is *ankylosing spondylitis*: 95% of patients with this condition are HLA-B27 positive. Cross-reactivity of *Klebsiella* antigens with HLA-B27 has been demonstrated. Patients affected by ankylosing spondylitis were found to have higher numbers of *Klebsiella* organism in their feces, and higher levels of cross-reacting IgG and IgA antibodies. Dietary modification was associated with a decline in antibody levels and a clinical improvement. The etiology of canine ankylosing spondylitis—which is not thought to be clinically significant—is not well understood.

Finally, recent work (Rose 2001) suggests that the *cardiomyopathy of Chagas' disease* (American trypanosomiasis), at least in people, may be caused by molecular mimicry. Although this mechanism of disease has not been proven in *T. cruzi*-infected dogs, it is noteworthy that they suffer from a rather similar cardiomyopathy. Figure 3.7 illustrates the concept of molecular mimicry.

CELLULAR IMMUNE RESPONSE. The central role of small lymphocytes in adaptive immunity has already been mentioned. Most small lymphocytes are B or T cells. B and T cells cannot be distinguished morphologically, but special stains and other methods reveal that 70% to 80% of lymphocytes circulating in the blood are T cells and 10% to 15% are B cells. The remaining non-B and non-T cells (so-called double-negative or *null* cells) represent a mixed bag of lymphocytes, including NK cells.

T cells are so named because they must undergo maturation in the thymus. T cells bear specific antigen receptors (TCRs, T-cell receptors) that are structurally quite distinct from the surface immunoglobulin-receptor complexes of B cells. TCRs are heterodimers composed of two chains: 95% are composed of α and β chains (*alpha-beta* ($\alpha\beta$) receptors) and 5% are *gamma-delta* ($\gamma\delta$) receptors. Although quite distinct from them, TCRs share with immunoglobulins the fact that their component chains are made up of one of many variable (V), diversity (D), and joining (J) segments together with a carboxy-terminal constant (C) region (however, the *gamma* (γ) chain does not have a D segment). The *beta* (β) chain, for example, is made from just one of 25 *V-beta* (V_β) regions, and there are about 100 *V-alpha* (V_α) genes to choose from. So, as with immunoglobulins, an enormous number of possible V(D)J permutations exist, and this is largely responsible for the huge diversity in TCR specificities. The way that the heterodimeric chains fold together further increases diversity.

The TCR complex includes another protein called CD3. Presence of CD3 on the surface of a small lym-

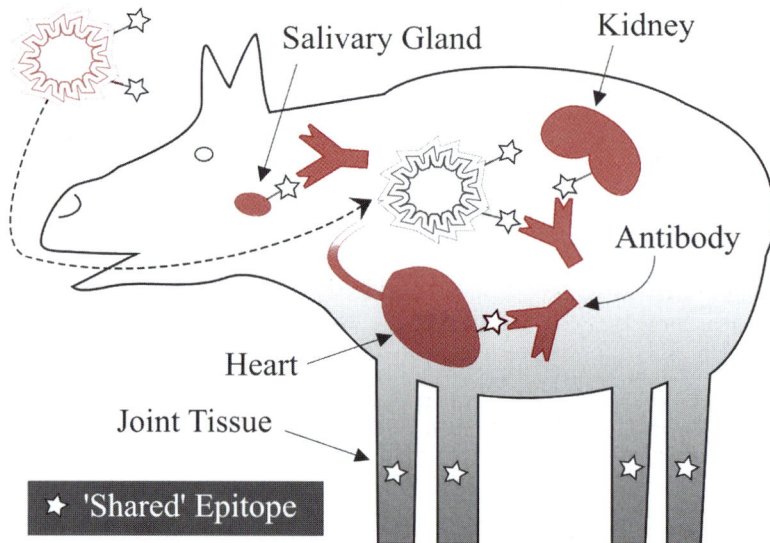

FIG. 3.7—Some pathogens have antigens that resemble host tissues (represented as white stars in this diagram). This is most unfortunate for the host, since an immune response directed against the invader may "wash over" to produce autoimmune disease. The resulting autoimmune disease may produce considerably more morbidity than the initiating infection. Heart, kidney, joint tissues, salivary glands, and lacrimal glands may be targeted. Certain breeds or individuals within a species may be more prone to the adverse effects of molecular mimicry.

phocyte can be detected and used to identify it as a T cell of some sort. T cells can be further divided into important functionally distinct subsets. *Helper/inducer T cells* aid in the generation of immune responses by other T cells and by B cells: they bear a marker called CD4 on their surfaces, as well as CD3, so are sometimes called CD4+ T cells. *Cytotoxic T cells* can lyse virus-infected cells and tumor cells: they bear CD8 as well as CD3 on their surfaces (and are therefore also called CD8+ T cells). To go one step further, it is now clear that CD4+ helper/inducer T cells can be functionally divided into at least three subsets: Th0, Th1, and Th2, which are distinguishable by the profile of lymphokines they secrete when stimulated. *Th1 T cells* secrete IL-2, interferon-gamma (IFN-γ), and lymphotoxin, but not Th2 lymphokines typified by IL-4. *Th2 T cells* have the opposite profile: they secrete IL-4, IL-5, IL-9, and IL-13, but not Th1 lymphokines. *Th0 T cells* have a mixed Th1-Th2 pattern of secretion. The lymphokines secreted by Th1 T cells tend to lead to delayed-type hypersensitivity and a cell-mediated immune response. The Th2-lymphokine profile favors an IgG1 and IgE antibody response. To some extent, a Th1 response suppresses a Th2 response and vice versa. Whether a given microbial invader will provoke a Th1 or Th2 response depends on the amount of certain cytokines secreted by T cells (particularly IL-4) and macrophages (particularly IL-12). It has been suggested that a Th1 response is attuned to deal with intracellular pathogens (such as viruses) and that a Th2 response is ideal for extracellular pathogens (e.g., many parasites and bacteria).

B cells can recognize and bind antigens in their native form via their surface immunoglobulins. However, T cells require antigen to be trapped, processed, and correctly presented to them. CD4+ helper T cells require antigen to be presented in association with MHC Class II molecules. This task is usually carried out by "professional" APCs. B cells can serve as APCs because they express MHC class II molecules on their cell surfaces. Other "professional" APCs include monocytes, macrophages, and their relatives (Langerhans' cells and dendritic cells). On the other hand, CD8+ cytotoxic T cells require antigen to be presented in association with MHC class I molecules. Essentially all mammalian cells express MHC class I molecules. Thus, CD8+ T cells, one role of which is to kill virus-infected cells, are barely restricted in the kinds of cells they can interact with and target.

Recognition of processed antigen by T helper cells (i.e., CD4+ T cells) is the most critical, central event in the immune response. This is because activated T helper cells control and modulate the activities of the other cells that are necessary for an effective immune response. The antigen fragment in the cleft of the MHC class II molecule on the surface of an APC represents the epitope that is recognized by the CD4+ TCR. Binding of the TCR to the antigen-MHC class II complex is not quite enough, however, to maximize activation of the T cell. *Costimulatory molecules* on the APC and T

helper cell must also interact. *B7* on the surface of the APC and *CD28* on the surface of the T cell bind to complete the stimulatory signal. Subsequently, the activated TCR complex conveys its signal via a transduction pathway to the interior of the cell. This signal upregulates CD40 ligand gene expression and leads to the expression of CD40 ligand on the surface of the CD4+ cell. The CD40 ligand binds to CD40 receptor on the surface of the APC. This interaction activates the APC to release IL-1, which in turn causes the release of both IFN-γ and IL-2 from CD4+ cells. Interestingly, secreted IL-2 then feeds back positively on the CD4+ cells to stimulate expression of more IL-2 receptors. Various cell growth and differentiation factors are also produced by stimulated CD4+ cells. The binding of secreted IL-2 to IL-2 receptor-bearing CD4+ T cells induces clonal proliferation. The requirement for both IL-2 secretion and IL-2 receptor expression for T cells to proliferate helps to ensure that only T cells specific for the antigen provoking the immune response become activated. Activated helper T cells subsequently stimulate immune effector cells, such as cytotoxic cells and B cells.

Cytotoxic CD8+ T cells bind to cells expressing their cognate antigen fragments in association with MHC class I molecules. For example, the cell might be virus infected and expressing viral protein fragments on its surface. The infected cell comes into direct contact with the CD8+ T cell, which is thought to transfer various enzymes (e.g., esterases and proteases) from within its granules to help kill the infected cell. Production of *perforin* molecules is important in the killing process. Perforin has some similarities in structure and function to complement membrane attack-complex components. It "punches" holes in the membrane of the targeted cell. Another mechanism of cell killing involves binding of Fas [also called Apo-1 (apolipoprotein 1)] on the target cell by Fas ligand on the CD8+ T cell. This interaction leads to programmed cell death (apoptosis) of the target cell.

NK cells are slightly larger than other lymphocytes and have a granular appearance; hence, they are sometimes called large granular lymphocytes rather than small lymphocytes. NK cells can bind IgG because they express membrane receptors for the constant region (i.e., stalk) of IgG. They cause ADCC by binding and killing IgG-coated organisms or infected cells. Again, this is a perforin-dependent process. Additionally, NK cells can destroy virally infected cells or tumor cells in a process that does not involve antibody at all. NK cells have been described as a rather primitive, multifunctional component of the immune system. They can be considered to straddle the boundary between innate and adaptive immunity.

INHERITED DISORDERS OF CELLULAR IMMUNITY. Recently, a number of primary disorders of cellular immunity have been well characterized in species of veterinary importance. Two examples of different kinds of severe combined immunodeficiency (SCID) will be cited: one involves a mutation in the IL-2 receptor gene, and the other involves a mutation that prevents proper V(D)J joining in immunoglobulins and TCRs.

X-linked SCID (X-SCID) has been reported in male Cardigan Welsh corgi puppies (Somberg et al. 1995). Affected puppies failed to thrive and had diarrhea, intermittent vomiting, and impalpable lymph nodes. The premature death of a male sibling, suspected to be affected, was noted. Serum immunoglobulin quantitation revealed a low concentration of IgG, undetectable IgA, and a normal concentration of IgM. A hemogram revealed mild anemia and lymphopenia. There was a normal percentage of T cells in the peripheral blood, with an increased CD4/CD8 ratio. However, peripheral blood T cells were unable to proliferate in response to the polyclonal T-cell mitogen phytohemagglutinin (PHA) and/or in response to IL-2. PHA-treated peripheral blood lymphocytes were unable to bind IL-2. These findings were identical to earlier findings from basset hounds with X-SCID. In that breed, the problem was due to a mutation in their IL-2 receptor γ chain (IL-2R γ). This γ chain is actually an essential part of several cytokine receptors, including those for IL-4, IL-7, IL-9, and IL-15; for this reason, it is called the common γ chain (or γc). Examination of the corgi's γc cDNA revealed the insertion of a cytosine residue following nucleotide 582, resulting in a premature stop codon. This new γc mutation in Cardigan Welsh corgi puppies results in X-SCID, with similar immunologic abnormalities to those observed earlier in basset hounds. In bassets, the same disease results from a different γ-chain mutation.

Autosomal recessive SCID of Arabian (Arab) foals (Shin et al. 2000), Jack Russell terriers (Meek et al. 2001), and CB17 mice is due to faulty V(D)J recombination in the genes encoding immunoglobulins and TCRs. In all three species, the mutation is not in the gene encoding the lymphocyte-specific endonuclease that recognizes and cleaves germline DNA at target sequences adjacent to V(D)J gene segments. Rather, the mutation is in one of the components necessary for double-stranded DNA repair, or religation. The molecular defect in SCID foals, terriers, and mice is in the catalytic subunit (CS) of the DNA-dependent protein kinase (DNA-PK). DNA-PK is an extremely large multiprotein complex. This large enzyme is specifically activated to phosphorylate its target proteins in the presence of DNA loose ends, which suggests that it has a role in DNA repair. In higher eukaryotes, deficiency of any of the component polypeptides of DNA-PK effectively disrupts the organism's ability to repair double-stranded DNA breaks efficiently, resulting in extreme sensitivity to ionizing radiation. However, it is not this radiation sensitivity that is usually lethal to the mutant organism. Rather, DNA-PK deficiencies are lethal traits because vertebrate immune systems are dependent on nonhomologous DNA end joining to complete V(D)J recombination. Mutants unable to complete V(D)J recombination die young of overwhelming infections secondary to profound immunodeficiency.

Interestingly, although all three species have a mutation in the gene encoding CS of DNA-PK, the severity of immunodeficiency is worst in Arabian foals and least severe in the mice. There seems to be significant species variation in how essential DNA-PK$_{CS}$ is for V(D)J recombination. The severity of the V(D)J recombination deficits in these three examples of inherited DNA-PK$_{CS}$ deficiency correlates inversely with the relative DNA-PK enzymatic activity expressed in normal fibroblasts derived from affected members of these three species.

ACQUIRED DISORDERS OF CELLULAR IMMUNITY. Acquired (or secondary) immunodeficiencies are much more common than primary forms. Infectious, neoplastic, metabolic, and environmental (including nutritional) causes predominate. Of these, infectious causes are probably the most important.

Canine distemper virus causes profound depression in cell-mediated immunity if the infection takes hold prenatally or in the first few weeks of a puppy's life. Older animals infected by virulent virus may experience transient depression of cell-mediated immunity. *Canine parvovirus* infection and *feline panleukopenia* cause pancytopenia, including lymphopenia. In utero infection can cause thymic atrophy and irreversible, profound immunosuppression. Lymphocyte-stimulation assays also show diminished lymphocyte responsiveness in parvovirus infected puppies and kittens; i.e., the virus causes qualitative as well as quantitative lymphocyte abnormalities.

FeLV infection and FIV infection cause similar immunodeficiency syndromes. FeLV-infected cats develop T-cell functional defects characterized by reduced in vitro lymphocyte responsiveness to stimuli, prolonged retention of skin allografts, and diminished delayed-type hypersensitivity reactions. Some FeLV strains are considerably more immunosuppressive than others. Differences in the SU surface glycoprotein molecules of different strains seem to explain this variability, although this is incompletely understood.

FIV causes profound abnormalities in cellular immunity (Sellon 1998). The thymus is a site of early replication of the virus; this depletes the T-cell pool. Virus later infects follicular dendritic cells in lymph nodes, gaining further access to naive T cells as they transit through the node. Early in the acute stage of infection, levels of FIV are high in circulating CD4+ T cells. Later on, more FIV is found in B cells than in CD4+ T cells. After the host mounts a humoral immune response to the virus, FIV levels in circulation decrease markedly. However, viral replication does continue at a lower level, so this is not a true example of a latent period.

The immunodeficiency caused by FIV is characterized by a decline in absolute number and relative proportion of CD4+ T cells. Possible causes for the decline in CD4+ T cells include failure of production (by marrow and/or thymus) and destruction of infected cells (either directly by the virus, by the immune system, or by apoptosis). In vitro, apoptosis (programmed cell death) can be seen in FIV-infected lymphocytes. The virus can cause cell fusion, so direct cytopathicity may be one mechanism of CD4+ T-cell loss. CD8+ cytotoxic T cells may destroy virus-infected CD4+ cells, further diminishing their number (Sellon 1998).

During the course of infection, lymphocytes of FIV-infected cats become progressively refractory to B-cell and T-cell mitogens; that is, they do not exhibit the expected proliferative responses. They express diminished or otherwise abnormal cell surface molecules; e.g., CD4 and IL-2 receptors. Cytokine production can be abnormal: IL-6 secretion may be increased and TNF-α may be either increased or decreased. NK cell function may also be adversely affected.

FIV causes substantial dysfunction of other immune system components, such as phagocytes and B cells. Hypocomplementemia and high concentrations of circulating immune complexes may be immunosuppressive. Eventually, despite a vigorous but ineffective immune response, FIV infection leads to profound immunodeficiency, and the patient succumbs to one or more opportunistic infections or neoplasms (Sellon 1998).

SUPERANTIGENS AND DISEASE. Superantigens are molecules that can stimulate T lymphocytes by a mechanism that differs from that employed by conventional antigens (see Figure 3.8). Conventional antigens are recognized by CD4+ T cells when a peptide fragment of the antigen is presented to the T cell on the surface of another cell. To be properly presented, the antigen fragment must be bound in the cleft of an MHC class II molecule on the surface of an APC. This complex ligand then interacts with variable elements of the TCR on the surface of the CD4+ T cell and leads ultimately to T helper cell stimulation. The specificity of T-cell antigen recognition depends upon the fact that only a small subset of T cells, with a compatible arrangement of variable elements in their receptors, will be able to bind to a particular antigen fragment in the cleft of a specific MHC molecule.

Superantigens also interact with CD4+ TCRs together with MHC class II molecules. However, the superantigen is not presented to the variable elements of the TCR in the cleft of the MHC molecule. Rather, it is bound elsewhere on the MHC molecule and interacts with part of the exposed exterior of the TCR molecule. Clearly, this sort of interaction is likely to be much less specific than that employed in conventional antigen recognition. The part of a TCR that can interact with a superantigen is encoded by the V_β segment of the TCR gene complex. For this reason, it has been suggested that superantigens might be better named V_β-selective elements. During T-cell development, TCR gene rearrangements occur, so that one V_β gene segment is chosen for use, essentially at random, from a selection of about twenty or so. This is one of the ways that diversity of immune responsiveness can be generated in a genetically parsimonious fashion. The super-

antigens that have been studied so far can each interact with one to seven different kinds of V_β gene products. Therefore, if we assume that the 20 or so different V_β gene segments are used equally by T cells, then about 5% to 35% of all CD4+ T cells might be able to interact with a particular superantigen. Some of these assumptions may be unreasonable, but the argument does make the point that superantigens can stimulate massive, somewhat directed, T-cell responses.

Two main types of superantigens have been identified so far. Firstly, there are bacterial superantigens such as the staphylococcal enterotoxins. *Staphylococcus aureus* enterotoxins are a major cause of food poisoning in people, responsible for about 25% of all outbreaks reported in the United States. Other staphylococcal superantigen toxins cause various toxic shock syndromes, including tampon-related toxic shock. Some streptococci and mycoplasma species can produce toxins with similar effects. These bacterial superantigens are generally proteins that are about 220 amino acids long. It is thought that the clinical signs produced by these toxins are in part due to massive, inappropriate, T-cell stimulation and subsequent

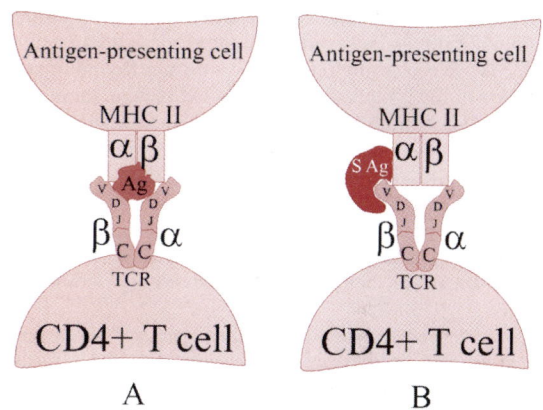

FIG. 3.8—Conventional antigens are recognized by CD4+ T cells when a peptide fragment of the antigen (Ag) is presented to the T cell on the surface of an antigen-presenting cell (as in **A**). To be properly presented, the antigen fragment must be bound in the cleft of a major histocompatibility complex class II (MHC II) molecule on the surface of the antigen-presenting cell. This complex ligand then interacts with variable elements (V) of the T-cell receptor (TCR) on the surface of the CD4+ T cell and leads ultimately to T helper cell stimulation. The specificity of T-cell antigen recognition arises because only a small subset of T cells, with compatible variable elements in their receptors, are able to bind to a particular antigen fragment. Like normal antigens, superantigens (S Ag) also interact with CD4+ TCRs and MHC II molecules. However, the superantigen is not presented to the TCR in the cleft of the MHC molecule. Rather, it interacts with an external V_β region of the TCR molecule (as in **B**). For this reason, it has been suggested that superantigens might alternatively be named V_β-selective elements. Superantigens can stimulate massive, somewhat directed, T-cell responses. (Adapted from Zumla 1992.)

release of lymphokines such as IL-2 and TNF. Interestingly, infection with several of the bacterial organisms that produce superantigen toxins has been associated with the development of probable autoimmune disorders, such as arthritis, rheumatic fever, and skin rash. It has been suggested that superantigens might be responsible for the development of these autoimmune manifestations. This could occur if autoreactive T cells, which are generally present in small, clinically insignificant numbers in normal individuals, were stimulated by the superantigen to proliferate massively and/or increase their activity.

A second type of superantigen is encoded in the mouse genome. For years, it has been known that certain strains of mice express antigens on some of their cells that stimulate CD4+ T cells from other strains of mice, even though the two strains might be identical at the MHC. These self-superantigens or endogenous superantigens were originally termed minor lymphocyte stimulating (Mls) antigens. At first, it was believed that endogenous superantigens were expressed from a single genetic locus, but subsequently it became clear that there are multiple different superantigens, expressed from nonlinked loci. Superantigens expressed from different genetic loci may differ in their V_β specificity. As one would expect, mice that endogenously express these superantigens delete autoreactive T cells that bear the relevant V_βs during thymic maturation of the lymphocytes. As a consequence, these animals lack significant portions of their potential T-cell repertoire, and they maintain tolerance to the endogenous superantigens. Interestingly, the lack of a whole swag of potential T cells does not seem to cause any increased susceptibility to infectious disease in Mls-expressing mice, and the phenomenon is extremely widespread in both wild and laboratory strains of mice.

The first strong hint that an endogenous superantigen gene and an endogenous mouse mammary tumor virus[1] (MMTV) might be one and the same thing came in 1990, when an Mls gene was mapped to chromosome 12 and tightly linked to a well-characterized endogenous MMTV provirus. Even more impressive was that cell lines of a particular MHC type that expressed an endogenous superantigen also transcribed the appropriate endogenous MMTV mRNA, whereas cell lines of the same MHC type that did not have superantigen activity lacked the retroviral mRNA.

Further evidence linking MMTV with superantigen activity concerns a conventionally transmissible (i.e., exogenous) form of the virus. C3H/HeJ mice are known to transmit MMTV vertically from mother to offspring in their milk. The offspring are infected for life and persistently express retroviral gene products to a variable degree. Mice of this strain were noticed to have fewer $V_\beta 14$ bearing T cells than other, closely related strains of mice. Suspecting that C3H/HeJ mice might express a $V_\beta 14$-specific endogenous superantigen, investigators carried out classical backcrossing genetic studies. They were surprised to discover that the superantigen was maternally inherited. By foster nursing experiments, they went on to show that a $V_\beta 14$-specific superantigen is transmitted to the offspring of C3H/HeJ mice, probably in milk. They suspected that a component of MMTV might be the $V_\beta 14$-specific superantigen, so they studied substrains of C3H/HeJ that do not have MMTV in their milk. Substrains that did not transmit MMTV also did not transmit $V_\beta 14$-specific superantigen activity. So it now seems clear that both endogenous and exogenous forms of MMTV encode a superantigen. Interest has focused upon the unusual open reading frames (ORFs) in the long terminal repeats (LTRs) of all MMTVs. Each ORF encodes a 320-amino-acid protein of unknown function. Recent experiments indicate that the 3' LTR ORF of MMTV encodes the superantigen.

What benefit would possession of a superantigen confer upon a milk-borne retrovirus? Superantigens can cause a paradoxical immunosuppression in vivo, so perhaps this provides an advantage to the virus. Another idea is that activation of T cells by viral superantigen might make cells susceptible to retroviral infection, facilitating spread of the virus. Conversely, mice may have evolved to counter the viral strategy by "endogenizing" MMTV, expressing self-superantigen and thereby ensuring the deletion of all those T cells capable of responding to the exogenous pathogen. Some recent experimental data support this last notion and offer the possibility of exciting approaches to antiviral therapy and immunization.

Environmental Influences on Infection. The environment in which an animal lives can have a profound influence on its likelihood of contracting and succumbing to an infection. Some of the reasons for this are relatively straightforward. For example, an environment that provides adequate, nutritious food will help to enable animals to grow to adulthood and meet their genetic potential. Conversely, if an animal suffers protein or caloric malnutrition, this can cause deficiencies of cell-mediated and humoral immunity, hypocomplementemia, and phagocyte dysfunction. In starved young animals, premature thymic atrophy may occur. Even in the face of adequate protein and calorie intake, vitamin A, vitamin E, zinc, and selenium deficiencies have been reported to cause various forms of immunodeficiency. Interestingly, overfeeding and obesity can also cause an increased susceptibility to infection.

Hypothermia is associated with reduced T-cell function in some species. Neonates are particularly prone to hypothermia in cold environments.

---

1. MMTV is a retrovirus. One of the unique features of retroviruses is that their genetic material may become integrated into the germline DNA of the host, so that retroviral sequences become part of the "genetic dowry" of the host animal. Eventually, these endogenous retroviral sequences may become fixed within the gene pool, so that all members of the host species have a complement of endogenous retroviral elements within their chromosomal DNA. There is compelling evidence that germline retroviral integration events of this kind have occurred repeatedly during vertebrate evolution.

Crowding and "stress" in housed animals can be associated with poor air quality, increased exposure to infectious agents, and immunodeficiency. Psychological stress may alter immune function through a number of different mechanisms. These include (a) direct innervation of lymphoid tissues by the central nervous system and (b) stress-induced release of hormones from the brain and other endocrine organs that bind to and alter the functions of cells of the immune system. In humans, adverse behavioral changes may occur in response to stress—for example, loss of sleep, increased smoking, increased alcohol intake, reduced exercise, a less "healthy" diet, and less adherence to medical advice. It is not clear what, if any, veterinary equivalent there may be to these behavioral changes, although some stressed animals certainly do alter their behavior significantly. Healthy people exposed to stressful tasks that lasted for only a few minutes—including difficult thinking tasks and tasks that caused anxiety—showed suppression of T-cell mitogenesis and an increase in the number of circulating CD8+ and NK cells in blood. Living near the Three Mile Island nuclear power plant at the time of the accident, taking care of a relative with Alzheimer's disease, taking medical school examinations, and suffering from clinical depression have all been associated with alterations in both the number and function of various subpopulations of lymphocytes. These alterations include a reduced proliferative response to mitogen stimulation, reduced NK cell cytotoxicity, and altered production of cytokines. Although the range of effects that stress can have on immune function is wide, the magnitude of the effects is small (Cohen and Rabin 1998).

Air quality can be a particularly important environmental factor in intensively reared farm animals such as pigs and chickens. Dust, aerosolized bacteria, and toxic gases (e.g., ammonia and hydrogen sulfide) are particularly important factors. In cold weather, farmers are sometimes tempted to reduce the speed of exhaust fans to maintain internal temperatures. This can dramatically increase the air humidity and ammonia concentrations inside.

Drummond and colleagues (1980) assigned 4-week-old piglets from each of two litters to one of four rooms, the environment of which could be tightly controlled. These rooms were randomly assigned to one of four aerial ammonia concentrations: 0 (control), 50, 100, and 150 ppm (parts per million) of ammonia. Exposure was maintained at a constant level for 4 weeks. Piglets breathing air containing 50 ppm ammonia showed a 12% less daily weight gain compared with the control group. The average daily weight gain of piglets in both the 100 ppm and 150 ppm ammonia chambers was 30% less than that of the control piglets. In addition, piglets exposed to 100 or 150 ppm of aerial ammonia were lethargic in comparison to the controls and those breathing 50 ppm ammonia. Coughing was only apparent among piglets at the 100-ppm and 150-ppm levels. Excessive lacrimation (i.e., tear production) was noted in all piglets exposed to aerial ammonia. This was associated with black skin discoloration at the medial canthi of the eyes. The size of the discolored areas was directly proportional to the ammonia concentration being breathed.

Exposure to aerial ammonia increases the nasal turbinate shrinkage seen in *Bordetella bronchiseptica*-infected pigs. This is a dose-dependent effect, with 100 ppm ammonia causing more shrinkage than 50 ppm.

REFERENCES

Addie DD, Jarrett O. 1998. Feline coronavirus infection. In: Greene CE, ed. Infectious Diseases of the Dog and Cat, 2nd ed. Philadelphia: WB Saunders, pp 58–69.

Ascenzi P, Visca P, Ippolito G, et al. 2002. Anthrax toxin: A tripartite lethal combination. FEBS Lett 531:384–388.

Boes M. 2000. Role of natural and immune IgM antibodies in immune responses. Mol Immunol 37:1141–1149.

Cohen S, Rabin BS. 1998. Psychologic stress, immunity, and cancer [Editorial]. J Natl Cancer Inst 90:30–36.

Collinge J. 2001. Prion diseases of humans and animals: Their causes and molecular basis. Ann Rev Neurosci 24:519–550.

Diener TO. 1999. Viroids and the nature of viroid diseases. Arch Virol (Suppl) 15:203–220.

Drummond JG, Curtis SE, Simon J, Morton HW. 1980. Effects of aerial ammonia on the growth and health of young pigs. J Anim Sci 50:1085.

Dunn JK, Greene CE. 1998. Fever. In: Greene CE, ed. Infectious Diseases of the Dog and Cat, 2nd ed. Philadelphia: WB Saunders, pp 693–701.

Giger U, Greene CE. 1998. Immunodeficiencies and infectious diseases. In: Greene CE, ed. Infectious Diseases of the Dog and Cat, 2nd ed. Philadelphia: WB Saunders, pp 683–693.

Gorham JR, Foreyt WJ. 1998. Salmon poisoning disease. In: Greene CE, ed. Infectious Diseases of the Dog and Cat, 2nd ed. Philadelphia: WB Saunders, pp 135–139.

Greene CE, ed. 1998. Infectious Diseases of the Dog and Cat, 2nd ed. Philadelphia: WB Saunders.

Haag J, O'hUigin C, Overpath P. 1998. The molecular phylogeny of trypanosomes: evidence for an early divergence of the Salivaria. Mol Biochem Parasitol 91:37–49.

Henderson B, Wilson M. 1998. Commensal communism and the oral cavity. J Dent Res 77:1674–1683.

Holton NJ, Goodwin TJ, Butler MI, Poulter RT. 2001. An active retrotransposon in *Candida albicans*. Nucleic Acids Res 29:4014–4024.

Isberg RR, Hamburger Z, Dersch P. 2000. Signaling and invasin-promoted uptake via integrin receptors. Microbes Infect 2:793–801.

Johnson JR, Stell AL, Delavari P, et al. 2001. Phylogenetic and pathotypic similarities between *Escherichia coli* isolates from urinary tract infections in dogs and extraintestinal infections in humans. J Infect Dis 183:897–906.

Klein BS. 2000. Molecular basis of pathogenicity in *Blastomyces dermatitidis*: The importance of adhesion. Curr Opin Microbiol 3:339–343.

Kohno S, Fujimura T, Rulong S, Kwon-Chung KJ. 1994. Double-stranded RNA virus in the human pathogenic fungus *Blastomyces dermatitidis*. J Virol 68:7554–7558.

Konsman JP, Cartmell T. 1997. Neural pathways from the immune system to the brain. Eur Cytokine Network 8:221–223.

Krohne SG. 2000. Canine systemic fungal infections. Vet Clin North Am Small Anim Pract 30:1063–1090.

Linial M. 2000. Why aren't foamy viruses pathogenic? Trends Microbiol 8:284–289.

Lotter H, Khajawa F, Stanley SL Jr, Tannich E. 2000. Protection of gerbils from amebic liver abscess by vaccination with a 25-mer peptide derived from the cysteine-rich region of *Entamoeba histolytica* galactose-specific adherence lectin. Infect Immun 68:4416–4421.

Mackowiak PA. 1994. Fever: Blessing or curse? A unifying hypothesis. Ann Intern Med 120:1037–1040.

Meek K, Kienker L, Dallas C, et al. 2001. SCID in Jack Russell terriers: A new animal model of DNA-PK$_{cs}$ deficiency. J Immunol 167:2142–2150.

Mi S, Lee X, Li X, et al. 2000. Syncytin is a captive retroviral envelope protein involved in human placental morphogenesis. Nature 403:785–789.

Mishra C, Lambert J. 1996. Production of anti-microbial substances by probiotics. Asia Pac J Clin Nutr 5:20–24.

Rose NR. 2001. Infection, mimics, and autoimmune disease [Commentary]. J Clin Invest 107:943–944.

Samuelson LC, Phillips RS, Swanberg LJ. 1996. Amylase gene structures in primates: Retroposon insertions and promoter evolution. Mol Biol Evol 13:767–779.

Sellon RK. 1998. Feline immunodeficiency virus infection. In: Greene CE, ed. Infectious Diseases of the Dog and Cat, 2nd ed. pp 84–96. Philadelphia: WB Saunders, pp 84–96.

Shin EK, Rijkers T, Pastink A, Meek K. 2000. Analyses of TCRB rearrangements substantiate a profound deficit in recombination signal sequence joining in SCID foals: Implications for the role of DNA-dependent protein kinase in V(D)J recombination. J Immunol 164:1416–1424.

Somberg RL, Pullen RP, Casal ML, et al. 1995. A single nucleotide insertion in the canine interleukin-2 receptor gamma chain results in X-linked severe combined immunodeficiency disease. Vet Immunol Immunopathol 47:203–213.

Späth GF, Epstein L, Leader B, et al. 2000. Lipophosphoglycan is a virulence factor distinct from related glycoconjugates in the protozoan parasite *Leishmania major*. Proc Natl Acad Sci USA 97:9258–9263.

Ting CN, Rosenberg MP, Snow CM, et al. 1992. Endogenous retroviral sequences are required for tissue-specific expression of a human salivary amylase gene. Genes Dev 6:1457–1465.

Tizard I. 2000. Veterinary Immunology: An Introduction, 6th ed. Philadelphia: WB Saunders.

Webster RG. 1997. Influenza virus: Transmission between species and relevance to emergence of the next human pandemic. Arch Virol (Suppl) 13:105–113.

Wilks D, Sissons JGP. 1997. Infection. In: Tomlinson S, Heargerty AM, Weetman AP, eds. Mechanisms of disease: An introduction to clinical science. Cambridge: Cambridge University Press, pp 160–201.

Willett BJ, Hosie MJ. 1999. The role of the chemokine receptor CXCR4 in infection with feline immunodeficiency virus. Mol Membrane Biol 16:67–72.

Winkelstein JA. 1998. The complement system. In: Gorbach SL, Bartlett JG, Blacklow NR, eds. Infectious diseases, 2nd ed. Philadelphia: WB Saunders, pp 35–41.

Woolf N. 2000. The Immune System. In: Cell, tissue and disease: The Basis of Pathology, 3rd ed. Edinburgh: WB Saunders, pp 137–181.

Zasloff M. 2002. Antimicrobial peptides of multicellular organisms. Nature 415:389–395.

Zumla A. 1992. Superantigens, T cells, and microbes. Clin Infect Dis 15:313–320.

4

PATHOPHYSIOLOGY OF THE GASTROINTESTINAL TRACT

Charles-Henri Malbert, Editor, and Anthony T. Blikslager, Samuel L. Jones, Marie-Louise Grondahl, Alfred M. Merritt

The origin of gastrointestinal dysfunctions involves disturbances in the neurohumoroimmune control of the gut function (Wood et al. 1999). All components of these mechanisms are so intermingled that it is virtually impossible to pinpoint the actual causal components affected by a pathological process. For instance, gastric ulceration affects the myenteric neurons through the production of calcitonin gene-related peptide (CGRP) by mast cells that are part of the immune system of the gut (Holzer 1998). In addition, the redundant nature of the control mechanisms explains why the occurrence of gastrointestinal symptoms is associated with massive disturbance of the regulatory systems. Indeed, in addition to the redundant nature of the control mechanisms supervising food absorption, processing, and transit, the overall capacity of the gut especially toward absorption is around 70% in excess (Weber and Ehrlein 1998).

DEFECTS IN TRANSIT. Whereas defects in transit might occur at different levels of the gastrointestinal tract, the most relevant for veterinary medicine are those located at the gastrointestinal level. Furthermore, transit defects affecting more distal parts of the gut, for example, the cecocolon, are most often a consequence of altered absorption and/or intestinal inflammatory processes.

Gastric emptying is a delicate mechanism prone to defects, since the stomach must accommodate and process a large quantity of food in a limited time (the meal) and regulate the outflow of chyme in relation to the absorbing capability of the small intestine. In contrast to this accommodation, the postprandial phase takes a significant portion of the day, especially in carnivores. The most important concept in gastrointestinal transit physiopathology is the inhibitory nature of the defects. Except after some surgery aimed specifically at facilitating gastric drainage, such as pyloroplasty or pylorectomy, altered gastric emptying reduces transit time (Malbert and Horowitz 1997).

In Monogastric Species. The reduction in gastric emptying—or gastroparesis—results in symptoms similar to those described in humans, such as functional dyspepsia, and includes nausea, vomiting, epigastric pain, abdominal bloating, and postprandial fullness. Symptoms are frequently reported to occur in connection with food intake, particularly following the ingestion of foods that contain fat. In addition, food consistency or preparation appears to be a determinant of symptoms; for instance, solid food containing fat is less likely to induce symptoms than are fat-containing liquids.

MECHANISMS OF GASTRIC EMPTYING

THE PROXIMAL STOMACH AFTER A MEAL. Peristaltic contractions are found in the distal stomach but not in the proximal stomach. The proximal stomach shows only tonic activity, which is modified by the arrival of food in the stomach and the duodenum. Immediately after a swallow, a *receptive relaxation* of the proximal stomach is triggered that lasts about 20 seconds. One receptive relaxation occurs for about each swallow during a meal. In contrast, *adaptive relaxation* is triggered by the arrival of the first nutrient molecules in the duodenum very early during gastric emptying and lasts about 1 hour. In response to the arrival of food in the duodenum, polymodal vagal sensory neurons located in the duodenal wall are activated and trigger a vagovagal reflex (Azpiroz and Malagelada 1986). The efferent limb of this reflex involves secretion by vagal efferent neurons of nitric oxide (NO), which is the most potent relaxant of the smooth muscle. Failure to induce an adaptive relaxation is a common cause of delayed emptying. Indeed, once the pressure within the stomach is above 30 mm Hg, a local intramural reflex acting in conjunction with a vagovagal inhibitory reflex inhibits distal stomach peristaltic contractions (Treacy et al. 1994). This amplifies the level of distension of the stomach, since acid secreted throughout the meal cannot be evacuated and contributes to build up the distending volume.

THE DISTAL STOMACH AND THE PYLORUS DURING AND AFTER A MEAL. Within a few minutes of the onset of a meal, a stable contraction pattern occurs: three contractions per minute travel through the stomach. The contractions of the distal part of the stomach correspond to phasic, peristaltic waves that mix and grind solid food and transport it to the pylorus. The peristaltic nature of the waves is critical to the pressurization of the most distal part of the stomach, which itself is the origin of the retropulsion that grinds food particles. Indeed, food transport throughout the gut is a consequence of the sole means of a positive pressure gradient, the pressure before the bolus being greater than the pressure after. Peristalsis represents the very basis of the generation of this pressure gradient. Since peristalsis relies on the integrity of myenteric neurons, systemic diseases—such as diabetes, hypergastrinemia, and hypoxemia—that affect the behavior of these neurons potently inhibit emptying (Pinna et al. 1995).

Most of the time, the pylorus is partially open and closes only sporadically. During *normal* emptying, the pylorus works in conjunction with the distal antrum and the proximal duodenum so that the pressure within the pyloric canal is not a barrier to aboral propulsion of gastric contents being pushed by a peristaltic antral contraction. The antropyloroduodenal unit may become dissociated especially during emptying of high-caloric lipid meals. The activation of a vagovagal reflex originating from duodenal vagal chemoreceptors is associated with suppression of antral and duodenal, but not pyloric, phasic contractions. The contractile pattern of contraction generated at the pyloric level only is called *isolated pyloric pressure waves* (Anvari et al. 2000). Similar contractile patterns have been observed not only during the emptying of a high-caloric meal but also in pathological situations associated with gastroparesis. Most of the pharmacological compounds that normalize defective emptying suppress isolated pyloric pressure waves (see Figure 4.1).

MOVEMENTS IN THE FASTING STATE. Some time after the meal, depending on its energy content and the animal species, antroduodenal contractions show a different pattern that is typical of the interdigestive period: the migrating motor complex (MMC). In dogs, for instance, the MMC replaces the postprandial pattern about 4 to 6 hours after the meal (Szurszewski 1998). For about 40 minutes, the stomach is quiescent (phase I). Then, peristaltic contractions gradually resume, but neither their amplitude nor frequency are maximal (phase II). Throughout phase II, which also lasts about 40 minutes, the frequency and amplitude of gastrointestinal peristaltic contractions rise steadily. Finally, for about 10 minutes, the contractions occur at maximal frequency and force (phase III). After this phase, the contractions dissipate, and the stomach is quiescent (phase I). The MMC is repeated about every 90 minutes.

The relevance of the MMC to functions of the gut is still unclear. It has been described as an intestinal housekeeper enabling the aboral transport of indigestible particles after the postprandial phase. It also acts as a master clock for gallbladder contractions and the exocrine pancreas. As a consequence, pancreatic secretion and bile content in the duodenum are maximal during phase III of the MMC. The bacteriostatic properties of pancreatic secretion and bile secretion combined with the propulsive component of the MMC explain the intricate relationship between intestinal bacterial overgrowth and the MMC (Husebye 1995). Suppression of the MMC leads to bacterial overgrowth, and, conversely, bacterial overgrowth is associated with suppression of the MMC pattern. Finally, the MMC is not present immediately after abdominal surgery. The reappearance of the MMC is an early sign that transit in the small intestine has resumed (Hotokezaka et al. 1996).

THE GASTRIC EMPTYING PROCESS. After a liquid meal, the food leaves the stomach at an approximately exponential rate. The transit time depends on, among other factors, the osmotic and calorific value of the meal (Mayer 1994). For healthy pigs or dogs, the mean half-emptying time for a 10% glucose solution—that is, the time required for 50% of the meal to leave the stomach—is 20 minutes. Emptying of a liquid meal begins immediately. Emptying of water is always maximal, and a dog can empty about 1 L of water within about 15 minutes.

After a solid or a semisolid meal, the food begins to leave the stomach only after several minutes, a delay called the lag *phase*. Once this lag phase occurs, a mean fixed quantity of food is evacuated from the stomach per unit of time. Therefore, gastric emptying is more or less linear in time. The lag phase for a semisolid meal is shorter than that for a solid meal. On average, a dog's stomach requires 3 hours to eliminate 250 g of meat (see Figure 4.2).

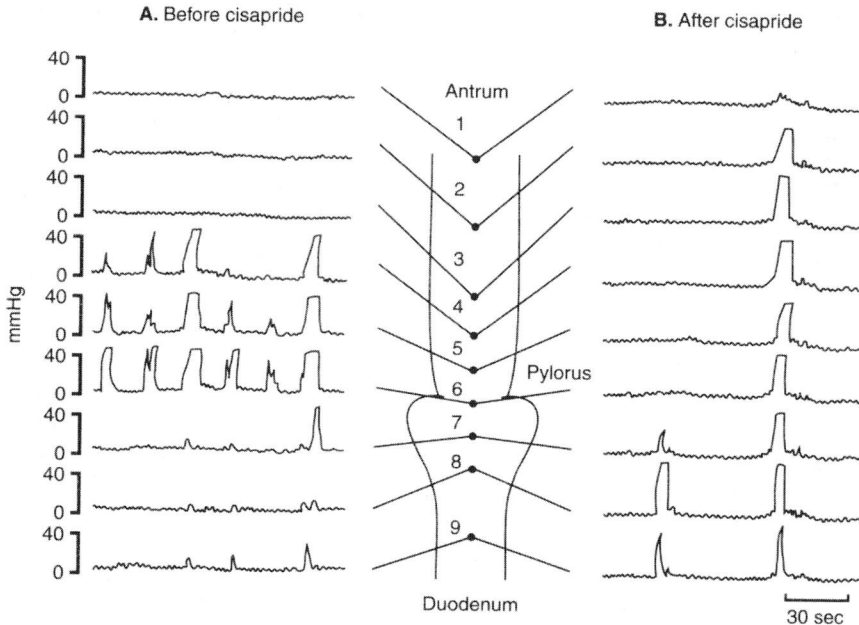

FIG. 4.1—Changes in intraluminal pressures at the gastroduodenal junction in a normal patient (**A**) and a diabetic patient (**B**) after a meal. Note the absence of antral and duodenal pressure events in the diabetic condition while the pylorus is still active producing isolated pyloric pressure waves (IPPWs). This pattern of contraction is always associated with reduced emptying rate in dogs, pigs, and people.

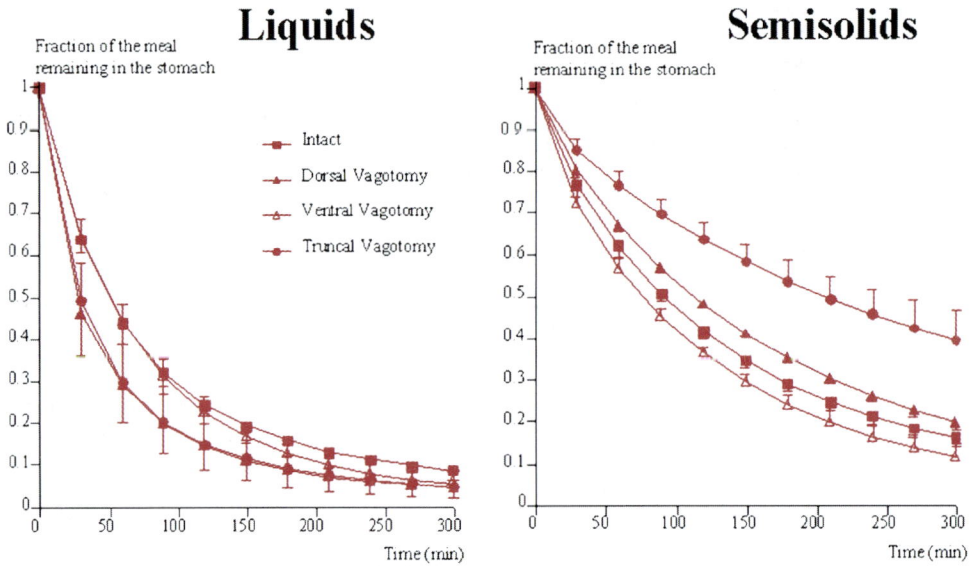

FIG. 4.2—Gastric emptying profiles of liquid (**left panel**) and semisolid (**right panel**) meals in intact pigs after dorsal or ventral vagal section and after truncal vagotomy. Time zero corresponded to the maximal amount of radioactive meal present in the stomach. Note the initially faster emptying of liquids after dorsal vagotomy. Semisolids emptying was drastically inhibited after truncal vagotomy.

Alterations in gastric emptying, in addition to those associated with actual gastrointestinal diseases, are classically described in diabetes, autoimmune diseases, and hyperthyroidism. Most of these diseases are related to altered enteric nervous system (ENS) function. Acute stresses are also most often associated with reduction in gastric emptying and intestinal transit. However, the nature of the stress affects the overall response, since restraint is associated with reduced emptying, whereas the emptying rate increases during thermal stress. One classical stress condition in veterinary abdominal surgery—diet restriction or long-term fasting—leads to reduced emptying upon realimentation (see Figure 4.3).

CONTROL OF GASTRIC MOTILITY AND EMPTYING

NEUROHUMORAL CONTROL OF GASTRIC MOTILITY. The gut is innervated by intrinsic and extrinsic neurons. Intrinsic neurons located within the gut wall act as a first stage for the integration of signals arising from the physical state of the gut wall and the chemicals present within the intestinal lumen. The nerve signals holding both types of information are transmitted to the brain via vagal afferent neurons, the majority of which are interconnected to the intrinsic neurons. Irrespective of the destination of the afferent signal (or the ultimate integration array), sensory neurons can detect a vast array of stimuli in the physiological and pathological ranges (Grundy and Scratcherd 1989).

Vagal sensory neurons can be classified as mechanosensitive, chemosensitive, or both (so-called polymodal) (Mei et al. 1996). For mechanosensitive afferents only, the nature of the response, while the mechanical stimulus remains constant, is either long-lasting (slow-adapting receptors, the discharge in response to increased luminal pressure lasts for 10 seconds or longer) or short-lived, with the pressure actually changing from one level to another (rapid-adapting

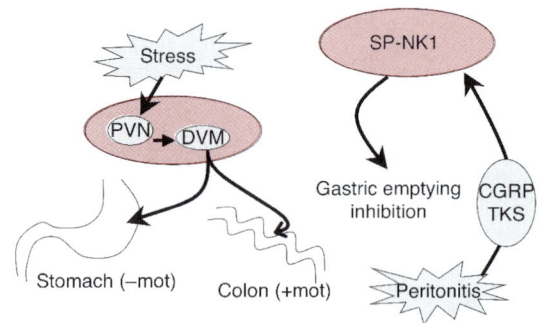

FIG. 4.3—Brain-gut axis interactions explaining the decreased emptying in various pathological conditions. Stress is acting via the paraventricular nucleus (PVN) that is supplying signals to the dorsal vagal nucleus (DVM) in which the cell bodies of vagal motoneurons are located. The activation of this nucleus is associated with decreased gastric motility and increased colonic motility. Peritonitis also triggers gastric stasis as a subsequent activation of the brain involving substance P (SP) and neurokinin 1 (NK1) receptors. An intermediate link is calcitonin gene-related peptide (CGRP) neurons probably located in the gut wall. TKS, thymidine kinase, soluble. (From Bueno et al. 1997.)

receptors with a discharge increase lasting about 1 second). Chemosensitive afferents behave always as slow-adapting receptors. Whereas all these receptor types participate in the control of emptying after a meal, perhaps the most relevant information in a pathophysiological perspective is the absence of chemoreceptors in the stomach. Since gastric adaptation is critical with respect to pain perception and in emptying and since it is generated primarily as a result of early activation of duodenal chemoreceptors, one may understand that viscous, large, and low-nutrient meals may be associated with gastroparesis and epigastric pain.

The activation mechanism of all chemosensitive and some mechanosensitive vagal afferents involves the integrity of the duodenal and jejunal mucosa, since vagal afferents are unable to sense directly the presence of food constituents or mucosal stretch. Endocrine cells located alongside the enterocytes synthesize, at their basolateral side, cholecystokinin (CCK) and 5-hydroxytryptamine (5-HT or serotonin),

which are afterward secreted by a paracrine route (Grundy et al. 1994). Vagal afferents support receptors for both CCK and 5-HT and are activated through binding of the ligand to the membrane receptor. This two-step activation process is why inhibition or reduction in the mucosal absorption of nutrients is associated with reduction in vagal input toward the control centers and with an accelerated gastric emptying rate. In contrast, a subtype of mechanoreceptor is directly activated by stretching after the spatial deformation of potassium ion (K^+) channels located in the afferent receptor membrane. The method of activation of these neurons might explain why high potassium content in a meal is associated with a reduction in gastric emptying (see Figure 4.4).

In addition to physiologically active vagal afferents, a subpopulation of mechanosensitive afferents is quiescent in normal situations (Michaelis et al. 1996). Their mechanical threshold is high (above 40 mm Hg). Since these pressures are obtained only in pathological con-

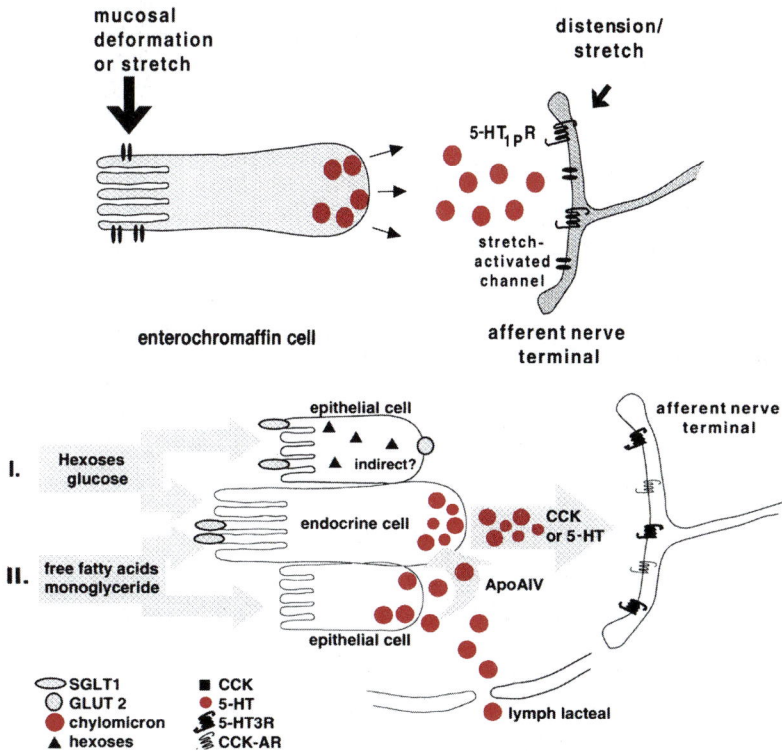

FIG. 4.4—Mechanisms involved in the mechanical and chemical transduction of the sensory events occurring in the gut by afferent neurons. **Top:** The transduction of the mechanical information occurs by two pathways. For mechanical stimulus located at the mucosal level only, the enterochromaffin cell releases 5-hydroxytryptamine (5-HT) via the paracrine route. Eventually, 5-HT will bind with a subtype of 5-HT receptor located on the neuronal membrane, hence depolarizing the neuron. Alternatively, strong mechanical stimulations are able to depolarize afferent neurons directly by activation of stretch-activated K^+ channels. **Bottom:** Chemical sensitivity is entirely dependent on endocrine cells located in the mucosa alongside the epithelial cell. Upon activation, this cell releases cholecystokinin (CCK) or/and 5-HT. Since nutrients require contact with the endocrine cell, absorption is a prerequisite for neuronal depolarization. ApoAIV, apolipoprotein AIV; CCK-AR, CCK-activated receptor; GLUT2, glucose transporter 2; 5HT1pR, 5HT1p receptor; 5-HT3R, 5HT3 receptor; and SGLT1, sodium glucose luminal transporter 1. (From H. Raybould, NIPS, 13:1998, with permission)

ditions, they supply nociceptive signals to the brain but cannot be considered as nociceptors, for instance, in the sense defined for skin. Most compounds used to suppress abdominal pain act on the compliance of the gut so that the pressure, at the level of the sensory endings, is less than the threshold for activating these receptors (see Figure 4.5).

CONTROL OF GASTRIC EMPTYING AND MOTILITY BY THE PHYSICAL AND CHEMICAL PROPERTIES OF A MEAL. Food is complex, being characterized by a number of variables: quantity, consistency, particle size, osmolarity, calorific content, and composition (carbohydrates, proteins, fats, vitamins, etc.) All of these factors affect gastric emptying. The volume of the food acts directly on stretch mechanoreceptors in the stomach to elicit adaptive relaxation in the proximal stomach and peristaltic contractions in the distal stomach. However, the size of the meal is not linearly related to gastric emptying rate since, above a threshold, the greater the volume, the less the emptying. For instance, in the 40-kg pig, the threshold is around 1 L. Liquids with the same osmolarity as that of the body fluid (i.e., isotonic liquids) are transported most rapidly into the duodenum. Gastric emptying is slower with hypertonic and hypotonic liquids. As a consequence, it is critical for rehydration solutes to supply isotonic fluid for their rapid access to the absorptive site, that is, the small intestine. The composition of a meal is of paramount importance with respect to emptying rate since only a limited quantity of carbohydrate, fat, and protein can be absorbed per unit of time by the small intestine (Malagelada and Azpiroz 1989). If the stomach delivered these substances more rapidly, they would reach the small intestine only partially absorbed and, as a result, would be converted by yeasts or bacteria (fermentation), ultimately leading to diarrhea. Moreover, unnecessary food would be lost. To adapt gastric emptying to the absorption capacity of the small intestine, the duodenal chemoreceptors together with hormonal secretions (mostly CCK and motilin) supply signals to delay gastric emptying. The quantitative importance of the inhibitory capabilities of different food constituents differs among species. In dogs (as in humans), lipids have greater inhibiting properties toward emptying than do carbohydrates or proteins. In contrast, in pigs, carbohydrates have greater inhibiting properties than do lipids and proteins. The size of the food particles is of primary importance in carnivorous species. Only small food particles can pass through the pylorus after a meal. Often a portion of the food must be broken down in the stomach into finer particles. The effect of particle size can be easily observed if the gastric emptying of pieces of liver is compared with that of liver that is ground into fine particles (homogenized). Homogenized liver leaves the stomach almost like a liquid, whereas pieces of

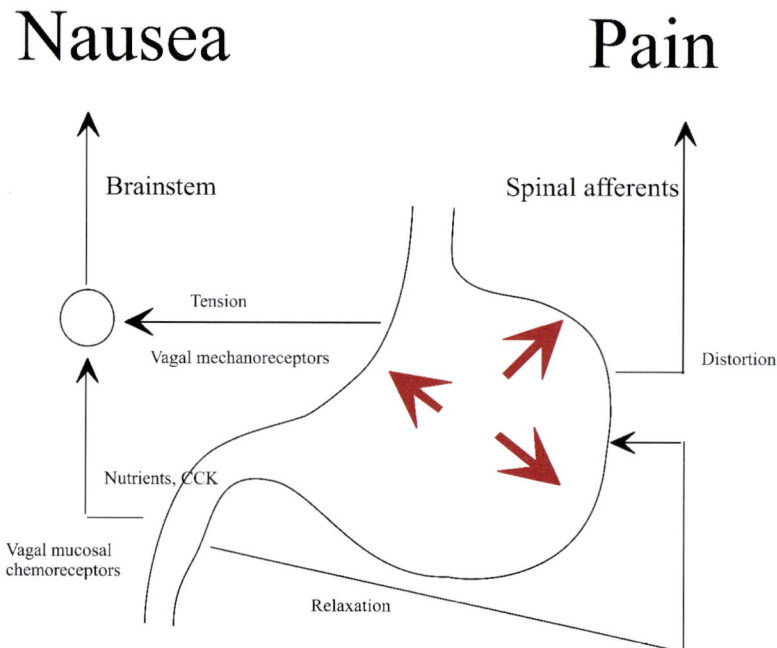

FIG. 4.5—The origin of symptoms associated with gastric distension. Pain is mainly mediated by spinal afferents, whereas nausea and food intake reduction are associated with vagal afferents. CCK, cholecystokinin.

liver create a lag phase. The other extreme is seen with indigestible pellets (such as capsules used for drug administration): in the fed state, all of these stay in the stomach, and, in phase III of the MMC, they are eliminated en masse (Akkermans and Vanisselt 1994).

ILEAL CONTROL OF GASTRIC EMPTYING. Unabsorbed nutrients arriving in the ileal lumen activate the so-called ileal brake that slows gastric emptying in most animals species evaluated thus far (Cuche and Malbert 1999). Together with a more distal (colonic) brake, this reflex enables a reduced rate of arrival of highly fermentable carbohydrates to the colon, where they could otherwise cause osmotic diarrhea. In animal species with a specialized colon (horses and pigs), the ileal brake is also activated by the reflux of short-chain fatty acids (SCFAs) from the colon into the distal ileum through the ileocecal sphincter. Irrespective of its origin, the ileal brake involves primarily the release of peptide YY (Wen et al. 1995) by ileal mucosa into the systemic blood (see Figure 4.6).

In Ruminants

RETICULORUMINAL DYSFUNCTION. The ruminant forestomach can be regarded as a versatile, but well-regulated, fermentation vat with anterior-to-posterior mixing contractions at approximately 1-minute intervals that decrease during feeding. The ruminoreticulum (RR) is the site of a symbiotic relationship between the host and the microbes that convert food that is indigestible to the host into volatile fatty acids (VFAs), microbial protein, and vitamins. As a consequence of the delay between eating and nutrient availability, chemical feed-intake stimulants can override the inhibition of feeding caused by stress, diet bulk, or adverse diets. A well-known alternative to appetite stimulation is the influence of orally administered drugs on various components of the ruminant ecosystem, i.e., the chemical control of rumen microbial metabolism to improve the feed/gain ratio. The RR, as a special pharmacokinetic compartment, with dilution in a very large volume and recirculation of active ingredients, also complicates the rate and degree of absorption, i.e., the bioavailability, of drugs. In addition, since the halftime for emptying through the reticulo-omasal orifice is a minimum of 5 to 7 hours, the RR may act as a reservoir for special pharmaceutical drug formulations that induce a continuous, slow release of active ingredients.

A basic motor activity cycle of the RR starts in the reticulum as a rapid biphasic contraction and ends in the rumen as a slower primary contraction that may be either uniphasic (dorsal sac) or biphasic (dorsal and ventral sacs). The reticulum also synchronizes or activates other forestomachs' motor events, such as relaxation of the reticulo-omasal orifice in cattle and sheep and relaxation of the omasum, followed by contraction of the omasal canal, in sheep. The biphasic reticular contraction is briefer in sheep than in cattle (Ruckebusch 1989).

The primary roles of extrinsic contractions are mixing and aborad propulsion of the contents of the forestomachs. The extrinsic system enables cyclic motor activity of the RR as vagovagal reflexes, and coordinates this cyclic activity with the processes of regurgitation and eructation. The outflow from the gastric centers by the vagal motor neurons is strictly related to the afferent neural input. Two additional interconnected neuronal networks act as vagal relays to and from the gastric centers. One network of interneurons controls the frequency of the cyclic ruminoreticular movements; the other regulates the amplitude of the forestomach contractions through vagal discharges, first in the reticulum and later in the rumen. The networks are evoked by an activity of the central nervous system (CNS), which is reflexly modified by sensory inputs coming largely from the alimentary tract itself. The frequency and amplitude of extrinsic contractions are inhibited by abomasal distension. The magnitude of the extrinsic contractions and their form (i.e., primary or secondary rumen motility, regurgitation, or eructation) are related to coarse particles or gas, which distends the reticulum or stretches the rumen pillars.

Two main alterations can be present at the reticulorumen, leading to indigestion:

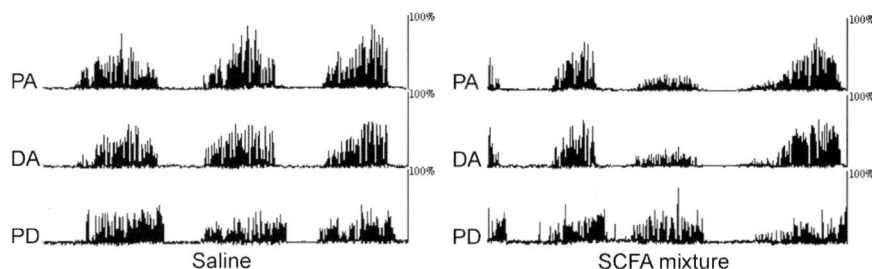

FIG. 4.6—Ileal brake toward gastric motility in a pig. Infusion of short-chain fatty acids (SCFAs) in pigs or carbohydrates and lipids in dogs within the distal ileum generates long-lasting inhibition of gastric phasic motility and a slow gastric emptying rate. DA, distal antrum; PA, proximal antrum; and PD, proximal duodenum.

- Motility-associated diseases (e.g., atony and paresis) with multiple origins such as iatrogenic, mechanical, alimentary, metabolic, and/or infections
- Fermentation-related diseases (acidosis and alkalosis) caused by or associated with excess carbohydrates (lactic acidosis), pyloric stenosis (hydrochloric acidosis), and hepatic alkalosis (ruminal alkalosis)

MOTILITY-ASSOCIATED DISEASES. The ability of the reticulorumen to contract rhythmically is the result of a vagovagal reflex system mediated by gastric centers located in the medulla within the dorsal motor nucleus. The role of the CNS is thus to integrate the activity conducted from separate regions by afferent fibers, in order to arrange their sequential contractile activity and to control the frequency and amplitude of contractions with feeding via tactile stimulation of the oral cavity (Leek and Harding 1975). The cyclic motor activity of the reticuloruminal and omasal muscular coat is impaired after section of the two vagus nerves or after anesthesia. Within 1 day of bilateral thoracic vagotomy, rhythmic periods of spike-burst discharges are seen, and, within 1 to 2 weeks, simultaneous contractions of the whole reticulorumen occur as group discharges (Gregory 1984). These contractions occur simultaneously over the whole reticulorumen in contrast to the progressive forward and backward spread of activity seen in intact animals. In part, they involve the activity of the ganglionic cells of the neural plexuses in the ENS. The intrinsic activity that develops in chronically vagotomized sheep also persists after bilateral section of the splanchnic nerves. The local activity is stimulated by distension, suggesting a major role for the ENS in basal smooth muscle tone. However, this intrinsic activity, since it is not propagated from the reticulum to the rumen, is unable to generate a significant transit of food and particle size reduction (see Figure 4.7).

FERMENTATION-RELATED DISEASES. The essential factor in the microbial activity within the reticulorumen is the stability of its pH. Three main pathologies are associated with variations in reticuloruminal pH.

Lactic Acidosis. This originates from explosive fermentation of carbohydrates (Telle and Preston 1971; Allinson et al. 1975). Through its undissociated form, lactic acid inhibits the reticuloruminal contractions that are essential for eructation (type 2 cycle). As a consequence, the amount of gas in the rumen increases, which increases reticuloruminal contractions and hence the amount of eructated gas. Besides a definite ruminal pressure, however, inhibitory vagovagal mechanisms amplify ruminal atony. A key phenomenon in understanding the origin of this aggravating mechanism is the action of lactic acid on the epithelial cells of the ruminal wall. Indeed, lactic acid opens the gap between epithelial cells, allowing a large quantity of unprocessed lactic acid to enter the submucosa (Crichlow and Leek 1981). These large quantities of

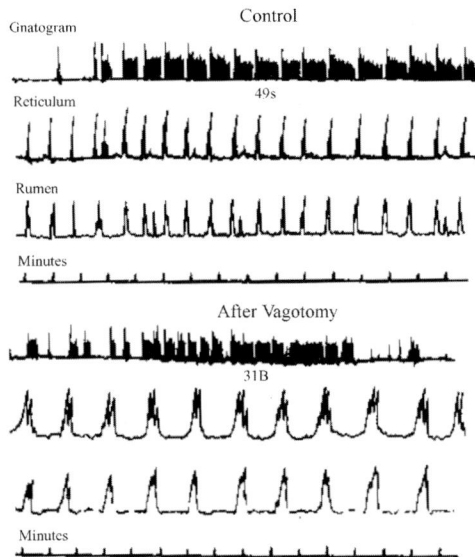

Intrinsic Activity

FIG. 4.7—Reticuloruminal motility in adult sheep with and without an intact vagal supply. In intact animals, reticuloruminal contractions occur about one per minute, are short-lived, and are propagated from the reticulum to the rumen. These contractions are modified by rumination (shown on the gnatogram). After vagotomy, reticuloruminal contractions disappear, but if the animal is sustained for several weeks by enteral feeding, the enteric nervous system is able to generate a contractile pattern. These contractions are long-lasting and nonpropagated. Sometimes, they are associated with a pseudorumination pattern.

lactic acid interact with vagal afferents that become inhibited (hence, the initial atony) and unable to react to an increase in ruminal pressure (hence, the inefficacy of the physiological regulatory mechanism).

Some ionophoric antibiotics can slow the rate of these fermentations. They inhibit the synthesis, from some amino acids (such as tryptophan), of toxic substances [3-methylindol (skatole)] within the lungs. Associated effects are (a) increased water intake and hence faster ruminal turnover, and (b) an increased propionate percentage among the VFAs. Propionate is a key factor for the hepatic metabolic regulation of food intake in ruminants (see Figure 4.8).

Hydrochloric Acidosis. This is the consequence of a drop in ruminal pH that is associated with abomasal reflux of hydrochloric acid (HCl) (Dirksen 1965). This reflux is facilitated by (a) pyloric stenosis (Kuiper and Breukink 1986) or defects in abomasal transit associated with partial abomasal displacement, and (b) abomasal and duodenal ulcers. The sequestration of chloride ions in the rumen triggers a large increase in the alkaline reserve of the blood with hypochloremia and hypokalemia. Consequently, the kidney tries to hold potassium in exchange for hydrogen ions (H^+). This form of acidosis is therefore associated with a paradoxical aciduria. Reticuloruminal atony involves suppression of tonic and phasic contractions that, in turn, trigger ruminal distension. The origin of reticuloruminal atony is not due to hypokalemia but rather to reduced ionization of the calcium, which is itself the consequence of blood alkalosis. If untreated, the outcome of the disease is often terminal, especially in cows with abomasal displacement, the hypokalemia being responsible for auricular fibrillation.

Ruminal Alkalosis. The early sign of suppression of ruminal transit is ruminal alkalosis associated with inhibition of VFA production. The origins of ruminal alkalosis are numerous but always related to a reduction or an absence of food intake. The increase in ruminal pH improves the absorption of ammonium hydroxide (NH_4OH) (pK_a, 8.8 to 9.1) in its nonionized form that will stress the metabolic capabilities of the liver. As a reminder, ruminal pH rising from 4.5 to 6.5 will triple the absorption of NH_4OH. The hyperammonemia is responsible for ruminal paresis that enhances the putrefaction of ruminal contents (see Figure 4.9).

ABOMASAL DISORDERS. The function of the abomasum of ruminants is essentially similar to that of the mammalian stomach of monogastric animals, that is, proteolytic digestion of food under acidic conditions. Nevertheless, abomasal function and, with it, abomasal motility, differs somewhat, depending on whether the animal is in the preruminant or the adult ruminant stage.

ABOMASAL MOTILITY AND TRANSIT. Abomasal motility is characterized at the level of the antral area by regular contractions at a frequency of approximately 7 per minute in sheep and 3 to 4 per minute in calves. The motility of the body (corpus) is much more irregular and mainly seems to involve tonic contractions. As in monogastric animals, the corpus is important as the food reservoir and for ensuring delivery of food to the antral pump. In general, some 18 to 20 times per day, the abomasal motility becomes inhibited for periods of 10 to 15 minutes at a time at the appearance in the duodenum of phase III activity of the migrating motor complex. Outflow of chyme from the abomasum, and

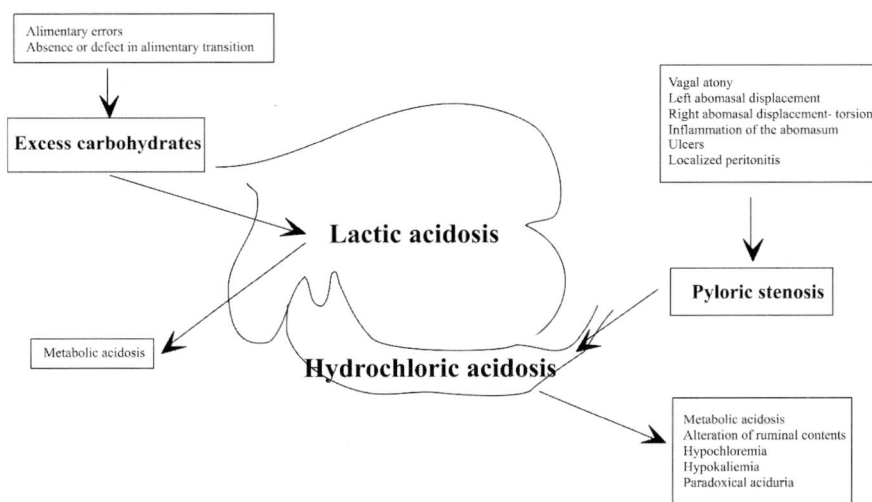

FIG. 4.8—Pathophysiology of ruminal acidosis.

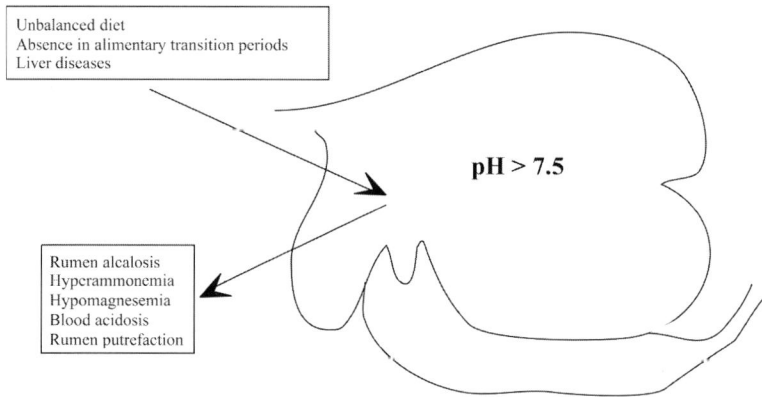

FIG. 4.9—Pathophysiology of ruminal alkalosis.

antral motility, tend to reach a maximum for about 20 minutes prior to a phase III and then cease until abomasal motility restarts. In adult ruminants and generally also in young suckling ruminants, this pattern of small intestinal motility—the migrating motor complex—occurs regularly throughout the day, independently of feeding (Malbert and Ruckebusch 1987). This contrasts with dogs or people, in which the MMC is seen only in the fasting state.

Factors Regulating Abomasal Emptying in Young Ruminants. Duodenal osmolality appears to be an important parameter in the regulation of abomasal emptying in young ruminants (Gregory et al. 1985). Inhibitory feedback signals are activated by duodenal infusions of hypo-osmolar and hyperosmolar sodium bicarbonate ($NaHCO_3$) and sodium chloride (NaCl) solutions. As a result, infusion of near-isotonic $NaHCO_3$ induces the maximal rate of abomasal emptying of a water meal in milk-fed calves, with isotonic NaCl slightly less effective. Water or hypertonic salt solution inhibits the rate of emptying. Abomasal emptying is not influenced by hypotonic ammonium chloride (NH_4Cl) but is inhibited by duodenal infusion of hypotonic to hypertonic solutions of potassium chloride (KCl) plus calcium chloride ($CaCl_2$) and by hypertonic NH_4Cl plus glucose.

Perhaps the strongest inhibitory influence of all on abomasal emptying is that of duodenal infusion with H^+ ions (Gregory et al. 1984). It was found that, with a duodenal infusion of isotonic NaCl from pH 2.0 to 12.0, there was no effect of pH per se on abomasal function. Rather, abomasal emptying and gastric juice secretion were inhibited according to the amount of titratable acid present in the infusate, such that complete abolition of abomasal emptying was seen with a duodenal infusion of about 37 mEq/h titratable acid, whereas a definite inhibition could already be seen at 18.5 mEq/h.

Factors Regulating Abomasal Emptying in Adult Ruminants. A variety of duodenal stimuli can affect abomasal motility and the rate of outflow (Malbert 1989). In contrast to young, milk-fed ruminants, osmolality of the duodenal chyme is not considered to exert any (physiological) control on abomasal outflow in adult ruminants. On the contrary, abomasal motility and outflow are inhibited by duodenal infusion of SCFAs, acetic propionic, or butyric acids (mainly) or lactic acid. The threshold dose for inhibition of the abomasum in sheep is about 4 mL/min of 0.1 mmol SCFA or 24 mmol/h, which together with the endogenous SCFA in the abomasal contents was calculated to represent a duodenal concentration of about 35 mmol. It seems unlikely that such concentrations will be reached except in exceptional circumstances.

MECHANISMS CONTROLLING ABOMASAL FUNCTION. In ruminants, vagotomy delays abomasal emptying. However, the situation is significantly different from that in the monogastric species. In ruminants, vagotomy increases the frequency and amplitude of the antrum so that all plateau potentials are superimposed with action potentials (Malbert and Ruckebusch 1989). In contrast, in monogastric species, vagotomy reduces or abolishes phasic contractions at the antral level. Therefore, the vagus carries inhibitory signals to the antrum in ruminants and excitatory ones in monogastric species. The therapeutic consequence is obvious: compounds used to treat vagal indigestion in monogastric species are not suitable for ruminants and will exacerbate their symptoms. A few studies have indicated that some of the gastrointestinal hormones—for example, cholecystokinin, gastrin, secretin, somatostatin, glucagon, and insulin—can exert a strong modulating role on abomasal motility and emptying/outflow, although the physiological significance of most of these effects remains to be determined (see Figure 4.10).

DISTURBANCES IN ABOMASAL FUNCTION WITH PARASITIC INFECTION. Parasitic infection can cause gross changes in the secretion of gastrointestinal hormones

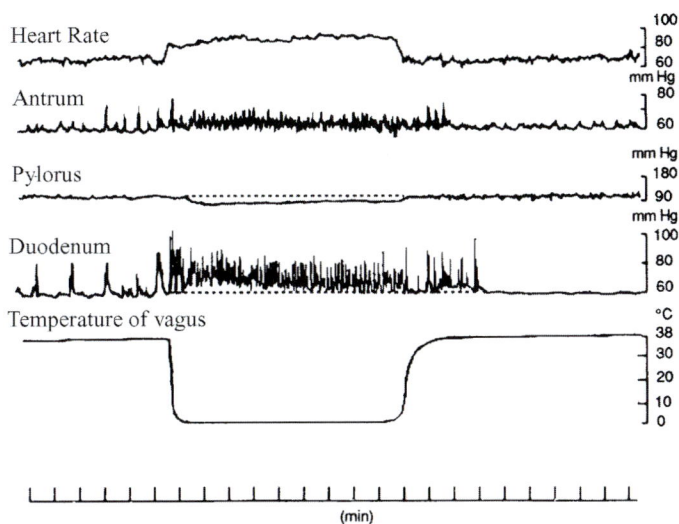

FIG. 4.10—Manometric recording of the gastroduodenal junction of the sheep during left vagal cooling while the right vagal trunk has been cut. During the 0°C period, equivalent to vagal section, the motility of the antrum and the duodenum was increased while the pyloric tone was decreased. The efficacy of vagal cooling is demonstrated by the change in heart rate.

that is likely to play a major role in at least some of the pathological responses observed (Titchen and Anderson 1977). Thus, hypergastrinemia (up to 10 times above normal levels) is caused by infections with *Ostertagia* and *Haemonchus contortus* in which raised somatostatin levels are also observed; no information is presently available for *Trichostrongylus axei*. The duodenal parasite *Trichostrongylus colubriformis* has no influence on gastrin levels, but rather it causes raised CCK levels. It is likely, but not yet proven, that these hormonal changes contribute to the disturbances in abomasal motility and outflow, gastrointestinal secretions, small intestinal transit, and anorexia observed in infected animals. Where tested, the raised hormone levels were due to increased secretion by the host rather than a secretion from the parasite. However, the mechanism of hormone stimulation has still to be clarified; for example, it could involve an immune response, a response to a parasite toxin, or stimulation (irritation) by the larvae of the ENS or extrinsic nerves. The paradoxical increase in gastrin levels despite a reduction in acid secretion with abomasal infection is partly a result of the destruction by the parasites of the acid-secreting parietal cells and their replacement by undifferentiated cells and perhaps partly due to the raised somatostatin levels. The parasites may also be able to secrete a toxin that inhibits acid secretion.

The inhibition of acid secretion results, in severe infections, in failure to activate pepsinogen. This lack of proteolysis can have severe consequences—apart from the nutritional aspects of lack of protein intake, it can result in bacterial overgrowth of the intestine, which can be a major factor in the diarrhea associated with parasite infection. The raised plasminogen levels found in infected animals are partly a result of this failure to activate pepsinogen but mainly due to the increased leakiness of the abomasum following the tissue damage inflicted by the parasites.

DEFECTS IN ABSORPTION AND SECRETION

Basic Mechanisms of Intestinal Absorption and Secretion. The electrogenic sodium ion (Na^+) absorption is the basic process for electrolyte, water, and nutrient absorption in the small intestine. The transport processes are driven by the basolateral sodium- and potassium-activated adenosine triphosphate (NaK-ATPase) that actively extrudes 3 Na^+ to the basolateral side and lets 2 K^+ into the cell for every ATP molecule hydrolyzed. This electrogenic pump, together with the differential permeabilities, generates a membrane potential of about −55 mV (extracellular fluid, 0 mV) and keeps the intracellular Na^+ concentration low at 12 mEq/L (interstitial fluid, 105 mEq/L) and K^+ concentration high at 93 mEq/L (interstitial fluid, 4 mEq/L). The Cl^- concentration is about 44 mEq/L in enterocytes and 93 mEq/L in the interstitial fluid (Siegenbeek van Heukelum 1986). Thus, there exists a steep electrochemical gradient for Na^+ entry into the cell. Electrolyte transport is controlled mainly by local neurohumoral regulation; that is, the epithelium is regulated by the local endocrine and immune cells and the ENS.

Absorption

ELECTROGENIC SUBSTRATE-COUPLED SODIUM ABSORPTION IN THE SMALL INTESTINE. In the small intestine, the sodium (Na) entry is coupled to glucose via the Na^+/glucose cotransporter in the luminal membrane of the enterocytes on the villi. This

Na$^+$/glucose cotransporter—named *sodium glucose luminal transporter 1* (SGLT-1)—is expressed in the mature/differentiated enterocytes of the villi. Two Na$^+$ ions followed by one glucose molecule bind to the protein, which internalizes the substrates to the inner surface of the membrane (Wright et al. 1994). Glucose crosses the basolateral membrane by facilitated diffusion by the protein *glucose transporter 2* (GLUT-2), and Na is extruded by the NaK ATPase generating a transepithelial electrical potential (5 to 10 mV) with the basolateral membrane positively charged in relation to the luminal surface. In this way, glucose is transported "uphill" (against a concentration gradient) by means of the active Na absorption, so the glucose transport is therefore termed *secondary active*. Secondary active transport also exists for other nutrients: for example, galactose uses SGLT-1, and several of the group-specific amino acid-transport systems in the enterocyte brush border are dependent on the Na$^+$ gradient (Ganapathy et al. 1994). In addition, some of these amino acid-transport systems are dependent on the presence of chloride (Cl$^-$).

Cl$^-$ is absorbed via the paracellular pathway with the transepithelial potential as the driving force. Cl$^-$ may also be absorbed through the cell. In the leaky small intestinal epithelium, there is some backleakage of Na through the paracellular route. This prevents the generation of steep gradients, like high transepithelial potentials, which would impair the transport properties for nutrients, and additionally the backleakage guarantees the presence of Na$^+$ near the brush-border membrane.

ELECTRONEUTRAL SODIUM CHLORIDE ABSORPTION. Electroneutral NaCl absorption takes place in the ileum and colon, and results from the combined action by two transporters: the Na$^+$/H$^+$ exchanger (NHE) and the Cl$^-$/HCO$_3^-$ (bicarbonate) exchanger (AE or anion exchanger). Na$^+$ and Cl$^-$ are absorbed in exchange for intracellular H$^+$ and HCO$_3^-$, respectively, thus maintaining both electroneutrality and pH homeostasis. This electroneutral NaCl transport, present in both the small intestine and the proximal colon, accounts for 20% of the total influx of Na and is the predominant mechanism of Na absorption in the absence of nutrients in the lumen.

L-Glutamine stimulates NaCl absorption in the small intestine, an effect mediated via metabolism of glutamine in the enterocyte, which is presumed to stimulate the Na$^+$/H$^+$ and Cl$^-$/HCO$_3^-$ exchange mechanisms. Other than from Na$^+$/H$^+$ and Cl$^-$/HCO$_3^-$ exchange, the basolateral membrane also takes up Na and Cl via the Na$^+$-K$^+$-2Cl$^-$ cotransporter energized by the low intracellular Na$^+$ and K$^+$ concentrations. The Na$^+$-K$^+$-2Cl$^-$ cotransporter has a central role in the ongoing Cl$^-$ secretion after the opening of the luminal Cl$^-$ channels (Cook and Young 1989) (see Figure 4.11).

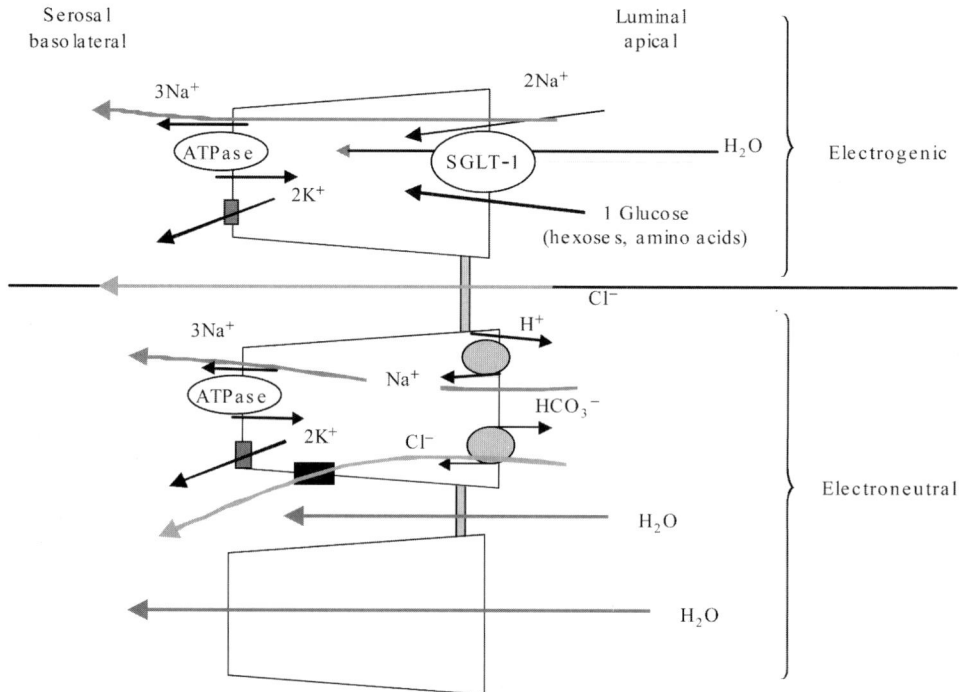

FIG. 4.11—Cell models of solute-coupled Na$^+$ absorption and electroneutral NaCl absorption. ATPase, adenosine triphosphatase; and SGLT-1, sodium glucose luminal transporter 1.

SECRETION

CHLORIDE SECRETION. Cl⁻ enters the enterocytes via the basolateral electroneutral Na^+-K^+-$2Cl^-$ cotransporter. Various secondary messengers [Ca^{2+}, cyclic adenosine monophosphate (cAMP), cyclic guanosine 3,5′-monophosphate (cGMP), and diacylglycerol] can induce opening of the chloride channels in the brush-border membrane, and thereby Cl⁻ secretion occurs driven by the transmembranous electrical gradient and sustained by the cotransporter. The basolateral K channels are also of importance in epithelial chloride secretion, since the exit of K keeps the cell membrane potential more negative than the Nernst potential for Cl⁻ and thus energizes the cotransporter by lowering intracellular K^+ (Greger and Kunzelmann 1990).

The cystic fibrosis transmembrane conductance regulator (CFTR) most likely represents one form of the Cl⁻ channel. The principal site of CFTR expression is in the crypts, and the level of CFTR messenger RNA (mRNA) decreases gradually as the cells differentiate and migrate from the crypt to the villus. In the colon, a distinct boundary is present two-thirds of the distance between the crypt and the surface epithelium. Along the length of the intestine, CFTR expression declines toward the distal colon. The Cl⁻ secretion generates a transepithelial potential difference, and Na^+ follows passively, presumably via the paracellular pathway with the transepithelial potential as the driving force.

BICARBONATE (HCO_3^-) SECRETION. HCO_3^- enters the enterocyte via an Na^+-driven secondary active transport in the basolateral membrane and is secreted through the CFTR and probably via a Cl^-/HCO_3^- exchanger (see Figure 4.12).

WATER TRANSPORT. The water transport is closely coupled with solute movements and is passive and iso-osmotic in the small intestine. The pathway and mechanism by which water is absorbed remain obscure. Prevailing evidence largely indicates that water transport by the small intestine occurs through the paracellular pathway (Chang and Rao 1994); for example, the paracellular pathway has been reported to grow wider during absorption. Evidence has not been found for specific water-channel-mediated water transport in the intestine. For the transcellular pathway, an interaction of SGLT-1 and water in the intestinal brush-border membrane is suggested by Hirayama and colleagues, who found the stoichiometry of 2 Na^+, 1 glucose. The route for the secretion of water is also uncertain. The assumption that the paracellular route is used has been questioned by several authors who have found the paracellular space diminished after cholera toxin (CT) and vasoactive intestinal polypeptide (VIP) stimulation.

Alterations in Secretion and/or Absorption

ENTEROTOXIGENIC DIARRHEA. The secretory diarrheas are induced by enterotoxigenic bacteria that colonize the small intestine and release enterotoxins, stimu-

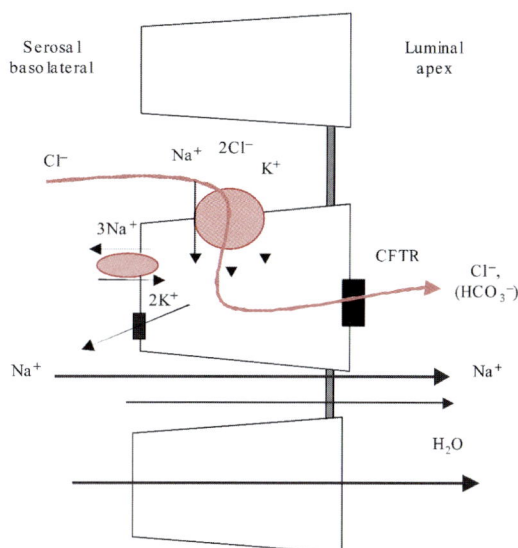

FIG. 4.12—Cell model for Cl^-/HCO_3^- secretion. CFTR, cystic fibrosis transmembrane conductance regulator.

lating electrolyte and fluid secretion without any initial damage to the intestinal mucosa. The average 50-kg pig ingests 5 L of fluid and secretes daily 18 L of salivary, gastric, biliary, pancreatic, and intestinal fluid. This volume is reduced during transit of the small intestine to about 5 L and during further passage of the colon to approximately 800 mL, which is excreted in feces. Alteration in active ion-transport mechanisms can result in excessive fluid and electrolyte accumulation in the intestinal lumen, which can lead to diarrhea if the absorptive capacity is exceeded. The enterotoxigenic diarrhea is primarily caused by active Cl⁻ and HCO_3^- secretion and inhibited electroneutral NaCl absorption in the small intestine. The spillover (active secretion and inhibited reabsorption) from the small intestine to colon can be compensated for by the latter to some extent where the absorptive capacity is exceeded. The absorptive capacity of the porcine colon is estimated to be 18 mL/kg body weight per hour, giving 3 and 22 L in weanling and 50-kg pigs, respectively (about 4.5 times a normal load). However, in neonates, sucklings, and weanlings, the bacterial flora has not yet been fully established in the colon, resulting in a lower absorptive capacity (Argenzio and Whipp 1979). In severe watery diarrhea, the daily loss of electrolytes and fluid can reach an amount several times the extracellular fluid. In per-acute incidence in piglets, the massive loss of fluid to the intestinal lumen can happen so fast that death due to hypovolemia occurs without any signs of diarrhea.

CT is the best-studied mediator of secretory diarrhea. It induces secretion by a direct stimulation of the enterocytes and an indirect stimulation via the ENS. It is a two-component toxin composed of a B domain, which binds to the GM′ receptor on the luminal enterocyte membrane, and an active A domain. After binding, the A domain enters the cell and activates via G protein the adenylate cyclase (located on the basolateral membrane) that may then stimulate the protein kinases, which in turn phosphorylate membrane proteins, resulting in both opening of the luminal chloride channel and the basolateral K channels, inhibition of the electroneutral NaCl absorption, and stimulation of HCO_3^- secretion (Rabbani 1996). Intraluminal CT also provokes, probably by the same intracellular pathway, enterochromaffin cells to degranulate and release 5-HT in several species (Grondahl et al. 1996, 2002). 5-HT initiates a cascade of reactions involving both the release of eicosanoids, such as prostaglandin E_2 (PGE_2) and activation of the secretomotor neurons in ENS. As already described, the secretory reflex arc is assumed to have a cholinergic interneuron, whereas the efferent neuron releases VIP to the epithelial cells. The source of the PGE_2 is supposed to be the fibroblasts, since cell cultures of porcine fibroblasts have been shown to produce PGE in response to 5-HT. PGE_2 also induces secretion by activation of the ENS, whereas both 5-HT and PGE_2 induce secretion by direct stimulation of the enterocytes. Additionally, CT stimulation induces a decrease in the tight junctional resistance, thereby increasing permeability and transport (secretion) via the paracellular pathway, which is the main action of another toxin from *Vibrio cholerae*, the zonula occludens toxin (see Figure 4.13).

Enterotoxins from enterotoxic *Escherichia coli* (ETEC) [heat-labile toxin (LT) and heat-stable toxin 1 and heat-stable toxin 2 (ST1 and ST2)] likewise induce secretion involving ENS, 5-HT, and PGE_2 (Reevesdarby et al. 1995). Involvement of ENS, prostaglandins, and 5-HT in the secretion induced by enterotoxigenic *Salmonella typhimurium* has also been demonstrated. The compensatory colonic absorption is impaired in enterotoxigen diarrhea, due to a reduction in luminal content of SCFA, but the capacity for SCFA and NaCl absorption is unaltered.

ENTEROINVASIVE DIARRHEA. The diarrheas caused by enteroinvasive organisms (bacterial, viral, and protozoal) have both an osmotic component and a secretory component. The osmotic part is induced by malabsorption, since the absorptive surface is markedly reduced due to mucosal lesions (from villus atrophy and relative crypt hyperplasia to leakage of the epithelial lining), while inflammatory mediators induce the secretory part. Neonatal calves with diarrhea involving both ETEC and virus (rotavirus or coronavirus) have, in addition to hypersecretion of electrolytes and fluid from the crypts, blunted villi often covered with rather immature epithelial cells with little absorptive capacity (Berschneider 1992).

NEURAL INJURY, REPAIR, AND ADAPTATION OF THE GASTROINTESTINAL TRACT

Mechanisms of Mucosal Injury and Repair

MUCOSAL BARRIER FUNCTION. Gut barrier function is vital because it prevents bacteria and associated tox-

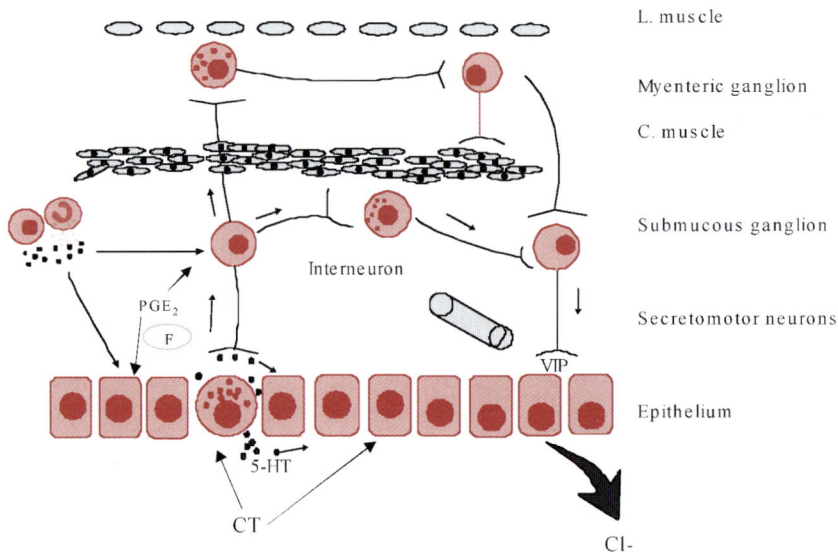

FIG. 4.13—Model for induced secretion illustrating enteroendocrine cells as sensory detectors in regulation of ion transport. Cholera toxin stimulates release of serotonin (5-HT or 5-hydroxytryptamine) from the enterochromaffin (EC) cells, which in turn initiates a cascade of secretory reactions. C. muscle, circular muscle; CT, cholera toxin; F, fibroblasts; L. muscle, longitudinal muscle; PGE_2, prostaglandin E_2; VIP, vasoactive intestinal polypeptide.

ins from gaining access to subepithelial tissues and the circulation. This is a particular concern in animals undergoing breakdown of the intestinal barrier, such as occurs during intestinal ischemia-reperfusion injury, because of the rapid and often irreversible onset of endotoxemia or sepsis. The luminal surface of the intestine is composed of a single layer of columnar epithelium that has two conflicting functions: it must serve as a protective barrier against luminal bacteria and toxins while absorbing solutes necessary to maintain the well-being of the host. This conflict is most notable at the intercellular space, which acts as a sieve that theoretically allows passage of select solutes and water (Pappenheimer 1990) but prevents the passage of bacterial toxins (Madara and Trier 1994). The intercellular space is regulated by the tight junction, which in turn appears to fluctuate in size depending on the degree to which the attached cytoskeleton contracts. Intestinal injury, such as that caused by intestinal ischemia or inflammatory cell infiltration, results in enlargement of the intercellular space, due initially to loosening of the tight junctions and subsequently to disruption of epithelial continuity.

Ions may follow two routes when traversing epithelium: transcellular and paracellular. The tight junctions regulate the paracellular flow of ions. Tight junctions differ in structure from different portions of the mucosa (Madara and Pappenheimer 1987). Intercellular tight junctions in the crypts are more leaky than those in the villus because of fewer and less organized tight junction strands associated with dividing and immature epithelium. Conversely, the villus tends to have a greater number of well-organized tight junction strands. In addition, the apical portion of enterocytes on the villus is wider than that of crypt enterocytes, so there are fewer tight junctions per unit area in the villus. Taking these factors into consideration, it has been estimated that 75% of the paracellular conductance is localized to the crypt. The structure of tight junctions also varies with the segment of intestine. For example, tight junctions have more strands in the ileum than in the jejunum.

GASTRIC ULCER DISEASE

INFLUENCE OF FORM AND FUNCTION ON GASTRIC ULCER DISEASE. The stomach is confronted by a remarkably hostile environment based on its dual roles of digestion and retention. In terms of digestion, the stomach is capable of dramatically lowering the pH and secreting pepsinogen in order to begin breaking down protein. However, both HCl and pepsinogen (which is converted to pepsin) are inherently damaging to mucosae, which have a number of mechanisms to prevent injury, depending on the region of the stomach. There are four regions of the stomach based on the type of mucosal lining (in an orad to aborad order): nonglandular stratified squamous epithelium, cardiac epithelium, proper gastric mucosa, and pyloric mucosa. The stratified squamous mucosa has no secretory function, but it does have an important Na+-absorptive

function in ruminants, partly because it is considerably thinner than that of other species such as horses (Blikslager et al. 1997b). The function of the stratified squamous mucosa in horses is unknown but may be related to protection from abrasion by roughage. The cardiac epithelium secretes bicarbonate and is particularly prominent in pigs. However, relatively little is known about this mucosal region. The proper gastric mucosa contains secretory glands containing HCl-secreting parietal cells and pepsinogen-secreting zymogen cells. In addition, this segment of mucosa contains enterochromaffin-like cells that secrete histamine in response to various stimuli, which in turn amplifies HCl secretion by the parietal cells. The pyloric mucosa contains both G cells and D cells, which secrete gastrin and somatostatin, respectively. These hormones serve to enhance or reduce gastric acid secretion, respectively (Merritt 1999).

The extent to which the stratified mucosa extends into the stomach from the esophagus varies widely with species. For example, in dogs, the stratified squamous mucosa ends at the gastroesophageal junction, whereas pigs have a small patch of squamous mucosa within the stomach that surrounds the gastroesophageal opening. On the other hand, the equine stomach has a very extensive region of stratified squamous mucosa that occupies approximately half of the stomach mucosal surface area and changes abruptly to cardiac glandular mucosa at a line of demarcation called the *margo plicatus*. Gastric ulcer disease in horses and pigs predominantly involves the stratified squamous epithelium. Conversely, ulceration in dogs is typically within the proper gastric mucosa.

An additional factor that likely affects development of gastric ulcer disease is the degree to which the pyloric sphincter allows reflux of contents from the small intestine. For example, in horses, gastric contents typically contain significant concentrations of bile salts, indicating that reflux from the duodenum is a frequent occurrence. Although refluxed duodenal contents have a relatively high pH, and therefore may aid in the buffering of gastric contents, the high concentrations of bile salts have been implicated in ulceration of the proximal portion of the equine stomach (Berschneider et al. 1999).

GASTRIC MUCOSAL RESISTANCE TO INJURY. Mechanisms by which the stratified squamous mucosa resists injury are critical in pigs and horses, where this type of ulceration is prevalent (Argenzio 1999). The stratified squamous mucosa is exceptionally impermeable. This, in effect, is the only mechanism this mucosa has to defend itself against injury. The stratified squamous epithelium consists of four layers: the outer *stratum corneum*, *stratum transitionale*, *stratum spinosum*, and the basal *stratum germinativum*. However, not all layers contribute equally to barrier function, which is largely composed of interepithelial tight junctions in the *stratum corneum* and mucosubstances secreted by the *stratum spinosum*.

The site of HCl secretion (proper gastric mucosa) is also protected from so-called backdiffusion of H+ ions by mechanisms similar to those that exist at the stratified mucosal level, but there are also a number of other critical mechanisms to prevent acid injury. The gastric mucosa secretes both mucus and bicarbonate, which together form a HCO_3^--containing gel that titrates acid before it reaches the lumen (Schreiber et al. 2000). This leaves the question as to how acid reaches the lumen in order to aid in digestion. Although this has not been fully resolved, it appears that channels immediately above gastric pits are formed by secretory-induced hydrostatic pressure (Holm et al. 1990). The mucus layer is principally formed by glycoproteins (mucins) secreted by goblet cells but also includes other gastric secretions and sloughed epithelial cells. Mucins consist of core peptides with a series of densely packed O-linked polysaccharide side chains that, once secreted, become hydrated and form a viscoelastic gel that is composed of two components: a firmly adherent gel and a loosely adherent layer, both of which are approximately 80- to 150-μm thick. Thus, although the loosely adherent layer is susceptible to shear forces imparted by gastrointestinal motility and the movement of microvilli, a mucus layer depth of at least 80 μm is always maintained. In addition, removal of the loosely adherent layer stimulates secretion of additional mucus. However, the mucus layer does not form an absolute barrier to backdiffusion of acid. Thus, for acid that does backdiffuse into the gastric mucosa, epithelial Na^+/H^+ exchangers are capable of expelling H^+ once the cell reaches a critical pH (Flemstrom 1994) (see Figure 4.14).

An additional mucosal function that serves to reduce the level of injury is *adaptive cytoprotection*, wherein application of topical irritants to gastric mucosa results in subsequent protection of mucosa in response to repeated exposure to damaging agents. For example, pretreatment with 10% ethanol protects against mucosal damage in response to a subsequent application of absolute ethanol, and this effect is abolished by treatment with the cyclooxygenase (COX) inhibitor indomethacin. Prostaglandins appear to be cytoprotective in the stomach at doses less than those used to inhibit gastric acid secretion, ruling out a simple antacid mechanism. Initially, cytoprotection was attributed to prostaglandin-stimulated mucus production. An associated beneficial effect of prostaglandins is the increased production of bicarbonate, which is trapped within mucus on the surface of the mucosa (Mutoh et al. 1995). Interestingly, PGE_2 appears to lose its cytoprotective activity in the presence of the mucolytic agent N-acetylcysteine. However, removal of the mucus layer in mucosa exposed to 70% ethanol did not reduce the protective effect of prior treatment with a mildly irritating dose of NaCl, casting doubt on the role of mucus in the prostaglandin cytoprotective response. Attention has also been directed at enhanced mucosal blood flow as a potential mechanism for prostaglandin-mediated cytoprotection. Pretreatment with prostaglandin I_2 (PGI_2) protects against such damage, possibly as a result of increased mucosal blood flow (Konturek and Robert 1982), although PGE_2, which is also cytoprotective, does not increase blood flow. Nonetheless, PGE_2 may prevent vascular stasis associated with irritant-induced vascular damage as a result of inhibition of neutrophil adherence to damaged endothelium (Suzuki et al. 1991).

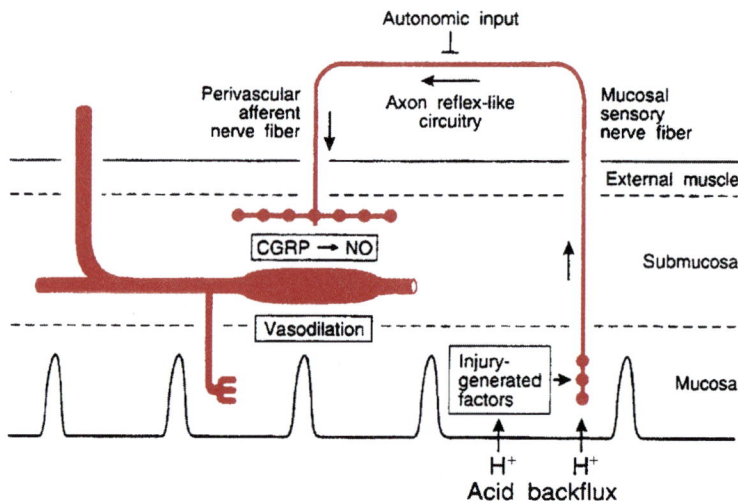

FIG. 4.14—Diagram showing the pathways and mediators of the hyperemic response to acid backdiffusion. Vasodilation is brought about by an axon reflexlike circuitry (*arrow*) that is under control of autonomic neurons in the splanchnic nerves. CGRP, calcitonin gene-related peptide; and NO, nitric oxide. (From Holzer et al. 1995.)

Sensory extrinsic and intrinsic neurons have also been implicated in cytoprotective mechanisms. For example, pretreatment of newborn rats with capsaicin (to which sensory nerves are sensitive) renders the mature rats more susceptible to gastric injury when exposed to damaging agents such as concentrated ethanol. Alternatively, use of a low dose of capsaicin, which stimulates rather than destroys sensory nerves, protects gastric mucosa against injurious agents (Holzer 1990, 1998; Holzer et al. 1995). Sensory nerves contain neuropeptides such as CGRP and substance P, which may play a protective role via vascular mechanisms. For example, CGRP stimulates increased gastric blood flow, which is theorized to reduce injury in much the same way as prostaglandins. In fact, recent studies suggest that the roles of prostaglandins and CGRP in gastric cytoprotection are intimately intertwined. In particular, PGI_2 is believed to sensitize sensory nerves following treatment with a mild irritant, with resultant increases in CGRP release and mucosal flow. This then results in adaptive cytoprotection against agents such as concentrated ethanol. Similar studies have shown that antagonists of CGRP inhibit the cytoprotective action of PGE_2. Another neural mediator, nitric oxide, has also been implicated in adaptive cytoprotection. Interestingly, nitric oxide has a number of actions that are similar to those of prostaglandins, including maintenance of mucosal blood flow (see Figure 4.15).

MECHANISMS OF GASTRIC INJURY. A breakdown in the aforementioned protective mechanisms results in gastric injury. For example, although stratified squamous epithelium is relatively impermeable to HCl, a number of factors can dramatically enhance the damaging effects of HCl in this epithelium. In particular, bile salts and SCFAs are capable of breaking down the squamous epithelial barrier at an acid pH, thereby exposing deep layers to HCl, with subsequent development of ulceration (Lang et al. 1998). Bile salts may also be present in the proximal porcine and equine stomach as a result of reflux from the duodenum. Although such reflux has a relatively high pH, it appears that bile salts adhere to stratified squamous epithelium, becoming lipid soluble and triggering damage once the pH falls below 4. Diet and management (e.g., periods of fasting) also play crucial roles in the development of conditions conducive to gastric ulceration. Fasting conditions increase the concentration of duodenal contents within the proximal stomach, particularly bile.

Whereas one of the major causes of ulcer disease in people is associated with the presence of *Helicobacter pylori*, such a relationship is not obvious in animals. Indeed, *H. pylori* has not been found in dogs, although it has been found on rare occasions in cats. Although other *Helicobacter* species are commonly found in the stomachs of these species, the presence of these organisms seems to have little influence on the prevalence or severity of gastric ulcers (Simpson et al. 1999; Strauss-Ayali and Simpson 1999; Neiger and Simpson 2000). This may relate to the relative lack of pathogenicity of *Helicobacter* species other than *H. pylori*, since infection with a variety of *Helicobacter* species has little effect on gastric function in dogs and cats.

The source of prostaglandins responsible for gastric protection was originally assumed to be cyclooxygenase

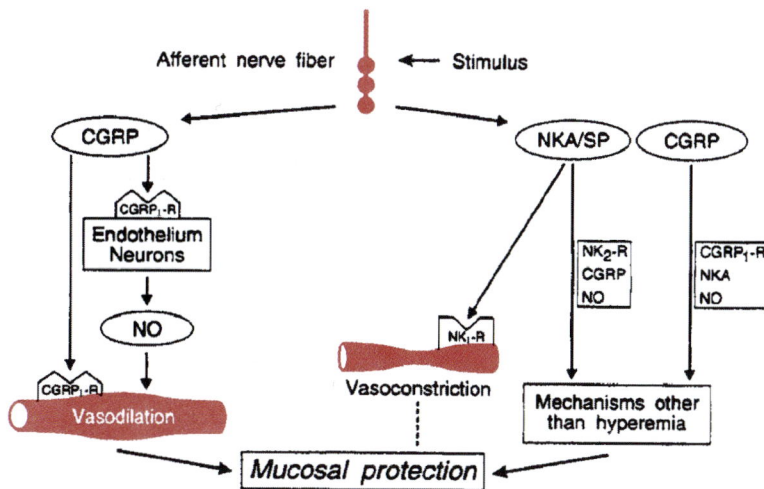

FIG. 4.15—Summary of the vasodilator and protective mechanisms that are initiated by stimulation of extrinsic afferent neurons and subsequent release of peptide transmitters. Whereas calcitonin gene-related peptide (CGRP) causes vasodilation, neurokinin A (NKA) and substance P (SP) elicit vasoconstriction. Both CGRP and NKA/SP stimulate hyperemia-independent mechanisms of protection. The protective action of CGRP involves NKA and nitric oxide (NO), whereas that of NKA/SP depends on CGRP and NO. (From Holzer et al. 1995.)

1 (COX-1), since this COX isoform is constitutively expressed in gastric mucosa, whereas COX-2 is not expressed in the stomach unless it is induced by inflammatory mediators. However, mice in which the COX-1 gene has been knocked out fail to develop spontaneous gastric lesions, possibly because of compensatory increases in prostaglandin production by COX-2. This concept agrees with recent data indicating that inhibition of both COX isoforms is required to induce gastric ulceration (Wallace and Miller 2000; Wallace 2001; Wallace and Ma 2001). In addition, COX-elaborated prostaglandins are important for repair of preexisting gastric ulcers. Interestingly, the COX isoform involved in repair appears to be COX-2 because, although prostanoids released by COX-2 likely contribute to early inflammatory events, induction of COX-2 at the site of the ulcer likely provides high local levels of prostanoids that facilitate gastric reparative mechanisms.

GASTRIC REPARATIVE MECHANISMS. Mechanisms of gastric repair are highly dependent on the extent of injury. For instance, superficial erosions can be rapidly covered by migration of epithelium adjacent to the wound, a process termed *epithelial restitution* (described in more depth under small intestinal mucosal repair in the *Intestinal Reparative Mechanisms* section). However, ulceration (full-thickness disruption of mucosa and penetration of the muscularis mucosa) requires repair of submucosal vasculature and matrix. This is initiated by formation of granulation tissue, which supplies connective tissue elements and microvasculature necessary for mucosal reconstruction. Connective tissue elements include proliferating fibroblasts that accompany newly produced capillaries that form from proliferating endothelium. Nitric oxide is critical to both of these processes (Wallace and Miller 2000), which likely explains the reparative properties of nitric oxide in the stomach.

Once an adequate granulation bed has been formed, newly proliferated epithelium at the edge of the wound begins to migrate across the wound. In addition, gastric glands at the base of the ulcer begin to bud and migrate across the granulation bed in a tubular fashion. Epidermal growth factor (EGF) is expressed by repairing epithelium and appears to facilitate these processes. In addition, these events are facilitated by a mucoid cap, which retains reparative factors and serum adjacent to the wound bed. Importantly, this cap maintains a neutral pH in order to facilitate healing. Once the ulcer crater has been filled with granulation tissue, and the wound has been reepithelialized, the subepithelial tissue remodels by altering the type and amount of collagen. Despite the remodeling process, ulceration tends to recur at sites of previous ulceration, and there is the concern that this aspect of repair can result in excessive deposition of collagen and fibrosis (Podolsky 1999).

INTESTINAL EPITHELIAL INJURY AND REPAIR

ISCHEMIA-REPERFUSION INJURY. Although intestinal reperfusion injury appears to be an important cause of mucosal damage in laboratory animals (Nilsson et al. 1994), studies in large animals such as pigs and horses (Blikslager and Roberts 1997; Blikslager et al. 1997a, b) have shown inconsistent results.

Reperfusion injury is initiated during ischemia when the enzyme xanthine dehydrogenase is converted to xanthine oxidase, and its substrate, hypoxanthine, accumulates simultaneously due to ATP utilization (Moore et al. 1995). However, there is little xanthine oxidase activity during ischemia, because oxygen is required as an electron acceptor. During reperfusion, xanthine oxidase rapidly degrades hypoxanthine in the presence of oxygen, producing the superoxide radical as a by-product. The superoxide radical contributes to oxidative tissue damage and, most importantly, activates neutrophil chemoattractants. Thus, inhibition of xanthine oxidase in feline studies of intestinal ischemia-reperfusion injury prevents infiltration of neutrophils, and subsequent mucosal injury.

What has been difficult to discern from the equine literature is whether the inconsistent presence of reperfusion injury is related to species-specific differences in mechanisms of reperfusion injury or attributable to the type of ischemia utilized. For instance, very little reperfusion injury was demonstrated in studies using various forms of strangulating obstruction, whereas separate studies in the equine jejunum and colon using low-flow ischemia have consistently demonstrated reperfusion injury (Dabareiner et al. 1995, 2001). However, the fact that inhibitors of xanthine oxidase had no effect on the level of reperfusion injury suggests that there may be alternate sources of reactive oxygen metabolites (ROMs) in horses. In fact, even in extensively studied feline models of ischemia-reperfusion injury, the source of a significant proportion of ROMs is unknown and independent of xanthine oxidase and neutrophils. In addition, the relationship between the levels of ROMs formed during ischemia-reperfusion and the level of mucosal injury is not linear, indicating that factors other than ROMs are responsible for triggering mucosal injury.

One aspect of intestinal reperfusion injury that has been universally agreed on is the critical role of neutrophils. For example, reperfusion injury was prevented without blocking xanthine oxidase by inhibiting activation of neutrophils. Studies in cats have shown that the most important population of neutrophils involved in mucosal reperfusion injury is resident tissue neutrophils and not neutrophils recruited from the circulation. Studies demonstrating reperfusion injury in the equine colon following low-flow ischemia have shown significant accumulation of neutrophils within the mucosa.

INTESTINAL REPARATIVE MECHANISMS. Once intestinal epithelium is disrupted, two events occur almost immediately to reduce the size of the denuded portion of the villus: contraction of the villus and epithelial restitution. For example, 1 to 2 hours after detergent-induced epithelial injury in guinea pig ileum, villi were 30% shorter, and epithelial restitution resulted in coverage of denuded villus tips. In porcine ileum subjected to 2 hours of ischemia, villi were 60% of their former height, and 50% of the denuded villus surface area was covered in flattened epithelium within 6 hours (Blikslager et al. 1999). Villus contraction appears to be regulated by intrinsic neurons, since inhibition of enteric nerve conduction prevents villus shortening after injury. The contractile component of the villus is a network of myofibroblasts distributed throughout the lamina propria of the villus and along the central lacteal. Inhibition of villus contraction results in retarded epithelial repair because of the larger denuded surface that remains to be covered by migrating epithelium compared with similarly injured villi that have contracted. As villi contract, as long as there is an intact basement membrane, epithelium from the margins of the wound migrates centripetally to resurface toward the tip of the villus, where injury associated with ischemia and toxic luminal substances is most profound. The process of restitution is similar in denuded colonic mucosa, except that it may proceed more rapidly because of the lack of villi. Epithelial restitution is solely a migratory event that does not depend on provision of new enterocytes by proliferation. Cellular migration is initiated by extension of cellular lamellipodia that receive signals from the basement membrane via integrins. Intracellular signaling converges on the actin cytoskeleton, which is responsible for movement of lamellipodia. Specific components of the basement membrane appear to be critical to the migratory process. Other elements of the basement membrane, including proteoglycans, hyaluronic acid, and noncollagenous proteins, such as fibronectin and laminin, may also provide important signals (McCormack et al. 1992). In addition, cells subjacent to epithelium, including myofibroblasts and immune cells, provide important signals for epithelial restitution.

Although epithelial restitution results in gross closure of previously denuded regions of gastrointestinal mucosa, closure of interepithelial spaces is ultimately required to restore normal epithelial barrier resistance. Since the tight junction is principally responsible for regulating the permeability of the interepithelial space, it is likely that repair and closure of this structure are critical to restore intestinal barrier function. Tight junctions consist of a group of transmembrane proteins that interdigitate from adjacent cells. Although occludin was originally thought to be the predominant tight junction transmembrane protein, a group of proteins termed *claudins* appear to be more critical (Kinugasa et al. 2000). These transmembrane proteins interact with the cytoskeleton via a series of intracellular proteins, including zonula occludens (ZO-1, ZO-2, and ZO-3), cingulin, and others. In addition, local regulatory proteins, such as the small GTPase Rho, are critical to tight junction function. In general, the relative contractile state of the actin cytoskeleton determines the degree to which tight junctions are open or closed, but the complexities of regulation of this process are poorly understood.

Once the epithelial barrier has been restored, normal mucosal architecture is reestablished to allow normal gut absorptive and digestive function. In porcine ileum subjected to 2 hours of ischemia, the epithelial barrier was restored within 18 hours, but villi were contracted and covered in epithelium with a squamous appearance. Restoration of normal villus architecture required a further 4 days. The flattened villus epithelium that characterizes restitution is replaced by newly proliferated crypt epithelium. Under normal circumstances, new enterocytes are formed by division of stem cells, of which there are approximately four at the base of each mucosal crypt. Newly divided enterocytes migrate from the crypt onto the villus. During migration, enterocytes differentiate and acquire specific absorptive and digestive functions. Fully differentiated enterocytes reside on the upper third of the villus for 2 to 3 days and are then sloughed into the intestinal lumen. This process is accelerated during mucosal repair, which requires increased proliferative rates. Increased proliferation may be stimulated within 12 to 18 hours by a variety of locally available gut-derived factors, including luminal nutrients, polyamines, and growth factors. The return of the normal leaflike shape of the villus occurs subsequent to the appearance of normal columnar epithelium.

MEDIATORS OF REPAIR

Prostaglandins. PGI$_2$ and PGE$_2$ rapidly restore the closure of the tight junctions during epithelial restitution. In addition, treatment of porcine ileum subjected to 1 hour of ischemia with the nonsteroidal anti-inflammatory agent indomethacin retarded the recovery of normal transepithelial resistance and exacerbated the mucosal-to-serosal flux of the polysaccharide inulin (molecular weight, 5500 daltons). This is of considerable importance to patients with intestinal injury who are treated with nonsteroidal anti-inflammatory agents, because reduced prostaglandin levels may prolong epithelial barrier repair and allow the passage of bacterial toxins from the intestinal lumen into subepithelial tissues.

Polyamines. The process of restitution is absolutely dependent on a group of compounds called *polyamines* (Wang et al. 1991, 1994; Banan et al. 1996). The rate-limiting enzyme in the formation of the polyamines spermine, spermidine, and putrescine is ornithine decarboxylase (ODC). In rats with stress-induced duodenal ulcers, systemic administration of the ODC inhibitor α-difluoromethylornithine significantly reduced polyamine levels and markedly reduced epithelial restitution. Furthermore, intragastric treatment of these same rats with putrescine, spermidine, and spermine prevented the delayed mucosal repair induced by α-difluoromethylornithine.

The mechanisms whereby polyamines stimulate epithelial restitution are not clear. McCormack and colleagues (1994) hypothesized that polyamines increased the activity of transglutaminase, an enzyme that catalyzes the crosslinking of cytoskeletal and basement membrane proteins. Polyamines regulate cytoskeletal cellular migration via activation of the small GTPase Rho-A by elevating intracellular Ca^{2+} levels. These elevations in Ca^{2+} result from polyamine regulation of expression of voltage gated K^+ channels and altered membrane electrical potential.

Polyamines also play a role in the normal physiological regulation of crypt cell proliferation and differentiation (Ray, Zimmerman et al. 1999). Polyamines are produced by fully differentiated enterocytes at the villus tip and may reach the crypt either within sloughed luminal epithelium or via local villus circulation. Following intestinal injury, polyamines appear to stimulate enhanced proliferation by increasing the expression of proto-oncogenes, which control the cell cycle. The mechanism whereby polyamines influence gene expression likely relates to the cationic nature of these compounds, which may influence the tertiary structure of negatively charged DNA and RNA.

Growth Factors. Locally produced growth factors, including EGF, transforming growth factors (TGF-α and TGF-β), and hepatocyte growth factor (HGF), also have the ability to stimulate both epithelial restitution and proliferation. EGF, produced by the salivary glands and duodenal Brunner's glands, and TGF-α produced by small intestinal enterocytes, are potent stimulants of enterocyte proliferation. These growth factors share approximately 30% of their amino acid structure, bind to the same receptor on the basolateral surface of enterocytes, and are not related to TGF-β. The physiological role of EGF is somewhat difficult to discern because it is present in the intestinal lumen, with no apparent access to its basally located receptor (Wright 1998). However, it has been proposed that EGF acts as a "surveillance agent" that gains access to its receptor during epithelial injury (when the EGF receptor would likely be exposed) to stimulate proliferation. TGF-α presumably has a similar role, but it is present in greater concentrations in the small intestine because it is produced by differentiated villus enterocytes. The mature peptide is cleaved from the extracellular component of the transmembrane TGF-α precursor and released into the lumen.

Intestinal Nutrients. The principal metabolic fuel of enterocytes is glutamine, and for colonocytes is butyrate. However, recent studies suggest that glutamine and butyrate have more specific proliferative actions aside from their role as nutrients. Because of such growth-promoting actions, glutamine was shown to prevent intestinal mucosal atrophy and dysfunction that accompany starvation and long-term total parental nutrition.

Visceral Pain

VISCERAL AFFERENTS AND NOCICEPTORS. Until relatively recently, the convention has been that the visceral sensory system pales in comparison to the somatic sensory system with regard to input into the CNS. Undoubtedly, this impression developed because of the diffuseness and generally poor localization of visceral pain, in contrast to human somatic pain, and the observation that insults such as pinching and cutting of normal gut rarely induce a pain sensation, whereas those types of insults are common causes of pain from skin and muscle. Within the last 10 years, however, it has become increasingly clear that the sensory innervation of the abdominal viscera, the hollow organs in particular, is extensive and complex, but a large proportion of this innervation is probably devoted to imperceptible activity, either because the activity is confined to the intestinal level or does not involve central mechanisms that are nociceptive. Thus, the visceral receptors and afferent fibers involved in generation and transmission of nociceptive stimuli to the CNS may be fewer in total number than their somatic counterparts, but they are, nonetheless, numerous.

Afferent sensory fibers travel to the CNS through one of two major routes: (a) the vagus nerve with cell bodies in the nodose ganglia and (b) the sympathetic trunk system of the thoracolumbar region of the spinal cord, with cell bodies in the dorsal root ganglia. There are also afferent pathways in the pelvic nerves that innervate the lower bowel from the sacral level of the spinal cord. These are referred to as the *extrinsic* primary afferent neurons, in contrast to those whose cell bodies and projections are confined within the gut wall that are referred to as *intrinsic* primary afferent neurons (IPANs). There is a third classification of sensory neurons, referred to as *intestinofugal* neurons, whose cell bodies are found within the gut wall but whose processes form synapses within the prevertebral sympathetic ganglia (Furness et al. 1999). Events within the gastrointestinal tract that induce a perception of discomfort or pain (i.e., nociception), and the associated pseudoaffective reflexes such as increased heart rate, decreased depth of breathing, and abdominal muscle cramping, naturally involve the *extrinsic* primary afferent neurons. These projections are, for the most part, unmyelinated, slow propagating, C-type fibers that are capsaicin sensitive, their respective receptors are primarily responsive to excessive stretch of the serosa, and they have a relatively high threshold of response. Certain chemical mediators, the production of which may be provoked by immune-mediated processes, also stimulate those extrinsic fibers that are transmitting a nociceptive message (see Figure 4.16).

In contrast, IPANs work locally and imperceptibly at the ENS level in response to stretch, mechanical, and chemical stimulation. Stretch reception in this context

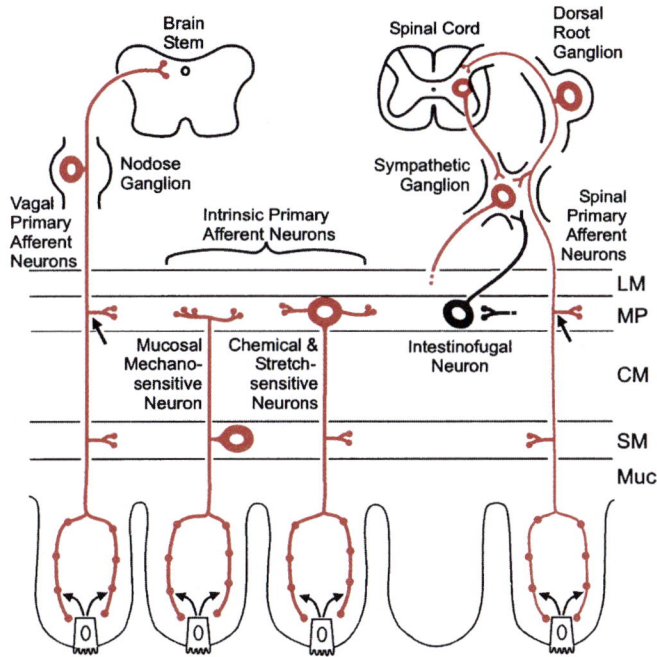

FIG. 4.16—Schematic representation of neural afferents involved in painful sensation. CM, circular muscle; LM, longitudinal muscle; Muc, mucosa; and SM, submucosa. (From Furness et al. 1999.)

is to smooth muscle tension rather than serosa, whereas the mechanical and chemical receptors are primarily involved in the constant monitoring of what is occurring at the mucosal surface. Thus, the IPANs are directly involved in influencing gastrointestinal motile, secretory, and vasodilatory activity. On the other hand, the main function of the intestinofugal neurons may be directed at controlling intraintestinal reflexes, where more aboral sections of the gastrointestinal tract influence the motor activity of more orad regions from which they receive digestive products, as exemplified by the documented duodenal and ileal "brakes" and the duodenogastric reflex.

ROLE OF THE VISCERAL AFFERENTS. The obvious role of the visceral afferent nerves is to continually sample what is occurring at the gut level and report the results to the ENS and CNS. As previously indicated, the majority of this activity is imperceptible, or nonnoxious if perceived at a central level through primary extrinsic nerve traffic. Stimulation of the extrinsic afferent neurons to the point of being noxious can become a very complex process. A wide range of chemical mediators has been described in the visceral afferent system. Activation of the afferents by these mediators has been broken down into three primary effects: (a) direct stimulation of primary afferents, (b) indirect stimulation of primary afferents through activation of other cells (e.g., immunocytes and enterochromaffin cells) that express the mediators, and (c) alteration of afferent nerve phenotype that results in

alteration of nerve mediator expression, or receptor types and/or their binding characteristics (Kirkup et al. 2001). At the intestinal level, direct stimulation can involve 5-HT (serotonin), capsaicin, ATP, adenosine, histamine, and prostaglandin. Indirectly stimulating mediators released through immunocyte and sympathetic varicosity activation include PGE_2, nerve growth factor, bradykinin, various interleukins, and adenosine. Threshold stimulation of nociceptive nerve terminals by one or a combination of the aforementioned mediators will promote tachykinin/substance P (SP), CGRP, and neurokinin release by specific gene expression in stimulated C fibers. Continued induction of mediator release can recruit high-threshold fibers that have been heretofore "silent" into transmitting nociceptive information to the CNS and eventually "sensitize" the receptors on those fibers to where they will respond to lower levels of stimulation, resulting in hyperalgesia (Gebhart 2000a, b). Prostaglandin and adenosine stimulation may be particularly prone to inducing sensitization (see Figure 4.17).

Stimulation of the majority of receptors on a nociceptor terminal induces depolarization through promotion of increased intracellular calcium concentration. On the other hand, the vanilloid (VR_1) receptor for capsaicin, $5-HT_3$ receptor for serotonin, and P2X receptor for ATP directly activate nonselective cation channels, which allows for Na^+ influx to induce depolarization. This latter finding has led to investigation of the potential antinociceptive properties of sodium channel blockers such as amiloride.

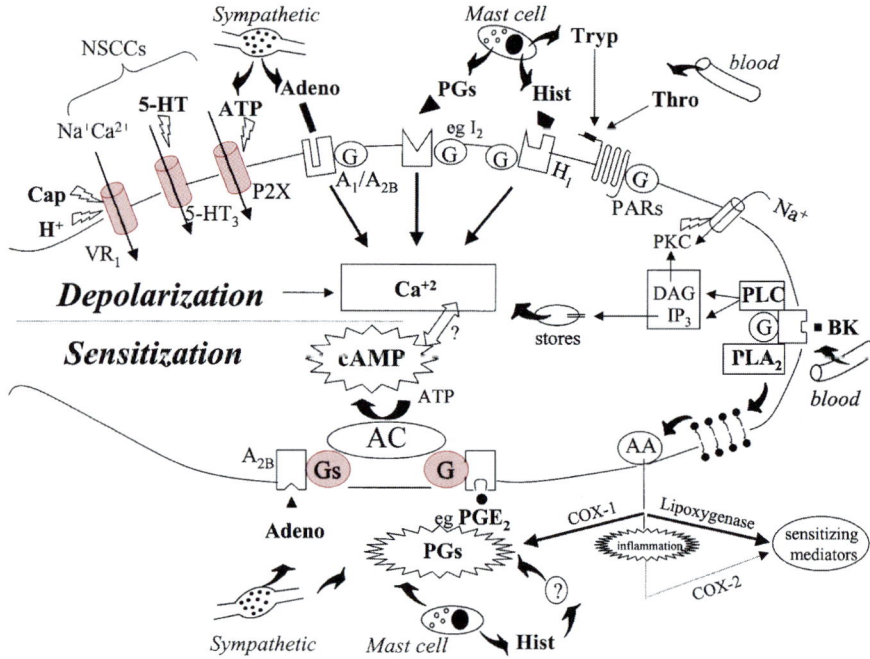

FIG. 4.17—Model of stimulation of neuron terminal. In addition to stimulation by 5-hydroxytryptamine (5-HT or serotonin) and cholecystokinin (CCK), the neuron can be activated by mast cell production. AA, arachidonic acid; AC, adenylate cyclase; Adeno, adenosine; ATP, adenosine triphosphate; BK, bradykinin; cAMP, cyclic adenosine monophosphate; Cap, capsaicin; COX-1 and COX-2, cyclooxygenase 1 and 2; DAG, diacylglycerol; Hist, histamine; IP3, inositol 1,4,5-trisphosphate; NSCCs, nonselective cation channels; PARs, protease activated receptors; PGE$_2$, prostaglandin E$_2$; PLA$_2$, phospholipase A$_2$; PGs, prostaglandins; PLC, phospholipase C; Thro, thrombin; Tryp, mast cell tryptase; and VR1, vanilloid receptor 1. (From Kirkup et al. 2001.)

NEUROPHYSIOLOGICAL BASIS OF VISCERAL PAIN. The sensory traffic generated by nociceptors activates neurons within the spinal cord and brain stem, which project to the cortex via the thalamus to elicit a painful sensation (Woolf and Salter 2000). It was long held that visceral pain is conveyed to the CNS strictly via spinal afferents, but increasing numbers of studies indicate the involvement of both spinal and vagal afferents. It appears that SP, in particular, plays a very important role in this process. SP belongs to the tachykinin family of peptides, along with CGRP and the neurokinins. The release of SP by CNS tissue in response to a nociceptive stimulus is well recognized. Peripheral noxious stimuli are transmitted to the spinal cord via capsaicin-sensitive afferent neurons that contain SP and are carried by the vagal and sympathetic trunks. The participation of SP release following neurokinin-1 receptor stimulation in the visceral nociceptive response has also been well documented, primarily through study of the rat colonic distension and intraperitoneal acetic acid models (Bueno et al. 1997).

As well, it is known that CGRP and SP coexist in primary afferent neurons and are likely to be coexpressed when these nerves are stimulated (Gay et al. 2000). Furthermore, CGRP potentiates several of the biological actions of SP. A further implication of CGRP in the visceral nociceptive response has been demonstrated in rats, where intrathecal treatment with the CGRP receptor antagonist, human CGRP (hCGRP)-(8-37), significantly reduced the response to colorectal distension in animals pretreated with intracolonic instillation of acetic acid (Plourde et al. 1997).

The concept of *neuronal plasticity* has opened up a whole new understanding of the development of hyperalgesia and allodynia, terms applied to states of respectively increased or acquired pain sensitivity to a given stimulus. Many of the mechanisms involved in neuronal adaptation that have been discovered to date have derived from studies in animals, primarily rodents. The implications for these, and continuing, discoveries for developing new strategies of pain management in human and veterinary medicine are obvious. Woolf and Salter (2000) describe three stages of neuronal plasticity—activation, modulation, and modification—that all alter the nociceptor peripheral terminal threshold. *Activation* is regarded as activity dependent in that it is induced by repeated stimulation. As applied to visceral sensitivity, it may occur at the nociceptor terminal or within the dorsal horn neurons of the spinal column. Nociceptor terminal activation can result in its decrease in threshold due to, for instance, autosensitization of its VR_1 receptors upon their repeated activation by capsaicin. Dorsal horn neuron activation may result from high-frequency input of sustained noxious stimulation, where the continual release of peptides such as SP and CGRP, and of glutamate, cause an upregulation of *N*-methyl-D-aspartate (NMDA) within the neurons, a condition referred to as *windup*. Effects of activation are reversible, pending control of the underlying cause. *Modulation* refers to alteration of intrinsic functional properties or cell surface expression of channels in primary extrinsic afferent or dorsal horn neurons. Peripherally, this occurs in the primary afferents secondary to sensitizing by inflammatory mediators such as 5-HT, SP, bradykinin, PGE_2, and neurotrophic factors released by inflammatory cells and tissue damage. Centrally, modulation is due to intracellular effects that result in a combination of facilitated excitatory and depressed inhibitory synaptic responses, which amplifies responses to both noxious (hyperalgesia) and innocuous (allodynia) stimuli. Upregulation of NMDA receptors within the dorsal horn (windup) is again considered to be a very important component of this central modulation. *Modification*, the most extreme of these changes, can be provoked by either inflammation or nerve damage. Its development may be mediated by loss (apoptosis) of inhibitory neurons, establishment of misdirected excitatory synapses, and induced expression of constitutive and novel gene products. This latter activity can result in the expression of inflammatory mediators by A-fiber neurons, which normally do not express such substances. The ultimate unfortunate effect of modification is persistent pathological pain that may be very difficult, at this stage of our knowledge, to control therapeutically.

An extremely important study by Ruda and coworkers (2000) clearly demonstrates how neuronal plasticity can lead to a persistent condition of hyperalgesia in adult rats, due to an unexpected cause, namely, their exposure as neonates to a severe, weeklong focal inflammation. The inflammation in this instance was somatic: injection of Freund's adjuvant into the hindpaw. The hyperalgesic condition was behaviorally demonstrated as well as marked by a significantly greater number of nociceptive unmyelinated and finely myelinated primary afferent neurons in the ipsilateral sciatic nerve and dorsal laminae of the spinal cord, and a significantly greater number of terminals within the ipsilateral dorsal root ganglion (DRG) in which CGRP was histochemically labeled. This concept is now starting to be explored with respect to visceral problems, as well. Thus, the message is that clinicians should never overlook an adult patient's history back to infancy when examining and evaluating a case of irritable bowel syndrome. A case in point is that of an adult horse that experiences repeated bouts of moderate to severe colic for which there is no etiologic explanation, even after exploratory laparotomy.

With regard to CNS processing of somatic and visceral sensory signals, current imaging technology has challenged earlier contentions that the cerebral cortex plays a minimal role in pain perception (Ladabaum et al. 2001). Of particular note has been the activation of the anterior cingulate cortex in nearly all pain studies. Other regions within the brain that have been associated with nociception include the insula, somatosensory cortices, prefrontal and inferior parietal cortices, lentiform nucleus, and hypothalamus.

Pathophysiology of Colic. The *Merriam-Webster's Collegiate Dictionary* describes *colic* as "a paroxysm of acute abdominal pain localized in a hollow organ and often caused by spasm, obstruction, or twisting." The operative phrase is "*abdominal* pain localized in a hollow organ," which, in modern parlance, is referred to as *visceral pain*, as opposed to *somatic pain*, which has a primarily musculoskeletal origin. Visceral pain has five important characteristics (Cervero and Laird 1999):

1. It is not evoked from all viscera, because the parenchyma of most solid viscera (e.g., liver, kidneys, and lung) are not sensitive to pain, *although their ducts may be*.
2. It is not always a result of visceral injury (e.g., sharp cutting of an intestine is not painful, whereas excessive stretching usually is).
3. It is diffuse and poorly localized.
4. It is referred to other locations (human experience).
5. It is accompanied by motor and autonomic reflexes that in themselves may or may not be perceived at a conscious level.

Probably the most common cause of visceral pain is excessive stretching of the serosal membrane of the intestinal tract. All three of the problems—spasm, obstruction, and twisting—just mentioned in the Merriam-Webster definition can evoke such a stretching due to focal entrapment of gas and/or contents, as can inflammation and its attendant subserosal edema.

SIGNS OF COLIC IN ANIMALS. A major diagnostic challenge for veterinarians is to recognize the clinical signs of visceral pain, commonly referred to as *colic* or *acute abdomen*. Such signs often go hand in hand with reflex responses such as increased heart rate, decreased depth of respiration, and tensing of abdominal musculature. A distinction between these reflex responses and true signs of nociception, defined here as conscious *perception* of a painful stimulus, needs to be emphasized (see Figure 4.18).

Among all of the domesticated animal species, the most frequent, and well-recognized, signs of colic occur in horses. These signs can range from uncharacteristic restlessness and looking around at the abdomen to violent thrashing and rolling. The relative accuracy of relating the pattern of clinical signs to the severity of the pain in a horse stems from the centuries of close interaction between people and horses, the fact that the beast is not reluctant to display such signs, and the

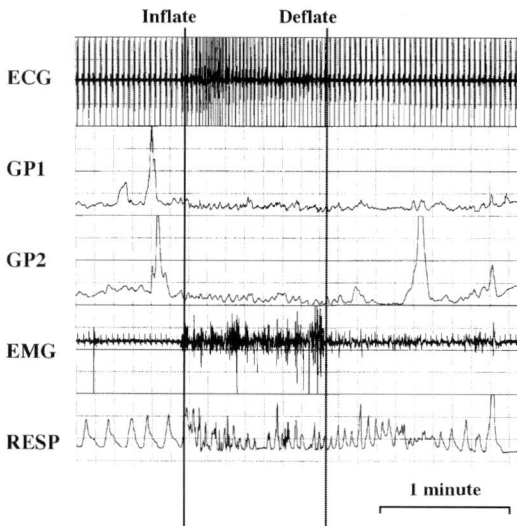

FIG. 4.18—Simultaneous recording of electrocardiogram (ECG), intra-gastric pressure (GP1 and GP2), abdominal muscle myoelectrical activity (EMG, electromyogram), and respiratory movement (RESP) from a horse before, during, and after a 1-minute inflation of a balloon within the duodenum that induced signs of colic. The increased heart rate, decreased gastric motility, increased EMG activity indicating tensing of abdominal muscles, and increased, shallow respiratory movement are all considered as reflex responses to the duodenal distension that could be seen without accompanying signs of nociception.

TABLE 4.2—Essential components of a full presurgical clinical evaluation of a colicky horse

Physical examination
    Assessment of degree and type (visceral vs parietal) of *pain*
    Shape of the *paunch*
        Rate and character of the *pulse*
    Mucous membrane *perfusion*
    Audibility of gut sounds—"*peristalsis*"
        Presence of *pings* on simultaneous auscultation–
        percussion of the abdomen
    Per rectal *palpation*
    Amount and character of gastric fluid after *passing a tube*
Basic clinical laboratory data
    Blood *packed cell volume* and *total protein*
    Peritoneal fluid cytology and *total protein*
Imaging alternatives according to case
    Endoscopy
    Ultrasonography
    Radiology

expanding opportunity over the last 40 years to relate signs to pathology through the application of surgical intervention and more and more sophisticated diagnostic imaging devices. This has resulted in a detailed algorithmic approach to a given case that is designed to cover the essentials of a complete clinical evaluation upon which further decisions concerning medical/surgical management, or euthanasia, are made (see Tables 4.1 and 4.2).

As for other domesticated species, signs of visceral pain have also been well documented in small animals, particularly dogs. Again, the accuracy of relating specific signs or patterns of behavior to specific

TABLE 4.1—Common clinical signs of colic in horses according to clinical assessment of severity

Mild	Restlessness
	Standing and looking at flank
	Shifting on hindlimbs
	Stretching neck
Moderate	Pawing
	Stretching body
	Kicking at abdomen
	Sternally recumbent and looking at flank
Severe	Recumbent and rolling
	Recumbent on back
	Dog sitting

pathological entities within the abdomen of dogs and cats is due in large part to the willingness of their owners to pay for diagnosis and treatment of the problem, thus providing veterinarians the opportunity to obtain a definitive diagnosis. Ruminants, on the other hand, appear to be more refractory to conditions that would induce signs of colic in horses or small animals. Perhaps the most common sign of visceral pain in ruminants is treading and kicking at the abdomen with the hindfeet, and this may occur only within a short time window early in the development of the problem, which is usually some sort of acute obstruction such as a volvulus or intussusception (see Table 4.3).

It is extremely important when examining an animal with signs indicative of abdominal distress to determine whether a component of the observed discomfort is emanating from the peritoneum rather than from the intestinal tract. That is, is there a *parietal* component or is the pain strictly visceral in origin? Reluctance to move and extreme tenseness of the abdominal muscles, commonly referred to as *splinting*, are strong indications of parietal involvement (i.e., peritonitis). With severe peritonitis, any attempt to palpate deeply into the abdomen will be met by strong avoidance behavior that may include biting or kicking at the hand doing the palpating. In less severe cases, some deeper palpation may be tolerated, but obvious discomfort can be induced when the palpating hand is quickly retracted, a phenomenon referred to as *rebound tenderness*, which is usually not seen if the source of the discomfort is strictly visceral.

Undoubtedly, there are situations where both visceral and parietal reactions come into play in causing abdominal discomfort. For instance, one of the most common causes of severe abdominal pain in dogs is acute pancreatitis, which is probably due to a combination of the direct effect of the inflammation on the serosa surrounding the gland and a secondary parietal peritonitis induced nearby.

TABLE 4.3—Some common clinical signs of colic in dogs

Pacing continually
Repeatedly assuming different positions
Repeatedly looking and licking at abdomen
Standing stretched out
Repeatedly whining and/or growling
Snapping if abdomen touched

PATHOPHYSIOLOGY OF COLIC OF GASTROINTESTINAL ORIGIN

EXCESSIVE GUT DISTENSION. As indicated earlier in this chapter, the most common cause of abdominal pain of visceral origin is the excessive stretching of the serosa overlying a hollow viscus. Again, in veterinary medicine, the horse provides the most useful model for illustrating the various conditions that can manifest as colic, since just about all of the wide range of problems that cause colic can happen in this species. Distension of a viscus by entrapped gas and/or ingesta is the most common cause of excessive serosal stretch. This entrapment and stretch can occur as a result of (a) physical obstruction due to a volvulus, incarceration, intussusception, or stricture; or (b) functional obstruction due to dysmotility caused by chemical or congenital disruption of the enteric muscular and/or nervous system. The serosa may be additionally stretched by edema of the intestinal wall, caused either by obstruction of the venous return from an incarcerated or twisted section of bowel where arterial supply is still intact, or by inflammation. Added to this in some cases is further distension due to extravasation of fluid into gut lumen as a result of the venous obstruction. Regarding vascular compromise, it should be pointed out that nociception occurs only so long as the arterial supply to the affected segment is still intact. Afferent nerves within the bowel that are responsible for transmitting nociceptive signals to the CNS quickly become inoperative under ischemic conditions and then die along with the rest of the tissues if the ischemia persists for very long. At this stage, patients may experience some relief from the pain but continue to show signs of severe toxemia.

GASTROENTERITIS. The previous discussion focused on stretch-sensitive neurons within the ENS, primarily those with a high threshold response that stimulate central nociceptive pathways. In this regard, the intramural edema associated with inflammation can also excite serosal stretch receptors. In addition, there is growing evidence that chemoreceptors may also be involved in nociception, and that both stretch and chemoreceptors use the same afferent pathways. Chemoreception within this context would be primarily related to stimulation by inflammatory mediators such as interleukins, tumor-necrosis factor, prostaglandins, bradykinin, and histamine. These substances may act directly to stimulate certain visceral afferents or evoke the release of chemical messengers such as SP, 5-HT, or CGRP that, through their specific receptors, stimulate the afferents (see the section *Neurophysiological Basis of Visceral Pain*). Also, when inflammation is involved, there are often systemic consequences reflective of cytokine production that are not seen if the colic is due strictly to an obstructive condition that has no attendant inflammatory component. These systemic consequences can include depression, fever, leukopenia, hypotension, and generalized intestinal stasis (ileus). Depending on species and extent of the inflammatory response, vomiting (gastric distension with fluid in the case of horses) and/or diarrhea may also be seen.

Gastroenteritis, in its broadest terms, refers to various types of immune, inflammatory cell recruiting responses within the submucosa to antigens for which the gut has no tolerance, either innate or acquired. Such antigens can be found as part of the makeup of viruses, bacteria, parasites, and foodstuffs to which the mucosa is constantly exposed. The chemical messengers subsequently expressed, such as the aforementioned SP and 5-HT, have been shown, primarily to date by in vitro studies, to disrupt normal gastrointestinal motility in a way that, theoretically, could either be responsible for initiating a condition that results in colic or provoke an already established situation. Undoubtedly, the documented in vivo effects of various foreign antigens on gastrointestinal motility are more complex in cause than simply being due to the expression of a single chemical messenger. However, the point is that a dysmotility, per se, could be the sole basis for the nociceptive stimulus in a given case. An example of this might be the so-called spasmodic colic in horses that has been attributed to, among other things, the active migration of ingested small strongyle larvae. The migratory activity of the larvae themselves is usually imperceptible. Yet, while the immune response that they induce by their presence within the submucosa may cause only minimal inflammation, it could, nonetheless, result in the expression of chemical mediators in sufficient amounts to provoke a dysmotility that entraps gas within intestinal segments and induces periodic bouts of severe discomfort.

In summary, *colic* in veterinary medicine refers to a broad range of clinical signs that we have come to recognize as indicators of visceral nociception. By convention, we make general assessments regarding the severity of the pain (i.e., mild, moderate, or severe) through the pattern of signs presented.

PATHOPHYSIOLOGY OF ACUTE GASTROINTESTINAL INFLAMMATION. The inflammatory response of the gastrointestinal tract is a mechanism ultimately aimed at eliminating pathogens, initiating tissue repair, and restoring the gastrointestinal barrier. Blood flow is altered, endothelial permeability increases, cells are rapidly recruited into the tissue, plasma protein cascades are activated, and a myriad of soluble products are released that coordinate the response, trigger innate and adaptive immunity, and mobilize reparative elements. Although the cellular and vascular response and the secreted mediators of inflammation are important for killing pathogens and limiting invasion of injured tissues by commensal organisms, they can be quite damaging to host cells and proteins if not tightly regulated. Thus, if the inciting stimulus is not eliminated quickly, the inflammatory response itself will cause significant tissue injury.

Initiation of the Inflammatory Response. Invasion of epithelial cells by *Salmonella* or other pathogenic organisms activates the synthesis of proinflammatory chemokines (chemoattractants) and cytokines by epithelial cells (Kagnoff and Eckmann 1997). Noninfectious injury to the mucosa also results in the production of chemokines stimulating an early and robust influx of neutrophils within hours of the damage. Of the chemoattractants produced by epithelium, interleukin 8 (IL-8) has a particularly important role in initiating inflammation by recruiting neutrophils from blood (Ina et al. 1997) and regulating migration of neutrophil migration through tissue matrix adjacent to epithelium (McCormick et al. 1997). Epithelial cells also produce TNF-α and arachidonic acid metabolites and other inflammatory mediators that activate recruited leukocytes (Jung et al. 1995). Once the inflammatory response has been initiated, TNF-α, IL-1β, and other cytokines produced by neutrophils, monocytes, mast cells, and epithelial cells continue to stimulate the production of chemokines by not only epithelial cells, but also other cells of the mucosa, thus potentiating the inflammatory response.

HOW DOES THE EPITHELIUM SENSE PATHOGENIC ORGANISMS AND DISTINGUISH BETWEEN PATHOGENS AND COMMENSAL FLORA? Epithelial damage induced by pathogen invasion and toxin-induced necrosis plus subsequent exposure of cells within the mucosa to not only the organism infecting the tissue, but also the contents of the gastrointestinal lumen, is a potent activator of inflammation. However, this brute-force mechanism of activating inflammation is not the only way the gastrointestinal epithelium can distinguish potential invaders. During invasion, many pathogens inject virulence gene products by a specific transport mechanism into the epithelial cell. This specialized system, called a type III secretory system, represents a virulence mechanism of bacteria that are important pathogens of a wide range of species from plants to people (Galan and Collmer 1999). Virulence proteins and toxins transported into the cytosol of the target cells subvert the cellular machinery to promote the ability of the pathogen to invade the cell. While doing so, chemokine and cytokine transcription is activated in the epithelial cell, signaling to the tissue that the cell has been invaded, and an inflammatory response is initiated.

Epithelial cells can also sense the presence of microorganisms via apical surface toll-like receptors that bind lipopolysaccharide, lipoproteins, lipoteichoic acid, and other microbial products, which when ligated stimulate IL-8 and TNF-α production (Cario and Podolsky 2000). However, these so-called pattern recognition receptors for bacterial products cannot distinguish between the products of pathogenic and commensal organisms.

WHAT PREVENTS THE NORMAL LUMINAL MILIEU FROM ACTIVATING A MUCOSAL INFLAMMATORY RESPONSE? One mechanism that regulates the response of epithelial cells is the expression of a coreceptor for toll-like receptors: CD14. CD14 is necessary for toll receptor signaling in response to lipopolysaccharide, for example. CD14 expression is generally very low except in inflamed mucosa (Podolsky 1999). Thus, inflammation upregulates an important sensor mechanism for microbial products. Epithelial cells also confine the localization of some receptors that sense microbial products to the basolateral membrane or to intracellular locations, where microbial products will be present only when the epithelial barrier has been breached (Gewirtz et al. 2001).

Vascular Response During Inflammation. Four important changes occur in the vasculature during inflammation: (a) alteration of blood flow, (b) increased vascular permeability, (c) increased adhesiveness of endothelial cells, leukocytes, and platelets, and (d) exposure of the basement membrane and activation of the complement, contact, and coagulation cascades.

A wide range of mediators alter blood flow during inflammation in the intestinal tract, ranging from gases such as nitric oxide (a major vasodilator of the intestinal vasculature) to lipids [prostaglandins, leukotrienes, thromboxanes, and platelet-activating factor (PAF)], cytokines, bradykinin, histamine, and others. The major sources for these mediators include activated leukocytes, endothelial cells, epithelial cells, and fibroblasts. The primary determinant of blood flow early in inflammation is vascular caliber, which initially decreases in arterioles but then quickly changes to vasodilation coincident with opening of new capillary beds, increasing net blood flow. The increase in blood flow is relatively short-lived, as the viscosity of the blood increases due to fluid loss and tissue edema through leaky capillaries. Leukocyte margination, platelet adhesion to endothelial cells and exposed matrix, and areas of coagulation protein accumulation further decrease local circulation.

Increased vascular permeability is initially caused by inflammatory mediator actions on the endothelial cells. Histamine, leukotrienes, PAF, prostaglandins, bradykinin, and other mediators stimulate endothelial cell contraction, and interendothelial gaps form (Joris et al. 1990). This stage of vascular permeability is readily reversible. Concurrently, mediators such as the cytokines TNF-α and IL-1β induce a structural reorganization of the interendothelial junctions, resulting in frank discontinuities in the endothelial monolayer. Cytokines also stimulate endothelial cells to express adhesion molecules that support adhesion of leukocytes and platelets (Springer 1994), leading to the next and perhaps most devastating event. Leukocytes (primarily neutrophils) and platelets adhere to exposed basement membranes and activated endothelial cells. Adherent neutrophils and platelets are then exposed to the mediators of inflammation present in the surrounding milieu. Thus, activated platelets and neutrophils release products such as oxidants and proteases (particularly elastase) that injure the endothelium and have the potential to cause irreparable harm to the microvasculature. Marginated neutrophils begin to transmigrate between endothelial cells. If in large enough numbers, this disrupts the integrity of the interendothelial junctions, worsening the vascular leakage (Rosengren et al. 1991).

Recruitment of Inflammatory Cells

NEUTROPHILS. Infection or injury to the gastrointestinal mucosa causes an influx of leukocytes from the blood that lays the foundation of the inflammatory response. Neutrophils, being the first to arrive during inflammation, have a dominant role in the acute response. Within minutes, neutrophils are recruited into the tissue, where they are activated to release products that are not only lethal to pathogens and proinflammatory but may also damage host cells and tissues. Not surprisingly, much attention has been paid to the role of neutrophils in the pathophysiology of many inflammatory conditions (Dallegri and Ottonello 1997). Moreover, neutrophil depletion is protective in many gastrointestinal diseases. Of interest to clinicians, blockade of neutrophil migration into inflamed tissues prevents many of the pathophysiological events associated with infectious enteritis, ischemia-reperfusion injury, and other gastrointestinal diseases (Elliott et al. 1994). Thus, the mechanism regulating the migration of blood neutrophils into inflamed tissues has been a focus of much research to identify therapeutic targets for clinical applications. Neutrophil transendothelial migration is a multistep process that is temporally and spatially regulated and has degrees of cell type specificity.

Of the activators of neutrophils at sites of inflammation, complement (C3-opsonized particles), cytokines (TNF-α and IL-1β), PAF, immune complexes, and bacterial products are among the most potent stimuli. Other mediators produced during inflammation may modify neutrophil activity, particularly formylated bacterial peptides, chemokines, complement fragments (C5a), leukotriene B$_4$, and prostaglandins. Activated neutrophils are highly phagocytic; produce large amounts of reactive oxygen intermediates; degranulate to release myeloperoxidase, cationic antimicrobial peptides (defensins), serine proteases (mainly elastase), and metalloproteinases; and secrete inflammatory mediators (TNF-α, IL-1β, prostaglandins, leukotrienes, and others). Activated neutrophils also produce some nitric oxide and other reactive nitrogen intermediates, albeit only a fraction of the amount produced by activated macrophages. Products of neutrophils and other inflam-

matory cells act in concert with the products of plasma protein cascades (the coagulation cascade, contact system, and complement cascade), activated in part by factors released by activated cells and in part by exposed matrix proteins and bacterial products. This network of responses amplifies the inflammatory response, alters blood flow, increases endothelial permeability, and sensitizes nociceptors (see Table 4.4).

MAST CELLS. Mast cells strategically reside in mucosal tissues, including the submucosa and lamina propria of the gastrointestinal tract, and constitute a crucial first line of defense at epithelial barriers. However, they are also important effector cells of the pathophysiology of inflammatory gastrointestinal diseases (Wershil 2000).

Mast cells are activated by a wide variety of microbial products and host-derived mediators (Galli et al. 1999). Among the activators of mast cells, the so-called anaphylatoxins (complement fragments C3a, C5a, and C4a) are extremely potent stimuli causing release of mediators of inflammation. In addition, mast cells are the primary effector cells of immunoglobulin E (IgE)-mediated anaphylaxis (type I hypersensitivity reactions) by virtue of their high-affinity receptors for IgE. Crosslinking of receptor-bound IgE on mast cell surface by antigens (i.e., food antigens) causes rapid degranulation, resulting in the explosive release of granule contents. Mast cells are also regulated by neural pathways in the intestine, responding to enteric pathogen invasion via neural reflexes that stimulate the release of inflammatory mediators.

Activated mast cells release preformed histamine, 5-HT, proteases, heparin, and cytokines from granules. Activation also stimulates de novo synthesis of a range of inflammatory mediators, including prostaglandins, PAF, and leukotrienes. Transcription of a number of peptide mediators, such as the cytokines TNF-α and IL-1β among many others, also increases upon stimu-

Table 4.4—Important activators of neutrophils

Class	Stimuli
Microbial products	Formylated peptides, lipopolysaccharide, peptidoglycan, lipoproteins, and lipoteichoic acid
Plasma proteins	Complement fragments C5a (soluble), C3b and C3bi (surface bound), immune complexes, and bradykinin
Cytokines	Tumor necrosis factor α, interleukin 1β, interferon-γ, interleukin 6, G-CSF, and GM-CSF
Chemokines	Interleukin 8, Gro-α, and NAP-2
Lipids	Leukotriene B$_4$, prostaglandin E$_2$, thromboxane B$_4$, and platelet-activating factor
Neuropeptides	Vasoactive intestinal peptide, substance P, and nociceptin
Biogenic amines	Histamine and serotonin

lation of mast cells. Mast cell products have profound effects on the vasculature, increasing endothelial permeability and causing vasodilation (Metcalfe et al. 1992). Moreover, mast cell-derived mediators enhance markedly epithelial secretion by a mechanism that involves the activation of neural pathways of epithelial secretion and direct stimulation of epithelial cells (Castro et al. 1987). Mast cell products significantly alter intestinal motility, generally increasing transit and expulsion of intestinal contents.

Mast cells have a newly identified role in host defense and inflammatory responses to bacterial pathogens (Malaviya and Abraham 2001). Their role is in part due to the release of proinflammatory mediators during bacterial infection, which is critical for recruiting and activating other innate host defense cells such as neutrophils. However, mast cells are also phagocytic, have microbicidal properties, and can act as antigen-presenting cells to the adaptive immune system. The role for mast cells in host protective responses appears to as a sensor of bacterial invasion. Unlike IgE-mediated responses, bacterial products seem to elicit a highly regulated and more selective response from mast cells. *Escherichia coli* stimulates mast cells to produce leukotrienes, TNF-α, and histamine. In contrast, endotoxin activates substantial IL-6 release with little degranulation.

Humoral Mediators of Inflammation

COMPLEMENT. The complement cascade is a fundamental part of the inflammatory response. Activation of the complement cascade—either by immune complexes (classical pathway) or by bacteria or bacterial products, polysaccharides, viruses, fungi, or host cells (alternative pathway)—results in the deposition of complement proteins on the activating surface and the release of soluble proteolytic fragments of several complement components (Goldstein 1992). In particular, activation of either pathway results in the deposition of fragments of the component C3, which are potent activators of neutrophils and monocytes. Opsonization of particles with C3 fragments constitutes a major mechanism of target recognition and phagocyte activation. During the activation of the complement cascade culminating in deposition of C3, soluble fragments of C3 (C3a), C5 (C5a), and C4 (C4a) are liberated. These fragments, termed *anaphylatoxins*, have potent effects on tissues and cells during inflammation. Perhaps most notably, they are chemotactic for neutrophils (particularly C5a), activate neutrophil and mast cell degranulation, and stimulate ROM release from neutrophils. The termination of the complement cascade results in the formation of a membrane-attack complex in membranes at the site of complement activation. If this occurs on host cells such as endothelium, the cell may be irreversibly injured. Although the primary source of complement is plasma, epithelial cells of the gastrointestinal tract also produce C3, suggesting that local production and activation of the complement cascade during inflammation occur in intestinal tissues (see Table 4.5).

Table 4.5. Biological responses to anaphylatoxins (Goldstein 1992)

Cell or tissue	Response
Blood vessels	Increased permeability
	Vasoconstriction
Mast cells	Degranulation (histamine, serotonin, and proteases)
Neutrophils and monocytes	Degranulation (proteases and cationic peptides)
	Chemotaxis
	Transendothelial migration
	Respiratory-burst activity
	Augmented phagocytosis
	Increased adhesion receptor expression
	Adhesion and aggregation
	Inflammatory mediator production: prostaglandins, thromboxane, leukotrienes, platelet-activating factor, cytokines, and chemokines

It is clear that if the regulatory mechanisms of the complement cascade fail, then the inflammatory response may be inappropriate and tissue injury can occur.

CONTACT SYSTEM. The contact system of plasma is initiated by four components: Hageman factor (HF), prekallikrein, factor XI, and high molecular weight kininogen. Bacterial cell walls, vascular basement membranes, heparin, glycosaminoglycans, and other negatively charged surfaces in the intestine capture HF and the other three important initiators of the contact system in a large multimolecular complex. The result is cleavage of HF by kallikrein and triggering of the contact system cascade, activation of intrinsic coagulation by factor XIa, activation of the alternative pathway by HF, and proteolytic cleavage of high molecular weight kininogen by kallikrein, releasing biologically active kinins.

The products of the contact system, particularly bradykinin, have several important biological properties that drive many of the vascular and leukocyte responses during inflammation (Kozin and Cochrane 1992). Bradykinin induces endothelial cell contracture and intracellular tight junction alterations that increase vascular permeability to fluid and macromolecules. Bradykinin also affects vascular smooth muscle contracture, resulting in either vasoconstriction or vasodilation, depending on the location. Bradykinin also increases intestinal motility, enhances chloride secretion by the intestinal mucosa, and intensifies gastrointestinal pain. In neutrophils, kinins stimulate the release of many inflammatory mediators, including cytokines, prostaglandins, leukotrienes, and reactive oxygen intermediates. Kallikrein cleaves C5 to release C5a, a potent chemotactic factor for neutrophils, and thus has a role in recruiting and activating inflammatory leukocytes.

Tissue Injury During Inflammation. Changes in blood flow to the mucosa and other regions of the intestine that reduce perfusion of the tissues can potentiate the initial damage caused by infection or injury.

Alterations in blood flow induced by products of the kinin cascade, by histamine, or by the myriad vasoactive lipids released by endothelial cells, platelets, mast cells, neutrophils, macrophages, and other cells in inflamed tissues can reduce tissue perfusion during inflammation. Nitric oxide, whether produced in endothelial cells or leukocytes (macrophages), is a potent regulator of blood flow and has a significant role in the control of perfusion during inflammation (Mashimo and Goyal 1999). Many of the mediators that affect perfusion also affect endothelial permeability, leading to altered osmotic and hydrostatic balance and tissue edema. In extreme cases, local and/or systemic coagulopathies initiated by vascular injury and absorption of microbial products and inflammatory mediators induce a hypercoagulable state, leading to microthrombus formation, which can reduce blood flow, or macrothrombus formation causing tissue infarction.

Neutrophils have a key role in tissue injury:

1. Neutrophils in inflamed tissues activated by potent host mediators (such as IL-1β and TNF-α) and bacterial products (LPS) release copious amounts of reactive oxygen intermediates.

2. Serine proteases (particularly elastase) and metalloproteinases released by degranulating neutrophils destroy tissue matrix proteins and cell surface proteins that make up intercellular junctions. These enzymes are particularly damaging to basement membranes and the cellular barriers of the endothelium and epithelium. Thus, they contribute to vascular permeability (and local tissue edema) and loss of the epithelial barrier function (increasing permeability and ulceration, which permits absorption of bacterial products and even invasion of luminal organisms).

3. Migration of neutrophils through endothelium during emigration into inflamed tissues is remarkable in that the permeability of the endothelial monolayer is preserved under most circumstances. However, there is a limit above which neutrophil migration alters the permeability characteristics of the endothelium. The effect is in part physical in that the mere movement of large numbers of neutrophils through the endothelium is sufficient to disrupt the tight junctions and in part due to toxic products of neutrophils that damage endothelial cells and basement membranes. The permeability may be affected to the extent that not only water but macromolecules (albumin, matrix proteins, complement, etc.) leak into the interstitium.

4. Similar to the endothelium of inflamed tissues, massive neutrophil transmigration occurs across the epithelium in response to infection or injury. Neutrophil transepithelial migration increases epithelial permeability by disrupting tight junctions. In addition, subepithelial accumulation of neutrophils can lead to ulceration (Nusrat et al. 1997). Neutrophil-induced damage to the epithelium contributes to protein-losing enteropathy associated with acute and chronic inflammatory diseases of the gastrointestinal tract.

Subepithelial mast cells also have an important role in altering epithelial permeability in inflamed intestine. During the intestinal hypersensitivity response, subepithelial mast cell release of protease II by degranulation increases epithelial permeability via an effect on tight junctions (Yang et al. 2001). This alteration in tight junction permeability results in enhanced transepithelial flux of macromolecules, including proteins and bacterial products. Cytokines released by mast cells and phagocytes also regulate tight junction permeability.

REFERENCES

Akkermans LMA, Vanisselt JW. 1994. Gastric motility and emptying studies with radionuclides in research and clinical settings. Dig Dis Sci 39(Suppl 12):S95–S96.

Allinson MJ, Robinson IM, Dougherty RW, Bucklin JA. 1975. Grain overload in cattle and sheep: Changes in microbial populations in the cecum and rumen. Am J Vet Res 36:181–185.

Anvari M, Myers J, Malbert C, et al. 2000. Antral compensation after proximal gastric vagotomy. J Gastrointest Surg 4:526–530.

Argenzio RA. 1999. Comparative pathophysiology of nonglandular ulcer disease: A review of experimental studies. Equine Vet J Suppl 29:19–23.

Argenzio RA, Whipp SC. 1979. Interrelationship of sodium, chloride, bicarbonate and acetate transport by the colon of the pig. J Physiol (Lond) 295:365–381.

Azpiroz F, Malagelada JR. 1986. Vagally mediated gastric relaxation induced by intestinal nutrients in the dog. Am J Physiol 251(6 Pt 1):G727–735.

Banan A, Wang JY, McCormack SA, Johnson LR. 1996. Relationship between polyamines, actin distribution, and gastric healing in rats. Am J Physiol 271(5 Pt 1):G893–G903.

Berschneider HM. 1992. Fibroblast modulation of intestinal secretory responses. In: Stead RH, ed. Neuro-immunophysiology of the Gastrointestinal Mucosa. New York: New York Academy of Sciences, pp 140–147.

Berschneider HM, Blikslager AT, Roberts MC. 1999. Role of duodenal reflux in nonglandular gastric ulcer disease of the mature horse. Equine Vet J Suppl 29:24–29.

Blikslager AT, Roberts MC. 1997. Mechanisms of intestinal mucosal repair. J Am Vet Med Assoc 211:1437–1441.

Blikslager AT, Roberts MC, Gerard MP, Argenzio RA. 1997a. How important is intestinal reperfusion injury in horses? J Am Vet Med Assoc 211:1387–1389.

Blikslager AT, Roberts MC, Rhoads JM, Argenzio RA. 1997b. Is reperfusion injury an important cause of mucosal damage after porcine intestinal ischemia? Surgery 121:526–534.

Blikslager AT, Rhoads JM, Bristol DG, et al. 1999. Glutamine and transforming growth factor-alpha stimulate extracellular regulated kinases and enhance recovery of villous surface area in porcine ischemic-injured intestine. Surgery 125:186–194.

Bueno L, Fioramonti J, Delvaux M, Frexinos J. 1997. Mediators and pharmacology of visceral sensitivity: From basic to clinical investigations. Gastroenterology 112:1714–1743.

Cario E, Podolsky DK. 2000. Differential alteration in intestinal epithelial cell expression of toll-like receptor 3 (TLR3) and TLR4 in inflammatory bowel disease. Infect Immun 68:7010–7017.

Castro GH, Harari Y, Russell D. 1987. Mediators of anaphylaxis-induced ion transport changes in small intestine. Am J Physiol 253(4 Pt 1):G540-548

Cervero F, Laird JM. 1999. Visceral pain. Lancet 353:2145–2148.

Chang EB, Rao MC. 1994. Intestinal water and electrolyte transport: Mechanisms of physiological and adaptive responses. In: Johnson LR, ed. Physiology of the Gastrointestinal Tract, 3rd ed. New York: Raven, pp 2027–2082.

Cook DI, Young JA. 1989. Effect of K+ channels in the apical plasma membrane on epithelial secretion based on secondary active Cl− transport. J Membr Biol 110:139–146.

Crichlow EC, Leek BF. 1981. The importance of pH in relation to the acid-excitation of epithelial receptors in the reticulo-rumen of the sheep. J Physiol (Lond) 310:60P.

Cuche G, Malbert CH. 1999. Ileal short-chain fatty acids inhibit transpyloric flow in pigs. Scand J Gastroenterol 34:149–155.

Dabareiner RM, Snyder JR, White NA, et al. 1995. Microvascular permeability and endothelial cell morphology associated with low-flow ischemia/reperfusion injury in the equine jejunum. Am J Vet Res 56:639–648.

Dabareiner RM, Sullins KE, White NA, Snyder JR. 2001. Serosal injury in the equine jejunum and ascending colon after ischemia-reperfusion or intraluminal distention and decompression. Vet Surg 30:114–125.

Dallegri F, Ottonello L. 1997. Tissue injury in neutrophilic inflammation. Inflamm Res 46:382–391.

Dirksen G. 1965. [Clinical observations on adipose tissue necrosis in cattle]. Wien Tierarztl Monatsschr 52:517–525.

Elliott E, Li Z, Bell C, et al. 1994. Modulation of host response to Escherichia coli o157:H7 infection by anti-CD18 antibody in rabbits. Gastroenterology 106:1554–1561.

Flemstrom G. 1994. Gastric and duodenal mucosal secretion of bicarbonate. In: Johnson LR, ed. Physiology of the Gastrointestinal Tract, 3rd ed. New York: Raven, pp 1285–1309.

Furness JB, Kunze WA, Clerc N. 1999. Nutrient tasting and signaling mechanisms in the gut: II. The intestine as a sensory organ: Neural, endocrine, and immune responses. Am J Physiol 277(5 Pt 1):G922–G928.

Galan JE, Collmer A. 1999. Type III secretion machines: Bacterial devices for protein delivery into host cells. Science 284:1322–1328.

Galli SJ, Maurer M, Lantz CS. 1999. Mast cells as sentinels of innate immunity. Curr Opin Immunol 11:53–59.

Ganapathy V, Brandsch M, Leibach FH. 1994. Intestinal transport of amino acids and peptides. In: Johnson LR, ed. Physiology of the Gastrointestinal Tract, 3rd ed. New York: Raven, pp 1773–1794.

Gay J, Fioramonti J, GarciaVillar R, Bueno L. 2000. Development and sequels of intestinal inflammation in nematode-infected rats: Role of mast cells and capsaicin-sensitive afferents. Neuroimmunomodulation 8:171–178.

Gebhart GF. 2000a. J.J. Bonica Lecture—2000: Physiology, pathophysiology, and pharmacology of visceral pain. Reg Anesth Pain Med 25:632–638.

Gebhart GF. 2000b. Visceral pain-peripheral sensitisation. Gut 47(Suppl 4):iv54–iv55 [Discussion, iv58].

Gewirtz AT, Simon POJ, Schmitt CK, et al. 2001. Salmonella typhimurium translocates flagellin across intestinal epithelia, inducing a proinflammatory response. J Clin Invest 107:99–109.

Goldstein IM. 1992. Complement: Biologically active products. In: Gallin JI, Goldstein IM, Snyderman R, eds. Inflammation: Basic Principles and Clinical Correlates. New York: Raven, pp 63–80.

Greger R, Kunzelmann K. 1990. Epithelial chloride channels. In: Young JA, Wong PYD, eds. Epithelial Secretion of Water and Electrolytes. Berlin: Springer-Verlag, pp 3–14.

Gregory PC. 1984. Control of intrinsic reticulo-ruminal motility in the vagotomized sheep. J Physiol (Lond) 346:379–393.

Gregory PC, Rayner DV, Wenham G. 1984. Initiation of migrating myoelectric complex in sheep by duodenal acidification and hyperosmolarity: Role of vagus nerves. J Physiol (Lond) 355:509–521.

Gregory PC, Miller SJ, Brewer AC. 1985. The relation between food intake and abomasal emptying and small intestinal transit time in sheep. Br J Nutr 53:373–380.

Grondahl ML, Hansen MB, Larsen IE, Skadhauge E. 1996. Age and segmental differences in 5-hydroxytryptamine-induced hypersecretion in the pig small intestine. J Comp Physiol [B] 166:21–29.

Grundy D, Scratcherd T. 1989. Sensory afferents from the gastrointestinal tract. In: Schultz SG, Wood JD, Rauner BB, eds. Handbook of Physiology. New York: Oxford University, 1:593–620.

Grundy D, Blackshaw LA, Hillsley K. 1994. Role of 5-hydroxytryptamine in gastrointestinal chemosensitivity. Dig Dis Sci 39(Suppl 12):S44–S47.

Hirayama BA, Lostao MP, Penayotova-Heiermann M., et al. 1996. Kinetic and specificity differences between rat, human, and rabbit Na+-glucose cotransporters (SGTL-1). Am J Physiol 270:6-919-26.

Holm L, Flemstrom G, Nylander O. 1990. Duodenal alkaline secretion in rabbits: Influence of artificial ventilation. Acta Physiol Scand 138:471–478.

Holzer P. 1990. Nerves and gastric mucosal protection. Dig Dis Sci 35:1048–1051.

Holzer P. 1998. Neural emergency system in the stomach. Gastroenterology 114:823–839.

Holzer P, Wachter C, Heinemann A, et al. 1995. Sensory nerves, nitric oxide and NANC vasodilatation. Arch Int Pharmacodyn Ther 329:67–79.

Hotokezaka M, Mentis EP, Schirmer BD. 1996. Gastric myoelectric activity changes following open abdominal surgery in humans. Dig Dis Sci 41:864–869.

Husebye E. 1995. Gastrointestinal motility disorders and bacterial overgrowth. J Intern Med 237:419–427.

Ina K, Kusugami K, Yamaguchi T, et al. 1997. Mucosal interleukin-8 is involved in neutrophil migration and binding to extracellular matrix in inflammatory bowel disease. Am J Gastroenterol 92:1342–1346.

Joris I, Cuenoud HF, Doern GV, et al. 1990. Capillary leakage in inflammation: A study by vascular labelling. Am J Pathol 137:1353–1363.

Jung HC, Eckmann L, Yang SK, et al. 1995. A distinct array of proinflammatory cytokines is expressed in human colon epithelial cells in response to bacterial invasion. J Clin Invest 95:55–65.

Kagnoff MF, Eckmann L. 1997. Epithelial cells as sensors for microbial infection. J Clin Invest 100:6–10.

Kinugasa T, Sakaguchi T, Gu X, Reinecker HC. 2000. Claudins regulate the intestinal barrier in response to immune mediators. Gastroenterology 118:1001–1011.

Kirkup AJ, Brunsden AM, Grundy D. 2001. Receptors and transmission in the brain-gut axis: Potential for novel therapies: I. Receptors on visceral afferents. Am J Physiol Gastrointest 280:G787–G794.

Kontukek SJ, Robert A. 1982. Cytoprotection of canine gastric mucosa by prostacyclin: Possible mediation by increased mucosal blood flow. Digestion 25:155–163.

Kozin F, Cochrane CG. 1992. The contact activation system of plasma: Biochemistry and pathophysiology. In: Gallin JI, Goldstein IM, Snyderman R, eds. Inflammation: Basic

Principles and Clinical Correlates. New York: Raven, pp 103–122.

Kuiper R, Breukink HJ. 1986. Secondary indigestion as a cause of functional pyloric stenosis in the cow. Vet Rec 119:404–406.

Ladabaum U, Minoshima S, Hasler WL, et al. 2001. Gastric distention correlates with activation of multiple cortical and subcortical regions. Gastroenterology 120:369–376.

Lang J, Blikslager A, Regina D, et al. 1998. Synergistic effect of hydrochloric acid and bile acids on the pars esophageal mucosa of the porcine stomach. Am J Vet Res 59:1170–1176.

Leek BF, Harding R. 1975. Sensory nervous receptors in the ruminant stomach and the reflex control of reticulo-ruminal motility. In: McDonald IW, Warner ACI, eds. Digestion and Metabolism in the Ruminant. Armidale, Australia: University of New England Publishing, pp 60–76.

Madara JL, Pappenheimer JR. 1987. Structural basis for physiological regulation of paracellular pathways in intestinal epithelia. J Membr Biol 100:149–164.

Madara JL, Trier JS. 1994. The functional morphology of the mucosa of the small intestine. In: Johnson LR, ed. Physiology of the Gastrointestinal Tract, 3rd ed. New York: Raven, pp 1577–1622.

Malagelada JR, Azpiroz F. 1989. Determinants of gastric emptying and transit in the small intestine. In: Wood JD, ed. Handbook of Physiology: The Gastrointestinal System. Bethesda: American Physiology Society, 1:909–937.

Malaviya R, Abraham SN. 2001. Mast cell modulation of immune responses to bacteria. Immunol Rev 179:16–24.

Malbert CH. 1989. Le rôle du pylore dans le contrôle de l'ingestion alimentaire chez les ruminants. INRA Prod Anim 2:23–29.

Malbert CH, Horowitz M. 1997. The pig as a model for human digestive motor activity. In: Laplace JP, Fevrier C, Barbeau A, eds. Digestive Physiology in Pigs. Paris, EAAP Publ 88, pp 3–13.

Malbert CH, Ruckebusch Y. 1987. Pyloric control of the MMC in sheep. Dig Dis Sci 32:920A.

Malbert CH, Ruckebusch Y. 1989. Vagal influences on the phasic and tonic components of the motility of the ovine stomach and gastroduodenal area. Int J Dig Motility 1:15–20.

Mashimo H, Goyal RK. 1999. Lessons from genetically engineered animal models: IV. Nitric oxide synthase gene knockout mice. Am J Physiol Gastrointest 277:G745–G750.

Mayer EA. 1994. The physiology of gastric storage and emptying. In: Johnson LR, ed. Physiology of the Gastrointestinal Tract, 3rd ed. New York: Raven, pp 929–976.

McCormack SA, Viar MJ, Johnson LR. 1992. Migration of IEC-6 cells: A model for mucosal healing. Am J Physiol 263(3 Pt 1):G426–G435.

McCormack SA, Wang JY, Johnson LR. 1994. Polyamine deficiency causes reorganization of F-actin and tropomyosin in IEC-6 cells. Am J Physiol 267(3 Pt 1):C715–C722.

McCormick BA, Nusrat A, Parkos CA, et al. 1997. Unmasking of intestinal epithelial lateral membrane beta1 integrin consequent to transepithelial neutrophil migration in vitro facilitates inv-mediated invasion by Yersinia pseudotuberculosis. Infect Immun 65:1414–1421.

Mei N, Coffin B, Lemann M, et al. 1996. Gastrointestinal sensitivity: Recent data in physiology, pathology, therapeutics—General introduction. In: Delvaux M, ed. Sensibilite Digestive. Paris: Elsevier Editions Scientifiques, pp 15–16.

Merritt AM. 1999. Normal equine gastroduodenal secretion and motility. Equine Vet J Suppl 29:7–13.

Metcalfe DD, Costa JJ, Burd PR. 1992. Mast cells and basophils. In: Gallin JI, Goldstein IM, Snyderman R, eds.

Inflammation: Basic Principles and Clinical Correlates. New York: Raven, pp 709–726.

Michaelis M, Habler HJ, Janig W. 1996. Silent afferents: A separate class of primary afferents? Clin Exp Pharmacol Physiol 23:99–105.

Moore RM, Muir WW, Granger DN. 1995. Mechanisms of gastrointestinal ischemia-reperfusion injury and potential therapeutic interventions: A review and its implications in the horse. J Vet Intern Med 9:115–132.

Mutoh H, Ota S, Hiraishi H, et al. 1995. Adaptative cytoprotection in cultured rat gastric mucus-producing cells: Role of mucus and prostaglandin synthesis. Dig Dis Sci 40:872–878.

Neiger R, Simpson KW. 2000. Helicobacter infection in dogs and cats: Facts and fiction. J Vet Intern Med 14:125–133.

Nilsson UA, Schoenberg MH, Aneman A, et al. 1994. Free radicals and pathogenesis during ischemia and reperfusion of the cat small intestine. Gastroenterology 106:629–636.

Nusrat A, Parkos CA, Liang TW, et al. 1997. Neutrophil migration across model intestinal epithelia: Monolayer disruption and subsequent events in epithelial repair. Gastroenterology 113:1489–1500.

Pappenheimer JR. 1990. Paracellular intestinal absorption of glucose, creatinine, and mannitol in normal animals: Relation to body size. Am J Physiol 259(2 Pt 1):G290–G299.

Pinna C, Bolego C, Puglisi L. 1995. Effect of substance P and capsaicin on stomach fundus and ileum of streptozotocin-diabetic rats. Eur J Pharmacol 276:61–69.

Plourde V, St-Pierre S, Quirion R. 1997. Calcitonin gene-related peptide in viscerosensitive response to colorectal distension in rats. Am J Physiol 273(1 Pt 1):G191–G196.

Podolsky DK. 1999. Mucosal immunity and inflammation: V. Innate mechanisms of mucosal defense and repair—The best offense is a good defense. Am J Physiol 277(3 Pt 1):G495–G499.

Rabbani GH. 1996. Mechanism and treatment of diarrhoea due to Vibrio cholerae and Escherichia coli: Roles of drugs and prostaglandins. Dan Med Bull 43:173–185.

Ray RM, Zimmerman BJ, McCormack SA, et al. 1999. Polyamine depletion arrests cell cycle and induces inhibitors p21(Waf1/Cip1), p27(Kip1), and p53 in IEC-6 cells. Am J Physiol 276(3 Pt 1):C684–C691.

Raybould H. 1998. Does your gut taste? Sensory transduction in the gastrointestinal tract. News Physiol Sci 13:275–280.

Reevesdarby VG, Turner JA, Prasad R, et al. 1995. Effect of cloned Salmonella typhimurium enterotoxin on rabbit intestinal motility. FEMS Microbiol Lett 134:239–244.

Rosengren S, Olofsson AM, Von Andrian UH, et al. 1991. Leukotriene B4-induced neutrophil-mediated endothelial leakage in vitro and in vivo. J Appl Physiol 71:1322–1330.

Ruckebusch Y. 1989. Gastrointestinal motor functions in ruminants. In: Schultz SG, ed. The Handbook of Physiology, sect 6: The Gastrointestinal System. New York: Oxford University Press, pp 1225–1282.

Ruda MA, Ling QD, Hohmann AG, et al. 2000. Altered nociceptive neuronal circuits after neonatal peripheral inflammation. Science 289:628–631.

Schreiber S, Hampe J, Eickhoff H, Lehrach H. 2000. Functional genomics in gastroenterology. Gut 47:601–607.

Siegenbeek van Heukelum J. 1986. Physiological aspects of absorption and secretion in intestine. Vet Res Commun 10:341–354.

Simpson KW, Strauss-Ayali D, McDonough PL, et al. 1999. Gastric function in dogs with naturally acquired gastric Helicobacter spp. infection. J Vet Intern Med 13:507–515.

Springer TA. 1994. Traffic signals for lymphocyte recirculation and leukocyte emigration: The multistep paradigm. Cell 76:301–314.

Strauss-Ayali D, Simpson KW. 1999. Gastric *Helicobacter* infection in dogs. Vet Clin North Am Small Anim Pract 29:397–414, vi.

Suzuki M, Asako H, Kubes P, et al. 1991. Neutrophil-derived oxidants promote leukocyte adherence in postcapillary venules. Microvasc Res 42:125–138.

Szurszewski JH. 1998. A 100-year perspective on gastrointestinal motility. Am J Physiol Gastrointest 37:G447–G453.

Telle PP, Preston RL. 1971. Ovine lactic acidosis: Intraluminal and systemic. J Anim Sci 33:698–704.

Titchen DA, Anderson N. 1977. Aspects of the physio-pathology of parasitic gastritis in the sheep. Aust Vet J 53:369–373.

Treacy PJ, Jamieson GG, Dent J. 1994. Pyloric motility and liquid gastric emptying during barostatic control of gastric pressure in pigs. J Physiol (Lond) 474:361–366.

Wallace JL. 2001. Nonsteroidal anti-inflammatory drugs and the gastrointestinal tract: Mechanisms of protection and healing—Current knowledge and future research. Am J Med 110(1A):19S–23S.

Wallace JL, Ma L. 2001. Inflammatory mediators in gastrointestinal defense and injury. Exp Biol Med 226:1003–1015.

Wallace JL, Miller MJS. 2000. Nitric oxide in mucosal defense: A little goes a long way. Gastroenterology 119:512–520.

Wang JY, McCormack SA, Viar MJ, Johnson LR. 1991. Stimulation of proximal small intestinal mucosal growth by luminal polyamines. Am J Physiol 261(3 Pt 1):G504–G511.

Wang JY, Viar MJ, Johnson LR. 1994. Regulation of transglutaminase activity by polyamines in the gastrointestinal mucosa of rats. Proc Soc Exp Biol Med 205:20–28.

Weber E, Ehrlein HJ. 1998. Relationships between gastric emptying and intestinal absorption of nutrients and energy in mini pigs. Dig Dis Sci 43:1141–1153.

Wen J, Phillips SF, Sarr MG, et al. 1995. PYY and GLP-1 contribute to feedback inhibition from the canine ileum and colon. Am J Physiol 269(6 Pt 1):G945–G952.

Wershil BK. 2000. Mast cell-deficient mice and intestinal biology. Am J Physiol 278:G343–G348.

Wood JD, Alpers DH, Andrews PLR. 1999. Fundamentals of neurogastroenterology. Gut 45:6–16.

Woolf CJ, Salter MW. 2000. Neuronal plasticity: Increasing the gain in pain. Science 288:1765–1769.

Wright EM, Hirayama BA, Loo DDF, et al. 1994. Intestinal sugar transport. In: Johnson LR, ed. Physiology of the Gastrointestinal Tract, 3rd ed. New York: Raven, pp 1751–1772.

Wright NA. 1998. Aspects of the biology of regeneration and repair in the human gastrointestinal tract. Philos Trans R Soc Lond [Biol] 353:925–933.

Yang PC, Berin MC, Yu LCH, Perdue MH. 2001. Mucosal pathophysiology and inflammatory changes in the late phase of the intestinal allergic reaction in the rat. Am J Pathol 158:681–690.

The main function of the respiratory system is to ensure appropriate gas exchanges (i.e., oxygen uptake and carbon dioxide production) are adequate to meet the metabolic requirements. This is the conceptual framework that provides a basis for understanding why some disorders unnoticed at rest may become a problem when the metabolic requirements are high, for example, during exercise.

Most of the respiratory disorders are directly or indirectly linked to one or several stresses that challenge its function:

- Biological stresses induced by viruses, bacteria, mycoplasma, fungi, and parasites
- Immunologic stresses induced by allergic reactions
- Mechanical stresses induced by trauma, abnormal structures, cardiac dysfunctions, and heavy exercise
- Chemical and physical stresses induced by air pollution with dusts, gases, the thermal environment, abnormal partial pressures of oxygen, and carbon dioxide in ambient air

When the respiratory system is challenged by one or several of these factors, it reacts by initiating several defense mechanisms, for example, sneeze, cough, bronchospasm, hypersecretion, and infiltration of inflammatory cells. Most of the time, these mechanisms are beneficial in order to protect the lung against injuries and restore the functional homeostasis. However, when these adaptations persist for too long or become recurrent, they may become deleterious for the pulmonary function and significantly impair gas exchange.

The dysfunction responsible for inadequate gas exchange may originate from different levels:

- Alveolar ventilation, or the movement of air between the environment and the alveoli
- Alveolocapillary diffusion, or the transfer of gases across the blood-gas barrier
- Lung perfusion, or the removal of gas by the pulmonary circulation
- Ventilation-perfusion adequation, or how alveolar ventilation is matched by alveolar perfusion for adequate gas transfer

The failure of the homeostatic processes induced by any aggression of the respiratory system will result in abnormal lung function, which in this chapter are arbitrarily divided into four categories:

- Obstructive disorders, which are mainly related to airway obstruction
- Restrictive disorders, which are mainly related to restricted expansion of the lung
- Vascular disorders, which are mainly related to impaired perfusion of the lung
- Environmental disorders, which are mainly related to inappropriate quality of inhaled air

PART 1: PHYSIOPATHOLOGY OF OBSTRUCTIVE RESPIRATORY DISORDERS

TATIANA ART AND PIERRE LEKEUX

During ventilation, air flows in and out of the respiratory tree. The respiratory muscles perform work to overcome lung elasticity, to generate airflow against frictional resistance between the air molecules and the wall of the airways and, to a lesser extent, against viscous resistance of the tissues. Inertia provided by the air and the tissue may also be overcome. In normal resting conditions, however, this factor is negligible. In quiet-breathing animals, the work of breathing serves mainly to overcome the elasticity of the lungs. When respiratory frequency increases, the energy devoted to overcome frictional resistance increases. An airway obstruction will nevertheless represent the major cause of the increase in energy spent to ensure an appropriate ventilation.

The airway resistance to airflow is directly proportional to its length (l) as well as to the physical properties of the breathed air (k), and inversely proportional to the radius (r) according to the following formula:

$$R = 8 \; l/r^4$$

While k and l are constant, at least in nonexperimental conditions, r may be modified by a lot of events. Any subobstruction may have dramatic consequences on the pulmonary function, especially on the total pulmonary resistance, because, when r is halved, resistance is multiplied by 16. Moreover, some kinds of localized obstructive processes may induce turbulent flow, which contributes to a further increase of resistance.

In veterinary medicine, obstructive respiratory disorders are of major importance as causes of economic losses in production animals and of poor performance, morbidity, and mortality in horses and pet animals. It is therefore important for students to have a basic knowledge of the possible causes of obstructions, their functional consequences on breathing, and the main species characteristics.

CLASSIFICATION OF OBSTRUCTIVE PROCESSES

According to the Location of the Obstruction Related to the Airway's Wall. The factors that affect the airway's radius may be related to conditions (a) inside the airway lumen, termed *intraluminal causes*, (b) within the wall of the airway, termed *intramural causes*, and (c) in the peripheral region of the airway, termed *extraluminal causes* (Figure 5.1).

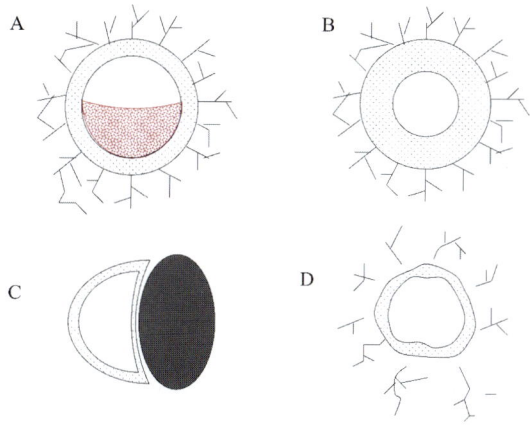

FIG. 5.1—Different types of airway obstruction: (**A**) intraluminal; (**B**) intramural; (**C**) extraluminal, related to an external compression; and (**D**) extraluminal, related to a loss of radial traction, as seen in pulmonary emphysema.

INTRALUMINAL CAUSES. The lumen may be partly obstructed by excessive secretions: this condition is frequent and generally related to excessive mucus production, or to impairment of mucus clearance when the mucociliary system is altered, or to the presence of purulent material in bacterial infection. Less frequently, obstruction may result from pulmonary edema, aspiration of fluids or foreign bodies, presence of blood in case of exercise-induced pulmonary hemorrhage, or postoperatively retained secretions.

INTRAMURAL CAUSES. Causes located within the wall of the airway include excessive contraction of small airway smooth muscle as in bronchial hyperreactivity, poor or no airway enlargement due to a lack of upper airway abductor muscle contraction as in laryngeal hemiplegia, and, lastly, thickening of the wall by muscle hypertrophy as in asthma, or by inflammation and edema as in laryngitis or bronchitis.

EXTRALUMINAL CAUSES. Any part of the respiratory tree may be subobstructed or obstructed by masses of various origins (polyps, lymph nodes hypertrophy, or neoplasia).

Lung volume has an important effect on small airway resistance. Bronchi are supported by the radial traction of the surrounding tissues, and their caliber enlarges as the lung expands. Consequently, reduction of lung volume or destruction of lung parenchyma, as seen in alveolar emphysema, may cause loss of radial traction and consequent narrowing of the airway.

Lastly, a dynamic partial collapse of some airway may occur when the surrounding pressure exceeds the pressure inside the lumen, creating a compressing transmural pressure.

According to the Location of the Obstruction Along the Respiratory Tree. Obstructions may be located at any part along the respiratory system and, according to their location, are classified either as *extrathoracic* or as *intrathoracic* obstructions. Extrathoracic obstructions include nasal, pharyngeal, laryngeal, and extrathoracic tracheal obstructions, whereas intrathoracic obstructions are related to problems at the level of the intrathoracic trachea, bronchi, and bronchioles.

The functional consequences of each are different. The first ones mainly induce increased inspiratory resistance and, when the subobstruction is serious or when the airflow is increased (during exercise or compensatory hyperventilation), they generally induce respiratory noises. The second ones induce increased expiratory airway resistance (e.g., heaves in horses) with active expiration and whistling audible at auscultation.

According to the Fact That the Obstruction Is Induced Either by Passive and/or Morphological Processes, or by Active and/or Functional Processes. Obstructive respiratory disorders may also be classified as either morphological or functional.

In the first case, the airway diameter is modified by a structural change caused by tumorous, infectious, inflammatory, repairing, collapsing, or other processes.

In the second case, the airway diameter is affected by an inappropriate function of respiratory muscles. Indeed, contraction and/or relaxation of ventilatory voluntary muscles and smooth muscles play a paramount role in the control of the cross-sectional area of the airway.

Firstly, at the level of the upper airway—that is, nostrils, pharynx, soft palate and larynx—the contraction of abductor skeletal muscles leads to airway enlarge-ment. Therefore, failure of these muscles (due to paresis, paralysis, or fatigue) will result in a rise in pulmonary resistance. This kind of dysfunction causes what is also termed *localized* obstruction.

Secondly, at the level of the lower airway, the smooth muscle in the trachea (where it connects both ends of the tracheal cartilage), the main bronchi (where it connects the cartilaginous plates), and the bronchiole (where it encircles the airway) is innervated by the autonomic nervous system and modulates the airway diameter by either contracting or relaxing. This kind of dysfunction causes a generalized airway obstruction.

FUNCTIONAL CONSEQUENCES OF OBSTRUC-TIVE PROCESSES. Conclusions about the possible origins of the lung mechanics and/or arterial blood-gas tension modifications in patients suffering from airway obstruction are often difficult. Indeed, because pathological changes usually are unevenly distributed, the measurement of overall function represents the summed characteristics of many lung compartments that have quite different mechanical properties.

Measurement of the mechanics of breathing allows one to assess general physical characteristics of the respiratory system such as the total pulmonary resistance, that is, the airway's permeability to airflow and the dynamic lung compliance, that is, an estimate of the lung elasticity and ventilatory asynchronism. The classic reference method of measurement is described in Figure 5.2.

Pulmonary scintigraphy may be useful to assess regional differences of the air distribution in the lung and consequently to point out some inhomogeneity in the resistance of the small airways (Figure 5.3) (Votion 1999).

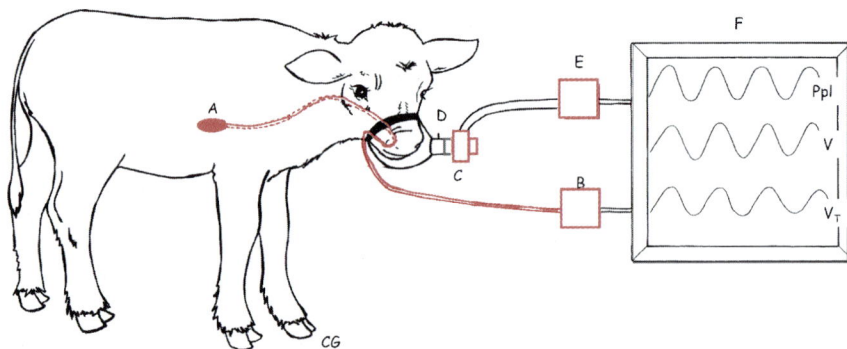

FIG. 5.2—Measurement of the mechanics of breathing in a calf. The pleural pressure changes (Ppl) are measured by means of an esophageal balloon catheter (A) positioned in the thoracic esophagus and connected to an external pressure transducer (B). The respiratory airflow (V) is measured by use of a pneumotachograph (C) placed in front of the nostril by means of a face mask (D) and connected to a differential pressure transducer (E). The tidal volume (V_T) is obtained by the integration of V. The respiratory signals are recorded by a computerized system and the respiratory parameters are calculated on-line and on a breath-by-breath basis.

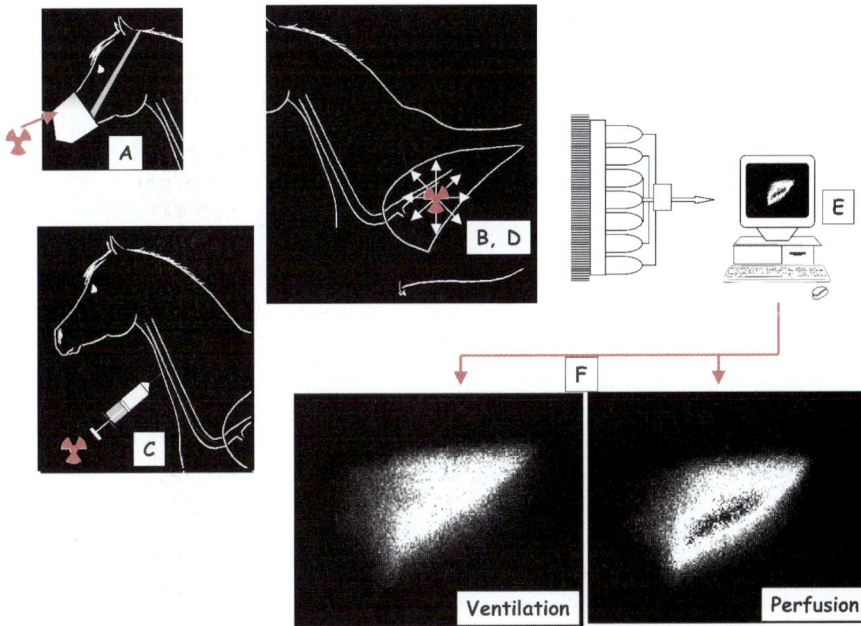

FIG. 5.3—The ventilation (V):perfusion (F) ratio evaluated by the use of scintigraphy. First, a radioactive aerosol is inhaled (**A**) and the functional image of the distribution of ventilation is recorded using a gamma-camera (**B**). Second, radioactivity is administered intravenously (**C**), and the image of the distribution of the lung perfusion is also recorded (**D**). Finally, a computerized program giving among multiple data the V/Q ratio (E) is used to analyze the ventilation and perfusion images (F).

Respiratory endoscopy enables morphological and sometimes functional examination of the airways and may help to assess some mechanisms of subobstruction, namely, at the level of the extrathoracic airways (Venker-van Haagen 1979).

Mechanics of Breathing

CHANGES IN TOTAL PULMONARY RESISTANCE AND DYNAMIC LUNG COMPLIANCE. Airways greater than 2 mm represent approximately 80% of the total pulmonary resistance (50% being due to the nasal passage), whereas small airway (2 mm and less) resistance contributes to the remaining 20%. This low contribution is explained by the fact that the summed cross-sectional area dramatically increases from the fourth generation bronchi up to the alveoli in regard to the total cross section of the upper airway.

As a consequence, during nasal breathing, upper airway resistance represents the major part of the total pulmonary resistance in most of the species. Therefore, an increase in the upper airway resistance will induce a greater increase in the total pulmonary resistance than will any increase in the lower airway resistance (Art et al. 1988). As already mentioned, a serious increase in upper airway resistance may lead to respiratory noises, especially when the airflow is high (i.e., during hyperpnea and during exercise), but more often it is clinically asymptomatic in quiet breathing and resting animals.

Whereas an upper airway obstruction mainly results in an increase in total pulmonary resistance, lower airway obstruction induces a proportionally weaker increase in total pulmonary resistance but will also induce a decrease in dynamic lung compliance. The reason why small airway subobstruction may have consequences on the lung compliance is explained by ventilatory asynchronism rather than by genuine changes in the lung elastic properties. Indeed, abnormally high resistance at the level of some intrathoracic airways induces inequalities in the regional ventilation; that is, inhaled air preferentially enters those areas of the lungs that have low-resistive airways. Consequently, for a given change in pleural pressure, the corresponding air volume entering the lungs will be reduced, and the value of the dynamic compliance will be lowered (Figure 5.4).

The functional significance of the ventilatory asynchronism is different according to the species considered. Indeed, two anatomic features may partially compensate for the subobstruction of the small airways: the interdependence between adjacent lung regions and the collateral ventilation. The interdependence tends to limit the nonuniform changes in regional ventilation. This mechanical interaction is the result of the intricate mesh of interconnecting elastic and collagenous tissue fibers in the lung (Mead et al. 1970). It has different importance according to the species: the interdependence seems to be consid-

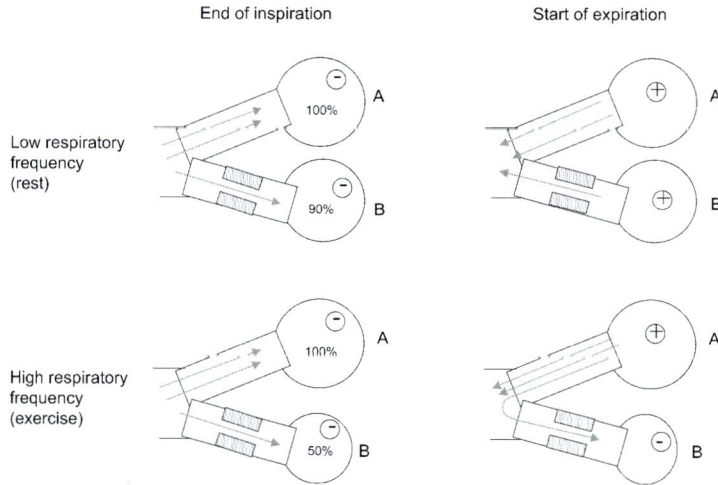

FIG. 5.4—The effect of ventilatory asynchronism on alveolar ventilation. The resistance of the bronchi serving the alveoli B is higher than normal; consequently, emptying of alveoli B is delayed with regard to the normal alveoli. Moreover, at high respiratory frequency (as in exercise or disease), alveoli B may "inhale" polluted air coming from alveoli A, impairing the gas exchange.

erable in dogs, weak in cattle, pigs, and goats, and intermediate in horses.

Collateral ventilation between adjacent lung areas—that is, transfer of air between adjacent lobules through collateral pathways—is also potentially able to reduce the nonuniformity of the ventilation distribution (Robinson and Sorenson 1978). The importance of collateral ventilation largely varies between species (Robinson 1982). Calf and pig lungs have no collateral pathways across interlobular septa. In contrast, collateral ventilation in dogs and cats is high. Lastly, horses have relatively low collateral ventilation, which is probably of limited usefulness at low respiratory frequencies and of no usefulness at all at high respiratory frequencies.

In exercise and disease, the increase in the resistance

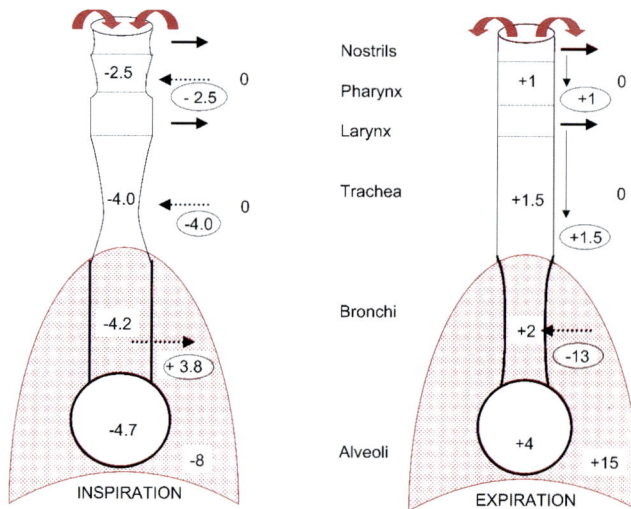

FIG. 5.5—Mechanism of occurrence of dynamic partial collapse in the respiratory tree. The data circled in red is the transmural pressure (TMP), that is, the pressure difference between the intraluminal and extraluminal pressures. When TMP is positive, the airway is passively dilated; when it is negative, the airway is passively compressed (what is called dynamic collapse). The phenomenon is negligible in sound airways at low respiratory frequency but is exacerbated by local airway obstruction, increase in respiratory frequency, or both factors.

to airflow in the airways may be exacerbated by the dynamic partial collapse that is observed once the pressure surrounding the airways exceeds the pressure within the lumen (Figure 5.5). This phenomenon is important in the airways because, except for the nasal cavities, they do not have bony support and therefore are especially subjected to this dynamic collapse. During inhalation, this occurs upstream from the obstruction in the extrathoracic airways. In this case, the pressure in the extrathoracic airways is strongly subatmospheric while the pressure in the surrounding tissues remains atmospheric. In the opposite case, during exhalation, dynamic partial collapse may occur in the intrathoracic airway downstream from the obstruction. In this case, because of the expiratory effort, the intrathoracic pressure becomes dramatically higher than the pressure prevailing inside some of the intrathoracic airways, and the section of the airway is narrowed. In both cases, this dynamic collapse further increases the airway resistance, creating a vicious circle.

WORK OF BREATHING AND BREATHING STRATEGY. Obstruction of the airways dramatically increases the mechanical work of breathing (Figure 5.6). To ensure (or try to ensure) appropriate ventilation, the sequence and intensity of respiratory muscle activation are modified. In animals suffering from lower airway obstruction, the expiration becomes active, with an important recruitment of the abdominal muscles. Abnormally high energy will be spent to maintain the ventilation. Therefore, such a phenomenon may lead to poor-performance syndrome in athletic animals, to reduction of the daily body gain or even weight loss in production animals, and to respiratory muscle fatigue or even failure in diseased animals.

Patients with lower airway obstruction often breathe at high lung volume and low respiratory frequency. This helps to reduce their airways' resistance by increasing radial traction exercised on them.

Gas Exchange. Gas-exchange impairment is less frequent in upper airway obstruction than in lower airway obstruction, except during exercise (e.g., idiopathic laryngeal hemiplegia in horses and dogs) or when the obstruction is severe (e.g., laryngitis in calves).

Patients with significant ventilatory asynchronism (i.e., due to small airway disease) associated or not with a high respiratory frequency (i.e., during exercise or compensatory hyperpnea) may frequently experience gas-exchange impairment (Figure 5.4). Under these conditions, the lobules that have a long time constant for filling do not fill adequately (during inspiration) before expiration begins. Consequently, regional ventilation-perfusion mismatching as well as a decrease in arterial partial pressure in oxygen (i.e., hypoxemia) and, in more severe cases, an increase in arterial partial pressure in carbon dioxide (i.e., hypercapnia) result. This impairment may be assessed by arterial blood-gas analysis.

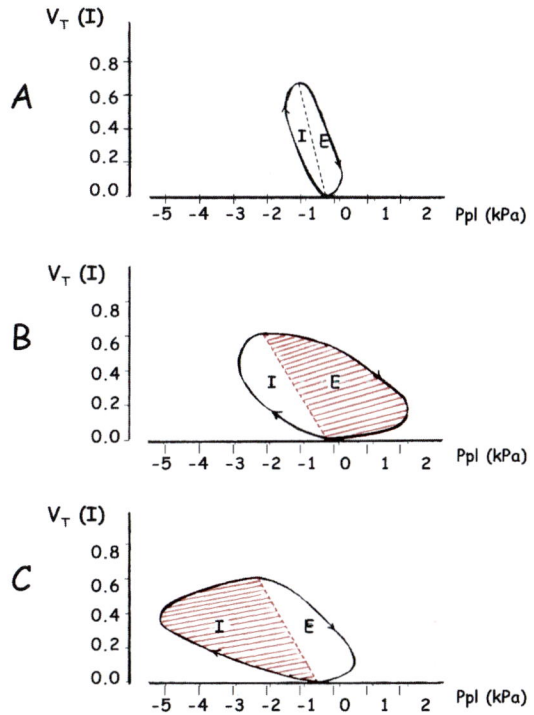

FIG. 5.6—Pressure-volume loop recorded during tidal breathing by the method described in Figure 5.2. The *dashed line* represents the lung dynamic compliance (Cdyn), the inspiratory (I) and expiratory (E) surfaces, and the work of breathing done during inspiration and expiration, respectively. These loops were recorded (**A**) in physiological conditions, (**B**) during severe intrathoracic airway obstructive disease, and (**C**) during severe extrathoracic airway obstruction. Note the increase in the expiratory and inspiratory work in conditions B and C, respectively. Ppl, pleural pressure changes; and V_T, tidal volume.

Other Changes. Obstruction of the lower airways may result in uneven ventilation distribution and ventilation-perfusion mismatching. Hypoxic vasoconstriction and vascular pulmonary hypertension may consequently occur.

Although the interdependence between adjacent lung areas may be favorable to compensate for the inhomogeneity of airway resistance in the lower airways, when the obstruction is too severe, the lobules with increased airflow resistance are abnormally stretched and compressed by the surrounding lung parts. This may induce deleterious stresses on the tissues of these lobules, eventually leading to emphysema or pulmonary hemorrhage.

In cows and pigs, where the interdependence between lobules is limited and the collateral ventilation is lacking, a definitive collapse of the alveoli, termed *atelectasis*, may occur when the air is totally absorbed out of a region distributed by a totally obstructed bronchi.

SPECIES PECULIARITIES. The variation in anatomic structures encountered between domestic species implies variation in their pulmonary function. This also influences the susceptibility to different respiratory problems, as well as the pathogenesis and the sequels of respiratory diseases. For example, a nasal obstruction may be life-threatening in a horse that is a compulsory nasal breather, but not in a dog that may breath through the mouth. Obstruction of the small airways has less functional impact in dogs, which have high collateral ventilation and lobar interdependence, than in cattle, which do not have these morphological specificities.

Some Frequent Obstructive Disorders in Horses. Respiratory disorders are frequent in equine practice. Whereas overt respiratory diseases are obvious and seldom cause a diagnostic challenge, most respiratory disorders in this species are subtle and insidious. They are liable to impair gas exchange during exercise and therefore limit a horse's performance primarily by increasing airway resistance to airflow and ventilatory asynchronism.

NASAL DISORDERS. During inspiration, pressure within the nostrils is subatmospheric, which, because they are poorly supported, tend to collapse. This dynamic collapse is prevented by the nasal muscles. In some horses with abnormal alar flaccidity, the use of nasal strips has been shown to be beneficial during exercise.

In case of damage to the motor pathways of the facial nerve, which is a common problem in horses, one of the nostrils may be paralyzed and the collapse is no longer prevented on this side. During exercise, the nasal resistance increases and, because the horse is limited to nasal breathing, and partial obstruction at this level will consequently result in exercise intolerance.

PHARYNGEAL DISORDERS. Pharyngeal lymphoid hyperplasia, which is very frequent in young horses, appears to result from the immaturity and hyperreactivity of the submucosal lymphoid tissue present throughout the pharynx. It has little effect on upper airway

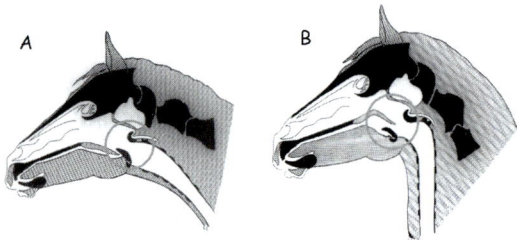

FIG. 5.7—Sagittal view of the pharynx/larynx region in physiological conditions (**A**) and showing how a dorsal displacement of the soft palate may obstruct the upper part of the trachea during inspiration (**B**).

function and does not impair gas exchange during exercise unless the hypertrophy is severe. In this case, pharyngitis may induce abnormal inspiratory noises during exercise, probably due to the reduction of the pharyngeal lumen by combination of the hypertrophied follicles and the dynamic collapse of the pharyngeal walls during inspiration.

Intermittent dorsal displacement of the soft palate— that is, a displacement of the caudal free border of the soft palate to a position above the epiglottis—is observed in sport horses in which it may induce narrowing of the nasopharyngeal airway with air turbulence during expiration and abnormal respiratory noises (gurgling), mouth breathing, and sometimes asphyxia and "choking down" at high speed (Figure 5.7) (Holcombe et al. 1997).

Diseases of the guttural pouches are rare but may potentially induce severe secondary problems. Indeed, several nerves pass along the guttural pouches: the motor nerves of the pharynx, the larynx, and other structures in the regions. Therefore, unilateral or bilateral infectious disorders—that is, empyema and mycosis—can cause obstructive disorders resulting from soft palate, pharyngeal, or laryngeal paresis.

LARYNGEAL DISORDERS. Left idiopathic laryngeal hemiplegia is common in horses. The primary lesion associated with this condition is damage to the left recurrent laryngeal nerve, resulting in the paresis or paralysis of the dorsal cricoarytenoid muscle. The horse cannot fully dilate the larynx on the affected side, and there is partial obstruction to airflow, inducing an increase in laryngeal resistance mainly during inspiration (Derksen et al. 1986). Most horses with laryngeal hemiplegia suffer exercise intolerance and abnormal inspiratory noise during exercise. The roaring is caused by turbulent airflow and sucking of the vocal cord into the lumen of the rima glottidis. In galloping horses, laryngeal hemiplegia has been shown to produce a severe hypercapnic hypoxemia.

Laryngeal hemiplegia is not a all-or-none disorder: endoscopic examination enables the examiner to determine that various stages of arytenoid cartilage movement exist, from normal function to paresis and paralysis (Tetens et al. 1996) (Figure 5.8).

Epiglottic entrapment is the envelopment of the apex and lateral margins of the epiglottis by the ventral epiglottic mucosa and aryepiglottic folds. This condition is sometimes found incidentally in horses with no history of respiratory problems, whereas severe respiratory distress is present in other cases. In these cases, endoscopy shows a significant reduction of pharyngeal diameter due to billowing of the entrapped fold during expiration, especially during exercise.

ACUTE AIRWAY DISORDERS. The etiology of acute airway disorders in horses is generally viral (mainly influenza and rhinopneumonia) but may also be bacterial (*Streptococcus equi*). The functional disorders are related to bronchoconstriction, mucosal edema, epithe-

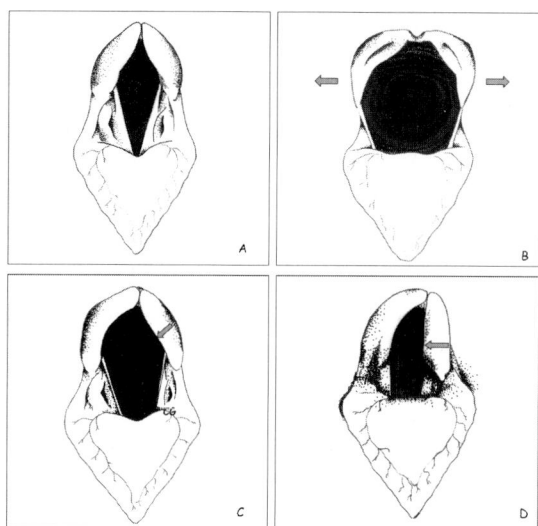

FIG. 5.8—Cranial view of the horse larynx at rest (**A**), in full abduction during exercise (**B**), suffering from a grade II/IV hemiparesis (asynchronism) (**C**), and suffering from grade IV/IV hemiplegia (complete paralysis) (**D**) of the left arytenoid cartilage. The last two conditions induce a partial subobstruction of the upper airways with a consequent increase in their resistance to airflow. They may result in occurrence of respiratory noises (roaring) and/or exercise intolerance.

lial necrosis, hypersecretion, and impaired mucociliar clearance caused by damage to the mucus and brush cells (Willoughby et al. 1992). These functional modifications are primarily moderate, but, when a horse's management is inadequate, they may predispose the horse to more deleterious effects caused by secondary bacterial infections.

HEAVES. This condition is the most common respiratory disease affecting mature horses. This syndrome is characterized by an airway hyperreactivity to inhaled allergens. Diet, previous airway infections, poor environmental conditions, and genetic predisposition probably are favoring or exacerbating factors (McGorum et al. 1998; Robinson 2001).

It is characterized by a chronic airway inflammation leading to an inhomogeneously distributed lower airway obstruction. Obstruction is caused by airway smooth muscle contraction, and the autonomic nervous system seems to play a major role in the pathophysiology of the disease. The decrease in the airway lumen may also partly be due to chronic bronchiolitis with hyperplastic epithelium. The alveoli subserved by completely or partially obstructed bronchioles are overinflated (alveolar emphysema). However, bullous interstitial emphysema created by rupture of the alveolar walls is rare in horses with heaves. Airway obstruction is also the result of plugging of airways with mucus, cellular debris, exudate, and purulent material from bacterial secondary infections. The accumulation of

this material is related to the mucociliary transport rate being significantly impaired: modification of the rheological properties of the bronchial secretions and loss of cilia due to epithelial lesions decrease the rate of transport of sputum.

Horses suffering from this lower airway disorder may be either in clinical remission (i.e., with no clinical signs) or in acute crisis. In the case of acute crisis, they have an increased airway resistance and a decreased dynamic lung compliance. The exacerbated regional differences in small airway resistance and lung compliance result in an uneven distribution of ventilation. The resulting inequalities in ventilation/perfusion ratio may in turn induce hypoxemia and sometimes hypercapnia. This phenomenon may sometimes induce an increase in pulmonary vascular resistance. Right ventricular hypertrophy and heart failure are, however, rarely reported.

The increase in total pulmonary resistance and the impaired gas exchange decrease the exercise tolerance of affected horses.

Some Frequent Obstructive Disorders in Dogs and Cats

NASAL DISORDERS. Obstructive nasal disorders are common in dogs and cats (Clercx et al. 1989a). Intranasal causes include nasal tumors, polyps, hypertrophic or inflammatory rhinitis, and ·foreign bodies. In dogs, most of the intranasal masses are malignant tumors, whereas, in cats, inflammatory nasopharyngeal polyps originating within the eustachian tube are more common. Extranasal causes include stenotic nares, which are anatomic abnormalities that are more specific to brachycephalic breeds of dogs and Persian cats, nasopharyngeal stenosis, cleft palate, soft-palate hypoplasia, oronasal fistula following dental disorder, or the presence of a foreign body behind the soft palate.

NASOPHARYNGEAL DISORDERS. The brachycephalic airway obstruction syndrome is a complex condition that results from varying degrees of upper airway obstruction. The signs consist of respiratory distress, stridor, reduced exercise tolerance and, in more severe cases, cyanosis and collapse. The inherent anatomy of the brachycephalic skull contributes to the development of these signs. Such anatomic features include a shortened and distorted nasopharynx, an overlong soft palate, bilateral stenosis and inspiratory collapse of the external nares, and everted laryngeal saccules. The increased negative pressure created in the pharyngolaryngeal region, as a result of these obstructing structures, ultimately results in distortion and collapse of the arytenoid cartilages of the larynx.

The obstructive dyspnea of the brachycephalic patients can be further complicated by severe restriction of the cranial laryngeal airway, which is caused by the displacement of the glossoepiglottic mucosal fold, the eversion of the mucosa lining the lateral ventricles, a subsequent inward and downward rotational distortion of parts of the arytenoid cartilages, and a dorsal scrolling of the epiglottis.

LARYNGEAL DISORDERS. Laryngeal disease is characterized by coughing, altered phonation, and varying degrees of obstructive dyspnea. Inspiratory stridor (or, in severe cases, both inspiratory and expiratory stridors) and exercise intolerance are additional features of obstructive dyspnea of laryngeal origin. This condition can lead to cyanosis and asphyxiation (Venker-van Haagen 1992).

Disorder conditions of the larynx include trauma, presence of foreign bodies, infection, laryngeal spasm, paralysis or collapse, and neoplasia. Congenital unilateral and bilateral paralysis has been reported in the Bouvier des Flandres and the Siberian husky breeds (Amis et al. 1986). Bilateral paralysis is most commonly encountered in elderly dogs of the larger breeds, as the result of neurogenic atrophy of the laryngeal musculature.

TRACHEAL DISORDERS. Obstructive pathologies of the canine trachea include essentially tracheal collapse, congenital hypoplasia, segmental stenosis, inflammatory diseases, tumors, and extraluminal compression (mediastinal or intrathoracic masses).

Tracheal collapse is an acquired disorder recognized in middle-aged to old dogs of toy and miniature breeds (Jerram and Fossum 1997). This syndrome is characterized by a chronic "goose honk" cough, associated with paroxysmal features of varying degrees of respiratory distress. During the phase of maximal inspiration, collapse of the cervical tracheal segment and dilation of the thoracic segment are imaged. Conversely, the study made during expiration usually shows a collapse of the thoracic segment, which is more frequently encountered.

Hypoplastic trachea is a congenital disorder recognized primarily in young brachycephalic dogs. The condition varies from mild to severe, the severity determining the prognosis for long-term survival of the patient. The condition is associated with chronic respiratory distress and coughing, intermittent acute bronchopneumonia, and recurrent episodes of upper respiratory tract infection.

LOWER AIRWAY DISORDERS. Patients with bronchial disease are commonly presented with coughing as the major complaint (Venker-van Haagen 1979). Other signs of pulmonary disease, such as exercise intolerance, increased respiratory effort, cyanosis, and systemic signs, can occur as well but are relatively uncommon unless pulmonary parenchyma is also involved (Clercx et al. 1989b). Pneumonia can occur secondary to diseased airways and decreased clearance mechanisms.

In feline allergic syndrome (feline asthma), symptoms result from bronchoconstriction, bronchial smooth muscle hypertrophy, inflammatory cell infiltration, increased mucus production, and decreased mucus clearance (Moise and Spaulding 1981).

Allergic bronchitis in dogs is not a well-defined clinical entity, because dogs suffering from this condition frequently have coexisting problems, such as chronic bronchitis, bacterial infection, or tracheal collapse. However, the dog has been used as an experimental model for allergic bronchitis with hypersensitivity responses created with ragweed and ascarid antigens.

Some Frequent Obstructive Disorders in Cattle. Obstructive syndromes in cattle are often associated to vascular and/or restrictive disorders.

STRIDULOUS LARYNGITIS. This is a severe obstructive laryngeal disorder observed during infectious rhinotracheitis or calf diphtheria. This syndrome is more frequent and more severe in double-muscled cattle, probably because of their morphological narrow rima glottidis and the higher airflow resistance of their larynx (Lekeux and Art 1987).

When compared with reference values for healthy cattle, infected animals show highly significant increases in total pulmonary resistance, in mechanical work of breathing, and in alveolar-arterial oxygen gradient, as well as highly significant decreases in dynamic compliance and arterial oxygen tension. The decrease in dynamic lung compliance in these animals suggests the presence of a concomitant ventilatory asynchronism caused by secondary lower airway disease, which is consistent with the postmortem findings, which show that bronchopneumonia frequently complicates the necrotic laryngitis.

The ratio of inspiratory to expiratory work of breathing is also significantly increased, probably because of a partial collapse of the extrathoracic part of the trachea during inspiration.

This clinical syndrome induces such important changes in pulmonary function that it disturbs the growing processes by increasing the energetic cost of breathing and by impairing normal feeding. This predisposes sick animals to secondary bronchopulmonary infections and to respiratory failure resulting from progressive respiratory muscle fatigue.

SHIPPING FEVER. Shipping fever is a respiratory syndrome caused by complex interactions between stress factors, environmental conditions, and several pathogens in which *Mannheimia* (*Pasteurella*) *hemolytica* plays an important role. Pulmonary function values recorded during the initial stage of this syndrome in feedlot cattle are consistent with an acute obstructive disease located mainly at the level of upper airways. The main dysfunctions are an increase in respiratory rate, total pulmonary resistance, work of breathing, and alveoloarterial oxygen gradient, and a decrease in tidal volume and arterial oxygen tension.

VERMINOUS BRONCHITIS. Lungworm infection with *Dictyocaulus viviparus* induces a reversible obstructive disease. When compared with normal animals, infected cattle present a significant increase in respiratory frequency, minute ventilation, total pulmonary resistance, and mechanical work of breathing, and a significant decrease in tidal volume, dynamic lung compliance, and arterial oxygen tension (Lekeux et al. 1985a). The hypoxemia during this obstructive disease is probably mainly due to an increase in ventilation-perfusion inequalities resulting from uneven distribution of ventilation.

Absolute intrapleural pressures are also more negative than in physiological conditions, suggesting an overdistension of the lung and/or the presence of trapped gas in this organ.

Clinical, functional, and pathological findings are all consistent with the picture of a lower airway obstructive disease.

ACUTE BOVINE RESPIRATORY SYNCYTIAL VIRUS INFECTION. This syndrome may vary from a moderate respiratory disorder to a severe respiratory distress syndrome, depending on the age, sensitivity, and immunologic status of the patient (Backer et al. 1997).

In the acute and early stages of the disease, this syndrome induces mainly a severe obstructive disease located at both large and small airways, as assessed by the large increase in respiratory frequency, an increase in maximal intrapleural changes, an increase in total pulmonary resistance, and an increase in alveoloarterial oxygen gradient, and the large decrease in tidal volume, dynamic compliance, and arterial oxygen tension (Lekeux et al. 1985c). These dysfunctions are partly reversed by inhalation of vagolytic and β-adrenergic drugs, suggesting the occurrence of diffuse bronchoconstriction.

Some Examples in Pigs

RHINITIS. Rhinitis, a common respiratory disorder in pigs, may be manifested as atrophic rhinitis, inclusion-body rhinitis, or necrotic rhinitis. Due to inflammatory processes and to local injuries during these disorders, the passage of air through the nasal cavities may be disturbed in some patients. The resulting increase in total pulmonary resistance and work of breathing could partly explain the negative effects of these syndromes on production parameters.

EXUDATIVE BRONCHOPNEUMONIA. Lower airway obstruction may also occur in pigs as a result of several bacterial, mycoplasmal, viral, and occupational diseases (more details are presented later in this chapter). The resulting peribronchiolar cuffing, airway mucosal edema, airway hypersecretion, and impaired mucociliary clearance increase the work of breathing and the ventilatory asynchronism because the porcine lung has no collateral ventilation. As a consequence, the physiological gas exchanges and production performances are impaired.

PART 2: FUNCTIONAL EFFECTS OF RESTRICTIVE PULMONARY DISEASES

TATIANA ART AND PIERRE LEKEUX

Restrictive pulmonary diseases are characterized by a limitation of the expansion of the lung because of alterations in the lung parenchyma itself or because of impairment in the pleural, chest wall, or respiratory muscle functions. The main functional consequences of restrictive lung diseases are a decrease in dynamic lung compliance and a reduction in lung volume—that is, vital capacity, residual volume, and total lung capacity. Nevertheless, abnormal gas transfer and extensive morphological changes detected in lung biopsies may occur with normal lung volumes. The respiratory airflow is generally well preserved, except when a patient suffers from a pulmonary disease with a combination of both restrictive and obstructive patterns.

Three classes of defects lead to a restrictive pattern: (a) alteration in lung parenchyma, (b) intraparenchymal changes, and (c) extraparenchymal changes (Figure 5.9).

PARENCHYMAL CHANGES. These troubles are rarely observed in animals but rather common in human medicine. They are generally characterized by cellular infiltrations and progressive pulmonary fibrosis. These alterations in lung tissue may be caused by conditions such as idiopathic pulmonary fibrosis or diffuse carcinomatosis. In other cases, pulmonary fibrosis may be secondary to severe infectious pulmonary diseases with the fibrosis being localized to the pulmonary lobes that have been affected by the acute disorders (Crystal et al. 1991; Hawkins 1998).

Physiopathology of Interstitial (Parenchymal) Lung Disorders. In human medicine, at least 130 different syndromes of interstitial lung disease, classified according to their physiopathological characteristics, have been described. Their etiology is unknown, although in some cases an inappropriate immunologic reaction is suspected. These fibrotic lung disorders include disorders of the lower respiratory tract characterized by injury to the lung parenchyma and by replacement of the normal architecture by mesenchymal cells and connective tissue matrix secreted by these cells. The name *interstitial* lung disorders reflects the concept that the fibrosis is confined to the interstitium of the alveolar walls. However, it has been demonstrated that most of the fibrotic disorders may also be alveolar. In this case, they are injuries of the epithelial surface often associated with (a) the interstitial contents moving through rents into the epithelial basement membrane and (b) mesenchymal cells and their products accumulating in spaces normally occupied by air (Hawkins 1998). The fundamental process underlying these modifications is relatively simple. The fibrotic lung disorders are chronic

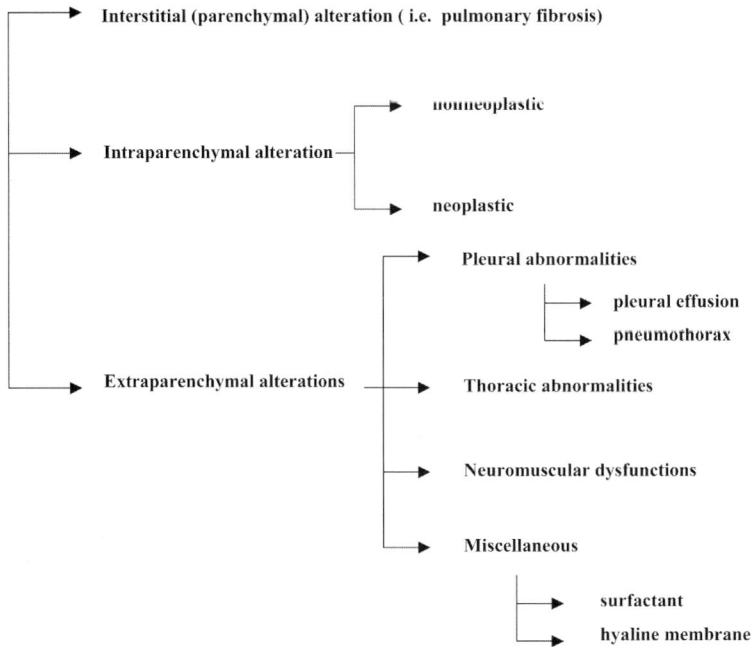

FIG. 5.9—Summary of the possible causes of restrictive pulmonary disease.

inflammatory disorders in which the inflammatory processes in the lower respiratory tract damage the lung and modulate the proliferation of mesenchymal cells that form the basis of the fibrotic scar. The pulmonary fibrosis is therefore similar to a normal wound-healing process, but whereas wound healing is normally localized in space and confined in time, the fibrotic lung disorders generally involve the entire organ and are chronic ongoing processes. Several mediators such as peptides and cytokines are involved in this condition (Crystal et al. 1991). Because it is inflammation that drives the mechanism of fibrosis, the differences between the various fibrotic disorders are explained by the differences between the types of inflammation. For instance, the inflammation of some interstitial lung disorders is dominated by alveolar macrophages, whereas in others the major components of inflammation are neutrophils, lymphocytes, and/or eosinophils.

Functional Effects of Interstitial (Parenchymal) Lung Disorders. The functional effects of these disorders depend on the stage of the condition. The pulmonary function may be normal despite the presence of histological lesions. As the condition worsens, the respiratory function is impaired. The main features are (a) an increased radial traction on the airway due to increased lung recoil, which promotes the airflow; and (b) an increase in thickness of the alveolar-capillary membrane, inducing a reduction in the diffusing capacity. The modifications generally observed include a decrease in the

total lung and vital capacity, a fall in dynamic and static lung compliance, an increase in maximal expiratory flow, a decrease in diffusing capacity, a widening in the alveolar-arterial differences for partial pressure in oxygen and carbon dioxide, an increased dead space volume/tidal volume ratio, and a ventilation/perfusion ratio inequality.

Pulmonary arterial hypertension has been also observed in patients suffering from diffuse interstitial fibrosis. The respiratory frequency is increased and the tidal volume and inspiratory time are decreased, whereas the expired minute volume and the ratio of inspiratory time to total breathing time remain unchanged (Lekeux et al. 1985c).

In large animals, the functional effects of the interstitial disorders are the same as those described in humans—that is, decreased arterial partial pressure in oxygen, decreased dynamic compliance, unchanged pulmonary resistance, and tachypnea (Derksen et al. 1982; Breeze 1985).

Interstitial (Parenchymal) Lung Diseases in Animals. These conditions are rarely described in large animals. One case of chronic restrictive pulmonary disease has been described in the equine species (Derksen et al. 1982.

Two types of chronic interstitial pneumonia of uncertain etiology have been identified in cattle: fibrosing alveolitis and bronchiolitis obliterans (Breeze 1985). The fibrosing alveolitis is characterized by diffuse inflammation of the lung tissue beyond the terminal bronchiole. Approximately 50% of cases are positive for precipitating antibodies to *Micropolyspora feani*, and these cases might represent chronic farmer's lung, whereas the others may be chronic stages of hypersensitivity to unidentified antigens. The etiology of the bronchiolitis obliterans is unknown and could be a sequel of viral infection or hypersensitive pneumonitis (Breeze 1985). It has been shown that respiratory syncytial virus pneumonia induces both restrictive and obstructive problems during the acute stage of the process (Table 5.1), and then is responsible for the occurrence of a subclinical restrictive disease during the chronic stage (Lekeux et al. 1985c).

Granulomatous pulmonary diseases described in dogs include eosinophilic granulomatosis, lymphomatoid granulomatosis, and granulomatosis associated with systemic lupus erythematosus.

INTRAPARENCHYMAL CHANGES. Intra-alveolar accumulation of fluid (as in edema) or cells (as in mycoplasma infection) and lack or immaturity of the surfactant also induce restrictive pulmonary problems.

Intraparenchymal disorders are frequently encountered in dogs and cats and include nonneoplastic and neoplastic disorders. Affected animals frequently present signs of coughing, dyspnea, or exercise intolerance. Thoracic radiographs are used to localize and characterize the disease process, certain patterns being suggestive of particular diseases. Cytological or histological evaluation is often required to obtain a definitive diagnosis; bronchoscopic collections, lung aspirates, or lung biopsies may be necessary. Less invasive tests, such as antibody titers for infectious diseases or fecal examinations for parasites, may be helpful in confirming a specific diagnosis.

Nonneoplastic Diseases. These disorders include viral, bacterial, protozoal, fungal, and parasitic diseases and lead to intraparenchymal accumulation of fluid and/or cells. The biological agents responsible for pulmonary diseases are numerous and generally specific according to the species.

With uncomplicated viral pneumonia, there is a loss of airway epithelial cells and influx of neutrophils into the airways, infiltration of peribronchial mononuclear cells, thickening and hyperhemia of alveolar septa, exudate with an increase in lymphocytes and neutrophils and fluid in alveoli, interstitial infiltrations with white blood cells, and capillary thrombosis.

In dogs, canine distemper virus infects epithelial tissue throughout the body. This viral infection is characterized by an interstitial pattern on thoracic radiographs and a lymphopenia. However, the secondary bacterial pneumonia commonly dominates the clinical image. In cats, calicivirus infection can result in an interstitial pneumonia. In horses, the most important viruses that cause equine respiratory diseases are equine influenza A2 and equine herpesvirus type 4 (or rhinopneumonitis). In all species, secondary bacterial infections are common sequels to viral infections.

Maedi, a chronic (several years' duration) progressive pneumonia that is described in sheep, is characterized by the gradual development of an interstitial pneumonia, without any evidence of a tissue-healing process. The pathogenesis of this problem is not well understood, but it seems that an unconventional immune response occurs and that the virus survives despite the production of antibodies. Gross abnormalities are localized in the lungs, where the bulk of the alveolar space is replaced by thickened alveolar walls. Generally, the lung is two to four times heavier than a normal lung (Figure 5.10). It is not known whether the lesions are due to the virus itself or due to the inappropriate antigen-antibody response (Pépin et al. 1998).

Bacterial pneumonia is a common cause of respiratory disease in dogs but is unusual in cats. Primary bacterial infection can occur as the result of *Bordetella*

TABLE 5.1—Respiratory function values from four Friesian calves suffering from bovine respiratory syncytial virus infection (RSV) and comparison with the values in healthy animals

Variables	RSV	Healthy
Arterial O_2 partial pressure (mm Hg)	59.3 + 6.0	101
Arterial CO_2 partial pressure (mm Hg)	45.8 + 3.0	43
Respiratory rate (min^{-1})	77 + 3	30.0
Tidal volume (L)	0.72 + 0.06	1.3
Maximal esophageal pressure (kPa)	−0.30 + 0.23	−0.57
Minimal esophageal pressure (kPa)	−1.55 + 0.16	−1.28
Maximal esophageal pressure changes (kPa)	1.24 + 0.15	0.71
Dynamic compliance (L/kPa)	0.84 + 0.1	3.5
Total pulmonary resistance (kPa/L/s)	0.21 + 0.03	0.14

The following points must be highlighted: The calves suffered from severe RSV. The respiratory effort was modified as assessed by the pressures recorded in the intrapleural space. Despite the increase in the intrathoracic pressure changes, tidal volume was lower than in healthy animals.

The mechanical characteristics of the lung and respiratory system (i.e., dynamic compliance and pulmonary resistance) were modified with regard to healthy animals, pointing out genuine parenchymal changes. Compare this result with those in Table 5.2. (From Lekeux et al. 1985c.)

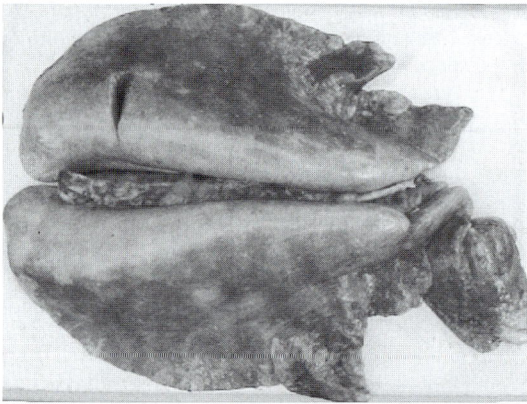

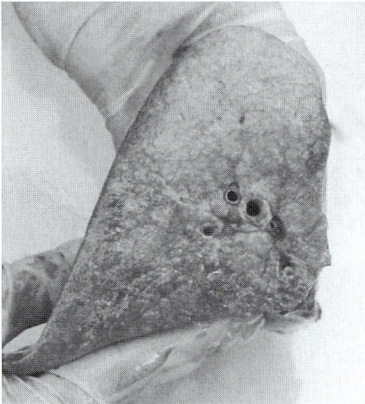

FIG. 5.10—Gross appearance of the lung from a sheep suffering from maedi. Note the increased lung volume as well as the pulmonary fibrosis and the disappearance of the air spaces obvious on the cross-sectional cut. (Courtesy of Prof. F. Schelcher, ENV Toulouse, France.)

bronchiseptica and possibly *Streptococcus zooepidemicus*. In horses, the two streptococcal species of primary importance in respiratory diseases are *S. zooepidemicus* and *S. equi.*

A wide variety of other bacteria can cause pneumonia, often as secondary invaders (Roudebush 1990). Possible primary etiologies should not be overlooked, since bacterial pneumonia is often a sequel of different clinical conditions, such as viral, mycoplasmal, or fungal respiratory infections, dysphagia, reduced levels of consciousness, severe metabolic disorders, immunosuppressive therapy, therapy with certain drugs like aspirin or digoxin, functional and anatomic disorders like tracheal hypoplasia or primary ciliary dyskinesia, immunodeficiency like phagocytic lymphocyte dysfunction, or intravenous catheterization.

Other *infectious bronchopneumonias* in animals include mycobacterial (tuberculosis) (Clercx et al. 1992), protozoal (toxoplasmosis), fungal, parasitic, and rickettsial diseases.

Neoplastic Diseases. Lung tissue can be affected by primary pulmonary neoplasia, metastatic neoplasia, lymphosarcoma, and neoplasia invading from adjacent tissues (Moulton et al. 1981).

Surveys of equine neoplasms indicate a very low incidence of thoracic neoplasia in this species (Sundberg et al. 1977).

In dogs and cats, neoplasia arising primarily from the lung is not very common, especially when compared with metastatic pulmonary neoplasia (Figure 5.11). The majority of lung neoplasms are carcinomas, which are most frequently adenocarcinomas (Moulton et al. 1981).

Lastly, the lung is a very common site of metastases. Tumor types with high incidences of pulmonary metastatic lesions include thyroid carcinomas and mammary carcinomas.

In sheep, the pulmonary adenomatosis is a contagious tumoral progressive and chronic process induced by a retrovirus that induces neoplastic cell proliferation in the alveoli and in the final stage of pulmonary edema (Palmarini et al. 1997).

EXTRAPARENCHYMAL CHANGES. In these cases, the lung is essentially normal. The restriction may be due to a large variety of conditions, such as

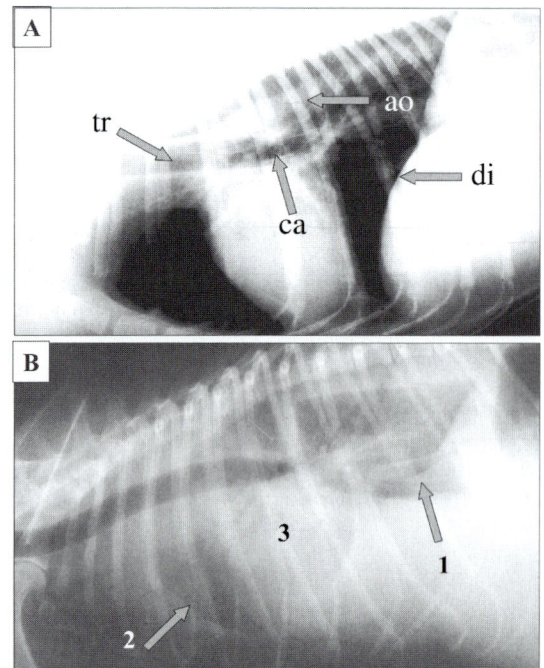

FIG. 5.11—**A:** A healthy dog, lateral view of the thorax: di, diaphragm; ca, carina; ao, aorta; and tr, trachea. **B:** A dog suffering from pleural effusion, lateral view: 1, displaced lung; 2, fluid line; and 3, reduced heart contrast. (Courtesy of the Medical Imaging Department, Liege, Belgium.)

abnormal pleural pressure or thoracic or neuromuscular dysfunction.

Early in the disease, the patients experience dyspnea, with little or no changes in the standard pulmonary function tests. Since the lungs are normal, the lung compliance and the capillary membrane diffusion capacity generally remain unmodified. These characteristics allow the differential diagnosis between parenchymal and extraparenchymal causes of restrictive diseases.

Abnormal Pleural Pressure. Accumulation of fluid (pleural effusion) or air (pneumothorax) in the intrapleural space may be responsible for restrictive phenomenon. These intrapleural disorders are frequent in dogs and cats (Noone 1985).

FUNCTIONAL EFFECTS. In these conditions, the absolute pleural pressure is no longer sufficiently negative. During inspiration, the pressure gradient is too weak to induce appropriate volume changes. During expiration, the pleural pressure may become positive, resulting in small airway collapse and/or alveolar atelectasis. During pneumothorax, active vasoconstriction may occur in the affected lung, and PaO_2 may fall (Anthonisen 1977).

PLEURAL EFFUSION. Pleural effusion is not a disease by itself, but a complication of severe pulmonary, cardiac, or other diseases. This condition may cause pleuritic pain, reduced movement of the chest, and absence of breath sounds, but the pulmonary mechanical parameters often remain unchanged.

Clinical signs of pleural effusion may occur acutely or develop insidiously. The degree of dyspnea does not directly correlate with the volume of pleural fluid. The most common sign is shortness of breath (i.e., tachypnea and shallow respiration). As pleural effusion is only the consequence of various diseases, other symptoms are often observed. Coughing, fever, and pleural pain are sometimes present.

The diagnosis of pleural effusion must be confirmed by thoracic radiography (Figure 5.12), which also demonstrates small effusions that are not detectable on physical examination. Further on, radiographic examination can reveal signs of the primary disease. Diagnostic ultrasound can be useful in detecting cardiac diseases or in locating pockets of pleural fluid.

Thoracocentesis is essential for establishing a definitive diagnosis. In addition, removal of fluid improves radiographic visualization and provides relief of associated dyspnea. Contraindications for thoracocentesis are a bleeding disorder and the presence of herniated abdominal content. Therapeutic thoracocentesis is frequently necessary when a large pleural effusion causes lung compression and hypoventilation.

PNEUMOTHORAX. A pneumothorax can either be closed (when air is trapped within the pleural space) or

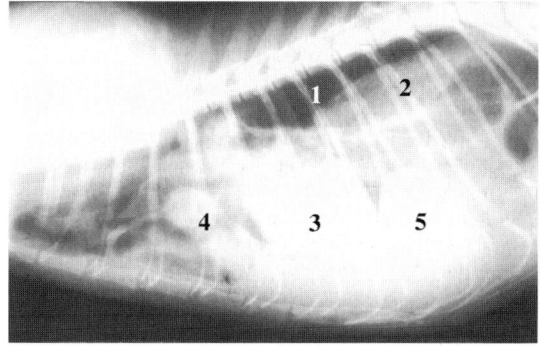

FIG. 5.12—A cat suffering from traumatic diaphragmatic hernia, lateral view: 1, normal lung; 2, collapsed lung; 3, reduced heart contrast; 4, abdominal content; and 5, liver. (Courtesy of the Medical Imaging Department, Liege, Belgium.)

open (when air can escape through the chest wall). When air enters the pleural space, the lung collapses, the rib cage overexpands and the diaphragm is depressed on the affected side. Although the pulmonary function tests show a reduced vital capacity, radiographs are most informative for diagnosing this disorder (Anthonisen 1977).

Blunt or penetrating trauma of the thorax or abdomen is the most frequent cause of pneumothorax in dogs and cats. Radiographic findings other than pneumothorax may include rib fractures, subcutaneous emphysema, pneumomediastinum, and pulmonary contusions. Other causes of pneumothorax include the rupture of pulmonary cysts, bullae or blebs, emphysema, and cavitations (infectious or neoplastic) (Clercx et al. 1992), or can be iatrogenic (thoracocentesis, biopsies) or spontaneous.

Tension pneumothorax is a severe condition that may occur if the lung or pleura acts as a one-way valve by which air is allowed to pump into the pleural space by respiratory motion while its flow back to the airway is prevented. In this case, the intrapleural pressures rise dramatically and become supra-atmospheric.

Abnormal Thorax. The pulmonary function may be influenced by the thoracic compliance. The latter may be too low (ankylosis) or too high, such as in newborn animals. The pulmonary capacity is reduced in the first case. A dramatic increase in the work of breathing and atelectasis results in the second condition.

Abnormal Neuromuscular Function. The diaphragm is the main inspiratory muscle. Therefore, a severe respiratory insufficiency will result from all problems impairing the diaphragmatic work. These problems include diaphragmatic hernia, dysfunction of the phrenic nerve, excessive abdominal pressure as in ruminal tympany in cattle, myopathy, muscle weakness in patients chronically treated by steroids, and muscle fatigue as in patients suffering from either acute or chronic respiratory disease. Lastly, pleural pain may also induce voluntary restricted thoracic movements.

TYMPANY IN RUMINANTS. Gastric tympany or bloat is an abnormal distension of the ruminant forestomach compartments with ingesta or gas. Cattle are more susceptible than sheep, but the disease does occur in the same conditions in small ruminants.

As the forestomach enlarges, the breathing is impaired because of the important cranial displacement of the diaphragm. Dyspnea is marked and accompanied by mouth breathing, protrusion of the tongue, salivation, and extension of the neck. The respiratory rate is increased up to 60 breaths/min. Death from asphyxia ultimately results when the distension is extreme enough to compromise the ventilation (Desmecht et al. 1995).

NUTRITIONAL MYODEGENERATION The so-called white muscle disease is a peracute to subacute myodegenerative disorder of cardiac and/or skeletal muscle. This syndrome occurs in most farm animal species but is most commonly found in young, rapidly growing calves, lambs, kids, and foals.

There are two distinct syndromes of nutritional myodegeneration: a cardiac form and a skeletal form. The cardiac form is associated with signs of myocardial decompensation, whereas the skeletal form is associated with skeletal myasthenia and difficult locomotion. The commonly affected muscles are those of the forelimbs and hindlimbs and of the neck region. In some cases, however, the diaphragm and the intercostal muscles may also be affected. In these cases, the animals show respiratory distress and evidence of abdominal effort when breathing. Cardiomyopathy often occurs along with the respiratory muscle disorders (Maas et al. 1996).

SYNDROME OF RESPIRATORY MUSCLE WEAKNESS OR FATIGUE. Fatigue is defined as the inability of a muscle to maintain a given force. The diaphragm is normally well adapted to resist fatigue, but some clinical situations in which a combination of adverse factors is present can lead to diaphragmatic fatigue. The clinical manifestations of inspiratory muscle fatigue include tachypnea, paradoxical abdominal motion, hypercapnia and, as a preterminal event, bradypnea.

From a functional point of view, the experimental setting demonstrates a reduced high/low ratio in the power spectrum of the electromyograph and a reduced rate of relaxation, together with a right shift of the force-frequency curve.

Respiratory muscle fatigue has been shown to occur in calves suffering from acute respiratory distress due to experimental pasteurellosis (Desmecht et al. 1996). A bilateral diaphragmatic paralysis of unknown origin has been also described in a pony (Table 5.2) (Amory et al. 1994).

Lastly, it has been suggested that respiratory muscle fatigue may occur in horses performing exhausting fast exercise and this may be partly responsible for the hypoxemia and hypercapnia observed in this specific condition.

DIAPHRAGMATIC DYSFUNCTION IN PET ANIMALS. Obesity (pickwickian syndrome) can affect the pulmonary function in a variety of ways. Intrathoracic and extrathoracic fat may interfere with expansion of the thoracic cavity and lungs during inspiration, resulting in hypoventilation.

Cranial displacement of the diaphragm may result from obesity, pregnancy, ascites, hepatomegaly, and intra-abdominal masses.

Herniation of abdominal contents through the diaphragm may occur at any level and may be congenital or acquired (Figure 5.13). Traumatic rupture of the

TABLE 5.2—Respiratory function values in a dyspneic pony with bilateral diaphragmatic paralysis (BDP) and comparison with the values in healthy ponies

Variables	BDP	Healthy
Arterial O_2 partial pressure (mm Hg)	49.4	95
Arterial CO_2 partial pressure (mm Hg)	49.0	44
Respiratory rate (min^{-1})	29.2 + 1.4	25.0
Tidal volume (L)	1.8 + 0.2	2.5
Peak inspiratory flow (L/s)	2.8 + 1	5.0
Peak expiratory flow (L/s)	3.2 + 0.2	4.3
Maximal esophageal pressure (kPa)	3.5 + 0.2	−0.2
Minimal esophageal pressure (kPa)	−3.1 + 0.1	−0.7
Maximal esophageal pressure changes(kPa)	6.6 + 0.2	0.56
Dynamic compliance (L/kPa)	8.1 + 0.9	9.5
Total pulmonary resistance (kPa/L/s)	0.058 + 0.05	0.051

The following points must be highlighted: This pony suffered from severe hypoxemia and from hypercapnia. Its respiratory effort was dramatically modified as assessed by the pressures recorded in the intrapleural space. Despite the increase in the intrathoracic pressure changes, tidal volume and peaks airflows were lower than in healthy animals.

In this case, the mechanical characteristics of the lung and respiratory system (i.e., dynamic compliance and pulmonary resistance) were unmodified with regard to healthy animals, pointing out that in this case the dysfunction was extraparenchymal. Compare this result with those in Table 5.1. (From Amory et al. 1994, with author permission.)

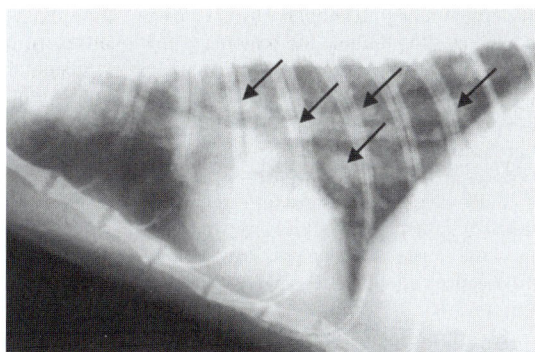

FIG. 5.13—Animal suffering from pulmonary metastases (*arrows*), lateral view. (Courtesy of the Medical Imaging Department, Liege, Belgium.)

diaphragm is usually the result of severe trauma (Wilson and Hayes 1986).

RESTRICTIVE DISORDERS LEADING TO NEONATE RESPIRATORY DISTRESS SYNDROME.
Maturation of the lung involves maturation of the surfactant system but also a thinning of the alveolar capillary barrier, a decrease in alveolar epithelial permeability, and the maturation of chest wall. Although the lack of surfactant is an important factor in the initiation of respiratory distress syndrome, the immaturity of both the lung and the chest wall, and the altered permeability characteristics of the lung, also play an important role in its expression.

Surfactant Deficiency. Pulmonary surfactant, a complex material composed mainly of phospholipids and proteins, has been shown that pulmonary surfactant is required to maintain alveolar stability and to prevent atelectasis. It reduces the work of breathing by increasing lung compliance and enhances alveolar fluid clearance. It is mainly produced and stored in alveolar epithelial type II cells. During fetal life, when there is no air-liquid interface within the lung, surfactant is not required. However, an adequate supply of pulmonary surfactant must be present at birth to enable lung stability and prevent atelectasis after the first breath. In the foal, surfactant has been detected as early as day 200 of gestation. Nevertheless, it has been suggested that pulmonary surfactant in the foal is insufficient to maintain lung stability before day 300 of gestation, with wide variability among individuals (Pattle et al. 1975). If the production of surfactant is delayed or if the birth is premature, the neonate is likely to suffer from neonatal respiratory distress syndrome (Clercx et al. 1989c). There is evidence that cortisol, thyroxine, adrenergic stimulation, and other agents stimulate maturation of the surfactant.

Altered Permeability Characteristics and Hyaline Membrane Formation. The neonate respiratory distress syndrome is frequently complicated by hyaline membrane formation, which is caused by aggregation of proteins and cellular debris accumulating in the alveoli as a result of increased alveolar permeability. This protein not only disrupts alveolar architecture but also interacts directly with the surfactant and inactivates the latter. Although hyaline membrane formation and atelectasis frequently complicate primary surfactant deficiency, they are not pathognomonic of this disorder.

Chest Wall Immaturity. The highly compliant chest wall of premature neonates predisposes them to a too low end-expiratory lung volume, even in the presence of surfactant. This results in a tendency for airway collapse and atelectasis, necessitates higher pressures to reopen closed airways, and consequently increases the work of breathing. When this condition is further complicated by a deficiency in lung surfactant, the work of breathing will further increase. The respiratory muscles must generate more pressure for inflation of the lungs, and respiratory muscle failure may result.

Neonate Respiratory Distress Syndrome in Large Animals. Neonate respiratory distress syndrome has been reported in premature lambs, pigs, calves, and foals (Gibson et al. 1976; Koterba and Paradis 1990). Piglets affected by the so-called barker syndrome present abnormally immature lungs and hyaline membranes, surfactant deficiency, and abnormal thyroid glands with clinical signs of hypothyroidism (Gibson et al. 1976). Calves and foals that are victims of complicated deliveries (dystocia and premature induction of labor) are usually more predisposed to develop respiratory distress syndrome (Koterba and Paradis 1990). As well, cesarean section seems to increase the risk of pulmonary troubles because of a lower production of surfactant when compared with calves born by vaginal delivery (Uystepruyst et al. 2002).

Neonate Respiratory Distress Syndrome in Small Animals. In dogs, age has been shown to influence the phospholipidic composition of the surfactant (Clercx et al. 1989c). Besides physiological changes, there is also a pathological condition in which the altered composition of surfactant from neonatal puppies is responsible for a syndrome (fading puppies complex) similar to the acute respiratory distress syndrome in human neonates. The role of surfactant changes in other clinical conditions has not yet been investigated in dogs and cats.

Conclusions. Interstitial pulmonary diseases, that is, parenchymal restrictive diseases, are uncommon in domestic animals. Intraparenchymal and extraparenchymal disorders induce most frequently restrictive diseases, either alone or in combination with obstructive or vascular diseases. The main functional difference between intraparenchymal and extraparenchymal disorders is that the latter do not impair the lung mechanisms.

PART 3: PHYSIOPATHOLOGY OF VASCULAR PULMONARY DISEASES

TATIANA ART AND PIERRE LEKEUX

The pulmonary circulation begins at the main pulmonary artery, which successively branches to form small arteries and finally form the capillary bed that lies in the wall of the alveoli. Each pulmonary capillary is lined by endothelial cells and surrounded by an interstitial space. On one side, this space is formed only by the two basal membranes of the alveolar and the capillary walls, whereas the interstitium is wider on the other side and contains collagen fibers. Airways and pulmonary vasculature are therefore closely related, and a disorder of the one may impair the function of the other. Some changes in pulmonary perfusion, either physiological or pathological, are schematically presented in Figure 5.14.

The vascular pulmonary disorders are most frequently related to (a) an increase in pressure in the pulmonary circulation due to either active (change in vascular tone) or passive (obstructive) mechanisms, (b) a vascular permeability alteration, or (c) a rupture of the vascular wall (Figure 5.15).

This section summarizes the mechanisms of the main pulmonary vascular disorders, their functional consequences, and some species peculiarities.

PULMONARY HYPERTENSION. The mean pulmonary artery pressure is maintained between narrow physiological limits that are specific for each species.

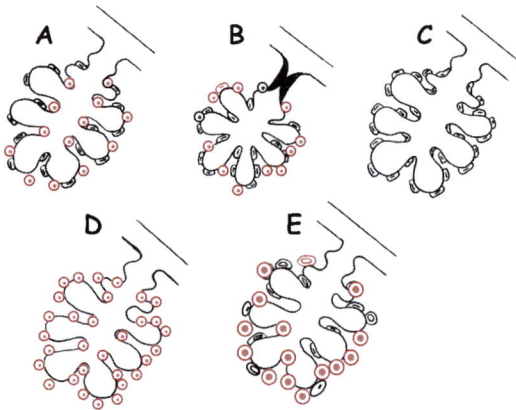

FIG. 5.14—Different kinds of problems that modify pulmonary perfusion and/or its efficiency for gas exchange. **(A)** Physiological conditions. Half of the capillaries are functional while the other half are closed. **(B)** Bronchial obstruction with a decrease in the surface exchange without modification of the pulmonary perfusion. **(C)** Pulmonary vascular obstruction. **(D)** Capillary recruitment during exercise. **(E)** Capillary dilatation as sometimes observed in cases of mitral insufficiency.

When the mean pulmonary artery pressure exceeds the normal resting values, the patient is said to suffer from pulmonary hypertension. The ultimate consequence of pulmonary hypertension is right-heart hypertrophy and failure. This so-called cor pulmonale refers to right-heart disease secondary to primary disease of the lung (Edwards 1988).

With persistent pulmonary hypertension, the pulmonary arterial wall thickens, inducing a secondary increase in the vascular pressure. This increase may be assessed by use of a Swan-Ganz catheter as shown in Figure 5.16.

The three main causes of pulmonary hypertension are increases in (a) pulmonary blood flow, (b) outflow pressure, generally left-atrial pressure, and (c) pulmonary vascular resistance.

Increase in Pulmonary Blood Flow. Congenital heart diseases with a left-to-right shunt through interventricular or interatrial septal defects cause an increase in pulmonary blood flow, which in turn induces a rise in pulmonary arterial pressure. This phenomenon is rather minor because of the ability of the pulmonary capillaries to sustain high blood flow. Sometimes, the pulmonary pressures may nevertheless reach systemic levels, causing right-to-left shunts and arterial hypoxemia.

Exercise induces a physiological increase in pulmonary blood flow. The pulmonary artery and the wedge pressures are increased approximately in the same proportion, while the pulmonary vascular resistance decreases because of the recruitment and/or dilation of the pulmonary vasculature. Mean pressure increase from 28 to 80 mm Hg has been reported in the pulmonary artery of fast-running horses (Erickson et al. 1992). Nevertheless, this hypertension is transient and has no deleterious consequences on the respiratory function.

Increase in Outflow Pressure. Increase in left-atrial pressure occurs by mitral stenosis, by a left ventricular failure, or by an increased preload induced, for instance, by aortic valve insufficiency. When pulmonary venous pressure is increased, pulmonary artery pressure also increases, but to a lesser extent, because pulmonary vascular resistance decreases. In acute conditions, the main consequence is pulmonary edema. By contrast, in chronic conditions, a sequence of changes occurs in both the lung parenchyma and the vasculature, leading to an increase in pulmonary vascular resistance and, hence, in pulmonary artery pressure. The consequent pulmonary hypertension is said to be *passive*.

In the early stage, the lung is congested and the interstitial spaces are expanded by edema. The basement membranes become thickened. With connective tissue proliferation, the lung becomes heavy and stiff. In later stages, these changes progress into alveolar fibrosis, local collection of macrophages and mast cells, scattered hemorrhages, and even patchy ossifications. As the pathology progresses, the vascular lumen is nar-

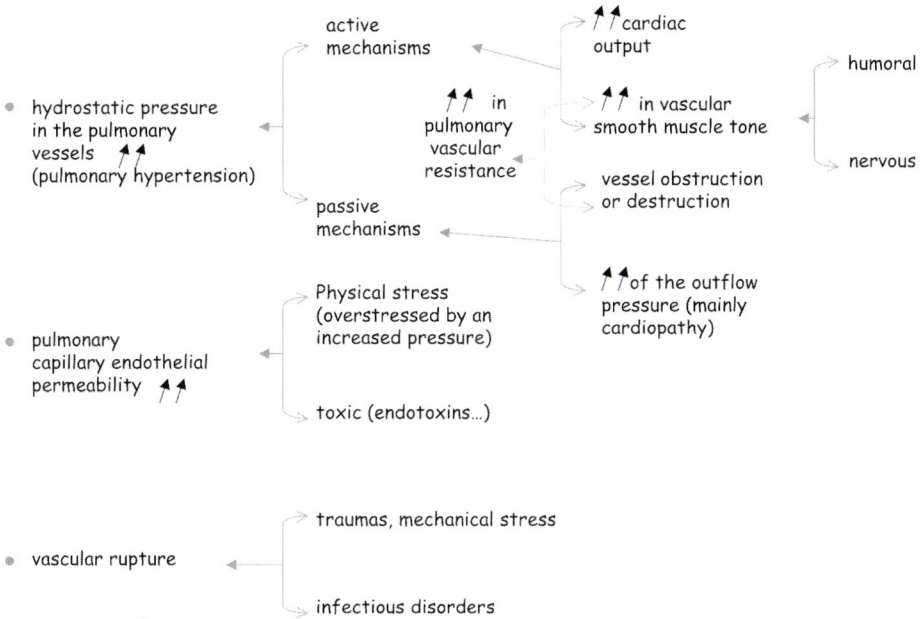

FIG. 5.15—Several causes of vascular pulmonary disorders (see the text for details).

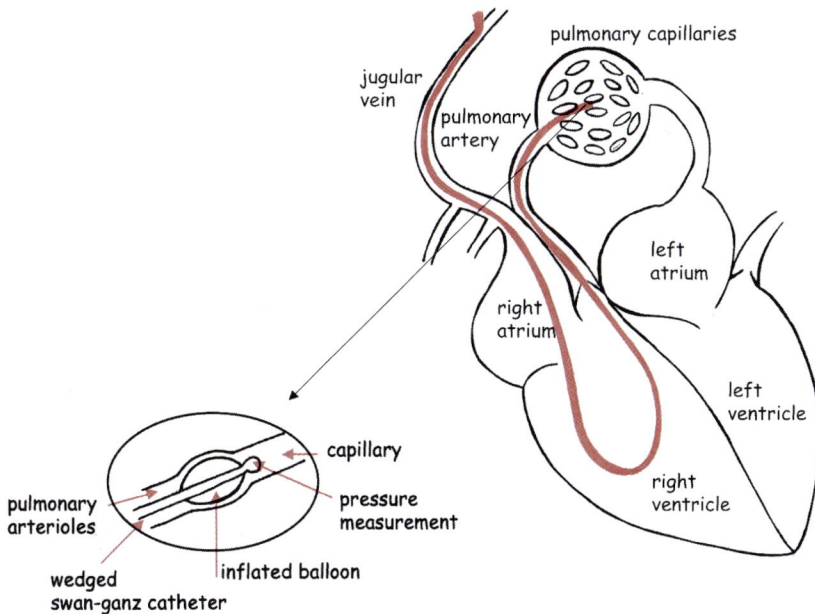

FIG. 5.16—Measurement of vascular pressures by means of a Swan-Ganz catheter. The catheter is introduced in the jugular vein by means of a cannula and progressively conducted into the right atrium, right ventricle, pulmonary artery, and pulmonary capillaries under pressure control. The pulmonary capillary pressure is estimated by wedging the distal end of the catheter and inflating the balloon in order to measure the pressure in the capillary.

rowed or even closed, and part of the increase in resistance is due to the reduction of the cross-sectional area of the vessels.

Increase in Pulmonary Vascular Resistance. Physiological variations in pulmonary vascular resistance are related to respiration as shown in Figure 5.17. Elastic fibers that compose the intra-alveolar septa include pulmonary capillaries. During inhalation, the elastic fibers are stretched and consequently the capillary lumens are narrowed, whereas the opposite occurs during exhalation. By contrast, the great pulmonary vessels on which these fibers are inserted are distended during inspiration and decrease their diameter during expiration.

The pathological and continuous increase in pulmonary vascular resistance is the most common cause of pulmonary hypertension. The resistance may increase following vasoconstriction, vascular obstruction, or tissue injury.

VASOCONSTRICTION. Acute vasoconstriction may occur in patients suffering from septicemia or endotoxemia. Indeed, one of the factors modulating the vascular caliber is the contraction (resulting in vasoconstriction) or relaxation (resulting in vasodilatation) of the smooth muscles in the pulmonary vessels. This may be induced by either nervous or humoral mechanisms. Substances such as autacoids, cytokines, and neuropeptides are potent vasomodulators of the pulmonary circulation. For instance, histamine, serotonin, thromboxane, tumor-necrosis factor, and endothelins are vasoconstric-

tors, whereas bradykinins, vasoactive intestinal peptide, and nitric oxide are vasodilators. Some mediators such as substance P, histamine, serotonin, bradykinin, platelet-activating factor, complement, leukotrienes, and tumor-necrosis factor are also able to modify vascular permeability (Linden et al. 1995).

In the diseased lung, there may be an increased effect of the vasoactive substances related to either an increased production or to a decreased deactivation, for instance, when the vascular endothelium is damaged, or to a disappearance of antagonistic vasoactive substances (Brigham et al. 1979).

Hypoxic pulmonary vasoconstriction results from alveolar hypoxia either in healthy animals transported at high altitude or in diseased patients suffering from respiratory disorders (Bisgard et al. 1975).

The mechanism for hypoxic vasoconstriction is related to both alveolar and mixed venous oxygen tensions. The greater the hypoxia and the larger the fraction of lung involved, the more the response shifts from the homeostatic maintenance promoting blood oxygenation toward the physiopathological end point of generalized pulmonary vasoconstriction with pulmonary hypertension and increased right-heart work.

The pulmonary hypertension resulting from hypoxia at high altitude induces a vasoconstriction response in the entire lung. The acute condition results in right-heart failure and pulmonary edema, whereas the chronic condition may induce progressive changes in the pulmonary vasculature. There is, however, a large variability in the responses among species. Cattle have a vigorous hypoxic constrictor response, causing a right-ventricular failure known as brisket disease. Pigs, ponies, and goats are slightly less reactive than cattle, whereas dogs, cats, and sheep do not develop pulmonary hypertension at altitude. These species also fail to develop right-heart failure at high altitude. It is interesting to note that the degree of right-ventricular insufficiency during chronic hypoxia is correlated with the thickness of the intermediate smooth muscle layer of the small pulmonary arteries prior to exposure to hypoxia.

VASCULAR OBSTRUCTION. Pulmonary hypertension may also result from mechanical obstruction generally resulting from thromboembolism, circulating fat, air, or parasites (Malik 1983).

VASCULAR OCCLUSION DUE TO TISSUE INJURY. Lastly, pulmonary hypertension may be induced by destruction of the vascular bed. Humoral factors released from leukocytes, platelets, plasma, lung endothelium, macrophages, and mast cells may contribute to vascular injury.

Obliterative lesions occur in emphysema, when the capillary bed is partly destroyed. Other pulmonary parenchymal diseases such as scleroderma, interstitial fibrosis, and granulomatous disease also increase pulmonary vascular resistance because they destroy blood vessels.

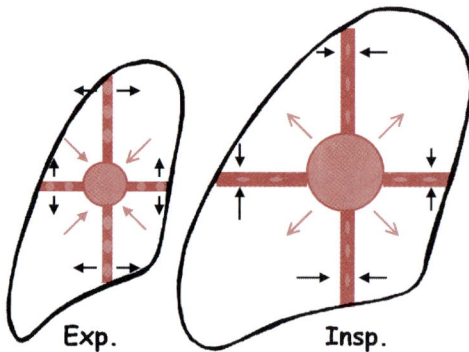

FIG. 5.17—Physiological variations in pulmonary vascular resistance, related to respiration. Elastic fibers are schematically represented by four branches (actually, there are several million fibers). They compose the intra-alveolar septae and include capillaries. During inhalation, the fibers are stretched, consequently, narrowing the capillary lumen, while the opposite occurs during exhalation. By contrast, the great pulmonary vessels on which these fibers are inserted are distended during inspiration and their diameter decreases during expiration.

PULMONARY EDEMA. Fluid is normally exchanged between the pulmonary circulation and the interstitium, between the interstitium and the pleural space, and between the airway interstitium and the epithelial surface (Aukland and Nicolaysen 1981) (Figure 5.18).

The fluid exchanges are well regulated so that excessive fluid does not accumulate in the pulmonary interstitium or in the pleural space. The accumulation of excessive fluid is also prevented by the extensive lymphatic system that drains these areas so that, in healthy lungs, fluid formation equals fluid removal so that excessive fluid cannot enter the lung interstitium, alveoli, or airways. Normally, transcapillary fluid exchange is controlled within very narrow limits, but in pathological conditions fluid may accumulate in the extravascular spaces and tissues of the lung. This phenomenon is called *pulmonary edema*. It may complicate a variety of heart and lung diseases, altering the gas exchange and the mechanics of breathing. Two stages of pulmonary edema are recognized, but the clinical differentiation may be difficult. The first phase is *interstitial edema*, which is characterized by engorgement of the perivascular and peribronchial interstitial tissues. The second phase is *alveolar edema*, when fluid moves into the alveoli (Figure 5.19) (Staub 1984).

Etiology

INCREASED CAPILLARY PRESSURE. This is the most common cause of edema and a frequent complication of heart diseases such as acute myocardial infarction, left-ventricular failure, and mitral valve disease. In all of these conditions, left-atrial pressure rises. The pressure at which pulmonary edema occurs depends on the magnitude and the rate of the pressure changes. In patients with chronic mitral failure, the pressure gradually increases, and a high left-atrial pressure may be reached without evidence of alveolar edema. This is partly due to the progressive adjustment of the lymphatic drainage by the increase in both the number and the caliber of lymph vessels. Nevertheless, these patients frequently present a marked interstitial edema. On the other hand, patients with acute myocardial failure have an alveolar edema with a smaller but more rapid increase in capillary pressure.

Less frequently, noncardiogenic causes, such as excessive intravenous saline perfusion or acute renal failure, can also induce pulmonary edema. In these conditions, the edema is partly caused by the rise in the hydrostatic pressure but also by an increase in capillary permeability apparently due to damage induced by the stretching of the endothelium that results from the condition.

INCREASED CAPILLARY PERMEABILITY. Inhaled toxins such as sulfur dioxide or nitrogen oxide, or circulating toxins such as endotoxin, cause pulmonary edema because they increase capillary permeability. Immunologically mediated processes such as purpura hemorrhagica also increase vascular permeability by complement activation.

LYMPHATIC INSUFFICIENCY. This occurs in diseases in which the normal lymphatic drainage is impaired because of obliteration, distortion, or compression of lymphatic vessels.

OTHERS. Decreased interstitial pressure, as may be observed in pneumothorax, or decreased osmotic pressure, as in hypoproteinemia, much more rarely provoke pulmonary edema.

Physiopathology. When left-atrial pressure is abnormally high, the rise in capillary pressure rapidly causes fluid accumulation in the pulmonary interstitium. Furthermore, the rate of edema formation is accelerated by an increased concentration of interstitial proteins or a disruption of the alveolar-capillary membrane. Moreover, when the endothelium of the capillary wall is damaged, the fluid begins to accumulate more rapidly in the lung tissue even at a low left-atrial pressure.

INTERSTITIAL EDEMA. Interstitial edema increases the alveolar-capillary membrane thickness by only 15% to 20%. This low increase is due to an expanded interstitial space. The tissue fluid moves rapidly from the gas-exchange sites into the more compliant perivascular spaces, preserving as long as possible a thin barrier for gas exchange. The modification of the alveolar-capillary membrane is so minimal that gas exchange remains unaffected. Once the capacity of fluid absorption of the interstitium has reached its maximum value and the interstitial space has expanded by approximately 50%, alveolar edema occurs.

ALVEOLAR EDEMA. Little is known about the mechanisms that lead to alveolar edema, but it seems to occur in an all-or-nothing fashion. The leaking site is supposed to be either the junction between the alveoli and the small alveolar ducts or at openings of the epithelial tight junctions. These leakage sites are clearly not selective and do not restrict the passage of plasma proteins.

ALVEOLAR SAFETY FACTORS. Edema formation is not detectable until left-atrial pressure exceeds a certain level. Research into knowing why has led to the concept of tissue edema safety factors, which prevent the formation of pulmonary edema when capillary pressure is elevated. The three tissue safety factors are (a) a decreased filtration pressure because the tissue hydrostatic pressure increases immediately, (b) a decreased tissue osmotic pressure because its protein concentration is diluted, and (c) a 5- to 10-fold increase in the lymph flow that carries away an important additional amount of fluid. These safety factors are less efficient when the pulmonary capillary endothelium is damaged. In this case, the inefficiency of the safety factors is due to the lymphatic vessels being less effective in fluid removal and the osmotic pressure in the tissues

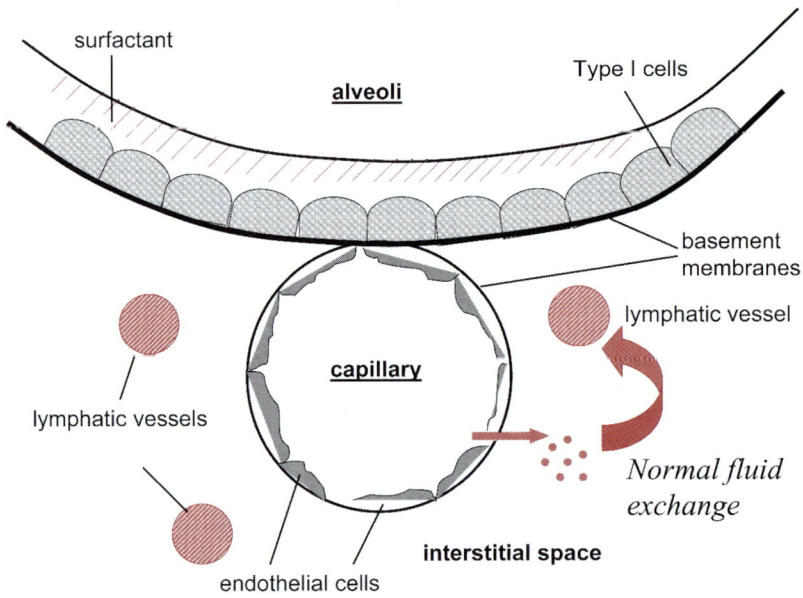

FIG. 5.18—Physiological fluid exchange between the pulmonary circulation, the interstitium, and the lymphatic vessels.

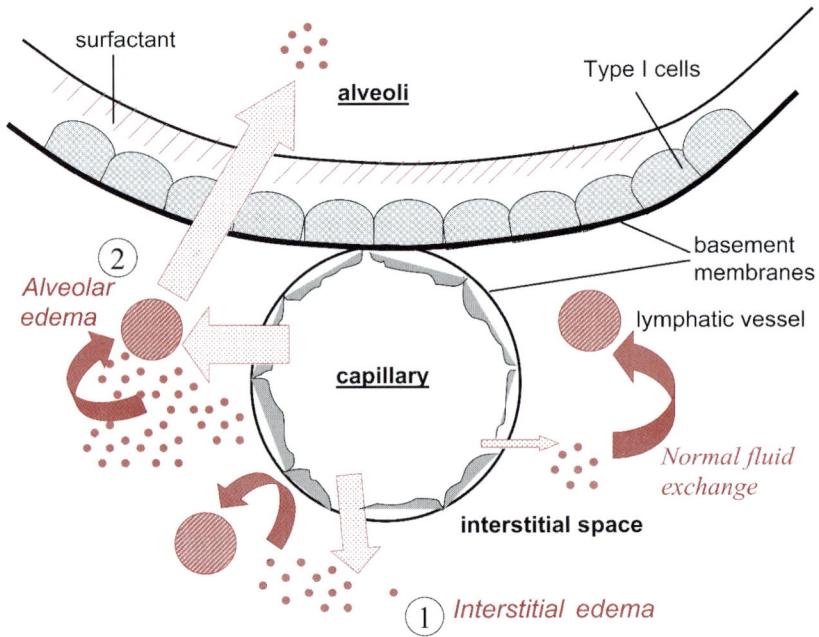

FIG. 5.19—Mechanisms of occurrence of (1) interstitial and (2) alveolar edema.

remaining high because the capillary wall is permeable to plasma proteins.

Functional Effects. When interstitial edema begins to develop, the dynamic lung compliance drops while arterial blood gases remain physiological in resting conditions. When alveolar edema occurs as the result of surface tension forces, the edematous alveoli shrink. The alveolar ventilation and alveoloarterial diffusion are impaired, and arterial partial pressure of oxygen drops dramatically while the alveoloarterial gradient of oxygen increases. The arterial partial pressure of carbon dioxide is generally normal because of increased ventilation of the nonedematous alveoli.

The alveolar edema induces a further decrease in lung compliance. This decrease is related to the reduced distensibility of the lung because of the fluid within the interstitium, to the changes in surface properties related to alveolar edema, and to the decreased lung volume.

Lower airway resistance may be increased in severe cases because the blood vessel engorgement and fluid in the airways reduce their cross-sectional area. Reflex bronchoconstriction following stimulation of irritant receptors in the bronchial wall may also play a role.

Administration of diuretics may help to resolve the edema by decreasing the hydrostatic pressure, while the impaired oxygenation may be improved by mechanical ventilation of the patient and/or by increasing the inspired oxygen concentration.

During vascular congestion and edema formation, the vascular resistance and consequently the pulmonary arterial pressure rise because cardiac output remains normal. Hypoxic vasoconstriction of the poorly ventilated or unventilated areas contributes to this phenomenon. In addition, perivascular "cuffing" probably also plays a role by compressing extra-alveolar vessels. Lastly, the collapse of the edematous alveoli and the edematous alveolar walls may compress the capillaries.

PULMONARY EMBOLISM

Definition and Pathophysiology. One of the functions of the lung is to filter the blood. The frequency of solid particles trapped in the blood vessels is unknown, but small emboli are probably very common and frequently undiagnosed. In contrast, larger emboli may induce pulmonary hemorrhage and atelectasis, and even pulmonary infarction, that are potentially fatal.

Most pulmonary emboli arise from venous thrombi formed in the deep veins of the lower extremities. Fat, air, and amniotic fluid are also potential thrombi, but this occurs more rarely. Factors that favor the formation of venous thrombi are stasis of the blood (local pressure, immobilization, and venous obstruction), alterations in the blood coagulation system (change in blood viscosity), and abnormalities of the vascular walls (trauma, inflammation, and phlebitis).

Functional Effects

EFFECT ON PULMONARY HEMODYNAMICS. The most obvious effect of pulmonary thromboemboli on pulmonary hemodynamics is an increase in pulmonary artery pressure. The pulmonary circulation normally has a large reserve capacity because many capillaries are unfilled. This reserve is so important that at least half of the pulmonary circulation may be obstructed by an embolus before a substantial rise in pulmonary artery pressure occurs. In addition to the purely mechanical effect of the embolus, there is some evidence that active vasoconstriction occurs in the remaining perfused area, lasting at least for some minutes after embolization. In experimentally embolized dog lungs, a local release of serotonin from platelets associated with the embolus, as well as a vasoconstriction reflex via the sympathetic nervous system, have been put forward to explain this phenomenon.

Right-ventricular failure may result from the pulmonary arterial pressure rise. In a few cases, pulmonary edema may occur, probably caused by leakage from those capillaries that are not protected from the raised pulmonary arterial pressure.

EFFECT ON THE RESPIRATORY AND LUNG MECHANICS. In experimental animals, the response to thromboemboli is an increase in pulmonary resistance and a fall in dynamic compliance. These changes occur immediately after the embolization and last for 30 to 40 minutes. Further on, the ventilation of the corresponding area is reduced. These phenomena are due to a local bronchoconstriction (responsible for the increase in pulmonary resistance) and alveolar duct constriction (responsible for the fall in lung dynamic compliance) and seem to be a direct consequence of the decrease in alveolar PCO_2. This bronchoconstriction can be reversed by adding carbon dioxide to the inhaled gas. The changes in elastic properties of the embolized area are probably also due to pulmonary edema and/or a loss of the pulmonary surfactant.

In patients suffering from pulmonary embolization, the respiration is rapid, shallow, and dyspneic. Stimulation of pulmonary chemoreflex via the activation of pulmonary C fibers by the release of prostaglandins as well as serotonin, and stimulation of irritant receptors, have been implicated in these modifications.

EFFECT ON GAS EXCHANGE. Moderate hypoxemia without carbon dioxide retention is often seen in cases of pulmonary embolism. Abnormal gas exchange in patients suffering from embolism results from a combination of several mechanisms, including ventilation-perfusion inhomogeneity (i.e., either a very high or a very low ventilation/perfusion ratio) as the main reason and physiological shunts, an increase in physiological dead space, and diffusion impairment as more minor reasons (Dantzker et al. 1978; Clercx et al. 1989a).

PULMONARY HEMORRHAGE. Most of the time, pulmonary hemorrhage is secondary to severe pulmonary lesions and generally originates in highly vascularized tissues, such as the wall of a necrotizing bacterial cavity, at the site of chronic bronchiectasis, in a bronchial adenoma or, very rarely, from venous varicosities due to chronic mitral stenosis. The majority of the bleeding sites are supplied by bronchial artery collaterals. Pulmonary hemorrhage is also encountered during chest trauma in all species and during strenuous exercise in the horses.

The functional effects of the hemorrhage itself are generally shaded by the effect of the primary cause of the bleeding. Nevertheless, when the hemorrhage is important, the presence of blood in the small and larger airways may induce obstructive disorders—that is, an increase in pulmonary resistance, ventilation asynchronism, and consequently impaired gas exchanges.

SPECIES PECULIARITIES. Although each species may suffer from the aforementioned different dysfunctions, some species are more susceptible than others to one of these pathological conditions, based on their morphological and/or functional characteristics.

Equine Species

EXERCISE-INDUCED PULMONARY HEMORRHAGE

DEFINITION. Exercise-induced pulmonary hemorrhage is defined as the presence of blood in the tracheobronchial tree following strenuous exercise in horses. Endoscopic surveys of the lower airways in racing horses have demonstrated that 95% of the horses examined bled on at least one occasion. There is no breed, age, or sex difference in exercise-induced pulmonary hemorrhage susceptibility, and no geographic variation is found in the incidence.

Most of the clinical signs are nonspecific. They include blood in the tracheobronchial airways and, much less frequently, epistaxis (10% of the cases). As far as its effect on performance is concerned, in some horses there is no influence at all whereas in others a definite exercise intolerance is observed.

Micropathological examination of end-stage exercise-induced pulmonary hemorrhage lesions shows destruction of alveolar tissue, extensive proliferation of bronchial blood vessels, and greatly increased numbers of anastomoses between the bronchial and pulmonary circulations. The pulmonary capillaries could consequently be submitted to the high systemic pressure and therefore be ruptured. However, it remains to be elucidated whether the bronchial neovascularization, which is a response to inflammation and is considered an integral part of pulmonary repair, occurs before or after the very first episode of exercise-induced pulmonary hemorrhage.

SITES OF BLEEDING. Most of the affected areas appear to be distributed in the caudodorsal bronchopulmonary segments. Some anatomic and functional characteristics of these regions could explain their predisposition to bleeding during exercise.

First, this segment is subtended by the terminal divisions of the principal bronchus, which could be a site that has a predilection for the deposition of inhaled particles. Secondly, because of the more negative intrapleural pressure at this level, the alveoli of these regions are fully dilated and consequently weakened. Thirdly, relatively smaller alveoli and thicker septa result in a regional difference in elastic properties and consequently in greater respiratory asynchronism. Moreover, the regional decrease in the distribution of the pores of Kohn and therefore in the collateral ventilation enhances the inhomogeneity of the distribution of ventilation. Lastly, the caudodorsal region of the lung is the least well perfused by the pulmonary circulation in the resting horse, whereas the opposite occurs during exercise (Figure 5.20) (Votion et al. 1999).

POSSIBLE ETIOLOGY. The occurrence of exercise-induced pulmonary hemorrhage following strenuous exercise and not after prolonged exercise of lower intensity suggests that the syndrome is the result of extreme mechanical forces applied to lung tissues and vessels. During heavy exercise, alveolar pressure is likely to become highly negative (Art et al. 1990), whereas intravascular pressure (both pulmonary and bronchial) increases greatly (Langsetmo et al. 2000). Transmural pressure—that is, the pressure gradient between airways and blood vessels—is expected to present important, irregular, and sudden variations (related to cardiogenic pressure increase in the vascular compartment and to respiration into the airway) that could cause the capillary rupture (West et al. 1993).

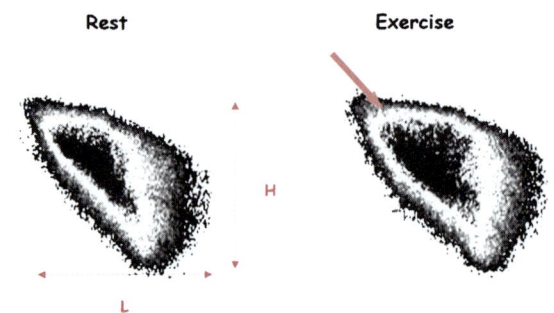

FIG. 5.20—Pulmonary perfusion in a horse, measured by pulmonary scintigraphy, showing the redistribution of blood flow induced by exercise. Both height and length are increased. Perfusion of the caudodorsal part of the lung is proportionally more increased than in the other parts, which could provide a partial explanation for the location of exercise-induced hemorrhages in this species.

HYPOXIC VASOCONSTRICTION IN CHRONIC OBSTRUC-
TIVE PULMONARY DISEASE. Pulmonary artery hypertension secondary to chronic pulmonary disease is of
major importance in human medicine. Chronic bronchiolitis is frequently observed in horses, and pulmonary hypertension due to a hypoxic vasoconstriction
may sometimes occur (Dixon 1978). In other species,
this could induce right-ventricular hypertrophy and
eventually right-heart failure, a complication that
seems to be uncommon in horses.

Bovine Species

BRISKET DISEASE. Brisket disease, also called high-
altitude disease, is a typical example of cor pulmonale. Clinical signs are tachycardia, jugular venous
distension, and subcutaneous edema of the brisket.
Cattle have a vigorous hypoxic pulmonary vasoconstrictor response, which explains their susceptibility
to this disorder (Tucker et al. 1975). When taken to
altitude, they develop pulmonary hypertension as a
result of increased pulmonary vascular resistance
(Will et al. 1962). The resulting pressure overload on
the right ventricle is responsible for the progressive
cardiac hypertrophy, dilation, and failure (Alexander
et al. 1960).

The severity of the disease depends on the level of
alveolar hypoxia, on the speed with which the condition develops, and on the individual reactivity to
chronic hypoxia. Indeed, some strains of cattle are less
sensitive to both acute and chronic hypoxia.

ACUTE ENDOTOXIC PASTEURELLOSIS. Intratracheal
or intravenous inoculation of high doses of
Mannheimia (*Pasteurella*) *haemolytica* organisms is
responsible for severe pulmonary vascular disease in
calves. The early changes in the mechanics of breathing consist of a decrease in lung dynamic compliance
without change in total pulmonary resistance. This suggests that respiratory tract injury in acute bovine pasteurellosis is initiated from the parenchyma and does
not result from extension of lesions from the conducting airways (Linden et al. 1995).

The gas-exchange impairments observed during this
syndrome result first from ventilation-perfusion mismatching in injured lung segments and later from pulmonary edema. This may result from increased pulmonary vascular permeability due to endothelial
damage generated by activated neutrophils and oxygen
radical release and from pulmonary hypertension due
to left-heart failure.

3-METHYLINDOL TOXICOSIS. Acute bovine pulmonary edema and emphysema may be caused by 3-
methylindol, a pneumotoxic compound that results
from the conversion of L-tryptophan ingested in lush
forage (Lekeux et al. 1985b). This leads to the development of acute pulmonary edema, alveolar epithelial
hyperplasia, and interstitial emphysema.

The functional disorders induced by 3-methylindol
in the early stage of the disease consist of large
decreases in dynamic lung compliance and arterial
oxygen tension and large increases in minute viscous
work and arterial carbon dioxide tension, without a
change in total pulmonary resistance. These dysfunctions are compatible with severe interstitial and pulmonary edema.

Canine Species

PULMONARY HYPERTENSION. The presence of *Dirofilaria immitis* in the pulmonary arteries and the right
heart, and the shedding of metabolic products and antigens by microfilariae and adult worms, are responsible
for the wide variety of changes then observed in the
pulmonary vascular bed and lung parenchyma (Thrall
et al. 1979). However, cor pulmonale is seen almost
exclusively in severe chronic infections.

The major vaso-occlusive effects are due to chronic
endarteritis and endothelial proliferation of the peripheral pulmonary branches.

The most common congenital cardiac defect causing
systemic to pulmonary shunting is patent ductus arteriosus. Females of certain small breeds are at greatest
risk for the development of this disorder, which is also
well recognized in cats (Bonagura and Darke 1995).

Due to the higher aortic than pulmonary blood
pressure, blood shunts continuously into the main
pulmonary artery. This results in a continuous cardiac
murmur, increased pulmonary flow, and increased
venous return to the left atrium and ventricle. Left-
ventricular failure with pulmonary edema develops
from volume overload. In a small percentage of
cases, the lumen of the patent ductus arteriosus is so
large that pulmonary vascular pressure markedly
increases.

Many other cardiac congenital defects are recognized and may lead to pulmonary hypertension. In
cases of interatrial or interventricular septal defects,
blood shunts from the left to the right. However, in conditions such as tricuspid or pulmonic stenosis that
increase right atrial or ventricular pressures, right-to-
left shunting may develop.

PULMONARY EDEMA. Most pulmonary edemas in
dogs and cats are cardiogenic in origin. Left-heart failure remains the most common cause of pulmonary
edema in dogs and cats. Left-heart failure is usually
evidenced by dyspnea, pulmonary rales, cough, and
exercise intolerance. In most patients with left-heart
failure, pulmonary congestion can be confirmed by thoracic radiography. The nature and distribution of
lesions on chest X-rays and the concurrent presence of
cardiomegaly associated with a systolic murmur usually implicate the failing heart as the cause of pulmonary congestion. When equivocal evidence of left-
heart failure is present in patients in which pulmonary
infiltrates of uncertain etiology are identified, left-atrial

pressure can be estimated by measurement of pulmonary artery wedge pressure using a Swan-Ganz catheter.

Noncardiogenic edema may be due to a great variety of pathogenetic mechanisms and are either high-pressure or high-permeability low-pressure edemas.

Acute respiratory failure with massive pulmonary edema, also called adult respiratory distress syndrome (ARDS) or shock lung syndrome, is the common response of the lung to a great variety of injuries. Pulmonary edema following pancreatitis in dogs is one of the many forms of this syndrome. In dogs and cats, aspiration of gastric content during anesthesia, unconsciousness, or dysphagic troubles, and inhalation of smoke or toxic inhalants, are common causes of permeability edema. Pulmonary edema in dogs and cats with terminal uremia is also common. Infectious diseases, including viral, bacterial, and parasitic pneumonia, may result in inflammatory lung edema.

PULMONARY THROMBOEMBOLISM. The best-recognized thromboemboli disease syndromes in companion animals are aortic thromboembolism associated with cardiomyopathy in cats and pulmonary thromboembolism due to heartworm disease and treatment in dogs.

Pulmonary thromboembolism is a common clinical disease in dogs but is frequently underdiagnosed. Postmortem diagnosis is complicated by the rapid dissolution of thrombi, and antemortem diagnosis requires specialized diagnostic techniques. Hypoxemia is a common but inconstant finding, and thoracic radiographic findings are frequently normal. Pulmonary scintigraphy is a noninvasive procedure that shows the combination of a normal ventilation scan and an abnormal perfusion scan, a ventilation-perfusion mismatch that aids in the diagnosis of thromboembolism (Clercx et al. 1989a). Pulmonary arteriography is the gold standard for diagnosis but is an invasive procedure that has potential limitations and complications.

LUNG HEMORRHAGE. Pulmonary injuries are common consequences of chest trauma, a condition that is frequently encountered in dogs and cats. Lung lacerations or contusions are associated with hemorrhage and edema. In lung contusion, intrapulmonary hemorrhage results from the tearing of capillaries and small blood vessels, and leads to alveolar wall disruption, interstitial hemorrhage, aspiration of blood, and atelectasis. The severity of the clinical signs depends on the extent of the lung injury and the type and severity of the concurrent lesions. Localized lung injury without pneumothorax or rib fracture may cause no overt clinical signs. When several lung lobes are involved, dyspnea, coughing, hemoptysis, and cyanosis may be observed. Except for hemoptysis and signs of hypovolemia, the clinical signs are nonspecific, and lung contusion needs to be confirmed radiographically.

Primary or secondary thrombocytopenia and a large number of primary or secondary coagulopathies can lead to diffuse, nontraumatic pulmonary hemorrhage. The etiologies are very diverse and include thrombocytopenia caused by bone marrow depression or immune-mediated diseases, and coagulopathies associated with congenital diseases, warfarin toxicity, and treatment with cytostatics and anticoagulants. The animals show a wide variety of nonspecific signs depending on the underlying primary disease and the degree of bleeding and anemia. Suspicious signs include prolonged bleeding time after venupuncture; subcutaneous, mucosal, or submucosal hemorrhage; and dyspnea. Hemoptysis often occurs but is not a consistent sign.

Conclusions. Even more than other respiratory dysfunctions, vascular pulmonary diseases present manifest species peculiarities. For instance, exercise-induced pulmonary hemorrhage, brisket disease, and pulmonary embolism are quite exclusively observed in horses, cattle, and dogs, respectively.

Therefore, these species peculiarities must be taken into account when dealing with the diagnosis, treatment, and prevention of vascular pulmonary diseases.

PART 4: ENVIRONMENTAL RESPIRATORY DISEASES: SOME EXAMPLES OF PHYSIOPATHOLOGICAL PROCESSES IN DOMESTIC ANIMALS

JULIEN HAMOIR AND PASCAL GUSTIN

Respiratory pathophysiological changes can arise from chemicals that are inhaled directly into the respiratory system from the ambient air or are absorbed into the circulatory system from the digestive tract (or via other tissues or systemic administration). Some solids or liquid pollutants can also be inhaled as particulate matter that can sometimes be the carrier of other potentially noxious agents. As there are enormous numbers of substances with this potential for harm, this section is restricted to a few important examples that can carry special risks for the respiratory processes of domestic animals.

Several xenobiotics (compounds that are foreign to the body) marketed as chemicals and drugs can induce respiratory pathophysiological changes following systemic administration and also after inhalation. In all animal species, as well as in people, chemical injuries are more and more often recognized as an important source of respiratory disorders. Pets live in essentially the same environmental conditions as people, and it is likely that these species can be vulnerable to similar respiratory disorders related to the pollution present in the human environment. Unfortunately, this aspect remains scarcely documented. Farm animals are also exposed to several atmospheric pollutants provoking or aggravating respiratory diseases induced by biological agents. For example, it is well known now that the morbidity of respiratory diseases observed in pigs and workers in piggeries, while very different, is closely related to atmospheric pollution in animal facilities. The aim of this section is thus to provide a brief overview of some environmental respiratory disorders relevant to veterinary medicine.

The first part is devoted to some examples of respiratory disorders associated with air pollutants in animals. The clearance of deposited particles and dissolved pollutants in mucus is then considered, followed by some examples of respiratory diseases induced by systemic chemicals.

INHALATION OF ATMOSPHERIC POLLUTANTS AND THEIR ROLES IN RESPIRATORY DISEASE.
The examples of respiratory disorders induced by atmospheric pollution in domestic animals that are discussed include ammonia (which is commonly detected in production-animal facilities), photochemical oxidants, and particulate matter, all of which are recognized as playing a major toxicological role in various environmental conditions.

Ammonia. Intensification of farming methods has led to an increase in animal density in animal facilities where several air pollutants can be concentrated. Animals are not the only targets of these pollutants, since a strong alteration in the results of pulmonary function tests by swine producers is well documented. Several substances that are potentially harmful for the respiratory system contaminate the air in animal facilities. Dust, endotoxins, and ammonia are among the most important. The deleterious effects of ammonia have been extensively investigated, mainly in pigs. Based on analysis of the dose-response curves established for each effect, it appears that ammonia at concentrations as low as 10 ppm or more can induce a marked inflammation in nasal cavities, a decrease in the ciliated surface of the turbinate mucosa, an epithelial and subepithelial inflammatory infiltrate in nasal cavities and sometimes in the trachea, hyperreactivity of the tracheal smooth muscle related to a deleterious effect on epithelial cells, stimulation of mucus production, changes in the permeability of the alveolocapillary barrier, and a modulation of the pulmonary vascular response to endotoxins. Due to the high water solubility of ammonia, a large amount of the inhaled gas can be absorbed by the mucus in the upper airways where the toxicity is first exerted. Ammonia can sensitize the nasal mucosa to other agents such as endotoxins. These data can be correlated with the high sensitivity of ammonia-exposed pigs to biological agents such as *Bordetella bronchseptica*.

Interactions between dust inhalation and ammonia have been identified. Dust can adsorb the gas, modulating its toxicity, depending on the experimental conditions and the considered segment in the respiratory tract. For example, the increase in the total cell counts in bronchoalveolar lavage fluids sampled in pigs exposed to organic dust can be modulated by a simultaneous exposure to ammonia. Ammonia can also induce systemic effects, such as lethargy, and have a negative impact on productivity. These considerations illustrate the necessity to control the level of pollution in animal facilities. It should also be noted that there are a lot of other potentially toxic gases, including carbon monoxide (CO), carbon dioxide (CO_2), sulfur dioxide (SO_2), hydrogen sulfide (H_2S), and oxides of nitrogen, such as nitrogen dioxide (NO_2) among others.

Photochemical Oxidants. *Photochemical air pollution* is the term given to the mixture of compounds produced as a result of the action of sunlight on pollutants produced in large part by the burning of fossil fuels. Among these photochemical oxidants potentially harmful for the respiratory tract, ozone plays an important toxicological role in all species. Photochemical products are not primary emissions but are produced by the action of sunlight on hydrocarbons and nitrogen oxides. They induce acute inflammation in the respiratory tract, leading to acute edema at high concentrations, for example, in cattle but also in other species. The toxicity of ozone, mainly detected in big cities with heavy traffic at concentrations as high as 0.3 ppm, involves functional and cellular effects, including epithelial damage, increased microvascular permeability, airway hyperresponsiveness and inflammation, and impaired respiratory and immunologic functions. The toxicological mechanisms explaining all of these effects are beyond the scope of this section. Many interactions between ozone and the effects, synthesis, release, and biotransformation of mediators as, for example, neurokinins, have been identified.

The biochemical mechanisms by which ozone exerts its toxicity are now better understood. Ozone can react with unsaturated fatty acids of cellular membranes to produce lipid ozonization products. These substances can lead to several effects, such as phospholipase activation and reactive oxygen species production. Ozone can also interact with the metabolic activity of pulmonary tissue. In rabbits, it has been demonstrated that ozone exposure can strongly inhibit two cytochrome P-450 activities in females with possible consequences for the pulmonary metabolism of xenobiotics. The cytochromes P-450 are hemoproteins that play important physiological functions as the oxygen-activating terminal oxidases in various oxygenation reactions. These particular structures have a wide distribution among various forms of life. They participate in steroid biosynthesis but also in the metabolism of various xenobiotics. Ozone could modulate their toxicity by blocking detoxification or bioactivation pathways.

Exposure to ozone also leads to activation of protective mechanisms, such as the stimulation of pulmonary adrenergic nerve fibers with a local release of neuropeptide Y (NPY), known for its protective role against edema in the lungs. Other protective mechanisms, such as superoxide dismutase (SOD) activity changes, decreased rate of release, and increased degradation of mediators, have also been investigated. These protective mechanisms could be involved in the tolerance to ozone appearing in animals chronically exposed to the gas. Many respiratory alterations induced by ozone have been found to diminish or disappear when this exposure is repeated for several days. This tolerance has been demonstrated for the ozone-induced anatomic changes as well as for the functionally deleterious effect and hyperresponsiveness to substance P. The real impact of ozone in domestic animals remains to be established.

Other photochemical compounds, such as peroxyacetyl nitrate (PAN), acrolein, and acetaldehyde, are present in photochemical smog. Another chemical oxidant is nitrogen dioxide produced in very large quantities by burning fossil fuels. Nitrogen dioxide is formed principally from nitric oxide emitted by combustion processes. Conversion of nitric oxide to nitrogen dioxide is rapid in the presence of ozone, as shown in Figure 5.21. As in the case of ozone, oxidant attack on components of cell membranes appears to be a major cause of lung injury.

Particulate Air Pollution. This includes particles with a very wide range of sizes, concentrations, and natures. These properties are very important because the pathophysiology processes associated with the particles' exposure depend on the physical, chemical, and biological characteristics of each one, so their size, their charge, their composition, and their ability to adsorb other pollutants play very important roles indeed and may influence their mechanism of toxicological damage. Indeed, as shown in Figure 5.22, the particle size dictates the quantities and regional deposition of the particle.

In human cases of professional occupational diseases, many have been related to inhalation of particles. The term *pneumoconiosis* refers to parenchymal lung disease induced by inorganic dust inhalation. In this category would fall diseases observed in coal workers, such as silicosis associated with inhalation of silica and asbestos-related diseases. A variety of other dusts cause pneumoconiosis: iron and its oxides causing siderosis, antimony, cadmium, and tin. Depending on the type of particles, their size, and their concentrations, deposition of aerosols in the lungs by impaction, sedimentation, and diffusion may vary considerably, inducing a wide range of pathological changes. Chronic bronchitis, emphy-

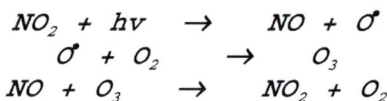

FIG. 5.22—Deposition pattern of particles in the respiratory tract. The size range of particles plays an important role. The larger particles are stopped in the upper respiratory tract, whereas the smaller particles are arrested in the terminal airway (bronchioles and alveoli) when the air velocity slows. The fraction of the atmospheric particles that is capable of entering the respiratory tract via the nose or mouth is defined as the *inhalable* fraction (<100 μm). If the size of particles decreases so they can penetrate farther into the respiratory tract and reach the alveolar region, this is the *respirable* fraction of the atmosphere. The upper size range of this fraction is 10 μm (<10 μm or PM_{10}). The finer part of PM_{10} (<2.5 μm) will penetrate easier to the alveoli, and this fraction is labeled $PM_{2.5}$. Note that these size ranges of the inhalable fraction and the respirable fraction can vary between species as a function of anatomic or physiological differences.

sema, and fibrosis with a reduction in arterial oxygen pressure, a rise in residual volume, and a reduction in forced expiratory volume due to a mixed obstructive and restrictive pattern can be variously combined.

In human cases of inhaled asbestos and cigarette smoke, bronchial carcinoma is a common complication. Pleural diseases are also recognized. Cigarette smoke contains particles but also many other agents, such as carbon monoxide, in a sufficient amount to raise the carboxyhemoglobin level in active or passive smoker's blood; nicotine, which stimulates the autonomic nervous system, causing tachycardia; hypertension; sweating; nausea; and aromatic hydrocarbons associated with bronchial carcinoma. Many pets, such as dogs and cats, are "passive smokers," but the real impact of this pollution in these species has not been determined.

Vehicle pollution and particularly diesel exhaust emissions, which contribute to particulate air pollution, adsorb trace amounts of heavy metals, such as iron, copper, chromium, and nickel, and a vast number of organic compounds, such as aliphatic hydrocarbons. These adsorbed organic compounds play an important role in the release of inflammatory mediators such as cytokines. It has also been shown that these diesel particles induce asthmatic symptoms in mice after intratracheal instillation. These diesel exhaust emissions contribute to formation of fine (<2.5 μm) and ultrafine (<100 nm) atmospheric particles.

Some examples can be cited to illustrate the implication of high levels of particulate air pollution in the alteration of human or animal health with excess morbidity and mortality. The first well-known episode is

$$NO_2 + h\nu \rightarrow NO + O$$
$$O + O_2 \rightarrow O_3$$
$$NO + O_3 \rightarrow NO_2 + O_2$$

FIG. 5.21—Reactions occurring when nitrogen dioxide absorbs solar radiation. First, the reaction may be driven to the right by the presence of catalysts such as volatile organic compounds. The rate of ozone production can increase greatly, especially in hot, sunny weather.

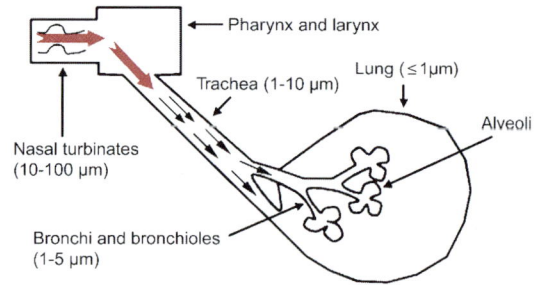

the 1930 Meuse Valley tragedy in Belgium. The next similar episodes occurred in London (1952–1962), where coal was widely used for domestic heating and industrial purposes, New York City, Paris, Rome, Mexico City, Steubenville (Ohio), and a lot of industrial megalopolises. These peaks of pollution were associated with the development of urban automotive transport (vehicle emission), manufacturing, and power generation, with often notable seasonal exposure.

Byssinosis is associated with inhaled organic dusts causing airway reactions. This is well known to occur from cotton-dust exposure. It leads to the release of mediators, such as histamine, resulting in bronchoconstriction and cough. After long-term exposure, permanent impairment of lung function similar to that observed in heaves-affected horses can develop. Occupational asthma can also be associated with allergenic organic dusts. Farmers' lung is a classic example of extrinsic allergic alveolitis. The role of biological particles like pollen are also well known because they produce hay fever every summer and spring.

Dust in animal facilities is a mostly organic mixture of animal and vegetable material. Animal dust derives from scales, fecal material, and dried urine, whereas vegetable dust derives from litter and feed. Feed particles are large and constitute the bulk of the dust, but there are many other constituents, such as bacteria, molds, other microorganisms, insect parts, chemical additives, and endotoxins. Inhalation of feed flour did not affect nasal mucosa but did induce bronchial airway inflammation in pigs with an increased number of macrophages and lymphocytes, as shown in Figure 5.23, without changes observed in CD4/CD8. A recent study demonstrated that dustborne endotoxins did not have effects attributable to endotoxin alone. However, the latter can enhance the sensitivity to biological agents. Another classic example of respiratory disease associated with dust in animal environments is heaves in horses.

RESPIRATORY CLEARANCE AND ATMOSPHERIC POLLUTANTS.

Particles that are deposited in bronchi and alveoli, and dissolved substances in the mucous layer, are efficiently removed from the lungs. Two distinct clearance mechanisms are involved: the mucociliary system and the alveolar macrophages. Coughing and sneezing are also two efficient mechanical mechanisms that assist in the process.

Bronchial seromucous glands and goblet cells produce the mucus. The superficial gel layer is viscous, allowing the deposited particles to be trapped. The deeper sol layer is less viscous, allowing the cilia to beat and the elimination of mucus to the pharynx, where it is swallowed. As previously mentioned, cough and expectoration can improve the clearance. Although the clearance may be stimulated in response to pollution in a first phase, many pollutants (e.g., ammonia, sulfur dioxide, nitrogen dioxide, and cigarette smoke) can paralyze or destroy the cilia. Some biological agents, such as *Mycoplasma hyopneumoniae*, can also

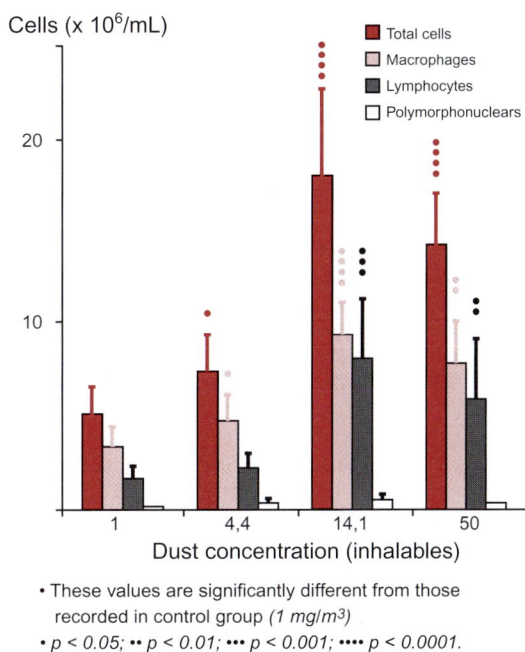

FIG. 5.23—Total cells, macrophages, lymphocytes, and neutrophils in pig bronchoalveolar lavage (BAL) after dust exposition versus control group. (From Urbain et al. 1999.)

adhere to porcine ciliated respiratory tract cells and seem to provoke the destruction of the cilia. Morphological alterations can also occur as observed in piglets exposed to ammonia. When acute airway inflammation is induced, bronchial epithelium may be denuded. Moreover, changes in mechanical properties of mucus and an increase in mucus production in response to airway inflammation are also well documented, leading to decreased clearance efficiency. All of these functional and morphological modifications can induce mucous plugging of bronchi, as in asthma, chronic obstructive pulmonary disease (COPD), and chronic bronchitis with alteration of gas exchanges in the lungs.

Drugs like clenbuterol can raise the mucus production and ciliary beats so that clearance is increased. However, when cilia are paralyzed or destroyed, this drug can alter gas exchanges due to mucous plugging of bronchi. Pollution is generally thought to induce cough by stimulating the mechanical and chemical receptors located in the larynx and airways. The coughing effect caused by ammonia at high concentration is well described in pigs, horses, and rabbits. However, by interacting with neurokinins released from C fibers in airways, ammonia, at low concentrations (30 ppm), can inhibit the reflex, illustrating the complexity of the mechanisms involved. The inhibiting effect of ammonia on bacterial clearance in young piglets exposed to 50 ppm for 2 hours has been described and known for over 20 years.

Macrophages also play an important role in clearing biological and particulate matter form the alveolar space. When they phagocytose a foreign body, they either migrate to the small bronchi, where they are eliminated by the mucociliary escalator, or they leave the lung by way of lymphatics or possibly the blood. This effective system can be overloaded when the dust burden is abnormally increased. Macrophages can migrate through the walls of respiratory bronchioles, where particles can exert their toxic effects through the release of inflammatory mediators. On the other hand, macrophagic activity can be inhibited by a great number of environmental factors, such as ozone, oxidant gases, ammonia, and drugs as inhaled and systemic steroidal anti-inflammatory compounds.

SOME SYSTEMIC POLLUTANTS

Toxic Bipyridyl Herbicides: Paraquat and Diquat. A classic example of a restrictive disorder after poisoning is paraquat toxicosis. Paraquat is a dipyridyl pesticide used as a contact herbicide for agriculture and for home use and horticulture. Paraquat exerts a selective lung toxicity producing fibrosis after acute alveolitis. Diquat, another dipyridyl herbicide, does not have a prominent pulmonary action because diquat pulmonary retention is lower than paraquat lung retention.

Paraquat disturbs normal biochemical processes and is able to initiate redox cycling and produce reactive oxygen species (free radicals). The latter can oxidize protein and deoxyribonucleic acid and facilitate lipid peroxidation. Depletion of NADPH may contribute to paraquat toxicity.

When cellular death occurs, the release of some cellular constituents may also lead to the generation of other reactive oxygen species. Some protective mechanisms shown in Figure 5.24 exist but are often insufficient cases of severe poisoning.

External exposure can give rise to mouth lesions, dermal irritation, and corneal opacity. After ingestion, the symptomatology of paraquat poisoning occurs in two phases. The first one begins with gastrointestinal symptoms and decreased kidney function but is often followed by a clinical improvement unless a massive dose has been ingested. In the second phase, occurring within about 7 days, severe pulmonary damage gradually develops. The targets are the type I and II pneumocytes, the capillaries, and the terminal bronchioles. This destructive stage is followed by a proliferative phase. At this point, the alveolar spaces are colonized by cells and fibroblasts producing abnormal collagen, which results in lung fibrosis. The macrophages appear to play an important role, although other inflammatory cells may be involved. The final reduction in compliance, a measure of the lung's elastic properties, and the impairment of gaseous diffusion alter the physiological lung function.

Ruminal Generation of Toxicants. The highly reducing environment created by anaerobic ruminal microbiota can give rise to toxic chemical agents in the forestomach and these may be absorbed from the digestive tract. Examples include

1. Accumulation of nitrate in crop and pasture plants and in weeds, especially where high levels of nitrogen fertilizer have been applied or herbicides are used. Often, runoff water and silo seepage are high in nitrates. In the bovine rumen, the nitrate is reduced to the much more toxic nitrite by bacterial nitrate reductase, a molybdenum-containing enzyme. Under normal circumstances, nitrite is rapidly utilized for ammonia synthesis, but, in cases of excessive acute intake of nitrate, the nitrite ion is absorbed into the bloodstream.

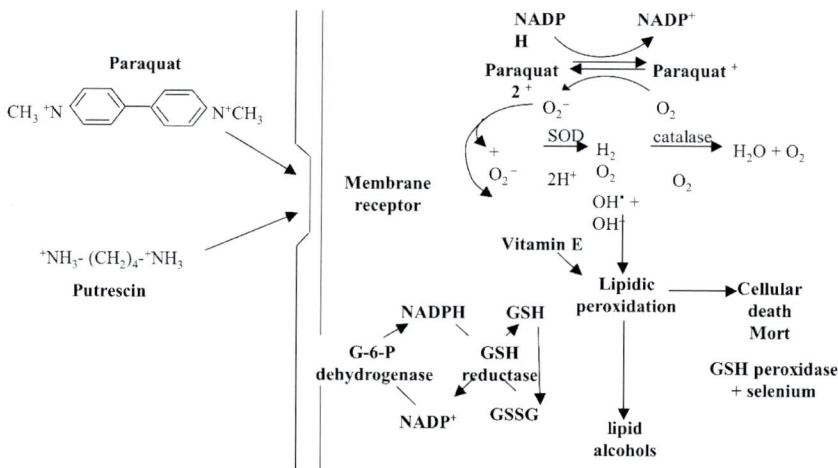

FIG. 5.24—Mechanism of toxicological damage caused by paraquat. The paraquat is bound together with a putrescine receptor. Next, the paraquat is able to initiate oxydo-redox cycling and produce reactive oxygen species. The protective effects of vitamin E, catalase, and glutathione peroxidase are also shown. G-6-P, glucose-6-phosphate; GSH, γ-glutamylcysteinylglycine; GSSG, oxidized form of glutathione; and SOD, superoxide dismutase.

When nitrite is absorbed, it reacts with hemoglobin (which contains ferrous iron), converting it to methemoglobin, in which the iron is in the ferric form and cannot carry oxygen. The outcome is brownish blood and severe hypoxia plus hypotension and tachycardia resulting from the vasodilation effect of the nitrite. Dyspnea and tachypnea are observed to compensate for the anoxia along with anxiety that can progress to anoxic convulsions and death.

2. 3-Methylindol toxicosis: Acute bovine pulmonary edema emphysema (ABPE), or fog fever, is an acute respiratory distress syndrome that may occur in maturing cattle when they are moved from dry-land pastures to lush, succulent forage, especially after hay or silage has been cut. The available evidence supports the view that fog fever is caused by 3-methylindol (3-MI), a ruminal fermentation product of ingested L-tryptophan in herbage. The 3-MI is absorbed into the bloodstream from the rumen and metabolized by a mixed-function oxidase (MFO) system in the lung to produce pneumotoxicity. 3-MI causes necrosis of type 1 pneumocytes and bronchial cells, followed by proliferation of type 2 alveolar cells plus the formation of a hyaline membrane. The 3-MI taken up by the lungs is metabolized by MFOs in type 1 pneumocytes or Clara cells and prostaglandin-H synthetase. This metabolic activation within the lung causes severe damage to epithelial cells.

The clinical signs include hyperpnea with severe dyspnea and an expiratory grunt, and a tendency to extend the head, protrude the tongue, and breathe orally, often with some frothing. Respiratory sounds are not pronounced. Mortality is high. On autopsy, the lungs are enlarged and edematous with emphysema. Calves treated experimentally with 3-MI develop signs of ABPE within 24 hours and show a large increase in respiratory frequency, minute viscous work, and $PaCO_2$ accompanied by a large decrease in tidal volume, dynamic compliance, and PaO_2. Pulmonary edema and alveolar damage are present on necropsy.

Plant Toxicosis. Some plants cause pulmonary toxicosis. *Ipomea batata* (sweet potato), sometimes used as livestock feed, can be infested by *Fusarium solani* that produces a substituted furan mycotoxin that causes acute pulmonary emphysema in cattle. Mixed function oxidases (MFOs) activate the substituted furans. Type 1 pneumocytes are damaged, producing emphysema and edema, and type 2 pneumocytes proliferate to replace type 1 cells, leading to the impairment of gaseous diffusion.

Organophosphate and Carbamate Poisoning. The organophosphate and carbamate families include several different chemical compounds widely used in agriculture and veterinary medicine as insecticides or as anthelmintics. Accidental or negligent poisoning has become a serious public health problem due to the severity of lesions and symptoms (3 million cases of severe poisoning and 22,000 deaths every year worldwide).

An identical chemical structure is shared by all organophosphate compounds. They are either aliphatic carbon, cyclic, or heterocyclic phosphate esters. In organothiophosphate, the double-bonded oxygen is replaced with a sulfur molecule. The chemical family of carbamates is comprised of cyclic or aliphatic derivatives of carbamic acid. These compounds have some proprieties analogous to those of organophosphates.

Their high liposolubility makes these compounds easily absorbed by different routes, and their slow organic degradation favors their accumulation in the body. In case of organothiophosphate, the pesticide must be biotransformed involving cytochrome P-450 activity in lung tissue into more active molecules in order to achieve biological activity. The difference in sensitivity to organophosphates between males and females may be due to sexually related differences in the cytochrome P-450 activity. The active form markedly inhibits cholinesterase activity, leading to an increase in acetylcholine effects.

Pulmonary edema involving acetylcholine and tachykinins, airway obstruction, and hyperreactivity to acetylcholine and histamine and mucus production are the main mechanisms involved in the toxicity of these substances (Figure 5.25). Administration of β-adrener-

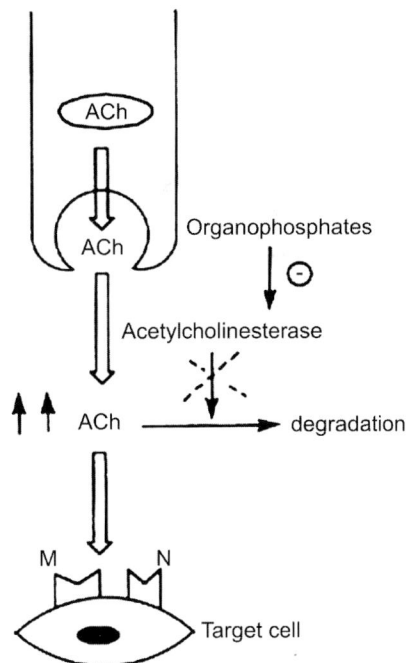

FIG. 5.25—Mechanism of toxicological action. This figure shows the inhibition of acetylcholinesterase by an organophosphorus or carbamate. This inhibition causes acetylcholine (ACh) accumulation and excessive synaptic neurotransmitter activity in the parasympathetic (cholinergic) nervous system and at neuromuscular (nicotinic) sites.

gic agonists seems to improve the airway obstruction only transiently, perhaps via a stimulation of prejunctional β_2-adrenoceptors enhancing acetylcholine release from cholinergic nerves. Atropine and other anticholinergic drugs remain the main antidotes. A decrease in dynamic compliance and arterial oxygen tension, and an increase in total pulmonary resistance and alveolar arterial oxygen gradient, are the main functional changes occurring in all animal species.

REFERENCES

Alexander AF, Will DH, Grover RF, Reeves JT. 1960. Pulmonary hypertension and right ventricular hypertrophy in cattle at high altitude. Am J Vet Res 21:199–204.

Amis TC, Smith MM, Gaber CE, Kurpershoek C. 1986. Upper airway obstruction in canine laryngeal paralysis. Am J Vet Res 47:1007–1010.

Amory H, Lomba F, Lekeux P, et al. 1994. Bilateral diaphragmatic paralysis of unknown origin in a pony. J Am Vet Med Assoc 205:587–591.

Anthonisen NR. 1977. Regional lung function in spontaneous pneumothorax. Am Rev Respir Dis 115:873–876.

Art T, Serteyn D, Lekeux P. 1988. Effect of exercise on the partitioning of equine respiratory resistance. Equine Vet J 20:268–273.

Art T, Anderson L, Woakes AJ, et al. 1990. Mechanics of breathing during strenuous exercise in thoroughbred horses. Respir Physiol 82:279–294.

Aukland K, Nicolaysen G. 1981. Interstitial fluid volume: Local regulation mechanism. Physiological Reviews 61:556–643.

Backer JC, Ellis JA, Clark EG. 1997. Bovine respiratory syncytial virus. Vet Clin North Am Food Anim Pract 13:425–454.

Bisgard GE, Orr JA, Will JA. 1975. Hypoxic pulmonary hypertension in the pony. Am J Vet Res 36:49–52.

Bonagura JD, Darke PGG. 1995. Congenital heart disease. In: Ettinger SJ, Feldman EC, eds. Veterinary Internal Medicine, 4th ed. Philadelphia: WB Saunders, pp 892–943.

Breeze RG. 1985. Respiratory disease in adult cattle. Vet Clin North Am Food Anim Pract 1:311–346.

Brigham KL, Bowers R, Haynes J. 1979. Increased sheep lung vascular permeability caused by *Escherichia coli* endotoxemia. Circ Res 45:292–297.

Clercx C, Van den Brom WE, Van den Ingh TSGAM, De Vries HW. 1989a. Scintigraphical analysis as a diagnostic tool in canine experimental lung embolism. Lung 167:225–236.

Clercx C, Van den Brom WE, Stokhof AA, De Vries HW. 1989b. Pulmonary scintigraphy in canine lobar and sublobar airway obstruction. Lung 167:213–224.

Clercx C, Venker-van Haagen AJ, Den Breejen JN, et al. 1989c. Effects of age and breed on the phospholipid composition of canine surfactant. Lung 167:351–357.

Clercx C, Coignoul F, Mainil J, et al. 1992. Canine tuberculosis: A case report and review of the literature. J Am Anim Hosp Assoc 28:207–211.

Crystal RG, Ferrans VJ, Basset F. 1991. Biologic basis of pulmonary fibrosis. In: Crystal RG, West JB, eds. The Lung: Scientific Foundations. New York: Raven, pp 2031–2046.

Dantzker DR, Wagner PD, Tornabene VM, et al. 1978. Gas exchange after pulmonary thromboembolism in dogs. Circ Res 42:92–103.

Derksen FJ, Slocombe RF, Brown CM, et al. 1982. Chronic restrictive pulmonary disease in a horse. J Am Vet Med Assoc 180:887–889.

Derksen FJ, Scott EA, Stick JA, et al. 1986. Effect of laryngeal hemiplegia and laryngoplasty on upper airway flow mechanics in exercising horses. Am J Vet Res 47:16–20.

Desmecht D, Linden A, Lekeux P. 1995. Pathophysiological response of bovine diaphragm function to gastric distension. J Appl Physiol 78:1537–1546.

Desmecht D, Linden A, Lekeux P. 1996. The relation of ventilatory failure to pulmonary, systemic, respiratory muscle, and central nervous system disturbances in calves with an experimentally produced pneumonia. J Comp Pathol 115:203–219.

Dixon PM. 1978. Pulmonary artery pressures in normal horses and in horses affected with chronic obstructive pulmonary disease. Equine Vet J 10:195–198.

Drummond JG, Curtis SE, Simon J. 1978. Effects of atmospheric ammonia on pulmonary bacterial clearance in the young pig. Am J Vet Res 39:211–212.

Edwards WD. 1988. Pathology of pulmonary hypertension. Cardiovasc Clin 18:321–359.

Erickson BK, Erickson HH, Coffman JR. 1992. Pulmonary artery and aortic pressure changes during high intensity treadmill exercise in the horse: Effect of furosemide and phentolamine. Equine Vet J 24:215–219.

Gibson EA, Blackmore RJJ, Wijeratne WVS, Wrathall AE. 1976. The "barker" (neonatal respiratory distress) syndrome in the pig: Its occurrence in the field. Vet Rec 98:476–479.

Hawkins EC. 1998. Disorders of the lung parenchyma. In: Nelson RW, Couto CG, eds. Small Animal Internal Medicine, 2nd ed. St Louis: CV Mosby, pp 297–305.

Holcombe SJ, Derksen FJ, Stick JA, Robinson NE. 1997. Effects of bilateral hypoglossal and glossopharyngeal nerve blocks on epiglottic and soft palate position in exercising horses. Am J Vet Res 58:1022–1026.

Jerram RM, Fossum TW. 1997. Tracheal collapse in dogs. Compend Continuing Educ Pract Vet 19:1049–1060.

Koterba AM, Paradis MR. 1990. Specific respiratory conditions. In: Koterba AM, Drummond WH, Kosch PC, eds. Equine Clinical Neonatalogy. Philadelphia: Lea and Febiger, pp 177–199.

Langsetmo I, Fedde MR, Meyer TS, Erickson HH. 2000. Relationship of pulmonary arterial pressure to pulmonary haemorrhage in exercising horses. Equine Vet J 32:379–384.

Lekeux P, Art T. 1987. Functional changes induced by necrotic laryngitis in double-muscled calves. Vet Rec 121:353–355.

Lekeux P, Hajer R, Breukink HJ. 1985a. Longitudinal study of the effects of lungworm infection on bovine pulmonary function. Am J Vet Res 46:1392–1395.

Lekeux P, Hajer R, Van den Ingh TS, Breukink HJ. 1985b. Pathophysiologic study of 3-methylindole-induced pulmonary toxicosis in immature cattle. Am J Vet Res 46:1629–1631.

Lekeux P, Verhoeff J, Hajer R, Breukink HJ. 1985c. Respiratory syncytial virus pneumonia in Friesian calves: Physiological findings. Res Vet Sci 39:324–327.

Linden A, Desmecht D, Amory H, et al. 1995. Pulmonary ventilation, mechanics, gas exchange and haemodynamics in calves following intratracheal inoculation of *Pasteurella haemolytica*. J Vet Med [A] 42:531–544.

Maas J, Parish SM, Hodgson DR, Valberg SJ. 1996. Nutritional myodegeneration. In: Smith BP, ed. Large Animal Internal Medicine. St Louis: Mosby Year Book, pp 1513–1518.

Malik AB. 1983. Pulmonary microembolism. Physiol Rev 63:1114–1207.

McGorum BC, Ellison J, Cullen RT. 1998. Total and respirable airborne dust endotoxin concentrations in three equine management systems. Equine Vet J 30:430–434.

Mead J, Takishima T, Leith D. 1970. Stress distribution in lungs: A model of pulmonary elasticity. J Appl Physiol 28:596–608.

Moise NS, Spaulding GL. 1981. Feline bronchial asthma:

Pathogenesis, pathophysiology, diagnostics, and therapeutic considerations. Compend Continuing Educ Pract Vet 3:1091–1102.

Moulton JE, Von Tscharner C, Schneider R. 1981. Classification of lung carcinomas in the dogs and cats. Vet Pathol 18:513–528.

Noone KE. 1985. Pleural effusions and diseases of the pleura. Vet Clin North Am Small Anim Pract 15:1069–1084.

Palmarani M, Fan H, Sharp JM. 1997. Sheep pulmonary adenomatosis: A unique model of retrovirus-associated lung cancer. Trends Microbiol 5:478–483.

Pattle RE, Rossdale PD, Schock C, Creasey JM. 1975. The development of the lung and its surfactant in the foal and in other species. J Reprod Fertil Suppl 23:651–657.

Pépin M, Vitu C, Russo P, et al. 1998. Maedi-visna virus infection in sheep: A review. Vet Res 29:341–367.

Robinson NE. 1982. Some functional consequences of species differences in lung anatomy. Adv Vet Sci Comp Med 26:1–33.

Robinson NE. 2001. International workshop on equine chronic airway disease. Equine Vet J 33:5–19.

Robinson NE, Sorenson PR. 1978. Collateral flow resistance and time constant in dog and horse lungs. J Appl Physiol 44:63–68.

Roudebush P. 1990. Bacterial infections of the respiratory system. In: GE Greene, ed. Infectious Diseases of the Dog and Cat. Philadelphia: WB Saunders, pp 114–125.

Staub NC. 1984. Pathophysiology of pulmonary edema. In: Staub NC, Taylor AE, eds. Edema. New York: Raven, pp 719–786.

Sundberg JP, Burstein T, Page EH, et al. 1977. Neoplasms of Equidae. J Am Vet Med Assoc 170:150–152.

Tetens J, Derksen FJ, Stick JA, et al. 1996. Efficacy of prosthetic laryngoplasty with and without bilateral ventriculocordectomy as treatments for laryngeal hemiplegia in horses. Am J Vet Res 57:1668–1673.

Thrall DE, Badertscher RR, McCall JW, Lewis RE. 1979. The pulmonary arterial circulation in dogs experimentally infected with *Dirofilaria immitis*: Its angiographic evaluation. J Am Vet Radiol Soc 20:74–78.

Tucker A, McMurtry IF, Reeves JT, et al. 1975. Lung vascular smooth muscle as a determinant of pulmonary hypertension at high altitude. Am J Physiol 228:762–767.

Uystepruyst C, Coghe J, Dorts T, et al. 2002. Optimal timing of elective caesarean section in Belgian White and Blue breed of cattle: the calf's point of view. Vet J 163:267–282.

Venker-van Haagen AJ. 1979. Bronchoscopy of the normal and abnormal canine. J Am Anim Hosp Assoc 15:397–410.

Venker-van Haagen AJ. 1992. Diseases of the larynx. Vet Clin North Am Small Anim Pract 22:1155–1174.

Votion D. 1999. Scintigraphy of the equine lung. Equine Vet Educ 11:300–309.

Votion D, Roberts C, Marlin D, Lekeux P. 1999. Feasibility of scintigraphy in exercise-induced pulmonary detection and quantification: Preliminary studies. Equine Vet J 30(Suppl):137–142.

West JB, Mathieu-Costello O, Jones JH, et al. 1993. Stress failure of pulmonaries in racehorses with exercise-induced pulmonary hemorrhage. J Appl Physiol 75:1097–1109.

Will DH, Alexander AF, Reeves JT, Grover RF. 1962. High altitude-induced pulmonary hypertension in normal cattle. Circ Res 10:172–177.

Willoughby R, Ecker G, McKee S, et al. 1992. The effects of equine rhinovirus, influenza virus and herpesvirus infection on tracheal clearance rate in horses. Can J Vet Res 56:115–121.

Wilson GP, Hayes HM. 1986. Diaphragmatic hernia in the dog and cat: A 25-year overview. Semin Vet Med Surg 1:318–326.

Additional Reading

Allen GK, Campbell-Beggs C, Robinson JA, et al. 1996. Induction of early-phase endotoxin tolerance in horses. Equine Vet J 28:269–274.

Chen JR, Lin JH, Weng CN, Lai SS. 1998. Identification of a novel adhesin-like glycoprotein from *Mycoplasma hyopneumoniae*. Vet Microbiol 62:97–110.

Clercx C, Gustin P, Landser FJ, Van de Woestijne KP. 1993. Measurement of total respiratory impedance in dogs by the forced oscillation technique. Vet Res Commun 17:227–239.

Delaunois A, Gustin P, Ansay M. 1992. Altered capillary filtration coefficient in parathion- and paraoxon-induced edema in isolated and perfused rabbit lungs. Toxicol Appl Pharmacol 116:161–169.

Dockery DW, Pope III CA. 1994. Acute respiratory effects of particulate air pollution. Annu Rev Public Health 15:107–132.

Doig PA, Willoughby RA. 1971. Response of swine to atmospheric ammonia and organic dust. J Am Vet Med Assoc 159:1353–1361.

Dosman JA, Graham BL, Hall D, et al. 1988. Respiratory symptoms and alterations in pulmonary function tests in swine producers in Saskatchewan: Results of a survey of farmers. J Occup Med 30:715–720.

Drummond J, Curtis S, Simon J, Norton H. 1980. Effects of aerial ammonia on growth and health of young pigs. J Anim Sci 50:1085.

Drummond JG, SE Curtis, RC Meyer, et al. 1981. Effects of atmospheric ammonia on young pigs experimentally infected with *Bordetella bronchiseptica*. Am J Vet Res 42:963–968.

Gustin P. 1997. Ozone-induced stimulation of pulmonary sympathetic fibers: A protective mechanism against edema. Toxicol Appl Pharmacol 147:71–82.

Gustin P, Urbain B, Prouvost JF, Ansay M. 1994. Effects of atmospheric ammonia on pulmonary hemodynamics and vascular permeability in pigs: Interaction with endotoxins. Toxicol Appl Pharmacol 125:17–26.

Kehrer JP. 1999. General and Applied Toxicology, 2 ed. London: Macmillan Reference.

Larsson K, Malmberg P, Eklund A, et al. 1988. Exposure to microorganisms, airway inflammatory changes and immune reactions in asymptomatic dairy farmers: Bronchoalveolar lavage evidence of macrophage activation and permeability changes in the airways. Int Arch Allergy Appl Immunol 87:127–133.

Lekeux P, Kyavu A, Clercx C, Ansay M. 1986. Pulmonary function changes induced by experimental dichlorvos toxicosis in calves. Res Vet Sci 40:318–321.

Lessire F, Gustin P, Delaunois A, et al. 1996. Relationship between parathion and paraoxon toxicokinetics, lung metabolic activity, and cholinesterase inhibition in guinea pig and rabbit lungs. Toxicol Appl Pharmacol 138:201–210.

Moreaux B, Nemmar A, Beerens D, Gustin P. 2000. Inhibiting effect of ammonia on citric acid-induced cough in pigs: Possible involvement of substance P. Pharmacol Toxicol 87:279–285.

Osweiler GD. 1996 Toxicology. Philadelphia: Williams and Wilkins.

Pope III CA, Thun MJ, Namboodiri MM, et al. 1995. Particulate air pollution as a predictor of mortality in a prospective study of U.S. adults. Am J Respir Crit Care Med 151:669–674.

Segura P, Chavez J, Montano LM, et al. 1999. Identification of mechanisms involved in the acute airway toxicity induced by parathion. Naunyn Schmiedebergs Arch Pharmacol 360:699–710.

Urbain B, Prouvost J, Beerens D, et al. 1996. Acute effects of endotoxin inhalation on the respiratory tract in pigs: Interaction with ammonia. Inhalation Toxicol 8:947–968.

Urbain B, Mast J, Beerens D, et al. 1999. Effects of inhalation of dust and endotoxin on respiratory tracts of pigs. Am J Vet Res 60:1055–1060.

Vargas MH, Romero L, Sommer B, et al. 1998. Chronic exposure to ozone causes tolerance to airway hyperresponsiveness in guinea pigs: Lack of SOD role. J Appl Physiol 84:1749–1755.

Zielinski GC, Ross RF. 1993. Adherence of *Mycoplasma hyopneumoniae* to porcine ciliated respiratory tract cells. Am J Vet Res 54:1262–1269.

PATHOPHYSIOLOGY OF CARDIOVASCULAR DISEASE

Robert L. Hamlin and Arnold A. Stokhof

The role of the cardiovascular system is to bring each of the trillions of cells comprising the body into contact with the outside environment so that (a) substrates and oxygen can be delivered to the cells to produce the adenosine triphosphate (ATP) necessary to fuel all life processes, (b) carbon dioxide, hydrogen ions, and nitrogenous wastes can be removed from the cells to sustain a constant internal milieu, and (c) calories produced by the cells can be released to the environment to sustain near constancy of temperature. It does this through a system of blood vessels, in which substances are carried by the blood, which moved by pressure differences generated by contraction of the heart.

PART 1: THE CARDIOVASCULAR SYSTEM AS A BIOLOGICAL CONTROL SYSTEM

ROBERT L. HAMLIN AND ARNOLD A. STOKHOF

The cardiovascular system achieves its goals when a number of physiological variables are controlled to within physiological limits (Figure 6.1). When one or more variables are outside of normal limits, cardiovascular disease is present, and the patient is showing signs or symptoms. These variables—termed controlled variables—are (a) systemic arterial blood pressure (sustained at approximately 100 mm Hg), (b) cardiac output (sustained at approximately 100 mL/kg/min), (c) blood volume (sustained at approximately 7% of body weight), and (d) stroke volume (sustained at approximately 1.5 mL/kg). The controllers of the levels of the controlled variables are (a) the force and rate of contraction of the heart, (b) the degree of constriction or relaxation of blood vessels, and (c) the thirst center determining water consumption and the kidneys determining water loss. Sensors of the levels of the controlled variables—the level detectors—are (a) high-pressure baroreceptors in the aortic and carotid sinuses, which measure the tension in the arterial walls, (b) the juxtaglomerular apparatus in the kidneys, which measures the amount of sodium delivered in the blood to the kidneys, (c) the low-pressure volume receptors principally in the left atrium, which measure the degree of stretch of the atrium, and (d) mechanoreceptors within the wall of the left ventricle, which measure the degree of motion of the wall. Information, principally in terms of neural signals, is sent (as a negative signal) from the level detectors to the medulla oblongata—considered the integrator of the biological control system—where comparisons are made with the levels (sent as a positive signal) of the controlled variable considered optimal for survival (the set-points). The summation of the negative input from the level detectors with the positive signal as the set-point is termed an *error signal*, a neuroendocrine signal that "instructs" the controllers what they should do to achieve or to sustain a proper value for the controlled variables. When a signal (termed an *etiologic factor*) perturbs the level of one or more of the controlled variables so that, despite activity of the controllers, the variable(s) is (are) outside of normal limits, the patient is said to have cardiovascular disease (Figure 6.1).

TRANSITION FROM FETAL TO NEONATAL CIRCULATION. Abnormalities in the transition from the fetal to the neonatal circulation result in a pathological circulation that often produces life-threatening or seriously impairing disease. An important example is patent ductus arteriosus, one of the more common congenital heart diseases.

Ventilation of a fetus submerged in amniotic fluid would not result in oxygenation of pulmonary capillary blood. Rather, fetal oxygenation occurs solely from the placental circulation. The umbilical vein from the placenta carries fully oxygenated blood from the placenta. Approximately half of this oxygenated umbilical venous blood returns to the fetus through the fetal liver while half bypasses the liver through the ductus venosus, but all enters the right atrium through the caudal vena cava. There the vast majority "streamlines" through the patent foramen ovale from right atrium to left atrium. The small volume of blood that does not traverse the foramen ovale, along with the fetal venous blood from the cranial vena cava, enters the right ventricle. From there, it is ejected into the pulmonary trunk, but bypasses the lungs by traversing the ductus arteriosus from the pulmonary trunk to the aorta. For this reason, very little blood actually traverses the pulmonary capillaries in the fetus.

The blood traverses both the foramen ovale and the ductus arteriosus from the right side of the circulation (i.e., right atrium, right ventricle, and pulmonary trunk) to the left side (i.e., left atrium, left ventricle, and aorta) because, in the fetus, pressures in the right side normally exceed those in the left side. Aortic pressure is lower than the pressure in the pulmonary trunk because the resistance to flow through the lungs is greater than the resistance to flow from the aorta through the systemic arterial circulation. The systemic resistance is low because of the placental circulation that serves as a low-resistance shunt.

At birth, ventilation decreases pulmonary vascular resistance and pulmonary arterial pressure; ligation of the umbilicus removes the placental circulation, thus

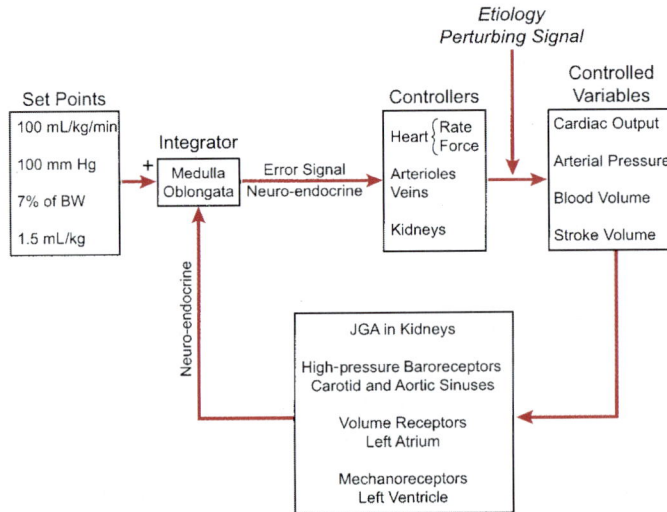

FIG. 6.1—Conceptual model of the cardiovascular system as a biological control system. Variables to be controlled are determined by activity of the controllers. The controllers are activated by the output of the medulla oblongata (the integrator). The output of the integrator is the result of input from the level detectors and the set-points—the desired levels of the controlled variables. The level detectors are placed strategically within the system so that they monitor the level of controlled variables where the values are most important. An etiologic force perturbs the level of the controlled variable, and activity of the biological control system returns the value of the controlled variable to a level not different from that in the set-point. The signals between the integrator and the controllers and between the level detectors and the integrator are either neural or endocrine. If levels of controlled variables approximate those of the set-point, cardiovascular health exists. BW, body weight; and JGA, juxtaglomerular apparatus.

increasing the systemic vascular resistance and pressure; and the flow of blood, which had been from right to left, reverses and becomes left to right through the ductus. Normally, however, soon after birth, both the foramen ovale and the ductus arteriosus close, thus terminating the shunts and isolating the left heart from the right heart except through the normal capillary circulations. The ductus arteriosus closes because the smooth muscle in its walls is stimulated by the elevation of the partial pressure of oxygen. Prostaglandins appear to be the messengers by which increased partial pressure of oxygen constricts smooth muscle in the ductus arteriosus. The elevation in partial pressure of oxygen results from the improved oxygenation of the blood by the efficient ventilation of the neonate, and by the fact that fully oxygenated blood is not mixed with venous blood as in the fetal circulation.

If, because of a hereditary deficiency in smooth muscle reactivity in the ductal wall, the ductus fails to close, then blood will flow continuously from the aorta to the pulmonary trunk through the patent ductus arteriosus. This results in the pulmonary circulation carrying much more blood (up to five times more) than the systemic circulation, and in dilatation of the left atrium, left ventricle, and the entire pulmonary circulation. If chronic distension of the left ventricle is severe, the ventricle may fail in its ability to empty blood from the lungs, and pulmonary venous and capillary pressures elevate, producing pulmonary congestion and/or edema. Patent ductus arteriosus is treated surgically by either ligating the communication or obstructing it with a coil inserted with a cardiac catheter.

OHM'S AND POISEUILLE'S LAWS. These two laws address the flow of a substance (e.g., electrons or blood) through a channel (e.g., copper wire or blood vessels). Ohm's law states that the amount of electrical current (I = amperes) flowing through a wire is equal to the difference in pressure (E = volts) between the input and output of the wire divided by the resistance (R = ohms) to flow through the wire: $I = E/R$, which is an equation with which almost everyone is familiar and which is intuitively obvious; for example, the greater the voltage difference is and the lesser the resistance is, the greater the flow is. Poiseuille's law states that the amount (CO or Q = cardiac output) of blood flowing through a blood vessel is equal to the difference in pressure (mm Hg) between the input and output of the vessel divided by the resistance to flow (dyne-seconds centimeters^{-5}) through the vessel. But for the flow of blood, to make the equation more useful, other factors were added by Poiseuille: the length (l) of the vessel, the radius (r), to the fourth power of the vessel, the viscosity (η) of blood. Poiseuille added the numbers 8 and π for mathematical correctness. His equation says that cardiac output (CO or Q) is equal to the pressure difference (ΔP) between the aorta (or pulmonary trunk) and the right atrium (or left atrium) times π times the radii of the sum total of all arterioles raised to the

fourth power, all divided by 8 times the viscosity (η) of blood times the length (l) of the vessel: $Q = [\Delta P\ \pi r^4]/[8\ \eta\ l]$. To make the equation still more useful, 8, l, and π can be omitted because they are always constant, and η can usually be excluded because viscosity is determined principally by the packed-cell volume, which seldom varies enough to alter cardiac output.[1] Thus Poiseuille's equation can be reduced to $Q = [\Delta P\ r^4]/\eta$. In the Poiseuille relationship, compared with Ohm's law, r^4 is placed in the numerator, since obviously radius is the reciprocal of resistance. But it is equally obvious that, as the pressure gradient or radius increases, flow increases; and, as viscosity increases (i.e., the blood becomes thicker), flow decreases. What is not obvious is why radius is taken to the 4th power. Don't worry about that exponent—just know that if vessel radius increases only 10%, flow increases almost 50%, whereas if the radius is decreased only 10%, flow decreases more than 33%.

FUNCTIONS OF THE CARDIOVASCULAR SYSTEM

Rhythmicity (Automaticity and Chronotropy). Rhythmicity is a property possessed by four or more regions of the heart (Figure 6.2), which enables them to discharge spontaneously, that is, without efferent neural volleys coming from the brain or without stimulation from other regions. It is this discharge that is responsible for initiating the waves of depolarization that stimulate the heart to contract, thus determining the heart rate (HR). These regions, in decreasing order of rhythmicity, are (a) the sinoatrial node (SAN), (b) the internodal pathways [ridges of myocardium extending from SAN to atrioventricular (AV) node], (c) the AV junction, the tissues within the right atrium just contacting the AV node, (d) the His-Purkinje fibers (specialized conductive tissue that expedites the wave of depolarization through the ventricles, and (e) mid-myocardial (M) fibers located approximately midway between in the endocardium and epicardium of the left ventricle. Normally, the dominant pacemaker is the SAN, and only if for some reason it is depressed will the subsidiary pacemakers discharge.

The SAN has an intrinsic rate of discharge determined by how rapidly potassium, calcium, and sodium ions build up in the SAN's cells and cause the inside to become relatively positive to the outside (depolarized). The rate of discharge of the SAN determines HR, so HR is used to monitor the chronotropic property. The normal SAN will discharge approximately 100 times per minute—slower in larger animals and faster in smaller animals.[2] The rate of discharge of the SAN, and

---

1. Of course when a patient is anemic, viscosity may be reduced, and the pressure difference required to pump blood through a vessel may be lower than normal. Contrariwise, if a patient is polycythemic and the blood viscosity is elevated, the pressure difference required to pump blood through the vessel may be greater than normal.

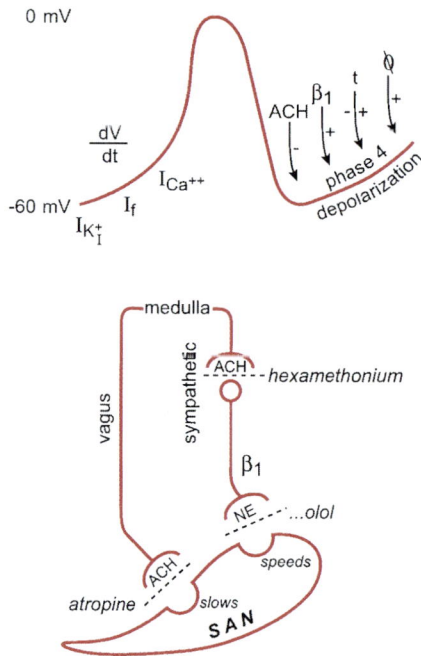

FIG. 6.2—Automaticity and chronotropy of the heart.
Bottom: The sinoatrial node (SAN) with autonomic, sympathetic, and parasympathetic (vagus) efferent nerves originating from the medulla oblongata. The SAN discharges automatically, but the rate of discharge can be accelerated when norepinephrine (NE) binds to β_1-adrenergic receptors, or decelerated when acetylcholine (ACH) binds to cholinergic receptors. The cholinergic receptors may be blocked by atropine (therefore, the rate of discharge of SAN increases) and adrenergic receptors may be blocked by drugs ending in …olol (therefore, the rate of discharge of SAN decreases). **Top:** The action potential from a typical SAN fiber that undergoes spontaneous, phase 4 depolarization—a drift in voltage from approximately 60 mV to a less negative value. This drift (dV/dt) occurs because positively charged ions (K^+, Na^+, and Ca^{++}) enter the cell through specific channels (IK^+, IF, and ICa^+) present in greatest density in the SAN. ACH decreases slope (slows heart rate), NE (the β_1-adrenergic mediator) increases slope (increases heart rate), an increase (+) in temperature (t) speeds heart rate, a decrease (−) in t decreases heart rate, an increase in tension (ϕ) speeds, and a decrease in ϕ slows rate of discharge.

therefore the HR, is influenced by the following factors (Shepherd and Vanhoutte 1979):

1. Stimulation of muscarinic cholinergic receptors[3] with acetylcholine produced by afferent volleys coming over the vagus nerves from the medulla oblongata slows the rate of discharge.

2. Stimulation of β_1-adrenergic receptors[4] with norepinephrine produced by afferent volleys coming over adrenergic nerves from the medulla oblongata speeds the rate of discharge.
3. Reduced temperature slows and increased temperature speeds rate of discharge.
4. Stretch of the SAN artery speeds rate of discharge of the SAN.
5. Hyperthyroidism accelerates and hypothyroidism decelerates the rate of discharge of the SAN.

An interesting relationship exists between HR and systemic arterial blood pressure (Figure 6.3). It is termed the *Marey reflex* because it was described first by the French veterinarian Etienne Marey (Wiggers 1975). The Marey reflex accounts for an inverse relationship between HR and arterial pressure—the lower the blood pressure is, the higher is the HR; the higher the blood pressure is, the lower is the HR. The reflex pathway is comprised of (a) high-pressure baroreceptors (tension receptors in the aortic and carotid sinuses) that discharge volleys of nervous impulses proportional with the height of the systemic arterial pressure, (b) afferent communications from the receptors to the medulla oblongata over the glossopharyngeal (from the carotid sinus) and the vagus (from the aortic sinus) nerves, (c) the cardioregulatory centers in the medulla oblongata that communicate with the hypothalamus to "compare" the pressure, "reported" by the baroreceptors, to the desired pressure (the set-point), and (d) efferent volleys emanating from the medullary cardioregulatory centers over the vagus nerves to the SAN.

When systemic arterial pressure is too high, the baroreceptors (Vattner and Boettcher 1975, 1978) send increased afferent volleys to the medulla, the medulla then sends an increased number of efferent volleys over the vagus nerve to the SAN, and the rate of discharge of the SAN—and, of course, the HR—decreases. The reduction in HR decreases cardiac output, which returns systemic arterial blood pressure toward normal. In addition, cardioregulatory centers decrease the number of volleys to the systemic arterioles sent over adrenergic nerves, the arterioles dilate, systemic vascular resistance decreases, and arterial pressure returns toward normal. If systemic arterial pressure is too low, the baroreceptors send fewer afferent volleys to the medulla, and the medulla, recognizing that the pressure is too low, decreases the number of efferent volleys to the SAN, the rate of discharge of the SAN, and of course the HR speed, and systemic arterial pressure elevates toward normal. In addition, the cardioregulatory centers send, over adrenergic nerves, increasing numbers of afferent volleys to the systemic arterioles. This causes them to constrict, systemic vascular resistance increases, and systemic arterial pressure returns toward normal. When a patient hemorrhages and sys-

---

2. In fact, the inverse relationship between rate of discharge of the SAN and body mass holds only among species but not within species; that is, small and large dogs have the same rates of discharge, but the SAN of a mouse discharges much more rapidly than the SAN of a horse.

3. These receptors may be blocked by parasympatholytic agents like atropine or glycopyrrolate.

4. These receptors may be blocked by β-adrenergic blocking agents usually ending in …olol (e.g., atenolol and propranolol).

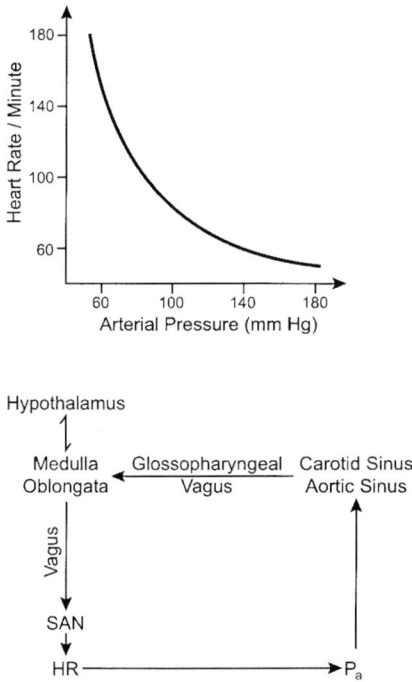

FIG. 6.3—Mechanism of the Marey reflex: heart rate and arterial pressure. **Top:** A graph of heart rate versus systemic arterial blood pressure, showing the inverse relationship between heart rate and pressure. This relationship is known as the Marey reflex, named after the French veterinarian Etienne Marey, who discovered it in the horse. **Bottom:** The Marey reflex begins with a change in systemic arterial pressure (P_a). This change is detected by high-pressure baroreceptors located in the carotid sinus and aortic sinus. The sinuses "report" the level detected in the sinuses over the glossopharyngeal and vagus nerves to the medulla oblongata. After "discussions" between the medulla oblongata and the hypothalamus, vagal efferent impulses are sent to the sinoatrial node (SAN), which either slows (if number of impulses increase) or speeds (if number of impulses decrease) the rate of discharge of the SAN. If P_a decreases, vagal efferent traffic to the SAN decreases, the rate of discharge of the SAN decreases, and the heart rate (HR) accelerates; if P_a increases, vagal traffic increases, the rate of discharge of the SAN decreases, and heart rate decreases.

temic arterial pressure decreases, the increase in HR is roughly parallel to the decrease in systemic arterial blood pressure.

Respiratory sinus arrhythmia (RSA) is a fluctuation in HR that occurs coincident with respiration. HR speeds during inspiration and slows during expiration. This waxing and waning of HR results from waxing and waning of vagal traffic, because of juxtaposition of cardioregulatory centers to respiratory centers in the medulla. For RSA to occur, the vagus nerve must be intact. Since one of the first features of heart failure is interference with vagal traffic, RSA either disappears or is attenuated in heart failure.

Chronotropic Inadequacy. Middle-aged to old-aged miniature schnauzers and cocker spaniels have a relatively high prevalence of a disease in which the SAN fails to discharge for rather long periods (Fox et al. 1998; Kittleson and Kienle 1998). This is termed *sick sinus syndrome*. It may be identified on the electrocardiogram (ECG) as the absence of deflections. Since the heart has stopped, there is no blood pumped, arterial pressure falls to a level not different from venous pressure, the pressure gradient across the capillary beds is zero, there is no cerebral blood flow, no oxygen reaches the brain, energy from ATP is unavailable to support cerebral function, and the dog faints. A reduction in chronotropy (i.e., the rate of discharge of the SAN decreases) also occurs with hypothyroidism and hypothermia. Chronotropic inadequacy also occurs with aging and heart failure.

Conductivity (the Dromotropic State). Conductivity (Sperelakis 1995; Zipes and Jalife 1995) refers to the property of the various tissues of the heart that allows them to propagate the wave of depolarization. The approximate velocities of propagation (i.e., conduction) of the waves are 1 m/s (meters per second) through the atrial myocardium, 0.025 m/s through the AV node, 2 to 5 m/s over the His-Purkinje system, and 0.5 m/s through the ventricular myocardium. Conductivity is independent of the size of the heart; that is, the velocity with which the wave of depolarization is approximately 1 m/s for either a mouse or an elephant. Therefore, it is of no surprise that durations of component deflections are much more brief for a mouse than for an elephant. The duration required for depolarization of a structure depends on the conduction velocity and the size of the structure (i.e., the lengths of the pathways). Conductivity (conduction velocity) can be estimated by recording the durations of various components of the ECG. Propagation through the atria—predominantly by muscle fiber to muscle fiber conduction—produces the P wave of the ECG. Propagation through the ventricles—expedited by the rapidly conducting Purkinje fibers—produces the QRS complex of the ECG. The time between the onset of atrial depolarization and the onset of ventricular depolarization is termed the PQ (or PR) interval. Approximately 70% of the PQ interval is spent by the wave of depolarization traversing the major portion of the AV node that conducts with the lowest velocity. If there is no cardiac enlargement, the durations (in milliseconds) for component deflections are approximately as listed in Table 6.1.

TABLE 6.1—Durations in milliseconds of component deflections seen on the electrocardiogram.

	Cat	Dog	Horse
P wave	40	50	130
QRS complex	40	60	120
PQ	70	100	360

DYSFUNCTION OF THE CARDIOVASCULAR SYSTEM

Diseases of Abnormal Conduction. With left atrial enlargement, as may be observed in dogs with mitral regurgitation (Buchanan 1979; Yoran et al. 1979a, b; Kleaveland et al. 1988; Darke 1987) or in cats with hypertrophic cardiomyopathy (Fox et al. 1995), the duration of the P wave lengthens, not because of decreased conductivity, but because of longer pathways caused by the atrial enlargement. With disease of AV conduction, or in response to drugs (e.g., digitalis glycosides, calcium channel blockers, or β-adrenergic blockers), the PQ interval of the ECG is prolonged (first-degree AV block) to over 140 ms in a dog or to over 360 ms in a horse. Occasionally an impulse fails to traverse the AV conduction system and some P waves are not followed by QRS complexes (second-degree AV block), and sometimes the impulse never traverses the AV conduction system and there is no relationship between P waves and QRS complexes (third-degree or complete AV block). Abnormal conduction occurs within the ventricles for a number of reasons: they are enlarged and the pathways of activation are longer, the specialized conductile tissue (His-Purkinje fibers) are diseased and fail to expedite the wave of depolarization to regions of the ventricles, the ventricular muscle is laden with scars or other regions that conduct poorly, or the velocity of conduction through the myocardial conduction velocity is depressed. This abnormal ventricular activation is identified on an ECG by a prolonged QRS complex (to over 65 ms in dogs) or by QRS complexes that are bizarre in configuration.

Currently, there is great interest in the area of cardiac resynchronization. With many heart diseases, the QRS complex is prolonged, indicating slow activation of the ventricles usually with some regions depolarized—and therefore contracting—earlier than other regions. This dyssynchrony reduces efficiency of contraction and leads to morbidity due to weakened contraction and mortality due to reentry of the wave of depolarization from tardy regions back into regions activated earlier. With modern pacemaker technology, the wave of depolarization may be picked up from an electrode placed within the earliest region depolarized, and delivered instantaneously to a tardy region next to which is placed an electrode. Thus, both regions are depolarized simultaneously—the ventricles are resynchronized—and efficiency of contraction is increased.

Premature Depolarizations. Occasionally (Antzelevitch and Sicouri 1994; Zipes and Jalife 1995), regions of the heart discharge (become pacemakers) prematurely without waiting to be stimulated in the normal course of activation that originates in the SAN. When this occurs, the events that follow are termed *premature depolarizations* (PDs), *premature beats* (PBs), *premature complexes* (PCs), or *premature systoles* (PSs). Pacemakers other than the SAN are termed *ectopic* (misplaced from the SAN) pacemakers, or latent pace-

makers since they discharge only after failure of the SAN to discharge on time. If a region possessing rhythmicity discharges because the SAN failed to discharge, the ectopic depolarization comes after a relatively long pause. The ectopic beat is termed an *escape beat*. This is in contradistinction to an ectopic depolarization that arises prematurely.

A region discharges prematurely because it is irritated. Two common causes of irritation are chronic stretch and oxygen deprivation; however, there are many drugs (including anesthetic agents) and electrolyte disturbances (in particular, hypokalemia or hyperkalemia and hypomagnesemia) that make fibers irritable enough to discharge prematurely. There are three general mechanisms by which a region may discharge prematurely. All require that the potential difference between the inside of the cell and the outside reaches threshold—a potential when the cell self-stimulates—before the cell would normally have been stimulated via the spread of activation originating at the SAN. The mechanisms are increased irritability (occurs least commonly), triggered activity (occurs most commonly due to drug effects), and reentry (the most common cause that occurs in the presence of stretch or oxygen deprivation).

Increased irritability—also termed increased *automaticity* or *rhyhmicity*—occurs when the resting membrane potential drifts so rapidly to the threshold value that it reaches threshold and causes the cell to discharge prematurely. This is termed *increased phase 4 depolarization*, because it is a depolarization (drift from negative to a less negative potential) that occurs during phase 4 between two action potentials. With triggered events, a cell becomes a pacemaker because an action potential develops oscillations after the action potential should have ended. These oscillations are termed *afterdepolarizations*, which may reach threshold very early [termed *early afterdepolarizations* (EADs)] or fairly late [termed *delayed afterdepolarizations* (DADs)] after the triggering action potential. When triggered activity produces premature depolarizations, the premature event occurs at a relatively fixed interval (termed *fixed coupling*) after the triggering event.

Reentry is a more difficult event to explain (Atkins et al. 1995). It occurs when a wave of depolarization reenters (or echoes out of) a normal pathway from a pathway that conducts slowly. Reentry requires either a long pathway, or two diverging pathways that conduct at different velocities and have effective refractory periods of different durations. Figure 6.4 shows the basis for reentry. Three regions (A, B, and C) in the heart are connected by three pathways (a, b, and c). Pathway b conducts relatively slowly but has a very short effective refractory period. The short refractory period means that it recovers soon after a previous wave has traversed it. Pathway c conducts relatively rapidly but has a relatively lengthy refractory period. The lengthy refractory period means that this pathway may not conduct another wave unless it follows the previous wave by a rather lengthy interval. A wave of depolarization travels down pathway a, and the wave splits and continues

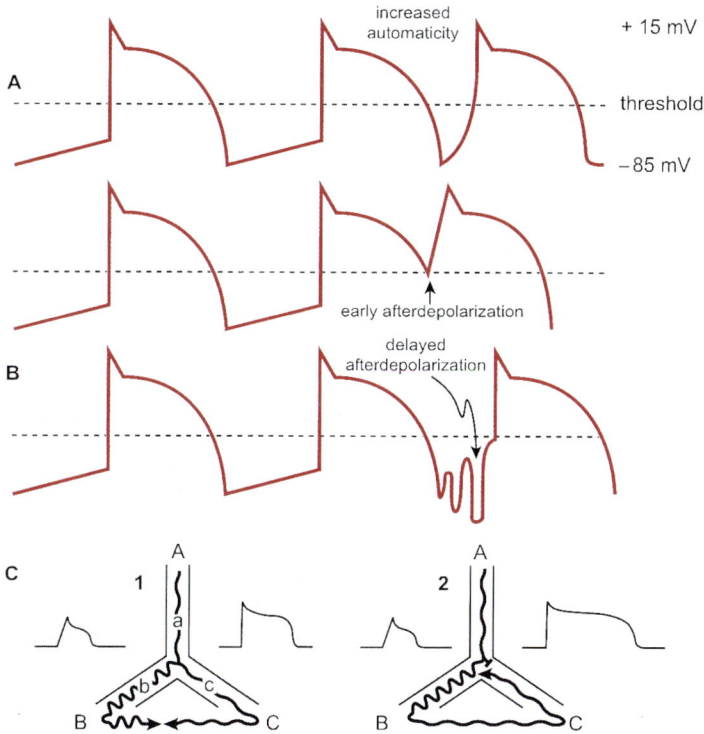

FIG. 6.4—Premature depolarization and circus movements. Schematic drawing showing (**A**) two normal action potentials followed by a premature action potential resulting from the cell reaching threshold—and firing spontaneously—due to an increased rate of early, slow diastolic depolarization. Notice that the membrane potential drills from −85 mV and reaches the threshold voltage (potential) at the dotted line. Schematic drawings (**B**) showing two normal action potentials followed by premature action potentials, one coming early after (**top**) and one coming rather later after (**bottom**) the triggering action potential. Triggered action potentials produce premature depolarizations because threshold is reached by afterdepolarizations triggered by the previous action potential. Schematic drawing (**C**) shows two forked pathways (1 and 2) and action potentials typical of each pathway located above. The action potential above pathway b is short (i.e., has a short refractory period), but its rise time is slow (i.e., it conducts slowly). The action potential above pathway c is long and has a rapid rise time (i.e. it has a long refractory period but conducts rapidly). In situation 1, a wave of depolarization originates in region A and travels down pathway a. The wave then splits and travels down pathways b and c toward regions B and C, respectively. Pathway b conducts slowly but has a short refractory period (i.e., it can accept another wave soon after the first one); pathway c conducts rapidly but has a rather long refractory period (i.e., it cannot accept another wave soon after the first one). The waves exit pathways b and c, travel through heart regions B and C, and then are extinguished when they collide closer to the exit point from pathway b. Of course, they collide closer to pathway b because that pathway conducts more slowly. In situation 2, however, for one reason or another, pathway c has an unusually lengthy refractory period. Notice how long the action potential is. The wave originates at A, travels down pathway a, and tries to enter pathways b and c; but because pathway c has such a long refractory period, the wave can only traverse—albeit slowly—pathway b. The wave then exits pathway b to region B, travels slowly through healthy myocardium to region C, and enters pathway c in the wrong direction—in a retrograde manner. Because so much time has elapsed that pathway c is now ready to accept the wave, the wave travels retrogradely through pathway c, and reenters and traverses pathway b. If this *circus movement* occurs only once, a single premature depolarization occurs, but if the circus movement continues, a tachycardia will develop. Sometimes a circus movement is termed an *echo*, implying that the impulse echoes out of pathway c into pathway b. Reentry is the most common mechanism for arrhythmias.

to travel down pathway b (slowly) and pathway c (rapidly). The waves emanate from pathways b and c, enter the myocardium at their outlets, and travel toward each other through the myocardium, but collide and are extinguished closer to the exit of pathway b. They collide closer to pathway b, because conduction down pathway b is slow, and the impulse has more time to travel from the exit of c to the exit of b (Figure 6.4).

Now suppose, for one reason or another, we prevent conduction down pathway c by lengthening its refractory period so that, when a wave reaches it, the wave cannot travel through. A wave travels down pathway a and tries to traverse pathways b and c, but it cannot traverse pathway c because the wave finds that pathway refractory to it. So the wave travels down pathway b, the slowly conducting pathway, but the pathway with a short refractory period. The wave exits pathway b, travels through the myocardium, and enters pathway c but traverses pathway c in a retrograde manner. It can traverse pathway c, because enough time has elapsed that this pathway has completed its refractory period by the time the wave has traveled down b and across the myocardium between the exits of b and c. The wave then ascends pathway c, reenters pathway b (which has completed its effective refractory period), and descends pathway b to reactivate the myocardium at its exit. This reentry constitutes a single premature depolarization. However, if the wave continues to descend b, ascend c, and reenter and descend b, in a circle (termed *circus movement*), there will be a stream of premature depolarizations—a tachycardia. If a region discharges rapidly for a short time, there is a paroxysmal (burst) tachycardia (period of rapid heart action) or, if continuously, merely a tachycardia.

Reentrant ectopic events may originate from within the atria, from within the ventricles, from within the AV node, or between the atria and the ventricles. Reentrant premature depolarizations also occur with fixed coupling; that is, the interval between the last normal depolarization and the premature depolarization is constant.

With a particularly dilated left atrium in dogs with mitral regurgitation or dilated cardiomyopathy, or in an ostensibly normal horse with a large left atrium because the horse is so large, multiple circus pathways may develop. This results in wavelets meandering through the atria, so that instead of a single wave traversing them from SAN to the most distal portion of the left atrium, hundreds of packets of atria are depolarized and contract independently of each other. This is known as *atrial fibrillation*. Instead of the atria contracting and ejecting blood into the ventricles. They "wiggle like a bag of worms" and do not eject blood. Of course, this is alright at rest, since the atria normally merely conduct blood from veins to ventricles, and their contraction is responsible, at rest, for only a trivial portion of ventricular filling.

Atrial fibrillation is recognized on an ECG by a rapid ventricular rate (many QRS complexes per minute) and irregular ventricular response (the intervals between QRS complexes are highly variable). As there are no P waves (since there is not a single wave traveling through the atria), there are tiny, irregular oscillations (f waves) in the baseline (produced by the hundreds of wavelets meandering through the atria).

FORCE OF CONTRACTION.

The force with which the left ventricle contracts is determined by three factors: (a) *myocardial contractility* (the inotropic state), (b) *preload* (the degree of stretch on the myocardial fibers just before they contract), (c) *afterload* (the interference to the ejection of blood from the left ventricle into and through the systemic arterial tree) (Braunwald et al. 1968; Katz 1993; Cannel and Lederer 1995; Lindemann and Watanabe 1995; Morgan and Morgan 1989).

Myocardial Contractility. Contraction of the myocardium (Braunwald et al. 1968) occurs when heavy meromyosin heads, extending from the myosin body, attach to binding sites on the actin filament and begin to swing. Myocardial contractility is determined as the velocity of cycling of the heavy meromyosin heads. Units of contractility are in muscle lengths per second: velocity. This cycling is fueled by energy released when ATP (located on the actin filament) is hydrolyzed by adenosine triphosphatase (ATPase, located on the myosin filament). Myocardial contractility can be measured best by (a) the velocity of cycling of heavy meromyosin heads; however, it can be estimated from (b) the rate of hydrolysis of ATP or by (c) the force of contraction of the ventricle if preload and afterload either are held constant or are accounted for if they happen to vary. On the other hand, contractility increases (albeit slightly) with increase in HR.

Under the impossible circumstances of the ventricle contracting against zero load (being massless in outer space), myocardial contractility can be measured as the velocity of fiber shortening, since, at zero load, neither preload nor afterload affects the function. The following experiment measures myocardial contractility (Figure 6.5). Hang a papillary muscle from a hook and stimulate the muscle with a current great enough to activate all portions of the muscle. Measure the velocity with which the papillary muscle shortens. If this is performed with an extremely heavy weight on the muscle, there will be no shortening . . . the velocity will be zero lengths per second. All of the energy of contraction will be dissipated in production of heat or in generation of tension—but no motion. For the subsequent stimulations, make the load on the papillary muscle lighter and lighter, and you will notice the tension generated will be less and less, but the velocity of fiber shortening will be greater and greater. When you have removed all of the weight, the velocity of shortening will be very rapid, but since the muscle must contract against itself, a maximal velocity will not be reached. However, notice the hyperbolic relationship between tension and velocity obtained over the experiment. That allows us to extrapolate the curve to the y-axis intercept, which occurs at zero load. This point of y-axis interception is the maximal velocity of fiber shortening, because it occurs at zero load. It is called the V_{max}. This maximal velocity depends solely on the velocity with which heavy meromyosin heads cycle; therefore, the y-axis intercept is the myocardial contractility or inotropic state. If you repeat the experiment on this muscle, and the y-axis intercept is lower, the muscle is under a negative inotropic influence as occurs in a failing heart. If you repeat the experiment and the y-axis intercept is greater than normal, the muscle is under a positive inotropic influence as occurs with exposure to digitalis or catecholamines.

The inotropic state is not determined by the number of heavy meromyosin heads that cycle, but only by the velocity with which any one cycles. The reason more heads cycling will not increase velocity is that there is zero load. If you (your arm representing a heavy

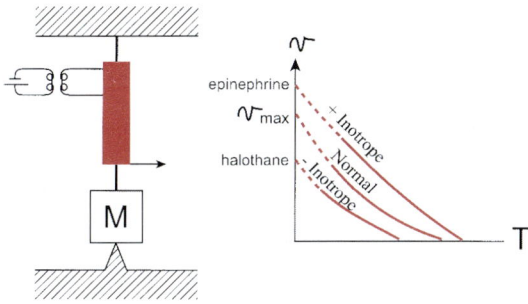

FIG. 6.5—Hang a portion of muscle (black bar) from the ceiling. A mass (M) is attached and is supported on a table below. A pointer is attached to the muscle to measure the velocity (*v*) with which it shortens as the load is lightened. A batter is attached to the muscle at the *top right*. The graph to the *right* shows plots of velocity of shortening versus the tension (T) developed by the muscle. The *middle curve* describes the function of a normal muscle. Notice that when the mass is too heavy to permit motion, a maximal tension is generated intersecting the abscissa. As the load is lightened more and more, the velocity increases. This curve is extrapolated to a point on the ordinate where the maximal velocity of shortening is shown. This occurs under the conditions of a "massless" muscle; therefore, this is an extrapolation. V_{max} is a measure of myocardial contractility and is defined as the velocity of fiber shortening when it shortens against no load. When a positive inotrope, epinephrine, is given, myocardial contractility increases; and when a negative inotrope, halothane, is given, contractility decreases. The maximal tension generated under all conditions is determined by both myocardial contractility (i.e., the rate of cycling of heavy meromyosin heads) and the preload.

meromyosin head) push a feather suspended by a string, you will achieve a maximal velocity, because the load, although not zero, is extremely light. By adding other persons (more arms representing more heavy meromyosin heads) to push the feather with you, you will not achieve any additional velocity.

With cardiomyopathy (Calvert et al. 1982; Calvert and Brown 1986; Katz 1990; Keene et al. 1991), or myocardial hypertrophy of any source (e.g., most volatile anesthetics or hypoxia) other than from exercise, myocardial contractility is reduced (Figure 6.6). The heart is under a negative inotropic influence (Figure 6.7). When this occurs, the heart is said to be failing; however, unless the patient is showing symptoms from the failing heart, the patient is not in heart failure. Myocardial contractility can be increased—even made supernormal—by administering positive inotropic agents (e.g., digitalis, catecholamines, dopamine, or milrinione), which increase the rate of cycling of heavy meromyosin heads.

Preload. The degree of stretch on the myocardial fibers just before they contract also determines the force of contraction (Sagawa 1978). Since the myocardial fibers surround the ventricular lumen, the degree of stretch of the fibers is determined by the volume of blood within

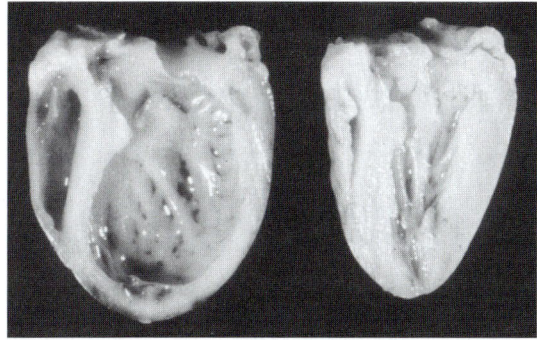

FIG. 6.6—Samples of hearts from twin turkey poults. The one on the **left** developed dilated cardiomyopathy due to exposure to furozolidone. The one at the **right** is normal. Notice the dilated left ventricle with thinning of both interventricular septum and left ventricular free wall in the cardiomyopathic heart.

LAP→	LVEDV	(WT)	− SV	= ESV,	P_a,	EF=$\frac{SV}{EDV}$,	T=AL
5	100	1	60	40	100	0.6	10,000
			2% halothane				
5	100	1	40	60	80	0.4	8,000
10	120	.8	60	60	100	0.5	15,000

FIG. 6.7—Response of the "left-side" of the heart to a negative inotrope: halothane [EF, ejection fraction; ESV, left ventricular end-systolic volume; LAP, left atrial pressure; LVEDV, left ventricular end-diastolic volume; P_a, systemic arterial pressure; SV, stroke volume; T, peak tension or afterload (AL); and WT, left ventricular wall thickness]. A LAP of 5 mm Hg fills the ventricle to an EDV of 100 mL with a wall 1 cm thick. A normal SV of 60 mL leaves an ESV of 40 mL (100 −60). This SV generated a P_a of 100 mm Hg from an EF of 0.6 and with an AL of 10,000 units. The 2% halothane weakens the force of contraction by decreasing the rate of cycling of heavy meromyosin heads. LAP remains at 5, LVEDV remains at 100, and WT remains at 1, but SV decreases to only 40 mL, leaving an ESV of 60. P_a decreased to 80 because of the reduction in SV, EF fell to 0.4, and AL decreased to 8000 units. But because the left ventricle removed less than the normal amount of blood from the pulmonary venous circulation, including the left atrium, LAP increased to 10 mm Hg. This doubling of filling pressure increased LVEDV to 120 and decreased WT to 0.8 (having stretched the same amount of myocardium around a larger chamber). Because of the increased preload (EDV increased from a normal of 100 to 120), SV returned to normal in accordance with the Frank-Starling mechanism. This occurred even though myocardial contractility was reduced by the halothane. P_a returned to 100 because SV normalized, EF increased to 0.5, and T increased to 15,000. Thus, a new steady state of function occurred during exposure to the negative inotrope, halothane, in which SV was normal, but in which LAP, EDV, and T were increased. Since SV and presumably cardiac output are normal, the patient should suffer no ill-effects of inadequate tissue perfusion, but since LAP, EDV, and T are elevated, the lung may be congested and the increased T increases myocardial oxygen demand.

the ventricle: the end-diastolic volume (EDV). The EDV is equal to the end-diastolic pressure (EDP) minus the pleural pressure (P_{pl}) all divided by the stiffness (E) of the ventricular wall:

$$PL = EDV = (EDP - P_{pl})/E$$

If that bothers you, you can understand it by using a balloon instead of a ventricle. The volume of gas in the balloon is equal to the pressure inside the balloon minus the pressure outside balloon, all divided by how stiff the balloon is.

The pleural pressure is usually −3 mm Hg, and if we assume that myocardial stiffness is constant,[5] then the EDV is linearly—actually curvilinearly—related to the EDP. This is shown as the bottom curve of Figure 6.8, which is a graph of resting pressure (PR) in the ventricle on the ordinate (y-axis) versus end-diastolic volume (V) of the ventricle on the abscissa (x-axis). Notice that, to increase volume from 50 to 100 mL (dV_1), only a slight increase in pressure of from 0 to 5 mm Hg (dP_1) was necessary; however, to increase volume from 100 to 150 mL (dV_2) a much larger increase in pressure of from 5 to 25 mm Hg (dP_2) was required. We can estimate the stiffness of the ventricle by dividing the changes in pressures (dP) by the changes in volumes (dV). The stiffness of the ventricle (dP/dV) from a volume of 50 mL to a volume of 100 mL was $(5 - 0)/(100 - 50)$ or 0.1 mm Hg/mL, whereas the stiffness of the ventricle from a volume of 100 to 150 was $(25 - 5)/(150 - 100)$ or 0.4 mm Hg/mL, four times stiffer. This also means that the ventricle was one-fourth as compliant, since compliance (the ease of filling) is the reciprocal of stiffness.

The compliance of the ventricle is termed the *lusitropic property*. In fact, relaxation of the ventricle occurs in two phases: isovolumetric and isotonic (Suga and Sugawa 1974; Brutsaert and Sys 1989; Gaasch 1994; Paulus and Shah 1999). Isovolumetric relaxation occurs as ventricular pressure falls rapidly immediately after the aortic valve closes and before the mitral valve opens. During this rather brief period, the fibers are relaxing and tension is decreasing, but the fibers are not lengthening. The ventricular volume is constant. This contribution to relaxation is a process that requires energy released from hydrolysis of ATP. This energy is used to drive calcium ions from the troponin-C molecule to the sarcoplasmic reticulum (SR). Because calcium ions are so concentrated in the SR, the process cannot be passive (i.e., moving down a concentration gradient). Thus, the rate of liberation of energy from ATP and the rate of resequestration of calcium ions by the SR are the prime determinants of dP/dt_{min}.

EDP, the prime determinant of EDV, is equal to the blood volume (determined by water drunk minus urine made) divided by the capacity of the veins (where 60%

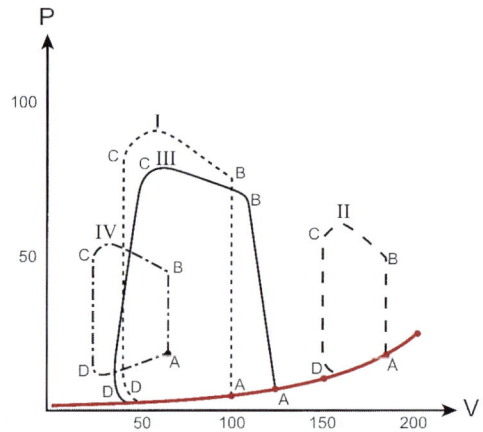

FIG. 6.8—Plots of pressure (P)-volume (V) loops of the left ventricle during normal physiology (I) and during various pathophysiological states (II, III, and IV). Units of the ordinate are pressure (mm Hg), and units of the abscissa are volume (mL). These curves are very useful in understanding why the ventricle may be unable to generate normal pressures, why preload may be greater than normal, and why stroke volume is reduced. The *heavy dark line* extending from the origin represents the filling pressure required to achieve a given end-diastolic volume without imposing pathological stiffness of the ventricle. The larger the ventricle is, the greater is the pressure required to fill it. The ventricle becomes physiologically stiffer the larger the chamber becomes.

A-B represents the contracting ventricle with a rapid increase in pressure but little change in volume—the so-called isovolumetric contraction period. The aortic valve opens at B, so pressure increases only slightly because the ventricle now is ejecting blood—the so-called period of isotonic contraction. B-C represents the ejection of blood principally into the aorta. C-D represents the precipitous fall of ventricular pressure with little change in volume—the so-called isovolumetric relaxation period. D-A represents the filling of the ventricle with little change in pressure—the so-called isotonic relaxation period. In the normal ventricle (I), pressure increases from A to B with no change in volume, and pressure decreases from C to D with no change in volume—truly isovolumetric (unchanging).

However, with mitral regurgitation (III), as pressure increases from A-B, volume decreases slightly proportional with blood regurgitating into the left atrium. This reduction in volume occurs before the ventricle ejects blood into the aorta. From C-D, volume continues to decrease as blood continues to regurgitate from ventricle into the atrium. Point A for curve III is larger than for the normal heart (I) because the regurgitation into the left atrium and pulmonary veins elevates pressures within those structures, and this increase in filling force overdistends the left ventricle.

Curve II represents ventricular function with a feebly contracting heart as in a patient with dilated cardiomyopathy. A-B is reduced because the ventricle generates less force, and B-C is reduced because stroke volume decreases—both consequences of the weakened ventricle. A is elevated because left atrial and pulmonary venous pressures elevate due to inadequate emptying by the weakened left ventricle.

Curve IV represents the left ventricle of hypertrophic cardiomyopathy. Because the left ventricle is so stiff. Point A occurs at a markedly elevated pressure and at a markedly reduced end-diastolic volume. Because of the reduced preload, force of contraction is reduced, so B-C is reduced. This is consistent with the Frank-Starling mechanism.

---

5. This is untrue in most heart diseases in which the heart becomes stiffer than normal.

to 70% of the blood resides). The venous capacity depends on the degree of constriction (which decreases venous capacity) or relaxation (which increases venous capacity) of venous smooth muscle; and the degree of constriction of smooth muscle depends on many of the same factors that influence afterload (to be discussed next). Actually, EDV is determined also by how vigorously the atrium is "kicking" blood into the ventricle just before the ventricle contracts. This atrial contribution, as a percentage of the total volume of blood ejected by each stroke of the ventricle, is only 15% at slow HRs and up to 35% at higher HRs.

The Frank-Starling curve is used to express the relationship between systolic function of the ventricle (as measured by developed pressure or tension, rate of rise of pressure or tension, stroke volume, and cardiac output) on the ordinate (y-axis) and EDV (milliliters) on the abscissa (x-axis). Since EDP is the prime determinant of EDV, EDP is often used as the units on the x-axis. Notice (top curve for Figure 6.9) that, as EDP increases, systolic function increases but

approaches a plateau at very high EDPs. The reason for this is that, as EDP increases, EDV increases; but, at very great EDVs, the ventricle becomes so stiff that further increments in EDP do not produce further increments in EDV.

The Frank-Starling law of the heart (Starling 1918) states that within physiological limits when all other factors are constant, the force of ventricular contraction is determined by the degree of stretch on the myocardial fibers just before they contract. There are two explanations for that relationship (Figure 6.10). First, the more the fibers are stretched (again within physiological limits), the more optimal is the interdigitation between actin and myosin, the greater the number of heavy meromyosin crossbridges that cycle, and the force of contraction increases. Secondly, as the fibers are stretched, calcium is bound more avidly to the troponin-C molecules, such binding permits attachment of more heavy meromyosin heads to actin, more heads cycle, and the force of contraction increases (Fuchs 1995).

Let's put together myocardial contractility and preload to explain why you survived your last anesthetic experience when you were anesthetized with isoflurane, an anesthetic that decreases myocardial contractility by approximately 50%. Refer to Figure 6.7, showing left atrial pressure (LAP), left ventricular end-diastolic volume or preload (EDV or PL), stroke volume (SV), end-systolic volume (ESV), and arterial pressure (P_a). (Also see Figure 6.10.)

Before you were anesthetized, your LAP was 5 mm Hg, a force that filled the left ventricle to an

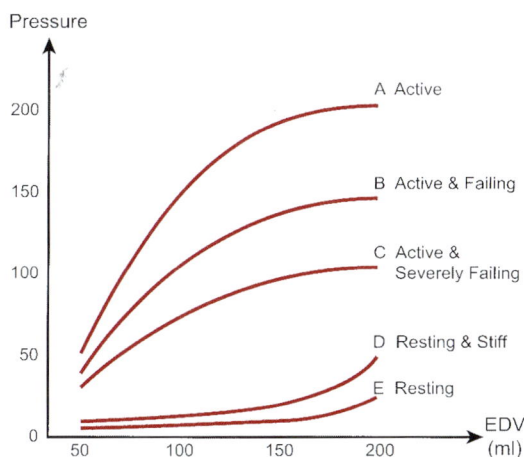

FIG. 6.9—Plot of either peak systolic (active: A, B, and C) or end-diastolic (resting: D and E) pressure within the left ventricle as a function of end-diastolic volume (EDV). Curves A and E represent the normal heart. Curves B and C represent systolic function during various degrees of myocardial failure. Curve D represents a relatively stiff ventricle. Notice that, as EDV increases, resting tension in the ventricular wall increases, more for the stiff ventricle (D) than for the normal ventricle (E). Notice that, as EDV increases from 50 to 150 mL, systolic function increases dramatically, but, as EDV increases from 150 to 200 mL, the systolic function still increases but to a much lesser degree. The lesser degree produces what is termed a relatively flat portion of the curve, such that if EDV decreases from 200 to 150 mL, systolic function does not decrease nearly so much. On the other hand, notice that in order for EDV to increase from 50 to 150 mL, the increase in resting wall tension is small, whereas to increase from 150 to 200 mL, resting wall tension must increase dramatically; i.e., the ventricle is much stiffer at larger volumes. The stiffness of the ventricle reflects the level of end-diastolic pressure required to achieve EDV.

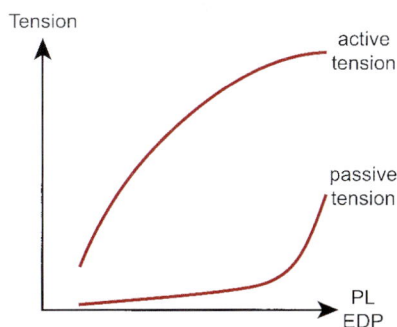

FIG. 6.10—Plots of active (systolic) and passive (resting or diastolic) tension versus preload (PL) or end-diastolic pressure (EDP)—the force principally responsible for preload. Notice that, in order for preload to increase, the tension on the ventricular wall in diastole (passive) must increase, and that, for particularly large preloads, the passive tension must be very great. Notice, also, that as preload increases, systolic force increases. Increasing preload optimizes the interdigitation between actin and myosin filaments, and increases the binding of calcium to troponin C. This is the classical curve representing the Frank-Starling law of the heart. See the next illustration for pathological conditions.

EDV of 100 mL, and from an EDV of 100 mL, the ventricle ejected an SV of 60 mL, leaving 40 mL behind—the ESV. The left ventricle was able to eject a SV of 60 mL because of its myocardial contractility (i.e., the velocity of cycling of heavy meromyosin heads) and because of its preload (the number of heavy meromyosin heads cycling). Now you breathe in 2% isoflurane that, in addition to putting you to sleep, decreases the velocity of cycling of heavy meromyosin heads (i.e., myocardial contractility) by 50%. This results in a reduced SV for the next contraction, so that instead of an SV of 60 mL, it falls to 40 mL. This results in a decrease in systemic arterial pressure and in a damming up of blood in the left atrium and pulmonary veins. LAP increases from a normal of 5 mm Hg to 10 mm Hg. This increased LAP results in an increase in EDV. The increase in EDV invokes the Frank-Starling mechanism, and the next force of contraction returns to normal and SV returns to 60 mL, even though the myocardial contractility has been reduced by 50%. Remember that this occurs because force of contraction is determined by both contractility (which determines the rate of cycling of heavy meromyosin heads) and preload (which determines the number of crossbridges cycling). Thus, SV and arterial pressure are normalized, even though contractility has been reduced by 50%, due to increased EDV produced by increased LAP, resulting from the failure of the left ventricle to remove blood normally from the left atrium and pulmonary veins. Therefore, you did not suffer from a reduction in cardiac output, but if you monitored your left atrial and pulmonary vascular volumes, you would find them increased. A little increase is alright, but if the increase is too much, then the left atrial stretch can be injurious, and increased pulmonary venous and possibly pulmonary capillary volumes can result in pulmonary distress. You will see this sequence repeated for common cardiovascular disorders.

Afterload. This is also a major determinant of left ventricular pressure (Suga and Sagawa 1974; Sagawa 1978; Taylor and Stevens 1983; Pedersen et al. 1995). If there is no interference to ejection of blood from the left ventricle, it must be obvious that no pressure could be generated.

Even if your arm muscles are big and strong, they cannot generate force if they push a feather across the room! In fact the maximal force will be generated when you attempt to push an immovable object.

Afterload is the interference perceived by the left ventricle as it ejects blood into and through the systemic arterial tree. It is expressed as the peak tension in the wall of the ventricle. The ventricle may be approximated as a thick-walled sphere, and, according to the law of Laplace, the tension (T) in the wall of a thick-walled sphere is equal to the pressure (P) inside times the radius (*r*), all divided by the wall thickness (WT):

$$T = P \times r/WT$$

But AL is the peak (p) tension, that is $(T = P \times r/WT)_p$. Peak tension almost always occurs at the instant just before the aortic valve opens, because, at that instant, the product of intraventricular pressure and ventricular radius divided by wall thickness is maximal. That is the instant when the systemic arterial pressure is its minimum—the diastolic arterial pressure (P_d), normally approximately 80 mm Hg. Even though the ventricular pressure increases from an arterial diastolic pressure of 80 mm Hg to a peak systolic pressure of 120 mm Hg, the tension in the wall of the left ventricle actually decreases because the radius becomes smaller and the wall becomes thicker.

Rather than measuring radius, it is customary to measure EDV (Figure 6.11). Since EDV = 4/3 π r^3, we often substitute EDV or PL in the equation for AL. Thus, AL is approximated as the product of P_d times PL divided by WT. Afterload is important not only because it estimates the toll contraction takes on the ventricle, but because it is also a prime determinant of myocardial oxygen consumption (MVO_2).

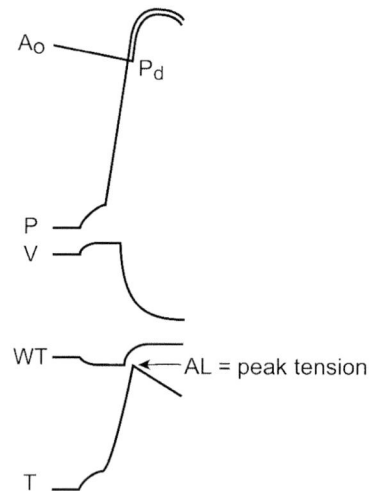

FIG. 6.11—Afterload is defined as the peak tension in the wall of the heart. The ventricle is commonly represented as a thick-walled sphere. According to the law of Laplace, the tension is approximated as the product of lumenal pressure times lumenal radius, all divided by wall thickness. This illustration shows aortic pressure (Ao), intraventricular pressure (P), ventricular volume which may be used interchangeably with radius (V ≈ r^3), thickness of the ventricular wall (WT), and the tension (T) in the wall. Tension is approximated as (P × V)/WT, but peak tension—afterload—occurs at the point marked AL. It occurs when aortic pressure is at its diastolic value (P_d). It is at this point that tension peaks. Even though pressure continues to rise, because volume (radius) decreases and the wall becomes thicker, tension actually decreases.

TOTAL INTERFERENCE TO EJECTION OF BLOOD FROM THE LEFT VENTRICLE INTO AND THROUGH THE SYSTEMIC ARTERIAL TREE. The total interference (Suga and Sagawa 1974; Sagawa 1978; Taylor and Stevens 1983; Eaton et al. 1993) to ejection of blood from the left ventricle into and through the systemic arterial tree is divided into impedance (Z) and systemic vascular resistance (SVR) (Figure 6.12). Normally, Z constitutes less than 10% of the interference, and of course SVR would then constitute more than 90%. In fact, the left ventricle does not pump blood through the SVR offered principally by the systemic arterioles, but rather ejects blood only into the initial portion of the aorta. Then, while the ventricle rests in diastole, the elastic recoil of the aorta squeezes its contents and moves blood back toward the left ventricle and through the systemic arterioles. However the aortic valve is slammed closed[6] by blood attempting to reenter the left ventricle; therefore, the blood is moved only through the systemic arterioles into the capillaries. *Impedance* is the effort needed to eject blood into the initial portion of the aorta. Impedance results from the necessity of the stroke volume to overcome the relative stiffness of the aorta. SVR is the effort spent to move blood through the systemic arterioles into the capillaries. Both Z and SVR depend on the degree of constriction or relaxation of the vascular smooth muscle. A partial list of endogenous affectors of vascular smooth muscle is presented in Table 6.2.

OXYGEN CONTENT IN THE MYOCARDIUM.
Most of the ATP used to fuel the heart is produced in its mitochondria as a result of a process requiring oxygen (Braunwald et al. 1968; Gibbs 1974). The amount of ATP necessary to fuel normal cardiac function would be used up very quickly, but, with adequate amounts of oxygen, ATP is rapidly and continuously produced. Adequate amounts of oxygen depend on a balance between oxygen delivery and oxygen utilization. Oxygen delivery depends on normal lung function, a normal amount of hemoglobin, and coronary blood flow adequate to carry the oxygenated blood. Coronary blood flow depends on the difference in pressure between the aorta (P_{Ao}) from which the coronary flow arises and the right atrium (P_{RA}) into which the coronary flow empties. Normal aortic pressure is approximately 100 mm Hg, and normal right atrial pressure is approximately 5 mm Hg (Figure 6.13). The aortic pressure (Milnor 1982) is sustained at 100 mm Hg as the product of cardiac output and SVR, and the right atrial pressure is sustained at 5 mm Hg by the right ventricle removing blood from the right atrium and pumping it into and through the pulmonary vascular tree. However, coronary blood flow (Q_{cor}) is affected by the coro-

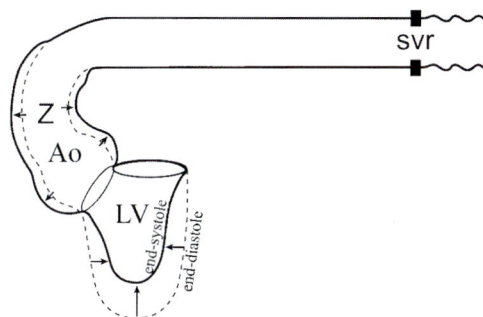

FIG. 6.12—A schematic diagram of the left ventricle (LV) and the aorta (Ao) arising from it. The *dashed lines* represent the ventricle and the aorta at their diastolic phases. When the ventricle ejects its stroke volume into the proximal portion of the aorta, notice that the ventricle becomes smaller (*dashed line to solid line*) and the aorta becomes larger (*dashed line to solid line*). In order for the aorta to accept the stroke volume, the smooth muscle and other components in the aortic wall must become stretched. The hindrance to blood flowing out of the ventricle and into the aorta is termed the *impedance*, and is denoted by a Z, and of course Z depends on the relative stiffness of the aorta. The energy stored due to elastic deformation of the aorta is manifested while the ventricle is resting, and sustains blood flow—particularly through the coronary circulation—even while the ventricle rests. The hindrance to blood flow out of the aorta is attributable to the systemic vascular resistance (SVR). The SVR depends on the degree of constriction or dilatation of the systemic arterioles that is attributable to the vascular smooth muscle. Of the total work performed by the ventricle, approximately 5% to 10% is required to overcome Z, whereas 90% to 9% must overcome SVR.

nary vascular resistance (CVR) to flow through the coronary vasculature. This resistance is altered by the degree of constriction or relaxation of smooth muscle in the coronary vessels (the coronary vascular resistance or CVR) and the compression of collapsible coronary vessels within the wall of the left ventricle. When the left ventricle contracts, the tension in its wall rises so much that it actually collapses the intramural vessels. Since elevated intramyocardial tension occurs only when the heart is contracting (during ventricular systole), coronary flow is obstructed only during systole; but since intramyocardial tension is low when the

TABLE 6.2—A partial list of endogenous affectors of vascular smooth muscle

Vasoconstrictors	Vasodilators
α_1-Adrenergic stimulation	β_2-Adrenergic stimulation
α_2-Adrenergic stimulation	Adenosine
Vasopressin/ADH	Atrial natriuretic factor
Angiotensin II	Nitric oxide
Thromboxane	Blood flow, itself
	Acetylcholine
	Dopamine
ADH, antidiuretic hormone.	

---

6. When the aortic valve slams closed and the column of blood within the aorta suddenly decelerates, cardiohemic structures are thrown into oscillations, which are heard as the second heart sound.

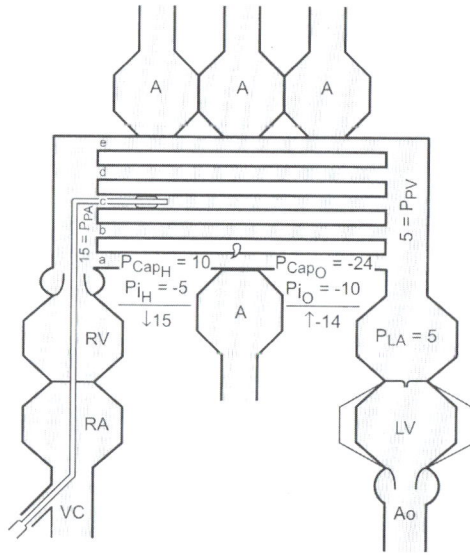

FIG. 6.13—A schematic illustration of the right side (RA, right atrium; and RV, right ventricle) and left side (LA and LV) of the heart, with the pulmonary capillary bed connecting the pulmonary trunk arising from the right ventricle to the pulmonary veins. Alveoli are labeled A. Of course, the lung contains millions of alveoli, and the pulmonary capillaries are "built" into the alveolar walls. Five pulmonary capillaries traversing the alveoli are labeled a, b, c, d, and e, and a balloon-tipped catheter is wedged in capillary c. When the balloon of this catheter is inflated and it wedges in a small pulmonary artery, the tip actually measures pressure in the pulmonary capillary (P_{capH}). The pressure in the pulmonary trunk (P_{pa}) is 15 mm Hg, caused by the right ventricle pumping blood into it, and the pressure in the pulmonary vein (P_{pv}) is 5 mm Hg, caused by the left ventricle removing blood from it and pumping it into the aorta (Ao). Observe the tiny drop of serum oozing out of capillary c into the interstices of the lung. The force producing this oozing is a balance between hydrostatic (H) and oncotic (O) pressures (P) within the capillary (cap) blood and within the interstices (i) of the lung. The net oncotic pressure is normally approximately −14 mm Hg in favor of serum being held in the capillary, whereas the net hydrostatic pressure is 15 mm Hg in favor of serum oozing from the capillary into the interstitium. Thus, there is a net of 1 mm Hg causing the oozing from capillary to interstitium. However no fluid accumulates in the interstitium because pulmonary lymphatics drain it back into the veins.

heart is resting (during ventricular diastole), coronary blood flows predominantly during diastole. When the HR speeds, the heart spends a greater percentage of time contracting, and when the HR slows, it spends a greater percentage of time in diastole. Thus, HR is a major determinant of coronary blood flow (Q_{cor}) and the delivery of oxygen to the myocardium. Put in the form of an equation,

$$Q_{cor} = (P_{Ao} - P_{RA})/CVR + HR$$

The amount of oxygen consumed by the heart (MVO_2) is determined, principally, by three factors: HR, myocardial contractility, and afterload. This is perfectly logical. The faster the HR is, the more oxygen is consumed. The greater the inotropic state is, the more oxygen is consumed. The greater the afterload—the maximal tension generated by the ventricle—is, the greater the oxygen is consumed. Remember that afterload is approximated as the product of intraventricular pressure times preload, all divided by wall thickness. Thus, increasing arterial pressure or preload or decreasing wall thickness will increase AL and MVO_2.

It should be emphasized that HR is an extremely important determinant of the amount of oxygen within the myocardium, since it increase MVO_2 and decreases Q_{cor} (Figure 6.14).

METHODS OF MONITORING CARDIAC FUNCTION. Cardiac function—most often left ventricular function—is a clinical description used to express how the heart, in its entirety, functions as a pump (Smith and Kampine 1990; Fox et al. 1998; Kittleson and Kienle 1998; Lilly 1998). In general, it addresses how well the heart removes blood from venous circuits (keeping venous pressures relatively low) and pumps it into and through arterial trees (keeping arterial pressure relatively high). Remember that it is the pressure gradient from artery to vein that is responsible for moving blood through the capillary beds so that the exchange of gasses, substrates, and calories can sustain constancy of the internal milieu. Cardiac function is often monitored, clinically, using (1) cardiac output (Q, CO), (2) ejection fraction (EF, which is the percent change in volume) or the echocar-

Determinants of O_2 Delivery→[O_2]→Determinants of O_2 Consumption

1. proper lung function	1. Heart rate (HR)
2. adequate healthy hemoglobin	2. Myocardial contractility
3. coronary blood flow (CBF)	3. Peak myocardial tension (afterload = AL)

$$CBF=(P_{Ao}-P_{RA})/(CVR+HR) \rightarrow [O_2] \rightarrow AL \approx PL \cdot Pa_{diast})/WT$$

FIG. 6.14—Energy for contraction and relaxation comes from adenosine triphosphate (ATP). Most ATP comes from aerobic metabolism in the mitochondria. Therefore, there must a balance between myocardial oxygen delivery and myocardial oxygen consumption. The determinants of each are shown. Notice that heart rate is a determinant of both oxygen delivery and utilization. An increase in heart rate decreases oxygen delivery, increases oxygen demand, and may lead to an oxygen deficit. If oxygen deficit leads to inadequate energy, both systolic function and diastolic function decrease. [O_2], myocardial oxygen content; P_{Ao}, mean aortic pressure diastolic pressure; P_{Ra}, mean right atrial pressure; CVR, coronary vascular resistance; PL, preload (end-diastolic volume); Pa_{diast}, arterial diastolic pressure; and WT, end-diastolic wall thickness.

diographic equivalent of EF, shortening fraction (SF, which is the percent change in diameter), (3) ESV, (4) the ratio of the preejection period (PEP) to the ejection time (ET) of the left ventricle, (5) the maximal rate of rise of the left ventricular pressure, and (6) left atrial or pulmonary capillary ("wedge") pressure (Fig. 6.13).

HR may be studied by auscultation of heart sounds or by palpation of arterial pulses or the point of maximal cardiac impulse against the thoracic wall; however, it can be studied most accurately by electrocardiography (ECG[7]) (Figure 6.15). The heartbeat originates in the SAN, the region of greatest rhythmicity, termed the *pacemaker*. When the SAN discharges, a wave of depolarization is sent through the atria from right atrium to left atrium. This wave does two things. It generates, on the torso surface, a voltage of approximately 0.3 mV and of approximately 50 ms in dogs or 130 ms in horses. It is termed the P wave of the ECG. This wave of depolarization stimulates (shocks) the atria into contraction, and the rate with which the SAN discharges determines the HR.

HR is usually expressed as the number of beats per minute, which may be determined by counting the number of beats or P waves in a minute, counting the number in 15 seconds and multiplying by 4, or counting the number in 6 seconds and multiplying by 10. An HR that is too slow (<100 in cats, <60 in dogs, and <20 in horses) is termed a *bradycardia*; an HR that is too fast (>220 cats, >160 in dogs, and >45 in horses) is termed *tachycardia*. Of course, an abnormal HR indicates an abnormal rate of discharge of the SAN.

It is quite obvious that CO is important, because the cardiovascular system could not possibly sustain constancy of the internal milieu without movement of adequate amounts of blood. EF, the ratio (nondimensional) of SV to EDV, is quite difficult to measure, but its approximation, shortening fraction, is measured quite easily by echocardiography (Figure 6.16). EF and SF express the ratio of how much blood is ejected during each stroke to the volume that is left behind in the ventricle. Because EF is nondimensional (mL/mL), it is almost independent of heart size. This is not true for SF, which is smaller in larger animals. EF is normally in excess of 0.55 (i.e., SV is more than 50% of EDV). SF is normally in excess of 0.25. SF is obtained echocardiographically as the ratio of (EDD − ESD)/EDD, where EDD is the end-diastolic internal diameter and ESD is the end-systolic internal diameter of the left ventricle. Since the volume of a sphere is the cube of radius (times $4/3 \mathrm{rd}\pi$), and radius is 50% of diameter, it is not too difficult to understand that EF and SF should provide a semiquantitatively similar description of ventricular function.

When EF falls below 50% and SF falls below 20%, the heart is said to be malfunctioning (Tidholm et al. 1997). Of course, this means that from a given EDV the

SV is less than anticipated. Exceptions to this are when the left ventricle ejects not only into the aorta but also into a low-pressure port, such as the left atrium (when mitral regurgitation is present), the right ventricle (when there is a hole in the interventricular septum), or the pulmonary trunk (when there is a communication between the aorta and pulmonary trunk). Thus, even a ventricle that has been weakened by a negative inotropic influence can sustain a normal or even elevated EF or SF because it has the opportunity of ejecting into a low-resistance circuit.

A corollary of EF is ESV (the volume of blood remaining in the left ventricle after it ejects a SV). Obviously if EF (SV/EDV) is great, and since ESV equals EDV minus SV, then ESV will be relatively small. Although ratios of volumes are nondimensional, each volume is measured in milliliters and of course depends on how large the body is. Thus, to use ESV as an index of ventricular function, it must be regressed to body size—usually to body surface area expressed in square meters (m^2). The larger the ESV/m^2 is and the greater the volume of blood left is behind in the ventricle after its stroke, the more compromised the ventricular function is. Many believe that ESV/m^2 is the most useful indicator of ventricular function and the best prognostic predictor.

The ratio of the duration between the onset of the QRS complex and the onset of left ventricular ejection (termed the *preejection period* or PEP) to the duration of left ventricular ejection (termed the *ejection time* or ET) is a nondimensional negative correlate of ventricular function (Figure 6.17). PEP is the time (milliseconds) spent by the left ventricle in generating enough force to open the aortic valve. ET is the time (milliseconds) spent ejecting. PEP may be considered "wasted" time, because no "useful" work (in a thermodynamic sense, ejection against a resistance) occurs. ET is considered "useful" time, because useful work is performed in terms of ejecting a volume of blood against the AL. A near linear inverse slope is produced when plotting ET against PEP/ET. Whereas both PEP and ET lengthen as heart weight increases, the ratio PEP/ET remains close to 0.3 for most mammals. Also both PEP and ET shorten as HR increases, however, as with the effects of heart size, PEP/ET remains quite independent of HR.

It is thought commonly that pressure developed by the left ventricle is a good measure of ventricular function—actually, it is more a measure of myocardial contractility. Systolic ventricular pressure approximates arterial pressure; clearly, arterial pressure can be no higher than left ventricular pressure. Furthermore, it is clear that systemic arterial pressure is the principal force driving blood through the systemic arterioles into and through the systemic capillaries. However, remembering Poiseuille's/Ohm's laws, the pressure/voltage is the product of blood/current flow times resistance. Thus, there might be an extremely forceful left ventricular contraction, but the systemic arterial pressure may not reflect it if the resistance to flow is low. Conversely, the

---

7. ECG stands for electrocardiography (the study), electrocardiograph (the instrument) or ECG (the tracing).

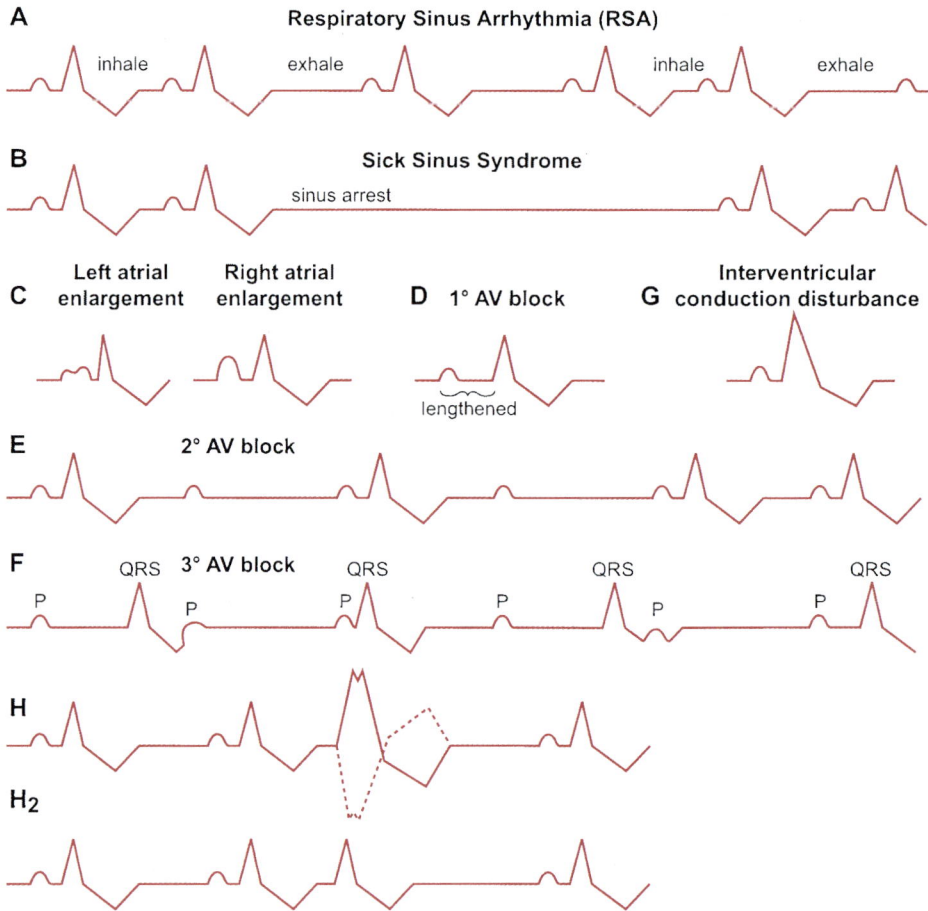

A Respiratory Sinus Arrhythmia (RSA)

inhale   exhale   inhale   exhale

B Sick Sinus Syndrome

sinus arrest

C Left atrial enlargement   Right atrial enlargement

D 1° AV block

lengthened

G Interventricular conduction disturbance

E 2° AV block

F 3° AV block

QRS   QRS   QRS   QRS

P   P   P   P   P   P

H

H₂

FIG. 6.15—Examples (B through H_2) of abnormal electrocardiograms (ECG) compared with a normal ECG (**A**). These are schematic representations of a typical lead II ECG from a dog:

A: Respiratory sinus arrhythmia showing heart rate speed during inspiration and slow during expiration. This is normal for quiet and/or sleeping dogs.

B: A period during which the sinoatrial node—the normal pacemaker—fails to discharge. This is termed *sinus arrest*.

C: Examples of left (broad, notched P wave) and right (peaked P wave) atrial enlargement. The broad, notched P wave results from delayed left atrial depolarization. The P waves of normal horses appear broad and notched because the atria of horses is so much larger than the atria of dogs.

D: With first-degree atrioventricular (AV) block, the QRS complex follows the P wave by a longer-than-expected duration. This is usually caused by retarded conduction over the AV node, which may be caused by high vagal (parasympathetic) tone or by disease of the AV conduction system.

E: With second-degree AV block, occasional P waves are not followed by QRS complexes, but all QRS complexes are preceded by P waves with a nearly normal and fixed interval. Some waves of atrial depolarization do not enter the ventricles because the impulse "dies" in the AV conduction system. This is usually caused by exaggeration of what causes first-degree AV block.

F: With third-degree AV block, P waves and QRS complexes appear with no fixed relationship between them. There is no electrical communication between atria and ventricles. This is usually caused by further aggravation of what caused second-degree AV block.

G: A "sloppy appearing," prolonged, or bizarre QRS complex preceded by a P wave indicates slow activation (depolarization) of the ventricles and is termed *interventricular conduction disturbance*. It may be caused by interruption of conduction over main bundles or the Purkinje fibers or by slow and/or circuitous conduction through the myocardium.

H: Two forms of ventricular premature depolarizations. Notice how after two normal beats the third beat arises prematurely. That makes it a premature depolarization. The fact that the QRS complex is bizarre makes it a ventricular premature depolarization. When the QRS complex is of the same polarity as the normal QRS complex the beat arises from regions of the right ventricle, but when the QRS is of opposite polarity (the *dotted line*), it arises from the left ventricle. Actually, the beat arises from specialized conductile tissue or M (midmyocardial) fibers in those ventricles, not from typical myocardial fibers.

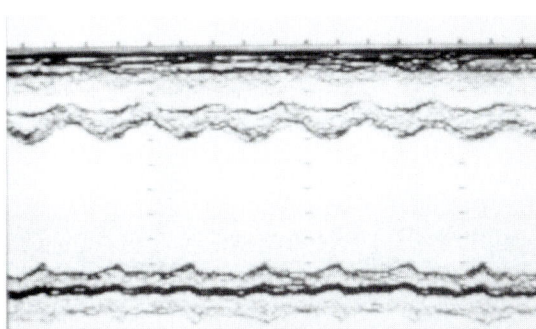

FIG. 6.16—An M-mode echocardiogram from a dog with dilated cardiomyopathy. The *dark black line* at the bottom is the pericardial sac, the *speckled band* above it is the left ventricular free wall, the *clear space* above that is the left ventricle, and the *band* above that is the interventricular septum. During systole, the free wall moves toward the septum. In this cardiomyopathic heart, notice how feeble the wall motion is. This indicates abnormal systolic function.

Thus, dP/dt$_{max}$ does not measure contractility, alone, but is also determined by preload. Therefore dP/dt$_{max}$ is termed a preload dependent estimate of contractility.

The maximal rate of decrease in left ventricular pressure (i.e., the maximal rate with which intraventricular pressure falls), dP/dt$_{min}$, has been proposed as an estimate of the lusitropic property (Figure 6.18).

EXAMPLES OF CARDIOVASCULAR DISEASES INVOLVING MECHANICAL MALFUNCTIONS

Mitral Regurgitation. Mitral regurgitation is the most common cardiovascular disorder in almost all animals but particularly so in dogs (Figure 6.19) (Buchanan 1979; Yoran et al. 1979a, b; Rowell 1986; Darke 1987; Paulus and Shah 1999). It occurs because the leaflets of the mitral valve—between the left atrium and left ventricle—are thickened and gnarled. The ventricles contract because of waves of depolarization traversing them, the waves generating the QRS complex of the ECG. Immediately after the onset of ventricular contraction, the pressure within the left ventricle slams closed the leaflets of the mitral valve. Closure of these valves suddenly decelerates the mass of blood within the left ventricle and frustrates the attempts of this blood from regurgitating (leaking) back into the left atrium. Sudden deceleration of this mass of blood throws cardiohemic structures into oscillations that constitute the first heart sound (S$_1$) described as *Lub*. Because of the diseased mitral leaflets, a portion of the blood within the left ventricle regurgitates through the mitral orifice into the left atrium. This regurgitation occurs under such a large pressure gradient (120 mm Hg in the left ventricle and only 5 mm Hg in the left atrium) that the velocity is great enough to produce disturbed flow (turbulent or eddy formation). Blood flowing in lamina is silent, whereas blood flowing with

force of left ventricular contraction may be quite modest, but the arterial pressure may be quite high if the SVR is high. However, left ventricular function can be monitored by the rate of change in intraventricular pressure. The maximal rate of rise of ventricular pressure (dP/dt$_{max}$) always occurs at the instant just before the aortic valve opens. At this instant, the left ventricle is a chamber closed by the mitral valve at one side and by the aortic valve at the other. Thus, the SVR is excluded from determining dP/dt$_{max}$. Rather, dP/dt$_{max}$ is determined only by the rate of force developed by the left ventricle. Remember that the rate of force development is determined by both the myocardial contractility (the velocity of cycling of heavy meromyosin heads) and the numbers of those heads that are cycling (determined by preload).

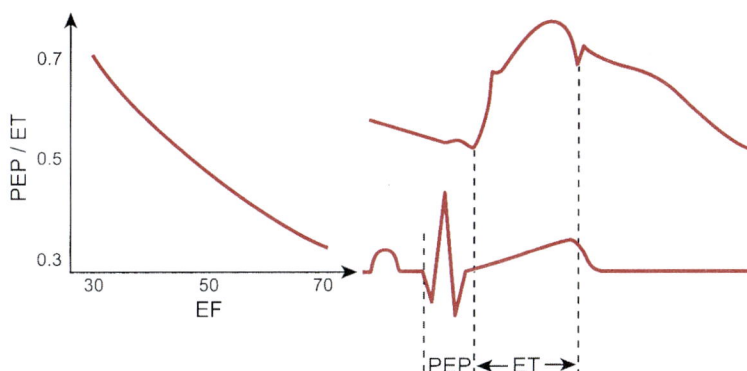

FIG. 6.17—Illustrations showing **(left)** the ratio PEP/ET versus EF, and **(right)** how systolic time intervals (PEP and ET) are measured. For the illustration on the right, the top curve is an aortic pressure curve and the bottom curve is the ECG. PEP extends from the onset of the QRS complex to the beginning of ventricular ejection. The ET extends from the beginning to the end of ventricular ejection. The PEP is relatively useless activity, since only pressure is generated but no blood is ejected. The ET is useful activity, since blood is ejected. The EF is the ratio of the amount of blood ejected (the stroke volume) to the volume of blood within the ventricle just before contraction (the preload or end-diastolic volume). Notice the inverse relationship between PEP/ET and EF. EF, ejection fraction; ET, ejection time; and PEP, preejection period.

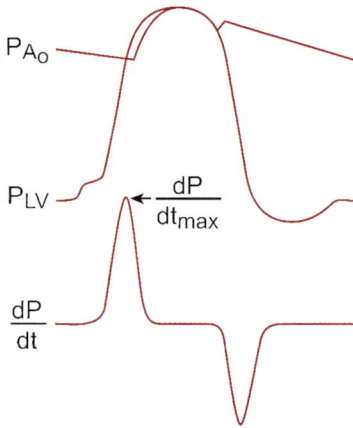

FIG. 6.18—Plots (*ordinate*) of aortic pressure (P_{Ao}), left ventricular pressure (P_{LV}), and rate of change of left ventricular pressure (dP/dt) versus time (*abscissa*). The maximal rate of rise of ventricular pressure (dP/dt$_{max}$) is shown. dP/dt$_{max}$ is used often as an estimate of myocardial contractility, but it is also determined by preload. dP/dt$_{max}$ almost always occurs at the instant just before ventricular pressure exceeds aortic pressure. When ventricular pressure exceeds aortic pressure, the leaflets of the aortic valve separate, blood is ejected from ventricle to aorta, and rate of rise of pressure decreases.

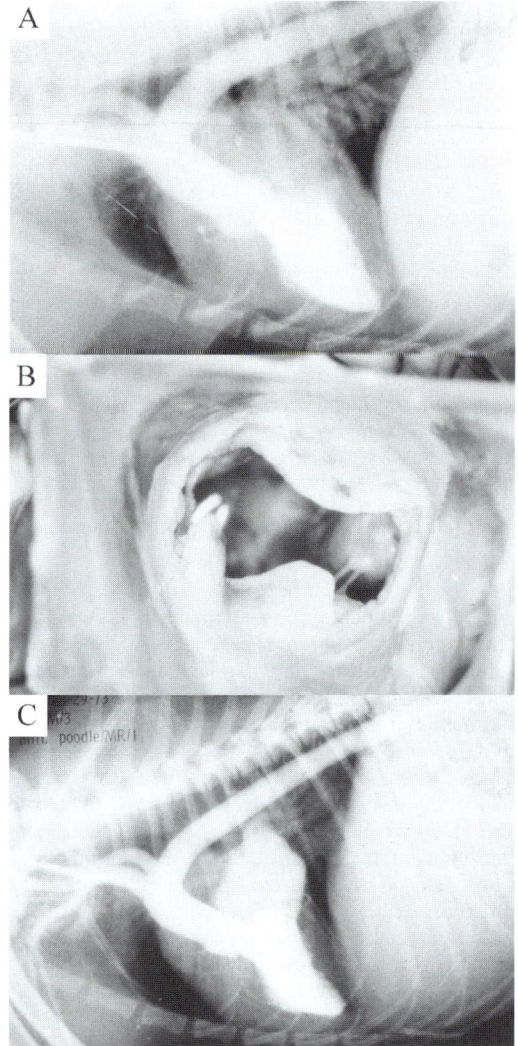

FIG. 6.19—**A:** A left lateral angiocardiogram obtained from a normal dog into whose left ventricle radiopaque dye was injected. Notice the dye fills the left ventricle and aller mixing with blood is ejected into the aorta. Because the leaflets of the mitral valve close properly, no dye regurgitates into the left atrium. **B:** Notice the thickened, gnarled leaflets of the mitral valve. You are looking through the incompletely closed mitral valve and can see the papillary muscles of the left ventricle. **C:** A left lateral angiocardiogram obtained from a dog with mitral regurgitation. Notice how dye mixed with blood is ejected into the aorta normally, but also leaks out of the left ventricle into the left atrium.

disturbance may impart oscillations of sufficient amplitude and of audiofrequency to be heard as murmurs. Blood regurgitates from the left ventricle into the left atrium whenever left ventricular pressure exceeds left atrial pressure. Regurgitation occurs during the entire period of ventricular systole (termed *holosystolic*) and usually extends from the first heart sound (Lub) to and slightly beyond the second heart sound (*dup*).

Below are values of cardiovascular function for the normal state (N), for the beat (albeit an imaginary one) after mitral regurgitation develops (MR_d), after initial compensations (MR_c), and after development of a new steady state (MR_{ns}), including hypertrophy. Notations are left atrial pressure (LAP), left ventricular end-diastolic volume (EDV) or preload (PL), thickness (WT) of the left ventricular free wall, the stroke volume (SV) that travels antegradely (a) into the aorta and retrogradely (r) into the left atrium, the end-systolic volume (ESV) which remains in the left ventricle after the SV is subtracted, the ratio of SV to PL [the ejection fraction (EF)], the aortic pressure (P_a), and the tension (T) in the wall of the left ventricle. Remember that tension is afterload, and that this equals the product of diastolic arterial pressure times PL all divided by WT. For the sake of these argu-

ments, mean aortic pressure will be used instead of diastolic arterial pressure, and EDV will be used instead of radius:

	LAP	EDV	(WT)	SV$_a$	SV$_r$	ESV	EF	P$_a$	T
Normal	5	100	1	60	0	40	0.6	100	10,000

The foregoing line states that under normal conditions with a filling force from the left atrium of 5 mm Hg, an EDV of 100 mL is achieved, the ventricular wall thickness is 1 cm, the SV into the aorta is 60 mL, the SV regurgitating into the left atrium is 0 mL (i.e., there is no mitral regurgitation), the ESV is 40 mL (EDV − SV = 100 − 60 = 40), the EF (SV/EDV) is 0.6, the P_a is 100 mm Hg, and the T (peak tension or AL) is 10,000 units.

We produce mitral regurgitation so that equal portions of the SV proceed antegradely and regurgitantly into the left atrium.

MR   5   100   1   40   40   20   0.8   80   8000

The foregoing line states that from a normal EDV of 100 mL, the SV increases to 80 mL (40 mL into the aorta and 40 mL regurgitantly into the left atrium), the ESV is only 20 mL (100 − 80), the EF increases to 0.8 (80/100), the P_a decreases to 80 mm Hg because the SV into the aorta (40 mL) decreases, and the T has reduced to 8000 [(100 × 80)/1]. Stroke volume increased when mitral regurgitation occurred, because the left ventricle could eject blood normally into the relatively high-pressure aorta and regurgitantly into the relatively low-pressure left atrium (a low-resistance port).

As a consequence of the previous ventricular contraction in which mitral regurgitation occurred, we observe the following:

MR_d 10   120   0.8   50   50   20   0.83   100   15,000

The foregoing line states that the LAP is elevated to 10 mm Hg because of the regurgitation from the previous beat. The EDV increases to 120 mL because of the added pressure in the left atrium filling the ventricle more completely. The WT is reduced to 0.8 cm because the same amount of muscle is stretched around a larger lumen. The SV increases to 100 mL (50 mL antegradely into the aorta, and 50 mL retrogradely into the left atrium). The fact that SV increased to 80 mL from a normal of 60 mL is explainable by increased EDV, which, invoking the Frank-Starling law of the heart, makes the ventricle contract more forcefully. The EF becomes 0.83 (100 mL/120 mL). The P_a returns to normal because SV_a (50 mL) is close to normal (60 mL). The T increases ($\uparrow$) to 15,000 [(P_a * EDV)/0.8].

As a consequence (Weber et al. 1987) of increased myocardial tension (T), a series of events is activated that causes myocardial hypertrophy. One sequence of events has been described as

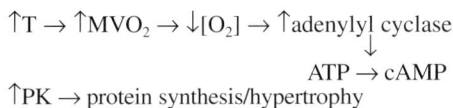

$$\uparrow T \rightarrow \uparrow MVO_2 \rightarrow \downarrow[O_2] \rightarrow \uparrow \text{adenylyl cyclase}$$
$$\downarrow$$
$$ATP \rightarrow cAMP$$
$$\uparrow PK \rightarrow \text{protein synthesis/hypertrophy}$$

As a result of increased protein synthesis and the resulting hypertrophy,

MR_{ns} 10   120   1.2   50   50   20   0.83   100   10,000

The foregoing line states that from the elevated LAP of 10 mm Hg, EDV remains at 120 mL. But, because of the hypertrophy, the wall thickens to 1.2 cm. This results in return of tension (AL) to 10,000 units—the normal value. As such, myocardial oxygen demand returns to normal.

It appears that the compensatory sequence is "designed" to sustain myocardial oxygen demand as close to normal as possible. Because antegrade SV and P_a are normal, the patient should not be manifesting signs or symptoms that might occur as a result of decreased SV or P_a.

But notice that, anatomically, the left atrium is enlarged and under greater pressure than normal. One would also anticipate that, if the left atrium is engorged, so might the pulmonary veins and pulmonary capillaries upstream from the left atrium be engorged. You will observe this morbid anatomy as we discuss many other prototypical cardiovascular disorders that lead to left-sided congestive heart failure.

Hypertrophic Cardiomyopathy. Hypertrophic cardiomyopathy (Fox et al. 1995; Kittleson Kienle 1998) is by far the most common cardiovascular disorder in cats. It is characterized by thickening and stiffening of the walls of the left ventricle. We will use the same presentation for hypertrophic cardiomyopathy as was used for mitral regurgitation. N is the normal state, hCMy is the state for the imaginary instant of production of hCMy, and $hCMy_{ns}$ is the new steady state of function for the cardiovascular system with hCMy. LAP stands for left atrial pressure, EDV stands for left ventricular end-diastolic volume or preload, SV stands for stroke volume, ESV stands for end-systolic volume (the volume of blood remaining within the left ventricle immediately after ejecting the SV), EF stands for the ejection fraction (SV/EDV), P_a stands for the systemic arterial pressure, and T stands for the peak myocardial tension (AL). Because there is no mitral regurgitation, the SV will represent only the stroke into the aorta:

	LAP	EDV	WT	SV	ESV	EF	P_a	T
N	5	100	1	60	40	0.6	100	10,000

For the foregoing line, notice that all values are as they were for the normal dog. Of course, since cats are much smaller than dogs, the volumes should be much smaller, but just assume we are dealing with a giant cat! This line states that from an LAP of 5 mm Hg, there is an EDV of 100 mL with a left ventricular wall thickness of 1 cm. The SV is 60 mL, giving an EF of 0.6. The P_a is 100 mm Hg, and peak myocardial tension is 10,000 units.

Now we are presented with a cat whose left ventricular wall has become massively hypertrophied (4 cm thick). The reason for this hypertrophy is unknown, but there is no doubt it has a genetic basis:

hCMy   5   50   4   40   20   0.8   80   1000

The foregoing line states that from an LAP of 5 mm Hg, the EDV is only 50 mL because the left ventricular walls are so thick (4 cm) and stiff. The SV decreases to only 40 mL because of the Frank-Starling law of the heart, which states that the force of contraction depends on the volume of blood in the ventricle (EDV or PL) just before it contracts. The EF is elevated to 0.8 even though the SV is reduced to 40 mL, because EDV is only 50 mL. The P_a decreases because the SV has decreased, and the T has decreased precipitously because the EDV (PL) is small, the P_a is reduced, and the WT is enormous.

Because of the fall in SV, blood dams up in the left atrium, pulmonary veins, and possibly pulmonary capillaries—just as it did with mitral regurgitation. Therefore the next line is observed:

$$hCMy_{ns} \quad 15 \quad 100 \quad 2.5 \quad 60 \quad 40 \quad 0.6 \quad 100 \quad 4000$$

In the foregoing line, notice that the EDV, SV, ESV, and P_a are all normal. This cat should not be feeling ill because of reduced cardiac output. But notice that in order to fill the ventricle, with the hypertrophied and stiff wall, the LAP must have been elevated.

Thus, we develop, in this cat with hCMy, engorgement of the left atrium, pulmonary veins, and pulmonary capillaries similar to what was observed in the dog with mitral regurgitation.

GOALS OF THERAPY BASED ON PATHOPHYSIOLOGY.

Goals of therapy (Cohn 1985; Smith and Kampine 1990; Fox et al. 1998; Kittleson and Kienle 1998; Lilly 1998) should be based on reversing the pathophysiological processes that result in death or incapacity. They are as follows:

1. Regulating heart rate (with digitalis, β-blockers like atenolol, and calcium channel blockers like diltiazem) is crucial to sustain cardiac output and ATP concentrations necessary for contraction, relaxation, and proper ionic fluxes across the cell membranes. A heart beating too rapidly consumes more oxygen and receives less oxygen because coronary blood flow (carrying oxygen to the heart) occurs predominantly when the heart is in diastole.

2. Minimizing chronic stretch (with afterload reducers like enalapril and positive inotropes like digitalis) of myocardium protects the cells from sustained injury. This decreases afterload and myocardial oxygen consumption.

3. Removing edema (with diuretics like furosemide and venodilators like nitroglycerine) enables the edematous organ to function better; for example, it decreases stiffness and effort of ventilation that occurs in pulmonary edema, and decreases the pendulous abdomen characteristic of ascites.

4. Improving baroreceptor function (with digitalis, spironolactone and angiotensin-converting enzyme inhibitors) so that these receptors "report" correct information to the medulla. There is abnormal function of high-pressure baroreceptors: the high-pressure baroreceptors located in the aortic and carotid sinuses serve to buffer changes in systemic arterial blood pressure. When blood pressure decreases, decreased tension in these receptors causes them to decrease afferent volleys over the vagus and glossopharyngeal nerves to the medulla. The medulla "interprets" the decreased afferent activity as indicating hypotension, and that the level of pressure is below the desired level. It then sends efferent volleys over the vagus to accelerate the heart rate and over α-adrenergic fibers to vasoconstrict arterioles. These two actions tend to return blood pressure toward normal. In heart failure, angiotensin II is thought to cause the release of aldosterone, and aldosterone loads the high-pressure baroreceptors with sodium-potassium ATPase. This loading injures the baroreceptors, which "think" that blood pressure is low even if it is not. Thus, the medulla responds by decreasing vagal efferent traffic and by stiffening arteries and arterioles by activating the smooth muscle in the media. Whereas these responses may be beneficial for a short-term fall in blood pressure as in acute hemorrhage, they are clearly injurious to the heart already injured by mitral regurgitation or dilated cardiomyopathy. Increasing heart rate increases myocardial oxygen consumption and shortens diastole—the period when most coronary blood flow occurs. Thus, the heart suffers an oxygen deficiency leading to further injury (Figure 6.20). Of course, the arterial and arteriolar vasoconstriction increases the afterload, which reduces further the systolic function of the heart (Bristow et al. 1982; Lefkowitz 1995; Dostal and Baker 1999; Brilla 2000; Melo et al. 2000; Swedberg 2000).

5. Upregulating β-adrenergic receptors (with low-dose β-blockers like carvedilol) is necessary for *fight or flight* responses to be reestablished. There is downregulation of $β_1$-adrenergic receptors in heart failure (Bristow et al. 1982; Muntz et al. 1994; Brilla 2000; Swedberg 2000). Patients in heart failure from almost any etiology have decreased activity of $β_1$-adrenergic receptors—termed *downregulation*. The mechanism is thought to involve high circulating levels of catecholamines precipitated by a reduction in systemic arterial pressure (invoking the baroreceptor reflex) and by a reduction in renal blood flow with increased production of angiotensin II (which both causes the release of and prevents the reuptake of norepinephrine). It is thought that this downregulation protects a "sick heart" from being "flogged" by high catecholamine activity that would produce more serious injury. Downregulation of the $β_1$-adrenergic receptors is manifested by the inability of a patient to mount an adequate fight-or-flight response and by the inability to increase heart rate (chronotropic incompetency) in response to either exogenous or endogenous catecholamines. This inability is manifested as both reduced cardiovascular function (due to downregulation of β-adrenergic receptors on the myocardium) and immune function (due to downregulation of β-adrenergic receptors on lymphocytes). Low-dose carvedilol (a nonspecific β-adrenergic blocking agent) is one of the drugs (the other two

A   atrial fibrillation

B   ventricular fibrillation

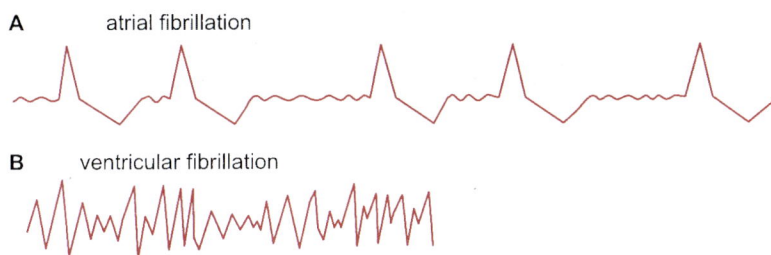

FIG. 6.20—Examples of atrial (**A**) and ventricular (**B**) fibrillation. With atrial fibrillation, the QRS complexes appear rapidly and irregularly, there are no P waves, and the baseline has coarse, low-amplitude oscillations termed *f waves*. Instead of the atria being depolarized by a wave originating from the sinoatrial node, hundreds of packets of atrial myocardium are stimulated independently by circus movements meandering through them. Since there is no uniform wave, there is no P wave. The meanderings produce the f waves. The ventricles are stimulated rapidly and irregularly because the meanderings from the atria enter the atrioventricular conduction systemic rapidly and irregularly. The fibrillating atria appear to wiggle like a bag of worms and eject no blood, but normal function of the ventricle does not depend on the atrial contribution except at high heart rates. With ventricular fibrillation, there are neither P waves nor QRS complexes, because the ventricles are depolarized with meanderings similar to those that occur in the atria with atrial fibrillation. This animal is clinically dead, because the ventricles wiggle like a bag of worms instead of beating.

being spironolactone and angiotensin-converting enzyme inhibitors) known to decrease severity of exercise intolerance and to prolong life; and it is thought that the mechanism of action is by *upregulation* of the β-adrenergic receptors. Upregulation of β-adrenergic receptors must be considered a primary goal of treatment of heart failure.

6. Terminating abnormal shunts (e.g., PDA) by ligation or inserting a coil prevents overcirculation of the lungs and left atrial and ventricular stretch.

7. Decreasing ventricular irritability (with an antiarrhythmic like sotalol) reduces premature depolarizations and tachycardia, and minimizes possibility of ventricular fibrillation (Antzelevitch and Sicouri 1994; Zipes and Jalife 1995) (Figure 6.20).

8. Slowing conduction through the AV node in atrial fibrillation (with diltiazem, digitalis, or atenolol) reduces the ventricular rate.

PART 2: THE EXTRACARDIAC PERIPHERAL CIRCULATION AND SHOCK

ARNOLD A. STOKHOF

DISTRIBUTIVE VESSELS. These link the aorta and pulmonary artery to capillaries and back via the venous funnel system to the atria (Mellander and Johansson 1968; Berne and Levy 2001) (Figure 6.21 and Table 6.3). This brilliant concise schematic condenses the major components of the system's circulation in mammals (Mellander and Johansson 1968).

CARDIOVASCULAR HEMODYNAMICS. Blood, the fluid inside the cardiovascular system, is a complex fluid. It is a suspension of red blood cells, white blood cells, and platelets in a liquid medium consisting of a colloidal solution of plasma proteins and suspended lipid globules in an aqueous solution. Veterinary students learn about the architecture of the cardiovascular system by dissection of embalmed cadavers that have been injected with colored latex. The students wonder at the extraordinary degree of branching as they follow the great vessels from the heart to the ends of the smallest arterial branches that are visible. As the capillaries are visible only under a suitable microscope, the next visible components are the venules that lead back to the veins. It requires a huge conceptual jump to grasp the transition between life and death. The amazing dynamism of the functional system in life calls for an awareness of the biophysics of things that are changing rapidly from moment to moment (Folkow and Neil 1971; Burton 1972; Milnor 1982; Taylor and Stevens 1983; Berne and Levy 2001). The term *flow* applied to the motion of blood in the various vessels and branches is complex. Starting with velocity, the term has the dimensions of distance per unit of time, for example,

TABLE 6.3—Approximate distribution of blood volume as it moves through the heart and the two major circuits

Example of percent distribution of blood volume pulmonary versus systemic circuits	
Heart	7.2%
Pulmonary circuit	8.8%
Systemic circuit	84 %

Note: Veins, 64%.
Hence, *capacitance* vessels.

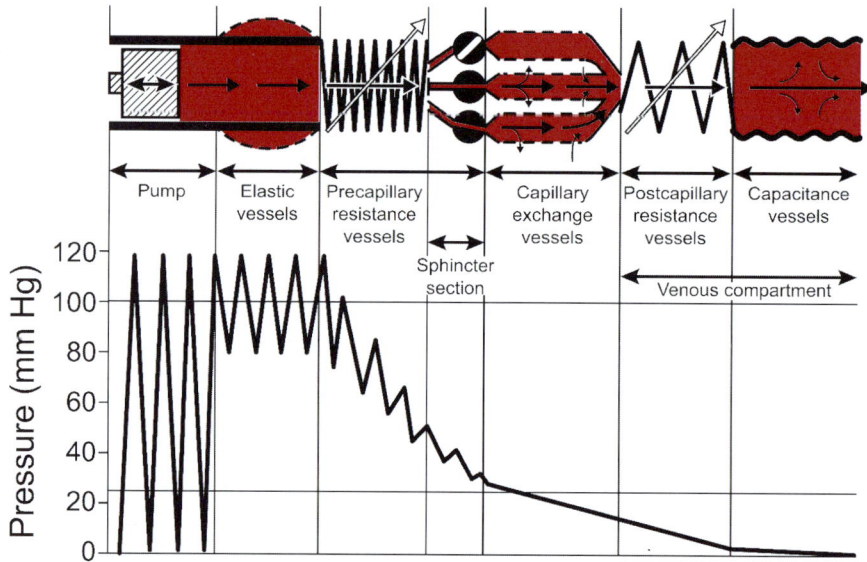

FIG. 6.21—Schematic diagram of the main features of the systemic circulatory system of mammals. The vertically divided sections represent (from left to right):
1. Left ventricle = pump
2. Aorta and large arteries = elastic vessels
3. Smaller arteries and arterioles = adjustable resistance vessels
4. Sphincters at ends of arterioles = regulators of capillary beds flow distribution
5. Capillaries = exchange vessels
6. Venules and smaller veins = postcapillary resistance vessels
7. Larger veins = capacitance vessels

From Mellander and Johansson, *Pharmacol. Rev.* 20:117–196, 1968, Am. Soc. Pharmacol & Exp. Therapeutics, with permission.

centimeters per second, which is linear velocity or the speed with which the fluid is moving through the tube. Flow is usually designated as volume flow or movement of volume per unit time. Because the blood vascular system varies in cross-sectional area, it is necessary to evaluate volume flow as a function of that area:

$$(v = Q/A) \text{ or } [Q = v \times A]$$

where A is area, Q is flow, and v is velocity.

If area is halved, velocity of flow will be doubled. What is it that imparts motion to the blood? It is the pressure gradient along the tubes but not the simple lateral pressure gradient. It is the *total pressure*, a combination of the lateral pressure and the dynamic pressure attributable to the kinetic energy of the flowing fluid. The latter is defined by this equation:

$$\rho \times v^2/2$$

where ρ is density and v is velocity.

As velocity is greater in narrower sections of the tubular system, the kinetic component of pressure is greater while the lateral pressure will be lower. In the canine ascending aorta, peak flow velocity is about 150 cm per second. It is significantly lower in the descending thoracic aorta. However, In the healthy cardiovas-

cular system in most arterial locations the kinetic component is but a negligible fraction of the total pressure. This changes dramatically if there is a constriction as in the case of aortic stenosis. Then the output of the powerful left ventricle is forced through a narrowed orifice of the aortic valve imparting a high kinetic energy because of the high velocity. The lateral pressure is reduced. This has the unfortunate consequence of reducing the fraction of the aortic flow that enters the coronary arteries.

The sheer complexity of the closed tubular system of the circulation is staggering (Smith and Kampine 1990) (Table 6.4). This is necessary to achieve the most remarkable feature of the system's design, namely, to bring oxygenated blood into close proximity with every active cell in the mammalian body. By *proximity* is meant close enough to be meaningful for function, for example, within about 100 microns between a capillary wall and a cell's membrane. After that closest capillary delivers bulk flow of blood by its pressure gradient, diffusion can effect the exchanges of solutes, gases, and water between the capillary wall and the adjacent cells. Any failure of this bulk flow delivery results in ischemia and progressive decline in cell function. One fail-safe feature of the vascular architecture is the multiple access via the network of interconnections among the capillaries. The density of capillary branches varies

TABLE 6.4—Detailed features of various vascular compartments and a glimpse of the extraordinary complexity of the circulatory system

Distribution of blood volume in dogs

Diameter of vessels (mm)	
Vena cava	12.5
Veins	1.5 up to 12.5
Venules	0.03
Aorta	10.0
Arteries	0.6 up to 10.00
Arterioles	0.02
Capillaries	0.008
Number of vessels	
Vena cava	1
Veins	2440
Venules	80 million
Aorta	1
Arteries	2440
Arterioles	40 million
Capillaries	1.2 billion
Length of vessels (cm)	
Capillaries	up to 0.1
Arterioles and venules	0.2
Arteries and veins	0.2 up to 40
Total blood volume[a] (mL)	
Capillaries	60
Arterioles	25
Arteries	145
Veins	570
Venules	110
Total cross-section area (cm²)	
Capillaries	600
Arterioles	125
Arteries	14
Veins	68
Venules	570

[a]Moving target.

with the priority of the cells of the organ served for (a) survival (e.g., brain, heart, and kidney) and (b) provision for huge increases of flow when needed (e.g., skeletal muscle for fight or flight).

The dual vascular system (Table 6.4) extends (a) through the systemic arterial tree to the systemic capillary beds, returning via the converging venous trunks to the right atrium, and (b) via the pulmonary arterial network and capillary beds to the pulmonary venous funnel to the left atrium. The cardiac chambers generate the motive force for the circulation of the blood. The capillary beds are the "business end" of the system, receiving the essential nutrients to pass on to the tissue cells and collect the waste products for return and redistribution to appropriate beds for disposal on the next circuit. An important role is played by the interstitium surrounding and interacting with the microvasculature, the setting for the capillary beds and their auxiliary drainage system: the lymphatics. The blood vessels and heart make up the "container" for the circulating fluid: the blood. In between heart and capillary beds are the distributive vessels: the arterial and venous "trees." The system is truly remarkable in that it is only partially closed as it allows for components of the noncellular medium to escape and return, including macromolecules such as albumin and globulins. The primary func-

tion of the peripheral vascular system is to distribute the blood to the tissues in a manner that allows for differential partitioning (shunting) of blood flow to meet the diverse needs of the various tissues (Berne and Levy 2001). This is accomplished by "gatemen" (smooth muscle sphincters at the ends of some arterioles) that modulate how much blood passes through each capillary network branch or subcircuit. Distribution is regulated by neurogenic, hormonal, and metabolic mechanisms under the influence of sensors that detect departures from homeostatic ranges (Wiggers 1975).

The distribution also involves some controls of vascular tone for general functions like thermoregulation. These controls include synthesis and secretion of vasoactive agents. The blood itself has some very specialized features that are the key to maintaining its fluidity and nonadhesiveness (Lilly 1998). These include antithrombotic substances that ensure that all the vascular branches stay patent. Since the tissues may be subjected to traumatic injury, there is always a risk of hemorrhage, so the system has to have a way to counteract this. The coagulation cascade is nature's solution (Figure 6.22). It is a way to trigger the clotting mechanism when a thrombus is needed to plug a damaged vessel. Another important role for the distributive system is to get cells with anti-infective and immune capabilities to areas where they are needed.

Pathophysiology of peripheral vascular disease occurs when infection or inflammation leads to degenerative changes in the arterial wall. Examples include various viruses, bacteria, and multicellular parasites:

1. *Strongylus vulgaris* larvae cross the intestinal epithelium and migrate up the cranial mesenteric artery in horses. They cause arteritis, intestinal dysfunction including colic, and sometimes lead to terminal aortic and iliac arterial thrombosis. This indicates the importance of using control measures against this noxious parasite.

2. After their intermediate host (typically a dung beetle) is ingested by dogs, *Spirocerca lupi* set up shop by forming nodules in the esophageal wall or further down the digestive tract. The worms' larvae migrate via the wall of the thoracic aorta. The damage they cause there can result in aneurysms that may rupture, resulting in lethal hemorrhage. Aortic thromboembolism is seen in cats, often in cases affected with a predisposing cardiomyopathy.

3. If the microfilaria of the canine heartworm, *Dirofilaria immitis*, introduced by the bite of an infected mosquito are allowed to develop to maturity, the adults become several inches long attached to the intimal wall of the pulmonary artery, a major obstructive and toxic crisis of pathophysiology.

4. The toxic agents in ergotism and fescue foot mycotoxicoses are numerous ergot alkaloids that are lysergic acid derivatives and cause severe vasoconstriction of arterioles, particularly in vessels in the extremities (tail and hooves). Their stimulant effect on smooth muscle includes actions on adrenoceptors and 5-HT

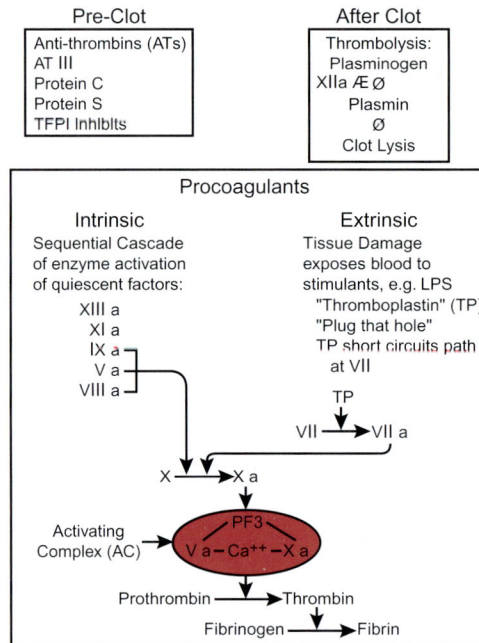

FIG. 6.22—The delicate balance of the clotting system. Various blood coagulation factors exist in plasma as quiescent inactive proenzyme proteins that require activation to become procoagulants. The inactive forms are represented by Roman numerals (but no longer in sequential order). When activated a small "a" is added after the number.

The endothelial cell (EC) surface is stimulated by a tissue factor (TF) to trigger the sequential cascade of enzyme activations that lead to coagulation and clot formation in the event of vascular trauma or release of activating agents, for example, by platelets or other cells.

1. The *intrinsic* (endogenous) *pathway* requires the full sequence of enzymatic activations to reach the culminating focus of an activating complex (AC) made up of a platelet factor (PF3), factor V_a, ionized calcium (Ca^{++}) and factor X_a. The AC forms proteolytic thrombokinase that cleaves prothrombin (factor II), forming thrombin (IIa) that converts fibrinogen to fibrin (factor I).

2. The *extrinsic pathway* is activated by tissue thromboplastin (TP), a lipoprotein that arises from damaged tissue cells and shortcuts the cascade by activating VII to VII_a that triggers AC formation as shown.

Activation of the intrinsic pathway (all components are intrinsic to the blood): A trigger is required to tip the balance, usually a biochemical stimulus that causes platelets (PLs) to adhere and degranulate at the EC surface. One milliliter of plasma has enough procoagulants to cleave all fibrinogen in blood in 1 minute if activated. The *pros* and *antis* are in balance to avoid this:

1. It restricts the AC to sites where it is needed: the factors need to be close together for activation (e.g., clumping of platelets).
2. The constant flow of blood dilutes them except at the active site.
3. Repair of the damage quickly covers the area to stop stimuli.
4. The *antis* are activated to provide protective blockade versus the *pros*.

Protection against coagulation: The vascular wall controls the anticoagulant factors. The ECs synthesize antithrombins (e.g., angiotensin III or AT-III) that bind to thrombin (T), inactivating it and arresting the cleavage of fibrinogen to fibrin. The AT-III plus T activate protein C (PC) in the presence of surface protein S (PS).

Complex interaction among these agents and others leads to inactivation of an inhibitor of plasminogen activation favoring lysis of clots. The anticoagulant potential of the ECs is regulated by

1. Protease inhibitors
2. Proteases that inactivate cofactors such as PC's effect on V_a and V-III_a
3. Inhibition of coagulation enzymes by competition with binding sites
4. Tissue factor pathway inhibitor (TFPI)

On the other hand, platelets, if activated, secrete endoglycosidases that degrade heparin sulfates and block thrombin inactivation, thereby having a procoagulant effect. Also, after aggregation, they change shape with villilike projections that adhere to the fibronectin. Later, fibrin forms and creates a network for the clot.

There is growing evidence supporting the concept that the endothelial cells are very important in pathophysiology. Reduced nitric oxide (NO) activity appears to contribute to subarachnoid hemorrhage, ischemia, vascular degeneration, and hypertension. It can result in a contractile response of the smooth muscle cells and even vasospasm.

receptors. The vascular changes may progress to dry gangrene because the vasoconstriction can become an arterial spasm with endothelial degeneration and dermal necrosis. Hooves may be sloughed. The feet are tender or painful, and knuckling of the pastern is sometimes seen. There is a neurological form with depression or excitability, loss of appetite, ataxia, weight loss, diarrhea, and clonic convulsions. In ergotism, the source of the toxins is a fungus, *Claviceps purpura*, which grows in the mature seeds of grains, such as rye, and certain grasses. In fescue foot, the source is a different fungus that affects the widely grown tall fescue (*Festuca arundinacea schreb*) at all stages of growth (Tor-Agbidye et al. 2001). The toxins, notably ergovaline, cause vasoconstriction and vascular spasm in the arteries of the feet, and some also antagonize prolactin. The latter effect can cause agalactia in sows, cows, and mares. Mares may develop prolonged gestation and thickened placentas, and may abort.

Aneurysm is a localized cylindrical or saccular dilation of an artery in excess of 50% of its normal diameter. It is fusiform if the entire circumference is dilated, but saccular if only part way round, in which case it is an outpouching rather than cylindrical. Since aneurysms may be asymptomatic, there is a risk of catastrophic hemorrhage into the retroperitoneal space, the abdominal cavity, or even the intestine (Berne and Levy 2001). The risk of wall rupture rises rapidly as radius increases, because wall tension is proportional to the product of pressure and radius (law of Laplace).

Inability to rise and stand that results in an immobile downer animal is a serious setting for pathophysiology, especially in large, heavy animals like cows. Even an alert downer cow often develops digestive disorders plus circulatory and neural dysfunction (Smith et al. 2002:1016–1018). The pressure imposed by the weight obstructs the flow of blood and lymph, and the ischemia can progress to necrosis over bony prominences that are intractable to therapy other than cushioning the affected areas and frequently changing the animal's position. These lesions are known as *decubitus ulcers*, and paraplegia predisposes animals to their onset. Devices, including flotation systems, have been developed to relieve the pressure.

Movement is very important for a healthy vascular system. *Veins* are thin-walled conduits for blood that convey blood from the capillaries back to the heart. They are distensible and collapsible. As such, they are capacitance vessels because they hold about 70% of the blood volume at rest. This compares with about 13% in the arteries and an estimated 7% in the capillaries. These estimates are subject to large variations, however, with changing physical activity and metabolic stimuli. Dramatic changes occur during vigorous exercise (Smith and Kampine 1990). Also, veins have smooth muscle in their walls that can increase venous pressure and cause the veins to shrink in diameter, reducing their capacity. Exercise increases venous return to the heart in part by increasing cardiac output,

partly by skeletal muscle contraction compressing some veins followed by relaxation with refilling, aided by one-way valves in some veins that direct flow toward the right atrium. Also, there are moderate fluid shifts from the vascular compartment to the interstitium with an increase in hematocrit. More capillaries are opened and active in exercising skeletal muscles, and there is considerable redistribution of blood flow among the various organs.

Pathophysiology sets in if exercise is pushed to exhaustion (Lilly 1998). At this point, maximal heart rate is reached, and stroke volume has plateaued and is starting to decline along with blood pressure. Dehydration is occurring, and vasoconstriction reduces heat loss. Hence, homeostatic regulation of body temperature is compromised, and severe hyperthermia can set in leading to malaise and incoordination. Anaerobic metabolism in the state of inadequate oxygenation of the tissues results in accumulation of L-lactate, a higher lactate/pyruvate ratio, and a marked fall in pH.

Vascular Blood Pressure and Flow: The Arterial Pulse. Arterial pulse pressure is a feature of the mammalian cardiovascular system (Berne and Levy 2001). The intermittent pumping of the ventricles gives rise to a strikingly pulsatile waveform in the arteries that is characterized by a steep rise followed by a slower decline. The dicrotic notch on the down slope is due to aortic valve closure that allows a transient retrograde surge of blood. The pulse is a dramatic pressure wave induced by the sudden entrance of the bolus or stroke volume of blood from the chamber of the left ventricle into the distensible tube of the aorta. The tube bulges, the pressure rises rapidly in the tube, and the pressure wave is propagated at high speed along the vessel. Note that the velocity of the pulse wave is about 10-fold greater than that of the velocity of the blood itself. The high velocity of the traveling pulse wave distends the vessel ahead of the blood, and the elastic recoil of the arterial wall maintains the initial momentum imparted to the blood as it entered the arterial tree. The pulse pressure is the difference between systolic and diastolic arterial pressures, about 35 to 60 mm Hg. It should be noted that the value for diastolic pressure is much higher in the arteries than in the ventricle. This is necessary to maintain the pressure head required for perfusion of the peripheral capillary beds through the diastolic phase. Wave reflection at major branching sites in the arterial tree (such as the aortic trifurcation at the iliac level) contributes to sustaining the diastolic pressure. The contour of the arterial pulse wave changes as it passes from the aorta along the arterial tree, the systolic wave becoming higher and more sharply peaked while the diastolic declines and acquires additional oscillations. Due to sinus arrhythmia, each inspiration increases heart rate and boosts systolic blood pressure about 15 mm Hg because inspiration promotes dilation of the intrathoracic blood chambers that increases filling and volume of blood ejected.

The level of the mean arterial pressure depends on cardiac output (CO) and peripheral resistance (R) whether or not any change in CO is a result of a rate change or stroke volume adjustment or of both (Smith and Kampine 1990). Peripheral resistance is the ratio of mean pressure and mean flow. Thus, for the systemic circulation, the total peripheral resistance (TPR) is the mean aortic pressure (MAP) minus the vena caval pressure (VCP) divided by the CO. A healthy dog might have a MAP of 87 mm Hg and a VCP of 3 mm Hg, with a CO at rest of 2.4 L/min (minute). The TPR is 35 mm Hg/L/min under these conditions. When challenged by vigorous exercise, the arterioles supplying skeletal musculature dilate maximally, which can be a 16-fold increase for the fraction of about one-fifth of the resting CO that supplies the muscles. To supply the extra oxygen needed, coronary artery flow will increase several fold. A dog with a failing heart, however, would be unable to attain these adaptive changes and would show exercise intolerance, becoming rapidly fatigued. Since the CO of the right side of the heart is the same as that of the left, similar calculations can be made for the pulmonary circuit by replacing the MAP and VCP with pulmonary artery and pulmonary venous mean pressures, for example, 13 − 5, yielding a total pulmonary resistance of 3.2 mm Hg/L/min at rest. At high exercise, the pulmonary circuit in horses can readily accommodate the changes required in health. However, in chronic obstructive pulmonary disease (COPD) with allergic bronchiolar constriction, the resulting hypoxia triggers pulmonary vasoconstriction, raising pulmonary vascular resistance. Then, to accomplish the increase in pulmonary arterial pressure (PAP) needed to maintain flow at the desired level, a substantial rise in PAP is needed, raising the workload on the right ventricle significantly. This can set the stage for right ventricle dysfunction and severe pathophysiology.

Chronic hypertension is a very common and important manifestation of pathophysiology in the human cardiovascular system (Deshmukh et al., cited in Lilly 1998:267–288). It has been much less studied in domesticated mammals because of the relative lack of pathophysiological research. In humans, the aortic and continuing arterial vascular compliance or elasticity decreases with age and the elastic modulus increases. The aortic pulse pressure is increased in the face of increased TPR and the heart's attempt to maintain CO. To pump the same volume into a less compliant vessel against a higher pressure head requires a significantly higher mean pressure with a greater rise in systolic than diastolic pressure. Progressive degenerative metabolic changes in the collagen and elastin of the arterial walls account for this arteriosclerotic stiffening. These progressive changes are linked to genetic and environmental (lifestyle) factors, including dietary excess of sodium and rich food, obesity, and neurogenic overstress. However, the major concern continues to be a more prevalent form of hypertension in which the underlying mechanisms are poorly understood, the so-called essential hypertension, which appears to be a multifactorial disease of dysregulation for which not all the key facts are known—a real pathophysiological enigma in which homeostatic controls fail to adjust vascular diameters to keep pressures within the desired range (Ganong 2003).

Dynamics of Capillary, Interstitial, and Lymphatic Exchange. For this topic, an excellent overview can be gleaned from an article by Hughes (2000).

The *pulse* is the pressure wave in the arteries that is physically palpable at certain anatomic locations. The pumping action of the left ventricle accounts for the intermittent surge and decline of arterial pulse pressure, characterized by a steep rise and a slower decline. Palpation of the pulse enables one to measure heart rate and other, more subtle, features of cardiovascular function. A sphygmomanometer enables an observer to measure systolic and diastolic arterial pressures that provide clues to the detection of pathophysiology. There is some evidence that the ventricles act as suction pumps (lusitropy) as well as their more obvious role as pressure pumps. The ventricular ejection dilates the aorta, raising the aortic pressure and speeding the blood on its way along the arterial tree. The expansion of the elastic walls of the arteries becomes the source of the energy that carries the blood out to the periphery. The diastolic pressure must be fairly high to ensure there is enough pressure to keep the capillaries functioning. As the diameter of the small arteries narrows on their way to the periphery, the proportion of the wall that is elastic tissue declines and that of smooth muscle increases. Between internal diameters of about 100 down to 30 microns, the pressure inside the vessels starts to drop steeply. Below this diameter, the pressure drop continues as the arterioles decline from about 30 to 10 microns. Many 8-micron-diameter capillaries arise from each arteriole, providing a huge increase in collective cross-sectional area of the vascular bed, slowing the velocity of blood flow, and dampening out the pulsatile nature of that flow. There are approximately 1000 capillaries per arteriole.

Starling proposed in 1896 that transvascular fluid transfers were governed by the gradients between hydrostatic pressure pushing out of the porous capillary walls and the osmotic concentration of large molecules drawing fluid back in (Starling 1918). He recognized that the balance changed as the blood passed through the capillaries from the arteriolar ends to the venular ends. At the arteriolar end, the hydrostatic pressure was paramount, so more fluid left than reentered from the interstitial fluid. The situation changed as the blood moved through toward the venular end, with the rising concentration of macromolecules (primarily plasma proteins) within the vascular compartment reversing the balance, causing a net reabsorption of fluid and solutes.

The structural basis of the microvascular barrier is a layer of endothelial cells surrounded by a capillary basement membrane and bounded on the inside by the glycocalyx as the luminal surface layer, which is composed of proteins, glycoproteins, and glycolipids that exert electrostatic forces attracting or repelling solutes. The selective permeability of the wall involves all of these factors, but albumin and orosomucoid may be most important. The typical capillary has a continuous wall and is permeable to water and small solutes but much less porous to macromolecules. However, tissues engaged in very large fluxes of water and solutes, such as the glomerulus and the intestine, have fenestrated capillaries with regions having a basement membrane but only a minimal endothelial layer that is dependent on electrostatic forces to maintain permeability at a low level. There are more porous discontinuous capillaries in organs such as liver, spleen, and bone marrow. These lack a basement membrane and have gaps up to 1 micron between their endothelial cells, allowing them to be permeable to plasma proteins. The interstitial matrix surrounding the capillary beds has a collagen framework containing glycosaminoglycans (GAGs), such as hyaluronan gel, along with proteins. The GAGs are high molecular weight long chains of disaccharide subunits that create a highly anionic environment that opposes compression, thereby helping resist edema on the one hand and contraction during dehydration on the other. Some components of the matrix may be mobilizable via the lymphatics.

Intracapillary hydrostatic pressure (HP) is the main determinant of fluid egress from the capillary networks. In most tissues, the site of greatest resistance to flow is the small arterioles antecedent to the capillary beds. In the lungs, however, the largest pressure drop occurs across the capillary bed. In the systemic circulation, the degree of modulation can be complete for certain beds that have precapillary sphincters that shunt all flow away from the affected bed. Alternatively, the modulators can be partial and adjustable, depending on neurogenic, myogenic, and humoral stimuli and interplay.

Offsetting the intracapillary HP is the interstitial HP, a parameter that has proved to be very hard to measure and varies greatly with the site. At many sites, it appears to be slightly subatmospheric, thereby favoring filtration from the vasculature to the interstitium. Some encapsulated organs have positive interstitial HPs (e.g., kidney) or variable ones (e.g., intestine between fasting and absorbing). Edema will accumulate where a tissue is most compliant (e.g., pulmonary edema accumulating peribronchially).

The colloid osmotic pressure (COP) is a consequence of macromolecular concentration in the solvent (plasma or interstitial fluid) (Figure 6.23). The biggest contributor (over 60%) to the COP of plasma is albumin. Only 40% of body albumin is intravascular. Furthermore, this 40% circulates through the interstitium every 24 hours. The COP of interstitial fluid is highly variable with location and activity. Skeletal muscle and subcutaneous capillaries are much less permeable to protein, while pulmonary capillaries are more permeable. As a result, protein concentration of lymph from skeletal muscle or skin is only about 50% of that in plasma, while, for pulmonary lymph, the estimate is

about 65%. The COP of healthy dog and cat plasma is typically between 16 and 24 mm Hg. Variations in COP in dogs is usually attributable to increases in globulin concentration that may be accompanied by reduced plasma albumin. Albumin synthesis occurs only in the liver and is regulated by the hepatic plasma COP. The COP and plasma colloids of various domesticated mammalian species have been studied (Zweifach and Intaglietta 1971; Thomas and Brown 1992).

FORMATION OF EDEMA. Edema occurs when excess interstitial fluid develops, and the tissues are said to be "waterlogged." With heart disease, edema develops because of elevation of capillary pressure to levels that drive serum out of the capillaries and into the interstitium faster than the lymphatics can remove it and redirect it back into the vascular system. The rate with which fluid moves across a capillary membrane depends on an imbalance of hydrostatic and oncotic forces across the membrane. For example, the normal dermal intracapillary hydrostatic pressure drops from about 32 mm Hg at its arteriolar end to about 15 mm Hg at the venular end of the capillary (at the level of the heart). The hydrostatic pressure of the interstitial fluid outside the capillary may be about 0 to −5 mm Hg, increasing the net outward hydrostatic pressure to about 27 mm Hg. Offsetting this outward push is the inward pull of the colloid osmotic pressure or oncotic pressure, which is constant within the capillary at about 25 mm Hg, abetted by a small but variable oncotic pressure of the interstitial fluid, depending on the concentration of nondiffusible proteins that have escaped from the capillary. The numbers vary with the different tissues of the body, their activities, and capillary permeability. The situation is very dynamic, but there is a net outward force on the order of only about 1 mm Hg, creating a need for collection of any surplus interstitial fluid into lymphatic microtubules for return to the vascular compartment. Normally, this fluid does not accumulate in the interstitium but only bathes it, because it is removed by the lymphatic channels and gradually pumped back into the vascular system, achieving intralymphatic pressures of up to 20 mm Hg. With heart failure, one side of the heart fails to remove the venous and capillary blood from circulation—the left ventricle from the pulmonary capillaries and the right ventricle from the systemic capillaries. Thus, with elevation of capillary hydrostatic pressure, there is an increase in the net force tending to drive fluid from the capillary into the interstitium. This imbalance may overwhelm the ability of the lymphatics to drain the interstitium, and excess fluid remains as edema. This is most marked in dependent parts where gravity adds to the problem, particularly where the subcutaneous tissue is relatively loose. Also, any increase in capillary permeability due to toxins or inappropriate mediators of capillary dilation can predispose to edema formation. It is important to recall that the situation for plasma proteins is very dynamic. Once they escape from a capillary, the only way they can return is via the lymph, and a

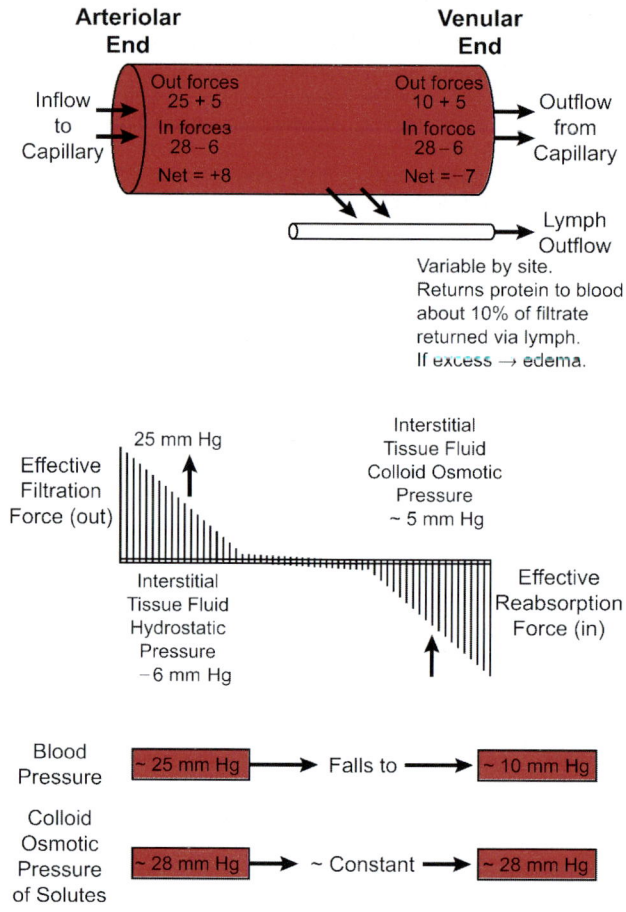

FIG. 6.23—Starling diagram of the forces involved in bidirectional fluid exchanges across the capillary wall of an example microvessel. This shows the hydrostatic pressure gradient from the arteriolar end causing blood flow through the capillary network and filtration of fluid and solutes to the interstitial fluid. Retention of the larger solutes in the vessel, particularly albumin, maintains the colloid osmolality of the plasma so that it progressively overcomes the declining hydrostatic pressure as blood passes along the capillary. It should be noted that the capillaries are not single tubes but part of more complex interconnecting networks. Also, the overall net effect is to have just a little more net outflow than net flow. Thus, there is a slow, gradual increase in interstitial fluid around the beds. This enters the fine lymphatic tubules that constrict to force any excess fluid toward the lymph vessels that convey it back, via lymph nodes, to the circulatory system, aided by skeletal muscle compression where applicable.

remarkably large proportion of circulating plasma proteins (estimates range between 25% and 50%) are returned to the bloodstream by the lymph every 24 hours. The pathophysiology of edema is complex and not easily explained (Berne and Levy 2001).

The "waterlogged" state of tissues impairs their function. If present in the lung (as so-called left-sided congestive heart failure), the lung becomes stiff, muscles of ventilation fatigue, regions of the lungs are poorly ventilated, and the patient may asphyxiate. If present in the limbs, udder, brisket, or liver (as so-called right-sided congestive heart failure), these structures become swollen; and, in the case of capillary congestion of the liver, serum "weeps" from the liver into the abdomen as ascites.

Interstitial edema is a significant risk factor as an outcome of cardiovascular pathophysiology that the body is designed to offset. If excess fluid moves to the relatively nondistensible interstitium, the HP in the latter rises and opposes further extravasation. At the same time, this increase in HP enhances lymphatic drainage. Also, exudation of low-protein fluid lowers interstitial COP, thereby maintaining the COP gradients across the capillary wall. The interstitium progressively opposes increasing distension up to a critical point when the structural resistance fails and fluid accumulates in the interstitium without the protective rise in HP or lymph flow. This stage is called *stress relaxation*, and the edema-forming processes gain the upper hand.

NEUROHUMORAL FACTORS THAT CONTRIBUTE TO PATHOPHYSIOLOGY. The overall function of the cardiovascular system is modulated by several systems, including neural and humoral regulatory factors. These influence both the healthy circulatory system during physiological interventions, such as exercise and during disease, as an essential contribution to their adaptation or to pathological changes (Muir and Lipowitz 1978; Swedberg 2000). Evidence has been provided that both the circulating neuroendocrines the renin-angiotensin-aldosterone system (RAAS) promote the development of myocardial fibrosis in hypertensive disease and chronic heart failure (Flood et al. 1999; Brilla 2000). Angiotensin II (AT-II) is the effector peptide of this system, and it regulates cellular growth. Several factors influence the healthy circulatory system during physiological events such as development, growth, environmental adaptation, and exercise. They also have profound effects during pathophysiological changes that result in disease. Components of the system have been identified in *cardiac tissue*, including *AT-II receptors*, suggesting an *autocrine* function *independent of AT-II derived from the circulatory system* (Dostal and Baker 1999). The biochemical pathway is as follows: the protein angiotensinogen is cleaved by the proteolytic enzyme renin to form the inactive decapeptide angiotensin I. This substance in turn is converted to the hormone AT-II by a specific enzyme: angiotensin-converting enzyme (ACE). AT-II activates plasma membrane receptors and is a potent vasoconstrictor with a half-life of several minutes. The release of antidiuretic hormone or arginine vasopressin (AVP) by AT-II from the pituitary gland causes a decreased urine production and an increased peripheral vascular resistance. Expansion of the blood volume is also stimulated by increased water consumption. The decreased norepinephrine uptake from preganglionic sympathetic synapses results in higher circulating catecholamine levels constricting vascular smooth muscle tissue and increasing afterload and heart rate. Myocardial oxygen demand increases, and the oxygenation of other tissues decreases. The development of arrhythmia is stimulated. If this stimulation goes on, the β_1-adrenergic myocardial receptors will be downregulated (i.e., the number of those receptors decreases). AT-II promotes vascular smooth muscle growth leading to arteriolar narrowing and myocardial hypertrophy. The production of free oxygen radicals by macrophages and neutrophils is stimulated and will result in lipid peroxidation and death of cardiac myocytes, which are replaced by fibrous tissue. In addi-

tion to this, the adrenal cortex is stimulated to release aldosterone, causing sodium retention by the distal convoluted tubules that induces decreased urine production and increases circulating volume. Edema and elevation of the arterial pressure may result. This effect is enhanced by a decreased vagal tone and vagus nerve activity, the resulting tachycardia increasing the myocardial oxygen demand. The action of ACE can be blocked with so-called ACE inhibitors that have a dual effect: they reduce the production of AT-II and raise the level of bradykinin, a potent vasodilator. Therefore, these drugs are useful to treat hypertension and congestive heart failure, and they have also been shown to prevent remodeling after myocardial infarction.

Atrial natriuretic peptide (ANP) or factor (ANF) is the most abundant of at least three related peptide hormones that exhibit extensive effects on cardiovascular and renal function. Under normal circumstances, ANP is predominantly synthesized by modified myocytes in both atria. Under pathological circumstances also ventricular synthesis of the peptide contributes significantly to the circulating pool (Pasternac and Cantin 1990). The biologically active form is cleaved from the carboxy end of a prohormone and released in response to stretch of the secretory myocytes following increased central venous pressure. Therefore, ANP is increased in patients with congestive heart failure, and it correlates with the filling pressure, for example, dilation of the atria. At the renal level, ANP shows a diuretic effect and a natriuretic effect, whereas, at the vascular level, it induces arteriolar vasodilation as well as venodilation. This vasoactive effect is similar to that of nitric oxide (NO) because ANP raises myocardial cyclic guanosine 5-monophosphate (cGMP) via stimulation of guanyl cyclase. In fact, ANP contributes to homeostasis and is a regulator of arterial blood pressure by acting as an antagonist of RAAS (Melo et al. 2000). Plasma levels of ANP, norepinephrine, and renin are clearly related to the severity of heart failure. Therefore, this hormonal cascade needs to be interrupted by pharmacological intervention in due time.

Growth hormone (somatotropin) is a peptide produced by the anterior pituitary in a pulsatile way. Its structure is species specific, and it has a short half-life (i.e., 20 to 30 minutes). It may act directly or indirectly by stimulating the production of IGF (insulin-like growth factor, or somatomedin) on target organs such as the heart. Myocardial function has been found to improve after giving growth hormone (Bogoyevitch 2000; Rajanayagam et al. 2000). It must be noted that the hormone is diabetogenic; therefore, monitoring blood glucose is recommended.

NO is a gaseous diffusible substance previously identified as an endothelium-derived relaxing factor after its discovery in 1979 by Furchgott. Together with two colleagues, he received in 1998 the Nobel Prize for his contribution to medicine and physiology. The substance is released from endothelial cells and cardiomyocytes, where the endothelial-type NO synthetase (eNOS) forms the major source of NO under physiological circumstances. In pathological conditions, NO is also available from an isoform, the so-called inducible-type

NO synthetase (iNOS). NO has a half-life of only a few seconds. It affects the vasculature by causing vasodilation and also modulates myocardial contractile function (Figure 6.24). The therapeutic application of sodium nitroprusside has been used for decades because of its known vasodilatory effects, which turned out to be based on the fact that the drug acts as an NO donor. This effect of sodium nitroprusside is inhibited by the NO scavenger, hemoglobin. L-N-monomethyl-arginine (L-NMMA) may inhibit eNOS.

NO acts in the heart in a variety of ways. End-diastolic distensibility is enhanced by the accelerating relaxation. In low doses it is a positive inotrope, but in higher doses negative, which also is the effect on the β-adrenergic response. It interacts with the Frank-Starling response and modulates the force-frequency relationship. The MVO_2 is modulated and influences both the heart rate and AV conduction (chronotropic and dromotropic effects). It has a chronic effect on myocardial growth, hypertrophy, and modeling and also on apoptosis (Paulus and Shah 1999).

ANGIOGENESIS. When small blood vessels are damaged by trauma or stimulated by tumor cells, the inflammatory cells and tumor cells release growth factors that activate endothelial cells of the capillary wall and adjacent macrophages outside it, causing the endothelial cells to divide, forming a growth cone directed toward the source of the stimulus. This creates new vascular branches (Figure 6.25). This is a very important factor in tumor growth because it increases its nutritional supply.

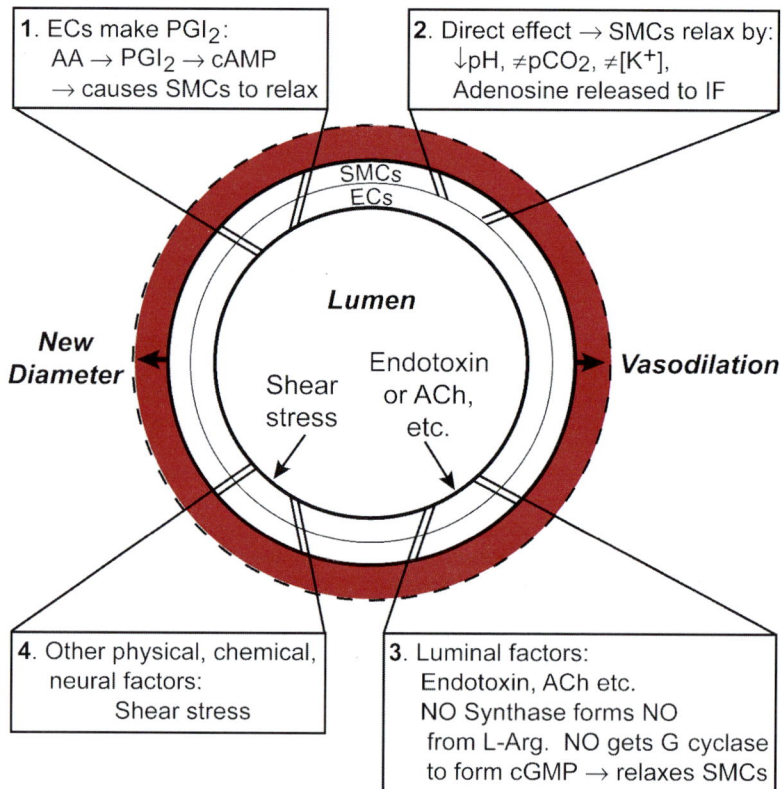

FIG. 6.24—Mediators of vasodilation (VD) in microvasculature. The diagram shows endothelial cells (ECs) of the capillary and other small microvascular vessels surrounded, in the case of arterioles and venules by smooth muscle cells (SMCs). The *dashed line* represents vasodilation. Four potential mechanisms are shown:

1. The ECs make prostacyclin (prostaglandin I_2 or PGI_2) that is formed from arachidonic acid (AA) and then forms cyclic AMP that relaxes the SMCs.
2. Increased: [H+], pCO_2, and [K+] lead to release of adenosine (AD) in the interstitial fluid (IF). AD is a potent vasodilator, and the SMCs lose tone, allowing VD to take place.
3. Luminal factors: Endotoxin and cholinergic agents such as acetyl cholinesterase (ACh) lead to formation of NO via action of the NO synthase enzyme on L-arginine. The NO causes G cyclase to form cyclic guanosine monophosphate (cGMP). The cGMP relaxes the SMCs.
4. Other physical (shear stress), chemical (endothelins cause VD in some circuits and some conditions, although they are vasoconstrictors in others), and neural factors.

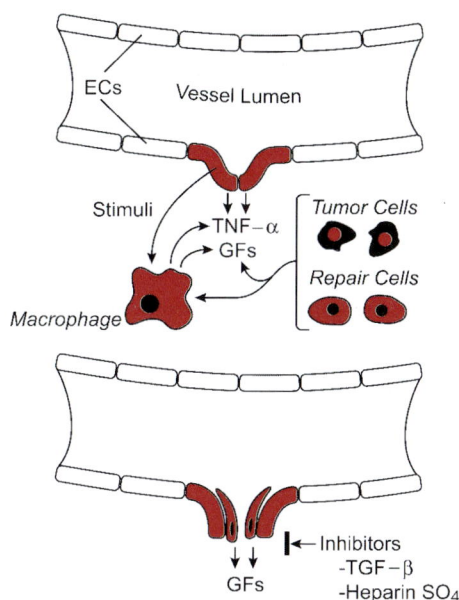

FIG. 6.25—Angiogenesis. This is triggered by stimulating cells such as tumor cells and/or repair cells at damaged sites. Such cells release growth factors (GFs) that activate endothelial cells (ECs) of the capillary wall and macrophages outside it. These various stimuli, including growth factors and tumor-necrosis factor (TNF-α), cause the ECs to expand and form a growth cone directed toward the source of the stimuli. The nodular cone of the vessel wall projects and divides, creating new vascular branches. This is a very important aspect of tumor growth because it increases its nutritional blood supply. Heparin sulfates and transforming growth factor β (TGF-β) inhibit the process.

PATHOPHYSIOLOGY OF SHOCK

The Nature of Shock. *Shock* is a circulatory crisis involving an imbalance between the intravascular capacity and the blood volume that results in inadequate tissue perfusion. Loss of thermal homeostasis, often expressed as hypothermia except in hot environments or when fever is present, is a common feature accompanied by hypotension, pale mucous membranes, and prolonged capillary refill time. The decline in peripheral circulation leads to hypoxia and metabolic dysfunction that can progress to cell and organ deterioration. At this stage, it becomes a medical emergency. Physical forces can trigger a shock state in a mammal—for example, electrocution by lightning strike or contact with a live electrical power source, traumatic stunning, other severe trauma to the central nervous system and/or peripheral nerves, or exposure to potent toxic chemicals. Also, extreme emotional stress or fear can result in paralyzing psychosomatic responses (Ganong 2003).

Cardiac Shock. The functional problem that leads to a shock response can start from cardiac dysfunction, in which case it is called *cardiogenic shock*:

1. The defective cardiac performance may be electrical in nature, for example, a rhythm that does not allow adequate tissue perfusion. The most extreme example of this is ventricular fibrillation in which there is no measurable arterial blood flow. Less extreme events are (a) ventricular tachycardia that does not allow enough time between beats for flow to be adequate, or (b) ventricular bradycardia where the interval is too long to sustain adequate flow. Alternatively, dysrhythmias such as atrial flutter or fibrillation interfere with cardiac rhythm and the effectiveness of ventricular systole.

2. The defective function may have a mechanical rather than an electrical origin. Typically, in humans, this would be a result of myocardial infarction causing significant loss of functional cardiac muscle. Alternatively, severe or sudden valvular dysfunctions or cardiac compression due to pericardial tamponade could compromise the heart's ability to sustain arterial blood pressure.

These are often life-threatening situations. Pathophysiological responses are complex. They include reflex sympathetic stimulation and vasoconstriction. Cardiac receptors send afferent stimuli up the vagus nerve that tend to evoke either pressor or depressor responses. Dorsal sympathetic fibers include pain fibers and other fibers that inhibit sympathetic vasoconstriction. Evidently, medullary centers must integrate conflicting signals in pathophysiological situations. The clinical signs are similar to those observed in hypovolemic shock plus progressive congestion of lungs and abdominal viscera as a result of the impaired systolic output and declining arterial blood pressure.

Noncardiac Shock. This category of shock includes the following:

1. Extracardiac *obstruction of blood flow*, as in massive pulmonary embolus or tension pneumothorax, pericardial tamponade, or cardiac tumor.

2. Massive *loss of circulating fluid volume* as a consequence of hemorrhage, protracted vomiting and/or diarrhea, blood loss, or severe burns that result in a large loss of plasma, including trauma or surgery.

3. Volume *maldistribution* with regional reduction in peripheral resistance, such as the massive vasodilation seen in histamine release in some acute allergic reactions and anaphylaxis. Septic shock is seen in acute systemic infections. The blood volume may be adequate, but there is a loss of vascular tone due to formation and release of potent mediators, including cytokines.

Hypovolemic shock is the prototypical example of noncardiac shock. This category of shock is a result of a major loss of body fluid from hemorrhage, trauma, burns, radiation, or acute pancreatitis. The fluid loss may be internal or external to the body. Mean pulmonary artery pressure may be very low with vascular pressures in the lung apices subatmospheric, allowing the alveolar pressure to compress and collapse the surrounding capillaries so that no blood can flow to those parts of the lungs from the pulmonary circulation.

Hemorrhagic Shock. In this example of hypovolemic shock, there is loss of both circulating fluid volume and of the vital oxygen-carrying capacity of hemoglobin in the erythrocytes. The resistance vessels in the pulmonary circulation constrict to compensate for the missing volume of blood. Also, interstitial fluid is mobilized by increased reabsorption into the capillaries as hydrostatic pressure falls, accompanied by a rapid, feeble pulse and a rapid respiratory rate. The initial fall in arterial blood pressure may be followed by a significant recovery within a few hours, but this may be transient and lead to a relapse into more serious pathophysiology that can progress to such irreversible damage accompanied by cardiac failure that even massive blood transfusions cannot reverse the functional decline. If hemorrhage is arrested soon enough, the homeostatic sensing and response systems provide negative feedback via baroreceptor and chemoreceptor reflexes, cerebral ischemic responses, release of vasoconstrictors, and renal conservation of Na, Cl, and H_2O. These responses increase the net volume of reabsorption. The combination of reduced vagal tone and increased sympathetic tone increases heart rate and venoconstriction. This is equivalent to an autotransfusion of blood from venocapacitance stores, including the spleen in dogs. Some species have constriction of the pulmonary and hepatic vasculature. Overall, the distribution of blood is modified in favor of maintaining cerebral and cardiac blood flow at the expense of renal, splanchnic, cutaneous, and muscular capillaries.

A serious outcome in affected dogs can be intestinal mucosal sloughing with swelling of centrolobular hepatic cells that obstruct the sinusoids, raising portal venous pressure. Also, renal ischemia can lead to kidney failure. If cerebral ischemia does occur, the medullary vagal centers are activated and produce bradycardia, worsening the hypotension and causing increased respiratory efforts to assist venous return. Typically, the cerebral ischemia becomes a problem when arterial blood pressure falls below 40 mm Hg and triggers a manyfold rise in sympathetic neural and adrenal medullary stimulations. The arterial hypotension coupled with arteriolar constriction and reduced venous pressure makes lower capillary hydrostatic pressure inevitable. This promotes net reabsorption from interstitial fluid accompanied by a decline in colloidal osmotic pressure. These findings were based on hemorrhagic shock in cats. There was also a shift of fluid from cells to interstitial fluid mediated by cortisol secretion.

Another significant change in hemorrhagic shock is a major increase in vasopressin secretion from the posterior pituitary as arterial blood pressure falls. This is a result of changing stimuli from the baroreceptors and left atrial stretch receptors after blood loss exceeds about 15 mL/kg body weight in dogs and pressure drops by over 20 mm Hg. Increased renin secretion gives rise to the potent vasoconstrictor AT-II, which also increases aldosterone secretion. The kidney increases reabsorption of sodium and water in the face of decreased renal blood flow.

The list of pathophysiological responses is an impressive saga of negative feedback designed to be protective to an animal challenged by extreme losses of circulating fluid (in this case, blood). The danger lies in the fact that a counterveiling positive-feedback train of events may be set in motion that has the opposite effect by exaggerating the primary event of the hemorrhage, namely, hypotension. These events include progressive cardiac failure, acidosis, central nervous system depression, activation of the coagulation cascade, and depression of the reticuloendothelial system. The weakening ventricles may be a consequence of decreased coronary artery perfusion and progressive vasodilation. Reduction of oxygen supply to the tissues has led to anaerobic glycolysis and acidosis with L-lactate accumulation. Homeostatic centers in the brain stem start to fail. Endogenous opioids are released that have a depressing effect on the nervous system. After an initial phase of hypercoagulability with platelet activation and leukocyte adhesion to endothelium promoting thrombus formation, there is a reversal to hypocoagulability and fibrinolysis.

Septic or Endotoxic Shock. This is typically Gram-negative bacterial septic shock with entry of endotoxins or lipopolysaccharides from the cell walls of gut organisms that are often part of the normal bacterial microflora of the bowel. After entry or absorption, they enter the reticuloendothelial system and accumulate in the liver, spleen, pulmonary alveoli, and leukocytes. The syndrome differs from that seen in cardiogenic or hypovolemic shock. There is often increased central venous pressure with increased cardiac output, hyperventilation with alkalosis, vasodilation with low peripheral resistance and hypotension, tachycardia, and fever. This is called a "warm" phase that may be followed by a "cool" phase with chilling, decreased central venous pressure and cardiac output, vasoconstriction, and cold cyanotic extremities. The clinical signs are attributable to the consequences of endotoxins:

1. Fever due to release of endogenous pyrogen
2. Release of prostaglandins, kinins, and β-endorphins
3. Activation of factor 12 and complement
4. Free radical damage to endothelium
5. Schwartzman reaction

A feature of endotoxin shock is volume maldistribution of the cardiac output; hence, the term *distributive shock* is applied. This is brought about by the local effects of microorganisms or fragments that induce serious local inflammation and immunologic disturbances (systemic inflammatory response syndrome or SIRS). This can progress to the multiorgan dysfunction syndrome (MODS). In late stages of septic shock, myocardial depressive factor (MDF) from the pancreas may depress myocardial contractility. Severe hypotension in septic shock has been attributed to NO formation in vascular smooth muscle. *Anaphylactic shock* is triggered by cytokines released in acute allergic reactions.

Neurogenic shock occurs when a sudden burst of autonomic excitation results in vasodilation with venous pooling of blood. The rapid loss of venous return to the heart causes a quick fall in cardiac output and syncope (fainting) with a loss of consciousness.

A similar phenomenon occurs in people in postural syncope from rising from the horizontal to the vertical position, particularly if they are taking certain adrenergic blocking drugs such as doxazocin. It would be very convenient and comforting if a technique could be devised to produce an immediate benign loss of consciousness at the moment just prior to slaughter for food animals.

Untreated, shock is a high-risk situation regardless of the cause, because it can turn the corner from efforts of self-regulatory homeostatic correction to a downward spiral of inappropriate pathophysiological responses. The outcome is progressive cell death with renal necrosis, cardiac failure, pulmonary edema, cerebrocortical hypoperfusion, and coma.

As our understanding of the complex processes responsible for the negative outcomes increases, we are becoming more able to reverse this pattern of *refractory shock*. Figure 6.26 summarizes the pathophysiology of the various categories of shock.

REFERENCES

Antzelevitch C, Sicouri S. 1994. Clinical relevance of cardiac arrhythmias generated by afterdepolarizations: Role of M cells in the generation of U waves, triggered activity and torsade de pointes. J Am Coll Cardiol 23:259–277.

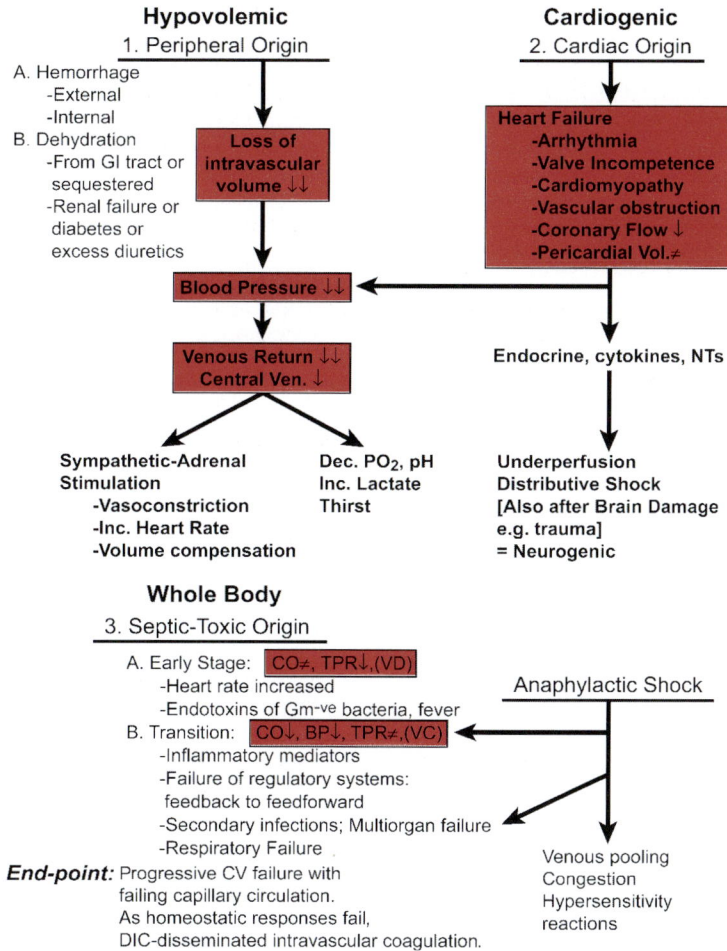

FIG. 6.26—Factors in the pathophysiology of shock. BP, blood pressure; CO, cardiac output; CV, cardiovascular; GI, gastrointestinal; TPR, total peripheral resistance; VC, vasoconstriction; and VD, vasodilation.

Atkins CE, Kanter R, Wright K, et al. 1995. Orthodromic reciprocating tachycardia and heart failure in a dog with a concealed posteroseptal accessory pathway. J Vet Intern Med 9:43–49.

Berne RM, Levy MN. 1998. Physiology, 4th ed. St Louis: CV Mosby.

Berne RM, Levy MN. 2001. Cardiovascular Physiology, 8th ed. St Louis: CV Mosby.

Bogoyevitch MA. 2000. Signalling via stress-activated mitogen-activated protein kinases in the cardiovascular system. Cardiovasc Res 45:826–842.

Braunwald E, Ross RJ, Sonnenblock EH. 1968. Mechanisms of Contraction of the Normal and Failing Heart. Boston: Little, Brown.

Brilla CG. 2000. Renin-angiotensin-aldosterone system and myocardial fibrosis. Cardiovasc Res 47:1–3.

Bristow MR, Ginsburg R, Minobe W. 1982. Decreased catecholamine sensitivity and beta-adrenergic receptor density in failing human hearts. N Engl J Med 307:205–211.

Brutsaert DL, Sys SU. 1989. Relaxation and diastole of the heart. Physiol Rev 69:1228–1297.

Buchanan J. 1979. Valvular disease (endocardiosis in dogs). Adv Vet Sci Comp Med 21:75–105.

Burton AC. 1972. Physiology and Biophysics of the Circulation. Chicago: Year Book Medical.

Calvert CA, Brown J. 1986. Use of M-mode echocardiography in the diagnosis of congestive cardiomyopathy in Doberman pinschers. J Am Vet Med Assoc 189:293–297.

Calvert CA, Chapman WL, Toal RL. 1982. Congestive cardiomyopathy in Doberman pinscher dogs. J Am Vet Med Assoc 181:598–602.

Cannel MB, Lederer WL. 1995. The control of calcium release in heart muscle. Science 268:1045–1049.

Cohn P. 1985. Clinical Cardiovascular Physiology. Philadelphia: WB Saunders.

Darke PG. 1987. Valvular incompetence in Cavalier King Charles spaniels. Vet Rec 120:365–366.

Dostal DE, Baker KM. 1999. The cardiac renin-angiotensin system: Conceptual, or a regulator of cardiac function? Circ Res 85:643–650.

Eaton GM, Cody RJ, Binkley PF. 1993. Increased aortic impedance precedes peripheral vasoconstriction at the early stage of ventricular failure in the paced canine model. Circulation 88:2714–2721.

Flood SM, Randolph JF, Gelzer AR, Refsal K. 1999. Primary hyperaldosteronism in two cats. J Am Anim Hosp Assoc 35:411–416.

Folkow B, Neil E. 1971. Circulation. London: Oxford University Press.

Fox PR, Liu SK, Maron BJ. 1995. Echocardiographic assessment of spontaneously occurring feline hypertrophic cardiomyopathy: An animal model of human disease. Circulation 92:2645–2651.

Fox P, Sisson D, Moise S. 1998. Textbook of Canine and Feline Cardiology. Philadelphia: WB Saunders.

Fuchs F. 1995. Mechanical modulation of the Ca^{++} regulatory protein complex in cardiac muscle. News Physiol Sci 10:6–12.

Furchgott RF, Vanhoutte PM. 1979. Endothelium-derived relaxing and contracting factors. FASEB J. 3:2007–2018.

Gaasch WH. 1994. Diagnosis and treatment of heart failure based on left ventricular systolic or diastolic dysfunction. J Am Med Assoc 271:1276–1280.

Ganong WF. 2003. Cardiovascular disorders: Vascular disease. In: McPhee SJ, Lingappa VR, Lange JD, eds. Pathophysiology of Disease: An Introduction to Clinical Medicine. 4th ed. New York: Lange Medical Books/McGraw Hill, pp 301–327.

Gibbs CL. 1974. Cardiac energetics. In: Langer GA, Brady AJ, eds. The Mammalian Myocardium. New York: John Wiley, pp 105–133.

Hughes D. 2000. Transvascular fluid dynamics. Vet Anaesth Analg 27:63–69.

Katz AM. 1990. Cardiomyopathy of overload: A major determinant of prognosis in congestive heart failure. N Engl J Med 322:100–110.

Katz AM. 1992. Physiology of the Heart. New York: Raven.

Katz AM. 1993. Cardiac ion channels. N Engl J Med 328:1244–1251.

Keene BW, Panciera DP, Atkins CE, et al. 1991. Myocardial L-carnitine deficiency in a family of dogs with dilated cardiomyopathy. J Am Vet Med Assoc 198:647–650.

Kittleson M, Kienle R. 1998. Small animal cardiovascular medicine. St Louis: Mosby.

Kleaveland JP, Kussmaul WG, Vinciguerra T, et al. 1988. Volume overload hypertrophy in a closed-chest model of mitral regurgitation. Am J Physiol 254:H1034–1041.

Lefkowitz RJ. 1995. Clinical implications of basic research: G proteins in medicine. N Engl J Med 332:186–187.

Lilly L. 1998. Pathophysiology of Heart Disease. Baltimore: Lippincott Williams and Wilkins.

Lindemann JP, Watanabe AM. 1995. Mechanisms of adrenergic and cholinergic regulation of myocardial contractility. In: Sperelakis N, ed. Physiology and Pathophysiology of the Heart. Boston: Kluwer Academic, pp 467–494.

Mellander S, Johansson B. 1968. Control of resistance, exchanges and capacitance functions in the peripheral circulation. Pharmacol Rev 20:117–196.

Melo LG, Pang SG, Ackerman U. 2000. Atrial natriuretic peptide: Regulator of chronic arterial blood pressure. News Physiol Sci 15:143–149.

Milnor WR. 1982. Hemodynamics. Baltimore: Williams and Wilkins.

Morgan JP, Morgan KG. 1989. Intracellular calcium and cardiovascular function in heart failure: Effects of pharmacologic agents. Cardiovasc Drug Ther 3:959–970.

Muir WW, Lipowitz AJ. 1978. Cardiac dysrhythmias associated with gastric dilatation-volvulus in the dog. J Am Vet Med Assoc 172:683–689.

Muntz KH, Zhao M, Miller JC. 1994. Downregulation of myocardial β-adrenergic receptors: Receptor subtype selectivity. Circ Res 74:369–376.

Opie L. 1998. The Heart Physiology, from Cell to Circulation. Philadelphia: Lippincott-Raven.

Pasternac A, Cantin M. 1990. Atrial natriuretic factor: A ventricular hormone. J Am Coll Cardiol 15:1446–1448.

Patterson DF, Pyle RL, Buchanan JW, et al. 1971. Hereditary patent ductus arteriosus and its sequelae in the dog. Circ Res 29:1–13.

Paulus WJ, Shah AM. 1999. NO and cardiac diastolic function. Cardiovasc Res 43:595–606.

Pedersen HD, Koch J, Poulsen K, et al. 1995. Activation of the renin angiotensin system in dogs with asymptomatic and mildly symptomatic mitral valvular insufficiency. J Vet Intern Med 9:328–331.

Rajanayagam MAS, Shou M, Thirumurti V, et al. 2000. Intracoronary basic fibroblast growth factor enhances myocardial collateral perfusion in dogs. J Am Coll Cardiol 35:519–526.

Rowell LB. 1986. Human Circulation: Regulation During Physical Stress. New York: Oxford University Press.

Sagawa K. 1978. The pressure-volume diagram revisited. Circ Res 43:677–688.

Shepherd JT, Vanhoutte PM. 1979. The Human Cardiovascular System: Facts and Concepts. New York: Raven.

Smith BB, Angelos J, George LW. 2002. Down cows (alert downers). In: Smith BP, ed. Large Animal Internal Medicine, 3rd ed. St Louis: CV Mosby, pp 1016–1018.

Smith JJ, Kampine JP. 1990. Circulatory Physiology: The Essentials, 3rd ed. Baltimore: Williams and Wilkins.

Sperelakis N. 1995. Physiology and Pathophysiology of the Heart. Boston: Kluwer Academic.

Starling EH. 1918. The Linacre Lecture on the Law of the Heart. London: Longmans, Green.

Suga H, Sugawa K. 1974. Instantaneous pressure-volume relationship and their ratio in the excised, supported canine left ventricle. Circ Res 35:117.

Swedberg K. 2000. Importance of neuroendocrine activation in chronic heart failure: Impact on treatment strategies. Eur J Heart Fail 2:229–233.

Taylor DEM, Stevens A. 1983. Blood Flow: Theory and Practice, New York: Academic Press.

Thomas LA, Brown SA. 1992. Relationship between colloid osmotic pressure and plasma protein concentration in cattle, horses, dogs, and cats. Am J Vet Res 53:2241–2243.

Tidholm A, Svensson H, Sylven C. 1997. Survival and prognostic factors in 189 dogs with dilated cardiomyopathy. J Am Anim Hosp Assoc 33:364.

Tor-Agbidye J, Blythe L, Craig AM. 2001. Correlation of endophyte toxins (ergovaline and lolitrem B) with clinical disease: Fescue foot and perennial ryegrass staggers. Vet Hum Toxicol 43:140–146.

Tsien R. 1986. Excitable tissues in the heart. In: Andreoli T, Hoffman JF, Fanestil DD, Schultz SG, eds. Physiology of Membrane Disorders. New York: Plenum, pp 475–493.

Vattner SF, Beottcher DH. 1975. Reduced baroreflex sensitivity with volume loading in conscious dogs. Circ Res 37:236–242.

Vattner SF, Boettcher DH. 1978. Regulation of cardiac output by stroke volume and heart rate in conscious dogs. Circ Res 42:557–561.

Weber KT, Clark WA, Janicki JS, Shroff SG. 1987. Physiological versus pathological hypertrophy and the pressure-overloaded myocardium. J Cardiovasc Pharmacol 10(Suppl):537–550.

Wiggers CJ. 1975. Modern Aspects of Circulation in Health and Disease. Philadelphia: Lea and Febiger.

Yoran C, Yellin EL, Becker RM, et al. 1979a. Dynamic aspects of acute mitral regurgitation: Effects of ventricular volume, pressure and contractility on the effective regurgitant area. Circulation 60:170–176.

Yoran C, Yellin EL, Gabbay S, et al. 1979b. Mechanisms of reduction of mitral regurgitation with vasodilator therapy. Am J Cardiol 43:773–777.

Zipes DP, Jalife J. 1995. Cardiac Electrophysiology: From Cell to Bedside. Philadelphia: WB Saunders.

Zweifach BW, Intaglietta M. 1971. Measurement of blood plasma colloid osmotic pressure: II. Comparative study of different species. Microvasc Res 3:83–88.

General References

Berne RM, Levy MN. 1998. Physiology, 4th ed. St Louis: CV Mosby.

Berne RM, Levy MN. 2001. Cardiovascular Physiology, 8th ed. St Louis: CV Mosby.

Braunwald E, Ross RJ, Sonnenblock EH. 1968. Mechanisms of Contraction of the Normal and Failing Heart. Boston: Little, Brown.

Burton AC. 1972. Physiology and Biophysics of the Circulation. Chicago: Year Book Medical.

Katz AM. 1992. Physiology of the Heart. New York: Raven.

Opie L. 1998. The Heart Physiology, from Cell to Circulation. Philadelphia: Lippincott-Raven.

Shepherd JT, Vanhoutte PM. 1979. The Human Cardiovascular System: Facts and Concepts. New York: Raven.

Smith JJ, Kampine JP. 1990. Circulatory Physiology: The Essentials, 3rd ed. Baltimore: Williams and Wilkins.

Wiggers CJ. 1975. Modern Aspects of Circulation in Health and Disease. Philadelphia: Lea and Febiger.

7

PATHOPHYSIOLOGY OF THE REPRODUCTIVE SYSTEM

Mats H.T. Troedsson and Scott Madill

MAMMALIAN SEX DETERMINATION

Defining How Sex Is Determined. Most recorded early ideas on embryonic development and sex determination come from the ancient Greek philosophers (Hunter 1995). They were men, and most of the ideas could be regarded as fairly sexist. Democritus of Abdera (460–370 BC) hypothesized that females originate from the left testis and males from the right. This theory led to a slew of philosophies where rightness/ righteousness/dexterous were associated with males. Later the uterus became involved in the theory of right-left sex determination. Dissected sows' uteri had more male fetuses in the right horn, suggested to be the result of more semen (male determining) having flowed into the right side of the uterus. The Greeks also focused on male (seminal) and female (menstrual) fluids (male and female sperm). Pythagoras (580–500 BC) was of the opinion that male sperm gave rise to the noble parts and female sperm to the gross parts of the fetus. Hippocrates believed that, if both male and female sperm were strong, it would result in a male baby, and that weak male and female sperm resulted in a female baby. If sperm from one individual was strong and weak from the other, it depended on which there was most of. Aristotle thought that sex of the embryo was determined by environmental conditions in the uterus. Heat and dryness in the uterus would result in a male embryo, and a damp and cold uterus resulted in a female embryo. Final sex of the embryo was deter-

mined by the interaction of warm versus cold winds, the side of the uterus the fetus was presumed to lie on and which of the father's testes the sperm originated from. The mechanism of sex determination did not advance much until sex chromosomes were identified at the start of the 20th century.

Different types or levels of sex can be defined (Short 1982). *Genetic sex* is defined by a specific chromosomal pattern. *Gonadal sex* is defined by the presence of ovaries versus testes. *Phenotypic sex* depends on internal and external genitalia, and secondary sex characteristics. In addition, germ cells (egg versus sperm), hormones [(estrogen, testosterone, and Müllerian inhibiting substance (MIS)], the brain, and behavior are all involved in sex determination and sexual differentiation.

OVERVIEW OF THE STEPS IN MAMMALIAN SEX DETERMINATION. Mammalian sex determination can be regarded as a three-step process (Capel 1998):

1. Genetic sex is determined at the time of fertilization. The X-containing oocyte is fertilized by either an X-bearing or a Y-bearing sperm.
2. Sex determination occurs when the bipotential or indifferent gonad is put on the male pathway by the action of a Y-chromosome gene in male embryos. In female embryos, the absence of this gene allows development of the ovary.
3. Sexual differentiation of male and female phenotypes results from the specific hormone secretions of the now determined testis or ovary.

Every indifferent embryo has the potential to be either male or female, developing male or female structures. During fetal life, either the Wolffian or the Müllerian ducts develop while the Müllerian ducts regress after differentiation of the indifferent or bipotential gonads into testes or ovaries. Removal of the indifferent gonads causes female development: the Wolffian ducts regress while the Müllerian ducts develop into oviducts, uterus, and upper vagina.

GENETIC SEX. In mammals, the genetic sex of the next generation is set at the time of fertilization and depends on whether an X-bearing or Y-bearing sperm fertilizes the oocyte, which invariably carries an X chromosome. In the absence of a Y chromosome, XX, XO (O = absence of one chromosome in a pair), and XXX individuals are all female, whereas, irrespective of how many X chromosomes an individual has, a single Y chromosome is sufficient to send development along the male pathway. The fact that the presence of a Y chromosome signaled the indifferent gonad to become a testicle stimulated a search for a testicular determining gene on the Y chromosome: the testis-determining factor (TDF). At various times, the Y chromosome, H-Y antigen (male-specific histocompatibility antigen), Bkm (banded krait minor satellite—sex-specific in banded krait), and ZFY (zinc-finger Y) have all been suggested to be the TDF (McLaren 1991). This has now been resolved with the discovery of *SRY/sry* (sex-determining region *Y* gene): *sry* is a single copy gene that is expressed in the urogenital ridge prior to gonadal differentiation, and expression is independent of the presence of primordial germ cells. Although *SRY* may be the master switch in the sex-determination cascade, it is far from the only gene involved (Koopman 1995; Haqq and Donahoe 1998).

HORMONAL SEX. Differentiation of the indifferent gonad as a testicle or an ovary determines its major hormonal products. These are important in determining further sexual differentiation of an individual. It does not matter what the chromosomal makeup of the individual is, functional testes will secrete testosterone and MIS, which are important for subsequent differentiation as a male during fetal life and for developing the male secondary sex characteristics seen following puberty. The ovarian product in this regard is estrogen. The ovary requires viable oocytes to form and maintain follicles and their associated steroidogenesis. In contrast, the testicle does not require germ cells to be present for formation or for active hormone production.

PHENOTYPIC SEX. To achieve either male or female gonads, the starting point is a single indifferent structure (albeit with cortical and medullary regions), which then differentiates as either male (testicle) or female (ovary).

The strategy for developing the male duct system and the female duct system is the opposite. All embryos start with the rudiments of both male and female systems, one of which will regress while the other develops under the influence of the now sexually differentiated gonads. In the early, sexually undifferentiated embryo, the rudimentary male ducts (Wolffian or mesonephric ducts) appear first, as the excretory ducts of the mesonephros. The rudimentary female ducts (Müllerian or paramesonephric ducts) develop only after the early indifferent gonad is visible. They develop adjacent to the Wolffian ducts, starting near the gonad and developing caudally, apparently using the Wolffian ducts as a guide (hence paramesonephric) (Wilson 1994; Hunter 1995). During fetal life, either the Wolffian or the Müllerian ducts develop while the other set of ducts regresses after differentiation of the indifferent or bipotential gonads into testes or ovaries. In males, testosterone secreted by testicular Leydig cells is required for maintenance and development of the Wolffian ducts, while secretion of MIS causes regression of Müllerian ducts. Conversion of testosterone to dihydrotestosterone (DHT) by 5α-reductase is needed for the urogenital sinus to develop into the male external genitalia. Removal of the indifferent gonads causes both genetically male and female embryos to undergo a female pattern of genital development: the Wolffian ducts regress while the Müllerian ducts develop into oviducts, uterus, and upper vagina. The origin of the mature organ structures is shown in Figure 7.1.

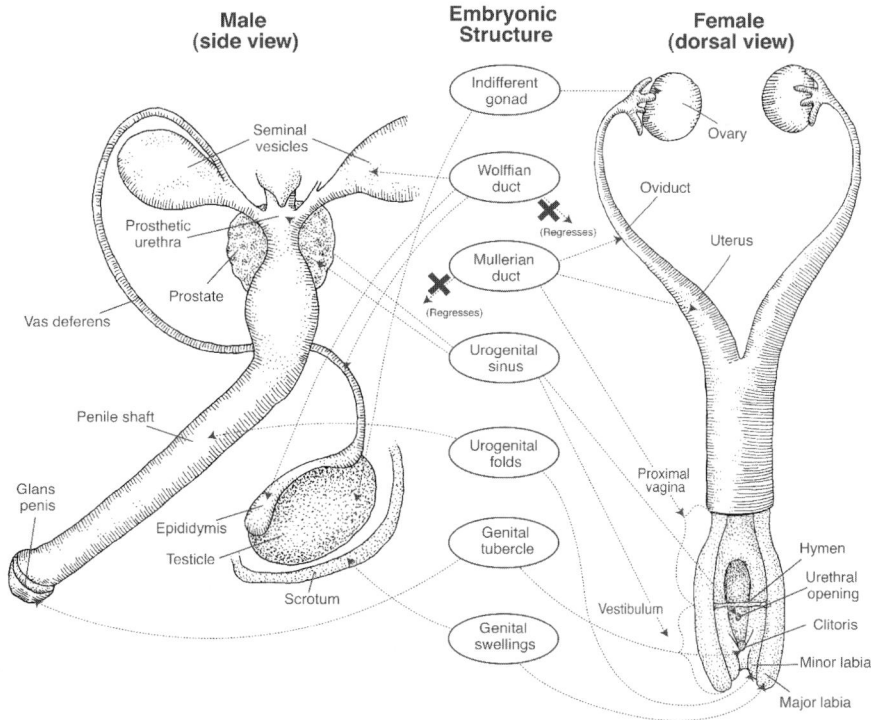

FIG 7.1—Origin of mature sexual structures.

GONADAL DESCENT. Testicular descent occurs only in mammals, and in those species where it does occur the testes require lower temperature present in the scrotum for successful spermatogenesis. The reason for evolution of this feature in most mammalian species but not in others, such as the elephants, is unknown (Hutson and Donahoe 1986).

Transabdominal Testicular Descent. In the early embryo, the gonad on the urogenital ridge is anchored to the body wall by cranial and caudal suspensory ligaments. The caudal suspensory ligament (the gubernaculum or genitoinguinal ligament) connects the gonad to the future inguinal region. During embryonic development, the cranial suspensory ligament regresses in the male, apparently under the influence of testosterone (Adham et al. 2000). In the female, the cranial ligament is retained while the gubernaculum regresses to a thin band of tissue. Thus, during early embryonic development, the female gonad is relatively tightly bound to the dorsal body wall while that of the male is relatively tightly bound to the inguinal region. In the male, the gubernaculum thickens, forming the gubernacular bulb as the cranial suspensory ligament regresses. This applies traction to the gonad. Instead of the testicle being pulled across the abdominal cavity by the gubernaculum, it is anchored to the inguinal region by a gubernaculum of constant length while the abdomen of the embryo elongates (Hutson et al. 1997). The identity of the hormone causing transabdominal descent of the testis has been unclear, with contradictory research results offering support for MIS. Recently, insulin-like factor 3 has been shown to perform this function, at least in mice (Adham et al. 2000).

Inguinoscrotal Testicular Descent. While the gubernaculum thickens, it also grows out through the internal inguinal ring and canal and moves through the external inguinal ring and into the future scrotum. It also hollows out to allow an outpouching of peritoneum, which will eventually form the vaginal tunic. The cremaster muscle forms from the outer rim of the gubernaculum (Hutson 1994). There is good evidence that the inguinoscrotal movement of the gubernaculum is controlled by androgens. There is less agreement on how these androgens act. The two sites currently proposed are direct action on the gubernaculum, and an indirect action via the spinal nucleus of the genitofemoral nerve (GFN). The spinal nucleus of the GFN is sexually dimorphic in rodents, containing more cells in males than females, and transection of the GFN inhibits migration of the gubernaculum into the scrotum. The putative neurotransmitter involved is calcitonin gene-related peptide (CGRP), binding sites for which have been demonstrated on the gubernaculum during the phase of its outgrowth. CGRP causes contraction of the gubernaculum in vitro, and blockade of its action in vivo causes delayed testicular descent (Hutson et al. 1997). Some time after it completes inguinoscrotal migration, the bulky gubernaculum regresses, allowing the epididymis and testicle to enter the scrotum (see Table 7.1).

CRYPTORCHIDISM. This is the failure of one testicle (unilateral) or both (bilateral) to descend into the scrotum at the normal time. Since testicular descent is a complex process, the condition could have multiple etiologies. It is often suspected in human medicine to be due to a defect in prenatal androgen secretion. Other causes could be mechanical (e.g., abdominal wall defect, so no increase in abdominal pressure) and neurological (e.g., GFN/CGRP anomalies). Aberrant migration of the gubernaculum is also postulated in some cases. Problems associated with cryptorchidism include infertility and tumor formation (Sertoli cell tumor in dogs and seminoma in humans) (Hutson 1994; Hutson et al. 1997). Cryptorchidism is generally considered not to be a simple genetic trait, but one that has a large genetic component. In most species, it has been thought to be autosomal recessive, or perhaps dominant with incomplete penetrance (Blanchard et al. 1990). Therefore, it has been recommended not to use affected animals for breeding. In horses, the genetic component is questioned, though a predisposition in some breeds was seen in one hospital based case-control study (Hayes 1986).

BRAIN SEX. Differences in behavior of the sexes first led to speculation that the areas that produce behavior—the central nervous system—may differ in construction and/or function. Numerous sexual dimorphisms in the brain have now been demonstrated from insects to mammals and vary from gross anatomic differences to ultrastructural, biochemical, and molecular mechanisms. The size of specific areas of the brain may vary by sex, as may clusters of neurons (nuclei), the projections and connections between different areas, concentrations and distributions of enzymes, neurotransmitters and their receptors, and the receptors for steroid hormones. The brain areas that will become sexually dimorphic start out as monomorphic in early development. The dimorphic changes are probably mediated by an interaction of genetic and epigenetic (the environment of the cell) factors, the most notable of the latter being the hormones. Of the hormones,

TABLE 7.1—Timing of testicular descent

Species	Time
Ram and bull	Halfway through gestation
Boar	Last quarter of gestation
Stallion	Just before birth to first 2 weeks postnatally
Tom	Usually by birth; should be easily palpable at first vaccination (6–8 weeks)
Dog	10–14 days of age, but may not be fully in scrotum until 6–8 weeks
Human	Prior to birth

those that appear important in sexual differentiation of the brain are not surprisingly the sex steroids, progesterone, testosterone, and estrogen, and especially the latter two. Steroids affect those cells that have receptors for them, which represent only a fraction of brain cells and are located in specific areas. The steroid may also secondarily affect cells lying in close proximity to these primary targets, as well as cells with which they have a connection (Gahr 1994; Forger 1998).

Sexually dimorphic nucleus of the preoptic area (SDN-POA) is one of the first sexually dimorphic areas described (in rats), and differences between sexes have been described in several species, including humans. The area is five to six times larger in males compared with females. A surge of testosterone around the time of birth is responsible for the difference (after it is aromatized locally to estrogen). Treatment of female neonates with testosterone will masculinize this area. Estrogens act to prevent cell death in the SDN-POA of males, whereas cell death reduces the number of SDN-POA neurons in females. Changes are permanent, but the functional significance of the area is unknown. It may be important for copulatory behavior.

Spinal nucleus of the bulbocavernosus (SNB) is the motor nucleus for the bulbocavernosus muscles, which are vital for penile erection. Both the muscles and the SNB are present and equal in size in male and female neonates, but degenerate during female development. In adulthood, the muscles cannot be found in females and the SNB nucleus has only one-third the number of neurons compared with that in males. Steroid treatment of neonatal females saves both the muscles and neurons. However, androgen receptors are found only in the muscles, not in the neurons. Steroid maintenance of the innervated target organ in the male is what prevents cell death in the neurons and leads to sexual dimorphism of the nucleus.

Anteroventral nucleus of the preoptic area (anteroventral periventricular nucleus-POA) is involved in the generation of the luteinizing hormone (LH) surge that causes ovulation. It is larger in females than in males, and testosterone treatment of neonatal females reduces its size to that of the male's. Testosterone acts by increasing neuronal death in this area.

Intersex

CHIMERA. Originally, a chimera was a mythological creature that had a lion's head, goat's body, and serpent's tail. However, the modern scientific definition of a chimera is an animal composed of a mixture of genetically different cells that originate from different zygotes (Hunter 1995; Rosnina et al. 2000). Usually thought to occur by amalgamation of (usually two) different early embryos that then continue development as a single individual, it can also be due to double fertilization of an oocyte containing two nuclei (one nucleus plus second polar body). The condition occurs rarely in nature. A readily detectable chimera would have XX/XY combinations of cells. They could also be XX/XX or XY/XY, but these are a bit more difficult to detect and usually would not result in an abnormal sexual differentiation. XX/XY chimeras may develop as fertile males or females, depending on the balance of XX and XY somatic cells in the early gonad. Males generally outnumber females by 3 to 1.

MOSAIC. Mosaic individuals are also composed of two (or more) cell lines but arise from a single zygote (Hunter 1995; Rosnina et al. 2000). Early in development, a chromosome may be lost from one cell, and all the cells in the lineage resulting from it (cell line) will be missing the same chromosome. The chromosome may be added to another line of cells. They arise from disorders of mitosis during cell division (mitotic nondisjunction) where the paired chromosomes do not separate normally. The condition is most likely to be seen in the sex chromosomes because all autosomal monosomies (one copy) and most autosomal trisomies (three copies) are lethal during embryonic development, resulting in death of the cell lines involved or the entire embryo.

TRUE HERMAPHRODITE. The term hermaphrodite originates from the Greek mythology. Hermaphroditus, the son of Hermes and Aphrodite, merged with the nymph Salmacis, and the resulting single body had both male and female features (Hunter 1995). True hermaphrodites have both ovarian and testicular tissue. There may be one ovary and one testicle, an ovotestis, or any combination (Rosnina et al. 2000). These are rare in mammals. When they do occur, the condition is thought to be due to the use of the master switch followed by a sex-specific cascade for sex determination. The resultant sexual phenotype may be male, female, or hermaphrodite, depending on the ratio of Y-containing cells to other types in the gonad.

PSEUDOHERMAPHRODITE. This is an abnormality of phenotypic sex. The chromosomal and gonadal sex are the same, but the phenotype of the internal and/or external genitalia shows some features of the opposite sex. Pseudohermaphrodites are classified on the basis of their gonadal sex (Hunter 1995; Rosnina et al. 2000). Male pseudohermaphrodites have XY chromosomes and testes but female characteristics of internal or external genitalia. Female pseudohermaphrodites have XX chromosomes and ovaries but masculinized genitalia.

SEX REVERSAL: XX MALES AND XY FEMALES. Both gonadal and phenotypic sex agree but are at odds with chromosomal sex. In both XX and XY sex reversal, true hermaphrodites may also occur. XX sex-reversed males have both testes and are phenotypically male though sterile since XX germ cells seem unable to survive in the testes. One cause of the condition is a translocation of *SRY* to X or an autosome.

XY sex-reversed females are phenotypically females with ovaries but chromosomally XY. In humans, the ovaries degenerate to streak gonads. The cause of the condition is often due to a deletion of *sry* from the Y chromosome or a mutation, causing its inactivation (Hunter 1995).

ANDROGEN-BASED DISORDERS. Genetic defects that decrease androgen action in genetic males or increase androgen action in genetic females are the most frequently diagnosed causes of disorders in sexual differentiation (Haqq and Donahoe 1998).

Androgen receptor is the product of an X-linked gene in humans. Complete deficiency leads to complete androgen insensitivity and testicular feminization (Haqq and Donahoe 1998). Affected individuals are XY and have testicles but phenotypically are taller than average females. Phenotypical alteration as a result of androgen receptor defects include Wolffian duct regression (no testosterone-androgen receptor activity), female external genitalia (DHT-androgen receptor activity), and Müllerian duct regression (normal MIS activity). The testes are most commonly located inguinally but occasionally labially (Short 1982). Some mutations of the receptor cause only partial inactivation with resulting partial masculinization (Haqq and Donahoe 1998).

5α-Reductase defects are also part of the testicular feminization syndrome. These individuals have testosterone but are not capable of producing DHT. The androgen receptors are normal, and testosterone can function normally. The affected individuals are XY and have bilateral testes and normally virilized Wolffian structures, but these terminate at a blind vagina. The external genitalia are female. Testes may be descended to the labia majora. An increase in testosterone after puberty can result in enlargement of the clitoris (Short 1982; Wilson 1994).

DISORDERS ASSOCIATED WITH MÜLLERIAN-INHIBITING SUBSTANCE

PERSISTENT MÜLLERIAN DUCT SYNDROME IN MALES. Affected individuals are relatively normal males that may have cryptorchidism but also have a uterus and oviducts. This can be the result of either deficiency of MIS or end-organ unresponsiveness. Some have no MIS, whereas others have normal MIS levels and presumably a receptor defect (Lee and Donahoe 1993). Cryptorchidism in patients with PMDS (persistent Müllerian duct syndrome) may have different mechanisms for failure of testicular descent. The testicles could be retained abdominally due to lack of MIS or receptors if MIS is important for the abdominal phase of descent, or may be due to restraint from retained Müllerian duct structures that would operate irrespective of importance of MIS in descent. In these individuals, the testis is tightly linked to the oviduct, and the observed phenotype depends on how mobile these are. In most cases, they are fairly mobile, and the testes descend, dragging the oviducts and a portion of the uterus along into the inguinal canal *hernia uteri inguinalis*. Less frequently, the round ligament restrains the uterus and oviducts, leading to bilateral cryptorchidism (Josso 1994).

MIS EXCESSES. Exposure of female fetuses to MIS during early embryogenesis causes regression or agenesis of Müllerian structures and an *endocrine sex reversal* of the ovaries (because MIS inhibits aromatase). Immature ovaries exposed to MIS have reduced aromatase activity and hence produce more testosterone. This may explain seminiferous tubule formation in freemartin heifers, fitting with a role for MIS in normal gonadal differentiation. In this hypothesis, an absence of MIS is critical for normal ovarian steroidogenesis, whereas the presence of MIS in developing testes of the male may increase testosterone and decrease estrone production (Lee and Donahoe 1993).

TURNER'S SYNDROME. Affected individuals have only a single X sex chromosome (XO). XO individuals tend to have streak gonads. The ovaries are normal early in gestation but have an accelerated rate of atresia. The XO germ cells are lost at an increased rate as they enter meiosis. By the time of birth, few oocytes are left in the ovaries. The explanation for this is that two X chromosomes are functional in female germ cells during oogenesis, and this seems normally to be a requirement. The ovaries of XO individuals degenerate to streaks of fibrous connective tissue, unable to generate follicles or perform steroid synthesis; hence, there are few secondary sex characteristics. Most of these individuals have a juvenile reproductive tract, and 97% have primary amenorrhea. The cause of most Turner's syndrome cases is paternal, a result of defective sperm. It is generally considered that the sperm are devoid of a sex chromosome due to errors in meiosis or mitosis (it has been suggested that the chromosome may be lost after the sperm penetrates the egg in affected mice).

KLEINFELTER'S SYNDROME. This is a condition where males have an extra X chromosome (XXY). The defect is due to errors in meiosis and arises approximately equally from the mother (XX oocyte) and the father (XY sperm). Germ cells are generally present in the testes prior to puberty but in reduced numbers. In humans, males tend to be tall but have delayed puberty, low testosterone production, sparse pubic and body hair and a relatively small penis, probably all secondary to the reduced testosterone production. Following puberty, affected males are generally sterile. The testes are small and atrophied and have no or few germ cells, and the majority of seminiferous tubules are atrophied. As with females, one of the two X chromosomes in these individuals is visible as a heterochromatic Barr body.

Examples of Intersexuality in Domestic Animals

CATTLE: FREEMARTINISM. This is the best-known syndrome causing derangement of sexual development in cattle (Echternkamp 1998). It affects female calves in twin pregnancies where the co-twin is a male. Over 90% of female calves from such pregnancies are affected. The disorder requires vascular anastomosis of chorioallantoic vessels between the two placentas. Affected females have a rudimentary ovary, with no or few germ cells, and may even have some testicle-like tissue. The ovary may have a tunica albuginea, similar to the covering of a normal testicle. The Müllerian duct is variably regressed, generally the oviducts are more regressed, and there is a rudimentary uterus. From the urogenital sinus, there is a small vulva present and a short blind-ending vagina (i.e., the Müllerian duct and urogenital sinus derivatives have not joined together). Masculinization of external genitalia is usually only slight and rarely is the clitoris enlarged. There may be testosterone-dependent growth of some Wolffian duct derivatives, seminal vesicles, epididymides, and prostate.

A generally accepted explanation for the condition is that indifferent gonads of the co-twinned bull calf start to develop as testicles at around 40 days. The female gonads are similar to normal presumptive ovaries until approximately day 50 of gestation. The male is producing appreciable MIS from about day 50, and his Müllerian ducts have commenced regression at this time. After day 50, the female gonads are inhibited by MIS transferred by anastomosed vessels from the male. This causes gonadal growth to cease, stops germ cell multiplication, and starts Müllerian duct regression. Müllerian regression is simultaneous in males and females. From 60 to 80 days, female gonadal regression and loss of germ cells continue. From 90 to 100 days (follicle formation in normal females), ovarian stunting is complete in freemartins. The affected female may develop Sertoli cells and seminiferous tubules in the ovarian medulla/rete region (about 50% of cases) with MIS production now from the female, but the damage is already done by circulating MIS from the male co-twin. Some Leydig cell formation may occur after 3 months. These sex-reversed gonads produce testosterone instead of estrogen due to inhibition of the aromatase enzyme. Since there is also passage of cells across the placental anastomoses, and germ cells and blood cell precursors are known to migrate, resultant calves (both male and female) are blood cell chimeras. These bull calves generally mature to have poorer fertility than do normal males, with poor-quality semen and low nonreturn rates. A low incidence of freemartinism is also reported in sheep, goats, and pigs. It is not reported in marmosets or people despite extensive vascular anastomoses.

GOATS. Intersex conditions are commonly reported in goats. The best described is associated with polled animals (Smith and Sherman 1994; Mickelsen and Memon 1997). Sex reversal in goats is caused by a recessive hermaphrodite (h) gene that is linked to the dominant polled (P) gene. It is more common in the dairy breeds—Saanen, Toggenburg, and Alpine—and appears to be the most common form of intersex in domestic animals. The affected animals are sex-reversed females being XX genetically but with testes. Phenotypically, they are mostly female at birth, but on attaining puberty they become larger than normal females, the head becomes masculine, erect hair develops on the neck,

and the clitoris enlarges and may be visible externally. They have small teats, develop buck odor, and become aggressive with male-type libido. Intersex animals are almost invariably 60, XX, P/P, and type positive for H-Y antigen. The polled gene also affects normal XY bucks. Bucks homozygous (PP—and therefore also hh) tend to become sterile due to blockage of the epididymal duct in the caput epididymis, resulting from poor differentiation of the duct. This leads in turn to palpable sperm granuloma formation.

HORSES. The most common syndrome is (63, XO) mares with gonadal dysgenesis (Turner's syndrome in people) (Trommerhausen Bowling et al. 1987). The second most common is the XY sex-reversal syndrome. Affected animals, though, of XY karyotype develop phenotypically as a spectrum from fertile mares to virilized intersexes with high testosterone, gonadal dysgenesis, variable Müllerian regression, and an enlarged clitoris. Two etiologies appear to be occurring: (a) The defect is transmitted by a carrier mare as an X-linked recessive or autosomal sex-limited dominant trait. (b) The transmission is via the stallion. Over several seasons, a stallion bred 22 mares, resulting in 8 normal XX females, 10 normal XY males, and 31 sex-reversed XY females. It is believed that a Y-chromosome incompatibility may be occurring, since the particular stallion also produced normal males in this period.

PIGS. Rarely is there evidence of vascular anastomosis in the developing placentas of early pig fetuses. When membranes abut at the tips, they generally become necrotic. Thus, freemartinism is rare. Other forms of intersex are, however, not unusual in genetically female pigs (Hunter 1995). These generally involve the presence of ovotestes or testes. The incidence of intersex in pigs varies from 0.1% to over 4%. The higher levels are associated with inbreeding and the use of particular boars. The ovotestes range from having approximately equal quantities of ovarian and testicular tissue to being more than 90% testicular. Some of these animals show cyclic activity on the normal ovary and occasionally became pregnant. A less common pattern is bilateral ovotestes and finally of bilateral testes with no ovarian tissue present. No germ cells are found in the testicular portion of such gonads. Phenotype varies, but all animals have a full uterus, though in those with more testicular tissue it is immature in appearance (no trophic female hormones). Fallopian tube regression or development is also dependent on the testicular content of the ipsilateral gonad. Conversely, animals with testicular tissue have a well-developed epididymis. The "brain sex" of the animals also correlates to their degree of masculinization. Those with one ovary and smaller amounts of testicular tissue have feminine brain modeling at least in that they can experience a surge of LH release. More masculinized individuals do not respond to estradiol injections with an LH surge. It is not clear why ovotestes develop in these pigs, and especially why the combination of one normal ovary and one ovotestis occurs. Possibilities explanations include the following (Hunter 1995):

• One possibility is failure of germ cell migration to the genital ridge. In the absence of germ cells, affected sections of the ovary may cease to develop, and supporting cells transmutate to Sertoli cells and sex cords. These animals may then develop some kind of uterus, because the Sertoli cells may require the presence of germ cells for full function and MIS production. Or transmutation to Sertoli cells might be too late, and the critical period of Müllerian duct sensitivity to MIS may be missed. This lack of migration could be due to lack of a chemotactic factor from the urogenital ridge to guide the migrating germ cells.

• It has been suggested that a genetic defect in affected animals causes the ovarian supporting cells to secrete MIS instead of the closely related inhibin, leading to loss of germ cells and virilization of the gonad. Variable effects are due to timing of onset and may also be affected by variations in the rate of development between left and right gonads.

• Chimerism of affected animals is also suggested.

DOGS

HYPOSPADIAS. In this condition, there is a partial failure of fusion of the urogenital folds. Thus, the urethra does not open at the end of the glans penis but further back, anywhere from the penile shaft to the perineal region. It is a mild form of male pseudohermaphroditism, which could be due to inadequate testosterone production, inadequate activity of 5α-reductase to convert testosterone to DHT, or a receptor problem (Meyers-Wallen and Patterson 1986; Feldman and Nelson 1996).

XX SEX REVERSAL. Affected animals are chromosomally female (78, XX) but have bilateral testes (usually cryptorchid) and are male externally, but with some abnormalities of the genitalia (hypospadias and other penile malformations). These animals have no oviducts but do have a small uterus. The condition may be due to the transfer of *Sry* to an X chromosome. It is seen in some families of cocker spaniels. XX hermaphrodites, with female genitalia that are variably masculinized, also result from this syndrome (Meyers-Wallen and Patterson 1986).

PMDS. This is a form of male pseudohermaphroditism. Affected dogs are 78 XY and have bilateral testes and usually bilateral or unilateral cryptorchids, but are otherwise normal males externally. Internally, in addition to male structures, they have full Müllerian structures: oviducts, uterus, cervix, and cranial vagina. The cranial uterine horns are attached to the testes (Meyers-Wallen and Patterson 1986). PMDS is inherited in miniature schnauzers, where it is transmitted as an autosomal recessive trait and is due to peripheral resistance (i.e., receptor defect). Homozygous affected dogs have normal levels of bioactive MIS (Lee and Donahoe 1993).

Since they are phenotypically normal (except for cryptorchidism) externally, they are typically not diagnosed until castrated, or they may present when older for signs associated with pyometra or Sertoli cell tumor.

CATS. The tortoiseshell cat is an example of X-chromosome inactivation. Its coat is a patchwork of orange and black. Black is produced by a dominant gene B, while yellow is produced by its recessive allele b. The locus involved is on the X chromosome (X linked). If a female cat receives an X chromosome with the B gene from one parent and an X with b from the other parent, random X inactivation of cells early in development will result in clones of daughter cells where B is active in some and b in others, resulting in the patchwork coat. Since an XX chromosome constitution is needed to be a tortoiseshell, males with this coat pattern are rare. Some are XXY and sterile, but most are chimeras with two cell populations (XX/XY or XY/XY), and some of these are fertile (Johnston et al. 2001).

PATHOPHYSIOLOGY OF FEMALE REPRODUCTION. Continuous or nonseasonal breeders go through repeated estrous cycles throughout the year in the absence of pregnancy. Examples are cows, sows, and people. Other species cycle at particular times of the year, usually designed so that birth occurs in the spring. Because of this, the time of year they breed will depend on the gestation length. Animals with very short pregnancies tend to breed in late winter or in the spring (mink and cats), animals with gestation periods of 5 to 6 months tend to breed in the fall (sheep and goats), and those with very long gestation periods breed in the spring so they can give birth at the same time next year (horses).

Monoestrous species have just one cycle, after which they become anestrus. Examples would be domestic dogs (which tend to be nonseasonal) and wolves, and roe deer, which are seasonal.

Most of the domestic species are polyestrous. In the absence of a pregnancy, they will have repeated, sequential cycles. They may do this continuously through the year (cows, sows, and people), or the sequence may eventually be interrupted by a seasonal anestrus in seasonally breeding animals (sheep and horses). Most domestic species are also spontaneous ovulators. When a large, mature follicle is present during estrus, the hypothalamic-pituitary-ovarian axis of hormonal feedback mechanisms allows a surge of LH to be released from the anterior pituitary, which triggers ovulation. Examples are sheep, pigs, cows, dogs, and horses. These species will go through cycles of estrus and diestrus irrespective of mating or the presence of a male. Other species, like house cats and most mustelids, will come into proestrus and estrus, but the trigger mechanism for LH release is coitus, and they may not ovulate if not mated. This repeated estrogen exposure can be harmful in some species, like ferrets. It causes severe suppression of bone marrow blood cell precursors, and these females often die if they are not bred or spayed.

Follicular Development and Ovulation

FOLLICULAR GROWTH. The mitotic phase of the oogonia terminates before birth or shortly thereafter. At this time, all oogonia have entered the first meiotic division and developed into primary oocytes. Because of this early meiosis, a female is born with all the oocytes within her ovary that she ever will have. The incidence of ovulated defect oocytes increases with age in women, and this has also been described in horses (Carnevale and Ginther 1995). The oocytes arrest in diplotene of the first meiotic prophase (dictyotene) and become surrounded by a primordial follicle. At puberty, follicular growth begins with the preantral phase, which includes growth of the primary oocyte without reactivation of meiosis. At this time, the surrounding granulosa cells divide into several layers and secrete a glycoprotein that forms an acellular layer—the zona pellucida—between the oocyte and granulosa cells. Gap junctions are established between granulosa cells and between granulosa cells and oocytes. Gap junctions are under the control of estrogen and follicle-stimulating hormone (FSH) (Erickson 1986). Ovarian stromal cells form the vascularized theca layer. In the presence of FSH, the follicle may develop into an antral follicle (Graafian follicle). Both granulosa and theca cells proliferate in response to FSH, LH, insulin-like growth factor I (IGF-I), and epidermal growth factor (EGF), resulting in further increase in follicular size. The proliferating theca cells divide into two layers—theca interna and theca externa—and fluid between dividing granulosa cells forms follicular fluid within the antrum. The Graafian follicles synthesize ovarian steroids that eventually is secreted into the circulation and become part of the endocrine hypothalamic-pituitary-ovarian feedback axis. Ovarian follicular growth and the timely release of an oocyte require a fine-tuned interaction between endocrine and paracrine factors of the central nervous system, pituitary gland, and ovary (Figure 7.2). In addition, follicular atresia or maturation to ovulation includes apoptosis, tissue remodeling, local changes in blood flow, growth factors, and immune products normally associated with an inflammation.

The release of FSH and LH from the anterior pituitary is controlled by gonadotropin-releasing hormone (GnRH). This hypothalamic peptide is produced and secreted from the medial basal hypothalamus in very small quantities and precisely timed bursts that can be coded for amplitude and frequency. If diluted in the general circulation, it would be largely ineffective because the burst signal would be lost. GnRH is transported by a specific pathway of blood vessels from the site of hormone release at the base of the hypothalamus (the median eminence) to the anterior pituitary gland: the hypothalamic-hypophyseal portal system. This system is unique in having a capillary plexus at both ends: one at the median eminence to pick up the hormones, and the second at the anterior pituitary to aid their transport into the relevant target cells. Thus, GnRH travels a very short distance in a small-volume blood system. Central regulation of GnRH release is believed to occur by a catecholaminergic mechanism that can be

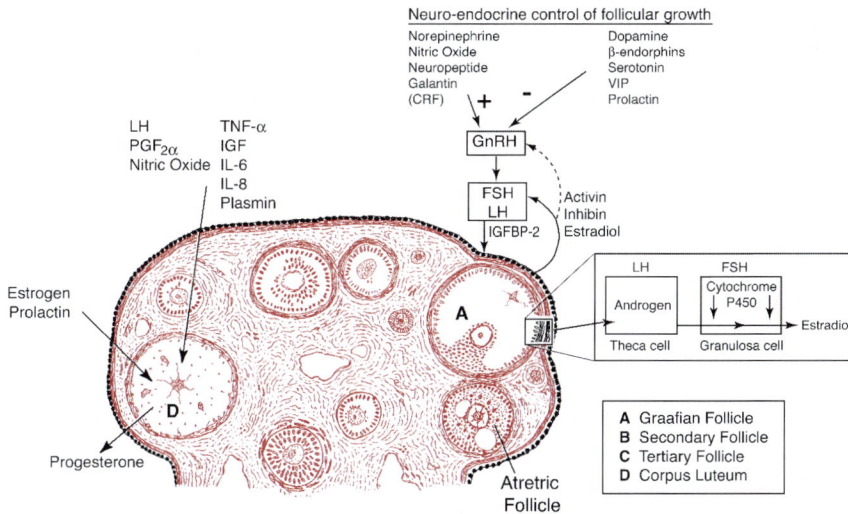

FIG 7.2—Ovulation: interaction between immune and endorphin systems. CRF, corticotropin-releasing factor; FSH, follicle-stimulating hormone; GnRH, gonadotropin-releasing hormone; IGF, insulin-like growth factor; IGFBP-2, insulin-like growth factor-binding protein 2; IL-6, interleukin 6; IL-8, interleukin 8; LH, luteinizing hormone; $PGF_{2\alpha}$, prostaglandin $F_{2\alpha}$; TNF-α, tumor-necrosis factor α; and VIP, vasoactive intestinal polypeptide.

modified by gonadal steroids and endorphins. Axons containing norepinephrine, dopamine, serotonin, γ-aminobutyric acid (GABA), pro-opiomelanocortin (POMC), corticotropin-releasing factor (CRF), vasopressin, substance P, neurotensin, galanin, and neuropeptide Y terminate on the GnRH neuron (Halasz 1993). Generally, dopamine, β-endorphins, serotonin, vasoactive intestinal peptide (VIP), and prolactin are believed to inhibit GnRH release, whereas norepinephrine, nitric oxide, neuropeptide Y, galanin, and maybe CRF are stimulatory. The exact neuroendocrine mechanism of GnRH release shows some species variation, and many of the GnRH modulators appear to be able both to stimulate and to inhibit GnRH secretion, dependent on the dose. At the level of the pituitary, GnRH stimulates synthesis and release of both FSH and LH. The differential release of FSH and LH can be explained in part by changes in the pulsatile pattern of GnRH release and by changes in steroid profiles, but also by the inhibitory effects of inhibin and the stimulatory effects of activin (Ying 1989; De Paolo et al. 1991). FSH receptors are localized on granulosa cells only, both mural and cumulus cells (Xu et al. 1995). Binding of FSH to granulosa cell receptors results in stimulation of aromatase that catalyzes the conversion of androgens to estrogens, production of LH receptors on the granulosa cells that enables the cells to respond to the preovulatory LH surge, and stimulation of granulosa cell mitosis that results in follicular growth. LH stimulates the theca interna cells to synthesize androgens (and, to a limited degree, estrogens) from acetate and cholesterol. Messenger RNA (mRNA) for the stereoidogenic enzymes cytochrome P-450, 17α-hydroxylase, 3β-hydroxysteroid dehydrogenase, and steroid acute regulatory protein are expressed on theca interna cells (Bao et al. 1977; Xu et al. 1995). LH also stimulates the theca cells to full differentiation in the developing follicle. The granulosa cells and the theca cells with their FSH and LH receptors combine to form the two-cell model of ovarian estrogen production. When LH binds to theca cells, production of thecal androgen is stimulated. The androgens move to the granulosa cells, which respond to FSH stimulation with production of cytochrome P-450, which aromatizes the androgens to estrogen. Increased estrogen concentrations and high FSH levels stimulate LH-binding sites on the outer layer of the granulosa cells, which is necessary for the Graafian follicle to reach its final maturation to a preovulatory follicle. The granulosa cells also synthesize inhibin, a hormone that inserts a negative-feedback effect on FSH at the pituitary level. Decreasing FSH concentrations result in follicular atresia unless LH is present. LH is suppressed by progesterone from the corpus luteum (CL) in diestrual animals and in species with a CL-dependent pregnancy, and from the fetal placental unit in species with CL-independent pregnancies. In the absence of progesterone, however, maturing Graafian follicles will respond to pituitary LH release and mature into preovulatory follicles. The LH surge stimulates growth in both follicular cells and the oocyte, and is also believed to stimulate the cellular, molecular, and circulatory changes that lead to ovulation.

OVULATION. This is the result of a complex paracrine/autocrine transmission of signals between hormones and the immune system, mediated via growth factors, and cytokines (Figure 7.2). Both apoptosis and necrosis (acute inflammation and vascular injury) contribute progressively to follicular stigma formation and follicular rupture (Murdoch et al. 1999a,b). As ovulation approaches, the number of apoptotic cells increases in the ovarian surface epithelium, tuna albuginea, and the apical follicular wall, resulting in a loss of surface or granulosa epithelium at the site of ovulation (Murdoch 1995). Several different mechanisms have been suggested to be responsible for ovulation. Brannstrom and colleagues (1998) suggested that changes in blood flow in the follicle resulting in increased flow in the base of the follicle and decreased flow in the apex may be essential for rupture of the follicle and the release of an oocyte. A shift in steroid production from estrogens to progesterone immediately before ovulation may regulate the expression of ovarian extracellular proteases that could act as matrix-degrading proteases inside the follicle prior to ovulation (Liu et al. 1998; Chaffin and Struffer 1999). Several studies have confirmed a role of plasmin in ovulation. Increased LH and prostaglandin concentrations stimulate plasminogen activator activity in thecal layers (Tilly and Johnson 1990). Plasmin cleaves tumor-necrosis factor α (TNF-α) exodomain from thecal endothelium, which has been shown to cause tissue dissolution at the time of ovulation in ewes (Murdoch et al. 1999a,b). Jackson and colleagues (1991) observed degradation of glycosaminoglycan specifically in the stigma region of the preovulatory follicle, which resulted in decreased collagen and a loss of tensile strength in this region. Recently, nitric oxide (NO) has been suggested to play a role in ovulation. An NO-generating system was found to be located in the stroma, theca cells, and the CL (Zachrisson et al. 1996). The role of insulin-like growth factor in follicular maturation and ovulation may differ between species but is generally considered to be important (Yoshimura et al. 1996; Mazerbourg et al. 2000). Prostaglandins and other eicosanoids play a fundamental role in the mechanism that causes follicular rupture and ovulation (Kranzfelder et al. 1996; Priddy and Killick 1993; Downey et al. 1998). Altered prostaglandin synthesis at the time of pending ovulation has been suggested to cause subfertility in women (Priddy and Killick 1993). Increased prostaglandin $F_{2\alpha}$ ($PGF_{2\alpha}$) concentrations have been observed in follicular fluid and in ovarian venous plasma acutely around the time of ovulation in cattle (Algire et al. 1992; Acosta et al. 2000). Induction of prostaglandin G/H-synthase 2 (PGHS-2), but not PGHS-1, was found in equine and bovine follicular fluid before ovulation (Liu et al. 1997; Sirois and Dore 1997).

The role of the immune system in ovulation is evident. Johnson and colleagues (1999) described ovulation as a cytokine [interleukin 6 (IL-6) and IL-8]-regulated inflammation, followed by anti-inflammatory reactions (IL-1-receptor antagonist). They suggested that an upregulation of collagenase expression is caused by TNF-α in preovulatory follicles. Chemokine activity and the presence of inflammatory cells also support ovulation as an inflammatory event (Watson et al. 1991; Murdoch and McCormick 1992; Araki et al. 1996; Arici et al. 1997; Karstrom-Encrantz et al. 1998).

Following ovulation, the collapsed follicle reorganizes, and the CL is formed. An extensive network of invading blood vessels is formed in the follicular antral space. The massive ingrowth of capillaries makes the CL one of the most vascular organs in the body. Thecal cells hypertrophy and become dispersed among luteinized granulosa cells. Granulosa and theca cells, respectively, form the large (>20 μm) and small (<20 μm) luteal cells (sometimes called granulosa lutein and theca lutein cells, respectively). Small and large luteal cells have been found in most, but not all, species examined.

Large luteal cells are responsible for most of the baseline progesterone secretion but do not respond to LH by increasing progesterone secretion. Small luteal cells do respond to LH with increased progesterone secretion. The function of the CL is to secrete progesterone to prepare the uterus for the ensuing pregnancy. Progesterone also prevents sexual receptivity. Further ovulations are prevented by the action of progesterone to suppress LH release from the hypothalamic-pituitary axis. FSH secretion and follicular growth may still occur.

The length of the estrous cycle depends on how long the CL is functional during the nonfertile estrous cycle. Induced ovulators have the shortest interval between behavioral estrous periods, but since they do not have a luteal phase, they could not be said to cycle. The CL requires hormonal support (luteotropins) for its function. Several luteotropins have been identified, and they vary in importance between species. They probably do not act in isolation but form a *luteotropic complex*. Furthermore, the luteotropic hormone in a species may also change over the estrous cycle or pregnancy. LH is found in all species examined and is responsible for at least the early changes of luteinization. As such, it has been termed the *universal luteotropin*. Prolactin (also from the anterior pituitary) is an important luteotropin in dogs, mice, rats, and hamsters, and may be important in other species. Estradiol is a vital luteotropin in rabbits, but in some other species may have the opposite action (be luteolytic). Although PGF$_{2\alpha}$ is the luteolytic hormone in all mammals examined, other prostaglandins may have luteotropic functions. Prostacyclin (PGI$_2$) in cattle and prostaglandin E$_2$ (PGE$_2$) in women are two examples.

Other hormones and substances that may have a role include FSH, growth hormone, progesterone, IGF-I, and EGF (see Table 7.2).

LUTEOLYSIS. In species with short cycles, there has to be a mechanism whereby, if the animal is not pregnant,

Table 7.2—Length (in days) of the estrous cycle in truly cycling animal species

Species	Length of cycle	Follicular phase	Luteal phase
Human	24–32	10–14	12–15
Cow	20–21	2–3	18–19
Swine	19–21	5–6	15–17
Horse	20–22	5–6	15–16
Sheep	16–17	1–2	14–15
Mouse and rat	4–5	2	2–3
Mouse and rat plus infertile mating	13–14	2	11–12

she is returned to estrus so another attempt at fertility can be made. Since the CL inhibits the hypothalamic-pituitary axis by its secretion of progesterone, in order for a new cycle to commence the influence of the CL must be removed. The natural life span of the CL is longer than the approximately 2 weeks of activity that is seen in a nonpregnant animal. To enable the next cycle to occur, the CL is therefore actively undergoing luteolysis in the absence of pregnancy. The sustained high levels of progesterone throughout the luteal phase finally cause downregulation of its own receptors in both the hypothalamus and endometrium. Increasing amounts of estrogen from developing follicles changes estrogen/progesterone ratio, resulting in an upregulation of receptors for oxytocin in the endometrium and an increase in the activity of the central oxytocin pulse generator (involving the hypothalamus and anterior pituitary). This increased oxytocin release and the increase in its number of receptors on the uterine endometrium cause PGF$_{2\alpha}$ release from the endometrium. The PGF$_{2\alpha}$ acts on the CL to cause luteolysis. PGF$_{2\alpha}$ entering the systemic circulation is rapidly and almost completely (99%) metabolized on passage through the lungs and thus may not be able to cause luteolysis. In many species, there is a specialized anatomy of the ovarian artery and uterine veins, in which they are tortuous and closely applied to each other. In these species, PGF$_{2\alpha}$ from the uterine endometrium passes up the uterine vein, and a portion of it is transferred across vessel walls into the ovarian artery (countercurrent exchange), from where it can directly access the CL. This strict system applies to sheep and guinea pigs. In horses and rabbits, there is no such system, and the PGF$_{2\alpha}$ is transferred via the systemic circulation. A less active metabolism in the lungs, or increased sensitivity of luteal cells to PGF$_{2\alpha}$, makes this possible. Although cows are generally considered to be in the countercurrent exchange group, there is some evidence that they and pigs may use a combination of both this local transfer mechanism and the systemic circulation route. In ruminants, the oxytocin release from the pituitary is backed up by release from the ovary, setting up a positive-feedback loop. The theory is that central oxytocin release acts on luteal oxytocin receptors, which induces local synthesis of PGF$_{2\alpha}$ within the CL. A positive-feedback loop is then established within the ovary between oxytocin and prostaglandin, which results in luteolysis. In primates, unlike all other species examined, there is apparently no role for the uterine endometrium in prostaglandin production that causes luteolysis.

Examples of Ovarian Diseases in Domestic Animals

PATHOLOGICAL ANESTRUS. Various systemic disorders can cause anestrus by suppression of the hypothalamic-pituitary axis. Excess cortisol secretion from the adrenal in Cushing's disease may cause anestrus, as may insufficient cortisol production in Addison's disease. Hypothyroidism is a relatively frequently cited cause of anestrus, especially in small-animal medicine. Achieving an exact diagnosis can be difficult. Disease directly affecting the reproductive organs can also be involved—for example, mares with ovarian granulosa-theca tumors may present for constant estrus, stallionlike behavior, or anestrus. Disorders of sexual differentiation, creating intersex conditions, can also present as anestrus. Examples include XO Turner's syndrome, XY sex reversal, testicular feminization syndromes, androgen receptor defects, and 5α-reductase deficiencies.

CYSTIC OVARIAN DEGENERATION. Cystic ovarian degeneration (COD) is a major cause of reproductive failure in cows. The condition is characterized by follicle-like ovarian structures that persist because of failure of ovulation (Seguin and Troedsson 2002). They are usually larger than 25 mm in diameter and persist in the absence of a CL for 10 days or more. Two types of cysts have been described. Follicular cysts have thin walls and may be single, multiple, or multilobular structures on one or both ovaries. Partially luteinized cysts tend to be single, unilateral structures with thicker walls because of the presence of luteal tissue. Follicular cysts can progress to become luteal cysts through luteinization. The mechanism by which ovulation fails and cysts develop is not known. The disease has been suggested to have a hereditary predisposition. Retained placenta, metritis, and hypocalcemia around the time of calving and postpartum ketosis have been associated with an increased prevalence of COD, but the pathophysiology of this association has not been established. Failure of ovulation may result from any of the paracrine/autocrine transmission signals between hormones and the immune system. Several researchers have suggested that LH is involved in cystic follicular degeneration, and the efficacy in treating cystic follicular degeneration with GnRH or gonadotropins supports this suggestion. Increased plasma concentrations of LH have been observed during the development of ovarian cysts (Peter 1997). This may inhibit the production of estradiol 17β by the preovulatory follicle, which could result in luteinization and/or a failure of the pituitary to secrete a well-timed preovulatory LH surge (Peter 1997). While most research on cystic follicular degeneration has focused on endocrine aspects of ovulation failure, little attention has been given to other factors that are involved in the normal mechanism of ovulation, such as apoptosis, blood flow and blood factors, NO, eicosanoids, and other immune mediators.

The diagnosis of COD is based on an accurate history and clinical examination. A history of constant or frequent estrus, short interestrous intervals, or anestrus may suggest COD. Examination of the ovaries by palpation per rectum reveals the presence of enlarged fluid-filled structures raised above the surface of the ovary that greatly increase total ovarian size. Ovarian cysts are larger than preovulatory follicles; structures larger than 50 mm in diameter are not uncommon. Differentiation between a single large cyst and several smaller cysts on the same ovary may not be possible nor may recognition of the presence of partially luteinized cysts (based on peripheral progesterone concentrations) unless ultrasonography is used. Ovarian cysts appear to be dynamic structures; those that develop early in the postpartum period may regress without treatment, and a normal estrous cycle may follow or another cystic structure may develop.

The management of cows with COD is directed toward inducing luteinization of the cyst and reestablishing normal estrous cycles. Spontaneous recovery from COD occurs in up to 60% of cows that develop it before the first ovulation after calving, but in only about 20% of cases that develop after the first postpartum ovulation. Evaluation of therapeutic agents for COD may be confounded by spontaneous recovery. Between 65% and 80% of cows treated with a single dose of human chorionic gonadotropin (hCG; which has a LH-like effect) establish a normal estrous cycle within 3 to 4 weeks. Currently, the most common treatment for ovarian cysts, especially follicular cysts, is an injection of GnRH. Therapeutic response is similar between hCG and GnRH. Cows responding to this treatment have an average interval to estrus of one estrous cycle (18 to 24 days). The treatment to breeding interval can be shortened by administering GnRH at the time of diagnosis, followed by a luteolytic dose of prostaglandin 10 days to 2 weeks later. With this regimen, it is not critical whether the cyst is follicular or luteal. Luteal-type cysts can be treated with the luteolytic activity of $PGF_{2\alpha}$. Cysts that luteinize in response to GnRH regress at a time similar to that of normal CLs; therefore, treatment with PGF may be used to reduce the interval from treatment with GnRH to estrus. Thin-walled follicular cysts may be inadvertently ruptured during examination of the ovaries, whereas others will intentionally attempt cyst rupture. Recovery rates following manual rupture have rarely been studied in well-designed controlled experiments but may be within the range reported for spontaneous recovery. Although it is conceptually possible that manual rupture of cysts may be followed by hemorrhage and adhesions between the ovary and surrounding structures, these complications appear to be much more common with the use of digital pressure to enucleate CLs than with manual rupture of ovarian cysts.

ANOVULATORY FOLLICLES IN MARES. Cystic follicular degeneration, as described in cows, does not occur in mares. Ovulation failure is normal in mares during the transition to and from seasonal cyclicity during the spring and fall. Ovulation failure during this time is physiological as a result of insufficient secretion of LH from the anterior pituitary. Large fluid-filled ovarian structures have been observed in mares during the fall transition (Knudsen 1964). These "autumn follicles" contained blood with liquid or gelatinous consistency. They were assumed to be the result of follicular development with declining exposure of LH. A similar condition in which anovulatory follicles develop has occasionally been observed during the breeding season (Ginther 1992). It was suggested that vascular accidents in association with failure of ovulation or at the time of follicular evacuation can result in the development of an anovulatory hemorrhagic follicle. The cause of ovulation failure is not known but has been suggested to be the result of insufficient pituitary gonadotropin stimulation or insufficient estrogen production from the follicle itself (Ginther 1992; McCue and Squires 2002). Follicular fluid has anticoagulatory properties, and the amount of follicular fluid at the site of follicular evacuation was proposed to determine the timing of coagulation (Ginther 1992).

Anovulatory hemorrhagic follicles are 50 to 150 mm in diameter. Ultrasonographic examination reveals scattered free-floating echogenic material within the follicular fluid. The particles swirl during ballottement of the abnormally enlarged follicular structure. Over time, fibrinous bands form, and the structure gives the impression of gelatinous consistency. Anovulatory hemorrhagic follicles regress spontaneously over 1 to 4 weeks, but they can persist for up to 2 months (McCue and Squires 2002). The structure often undergoes luteinization, and plasma progesterone concentrations may be elevated. Most persistent hemorrhagic anovulatory follicles do not respond to hCG or GnRH therapy. Elevated progesterone concentrations indicate that the structure is luteinized, and these mares may be treated with $PGF_{2\alpha}$ to lyse the luteal tissue and bring the mare into estrus.

GRANULOSA-THECA CELL TUMOR IN MARES. Granulosa-theca cell tumor (GTCT) is of sex cord-stromal origin. It has been described in a variety of species (people, cows, and dogs), and it is by far the most common ovarian neoplasm in mares. In horses, the tumor is usually unilateral, benign, and hormonally active. GTCT secretes inhibin, testosterone, and estradiol. The pathophysiology leading to the formation of a GTCT is not well understood. Data from people and mice indicate that hormonal and genetic factors are involved in the formation of the tumor (Jager et al. 1995; Risma et al. 1995; Glud et al. 1998; Keri et al. 2000). Excess gonadotropin secretion has been suggested to be an initiating signal in the formation of GTCT. Also, inhibin has been suggested to be involved in the formation of ovarian tumors. It was observed that mice deficient in inhibin developed a spontaneous form of granulosa cell tumor (Matzuk et al. 1992). The histological similarity between GTCTs in mares and granulosa cell tumors in women suggests that endocrine factors also could be implicated in the formation and progression of GTCT in mares (Bailey et al. 2002).

Abnormally increased synthesis and secretion of inhibin by the granulosa cells result in consistently elevated α-inhibin subunit concentrations in the circulation of mares with GTCTs (McCue 1992; Bailey et al. 2002). Inhibin suppresses FSH secretion from the anterior pituitary, which results in a suppression of follicular growth and maturation of the otherwise healthy contralateral ovary, and the mare becomes acyclic. Testosterone concentrations are often, but not always, elevated in mares with GTCT, and estradiol concentrations are variable (Stabenfeldt et al. 1979). Increased testosterone concentrations may be the result of a failure of the tumor to convert testosterone to estradiol because of lower than normal expression of aromatase P-450 in mares with GTCT (Watson and Thomson 1996).

A recent study showed that peripheral blood concentrations of LH were elevated in mares with GTCT (Bailey et al. 2001). Mares with GTCT had LH concentrations that were higher than concentrations measured in cycling mares. The cause of elevated LH concentrations in mares with GTCT is not known, but a lack of a positive relationship between LH and estradiol suggests that a positive-feedback mechanism by estradiol on the anterior pituitary is not involved (Bailey et al. 2002). Increased LH production could be the result of an absence of a negative feedback of progesterone in the pituitary in mares with GTCT, since no normal ovarian activity is present in these mares. However, elevated LH concentrations in mares with GTCT is interesting in the light of studies of the pathophysiology of granulosa cell tumors in other species. Deletion of a subunit of the inhibin gene in mice resulted in the formation of mixed sex cord-stromal tumors (Matzuk et al. 1992). Subsequent studies demonstrated that the loss of inhibin was more important in the development of tumors than was increased secretion of activin (Coerver et al. 1996). Inhibin-deficient mice that lack a functional GnRH gene showed suppressed circulating concentrations of FSH and LH. These mice did not form granulosa cell tumors, suggesting that gonadotropins are involved in the formation of these tumors (Kumar et al. 1996). Subsequent studies demonstrated that LH was required in the formation of granulosa cell tumors in mice (Jager et al. 1995; Risma et al. 1995). In a proposed equine model of the pathophysiology of GTCT, Bailey (2000) suggested that increased circular concentrations of LH could have a central role in the formation and regulation of equine GTCT.

Interaction Between Semen and the Female Reproductive Tract. For sperm to achieve fertilization of a viable ovum, spermatozoa must be transported to the site of fertilization in the oviduct, they must be maintained in the female tract until the ovum arrives, and they must be prepared to penetrate the egg. To accomplish this, spermatozoa of most species undergo capacitation. Spermatozoa motility is believed to be necessary for penetration of the ovum, and enzymes must be liberated through the acrosome reaction. After sperm penetration of the corona radiata and the zona pellucida of the ovum, the equatorial segment of the sperm must be able to fuse with the cell membrane of the oocyte, which then will pinocytose the sperm. Studies on sperm physiology in vivo is difficult because an ejaculate contains many subpopulations of spermatozoa with heterogeneous characteristics. Coitus/insemination and ovulation do not necessarily happen at exactly the same time. Heterogeneity within an ejaculate may therefore be required to ensure that fertile spermatozoa are present for an extended time in the female tract. At any given time, it is not possible to distinguish which spermatozoa are capable of fertilization from those that are not yet competent to fertilize an egg or from those that may never be capable of fertilization. Much consideration has been given to factors that are necessary for maintaining sperm motility and metabolism in assessing the quality of semen. However, factors such as biochemical characteristics and changes in spermatozoa and seminal plasma, uterine contractility, and the microenvironment of the female reproductive tract might also be essential components for successful fertilization to take place. For example, the integrity of the macromolecules of the sperm membrane may be an important component of sperm longevity; uterine motility during estrus and in response to semen is likely to be important factor for sperm transport; sperm transport may be affected by some seminal constituent, such as prostaglandin in ram semen; and membrane biochemistry is important for sperm capacitation, acrosome reaction, and the final steps of fertilization. All these factors may affect transport and survival of spermatozoa in the female reproductive tract.

The interaction between spermatozoa and the uterus involves both transport of spermatozoa to the oviduct and elimination by physical and immunologic means.

SPERM TRANSPORT. Spermatozoa are deposited in the vagina in cows, small ruminants, cats, rabbits, and people, and directly into the uterus in mares, sows, llamas, and maybe dogs. The cervix serves as a sperm barrier and storage site of sperm in species with vaginal ejaculation. In contrast, the uterotubal junction serves as the major barrier for the sperm cells to reach the fertilization site in the oviductal ampulla in mares (Scott et al. 1995). Rapid transport of a small number of sperm through the entire female reproductive tract into the peritoneal cavity has been described, but there may be some species variation (Phillips and Andrews 1937; Van Demark and Moeller 1950, 1951; First et al. 1968; Overstreet and Cooper 1978). It is believed that fertile spermatozoa are sequestered at a specific storage site in the oviduct until ovulation occurs. The caudal isthmus of most species is believed to be the site of sperm storage (Bader 1982; Scott et al. 1994; Thomas et al. 1994). The release of spermatozoa from their storage site is influenced by the time of ovulation, but the

mechanism for this is not fully understood. Sperm transport and survival of spermatozoa in the female reproductive tract have been studied in horses. Differences were found between fertile and subfertile stallions, and between fertile and some infertile mares.

SUBFERTILE STALLIONS. The total number of spermatozoa that reach the oviduct at 4 hours after insemination with fresh extended semen is significantly greater from fertile stallions compared with subfertile stallions. In addition, a greater fraction of motile and morphologically normal spermatozoa have been found in the oviducts of mares inseminated with semen from fertile compared with subfertile stallions. For example, more than 90% compared with 25% motile sperm were recovered from the oviducts of mares inseminated with semen from fertile and subfertile stallions, respectively (Scott et al. 1995).

SUBFERTILE MARES. When mares were inseminated with semen from normal fertile stallions, more spermatozoa of greater motility are observed in the caudal isthmus of reproductively normal mares, compared with subfertile mares that were susceptible to chronic uterine infection. Scanning electron microscopy of the oviducts has revealed pathological changes in the caudal isthmic epithelium in susceptible, but not in normal, mares (Scott et al. 1995). It is not clear whether the lower sperm numbers in the isthmus of susceptible mares are caused by a dysfunctional sperm transport to the oviduct or an impaired attachment of spermatozoa to the isthmic epithelium.

UTERINE CONTRACTILITY. Mating stimulates coordinated contractions in the uterine and oviductal smooth muscle layers (Fuchs 1972; Drobnis and Overstreet 1992). Although spermatozoa actively participate in the transport through the female reproductive tract, contractions of the myometrium and myosalpinx may be more important in regulating the transport of spermatozoa to the site of fertilization (Katila et al. 2000). It has been suggested that postcopulatory oxytocin release may serve to facilitate sperm transport, but a functional relationship between the oxytocin coital reflex and sperm transport has not been established (Wathes 1984; Carmichael et al. 1987). Using electromyography, myoelectric activity has been investigated in mares following insemination with fresh semen (Troedsson et al. 1998). An immediate increase in the myoelectric activity that lasted for 0.5 hours occurred following insemination. The mechanism of this rapid myometrial response to insemination is not fully understood. Equine seminal plasma, in contrast to the ram's, contains very little prostaglandin, but pituitary oxytocin release in response to teasing of estrous mares by a stallion was recently observed (Mann and Lutwak-Mann 1981; Alexander et al. 1995). Sexual stimulation and mating increase plasma concentrations of oxytocin in women, sows, ewes, and cows (Schams et al. 1982; Carmichael et al. 1987; Claus and Schams 1990;

Kendrick et al. 1993). A second phase of myoelectric activity was observed in mares after insemination with fresh semen (Troedsson et al. 1998). The initial activity that lasted only for 0.5 hours normalized to baseline myoelectric activity, and then the uterine activity increased again from 4 hours after insemination up to at least 12 hours after insemination. The second phase of myoelectric activity following insemination was similar to myometrial activity following a bacterial inoculation in normal mares and may therefore be the result of an inflammatory reaction to semen. Uterine contractions during the second phase of myoelectric activity are likely to be more important for sperm removal from the reproductive tract than for transport of a fertile population of spermatozoa to the fertilization site. The myoelectric response of the uterus to a bacterial challenge differed between young resistant mares and older mares with confirmed susceptibility to chronic uterine infection (Troedsson et al. 1993a). Resistant mares responded to a bacterial inoculation with an immediate increase in the myoelectric activity. The increased activity was sustained for 12 hours and followed by intermittently increased uterine activity for up to 20 hours after the inoculation. In contrast, susceptible mares had a significant delay for 3 hours in the myoelectric response to a bacterial intrauterine inoculation. It is not known whether, in susceptible mares, a delayed myometrial response is present after insemination, but, if this is the case, it may explain the lower number of spermatozoa that were found in the oviduct in susceptible compared with resistant mares as demonstrated by Scott and colleagues (1995).

SPERM SURVIVAL. The spermatozoa trigger an inflammatory reaction in the uterus (Troedsson et al. 1995). Only a very small portions of ejaculated/inseminated spermatozoa migrate successfully to the site of fertilization. Semen are eliminated through the vagina within hours of insemination. This rapid elimination of sperm from the uterus coincides with an increased myoelectric activity following insemination and may therefore be the result of uterine activity in response to insemination (Troedsson et al. 1998). When mares were inseminated with fresh semen, a 25% loss of spermatozoa into the vagina was observed within a few hours after insemination. The retrograde loss of spermatozoa was higher after insemination with extended semen (74%) or frozen/thawed semen (96%) (Bader and Krause 1980). No mechanism was determined that could explain these differences between fresh and extended and frozen/thawed semen, but cell-membrane alteration and damage during handling of the semen were suggested by the authors as potential causes. Sperm migration from frozen boar semen thawed in seminal plasma versus a glucose buffer was similar at 1 hour after insemination, but the number of spermatozoa found in the oviduct at 4 hours after insemination was significantly higher when spermatozoa were thawed in seminal plasma (Einarsson and Viring 1973). The authors concluded that some factor in the seminal plasma provided ways for the spermatozoa to survive for an extended time in the female reproductive tract. At the time of ejaculation, seminal plasma proteins are coating the spermatozoa, some of which protect the sperm cells from premature capacitation (Oliphant et al. 1985). In addition to a decapacitating function, sperm-coating proteins may protect the spermatozoa against selective phagocytosis and elimination from the uterus. The female tract tends to prevent morphological abnormal spermatozoa from reaching the site of fertilization (Yanagimachi 1994). The life span of acrosome-reacted or acrosome-damaged spermatozoa is very brief, and damaged or dead spermatozoa are eliminated more rapidly from the reproductive tract by phagocytosis than are intact spermatozoa.

An influx of leukocytes has consistently been found in the equine uterus within a few hours of insemination (Bader and Krause 1980; Kotilainen et al. 1994; Scott et al. 1994, 1995; Troedsson 1995). Up to 60% of spermatozoa recovered from the uterus have been observed to be phagocytosed (Phillips and Andrews 1937). Clinical observations suggest that insemination with frozen/thawed semen causes a marked uterine inflammation. A similar transient reaction, but of lower magnitude, can be observed in most mares following natural breeding or insemination with fresh semen. Spermatozoa alone (separated from seminal plasma and bacterial contaminants), cause an influx of polymorphonuclear neutrophils (PMNs) into the uterus. The number of PMNs recovered from the uterus at 4 hours after insemination with spermatozoa was comparable with the number of recovered PMNs at 5 hours after inoculation with *Streptococcus zooepidemicus* (Troedsson 1995). Further in vitro studies have suggested that both spermatozoa and seminal plasma play active but different roles in the inflammatory response to mating (Troedsson 1995; Troedsson et al. 1995, 1999, 2000). Equine spermatozoa induce PMN chemotaxis via complement activation (Troedsson et al. 1995; Rozeboom et al. 2001). In contrast to spermatozoa, seminal plasma markedly suppresses both chemotaxis and random migration of PMNs (Troedsson et al. 1995). It seems therefore likely that a transient postmating endometritis is physiological, with the purpose of eliminating excess spermatozoa, seminal products, and contaminants from the uterus. This would aid the uterus in providing an environment that is compatible with survival of an embryo when it descends into the uterine lumen at 5 days after fertilization. A function of seminal plasma may be to act as an inflammatory modulator in the uterus and, at least in part, be responsible for the transient nature of a mating-induced inflammation. Although most normal mares should be fully capable of eliminating a uterine inflammation within 5 days after contamination of the uterus, mares with compromised resistance to persistent uterine inflammation may be unable to control a uterine inflammatory response without seminal plasma as a modulator. If the mares ability to clear an inflammation physically from the uterus is impaired, the inflammation will persist and turn into a pathological condition with lower fertility as a result. In addition, sperm motion characteristics (motility, progressive motility, and velocity) were impaired when spermatozoa were exposed to an inflammatory uterine environment (Alghamdi et al. 2001). The impaired motion characteristics appeared to be the result of an excessive binding of spermatozoa to PMNs. Binding of spermatozoa to PMNs, opsonization of spermatozoa, and phagocytosis of opsonized spermatozoa were suppressed in the presence of seminal plasma (Alghamdi et al. 2001; Dahms and Troedsson 2002). These results suggest that seminal plasma is capable of protecting spermatozoa from a hostile inflammatory environment. This is further suggested by the finding that fertility was improved when seminal plasma was added to the insemination dose in sows and mares inseminated in the presence of a breeding-induced uterine inflammation (Rozeboom et al. 2000; Troedsson et al. 2002).

Uterine Defense Mechanisms

POLYMORPHONUCLEAR NEUTROPHILS. PMNs are the first inflammatory cells to enter an inflamed site. Chemoattractive properties of uterine fluid have been described in vitro, and the uterus responds quickly to an antigen by releasing PMN chemotactic mediators, resulting in a rapid migration of PMNs into the uterine lumen (Pycock and Allen 1988; Troedsson et al. 1990). Complement products, as well as leukotriene B (LTB$_4$), PGE, and PGF$_{2\alpha}$, may all serve as chemoattractants for PMNs in the uterus (Lees et al. 1997; Watson et al. 1987a, b; Pycock and Allen 1988, 1990). The complement cascade mediates a series of biological reactions, all of which serve in the defense against a "foreign agent." They include increased vascular permeability, chemotaxis, opsonization prior to phagocytosis, activation of membrane lipases, and lysis of target organisms. Complement activity as well as isolation of complement cleavage products has been demonstrated in the equine reproductive tract (Asbury et al. 1982; Watson et al. 1987a; Troedsson et al. 1993c). There are reports of both enhanced and depressed uterine PMN function in animals that develop a chronic form of endometritis. These conflicting results may be explained by different experimental designs and different stages of the estrous cycle during the experiments. Studies on the role of local uterine factors on PMN function have suggested that an impaired phagocytosis by uterine PMNs in susceptible mares is the result of insufficient opsonization in uterine secretion rather than a primary dysfunction of the PMNs (Troedsson et al. 1993c). Uterine PMNs from mares susceptible to chronic endometritis were found to be fully functional if given the right environment, but dysfunctional when uterine secretion from susceptible mares was used as a source of opsonin.

IMMUNOGLOBULINS. Several classes of immunoglobulins (IgGa, IgGb, IgGc, IgGT, IgA, and IgM) have been isolated from the uterus. Widders and coworkers

(1984) found that passive transudation of immunoglobulins into the uterine lumen was minimal and that IgG and IgA are produced locally by the genital tract (Widders et al. 1985). The uterus can therefore be classified as having a local immune system. Immunohistochemical studies of the endometrium have suggested that the concentration of free immunoglobulins and the number of immunoglobulin-containing cells remain at a constant level throughout the estrous cycle. Mares with persistent endometritis had increased numbers of immunoglobulin-containing cells when compared with reproductively normal mares (Waelchli and Winder 1991). Antibody-mediated uterine defense is without doubt important for effective elimination of bacterial contaminants from the uterus. However, the antibody-mediated uterine defense is fully functional in individuals that develop chronic endometritis, and the pathophysiology of susceptibility to persistent endometritis is caused by other factors.

PHYSICAL CLEARANCE. Mechanical aspects of the uterine defense system have recently been recognized as a major contributor in uterine clearance of bacteria and inflammatory products (Allen and Pycock 1988; Troedsson and Liu 1991; Troedsson et al. 1993a; LeBlanc et al. 1994). In an experiment on rabbit uterine defense mechanisms, Winter and colleagues (1960) concluded that cervical drainage from the uterus was involved in eliminating bacteria after a uterine infection. Knudsen (1964) found that older multiparous mares with partial dilation of the uterus accumulated intrauterine fluids after breeding. Hughes and Loy (1965) observed a relaxation of the cervix in young diestrous mares within 12 hours of the induction of a uterine infection. The relaxation of the cervix was associated with a vaginal discharge. Four days after the inoculation of bacteria, the cervical tone had returned to its original state. The authors concluded that mechanical drainage of the uterus through a relaxed cervix may be an important factor in the uterine ability to clear a bacterial infection. Using radioactive-labeled microspheres as markers, Evans and coworkers (1987) found that these were eliminated more effectively by young nulliparous mares compared with old multiparous mares. Several reports of fluid accumulation in the uterus following experimentally induced endometritis in susceptible mares suggested physical clearance to be an important part of the uterine defense system. Subsequent studies, using intrauterine inoculations of a combination of radioactive-labeled microspheres and bacteria, demonstrated impaired clearance in susceptible, but not resistant, mares (Troedsson and Lui 1991). Whereas resistant mares cleared the uterus of microspheres within 24 hours, susceptible mares retained them within the uterine lumen for up to 96 hours after inoculation. This time is close to the time when an embryo would enter the uterus if the mares had been bred (5 to 6 days after ovulation). Using electromyography to register myometrial activity, it has been observed that the impaired uterine clearance in susceptible mares is caused by reduced myometrial activity in response to the inflammation (Troedsson et al. 1993a). Myometrial contractility has been concluded to be an essential part of the uterine defense mechanisms. Uterine contractions are necessary for an effective physical clearance via cervical and lymphatic drainage. Studies using scintigraphic measurements of intrauterine clearance of radioactive colloids have further defined a delayed physical clearance in susceptible mares (LeBlanc et al. 1994a). In subsequent studies, the importance of physical uterine clearance was confirmed by the observations that administration of uterotonic drugs to mares with delayed uterine clearance resulted in normal clearance of colloids from the uterus, and treatment of mares with normal uterine clearance with prostaglandin inhibitors made them susceptible to delayed uterine clearance (LeBlanc et al. 1994b). These results suggest an important role of $PGF_{2\alpha}$ in physical clearance, but further studies are needed to clarify the mechanism of impaired uterine contractility in mares with delayed uterine clearance. Nikolakopoulos and coworkers (2000) suggested that susceptible mares had a defect in $PGF_2\alpha$ release in response to an inflammation. It has been suggested that mares susceptible to delayed uterine clearance have an intrinsic contractile defect of the myometrium (Rigby et al. 2001; Von Reitzenstein et al. 2002). A recent study found that susceptible mares had an increased uterine accumulation of nitric oxide in the uterine lumen 13 hours after insemination (Alghamdi and Troedsson 2007). Nitric oxide mediates smooth muscle relaxation, and the authors offered this effect as a possible explanation for the subnormal levels of myoelectrical activity between 6 and 19 hours into an inflammation in susceptible mares. Factors beside impaired uterine contractility that can predispose to delayed uterine clearance include anatomic abnormalities of the reproductive tract. Mares with delayed uterine clearance often suffer from a forward tilt of the uterus over the pelvic brim. This may be a contributing factor in an abnormal accumulation of fluid and inflammatory products after breeding. A failure of the cervix to relax during estrus, or insufficient lymphatic drainage, may also contribute to delayed clearance (Pycock 1994).

HORMONAL REGULATION OF THE UTERINE DEFENSE MECHANISM. The influence of the estrous cycle on intrauterine concentrations of immunoglobulins has been investigated in horses (Asbury et al. 1980; Mitchell et al. 1982). A selective increase in the concentration of IgG, but not IgA, IgGT, or IgM, was found in the presence of elevated blood progesterone concentrations (diestrus). In contrast, progesterone is believed to suppress PMN function, whereas estrogen has been proposed to have the opposite effect (Asbury and Hansen 1987; Colbern et al. 1987; Watson et al. 1987a). Endocrine stimulation of myometrial contractility is caused by oxytocin and $PGF_{2\alpha}$. However, progesterone and estrogen have a regulatory effect on myometrial contractility. Estrogen increases the concentration of oxytocin receptors, whereas progesterone is believed to have the opposite effect (Roberts et al. 1976; Fuchs et al. 1983; Soloff et al. 1983). Furthermore, estrogen stimulates prostaglandin synthesis by the epithelial cells of the endometrium (Demers et al. 1974; Schatz et al. 1987). Progesterone is believed to suppress prostaglandin synthesis (Abel and Baird 1980; Schatz et al. 1985; Gurpide et al. 1986). In addition to a regulatory role on myometrium, mediated by the regulation of oxytocin and prostaglandin receptors, steroid hormones may have a direct effect on the membrane potential of the myometrial cells (Rossier et al. 1987; Parkington and Coleman 1990). Another important regulatory role of steroid hormones on myometrial contraction is the control of myometrial gap junctions. Estrogen has a stimulatory effect, whereas progesterone is a potent inhibitor of myometrial gap junctions (Frank et al. 1925; Reynolds and Allen 1932; Csapo 1956; Garfield et al. 1977, 1980, 1982; Burghardt et al. 1984a, 1987; McKenzie and Garfield 1985).

A model of uterine defense has been proposed in horses (Figure 7.3) (Troedsson 1999). Humoral, as well as cellular and physical, components of the uterine defense system are involved in resistance to a persistent uterine inflammation. Within 2 hours of contamination (bacteria or semen), PMNs respond to a chemotactic signal, resulting in their massive migration to the uterine lumen. Activated uterine PMNs phagocytose bacteria, spermatozoa, and debris in the presence of opsonins. These opsonins include immunoglobulins, as well as complement factor C3b. During the activation of PMNs, $PGF_{2\alpha}$ is released, which causes myometrial contractions. Myometrial contractions are regulated by $PGF_{2\alpha}$ together with oxytocin in mares. Using phenylbutazone to inhibit $PGF_{2\alpha}$ induced myometrial contractions, Cadario and colleagues (1995) observed a delayed clearance of radiocolloids from the uteri of reproductively normal mares. The role of uterine contractions is to remove harmful inflammatory products that are released during PMN phagocytosis and during programmed cell death of PMNs. This physical or mechanical uterine defense is a key factor in the prevention of persistent inflammation and endometrial damage. In mares with a functional defense system, the majority of inflammatory products are cleared from the uterus within 24 to 36 hours of contamination. In contrast to resistant mares, susceptible mares fail to clear the uterus from contaminants and inflammatory products. An initial PMN migration into the uterus also occurs in susceptible mares, and the freshly migrated PMNs are activated and fully functional. In addition, antibody concentrations in the uterus are normal or elevated. However, the physical clearance of inflammatory products is impaired in susceptible mares. Inflammatory enzymes accumulating in the uterus may break down beneficial inflammatory mediators, possibly resulting in insufficient opsonization of antigens that thus escape phagocytosis by the PMNs. This results in a sustained inflammatory response in the uterus, with

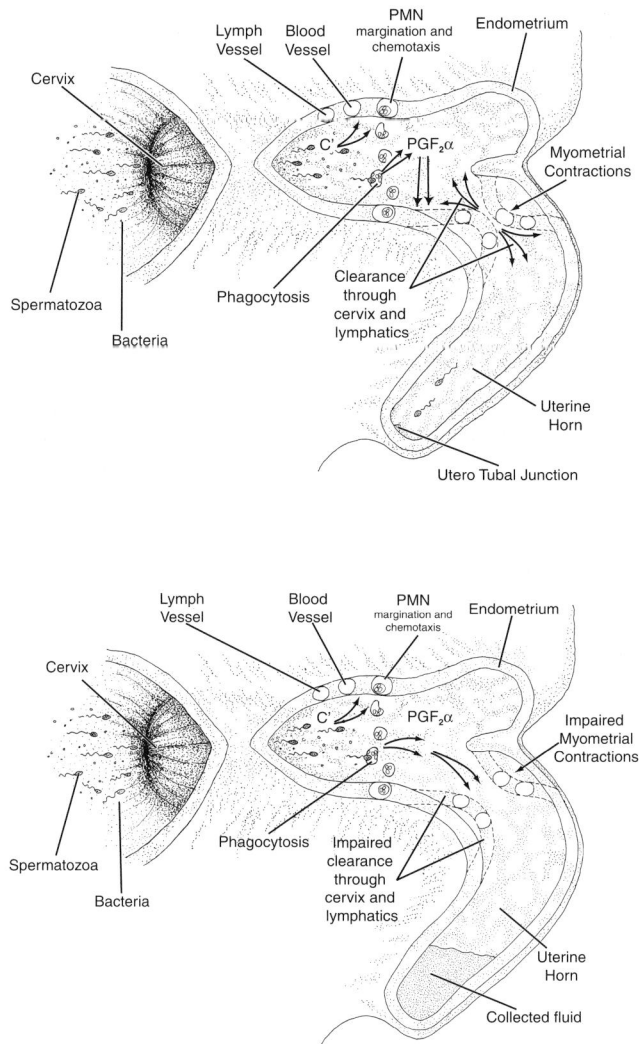

FIG 7.3—Proposed model of local uterine defense mechanisms in mares. A bacterial or seminal contamination triggers a massive invasion of polymorphonuclear neutrophils (PMNs) into the uterine lumen. The PMNs phagocytose the bacteria/spermatozoa, and the inflammation results in the release of prostaglandin $F_{2\alpha}$ ($PGF_{2\alpha}$). $PGF_{2\alpha}$ causes myometrial contractions, which are essential for uterine clearance via the cervix or the lymphatics. Mares susceptible to persistent endometritis have impaired myometrial contractions resulting in insufficient uterine clearance.

continuing migration of PMNs rendering the environment incompatible with pregnancy if conception has taken place. Furthermore, an enzymatic degradation of tissue enzymes may cause degenerative fibrotic changes to the endometrium.

Retained Fetal Membranes. The placenta serves as an interface between the fetus and the uterus. *Placenta* means "flat cake" in Latin and was so named because of the characteristic shape of the human placenta. Although the general function of the placenta is similar between domestic species, both the normal anatomy and physiology differ between species. The

placentae of domestic animals are classified based on their shape, origin, degree of invasiveness, structure of the fetal placental vasculature, and the degree of intimacy of attachment to the endometrium. The placenta is of embryonic trophoblastic origin and consists of the amnion, the yolk sac, the chorion, the allantois, and the umbilical vessels. The function of the placenta is to act as a physical and immunologic barrier between the fetus and the mother, to supply nutrition to the fetus, to exchange oxygen and carbon dioxide between the mother and the fetus, and to remove waste products from the fetus. In addition, the placenta is an endocrine active organ with hormone synthesis and metabolism of importance for maintenance and normal development of the fetus in many species.

Retained fetal membranes are defined as the failure of the entire or partial fetal membranes to be expelled after parturition. The actual separation and expulsion of the fetal membranes from the uterus occurs during the third stage of labor, but important cellular and biochemical events that involve maturation and separation of the placenta from the endometrium begin before parturition. Most research on the normal events that lead to expulsion of the placenta, and to placenta being retained, in domestic animals has been conducted on cows. Detachment of the placenta in the cow is initiated by a progressive collagenolysis of the maternal and fetal connective tissue of the placentome during the last month of gestation. The successive weakening of the interface between maternal and fetal tissue includes remodeling of connective tissue and influx of leukocytes to the site (Gunnick 1984; Heuweiser and Grunert 1987). Decreased collagenase activity has been associated with retained fetal membranes (Eiler 1997). The source of collagenase and proteolytic enzymes may be myometrial cells, fibroblasts, and leukocytes. Rupture of the umbilical cord in association with parturition is believed to cause collapse of the fetal placental vessels, with subsequent shrinkage of the chorionic villi (Roberts 1986). The final separation of the interdigitating components of the cotyledons is most likely the result of myometrial contractions induced by oxytocin and prostaglandin. During late gestation and parturition, the inducible prostaglandin enzyme COX-2 (cyclooxygenase 2) increases in fetal cotyledonary epithelium and maternal caruncular epithelium (Fuchs et al. 1999; Ivell et al. 2000). Myometrial contractions reduce the uterine size and the amount of circulating blood in the endometrium, resulting in relaxation of the endometrial crypts, which allows the chorionic villi to be released. Impaired collagenolysis appears to be the underlying cause of retained placenta in cows. Both infectious and noninfectious causes have been identified. Immature palcentomes, edema of the villi, and placentitis can cause retention of the fetal membranes. Uterine atony is not believed to be a common cause of retained placenta in cows, but an endocrine imbalance or disturbance in normal uterine contractions has been suggested to be a common cause of retained fetal membranes in mares (Haluska et al. 1987). Similar to cows, any swelling at the site of the microcotyledons can cause retention of the fetal membranes in mares. The most common site of partial retention in mares is the previously nongravid horn (Vanderplassche et al. 1971).

Delayed uterine involution in association with autolysis of the placenta (or part of the placenta) promotes the development of a uterine infection. Rapid bacterial growth within the uterine lumen during the immediate postpartum and resorption of toxins from the uterus may result in metritis. Postpartum endometritis is an important sequel to retained placenta in cows (Fredriksson et al. 1985). Absorption of Gram-negative bacteria and endotoxins may cause endotoxemia and peripheral vascular changes resulting in laminitis in mares (Blanchard et al. 1985).

PHYSIOLOGY AND PATHOPHYSIOLOGY OF MALE REPRODUCTION.

To pass his genes to the next generation, a male must be able to attract a mate, successfully defend a territory or harem, identify females at the receptive stage of their ovulatory cycle, and produce sufficient quantities of fertile spermatozoa and deliver them to the female by possessing the desire (libido) and physical ability to copulate. Many systems both within and outside the strict anatomic boundaries of the reproductive tract have profound influences on the success of this endeavor.

The male reproductive tract includes the paired testes, which are responsible for production of spermatozoa and male steroid hormones. In the vast majority of mammals, and in all the domestic species, the testes are held outside of the abdomen in a scrotum. Within each testis, a system of ducts drain the sperm out of the organ and into an epididymis, where they are matured and stored. The paired vas deferens run from the scrotum into the abdominal cavity, connecting the epididymis with the pelvic urethra. Ducts from the accessory sex glands join the urethra at this point, providing fluids that form the major volume of the ejaculate. From this point, the urethra continues distally as the penile urethra and opens at the glans (Setchell 1991; Amann 1993a; Hafez 2000).

Physiology of Testicular Function

THE TESTICLE. Testes consist of the seminiferous tubules, interstitial tissue, and a fibrous skeleton.

The seminiferous tubules comprise the majority of testicular volume where the sperm are made (approximately 85% of total volume in ruminants; 72% horse and 65% boar) and where the sperm are formed (see Figure 7.4).

Interstitial tissue lies between the tubules (about 15% of testicular volume in ruminants; 28% horse and 37% boar) and consists of blood vessels, nerves, lymphatics, macrophages and mast cells, and the Leydig cells that are responsible for testosterone production.

The remainder of the testis, contained in the interstitial tissue, consists of the fibrous skeleton and a system of ducts for sperm transport. In order from the seminiferous tubule, they are termed the straight tubules, the rete testis, and the efferent ducts.

SEMINIFEROUS TUBULES. These convoluted, hollow, fluid-filled tubes are open at both ends and empty via their short terminal segments—the straight tubules—into the rete testis. Approximate total lengths of the tubules in mature animals are 3000 m/testis in rams and 2800 m in the stallion. The tubules are not penetrated

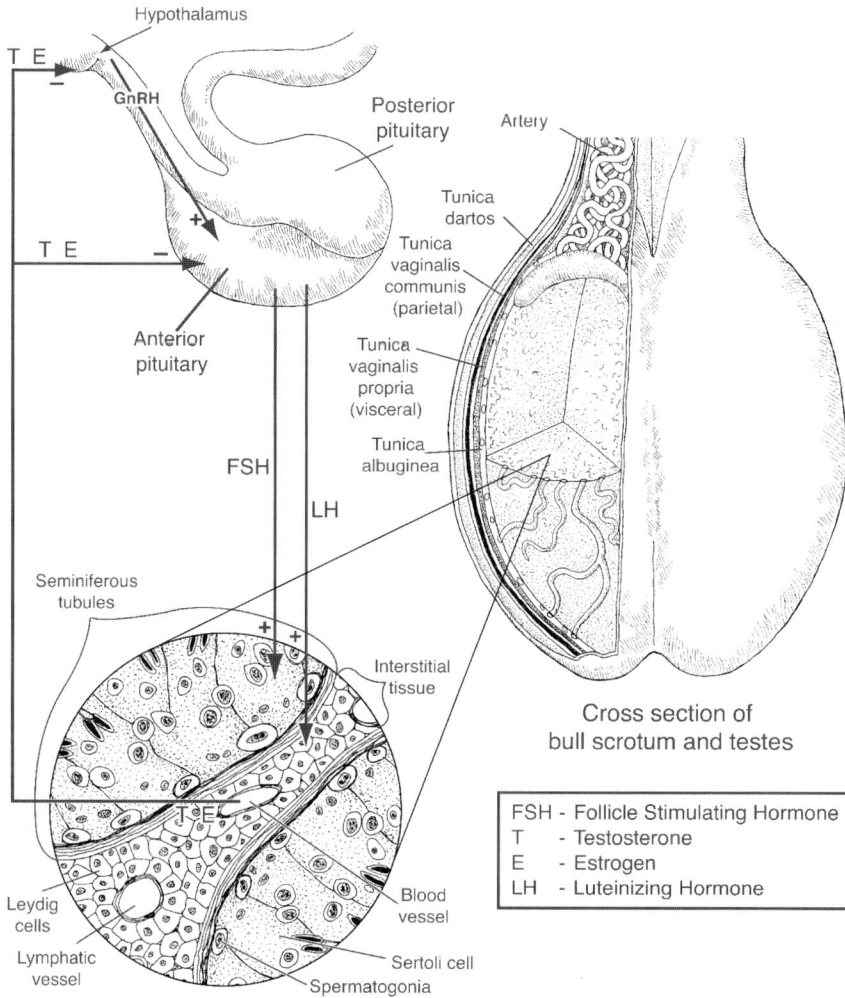

FIG 7.4—**Left:** Interstitial tissue and seminiferous tubules of the testes. E, estrogen; FSH, follicle-stimulating hormone; LH, luteinizing hormone; and T, testosterone. **Right:** Cross section of bull scrotum and testes. GnRH, gonadotropin-releasing hormone.

by blood vessels or lymphatics. The basement membrane is surrounded by a layer of myoid cells, which provide peristaltic contractions to move fluid and sperm along the tubules and into the duct system.

The tubule is lined by the seminiferous epithelium, which consists of Sertoli cells and the germ cells that will form spermatozoa. Germ cells at various stages of development occupy all levels of the epithelium, least differentiated at the basement membrane (spermatogonia) and most differentiated near the lumen (spermatids), into which sperm will be released as they finish development.

Individual Sertoli cells extend from the basement membrane to the lumen. They totally surround and serve to nurture the developing germ cells. Because of this, the Sertoli cells are also known as nurse cells.

As the germ cells divide and become more developed, they move gradually away from the basement membrane toward the lumen of the tubule (and apex of the Sertoli cell). The germ cells resulting from the division of a single spermatogonia develop as a clone, all joined together by intercellular bridges. This results in the synchronous development of large numbers of germ cells.

SPERMATOGENESIS: THE FORMATION OF SPERM. Spermatogenesis is the process that results in formation of highly specialized cells: the spermatozoa (Johnson 1991; Amann 1993b). It consists of the following:

1. Cellular proliferation by repeated mitotic divisions
2. Entry into meiosis with chromosome duplication, genetic recombination by crossing over, and then

meiotic reduction divisions to give haploid spermatids
3. Terminal differentiation of spermatids to spermatozoa

These three stages are associated with differently named intermediate cell types:

1. Proliferation: spermatogonia
2. Meiosis: spermatocytes
3. Differentiation: spermatids

PROLIFERATION. The germ cells adjacent to the basement membrane are the most primitive and are termed type A spermatogonia. When one of these cells divides, one of the daughter cells stays on the basement membrane to keep renewing the numbers. The other daughter cell becomes committed to the spermatogenic pathway and, once it does so, its course is irreversible. This committed cell continues to divide by mitosis, and all members of the clone remain linked so they keep dividing synchronously. The number of mitotic divisions depends on the species; usually, they will go through several divisions, multiplying their numbers each time (A_1 to A_4) before becoming a type B spermatogonia. This is usually the last one that divides by mitosis to produce the preleptotene spermatocyte and entry to meiosis.

Once the committed clone enters meiosis, the resting spermatogonia on the basement membrane will again divide by mitosis, and the process starts again. This new clone pushes the cells of the previous clone closer to the lumen. This precise interval between generations gives a timed repeat of different cell-type associations when the seminiferous epithelium is examined microscopically from basement membrane to lumen: every time you have an A_2 spermatogonia next to the basement membrane, then you will have cell types w, x, y, and z above it in order, and whenever you have an A_3 spermatogonia, then above it you will have l, m, n, o, and so on. This clonal division and orderly entry gives what is called the spermatogenic cycle: a timed repeat of cell associations. To complete the cycle (from A_2, w, x, y, and z to the next A_2, w, x, y, and z cell association at the same location of the seminiferous epithelium) takes a species-specific number of days. Depending on the species, it will take four to five of these cycles for a type A spermatogonia that started on the spermatogenic pathway to finish it and be released into the lumen of the tubule as a sperm.

MEIOSIS. Each diploid primary spermatocyte undergoes meiosis (one round of DNA replication followed by two sequential divisions), at the end of which it will have generated four haploid spermatids. The first meiosis is long and results in the secondary spermatocyte. The second meiosis is quicker, resulting in a haploid spermatid that still looks fairly much like a regular round cell.

The combination of mitosis and meiosis that leads to formation of the spermatid is called spermatocytogenesis (proliferation + meiosis). Some authors prefer to use the term spermatocytogenesis only for mitotic divisions of the spermatogonia and refer to spermatocyte development simply as meiosis (Johnson 1991).

Since there may be five or six rounds of mitotic division (2^6: 1 cell becomes 64), and then each of these forms four haploid cells at meiosis, 256 sperm could develop from a single spermatogonia. In reality, many are lost along the way to the process of apoptosis: programmed cell death. The stage of germ cell experiencing maximum apoptotic losses varies with species and by season for seasonal breeders. Thus, whereas boars and people have a 30% to 40% loss of spermatocytes near the end of meiosis, bulls and stallions experience maximum losses in the latter stages of spermatogonial mitosis (Johnson et al. 2000).

DIFFERENTIATION (SPERMIOGENESIS). The newly formed haploid round spermatid now undergoes a long phase of terminal differentiation involving dramatic cellular changes to form the spermatozoa.

The nucleus elongates and chromatin condenses. Final nuclear shape is species specific.

The Golgi apparatus produces small granules that coalesce to form a large acrosomic vesicle that moves over the nucleus to form the acrosome. This structure is full of enzymes that become important at the time of fertilization.

The pair of centrioles migrate to the nucleus and bind to it while at the same time forming the axoneme, which rapidly elongates to form the core of the tail. Other cytoskeletal elements migrate to the tail to form the characteristic structure. Mitochondria migrate to the developing tail, line up, and later condense and form a spiral pattern in the midpiece region. These mitochondria will provide the energy for sperm motility.

The spermatid loses large amounts of its cytoplasm during this stage. This forms the residual body, which is phagocytosed by the Sertoli cell. The developing spermatid is tethered to its residual body by a cytoplasmic stalk attached to its neck region (Oko and Clermont 1998).

SPERMIATION: RELEASE OF SPERMATIDS. The release of the spermatid from its tether is known as spermiation, and the released cell is now a spermatozoa. The remnant of cytoplasm where it was tethered to the Sertoli cell is located in the midpiece region and is known as the cytoplasmic droplet. The duration of spermatogenesis is presented in Table 7.3.

TABLE 7.3—Duration (in days) of spermatogenesis

Human	72
Bull	61
Dog	61
Stallion	57
Ram	47
Boar	39

HOW MANY SPERM ARE PRODUCED?. The efficiency of spermatozoal production as measured by sperm production per gram of testicular parenchyma varies greatly across species, from 4 to 6×10^6/g in humans to 25×10^6/g in rabbits. Variations in efficiency are accounted for by variations in the length of spermatogenesis and in germ cell density (Johnson et al. 2000). The combined production from the two testicles of an adult stallion during the breeding season is estimated at 70,000 per second.

FUNCTIONS OF THE SERTOLI CELL. Sertoli cells organize the clones of germ cells in the seminiferous epithelium, support the cells, and ensure their timely release as spermatozoa. The maximum number of germ cells that can be supported by each Sertoli cell is fixed for each species, as is the number of Sertoli cells per testis, but the latter is highly heritable (Johnson 1991). They secrete controlling factors that regulate germ cell differentiation and maturation and phagocytose degenerating cells. Since each Sertoli cell can support only a certain number of germ cells, they promote apoptosis of excess and abnormal germ cells, apparently via the Fas system. In this apoptotic pathway, the Sertoli cells produce Fas ligand (Fas L), which binds to Fas molecules expressed on the surface of certain germ cells (perhaps those that are not being supported, as well), where it triggers the apoptotic pathway (Zirkin 1998; Huhtaniemi and Bartke 2001).

Sertoli cells also produce androgen-binding protein that is secreted into the lumen of the seminiferous tubule, where it binds androgens. This complex may be important in regulating epididymal function.

They form the tight junctions that form the blood-testis barrier, and they are the major source of estrogen in the males of many species.

HORMONAL CONTROL OF TESTICULAR FUNCTION: THE HYPOTHALAMIC-PITUITARY TESTICULAR AXIS. A similar system to the female system is at work. Hypothalamic GnRH releases FSH and LH from the anterior pituitary gland, with LH being more GnRH dependent than is FSH.

FSH acts on Sertoli cells and stimulates them in their supporting role for the developing germ cells and promotes seminiferous tubule growth and androgen-binding protein production by Sertoli cells.

LH acts on Leydig cells to increase testosterone synthesis and secretion. Some species (e.g., stallions) actually produce more estrogens then testosterone.

There appear to be minor species differences in the feedback regulation of the hypothalamic-pituitary-gonadal axis. In general, testosterone from the testicle feeds back on the hypothalamus to reduce GnRH secretion. There may also be some inhibitory function at the hypothalamus for the testosterone metabolites estradiol and dihydrotestosterone, but the extent of this is presently unclear (Tilbrook and Clarke 2001).

Inhibin is the other testicular hormone that has an important feedback loop to the hypothalamic-pituitary axis. Inhibin B is the physiologically important form of this hormone in the male for all species examined thus far, and its site of production is considered to be the Sertoli cell, though there is evidence in the stallion for considerable Leydig cell secretion (Taya et al. 2000; Tilbrook and Clarke 2001). Circulating inhibin acts directly at the level of the pituitary to specifically inhibit FSH secretion. At least in some species, testosterone has a synergistic action with inhibin in this regard, the extent of which is seasonally variable, at least in rams (Tilbrook and Clarke 2001).

HORMONAL CONTROL OF SPERMATOGENESIS. Testosterone levels in the testicular interstitial fluid and the seminiferous tubule are 25- to 30-fold higher than in peripheral blood. These high levels of testosterone are required in the testicle (at least 10-fold greater than peripheral blood) for normal spermatogenesis to occur.

Cells at the pachytene spermatocyte and early spermatid stages are particularly vulnerable to decreased testosterone levels. Testosterone works via the Sertoli cells by maintaining binding of the Sertoli cell to these developing sperm cell stages. There appears to be a synergistic role for FSH in this process. In the absence of this intimate binding to the Sertoli cell, the germ cells die.

FSH is required for the initiation of spermatogenesis at puberty. Whether it is required for continued spermatogenesis in mature animals *if testosterone levels are normal* is under debate. It is required if testosterone levels drop, but if they drop too far, FSH cannot maintain spermatogenesis alone. It appears that FSH is able to maintain spermatogenesis by increasing the number of spermatogonia and promoting maturation through meiosis to the round spermatid stage, but it cannot take the germ cells beyond this point (i.e., cannot do spermiogenesis). Testosterone is required to complete this process.

During spermatogenesis, many sperm cells are lost along the way by apoptosis. It appears there may be roles for both FSH and testosterone actions in preventing this cell death (Zirkin 1998).

The hypothalamic-pituitary-gonadal axis with its tropic hormones and feedback mechanisms is the main regulator of testicular function. Subservient to this endocrine system, but intrinsic to the successful functioning of the testicle for both steroid and sperm production, is a local control system. At this level, a vital dialogue among Leydig and Sertoli cells, peritubular myoid cells, interstitial tissue macrophages and the developing germ cells, among others, is constantly integrating the information received from the endocrine axis with local inputs. The local control system in the testicle is still poorly understood but under intense investigation. It involves paracrine, autocrine, juxtacrine, cryptocrine, and intracrine communication between and within the cellular populations of the testicle using growth factors, inhibin, activin, cytokines, and locally produced peptide hormones. This system adjusts steroidogenesis and is vitally important in the successful completion of spermatogenesis (Saez 1994; Gnessi et al. 1997).

BLOOD-TESTIS BARRIER. Fluid within the seminiferous tubules and rete testis is vastly different from blood plasma or interstitial fluid. Additionally, the more developmentally advanced germ cell stages express protein antigens that the immune system does not recognize as self (because they are first produced after puberty). To maintain these fluid differences and the immune compartmentalization, there is the blood-testis barrier, formed by tight junctions between adjacent Sertoli cells (Setchell 1991).

As germ cells divide and enter meiosis on their pathway to becoming sperm, they progressively move away from the basement membrane toward the lumen of the tubule. The tight junctions between adjacent Sertoli cells thus divide the seminiferous epithelium into basal and adluminal compartments. Stages up to preleptotene spermatocytes are in the basal compartment, whereas stages from pachytene spermatocytes on to spermatids and spermatozoa are in the adluminal compartment. Leptotene spermatocytes pass through the barrier, somewhat like a boat going through a lock: new junctions form on their basal side and then those on the luminal side open up (Setchell 1991).

The barrier blocks antibody entry to the adluminal compartment. Additionally, expression of Fas L by the Sertoli cell may have a role in destruction of Fas-expressing leukocytes that attempt to gain access to the seminiferous tubule (Zirkin 1998).

TESTICULAR TEMPERATURE CONTROL. In most mammals, the testes are extra-abdominal in an effort to maintain them below body temperature. This reduced temperature is required for normal spermatogenesis in the vast majority of species, as evidenced by failure of spermatogenesis in cases of cryptorchidism, despite relatively normal testosterone levels (Setchell 1991).

In addition to this external location, several anatomic features aid in testicular temperature regulation:

- The scrotal skin of many species is free of hair or only sparsely covered compared with the remainder of the body. The scrotum may contain abundant sweat glands to aid heat loss by evaporation.
- A smooth muscle layer beneath the skin of the scrotum, the tunica dartos, can raise and lower the testes to take them closer to the body in cold weather or away from it in warmer conditions.
- The arterial supply and vascular drainage of the testicle form a countercurrent heat-exchange system. The artery is very coiled after leaving the body, whereas the veins form a plexus (pampiniform plexus) of interconnected vessels. The relatively cool blood returning from the scrotum is used to cool the blood in the artery prior to it entering the testicle.

Testicular Degeneration. Testicular degeneration can be the result of direct trauma to the testicle, a toxic insult, an infection, or an alteration in testicular homeostasis—either nutritional (oxygen or nutrient), thermoregulatory, or by withdrawal of tropic hormone support.

Macroscopic and microscopic changes seen in the testicle undergoing degeneration have been well described (Ladds 1993). Depending on the inciting agent, there may be a transitory swelling and edema of the testicle, which is followed by a reduction in tone and then size. Depending on the degree and length of the insult, the testes may recover partially or fully, or may eventually become small and firm with fibrotic changes. The tunica-albuginea may become wrinkled as the testis shrinks, and this is considered a method of differentiating degeneration from atrophy in a case with little history. As the testicular parenchyma shrinks, the fibrous supporting skeleton of the testis remains, and the organ may take on a characteristic ribbed feel in some species (similar less marked changes may be discerned in the nonbreeding season of seasonally active males).

The microscopic changes seen in the degenerating seminiferous epithelium are similar irrespective of the cause. Variations are seen only in the extent and severity of the changes (Ladds 1993). Initially, degeneration occurs in some spermatids, while others form multinucleated giant cells. Spermatocytes show cytoplasmic vacuolation and nuclear degeneration, and finally all cells of the germline may be absent, leaving only Sertoli cells lining the tubule lumen. With a severe-enough insult, even these may be absent, with collapse of the tubule resulting.

DEGENERATION DUE TO LACK OF TROPHIC HORMONE SUPPORT. Since spermatogenesis depends on high intratesticular testosterone levels, anything lowering testosterone production can have adverse consequences for fertility. Disorders may arise at any level of the hypothalamic-pituitary-gonadal axis, involving levels and patterns of hormone secretion and alteration in hormone bioactivity, receptor function, and postreceptor effector mechanisms. Many of these problems are rare and involve genetic mutations; to others, such as strenuous physical exercise and emaciation, males appear more resistant than females. In domestic species, the most common cause of *hypogonadotrophic hypogonadism* is probably the use of exogenous anabolic steroid hormones and testosterone.

Anabolic steroids are chemically modified androgens. The aim of the modifications is to remove various amounts of the androgenic activity while maintaining their anabolic effects. However, all anabolic steroids maintain some androgenic activity. Such drugs may be administered to aid recovery from a debilitating illness or to increase the growth rate of food animals. They are perhaps most frequently associated with reproductive problems when they are given to show or performance animals to increase training effects on muscle mass and stamina and to increase competitive aggression.

The administered steroid acts as testosterone would on the hypothalamic-pituitary axis, providing feedback inhibition of GnRH and gonadotropin secretion. This results in loss of trophic support for the testicular Leydig cells, with a dramatic reduction in testosterone secretion. The androgenic component of the administered steroid is sufficient to maintain or even enhance some male secondary sexual characteristics. However, spermatogenesis suffers because of the requirement for very high testosterone levels locally within the testis. Treatment of stallions with testosterone and the anabolic steroids boldenone undecylenate and nandrolone decanoate causes dramatic reductions in testicular size and sperm production, and reductions in the percentage of morphologically normal sperm (Squires et al. 1982). Other administered sex steroids may have similar effects to testosterone by feedback inhibition of the hypothalamic-pituitary axis. Stallions are frequently treated with progestagens in an effort to modify their behavior for show or competition. Such treatment with twice the label dosage of altrenogest (Regumate) has been shown to decrease serum LH and testosterone levels and testicular size, with a parallel reduction in daily sperm production and an increase in morphologically abnormal sperm (Squires et al. 1997; Johnson et al. 1998b).

Stress is another factor that is thought to influence reproduction by its effects on the hypothalamic-pituitary gonadal axis. The effects of stress on secretion of pituitary and gonadal hormones, and the consequences for reproductive function, are best described in females (see Dobson and Smith 1995), but some work has also been performed in males. In unstressed bulls, episodic release of cortisol is negatively correlated with that of LH and testosterone (Welsh et al. 1979). Elevations in endogenous corticosteroid levels in response to stress are associated with reductions in circulating LH and testosterone in bulls (Welsh and Johnson 1981), as is administration of the synthetic corticosteroid dexamethasone (Thibier and Rolland 1976; Barth and Bowman 1994). Bulls treated with dexamethasone had a progression of sperm abnormalities indicating adverse affects on both epididymal maturation functions and testicular spermiogenesis (Barth and Bowman 1994). Stress is thought to suppress all levels of the hypothalamic-pituitary gonadal axis, with actions proposed for corticotropin-releasing hormone, adrenocorticotropic hormone, and cortisol (Tilbrook et al. 2000). As the lines between endocrinology and immunology become increasingly blurred, other mechanisms involved in the pathogenesis of stress on reproduction will likely become evident.

Loss of germline cells due to loss of trophic hormone support is by increased apoptosis, and, as with several other inciting agents, the stage of cell differentiation influences susceptibility. Experimentally, treatment of male rats with a potent GnRH antagonist or Leydig cell-specific toxins causes testosterone levels to decrease dramatically within 2 days. This reduction precedes a massive stage-specific increase in germ cell apoptosis involving spermatocytes and early spermatids. The apoptotic pathway involves members of the Bcl-2 family of proteins, with potential involvement of the Fas pathway (Sinha Hikim et al. 1995; Woolveridge et al. 1999).

The final stage of sperm formation is also affected by hormone withdrawal. Suppression of FSH or testosterone both lead to a mild reduction in spermiation. Simultaneous removal of both hormones has a synergistic effect, with half of mature spermatids not being released (Saito et al. 2000). This synergism probably reflects the ability of one of the hormones to compensate for the loss of the other, removal of both preventing this backup mechanism.

THERMALLY INDUCED DEGENERATION. Elevation of the testicular temperature to or above the normal core body temperature of an animal can cause degeneration of the seminiferous epithelium. Such changes would include a generalized febrile episode, such as response to a viremia, or an alteration in the ability of the animal to maintain a cooler testicular temperature. Scrotal dermatitis may actively raise scrotal temperature in the acute stages. In more chronic cases, the thickening of the scrotal skin acts to prevent heat loss. Similar insulation-type effects may be seen with scrotal edema and fat infiltration. Adhesions between the vaginal tunics can prevent testicular movement in response to changing environmental conditions and thus affect thermoregulation. Direct trauma to the scrotum and its contents, or infections involving the same structures, will cause an inflammation that results in thermal injury in addition to any direct effect on the testicle (McEntee 1990; Ladds 1993).

In all species studied, experimentally raising the temperature of the scrotum and its contents alone or raising the body temperature of the whole animal has resulted in spermatozoal abnormalities and eventually testicular degeneration [see Setchell (1998) for a review]. Sperm stored in the epididymis seem to be fairly resistant to these insults, with normal sperm being present in the ejaculate until sperm that were being formed in the testes during the heating episode appear, generally after 7 to 10 days. Depending on length and degree of scrotal hyperthermia and the species involved, the initial change is a reduction in motility of ejaculated sperm, followed by increases in morphologically abnormal sperm and finally a reduction in cell numbers. The changes reflect the sensitivity of different cell types to hyperthermia, with pachytene spermatocytes and spermatids being most susceptible. However, if the insult is of sufficient magnitude and duration, further cells in the germ lineage are affected, and eventually even Sertoli cells may succumb (Setchell 1998). There is evidence that germ cell stages that are most sensitive to testosterone withdrawal (androgen-dependent stages) are protected from damage during heat stress by the presence of normal testosterone levels (Lue et al. 1999).

Thermal damage also has direct effects on the spermatozoa that are not morphologically obvious but may have significant effects on fertility. Experimental scrotal insulation of ponies that results in a mild temperature increase (2° to 3°C) decreased the formation of disulfide bonds that stabilize the sperm chromatin (Love and Kenney 1999). Most susceptible in this regard were primary spermatocytes, leading the authors to speculate that the heating altered a factor that is later involved in protamine configuration or disulfide-bond formation, since these are not formed until well after the primary spermatocyte stage. Similar influences on sperm DNA synthesis and structure have been observed in other species. The effects of these alterations may not be seen until fertilization, when sperm chromatin is required to decondense. Other induced abnormalities of sperm may not become apparent until the resulting embryos fail to develop (Setchell 1998).

During testicular heating, oxygen consumption by the organ increases, but, compared with other tissues, there is little increase in blood supply. This leads to a potentially ischemic condition within the testicular parenchyma. Other possible mechanisms for thermal damage include enzymatic leakage and reduced detoxification of reactive oxygen species (ROS), leading to increased oxidative damage (Setchell 1998). The molecular mechanisms for thermally induced injury are beginning to be unraveled. Induction of apoptosis in developing germ cells following scrotal heating has been shown to involve the Bcl-2 family of proteins, with redistribution of Bax from cytosol to nucleus and upregulation of Bcl-2 (Yamamoto et al. 2000).

Febrile episodes caused by bacterial infection are not uncommon in veterinary medicine, but thermally induced testicular degeneration may not be the only problem facing such patients. Circulating endotoxins from Gram-negative infections have been shown to immobilize spermatozoa of domestic species and increase apoptosis of mature spermatozoa in people (Dennis 1962; Gorga et al. 2001).

VARICOCELE: A SPECIAL CASE OF THERMALLY INDUCED DEGENERATION?. Varicocele refers to abnormal dilation of the veins in the pampiniform plexus. The vast majority of information on the pathophysiology of the lesion comes from the human literature and animal models aimed at furthering understanding the human disease. Despite these studies, the condition in humans remains highly controversial with regard to its actual effect on fertility, its optimal method of diagnosis, whether treatment is beneficial, and its pathophysiology (Benoff and Gilbert 2001; Kamischke and Nieschlag 2001). The condition is of great interest to pathophysiologists because a currently proposed model for the effects of the condition on the testicle involves several of the previously discussed pathways (Benoff and Gilbert 2001).

In human medicine, varicocele is estimated to affect 15% of the general male population, with a preponderance of left-sided lesions (Takihara ct al. 1991). Detailed studies of the incidence in other species are unavailable, but it is assumed to be much lower (Turner 2001). The disease in humans is divided into primary and secondary categories. A secondary varicosity develops in response to partial occlusion of the spermatic veins by a pelvic tumor or similar space-occupying lesion that raises the intravascular pressure, but these are very uncommon. Primary varicosities are more difficult to explain, but two major hypotheses have been forwarded (Takihara et al. 1991). The first is that a valvular incompetence of the spermatic veins allows pooling of blood and increased pressure. This does not explain the preponderance of left-sided lesions, and it is now considered that any valvular incompetence is likely the result of vessel dilation rather than the cause. The second proposal is the gloriously named *nutcracker phenomenon*. In this scenario, the upright posture of *Homo sapiens* permits the left renal vein to be compressed between the abdominal aorta and superior mesenteric arteries; the internal spermatic vein joins the renal vein distal to the compression and thus has its resistance increased. Although this is the favored explanation in humans, its applicability to other species is doubtful.

A number of models for the pathophysiology of varicocele on the testis have been proposed: raised testicular temperature, testicular hypoxia, increased testicular pressure, backflow of renal and adrenal metabolites, an induced abnormality of the hypothalamic-pituitary-gonadal axis, and testosterone washout from the testis, among others (Takihara et al. 1991; Benoff and Gilbert 2001; Kamischke and Nieschlag 2001; Turner 2001). The most favored of the single hypotheses is elevation of testicular temperature.

Experimentally induced unilateral varicocele in animal models paradoxically results in an increase in blood flow through the testis (Turner 2001). This results in an increase in testicular temperature in both the ipsilateral testis and the contralateral testis, presumably due to reduced efficiency of the countercurrent heat-exchange mechanism between the testicular artery and pampiniform plexus under conditions of increased flow. Another mechanism postulated is retrograde flow of warmed abdominal blood down the dilated vessels, but this has less experimental support. Recently, a model that involves three pathways for the induction of germ cell apoptosis in varicocele has been proposed (Benoff and Gilbert 2001). The pathways are (a) increased testicular temperature, (b) increased cadmium ion (Cd^{2+}) concentrations in the testicle, and (c) reduced testicular androgen concentration. Temperature and testosterone effects have already been discussed. In the Cd^{2+} hypothesis, it is speculated that because varicocele increases intratesticular venous pressure, it increases the formation of interstitial fluid (which is a plasma filtrate). Since Cd^{2+} is a component of plasma, its level in the tissue spaces of the testicle increases. This Cd^{2+} is transported via calcium channels into the seminiferous tubule, where it has effects on both Sertoli cells and germ cells. In Sertoli cells, the effect would be on the cytoskeleton, which is important in tethering to the germ cells and movement of the developing germ cell stages from the base of the tubule toward its lumen and final release. In the germ cells, the effect of Cd^{2+} would be on the cytoskeleton and potentially by DNA fragmentation via direct Cd^{2+} induction of a calcium-dependent endonuclease. Much of this hypothesis needs to be confirmed.

DEGENERATION DUE TO ISCHEMIA. Staggering numbers of spermatozoa and large quantities of steroid and other hormones are produced by the testes of adult animals. The metabolic demands to maintain these production levels are commensurately high, but blood flow to the organ is relatively low. This means that there is little safety margin should the metabolic requirement increase (e.g., raised testicular temperature) or blood supply fall (Ladds 1993).

Testicular ischemia may arise in several ways. Older animals may suffer hyaline degeneration of vessel walls supplying small parts (arterioles) or large portions of the testicular parenchyma, with degeneration following infarction (Ladds 1993). Thrombosis of testicular artery branches has also been observed in domestic species, though the mild degree of resulting degeneration of the seminiferous epithelium is taken as evidence of adequate collateral circulation. The reason for thrombosis in most cases is unknown. The most spectacular cause of ischemia is testicular torsion, where the twisting of the spermatic cord occludes both the testicular veins and the artery. Affected animals frequently are in a great deal of pain. There is evidence that 1 hour of ischemia is enough to cause severe changes to the seminiferous epithelium (Ladds 1993). In cases of long-standing testicular torsion, cell death is by infarction, and the testis becomes necrotic. Much of the research into pathophysiology involves models that explore the effects of short-term torsion followed by surgical correction.

Using an experimental torsion and reperfusion model in rats, it has been shown that, following a 1-hour ischemic period, there was increased evidence of germ cell apoptosis within 4 hours (Turner et al. 1997). The injury was confined to the germ cells, with Sertoli and Leydig cells being unaffected. Increased PMN margination and lipid peroxidation in the testes after reperfusion imply that the apoptosis is a classic ischemia-reperfusion injury induced by increased ROS production from invading PMNs. Furthermore, the germ cell apoptosis in this study was prevented by infusion of superoxide radical scavengers prior to testicular detorsion and reperfusion (Turner et al. 1997). Subsequent work by the same group has suggested two gene-activation pathways for the induction of germ cell apoptosis during ischemia-reperfusion injury (Lysiak et al. 2000). It was proposed that in a selective pathway secretion of Fas L by invading PMNs could trigger apoptosis in those germ cells expressing Fas on their surfaces. Additionally, increased ROS levels in the tissue derived from the PMNs would elevate levels of Bax and in turn cause an indiscriminate release of cytochrome c from mitochondria.

Other investigators have also demonstrated the involvement of the Fas system in the induction of apoptosis following experimentally induced testicular ischemia (Koji et al. 2001). Interestingly, these authors found no evidence for involvement of the Fas system in the huge loss of developing germ cells to apoptosis in normal males.

While the end result of testicular injury from many causes appears the same, there is evidence that the pathophysiology has subtle variations. Thus, in rats, the stage of the germ cell lineage most sensitive to ischemia-reperfusion injury is slightly different from that most sensitive to withdrawal of trophic hormone support (Sinha Hikim et al. 1997; Lysiak et al. 2000).

Similarly, the apoptotic pathways involved may vary. Sertoli cells are thought to express Fas L, whereas damaged germ cells express Fas. The expression of Fas L by Sertoli cells may also have a role in maintaining the blood-testis barrier by eliminating Fas-expressing leukocytes attempting to gain access to the seminiferous tubule. In the Fas system, it is postulated that direct injury to germ cells causes them to increase expression of Fas, and they are then destroyed by Sertoli cells expressing normal levels of Fas L—normal Sertoli cells doing their job by removing damaged germ cells. By contrast, when the Sertoli cells alone are damaged, initially they cannot support the same number of germ cells, so they increase Fas-L expression that then eliminates those germ cells they cannot support, which have secondarily increased their Fas expression (Lee et al. 1999).

DEGENERATION DUE TO OUTFLOW OBSTRUCTION. Spermatoceles are cystic accumulations of sperm within the excurrent duct system. They are commonly described in the epididymis but may also involve the duct system within the testis itself. While frequently considered as secondary to trauma or inflammation, there is evidence that they may be due to a senile change of the seminiferous epithelium. In this situation, the epithelium sloughs immature germ cell forms, and these sloughed cells aggregate in the rete testis and excurrent duct system, blocking the lumen and resulting in the spermatocele (Itoh et al. 1999). In this case, degenerative changes to the seminiferous epithelium are the cause rather than the result of the outflow obstruction, or, depending on the location of the blockage, degenerative changes in some tubules could cause an outflow obstruction that then causes degeneration in other parts of the testicle.

Obstruction of the duct system may also be due to congenital malformation or a traumatic or infectious process. These conditions frequently result in inflammatory changes from sperm leakage or the infection itself, and obstruction follows the formation of a sperm granuloma (Blanchard et al. 1991; Althouse et al. 1993). Sperm and fluids accumulate and the intraseminiferous tubule pressure increases, resulting in degeneration. The testicular effects are more severe when the obstruction involves more proximal portions of the duct system: the rete testis, efferent ducts, and head of the epididymis (Blanchard et al. 1991). When the obstruction is located distally in the epididymis or in the vas deferens (such as follows vasectomy), long-term testicular effects may be milder after the early pressure increases. This is because epithelial cells lining the epididymis have considerable capacity to absorb fluids and phagocytose spermatozoa. The sperm-obstructing granuloma itself contains large numbers of macrophages that actively phagocytose spermatozoa, while within the duct system intraluminal macrophages break down the sperm, leaving mainly degradation products to be absorbed by the epithelial cells (McDonald 2000). Lymphocytes are also found near such granulomas (Caldwell et al. 1996), and part of the continued testicular degeneration following obstructions may have an immune component mediated by antisperm antibody formation, where the initial seminiferous tubule pressure increase disrupts the blood-testis barrier. The significance of this in the pathogenesis of testicular degeneration following excurrent duct obstruction is still unclear (McDonald 2000)

OTHER CAUSES OF TESTICULAR DEGENERATION. There are numerous other causes of testicular degeneration, including infection, blunt or penetrating trauma, radiation, plant and chemical toxins, nutritional excesses or deficiencies, diabetes, and senile degeneration in bulls. Several of the testicular toxins are specific to either Sertoli, Leydig, or germ cells within the testis and have been used to define physiological relationships between them. Nutritional causes may involve deficiencies or excesses, and vary depending on the particular metabolism of the species involved. They are rare in domestic species under normal conditions (McEntee 1990; Ladds 1993). Two examples are given next to illustrate mechanisms of pathophysiology.

Zinc is an essential enzyme cofactor that is involved in the integrity of many basic cellular processes, including nucleic acid metabolism, protein synthesis, carbohydrate metabolism, and membrane stability. Adequate levels are required for the synthesis of testosterone by Leydig cells and the conversion of testosterone to the more biologically potent 5α-dihydrotestosterone. Zinc is important for spermatogenesis and sperm motility. Deficiencies can arise due to lack of intake during starvation or from incorrectly formulated rations, or in cases of increased use such as chronic disease. Zinc deficiency results in lowered sperm production, reduced motility, testicular degeneration, and reduced testosterone secretion. The effects are thought to be mediated by a combination of reduced steroidogenesis and altered carbohydrate and protein metabolism (Smith and Akinbamijo 2000; Wong et al. 2000).

Gossypol, a pigment produced by the cotton plant, is found at high levels in cottonseed and its feed byproducts, depending on the processing method and cultivar involved. Monogastric animals are very sensitive to the toxic effects, and systemic signs and death may result. It has also been explored at low doses as a possible male contraceptive in humans. Ruminants are relatively resistant to its effects, being able to detoxify the molecule in the rumen by binding it to proteins and by a variety of other mechanisms. However, ingestion of high levels of free gossypol can overcome these defenses, and toxicity may result (Randel et al. 1992). Gossypol initially appears to lower sperm motility, and evidence in vitro suggests that this occurs by inhibition of cyclic adenosine monophosphate (cAMP) formation (Zavos et al. 1996). Spermatogenesis is then affected at the late spermatid stage, where a segmental aplasia of the mitochondrial sheath is observed in the midpiece, again with detrimental effects on motility. In laboratory rodents, the lesions progress at higher doses to severe losses of the seminiferous epithelium, affecting mainly the germ cell line (Randel et al. 1992). Results in ruminants are less consistent, but most studies find a reduction in sperm motility that takes approximately 1 month to develop and a corresponding increase in sperm midpiece abnormalities. Interestingly, some of these effects can be prevented by increased vitamin E supplementation (Velasquez-Pereira et al. 1998; Chenoweth et al. 2000).

Physiology of Erectile Function. For animals, it seems generally necessary for fertilization to occur in some form of aqueous environment. For water dwellers, this was not a problem, and many continue to broadcast eggs and sperm to the environment for fertilization to occur externally. Animals that moved onto the land resorted to internal fertilization as a way of overcoming their dry terrestrial environment. As part of this process, there had to be a way of transferring sperm from the male and into the female, and many developed some form of intromittent organ, or penis.

PENILE ANATOMY. In mammals, there are basically two penis types: musculocavernous and fibroelastic. The musculocavernous-type penis has a large amount of erectile tissue and is found in species such as horses, dogs, cats, and people. The fibroelastic type is seen in most artiodactyls (e.g., ruminants and pigs), and this type is predominated by fibroelastic tissue with smaller amounts of erectile tissue. The penis in these species has a sigmoid flexure, and the function of erectile tissue is to straighten this out so that the penis protrudes, with only modest (15% to 16%) increases in length and diameter (Beckett et al. 1974a; Johnson et al. 1998a).

Within the penis are three erectile bodies: the paired corpora cavernosa located dorsally and the corpus spongiosum ventrally. The base of the penis (proximal) is attached to the pelvic bone and is formed by the crura of the corpora cavernosa and the penile bulb, which is the proximal part of the corpus spongiosum. This area is surrounded by striated muscle, with the paired ischiocavernosus muscles covering the crura while the bulbocavernosus (aka bulbospongiosus) muscle surrounds the penile bulb.

The corpora cavernosa are enclosed in a thick fibrous tissue jacket: the tunica albuginea. They consist of a spongelike network of vascular sinuses and lacunae supplied by small arteries. Beyond the endothelium, the bulk of the wall of these vascular spaces is composed of smooth muscle cells in a collagen matrix through which run arterial and nerve supplies. The separation of the two corpora cavernosa is variably incomplete, with the degree of fusion varying between species. This is the high-pressure system that supplies rigidity to the penis for intromission (Andersson and Wagner 1995; Johnson et al. 1998a; Kandeel et al. 2001). Some species (dogs, raccoons, and seals) have an os penis, or baculum, which originates as a calcification of the fused ends of the corpora cavernosa. Intromission in these species may be initiated prior to the attainment of full erection, with full engorgement of the corpora cavernosa being relatively less important.

The corpus spongiosum surrounds the urethra and terminates at the glans penis. It is a low-pressure system that functions to increase penile volume. This system also forms the bulbus glandis at the base of the canine penis. An additional muscle, the ischiourethralis, is found in dogs. At the base of the penis, it inserts on a fibrous tissue ring that encircles the dorsal veins draining the corpus spongiosum. Contraction of this muscle restricts blood flow through these vessels, directing it instead through shunts into the bulbus glandis, which then swells. This swelling combined with contraction of the vestibular muscles of the female prevent withdrawal of the penis, resulting in the "tie" (Christensen 1954).

In other species, especially those where the female is an induced ovulator (rabbits, cats, and ferrets), the penis may have a series of barbs on the glans to enhance mechanical stimulation of the vagina at mating (Johnson et al. 1998a).

The paired retractor penis muscles are responsible for keeping the nonerect penis within the prepuce but are not present in all species. These smooth muscles are normally contracted but relax during erection to enable penile protrusion. During the juvenile period, the penis is attached to the prepuce and cannot be fully extended. This attachment later breaks down, though occasionally a remnant persists, a condition known as persistent penile frenulum, which results in a curved deviation of the penis on erection.

The blood supply to the penis in most species arises from branches of the internal pudendal artery, some supplying superficial areas while another division, the penile artery, eventually supplies the cavernous structures. Numerous arteriovenous anastomoses exist at all levels of the arterial tree and function to shunt blood away from cavernous structures when the penis is nonerect. Penile innervation is both autonomic and somatic. Autonomic supply is sympathetic and parasympathetic, whereas the somatic supply consists of sensory fibers to the skin and motor supply to perineal musculature (Andersson and Wagner 1995; Johnson et al. 1998a; Kandeel et al. 2001).

ERECTION. The normal flaccid state of the penis is maintained by tonic contraction of smooth muscle in the corpora cavernosa and spongiosum and arteries supplying them under the influence of sympathetic adrenergic input, involving norepinephrine as the neurotransmitter. Both α_1-adrenergic and α_2-adrenergic receptors are involved. Blood pressures within the erectile bodies in the flaccid state are actually much lower than are systemic blood pressures (Table 7.4). This is due to the tonic constriction and the use of numerous shunts that divert blood directly into draining vessels before it enters the penis (Andersson and Wagner 1995; Kandeel et al. 2001) (see Figure 7.5).

During erection, psychic stimuli acting on brain and tactile stimuli on penis (transmitted both to the local spinal cord reflex and to the brain) result in increased parasympathetic tone and relaxation of smooth muscle in arteries supplying the penis. Within the corpora, the increased parasympathetic tone results in the production of NO from endothelial cells lining the sinusoids and from the parasympathetic nerve terminals themselves. The NO then moves into smooth muscle cells of the surrounding trabeculae, where it causes relaxation by activation of guanylate cyclase and a subsequent increase in cGMP levels. The smooth muscle cells of the corpora are interconnected by gap junctions that enable a synchronized response. Arterial dilation and relaxation of the corporal sinusoids cause increased blood flow to the erectile corpora, and erection results (Andersson and Wagner 1995; Kandeel et al. 2001). Cyclic guanosine 3,5'-monophosphate (cGMP) within the smooth muscle cells is inactivated by the phosphodiesterase enzyme (PDE). In humans, the major subtype of PDE in the corpus cavernosum is PDE_5, and it is this enzyme that is targeted for inhibition by the drug sildenafil (Viagra), resulting in increased cGMP levels, continued cavernosal smooth muscle relaxation, and erection (Kandeel et al. 2001).

Following increased compliance and blood flow into the vascular spaces of the penis, the venous drainage is compressed, partly passively by expansion of the corpora and partly by contraction of bulbospongiosus and ischiocavernosus muscles. Evidence from several species indicates that contraction of the ischiocavernosus muscles occludes venous outflow and compresses arterial input to the corpus cavernosum penis during peak erection. Effectively, this makes the cavernosa a temporarily closed system. Continued contraction of the ischiocavernosus muscles compresses the crura of the corpus cavernosum against the ischium, forcing this blood into the body of the penis, resulting in the extraordinarily high peak pressures (Table 7.4).

TABLE 7.4—Comparison of resting and peak erectile pressures in the corpus cavernosum penis (CCP) and corpus spongiosum penis (CSP) of domestic species

Species	CCP Resting	Peak	CSP Resting	Peak
Dog	26	7435	19	1280[a]
Goat	19	7003[f]	16	1031[b]
Stallion	13	6530[c]	17	994[d]
Bull	16	14,198[e]		

All measurements in mm Hg (51.7 mm Hg = 1 psi).
[a]Purohit and Beckett (1976), [b]Beckett et al. (1975a), [c]Beckett et al. (1973), [d]Beckett et al. (1975b), [e]Beckett et al. (1974b), and [f]Beckett et al. (1972).

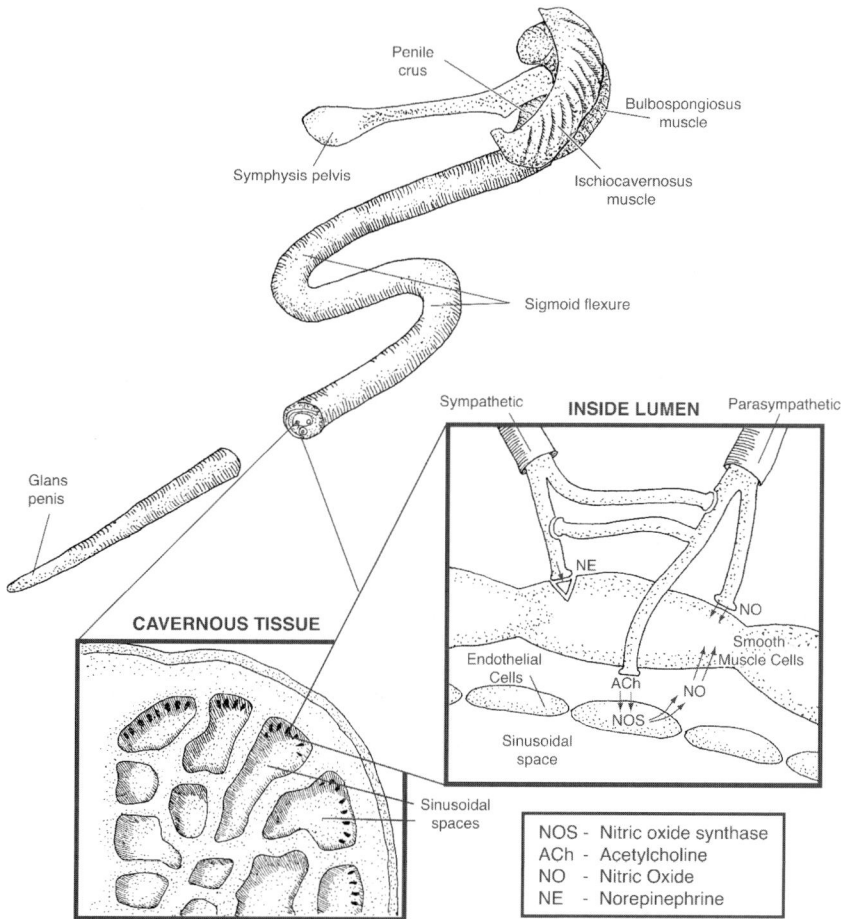

FIG 7.5—Mechanisms of erection. ACh, acetylcholine; NE, norepinephrine; NO, nitric oxide; and NOS, nitric oxide synthase.

In contrast, rhythmic contraction of the bulbospongiosus muscles is associated with achievement of peak pressures within the corpus spongiosum. Angiographic studies show that, unlike in the corpus cavernosum, blood flow continues through this compartment even at peak erection. The pressures achieved are thus somewhat lower because this system is not closed (Beckett et al. 1978; Bartels et al. 1984).

The two vascular bodies appear to operate at least partly independently during erection. In rams, bucks, and dogs, the corpus spongiosum commences filling before the corpus cavernosum (Becket et al. 1978; Carati et al. 1988). However, at least in bucks, peak pressures in the corpus spongiosum are not attained until the ejaculatory thrust, immediately after the peak pressures in the corpus cavernosum (Beckett et al. 1975a). This is clinically true in other species, as well; the glans of stallions and bulbus glandis of dogs do not achieve their full size until after intromission.

Circulating androgens, especially the cavernosal NO system, appear to have an important role in main-taining the full erectile capacity of the penis. Castration reduces the peak pressures attained in the corpus cavernosum of rats at erection, whereas androgen treatment of the animals restores full function (Mills et al. 1992). These changes are associated with alterations in blood flow both into and out of the penis and are at least partly mediated by alterations in the inducible NO synthase system within the corpus cavernosum (Mills et al. 1998). Since these experiments were performed using electrical stimulation of anesthetized animals, the changes are independent of any androgen effects on libido.

Failure of Erection/Erectile Dysfunction. Erectile dysfunction might be defined as the failure to achieve or maintain an erection of sufficient rigidity for intromission in the face of adequate libido. It is currently a hot topic in human andrology, a prominence coinciding with the development of the drug Viagra (from Pfizer). In men, the cause of erectile dysfunction may be psychogenic, drug induced, or associated with a systemic disease, neurological disorder, vascular disease, androgen deficiency, or primary penile disease (Kandeel et al. 2001). In the author's experience, lack of libido or poor breeding behavior is a more common presenting complaint in domestic animals with cases of androgen deficiency or apparent psychogenically based problems. At least in stallions, psychogenic problems may also manifest as failure of ejaculation (McDonnell 1992).

True failures of erection in the face of adequate libido are generally uncommon in domestic species. Those instances when they do occur are usually the result of direct injury to the penis, compromising the vascular erectile mechanism either by preventing the inflow of blood to the corpora cavernosa or by creating a pathway for egress of blood during erection that prevents the creation of a closed system and compromises the cavernosal pressure required for erection and intromission. Such injuries may be accompanied by desensitization of the penis, which can further compromise the attainment of full erection and may additionally prevent ejaculation.

Primary failure of erection in the presence of good libido has been best characterized in bulls. In young bulls that had never achieved an erection, congenital anomalies of blood vessels draining the corpus cavernosum have been reported. These vessels traverse the tunica albuginea and may either drain into the corpus spongiosum or directly into the dorsal penile veins (Ashdown et al. 1979a).

Proximal occlusion of the dorsal canal of the corpus cavernosum penis with hematoma or fibrous tissue has been identified in a series of bulls with failure of erection (Ashdown et al. 1979b). The authors speculate that turbulent flow and high intracorporeal pressures at this level may be causally associated with development of these lesions. In some cases, they might conceivably be the result of cavernosal clots developing after penile rupture rather than a cause of such a rupture, or from damage during mating that was insufficient to result in total tunica rupture. In this series, a number of animals had associated abnormalities of venous drainage from the corpus cavernosum. Intracorporeal clotting and fibrotic changes to the cavernous bodies that interfere with erection have been described in other species as sequelae to priapism (Love et al. 1992). Iatrogenic occlusion of the corpus cavernosum by local injection of acrylic is used as a highly successful method of preventing intromission when creating teaser bulls for use in breeding management programs (Claxton 1989).

Rupture of the corpus cavernosum penis, resulting in extravasation of blood and the formation of a large hematoma, may occur either proximal or distal to the sigmoid flexure of the penis. Proximal ruptures are less common and occur within approximately 10 cm of the ischiocavernosus muscles. It is postulated that these ruptures are secondary to occlusion of the dorsal canal of the corpus cavernosum (Ashdown and Glossop 1983). The proposed pathogenesis of these lesions involves turbulent flow and high corporeal pressures in this region at the time of erection due to vessel anatomy and proximity of the ischiocavernous muscles. Over

time, this results in subendothelial thickening and eventual clot formation in the area that occludes the dorsal cavernosal canal. Further sexual excitement generates extremely high pressures proximal to the obstruction, which results in rupture of the dorsal canal and hematoma formation that dissects within the tunica albuginea. Continued high pressures result finally in the explosive rupture of this tunic and formation of a hematoma in tissues caudal to the scrotum. Failure of erection becomes a combination of occlusion of the canal within the corpus cavernosum, loss of integrity of the tunica albuginea, and chronically by the formation vessels traversing the healing tunica at the site of the rupture. The difficulty with such a pathogenesis is accurately defining the sequence of changes: Did the canal occlusion truly occur prior to rupture of the tunica?

The more common site of rupture is the distal penis, generally cranial to the distal bend of the sigmoid flexure and adjacent to the insertion of the retractor penis muscles. A lower number of ruptures occur in the region of the preputial attachment (Pattridge 1953). This site is the same as that found in experimental studies using excised bull penises: the dorsal aspect of the distal sigmoid flexure opposite attachment of the retractor penis muscles (Beckett et al. 1974b). The resultant hematoma appears as a swelling cranial to the scrotum. Not all such hematomas are associated with a rupture of the corpus cavernosum; some may be due to injury of the dorsal penile veins (Pattridge 1953; Noordsy et al. 1970; Noordsy 1981). Experimentally, the mean pressure required to rupture the corpus cavernosum of excised bull penises was 1486 psi (>76,000 mm Hg), far greater than the 275 psi (14,198 mm Hg) maximal pressures attained at intromission by the same group (Beckett et al. 1974a, b). These authors and others speculate that pressures required to rupture the corpus cavernosum are generated when the fully erect penis is bent either by the bull thrusting against the perineal area of the cow or by movement of the cow following intromission. Bending this closed system could conceivably raise local pressures above the failure point of the tissues, resulting in rupture. As the rupture heals, vascular shunts may develop between the corpus cavernosum and corpus spongiosum or dorsal penile veins. In either case, blood can continue to drain from the corpus cavernosum during sexual excitement, which can prevent full erection and intromission (Young et al. 1977).

In contrast to bulls, rupture of the tunica albuginea in other species is rarely reported. Injuries to the penis of stallions, with hematoma formation, do occur at breeding. However, these are generally caused by a kick from the mare and rupture of more superficial vessels, resulting in varying degrees of preputial swelling, prolapse, and paraphimosis (Gatewood et al. 1989). There is no short-term or long-term compromise of the corpus cavernosum, and prompt aggressive treatment generally results in full return of erectile function. Nerve damage or delayed treatment that permits continued tissue damage and scarring may result in erectile or ejaculatory dysfunction.

Interestingly, stallions with surgically created shunts between the corpus cavernosum and corpus spongiosum are still fully capable of erection and ejaculation (Schumacher et al. 1999). The difference between species may be due to the penile type and blood volume involved in the erectile process. The excised stallion penises required infusion of 0.5 to 1.0 L of saline into the corpus cavernosum to cause rigid erection (Schumacher et al. 1999), whereas similar results are obtained in the fibroelastic bull penis with less than 28 mL (Beckett et al. 1974a), making leakage in bulls of relatively far greater importance.

DETUMESCENCE. Following full erection, the penis goes through a brief transition phase where sympathetic tone increases, initially resulting in arterial constriction and reduction of inflow. Detumescence follows as the venous outflow of the corpora cavernosa is reestablished. Increased norepinephrine release from local sympathetic nerves acts at α-adrenoreceptors (primarily α_1) on cavernosal smooth muscle cells to cause contraction, expelling blood from the cavernous sinuses, and the penis loses rigidity. There is accumulating evidence that endothelin 1 from cells lining the cavernous spaces aids norepinephrine in achieving penile detumescence and maintaining the resting flaccid state (Andersson and Wagner 1995).

FAILURE OF DETUMESCENCE/PRIAPISM. Priapism refers to a prolonged erection of the penis that is not associated with sexual excitement or stimulation and generally only involves the corpus cavernosum (Pautler and Brock 2001). The condition is uncommon, and among the domestic species it is most often reported in horses (Wheat 1966; Pearson and Weaver 1978; Wilson et al. 1991) but also occurs in cats (Swalec and Smeak 1989; Gunn-Moore et al. 1995) and dogs (Johnston et al. 2001). Etiology of the condition includes chronic stimulation of parasympathetic supply, failure of α-adrenergic mechanisms of detumescence, and states of hypercoagulation. These may have their roots in spinal cord injury or neoplasia, genitourinary neoplasia or inflammation, constipation, and direct injury to the erectile tissues. By far the most common situation in men and animals is as a side effect of drug therapy. Generally, this is due to psychotropic-type or anesthetic-type drugs, especially the phenothiazine tranquilizers, which have α-adrenergic blocking activity.

In men, the condition is broadly divided into high-flow and low-flow priapism (Pautler and Brock 2001). All cases start as high flow, with increased arterial input to the corpus cavernosum to give erection. In cases where venous outflow is maintained, the intracorporeal pressures remain below arterial blood pressure, and blood continues to flow into and through the tissue. The condition remains high flow, sinusoidal blood stasis does not occur, and tissues remain well oxygenated. This is most common after a direct pelvic injury where the normal arteriovenous shunting mechanism that causes blood to bypass the corpus cavernosum at rest is compromised.

Low-flow priapism is more common and is a true emergency condition. Here, following the initial high-flow state, the venous outflow is occluded (as occurs normally at peak erection). However, drainage is not reestablished, cavernosal sinusoids fail to contract and expel blood at the normal time, or, in cases of leukemia or hypercoagulation, blood viscosity may be altered preventing outflow. Intracorporeal oxygen levels and pH fall and carbon dioxide level rises, and eventually this blood sludges and clots form. Tissue hypoxia reduces the corporeal smooth muscle activity and response to contractile α-adrenergic stimuli. Ischemic injury to tissues is furthered by release of oxygen free radicals. Studies in men indicate a 12-hour window following commencement of the priapism where histological damage is minimal and treatment may be most effective. After this time, smooth muscle cells transform into a more fibroblastic character, and cellular destruction commences and is widespread by 48 hours (Pautler and Brock 2001). Longer term, the corpora become fibrotic, a process in which transforming growth factor β (TGF-β) appears to play an important role, and erectile function may be compromised. In severe cases or those where treatment is delayed, penile necrosis may necessitate amputation.

MAMMOGENESIS, LACTOGENESIS, AND PASSIVE IMMUNITY. Mammary glands are the defining characteristic of mammals and are found in the monotremes, marsupials, and eutherians. By continuing maternal investment in the offspring beyond parturition, they have permitted the young to be born at a stage of development where they would otherwise not survive. Monotremes (platypus and echidna) are regarded as the most primitive members of the mammals. Their mammary glands do not have nipples, discharging directly onto a specialized area of skin—the areola—from where the young ingest it. Marsupials have a short gestation period (usually just the length of the luteal phase of the estrous cycle), and the young are born at an immature, almost embryonic, stage. Following birth, they climb unaided to the pouch and attach to a nipple that subsequently swells and they become fixed to it, unable to detach until they have achieved sufficient growth. Within the eutherians, neonatal development varies from the blind and helpless, such as mice, puppies, and kittens, through the ruminants, which are capable of following their mother in a day, to guinea pigs, which are so highly developed at birth that they can actually get by without mother's milk at all. Most, however, are totally dependent on milk for the early part of postuterine life (Cowie 1984).

Physiology and Pathophysiology of Lactation

INTERNAL ANATOMY. Although externally highly variable, internally the mammary gland consists of just two basic types of tissue: parenchyma and stroma (Cowie 1984). The structure of the parenchyma is very similar across species. The basic milk-secreting structure is the alveolus, a sack lined by a single layer of secretory epithelial cells outside of which is a myoepithelial layer—the basket cells—which has contractile properties important for milk letdown. Beyond this is a basement membrane, and outside the basement membrane is a network of capillaries that brings in raw materials for milk synthesis.

Outside the glandular tissue is the stroma, a mixture of connective tissue and fat cells, termed the mammary fat pad. It functions as a supporting tissue, and recently it has been shown to be essential for normal development of the parenchyma: the mammary epithelial cells will not grow unless placed in adipose tissue (Forsyth 1998).

Alveoli are arranged in groups or clusters termed lobules (like grapes in a bunch), and groups of lobules are further arranged into lobes. Each alveolus discharges its secretion through a capillary milk duct, and individual capillary milk ducts empty into the intralobular ducts. These merge into progressively larger ducts to provide the route for milk removal.

Whereas the secretory tissue is similar across species, differences are present in the anatomy and arrangement of the duct system. In the monotremes, the major ducts discharge directly onto the skin of the alveolus or mammary patch. Each nipple has 12 to 20 major duct openings for dogs and humans. In the cows, goats, and sheep, major ducts empty into a large gland cistern, continuous with the teat cistern, which is then drained via the single streak canal. The mare and sow have two or three gland systems associated with each nipple, which has a separate streak canal for each gland system opening on it (Cowie 1984; Kainer 1993).

Supporting structures for the mammary gland are best described in cows. Here the udder is divided into distinct left and right halves by the major supporting structure, the median suspensory ligament. This is composed of elastin and collagen. In mature lactating cows, the elastin predominates, acting as a shock absorber for the gland during movement.

Other supporting structures are the lateral suspensory ligaments and their extensions, the lamellar plates. These project into the parenchyma of the gland and are interspersed with it.

MAMMARY DEVELOPMENT PRIOR TO PREGNANCY. At birth, the mammary gland consists of a rudimentary duct system that opens at a small nipple, and during the juvenile period the gland shows growth at the same rate as the rest of the body. Several weeks prior to puberty, depending on species, the growth of the mammary gland becomes allometric—faster than general body growth. This is in response to increased secretion of estrogen from ovarian follicles developing at this time (Forsyth 1998).

Following puberty, differential growth of the mammary tissue occurs. The smaller ducts proliferate quickly during estrus, while estrogen levels are high, and regress during the luteal phase, but at a slower rate than they grew in estrus. This is repeated so that in each subsequent cycle there is more duct proliferation during the growth phase than there is regression, resulting in a highly branched duct system. Duct proliferation is accompanied by development of connective and adipose tissue and vascular and lymphatic systems.

The extent of mammary development during cyclicity depends on the type of cycle an animal has. Thus, animals with ultrashort cycles and virtually nonexistent luteal phases (mice and rats) show mostly duct growth, and alveoli are rarely formed. Primates and most farm species have a longer cycle and full luteal phase, so duct development is almost full. Finally, in bitches, with a long luteal phase that can be considered a pseudopregnancy, duct growth is accompanied by considerable lobuloalveolar development. This degree of development occurs only during pregnancy in other species. Indeed, many of these nonpregnant bitches may lactate on demise of the corpora lutea (Forsyth 1998).

FINAL DEVELOPMENT OF THE MAMMARY GLAND. Exactly when mammary development to the stage that it is competent to secrete milk is completed (full alveolar development) depends on species. In monotremes, full development occurs in response to egg incubation. Mammary development of marsupials is identical in pregnant and nonpregnant females, and full development depends on the suckling stimulus of permanently attached pouch young. In eutherian mammals, full development of the mammary gland is completed during pregnancy or even early lactation (Forsyth 1998). The growth of the gland during pregnancy in nearly all species fits an exponential curve where the overall rate of growth is inversely proportional to gestation length for that species. Usually, it is not until the second half of gestation that lobuloalveolar development becomes rapid.

CONTROL OF MAMMARY GROWTH IN THE POSTNATAL PERIOD. Mammary growth and differentiation are controlled by ovarian, pituitary, adrenal, and placental hormones and locally produced growth factors, although the contribution of each hormone appears to vary with species. Most research has been performed in laboratory rodents, with a lesser amount in ruminants.

In general, duct growth depends on estrogen, adrenal steroids, and growth hormone (via the IGFs), whereas lobuloalveolar growth requires these three and the addition of progesterone and prolactin. Placental lactogens (prolactin-like hormones produced in the placenta) are found in many species and appear to have important roles in mammary growth during pregnancy. Relaxin, which is responsible for remodeling the connective tissue in the cervix and pelvic ligaments in preparation for birth, may also have a role in remodeling the mammary connective tissue. This may be required before the mammary ducts can achieve their full development. To the foregoing mix can be added insulin and thyroid hormone, although the older evidence for insulin involvement may actually be related more to its ability to act via the IGF system. Local growth factors known to play a role in stimulating mammary growth are IGF-I and IGF-II, EGF, and fibroblast growth factor (FGF). TGF-β has an inhibitory role that influences the pattern of the ductal tree (Cowie 1984; Akers 1998; Forsyth 1998).

EFFECT OF NUTRITION ON MAMMARY DEVELOPMENT. The lactation potential of an animal is determined by the number of secretory epithelial cells (alveolar cells) and the secretory activity of each cell. Cell number is considered the ultimate limiting factor. Correlations between total mammary cell numbers and milk yield range from 0.5 to 0.85. Thus, anything that reduces the number of cells (mammary parenchyma) will have a negative impact on lactational performance (Knight 2000).

Young replacement stock are often grown rapidly so that targets for early puberty and pregnancy can be met to maximize economic returns and reduce costs within a livestock operation. There is considerable, though often contradictory, evidence that excessive growth rates can reduce later milk yields. In both dairy cattle (Sejrsen et al. 1982) and beef cattle (Buskirk et al. 1996), sheep (McCann et al. 1989), goats (Bowden et al. 1995), and swine (Weldon et al. 1991), excessive growth rates in prepubertal animals have been shown to be detrimental to mammary parenchymal development. The critical time appears to be the allometric phase of mammary growth, just prior to puberty, when the gland may be growing at over three times the general body rate. This phenomenon is hormonally mediated. Rapidly grown animals have lower circulating growth hormone levels than do control animals. It appears that growth hormone, acting at the mammary gland via IGFs, is strongly mitogenic for the mammary tissue, and reducing its level at such a critical mammary growth stage is the cause of ultimately reduced production (Sejrsen et al. 1983; Knight 2000).

Initiation of Lactation: Lactogenesis. Lactogenesis is sometimes divided into two stages (Akers 1998): *lactogenesis I* is a limited degree of structural and functional differentiation of the secretory epithelium during pregnancy, whereas *lactogenesis II* is the completion of this differentiation in the peripartum period and the onset of copious milk production postpartum.

The model of limited, gradual differentiation during late pregnancy and then a sudden final differentiation to the stage of secretion around the time of parturition appears true of laboratory rodents and many other species. In ruminants, it appears that differentiation is essentially completed several weeks prior to parturition. In these species, all of the mechanisms for lactation are in place early, but the onset of large-scale synthesis and copious secretion of milk (lactation itself) is suppressed. This is accomplished by limiting the activities of key enzymes in the milk biosynthetic pathway. The main inhibitor of these enzymes is considered to be progesterone, and the decline in progesterone at the time of parturition triggers the onset of lactation (Cowie 1984; Lee and Oka 1992; Tucker 2000).

CONTROL OF LACTOGENESIS. Species differences exist in the timing of events and the relative importance of some hormones in the onset of milk production. However, taken together, the data indicate that lactogenesis is due to increases in circulating hormones that promote the process—prolactin, glucocorticoids, estrogens, growth hormone (and thus IGFs)—and an increase in the mammary tissue sensitivity to them, coupled with a decline in the negative influence of progesterone (Akers 1998). Based on recent evidence, placental lactogen also appears to promote lactogenesis in cattle, but it is not as potent as prolactin. In some species, the stimulus of suckling from the newborn appears important in giving full expression of synthetic and secretory activity (in addition to milk letdown).

CELLULAR SECRETION OF MILK CONSTITUENTS. There are five pathways for secretion of components into milk from the alveolar epithelial cells (Neville 1998; Shennan and Peaker 2000):

1. Proteins, lactose, some salts, and other nonfat components of milk are packaged into secretory vesicles in the Golgi apparatus. The presence of the lactose also draws water into these vesicles, which bud off from the Golgi and move to the apex of the cell. At the apical surface (i.e., adjacent to the lumen of the alveolus), the membrane surrounding the secretory vesicle fuses with the plasma membrane of the cell, and the contents are released into the alveolar lumen. This is a process of exocytosis.

2. Lipid droplets form near the endoplasmic reticulum and are transported to the apical membrane for secretion. Here there is lots of spare membrane left over after secretion of the lactose/protein/mineral/water by exocytosis from the Golgi secretory vesicle. This membrane surrounds the droplet and forms the milk fat-globule membrane. The portion of membrane beneath the fat globule pinches off, and the globule is secreted into the alveolar lumen. The membrane around each droplet of fat prevents them from coalescing, and the membrane itself provides a useful source of phospholipids to the offspring.

3. After lactose, fat, and secretory proteins, the next major components of milk to be secreted are the minerals that contribute to the ash content. Calcium and phosphate are secreted with proteins and lactose in the Golgi vesicles. Other salts may be pumped into the cell at its base, and some may then diffuse passively into the alveolus. The apical plasma membrane is permeable to monovalent ions (sodium, chloride, and potassium) and glucose. It is impermeable to divalent cations and disaccharides. This diffusion and pumping across basal and apical membranes is termed transmembrane transport. The cell membranes are also per-

meable to many pharmacological agents, such as some systemically administered antibiotics, which will then appear in milk.

4. Transcytosis is a mechanism for proteins that are not synthesized in the alveolar epithelial cell to enter the milk. This includes secretory immunoglobulin (IgA), hormones such as insulin and prolactin, growth factors such as IGF-I, and serum albumin. In this process, the protein interacts with a specific receptor at the basal membrane of the cell. The protein-receptor complex is internalized and transported across the cell to the apical membrane, where both protein and receptor are released into the alveolar lumen.

5. The final pathway is paracellular transport. During lactation, tight junctions form between adjacent mammary epithelial cells, which serve to separate the interstitial spaces and the alveolar lumen, effectively closing the paracellular transport pathway. During normal lactation, white blood cells appear to be able to pass into the alveolar lumen via this route without opening it to other substances. During pregnancy, mammary involution, and mastitis, the tight junctions open, and large proteins and other constituents can be transported via this route.

Maintenance of Lactation. Much of the information available on the maintenance of milk secretion comes from research in laboratory rodents. In these species, the minimum requirements for continued lactation are prolactin, corticosteroids, and oxytocin. Additional production is obtained by adding estrogens, insulin, and thyroid hormone, but some effects may be indirect via effects on general metabolic function.

Prolactin acts in a general fashion to maintain enzyme levels and protein synthesis. It increases gene-transcription rates and the half-lives of the resulting mRNAs. The effect of prolactin on some enzymes is enhanced by glucocorticoids. Prolactin also functions to prevent cell death (apoptosis) of mammary epithelium and maintains tight junctions between the cells.

Glucocorticoids regulate the activity of several enzymes in the milk-synthesis pathway by controlling their transcription rates. Adrenalectomy causes a 40% to 50% decrease in milk production in these species. Oxytocin is required for removal of milk from the alveolus. In its absence, the mammary glands degenerate due to milk accumulation. Although prolactin is the dominant player in maintenance of rodent lactation, a small role for somatotropin also appears to exist.

Ruminants are the most widely studied group outside of laboratory rodents, and there are several differences in their physiology. Once lactation is established, prolactin is not required for maintenance, though it does support maximal production levels. There is no effect of adrenalectomy on maintenance of lactation or production levels, so there is no requirement for glucocorticoids. Ruminants, however, do have a requirement for somatotropin for the maintenance of lactation. Somatotropin has been shown to maintain mammary secretory cell numbers and enhances the rate of milk synthesis.

LOCAL CONTROL OF MILK SYNTHESIS. Increasing the frequency of milk removal increases milk production, while decreasing milking frequency reduces production. In dairy cows, increasing milking frequency from two to three times daily increases production about 10%. Increasing to six times daily provides a 21% increase. Conversely, reducing frequency from two times to once daily reduces yield by up to 20%. A search for a component of milk that is inhibitory for milk production revealed a glycoprotein found in the whey fraction. This has now been called *feedback inhibitor of lactation* (FIL), and it has been isolated from several species. FIL is secreted by the epithelial cells of the mammary alveoli and acts as an autocrine regulator. After likely binding to a receptor on the cell membrane at the apex of the cell, it has immediate effects to inhibit protein and lactose secretion (Knight et al. 1998).

MILK EJECTION (LETDOWN). This is the process whereby milk that has been synthesized and stored in the mammary alveoli is released in response to the suckling stimulus of the offspring (Wakerley 1998). Milk is secreted relatively continuously into the lumen of the alveoli from the epithelium. Storage occurs within the lumen of the alveolus or in expansions of the duct system in species where these exist. In some species, a minor portion of milk in the mammary gland is stored in large dilations of the duct system, such as the large gland and teat cisterns of the ruminants. Other species may have only small collecting sinuses or no such collecting areas at all. Although milk within the storage ducts may be available passively to the suckling offspring, or, in the case of cows, to the milking machine, the majority of milk is stored within the alveoli. Here the effects of surface tension mean the milk cannot be removed solely by suckling, and access to this larger store requires that it is actively ejected.

Milk ejection is controlled by a neuroendocrine reflex that results in contraction of the myoepithelial cells underlying the alveolar epithelium, which overcomes the surface tension and forces milk into the duct system.

The nipple is densely innervated with intradermal sensory afferent nerves. Stimulation of these nerve endings by suckling results in a nerve impulse. These peripheral nerves synapse with nerves in the dorsal horn of the spinal cord that ascend the cord. After going through several synaptic relays, the stimulus arrives at the hypothalamus, where the information passes to the paraventricular and supraoptic nuclei, which contain oxytocin-producing neurons. Groups of cells are synchronously activated, resulting in release of oxytocin pulses from nerve endings located in the posterior pituitary gland. Oxytocin circulates in the blood and binds to receptors on the cell membrane of the alveolar myoepithelial cells, which contract, ejecting milk from the alveoli into the duct system, from where it is available for removal.

The milk-ejection reflex may be conditioned; thus, many dairy cows will let down in response to the sight and sounds of the milking parlor. A similar phenomenon occurs in women who are preparing to nurse. Frequency of nursing by offspring varies from the continuous attachment in the marsupials to once a week in the seals. The pattern of letdown during nursing also varies. In most domestic species, there is a single episode of letdown in response to suckling. In rats, the young may stay attached for hours, and during this time there are regular episodes of oxytocin secretion and milk letdown. The milk-ejection reflex can be abolished by fear or stress. These cause activation of inhibitory pathways, which stop oxytocin release even in the presence of suckling stimuli. This effect is mediated centrally, at least in part by using opioid inhibitory neurotransmitters (Wakerley 1998).

Passive Transfer of Immunity. Neonates are considered to have an active innate immunity but an undeveloped adaptive (acquired or antigen driven) response (Kelly and Coutts 2000). In species commonly encountered in veterinary practice, the fetal immune system becomes capable of responding to specific microbial invasion during gestation. The timing of this development of the specific immune system varies with species and the particular invading organism, but is generally not as powerful as that found in mature animals (Tizard 1996). While neonatal macrophages, neutrophils, and natural killer cells of the innate immune system function to remove large numbers of invading foreign cells, compared with the adult their numbers are few and their chemotactic and enzyme activities are lower. Deficits in adaptive immunity appear to involve poor function of antigen-presenting cells, which leads to defective T cell and B cell responses and lack of appropriate antibody response to intestinal pathogens, which can then colonize intestinal mucosa (Kelly and Coutts 2000). Generally, the uterine environment during pregnancy is sterile, and the fetus is not exposed to outside antigens. Because of this, the immune response of the neonate is a primary response that takes longer to develop and results in a lower concentration of circulating antibodies (Tizard 1996). Additionally, the neonatal intestinal epithelium, a major site of microbial exposure, is more permeable than that of the adult (Kelly and Coutts 2000). Thus, neonates, by several mechanisms, are more susceptible to infection than are adults (Tizard 1996).

Protection from attack during this vulnerable period is provided by antibodies, mainly IgG, transferred from the mother, a process termed transfer of passive immunity. This exchange may occur either in utero by transfer of immunoglobulin across the placenta or following birth via the early mammary secretion—the immunoglobulin-rich colostrum. Which strategy is employed depends on the placental barrier to immunoglobulin transfer (Tizard 1996).

COLOSTRUM. After alveoli appear during mammary development in late pregnancy, the lumen begins to accumulate the fluid that will form colostrum, the first milk. Compared with milk, colostrum is thicker and sticky,

with a more yellow/tan hue. It consists of secretions from the alveolar epithelial cells and proteins that are actively transported to the gland from blood. The most important of these proteins are the immunoglobulins that will be transferred to neonates when they first suckle. In domestic species, there is a preferential transport of IgG into colostrum when compared with other immunoglobulin classes. The mechanism is similar (though reversed) to that of absorption across the intestinal epithelium of neonates. Following binding to a specific membrane receptor on the basolateral surface of the acinar cell, the IgG-receptor complex is internalized, transported across the cytoplasm, and discharged into the alveolar lumen at the cell apex. The specificity for IgG transport is reduced once lactation starts, due to downregulation of the specific IgG receptor in alveolar cells by prolactin (Watson 1980; Barrington et al. 1997). The systemic and local mechanisms that control colostrum formation itself (colostrogenesis) are poorly understood.

Swine, camelids, and horses possess an epitheliochorial placenta, with six tissue layers between maternal and fetal circulations, whereas domestic ruminants have a syndesmochorial placenta. Offspring of all these species are born agammaglobulinemic, and passive immunity is transferred entirely by ingestion of colostrum after birth. The colostrum of sows contains mainly IgG and lesser quantities of IgA and IgM. When milk secretion commences, the serum-derived IgG is supplanted by IgA synthesized in the mammary gland as the predominant immunoglobulin (Stokes and Bailey 1998). A similar pattern is observed in horses (Kohn et al. 1989; Sheoran et al. 2000). In the domestic ruminants, however, IgG remains the dominant form throughout lactation. The source of immunoglobulin changes through the lactation. Colostral IgG, most IgM, and 50% of IgA are derived from circulating immunoglobulins. Later in lactation, the number of mammary plasma cells increases, raising the portion of immunoglobulin that is locally produced to around 70% for IgG and 90% for IgA (Tizard 1996; Husband 1998).

Puppies develop in an endotheliochorial placenta, with four tissue layers between fetal and maternal bloodstreams. Even with this reduction in the tissue barrier, puppies receive only 5% to 10% of their passively transferred immunoglobulin in utero, the remainder coming from colostrum. Canine colostrum is mainly IgG, with lesser quantities of IgM and IgA. This situation is reversed in canine milk, where IgA predominates (Felsburg 1998). Placentation type in cats is also endotheliochorial, and a similar proportion of immunoglobulin (mainly IgG) is transmitted to kittens prior to birth. Thus, colostrum supplies the majority of neonatal requirements. Feline colostrum also contains mainly IgG, with smaller amounts of IgA and IgM. Like other species, levels of all immunoglobulins fall when milk secretion begins, but in cats, as in ruminants, IgG remains the predominant type (Pu and Yamamoto 1998). In contrast, other researchers have found minimal differences between immunoglobulin content of feline colostrum and milk and no evidence of transplacental IgG transfer (Casal et al. 1996).

This sourcing of maternal immunoglobulins is of great survival advantage to newborns. Enteric pathogens are a major cause of neonatal morbidity and mortality, but dams protect their offspring by sharing their own immune system's knowledge of the local microorganism milieu. Antigens from pathogens that dams sample from the environment and present in the gut are taken up by the intestinal M cells and transported to gut-associated lymphoid tissue (GALT), where the antigens are presented to T and B lymphocytes, which become activated. Activated B cells will secrete immunoglobulins specific to the antigens against which they were activated, and both cell types may leave the GALT. On leaving the GALT, these cells move systemically and localize in various sites, including the mammary gland (Kelly and Coutts 2000)

The duration of maternal antibody persistence in the offspring is important from a disease-protection standpoint and also for practicing veterinarians in designing vaccination protocols. While passively derived immunoglobulins are present, they reduce immunoglobulin synthesis by neonates and reduce the response to vaccines. The persistence of these colostral antibodies varies between species, with the particular disease organism involved, and with the amount transferred from the mother. Duration of persistence in foals can vary from 2 weeks to 6 months, and in calves up to 9 months of age (Tizard 1996). A half-life of 15.7 days has been calculated for IgG in South American camelids (Weaver et al. 2000a). Transferred IgG has a half-life of 18 to 24 days in lambs, and the duration of protection depends on the pathogen involved. Gastrointestinal parasite immunity is negligible after 10 weeks, whereas that to bacteria ranges from 6 weeks to 6 months (Watson 1998). The half-life of maternally acquired immunoglobulins in puppies is approximately 8.4 days, providing a protection period of 8 to 16 weeks (Felsburg 1998), whereas circulating half-lives of transferred IgG and IgA in kittens have been estimated at 4.4 and 1.9 days, respectively (Casal et al. 1996).

IMMUNOGLOBULIN ABSORPTION. The ability to absorb intact macromolecules from the intestine and transfer them into the circulation is only developed late in gestation. In farm animals, it appears that this ability develops in response to the increased fetal cortisol levels that are associated with maturation of the hypothalamic-pituitary-adrenal axis. Since this change is also the trigger for birth in at least some of these species, the development of this specific intestinal function is precisely timed to maximize macromolecule transfer from colostrum immediately after birth (Sangild et al. 2000).

The immunoglobulins are proteins and, as such, would normally be subject to digestion. However, the proteolytic activity of the early neonate stomach is low, and this combined with the presence of trypsin inhibitors in colostrum ensures that the IgG passes rapidly and with limited degradation into the small intestine (Kruse 1983). Within the intestine, IgG passes through the epithelium by a process of transcytosis. The apical surface of small intestinal enterocytes express an Fc receptor to which the IgG binds. The receptor-IgG complex is then internalized by endocytosis and placed into transcytotic vesicles in the Golgi apparatus. These vesicles are transported to the basolateral cell surface, where they fuse to the plasma membrane, the receptor and IgG dissociate, and the IgG is released, passing into the lymphatics and intestinal capillaries (Mostov 1994; Tizard 1996). IgG binding to the receptor at the cell apex and then release at the basolateral surface may occur in response to pH changes between the two cell surfaces, being relatively more acidotic at the apex and neutral at the base (Mostov 1994). A similar mechanism is likely involved in passage of IgG across the hemochorial placenta of the human.

The specificity of the transport of macromolecules across the neonatal intestinal epithelium varies. It is nonspecific in ruminants, with all classes of immunoglobulins and many other large molecules being capable of transit. The resulting proportion of immunoglobulin classes in the neonatal bloodstream is thus directly proportional to their colostral content, though IgA is reexcreted. In contrast, foals and piglets selectively absorb IgG and IgM (Kruse 1983; Tizard 1996).

GUT CLOSURE. Intestinal closure is the time after which macromolecules are not absorbed intact across the intestinal epithelium. Timing varies with species but is generally considered to occur within 24 to 36 hours after birth. However, significant reductions in absorption occur within 6 hours, prior to formally defined closure, so earlier feedings of colostrum within this period result in better immunoglobulin transfer. Closure also occurs more rapidly in animals fed colostrum earlier (Weaver et al. 2000b).

The precise mechanism of closure is unknown but involves cessation of pinocytosis by neonatal intestinal epithelial cells and replacement of these cells by those of a more mature type (Weaver et al. 2000b). In piglets, macromolecules continue to be taken up into intestinal epithelial cells for approximately 3 weeks after birth, but closure occurs within 12 to 36 hours. Although the molecules are still absorbed into the cells after this time, they are not transferred into the bloodstream (Sangild et al. 2000).

This timing of closure does not appear to be universal. Intestinal closure in rodents does not occur until 2 to 3 weeks of age when there is an increased rate of cell replacement in the intestinal mucosa, and it appears to be hastened by elevations of the cortisol level in these species (Sangild et al. 2000).

Failure of Passive Transfer. The definition of successful passive transfer versus failure of passive transfer (FPT) and partial failure is variable, sometimes relying on 1 or 2 standard deviations below the population mean value and at others on a predetermined benchmark. The latter is now more common, but the immunoglobulin level required in neonatal plasma occasionally changes, and differences in the accuracy of measurement methods must be kept in mind (Weaver et al. 2000b).

Inadequate transfer of passive immunity to neonates predisposes them to development of infectious diseases, but not all such neonates will become ill. The development of disease still depends on the interaction of environmental and pathogen factors along with host factors, of which FPT is only one. It was reported that 23% of calves with FPT died versus 5% of those with adequate transfer, and the effect of FPT was not confined to the neonatal period. Calves with FPT had lower average daily gains, higher postweaning mortality, reduced first lactation production, and increased culling rate (Weaver et al. 2000b). Similarly, 39% of the 8.2% mortality rate in dairy calves up to 4 months old was attributable to FPT (Tyler et al. 1999), and 85% of beef calf mortality was associated with FPT (McGuire et al. 1976). However, other large field studies have reported no significant effect of adequate versus inadequate passive transfer on morbidity or mortality in dairy heifer calves (Sivula et al. 1996). In a study of 590 lambs, the death rate by 3 weeks of age was 45% for lambs with FPT and only 5% in those with adequate IgG transfer (McGuire et al. 1983). Most studies of foals have found a strong association between FPT and neonatal infection (McGuire et al. 1977; Raidal 1996) By contrast, there was no difference in morbidity or mortality rates in standardbred foals with adequate or inadequate immunoglobulin transfer under conditions of good management (Baldwin et al. 1991). Experimentally, piglets made deficient in immunoglobulin by deliberate withholding of colostrum are highly susceptible to neonatal sepsis. However, regression modeling has shown that FPT may be a minor influence on neonatal piglet mortality in some commercial situations under good management (Tyler et al. 1990). Thus, although FPT increases the risk of neonatal sepsis, it does not guarantee disease nor does adequate transfer preclude it.

Field trials indicate the prevalence of FPT in foals is between 2.9 and 24% (McGuire et al. 1977; Morris et al. 1985; LeBlanc et al. 1992). The incidence is from 10% to 60% in dairy calves and 11% to 31% in well-managed beef calves (Rogers and Capucille 2000; Weaver et al. 2000b). The overall prevalence of FPT in lambs ranges from 10% to 20%, with highest immunoglobulin levels found in singletons and progressively lower levels observed in twins and triplets (Logan and Irwin 1977). Little information is available on the incidence of this problem in puppies and kittens, but it may be less important than in the farm species. Kittens are thought to be able to survive reasonably well in the absence of colostrum ingestion provided their surroundings are sanitary and nutrition is good (Pu and Yamamoto 1998).

There is a generally linear relationship between intake of colostral IgG by the neonate and serum IgG levels, whereas the relationship for IgM is quadratic (Stott and Fellah 1983). Thus, adequate and early intake of high-quality colostrum is of the utmost importance in transfer of passive immunity. The causes of FPT can be broadly classified as failure of production, failure of ingestion, and failure of absorption. In some cases, the specific cause will fit into more than one of these categories.

FAILURE OF PRODUCTION. Dairy cows may produce colostrum with reduced immunoglobulin concentration because it becomes diluted by the rapid onset of lactogenesis around parturition, and calves may not voluntarily drink sufficient quantities of this dilute colostrum to achieve adequate transfer (Weaver et al. 2000b). Poor maternal nutrition in late pregnancy has been shown to decrease colostrum production. For ewes, this reduced level was below the requirements of twin lambs (Mellor and Murray 1986). Experimental data on the effect of restricted nutrition on colostrum production in cattle are less clear, with results indicating both reductions and no effect (Quigley and Drewry 1998).

Other factors reported to affect colostral IgG concentration include parity of the dam, length of the dry period, maternal vaccination program, and heat stress in late gestation, though some of these are controversial (Quigley and Drewry 1998; Weaver et al. 2000b). Another consideration is that, although colostral IgG may be adequate on laboratory measurements, the immunoglobulin may not be specific to pathogens encountered by the neonate. This may be a problem where dams are moved just prior to parturition and are not exposed to certain pathogens in the new environment for sufficient time to mount a response and transfer this to the colostrum. Moving dams at a suitable stage of gestation and/or assisting them with a vaccination program would help ensure that both sufficient and appropriate immunoglobulin is transferred (Aldridge et al. 1992).

FAILURE OF INGESTION. Failure of ingestion can be due to either maternal or neonatal factors. The importance of different causes varies with species, depending on offspring number and size, and the physiology of the peripartum period. Examples are presented next, many of which will also apply to other species.

CATTLE. Anything that prolongs the time it takes for a dam to rise following parturition will delay or reduce colostral intake by its calf. This would include injuries such as obturator paralysis in heifers and hypocalcemia in older cows. The pendulous udders and large teats of older dairy cows may interfere with suckling, and painful teat lesions or mastitis may cause the dams to avoid or actively discourage their calves. Offspring may occasionally be rejected for no apparent reason, especially by first-time mothers. When many animals are giving birth in close proximity, offspring are sometimes "stolen," and the neonate may be unable to obtain colostrum from its adoptive mother. Twin calves are at increased risk of FPT, presumably due to a combination of competition for available colostrum and an apparent increase in failure of absorption. Dystocia, especially if prolonged, may result in fetal asphyxia and a delay in the time taken for a calf to stand and suckle. Fetal malformations or injuries received during parturition will also prolong the time taken to ingest colostrum, and premature onset of lactation may result at worst in outright loss of colostrum prior to parturition or at least in dilution of IgG content (Broom 1983; Aldridge et al. 1992; Rogers and Capucille 2000).

SWINE. Piglets have a higher incidence of maternal rejection or attack than do ungulates, especially by farrowing gilts. Large litter sizes and the time taken to finish birth mean that early piglets have the opportunity to drink colostrum from multiple glands, leaving less for those later in the birth order. Large litters are also associated with more small and weak piglets, which take longer to find a teat and do not compete well with larger siblings. Not all teats on a sow may be fully functional, which exacerbates competition problems with large litters. Additionally, milk letdown in sows occurs only in short bursts, so piglets unable to ingest colostrum at this time are unable to supplement themselves at times of low competition. As in other species, neonate injury or malformation will negatively impact colostrum consumption (Broom 1983).

HORSES. Foals provide an illustration of the importance of colostral IgG concentration, which in practice is generally assessed by measuring specific gravity. Of foals with FPT, 81% ingested colostrum with a specific gravity of less than 1.06, whereas the incidence of FPT in foals ingesting colostrum with a specific gravity of greater than 1.06 was 0.006%; 23% of mares produced colostrum with a specific gravity of less than 1.06 (LeBlanc et al. 1992). Other important factors were age and breed of mare, with mares over 15 years producing more dilute colostrum resulting in an increased rate of FPT among their offspring. Colostral immunoglobulin concentration also followed a bell-shaped curve when plotted against length of gestation; both short and long gestations are associated with reductions in IgG concentration (LeBlanc et al. 1992). Mares that run milk prior to foaling have significantly lower colostral IgG concentrations and are more likely to be associated with an FPT foal (Morris et al. 1985).

FAILURE OF ABSORPTION. Delaying ingestion of colostrum until after gut closure has commenced will reduce the levels of immunoglobulin transferred to the neonatal circulation. The process of closure commences rapidly after birth, and reductions in the efficiency of immunoglobulin absorption occur within 1 hour in calves. Animals born in unsanitary conditions are more likely to rapidly establish a population of gut bacteria, and exposure to bacteria may also hasten gut closure. These animals are thus doubly at risk by being exposed to potentially infectious organisms and having an increased likelihood of FPT. Within 12 hours of birth, the secretion of gastrointestinal enzymes has risen, which increases IgG degradation, leaving less available for absorption (Quigley and Drewry 1998).

It has been observed that dilute colostrum may cause FPT by preventing adequate intake of IgG. Additionally, it has been shown that, even if identical amounts of IgG are fed, absorption of immunoglobulin from the more dilute colostrum is less efficient (Quigley and Drewry 1998). Calves left in contact with their mother actually absorb a greater proportion of ingested immunoglobulin, resulting in higher circulating IgG levels than in those fed an equal amount of colostrum either artificially or by suckling. However, this increased efficiency of absorption cannot overcome the lower intake of colostrum by naturally mothered dairy calves compared with artificially reared controls, and thus has not been recommended as a management practice (Weaver et al. 2000b). Extreme cold also reduces the efficiency of colostrum absorption, a factor that is further complicated by the reduced ability of chilled calves to ingest adequate quantities (Quigley and Drewry 1998).

Other factors reported to reduce immunoglobulin absorption include respiratory or metabolic acidosis, which generally results from dystocia, the feeding of acidotic transition diets to the mother, and the sex and breed of the calf (Quigley and Drewry 1998). Many of these areas are still controversial.

OTHER FUNCTIONS OF COLOSTRUM. Beyond its immunoglobulin content, colostrum contains other proteins, essential and nonessential amino acids, lipids, lactose, fat-soluble and water-soluble vitamins, peptide hormones, growth factors, cytokines, thyroid and steroid hormones, nucleotides, enzymes, and maternal cells, especially leukocytes (Blum and Hammon 2000).

Each milliliter of colostrum contains over 1 million cells of maternal origin. These cells in maternal colostrum are specifically recognized by epithelial cells of the neonatal small intestine and can be transported across it to appear systemically. With the exception of swine, which have large numbers of epithelial cells, the predominant cell types are neutrophils and macrophages. The functional capabilities of transferred neutrophils are questionable and appear to be mainly a by-product of mammary-gland defenses. The macrophages may act as antigen presenters, are functionally phagocytic, and secrete cytokines. Depending on the species, lymphocytes comprise from 5% to 40% of the total and arise from maternal mesenteric lymph nodes. The majority of these lymphocytes are T cells of the memory-activated subset. They are thought to be involved in the transfer of cell-mediated immunity to neonates, secretion of cytokines, and function in immunosuppression to enable gradual activation of the immune system (Le Jan 1996).

In the immediate postnatal period, the neonatal gastrointestinal tract goes through a rapid period of growth, differentiation, and functional maturation. Ingestion of colostrum has significant effects on the structure and functional development of the neonatal gastrointestinal tract. There is evidence that many of these effects are mediated by colostral EGF and IGF-I, though much of this work is controversial (Xu 1996; Blum and Hammon 2000). Colostrum causes maturation of intestinal epithelial cells shown by a change in the glycosylation pattern on the cell surface. Some of these molecules function as receptors for bacteria, and a change in their type leads to changes in the type of organisms that can adhere (Kelly and Coutts 2000).

Finally, the simple behavioral reward of colostrum ingestion also plays a role. The development of the mother-offspring bond is vital for survival of a newborn. The advantages extend beyond the neonatal period and immediate needs for nutrition and passive transfer of immunity to include the learning of lifelong survival strategies for foraging, shelter seeking, and predator avoidance (Nowak et al. 2000). While hormonal changes in parturition, passage of the fetus through the vagina, and presence of fetal fluids all appear important in establishing maternal behavior, bonding of the neonate to the mother appears to be reinforced by the ingestion of colostrum and later by milk (Goursaud and Nowak 1999).

For animals born into cold, wet, and windy environments, the nutritional aspect of colostrum intake is of greater importance to their immediate survival than is the absorption of adequate levels of immunoglobulin. Neonates are born with limited reserves of brown adipose tissue and carbohydrate stores that can be used for nonshivering thermogenesis. In cold climates, these are exhausted within a few hours, and, without ingestion of colostrum, hypothermia sets in, and the neonate will rapidly succumb. This is especially true for smaller offspring, where low body mass and high surface area to mass ratios can lead to rapid onset of hypothermia. Of the domestic species, this is probably most critical in lambs, especially those resulting from twin and triplet litters, due to body size reductions, and those from primiparous ewes that have poorer maternal abilities (Randall et al. 1997; Henderson 2000).

Energy is thus critical, and although its lactose levels are lower than milk, colostrum has much higher gross energy, due to higher content of fats and proteins. Colostrum ingestion raises circulating glucose, triglyceride, fatty-acid, and cholesterol levels in neonates not only because of its fat content but also because other factors in the colostrum appear to enhance digestion and absorption of the dietary fats. Cold-exposed lambs that ingest colostrum not only show these energy enhancements but also maintain a higher body temperature (Quigley and Drewry 1998; Blum and Hammon 2000; Hamadeh et al. 2000).

While colostrum has lower lactose levels than milk, the ingestion of colostrum has prolonged beneficial effects on glucose metabolism and enhances carbohydrate absorption. Protein content of neonates is raised by absorption of immunoglobulins, essential and nonessential amino acids, and other proteins. These are used for both protein synthesis and in gluconeogenesis.

Other components of colostrum, possibly IGF-I, appear to have anabolic affects (Quigley and Drewry 1998; Blum and Hammon 2000). Vitamins A, D, and E do not cross the placenta in adequate amounts and are absorbed from the colostrum to supply neonatal requirements. It is important that maternal diets be adequate in these nutrients to ensure their transfer into the colostrum (Quigley and Drewry 1998).

REFERENCES

Abel MH, Baird DT. 1980. The effect of 17β estradiol progesterone on prostaglandin production by human endometrium maintained in organ culture. Endocrinology 106:1599–1606.

Acosta TJ, Ozawa T, Kobayashi S, et al. 2000. Periovulatory changes in the local release of vasoactive peptides, prostaglandin $F_{2\alpha}$ and steroid hormones from bovine mature follicles in vivo. Biol Reprod 63:1253–1261.

Adham IM, Emmen JMA, Engel W. 2000. The role of the testicular factor INSL3 in establishing the gonadal position. Mol Cell Endocrinol 160:11–16.

Akers RM. 1998. Lactogenesis. In: Knobil E, Neill JD, eds. Encyclopedia of Reproduction. San Diego: Academic, 2:979–985.

Aldridge B, Garry F, Adams R. 1992. Role of colostral transfer in neonatal calf management: Failure of acquisition of passive immunity. Compend Continuing Educ Pract Vet 14:265–270.

Alexander SL, Irvine CHG, Shand N, Evans MJ. 1995. Is luteinizing hormone secretion modulated by endogenous oxytocin in the mare? Studies on the role of oxytocin and factors affecting its secretion in estrous mares. Biol Reprod Monogr 1:361–371.

Alghamdi A, Troedsson MHT, Laaschewitsch T, Xue J-L. 2001. Uterine secretion from mares with post-breeding endometritis alters sperm motion characteristics in vitro. Theriogenology 55:1019–1028.

Alghamdi A, Troedsson MHT. 2002. Concentration of nitric oxide in uterine secretion from mares susceptible and resistant to chronic post-breeding endometritis. Theriogenology 58:445–448.

Algire JE, Srikandakumar A, Guilbault LA, Downey BR. 1992. Preovulatory changes in follicular prostaglandins and their role in ovulation in cattle. Can J Vet Res 56:67–69.

Allen WE, Pycock JF. 1988. Cyclical accumulation of uterine fluid in mares with lowered resistance to endometritis. Vet Rec 122:489–490.

Althouse GC, Evans LE, Hopkins SM. 1993. Episodic scrotal mutilation with concurrent bilateral sperm granuloma in a dog. J Am Vet Med Assoc 202:776–778.

Amann RP. 1993a. Functional anatomy of the adult male. In: McKinnon AO, Voss JL, eds. Equine Reproduction. Philadelphia: Lea and Febiger, pp 645–657.

Amann RP. 1993b. Physiology and endocrinology. In: McKinnon AO, Voss JL, eds. Equine Reproduction. Philadelphia: Lea and Febiger, pp 658–685.

Andersson K-E, Wagner G. 1995. Physiology of penile erection. Physiol Rev 75:191–236.

Araki M, Fukumatsu Y, Katabuchi H, et al. 1996. Follicular development and ovulation in macrophage colony-stimulating factor-deficient mice homozygous for the osteopetrosis (op) mutation. Biol Reprod 54:478–484.

Arici A, Oral E, Bukulmez O, et al. 1997. Monocyte chemotactic protein-1 expression in human preovulatory follicles and ovarian cells. J Reprod Immunol 32:201–219.

Asbury AC, Hansen PJ. 1987. Effects of susceptibility to endometritis and stage of cycle on phagocytic activity of uterine derived neutrophils. J Reprod Fertil Suppl 35:311–316.

Asbury AC, Halliwell REV, Foster GW, Longino SJ. 1980. Immunoglobulins in uterine secretion of mares with differing resistance to endometritis. Theriogenology 14:299–308.

Asbury AC, Schultz KT, Klesius PH, et al. 1982. Factors affecting phagocytosis of bacteria and neutrophils in the mare's uterus. J Reprod Fertil Suppl 32:151–159.

Ashdown RR, Glossop CE. 1983. Impotence in the bull: 3. Rupture of the corpus cavernosum penis proximal to the sigmoid flexure. Vet Rec 113:30–37.

Ashdown RR, David JSE, Gibbs C. 1979a. Impotence in the bull: 1. Abnormal venous drainage of the corpus cavernosum penis. Vet Rec 104:423–428.

Ashdown RR, Gilanpour H, David JSE, Gibbs C. 1979b. Impotence in the bull: 2. Occlusion of the longitudinal canals of the corpus cavernosum penis. Vet Rec 104:598–603.

Bader H. 1982. An investigation of sperm migration into the oviducts of the mare. J Reprod Fertil Suppl 32:59–64.

Bader H, Krause A. 1980. Investigation about the transport, distribution and the fate of spermatozoa in the genital tract of the mare. In: Proceedings of the Ninth International Congress on Animal Reproduction and AI. Madrid: Londres, 5:197–205.

Bailey MT. 2000. Inhibin production and secretion in mares with granulosa cell tumors [PhD thesis]. St Paul: University of Minnesota, pp 96–143.

Bailey MT, Christman SA, Wheaton JE, et al. 2000. Inhibin localization in equine granulosa-cell tumors and inhibin forms in tumor fluid. J Reprod Fertil Suppl 56:247–255.

Bailey MT, Wheaton JE, Troedsson MHT. 2002. Inhibin concentrations in mares with granulosa-thecal cell tumors. Theriogenology 57:1885–1895.

Baldwin JL, Cooper WL, Vanderwall DK, Erb HN. 1991. Prevalence (treatment days) and severity of illness in hypogammaglobulinemic and normogammaglobulinemic foals. J Am Vet Med Assoc 198:423–428.

Bao B, Garverick HA, Smith GW, et al. 1997. Expression of messenger RNA encoding 3α-hydroxysteroid dehydrogenase isomerase during recruitment and selection of bovine follicles: Identification of dominant follicles by expression of sα-HSD mRNA within the granulosa cell layer. Biol Reprod 56:1466–1473.

Barrington GM, Besser TE, Gay CC, et al. 1997. Effect of prolactin on in vitro expression of the bovine mammary immunoglobulin G_1 receptor. J Dairy Sci 80:94–100.

Bartels JE, Beckett SD, Brown BG. 1984. Angiography of the corpus cavernosum penis in the pony stallion during erection and quiescence. Am J Vet Res 45:1464–1468.

Barth AD, Bowman PA. 1994. The sequential appearance of sperm abnormalities after scrotal insulation or dexamethasone treatment in bulls. Can Vet J 34:93–102.

Beckett SD, Hudson RS, Walker DF, et al. 1972. Corpus cavernosum pressure and external penile muscle activity during erection in the goat. Biol Reprod 7:359–364.

Beckett SD, Hudson RS, Walker DF, et al. 1973. Blood pressure and penile muscle activity in the stallion during coitus. Am J Physiol 225:1072–1075.

Beckett SD, Reynolds TM, Walker DF, et al. 1974a. Experimentally induced rupture of the corpus cavernosum penis of the bull. Am J Vet Res 35:765–767.

Beckett SD, Walker DF, Hudson RS, et al. 1974b. Corpus cavernosum penis pressure and penile muscle activity in the bull during coitus. Am J Vet Res 35:761–764.

Beckett SD, Purohit RC, Reynolds TM. 1975a. The corpus spongiosum penis pressure and external penile muscle activity in the goat during coitus. Biol Reprod 12:289–292.

Beckett SD, Walker DF, Hudson RS, et al. 1975b. Corpus spongiosum penis pressure and penile muscle activity in the stallion during coitus. Am J Vet Res 36:431–433.

Beckett SD, Reynolds TM, Bartels JE. 1978. Angiography of the crus penis of the ram and buck during erection. Am J Vet Res 39:1950–1954.

Benoff S, Gilbert BR. 2001. Varicocele and male infertility: Part 1. Preface. Hum Reprod Update 7:47–54.

Blanchard TL, Elmore RG, Kinden PA, et al. 1985. Effect of intrauterine infusion of *Escherichia coli* endotoxin in postpartum pony mares. Am J Vet Res 46:2157–2162.

Blanchard TL, Schumacher J, Taylor TS, Varner DD. 1990. Detecting unilateral and bilateral cryptorchidism in large animals. Vet Med 85:395–403.

Blanchard TL, Varner DD, Bretzlaff KN, Elmore RG. 1991. The causes and pathologic changes of testicular degeneration in large animals. Vet Med Small Anim Clin 86:531–536.

Blum JW, Hammon H. 2000. Colostrum effects on the gastrointestinal tract, and on nutritional, endocrine and metabolic parameters in neonatal calves. Livest Prod Sci 66:151–159.

Bowden CE, Plaut K, Maple RL, Caler W. 1995. Negative effects of a high level of nutrient intake on mammary gland development of prepubertal goats. J Dairy Sci 78:1728–1733.

Brannstrom TL, Zackrisson U, Hagstrom HG, et al. 1998. Preovulatory changes of blood flow in different regions of the human. Fertil Steril 69:435–442.

Broom DM. 1983. Cow-calf, sow-piglet behaviour in relation to colostrum ingestion. Ann Rech Vet 14:342–348.

Burghardt RC, Matheson RL, Gaddy D. 1984a. Gap junction modulation in rat uterus: I. Effects of estrogen on myometrial and serosal cells. Biol Reprod 30:239–248.

Burghardt RC, Mitchell PA, Kurten RC. 1984b. Gap junction modulation in rat uterus: II. Effects on antiestrogens on myometrial, serosal cells. Biol Reprod 30:249–255.

Burghardt RC, Gaddy-Kurten D, Burghardt RL, et al. 1987. Gap junction modulation in rat uterus: III. Structure-activity relationships of estrogen receptor binding ligands on myometrial and serosal cells. Biol Reprod 36:741–751.

Buskirk DD, Faulkner DB, Hurley WL, et al. 1996. Growth, reproductive performance, mammary development, and milk production of beef heifers as influenced by prepubertal dietary energy and administration of bovine somatotropin. J Anim Sci 74:2649–2662.

Cadario ME, Thatcher MJD, LeBlanc MM. 1995. Relationship between prostaglandin and uterine clearance of radiocolloid in the mare. Biol Reprod Monogr 1:495–500.

Caldwell JC, McGadey J, Kerr R, et al. 1996. Cell recruitment to the sperm granuloma which follows vasectomy in the rat. Clin Anat 9:302–308.

Capel B. 1998. Sex in the 90s: SRY and the switch to the male pathway. Annu Rev Physiol 60:497–523.

Carati CJ, Creed KE, Keogh EJ. 1988. Vascular changes during penile erection in the dog. J Physiol 400:75–88.

Carmichael MS, Humbert R, Dixen J, et al. 1987. Plasma oxytocin increases in the human sexual response. J Clin Endocrinol Metab 64:27–31.

Carnevale EM, Ginther OJ. 1995. Defective oocytes as a cause of subfertility in old mares. Biol Reprod Monogr 1:209–214.

Casal ML, Jezyk PF, Giger U. 1996. Transfer of colostral antibodies from queens to their kittens. Am J Vet Res 57:1653–1658.

Chaffin CL, Stouffer RL. 1999. Expression of matrix metalloproteinases and their tissue inhibitor messenger ribonucleic acid in macaque periovulatory granulosa cells:

Time course and steroid regulation. Biol Reprod 61:14–21.

Chenoweth PJ, Chase CC, Risco CA, Larsen RE. 2000. Characterization of gossypol-induced sperm abnormalities in bulls. Theriogenology 53:1193–1203.

Christensen GC. 1954. Angioarchitecture of the canine penis and the process of erection. Am J Anat 95:227–261.

Claus R, Schams D. 1990. Influence of mating and intrauterine oestradiol infusion on peripheral oxytocin concentrations in the sow. J Endocrinol 126:361–365.

Claxton MS. 1989. Methods of surgical preparation of teaser bulls. Compend Continuing Educ Pract Vet 11:974–990.

Coerver KA, Woodruff TK, Finegold MJ, et al. 1996. Activin signaling through activin receptor type II causes cachexia-like symptoms in inhibin-deficient mice. Mol Endocrinol 10:534–543.

Colbern GT, Voss JL, Squires EL, et al. 1987. Development of a model to study endometritis in mares. Equine Vet Sci 7:73–76.

Cowie AT. 1984. Lactation. In: Austin CR, Short RV, eds. Hormonal Control of Reproduction. Cambridge: Cambridge University Press, pp 195–231.

Csapo AI. 1956. Progesterone "block." Am J Anat 98:273–291.

Dahms BJ, Troedsson MHT. 2002. The effect of seminal plasma components on opsonisation and PMN-phagocytosis of equine spermatozoa. Theriogenology 58:457–460.

Demers IM, Yoshuga K, Greep RO. 1974. Prostaglandin F in monkey uterine fluid during menstrual cycle and following steroid treatment. Prostaglandin 5:513–520.

Dennis SM. 1962. Spermicidal activity of bacterial endotoxin. Nature 195:1227–1228.

De Paolo LV, Bicsak TA, Erickson GF, et al. 1991. Follostatin and activin: A potential intrinsic regulatory system within diverse tissues [Minireview]. Proc Soc Exp Biol Med 198:500–512.

Dobson H, Smith RF. 1995. Stress and reproduction in farm animals. J Reprod Fertil Suppl 49:451–461.

Downey BR, Mootoo JE, Doyle SE. 1998. A role for lipoxygenase metabolites of arachidonic acid in porcine ovulation. Ann Reprod Sci 49:269–279.

Drobnis EZ, Overstreet JW. 1992. Natural history of mammalian spermatozoa in the female reproductive tract. Oxf Rev Reprod Biol 14:1–45.

Echternkamp SE. 1998. Freemartin. In: Knobil E, Neill JD, eds. Encyclopedia of Reproduction. San Diego: Academic, 2:406–417.

Einarsson S, Viring S. 1973. Distribution of frozen-thawed spermatozoa in the reproductive tract of gilts at different time intervals after insemination. J Reprod Fertil 32:117–120.

Eiler H. 1997. Retained placenta. In: Youngquist RS, ed. Current Therapy in Large Animal Theriogenology. Philadelphia: WB Saunders, pp 340–348.

Erickson G. 1986 An analysis of follicle development and ovum maturation. Semin Reprod Endocrinol 4:233–254.

Evans MJ, Hamer JM, Gason LM, Irwine GHC. 1987. Factors affecting uterine clearance on inoculated materials. J Reprod Fertil Suppl 35:327–334.

Feldman EC, Nelson RW. 1996. Canine and Feline Endocrinology and Reproduction. Philadelphia: WB Saunders, pp 619–648.

Felsburg PJ. 1998. Passive transfer of immunity. In: Pastoret P-P, Griebel P, Bazin H, Govaerts A, eds. Handbook of Vertebrate Immunology. San Diego: Academic, pp 271–272.

First NL, Short RE, Peters JB, Stratman FW. 1968. Transport of boar spermatozoa in estrual and luteal sows. J Anim Sci 27:1032–1036.

Forger NG. 1998. Sex differentiation, psychological. In: Knobil E, Neill JD, eds. Encyclopedia of Reproduction. San Diego: Academic, 4:421–430.

Forsyth I. 1998. Mammary gland, overview. In: Knobil E, Neill JD, eds. Encyclopedia of Reproduction. San Diego: Academic, 3:81–88.

Frank RT, Bonham C, Gustavson RG. 1925. A new method of assaying the potency of female sex hormone based upon its effect on spontaneous contraction of the uterus of the white rat. Am J Physiol 74:395–399.

Fredriksson G, Kindahl H, Sandstedt K Edqvist LE. 1985. Intrauterine bacterial findings and release of $PGF_2\alpha$ in the postpartum dairy cow. Zentralbl Vet Med 32:368–380.

Fuchs AR. 1972. Uterine activity during and after mating in the rabbit. Fertil Steril 23:915–923.

Fuchs AR, Periyasamy S, Alexandrova M, Soloff MS. 1983. Correlation between oxytocin receptor concentration and responsiveness to oxytocin in pregnant rat myometrium: Effect of ovarian steroids. Endocrinology 113:742–749.

Fuchs AR, Rust W, Fields MJ. 1999. Accumulation of cycloxygenase-2 gene transcripts in uterine tissues of pregnant and parturient cows: Stimulation by oxytocin. Biol Reprod 60:341–348.

Garfield RE, Sims SM, Daniel EE. 1977. Gap junctions: Their presence and necessity in myometrium during parturition. Science 198:958–960.

Garfield RE, Kannan MS, Daniel EE. 1980. Gap junction formation in the myometrium: Control by estrogens, progesterone, and prostaglandins. Am J Physiol 238:C81–C89.

Garfield RE, Puri CP, Casapo AI. 1982. Endocrine, structural and functional changes in uterus during premature labor. Am J Obstet Gynecol 142:21–27.

Gahr M. 1994. Brain structure: Causes and consequences of brain sex. In: Short RV, Balaban E, eds. The Differences Between the Sexes. Cambridge: Cambridge University Press, pp 273–300.

Gatewood DM, Cox JH, De Bowes RM. 1989. Diagnosis and treatment of acquired pathologic conditions of the equine penis and prepuce. Compend Continuing Educ Pract Vet 11:1498–1504.

Ginther OJ. 1992. Characteristics of the ovulatory season. In: Reproductive Biology of the Mare, 2nd ed. Cross Plains, WI: Equiservices, pp 217–229.

Glud E, Kjaer S, Troisi R, Brinton LA. 1998. Fertility drugs and ovarian cancer. Epidemiol Rev 20:237–257.

Gnessi L, Fabbri A, Spera G. 1997. Gonadal peptides as mediators of development and functional control of the testis: An integrated system with hormones and the local environment. Endocr Rev 18:541–609.

Gorga F, Galdiero M, Buommino E, Galdiero E. 2001. Porins and lipopolysaccharide induce apoptosis in human spermatozoa. Clin Diagn Lab Immunol 8:206–208.

Goursaud A-P, Nowak R. 1999. Colostrum mediates the development of mother preference by newborn lambs. Physiol Behav 67:49–56.

Gunn-Moore DA, Brown PJ, Holt PE, Gruffydd-Jones TJ. 1995. Priapism in seven cats. J Small Anim Pract 36:262–266.

Gunnick JW. 1984. Pre-partum leukocytic activity and retained placenta. Vet Q 6:52–54.

Gurpide E, Markiewicz I, Schatz F, Hirata F. 1986. Lipocortin output by human endometrium in vitro. J Clin Endocrinol Metab 63:162–166.

Hafez ESE. 2000. Anatomy of male reproduction. In: Hafez B, Hafez ESE, eds. Reproduction in Farm Animals, 7th ed. Philadelphia: Lippincott, Williams and Wilkins, pp 3–12.

Halasz B. 1993. Neuroendocrinology in 1992. Neuroendocrinology 57:1196–1207.

Haluska GJ, Lowe JE, Currie WB. 1987. Electromyographic properties of the myometrium correlated with the endocrinology of the pre-partum and post-partum periods and parturition in pony mares. J Reprod Fertil Suppl 35:553–564.

Hamadeh SK, Hatfield PG, Kott RW, et al. 2000. Effects of breed, sex, birth type and colostrum intake on cold tolerance in newborn lambs. Sheep Goat Res J 16:46–51.

Haqq CM, Donahoe PK. 1998. Regulation of sexual dimorphism in mammals. Physiol Rev 78:1–33.

Hayes HM. 1986. Epidemiological features of 5009 cases of equine cryptorchism. Equine Vet J 18:467–471.

Henderson DC. 2000. Neonatal conditions. In: Martin WB, Aitken ID, eds. Diseases of Sheep, 3rd ed. Oxford: Blackwell Science, pp 58–65.

Heuweiser W, Grunert E. 1987. Significance of chemotactic activity for placental expulsion in cattle. Theriogenology 27:907–912.

Hughes JP, Loy RG. 1965. Investigations on the effect of intrauterine inoculations of *Streptococcus zooepidemicus* in the mare. Proc Am Assoc Equine Pract 15:289–292.

Huhtaniem I, Bartke A. 2001. Perspective: Male reproduction? Endrocrinology 142:2178–2183.

Hunter RHF. 1995. Sex Determination, Differentiation and Intersexuality in Placental Mammals. Cambridge: Cambridge University Press, 1995.

Husband A. 1998. Passive transfer of Immunity. In: Pastoret P-P, Griebel P, Bazin H, Govaerts A, eds. Handbook of Vertebrate Immunology. San Diego: Academic, pp 464–466.

Hutson JM. 1994. Testicular descent: The first step towards fertility. Int J Androl 17:281–288.

Hutson JM, Donahoe PK. 1986. The hormonal control of testicular descent. Endocr Rev 7:270–283.

Hutson JM, Hasthorpe S, Heyns CF. 1997. Anatomical and functional aspects of testicular descent and cryptorchidism. Endocr Rev 18:259–280.

Itoh M, Li X-Q, Miyamoto K, Takeuchi Y. 1999. Degeneration of the seminiferous epithelium with ageing is a cause of spermatoceles? Int J Androl 22:91–96.

Ivell R, Fuchs AR, Bathgate R, et al. 2000. Regulation of the oxytocin receptor in bovine reproductive tissues and the role of steroids. Reprod Domest Anim 35:134–141.

Jackson JA, Friberg AC, Bahr JM. 1991. Preovulatory changes in glycosaminoglycans and collagen content in the stigma region of the follicle of the domestic hen. Biol Reprod 45:301–307.

Jager W, Dittrich R, Recabarren S, et al. 1995. Induction of ovarian tumors by endogenous gonadotropins in rats bearing intrasplenic ovarian grafts. Tumor Biol 16:268–280.

Johnson L. 1991. Spermatogenesis. In: Cupps PT, ed. Reproduction in Domestic Animals, 4th ed. San Diego: Academic, pp 173–219.

Johnson L, Falk GU, Spoede GE. 1998a. Male reproductive system, nonhuman mammals. In: Knobil E, Neill JD, eds. Encyclopedia of Reproduction. San Diego: Academic, 3:49–60.

Johnson NN, Brady HA, Whisnant CS, La Casha PA. 1998b. Effects of oral altrenogest on sexual and aggressive behaviors and seminal parameters in young stallions. J Equine Vet Sci 18:249–253.

Johnson ML, Murdoch J, Van Kirk EA, et al. 1999. Tumor necrosis factor alpha regulates collagenolytic activity in preovulatory ovine follicles: Relationship to cytokine secretion by oocyte-cumulus cell complex. Biol Reprod 61:1581–1585.

Johnson L, Varner DD, Roberts ME, et al. 2000. Efficiency of spermatogenesis: A comparative approach. Anim Reprod Sci 60–61:471–480.

Johnston SD, Root Kustritz MV, Olson PNS. 2001. Canine and Feline Theriogenology. Philadelphia: WB Saunders, pp 525–536.

Josso N. 1994. Anti-Mullerian hormone: A masculinizing relative of TGF-β. Oxf Rev Reprod Biol 16:139–163.

Kainer RA. 1993. Reproductive organs of the mare. In: McKinnon AO, Voss JL, eds. Equine Reproduction. Philadelphia: Lea and Febiger, pp 5–19.

Kamischke A, Nieschlag E. 2001. Varicocoele treatment in the light of evidence-based andrology. Hum Reprod Update 7:65–69.

Kandeel FR, Koussa VKT, Swerdloff RS. 2001. Male sexual function and its disorders: Physiology, pathophysiology, clinical investigation, and treatment. Endocr Rev 22:342–388.

Karstrom-Encrantz L, Runesson E, Bostrom EK, Brannstrom M. 1998. Selective presence of the chemokine growth-regulated oncogene alpha (GROalpha) in the human follicle and secretion from cultured granulosa-lutein cells at ovulation. Mol Hum Reprod 4:1077–1083.

Katila T, Sankari S, Mäkelä O. 2000. Transport of spermatozoa in the reproductive tracts of mares. J Reprod Fertil Suppl 56:571–578.

Kelly D, Coutts AGP. 2000. Development of digestive, immunological function in neonates: Role of early nutrition. Livest Prod Sci 66:161–167.

Kendrick KM, Fabre-Nys C, Blache D, et al. 1993. The role of oxytocin release in the mediobasal hypothalamus of the sheep in relation to female sexual receptivity. J Neuroendocrinol 5:13–21.

Keri RA, Lozada KL, Abdul-Karim FW, et al. 2000. Luteinizing hormone induction of ovarian tumors: Oligogenic differences between mouse strains dictate tumor disposition. Proc Natl Acad Sci USA 97:383–387.

Knight CH. 2000. The importance of cell division in udder development and lactation. Livest Prod Sci 66:169–176.

Knight CH, Peaker M, Wilde CJ. 1998. Local control of mammary development and function. Rev Reprod 3:104–112.

Knudsen O. 1964. Partial dilatation of the uterus as a cause of sterility in the mare. Cornell Vet 54:423–438.

Kohn CW, Knight D, Hueston W, et al. 1989. Colostral and serum IgG, IgA, and IgM concentrations in standardbred mares and their foals at parturition. J Am Vet Med Assoc 195:64–68.

Koji T, Hishikawa Y, Ando H, et al. 2001. Expression of Fas and Fas ligand in normal and ischemia-reperfusion testes: Involvement of the Fas system in the induction of germ cell apoptosis in the damaged mouse testis. Biol Reprod 64:946–954.

Koopman P. 1995. The molecular biology of SRY and its role in sex determination in mammals. Reprod Fertil Dev 7:713–722.

Kotilainen T, Huhtinen M, Katila T. 1994. Sperm-induced leukocytosis in the equine uterus. Theriogenology 41:629–636.

Kranzfelder D, Reich R, Abisogun AO, Tsafriri A. 1996. Preovulatory changes in the perifollicular capillary network in the rat: Role of eicosanoids. Biol Reprod 42:379–385.

Kruse PE. 1983. The importance of colostral immunoglobulins and their absorption from the intestine of the newborn animals Ann Rech Vet 14:349–353.

Kumar TR, Wang Y, Matzuk MM. 1996. Gonadotropins are essential modifier factors for gonadal tumor development in inhibin-deficient mice. Endocrinology 137:4210–4216.

Ladds PW. 1993. The male genital system. In: Jubb KVF, Kennedy PC, Palmer NC, eds. Pathology of Domestic Animals, 4th ed. San Diego: Academic, 3:471–529.

LeBlanc MM, Tran T, Baldwin JL, Pritchard EL. 1992. Factors that influence passive transfer of immunoglobulins in foals. J Am Vet Med Assoc 200:179–183.

LeBlanc MM, Neuwirth L, Asbury AC, et al. 1994a. Scintigraphic measurement of uterine clearance in normal mares and mares with recurrent endometritis. Equine Vet J a26:109–113.

LeBlanc MM, Neuwirth L, Mauragis D, et al. 1994b. Oxytocin enhances clearance of radiocolloid from the uterine lumen of reproductively normal mares and mares susceptible to endometritis. Equine Vet J 26:279–282.

Le Jan C. 1996. Cellular components of mammary secretions and neonatal immunity: A review. Vet Res 27:403–417.

Lee MM, Donahoe PK. 1993. Mullerian inhibiting substance: A gonadal hormone with multiple functions. Endocr Rev 14:152–164.

Lee CS, Oka T. 1992. Progesterone regulation of a pregnancy-specific transcription repressor to beta-casein gene promoter in mouse mammary gland. Endocrinology 131:2257–2262.

Lee J, Richburg JH, Shipp EB, et al. 1999. The Fas system, a regulator of testicular germ cell apoptosis, is differentially up-regulated in Sertoli cell versus germ cell injury of the testis. Endocrinology 140:852–858.

Lees J, Carriere PD, Dore M, Sirois J. 1997. Prostaglandin G/H synthase-2 is expressed in bovine preovulatory follicles after the endogenous surge of luteinizing hormone. Biol Reprod 57:1524–1531.

Liu K, Wahlberg P, Ny T. 1998. Coordinated and cell-specific regulation of membrane type matrix metalloproteinase 1 (MT1-MMP) and its substance matrix metalloproteinase 2 (MMP-2) by physiological signals during follicular development and ovulation. Endocrinology 139:4735–4738.

Logan EF, Irwin D. 1977. Serum immunoglobulin levels in neonatal lambs. Res Vet Sci 23:389–390.

Love CC, Kenney RM. 1999. Scrotal heat stress induces altered sperm chromatin structure associated with a decrease in protamine disulfide bonding in the stallion. Biol Reprod 60:615–620.

Love CC, McDonnell SM, Kenney RM. 1992. Manually assisted ejaculation in a stallion with erectile dysfunction subsequent to paraphimosis. J Am Vet Med Assoc 200:1357–1359.

Lue Y-H, Sinha Hikim AP, Swerdloff RS, et al. 1999. Single exposure to heat induces stage-specific germ cell apoptosis in rats: Role of intratesticular testosterone on stage specificity. Endocrinology 140:1709–1717.

Lysiak JL, Turner SD, Turner TT. 2000. Molecular pathway of germ cell apoptosis following ischemia/reperfusion of the rat testis. Biol Reprod 63:1465–1472.

Mann T, Lutwak-Mann C. 1981. Biochemistry of seminal plasma and male accessory fluids: Application to andrological problems. In: Male Reproductive Function and Semen. Berlin: Springer-Verlag, pp 269–336.

Matzuk MM, Finegold MJ, Su J-GJ, et al. 1992. A α–inhibin is a tumor-suppressor gene with gonadal specificity in mice. Nature 360:313–316.

Mazerbourg S, Zapf J, Bar RS, et al. 2000. Insulin-like growth factor (IGF)-binding protein-4 proteolytic degradation in bovine, equine, and porcine preovulatory follicles: Regulation by IGFs and heparin-binding domain-containing peptides. Biol Reprod 63:390–400.

McCann MA, Goode L, Harvey RW, et al. 1989. Effect of rapid weight gain to puberty on reproduction, mammary development and lactation in ewe lambs. Theriogenology 32:55–68.

McCue PM. 1992. Equine granulosa cell tumors. Proc Assoc Am Equine Pract 38:587–593.

McCue PM, Squires EL. 2002. Persistent anovulatory follicles in the mare. Theriogenology 58:541–543.

McDonald SW. 2000. Cellular responses to vasectomy. Int Rev Cytol 199:295–339.

McDonnell SM. 1992. Ejaculation physiology and dysfunction. Vet Clin North Am Equine Pract 8:57–70.

McEntee K. 1990. Reproductive Pathology of Domestic Animals. San Diego: Academic, pp 252–278.

McKenzie LW, Garfield RE. 1985. Hormonal control of gap junctions in the myometrium. Am J Physiol 248:C296–C308.

McGuire TC, Pfeiffer NE, Weikel JM, Bartsch RC. 1976. Failure of colostral immunoglobulin transfer in calves dying from infectious disease. J Am Vet Med Assoc 169:713–718.

McGuire TC, Crawford TB, Hallowell AL, Macomber LE. 1977. Failure of colostral immunoglobulin transfer as an explanation for most infections and deaths in neonatal foals. J Am Vet Med Assoc 170:1302–1304.

McGuire TC, Regnier J, Kellom T, Gates NL. 1983. Failure of passive transfer of immunoglobulin G_1 to lambs: Measurement of immunoglobulin G_1 in ewe colostrum. Am J Vet Res 44:1064–1067.

McLaren A. 1991. Sex determination in mammals. Oxf Rev Reprod Biol 13:1–33.

Mellor DJ, Murray L. 1986. Making the most of colostrum at lambing. Vet Rec 118:351–353.

Meyers-Wallen VN, Patterson DF. 1986. Disorders of sexual development in the dog. In: Morrow DA, ed. Current Therapy in Theriogenology, 2nd ed. Philadelphia: WB Saunders, pp 567–574.

Mickelsen WD, Memon MA. 1997. Infertility and diseases of the reproductive organs of bucks. In: Youngquist RS, ed. Current Therapy in Large Animal Theriogenology. Philadelphia: WB Saunders, pp 489–493.

Mills TM, Wiedemeier VT, Stopper VS. 1992. Androgen maintenance of erectile function in the rat penis. Biol Reprod 46:342–348.

Mills TM, Lewis RW, Stopper VS. 1998. Androgenic maintenance of inflow and veno-occlusion during erection in the rat. Biol Reprod 59:1413–1418.

Mitchell G, Liu IKM, Perryman LE, et al. 1982. Preferential production and secretion of immunoglobulins by the equine endometrium: A mucosal immune system. J Reprod Fertil Suppl 32:161–168.

Morris DD, Meirs DA, Merryman GS. 1985. Passive transfer failure in horses: Incidence and causative factors on a breeding farm. Am J Vet Res 46:2294–2299.

Mostov KE. 1994. Transepithelial transport of immunoglobulins. Annu Rev Immunol 12:63–84.

Murdoch WJ. 1995. Programmed cell death in preovulatory follicles. Biol Reprod 53:8–12.

Murdoch WJ, McCormick RJ. 1992. Sequence analysis of leukocyte chemoattractant peptides secreted by preovulatory ovine follicles. Biochem Biophys Res Commun 184:848–852.

Murdoch WJ, Van Kirk EA, Murdoch J. 1999a. Plasmin cleaves tumor necrosis factor-α exodomain from sheep follicular endothelium: Implication in the ovulatory process. Biol Reprod 60:1166–1171.

Murdoch WJ, Wilken C, Young DA. 1999b. Sequence apoptosis and inflammatory necrosis within the formative ovulatory site of sheep follicles. J Reprod Fertil 117:325–329.

Neville MC. 1998. Lactation, human. In: Knobil E, Neill JD, eds. Encyclopedia of Reproduction. San Diego: Academic, 2:963–972.

Nikolakopoulos E, Kindahl H, Watson ED. 2000. Oxytocin and $PGF_2\alpha$ release in mares resistant and susceptible to persistent mating-induced endometritis. J Reprod Fertil Suppl 56:363–372.

Noordsy JL. 1981. Hematoma of the bovine penis: A technique for predicting successful surgical correction. Vet Med Small Anim Clin 76:1581–1590.

Noordsy JL, Trotter DM, Carnahan DL, Vestweber JG. 1970. Etiology of hematoma of the penis in beef bulls: A clinical survey. In: McFeely RA, Morse GE, Williams EI, eds. Proceedings of the 6th International Conference on Cattle Diseases. Stillwater, OK: Heritage, pp 333–338.

Nowak R, Porter RH, Levy F, et al. 2000. Role of mother-young interactions in the survival of offspring in domestic animals. Rev Reprod 5:153–163.

Oko R, Clermont Y. 1998. Spermiogenesis. In: Knobil E, Neill JD, eds. Encyclopedia of Reproduction. San Diego: Academic, 4:602–609.

Oliphant G, Reynolds AB, Thomas TS. 1985. Sperm surface components involved in the control of the acrosome reaction. Am J Anat 174:269–283.

Overstreet JW, Cooper GW. 1978. Sperm transport in the reproductive tract of the female rabbit: I. The rapid transit phase of transport. Biol Reprod 19:101–114.

Parkington HC, Coleman HA. 1990. The role of membrane potential in the control of uterine motility. In: Carsten ME, Miller JD, eds. Uterine function, molecular and cellular aspects. New York: Plenum Press, pp 195–238.

Pattridge PD. 1953. Surgical repair of the fractured penis in the bull. Southwest Vet 7:31–33.

Pautler SE, Brock GB. 2001. Priapism from Priapus to the present time. Urol Clin North Am 28:391–403.

Pearson H, Weaver BMQ. 1978. Priapism after sedation, neuroleptanalgesia and anaesthesia in the horse. Equine Vet J 10:85–90.

Peter AT. 1997. Infertility due to abnormalities of the ovaries. In: Youngquist RS, ed. Current Therapy in Large Animal Theriogenology. Philadelphia: WB Saunders, pp 349–354.

Phillips RW, Andrews F. 1937. The speed of travel of ram spermatozoa. Anat Rec 68:127–132.

Priddy AR, Killick SR. 1993. Eicosanoids and ovulation. Prostaglandins Leukot Essent Fatty Acids 49:827–831.

Pu R, Yamamoto JK. 1998. Passive transfer of maternal immunity In: Pastoret P-P, Griebel P, Bazin H, Govaerts A, eds. Handbook of Vertebrate Immunology. San Diego: Academic, pp 305–308.

Purohit RC, Beckett SD. 1976. Penile pressures and muscle activity associated with erection and ejaculation in the dog. Am J Physiol 231:1343–1348.

Pycock JF. 1994. Assessment of oxytocin and intrauterine antibiotics on intrauterine fluid and pregnancy rates in the mare. Proc Am Assoc Equine Pract 40:19–20.

Pycock JF, Allen WE. 1988. Pre-chemotactic and chemotactic properties of uterine fluid from mares with experimentally induced bacteria endometritis. Vet Rec 123:193–195.

Pycock JF, Allen WE. 1990. Inflammatory component in uterine fluid from mares with experimentally induced bacterial endometritis. Equine Vet J 22:422–425.

Quigley JD, Drewry JJ. 1998. Nutrient and immunity transfer from cow to calf pre- and postcalving. J Dairy Sci 81:2779–2790.

Raidal SL. 1996. The incidence and consequences of failure of passive transfer of immunity on a thoroughbred breeding farm. Aust Vet J 73:201–206.

Randall D, Burggren W, French K. 1997. Animal Physiology, 4th ed. New York: WH Freeman, pp 693–694.

Randel RD, Chase CC, Wyse SJ. 1992. Effects of gossypol and cottonseed products on reproduction of mammals. J Anim Sci 70:1628–1638.

Reynolds SRM, Allen WM. 1932. The effect of progestin-containing extracts of corpora lutea on uterine motility in the unanesthetized rabbit, with observations with pseudopregancy. Am J Physiol 102:39–55.

Rigby SL, Barhoumi R, Burghardt RC, et al. 2001. Mares with delayed uterine clearance have an intrinsic defect in myometrial function. Biol Reprod 65:740–747.

Risma KA, Clay CM, Nett TM, et al. 1995. Targeted overexpression of luteinizing hormone in transgenic mice leads to infertility, polycystic ovaries and ovarian tumors. Proc Natl Acad Sci USA 92:1322–1326.

Roberts JS. 1986. Veterinary Obstetrics and Genital Diseases, 3rd ed. Woodstock, VT: published by the author.

Roberts JS, Barcikowski B, Wilson, I, et al. 1976. Hormonal and related factors affecting the release of prostaglandin $F_{2\alpha}$ from ovine endometrium in vitro: Correlation with estrus cycle and oxytocin-receptor binding. Endocrinology 99:1107–1114.

Rogers GM, Capucille DJ. 2000. Colostrum management: Keeping beef calves alive and performing. Compend Continuing Educ Pract Vet 22:S6–S13.

Rosnina Y, Jainudeen MR, Hafez ESE. 2000. Genetics of reproductive failure. In: Hafez ESE, Hafez B, eds. Reproduction in Farm Animals, 7th ed. Philadelphia: Lippincott, Williams, and Wilkins, pp 307–317.

Rossier BC, Geering K, Krachenbuhl JP. 1987. Regulation of the sodium pump: How and why? Trends Biochem 12:483–487.

Rozeboom KJ, Troedsson MHT, Rocha GR, Crabo BG. 2000. The importance of seminal plasma on spermatozoa viability of subsequent artificial inseminations in swine. J Anim Sci 78:443–448.

Saez JM. 1994. Leydig cells: Endocrine, paracrine, and autocrine regulation. Endocr Rev 15:574–626.

Saito K, O'Donnell L, McLachlan RI, Robertson DM. 2000. Spermiation failure is a major contributor to early spermatogenic suppression caused by hormone withdrawal in adult rats. Endocrinology 141:2779–2785.

Sangild PT, Fowden AL, Trahair JF. 2000. How does the foetal gastrointestinal tract develop in preparation for enteral nutrition after birth? Livest Prod Sci 66:141–150.

Schams D, Baumann G, Leidl W. 1982. Oxytocin determination by radioimmunoassay in cattle: II. Effect of mating and stimulation of the genital tract in bulls, cows and heifers. Acta Endocrinol 99:218–223.

Schatz F, Markiewicz L, Berg P, Gurpide E. 1985. In vitro effect of ovarian steroids on prostaglandin output by human endometrium and endometrial epithelial cells. J Clin Endocrinol Metab 61:361–367.

Schatz F, Markiewicz L, Gurpide E. 1987. Differential effects of estradiol, arachidonic acid and A-23187 on prostaglandin $F_{2\alpha}$ output by epithelial and stromal cells of human endometrium. Endocrinology 120:1465–1471.

Schumacher J, Varner DD, Crabill MR, Blanchard TL. 1999. The effect of a surgically created shunt between the corpus cavernosum penis and corpus spongiosum penis of stallions on erectile and ejaculatory function. Vet Surg 28:21–24.

Scott MA, Liu IKM, Robertson KR, et al. 1994. Acrosomal status and movement characteristics of sperm in the oviducts of normal mares. In: Proceedings of the 6th International Symposium of Equine Reproduction, Caxambu, Brazil, pp 173–174.

Scott MA, Liu IKM, Overstreet JW. 1995. Sperm transport to the oviducts: Abnormalities and their clinical implications. Proc Am Assoc Equine Pract 41:1–2.

Sejrsen K, Huber JT, Tucker HA, Akers RM. 1982. Influence of nutrition on mammary development in pre- and postpubertal heifers. J Dairy Sci 65:793–800.

Sejrsen K, Huber JT, Tucker HA. 1983. Influence of amount fed on hormone concentrations and their relationship to mammary growth in heifers. J Dairy Sci 66:845–855.

Seguin B, Troedsson MHT. 2002. Diseases of the reproductive system. In: Smith BP, ed. Large Animal Internal Medicine. St Louis: CV Mosby, pp 1293–1295.

Setchell BP. 1991. Male reproductive organs and Semen. In: Cupps PT, ed. Reproduction in Domestic Animals, 4th ed. San Diego: Academic, pp 221–249.

Setchell BP. 1998. Heat and the testis. J Reprod Fertil 114:179–194.

Shennan DB, Peaker M. 2000. Transport of milk constituents by the mammary gland. Physiol Rev 80:925–951.

Sheoran AS, Timoney JF, Holmes MA, et al. 2000. Immunoglobulin isotypes in sera and nasal mucosal secretions and their neonatal transfer and distribution in horses. Am J Vet Res 61:1099–1105.

Short RV. 1982. Sex determination and differentiation. In: Austin CR, Short RV, eds. Reproduction in Mammals, 2nd ed. Cambridge: Cambridge University Press 2:70–113.

Sinha Hikim AP, Wang C, Leung A, Swerdloff RS. 1995. Involvement of apoptosis in the induction of germ cell degeneration in adult rats after gonadotropin-releasing hormone antagonist treatment. Endocrinology 136:2770–2775.

Sinha Hikim AP, Rajavashisth TB, Sinha Hikim I, et al. 1997. Significance of apoptosis in the temporal and stage-specific loss of germ cells in the adult rat after gonadotropin deprivation. Biol Reprod 57:1193–1201.

Sirois J, Dore M. 1997. The late induction of prostaglandin G/H synthase-2 in equine preovulatory follicles supports its role as a determinant of the ovulatory process. Endocrinology 138:4047–4048.

Sivula NJ, Ames TR, Marsh WE, Werdin RE. 1996. Descriptive epidemiology of morbidity and mortality in Minnesota dairy heifer calves. Prev Vet Med 27:155–171.

Smith OB, Akinbamijo OO. 2000. Micronutrients and reproduction in farm animals. Anim Reprod Sci 60–61:549–560.

Smith MC, Sherman DM. 1994. Goat Medicine. Philadelphia: Lea and Febiger, pp 438–439.

Soloff MS, Fernstrom MA, Periyasamy S, et al. 1983. Regulation of oxytocin receptor concentration in rat uterine explants by estrogen and progesterone. Can J Biochem Cell Biol 61:625–630.

Squires EL, Todter GE, Berndtson WE, Pickett BW. 1982. Effect of anabolic steroids on reproductive function of young stallions. J Anim Sci 54:576–582.

Squires EL, Badzinski SL, Amman RP, et al. 1997. Effects of altrenogest on total scrotal width, seminal characteristics, concentrations of LH and testosterone and sexual behavior in stallions. Theriogenology 48:313–328.

Stabenfeldt GH, Hughes JP, Kennedy PC, et al. 1979. Clinical findings, pathological changes and endocrinological secretory patterns in mares with ovarian tumors. J Reprod Fertil Suppl 27:277–285.

Stokes C, Bailey M. 1998. Passive transfer of immunity. In: Pastoret P-P, Griebel P, Bazin H, Govaerts A, eds. Handbook of Vertebrate Immunology. San Diego: Academic, pp 395–397.

Stott GH, Fellah A. 1983. Colostral immunoglobulin absorption linearly related to concentration for calves. J Dairy Sci 66:1319–1328.

Swalec KM, Smeak DD. 1989. Priapism after castration in a cat. J Am Vet Med Assoc 195:963–964.

Takihara H, Sakatoku J, Cockett ATK. 1991. The pathophysiology of varicocele in male infertility. Fertil Steril 55:861–868.

Taya K, Nagata S, Tsunoda N, et al. 2000. Testicular secretion of inhibin in stallions. J Reprod Fertil Suppl 56:43–50.

Thibier M, Rolland O. 1976. The effect of dexamethasone (DXM) on circulating testosterone (T) and luteinizing hormone (LH) in young postpubertal bulls. Theriogenology 5:53–60.

Thomas PGA, Ball BA, Miller PG, et al. 1994. A subpopulation of morphologically normal, motile spermatozoa attach to equine oviductal epithelial cell monolayers. Biol Reprod 51:303–309.

Tilbrook AJ, Clarke IJ. 2001. Negative feedback regulation of the secretion and actions of gonadotropin-releasing hormone in males. Biol Reprod 64:735–742.

Tilbrook AJ, Turner AI, Clarke IJ. 2000. Effects of stress on reproduction in non-rodent mammals: The role of glucocorticoids and sex differences. Rev Reprod 5:105–113.

Tilly JL, Johnson AL. 1990. Control of plasminogen activator in the thecal layer of the largest preovulatory follicle in the hen ovary. Endocrinology 126:2079–2087.

Tizard IR. 1996. Immunity in the fetus and newborn. In: Veterinary Immunology: An Introduction. Philadelphia: WB Saunders, pp 237–250.

Troedsson MHT. 1995. Uterine response to semen deposition in the mare. In: Proceedings of the Annual Meeting of the Society of Theriogenology. Hastings, NE: SFT, pp 130–135.

Troedsson MHT. 1999. Uterine clearance and resistance to persistent endometritis in the mare. Theriogenology 52:461–471.

Troedsson MHT, Liu IKM. 1991. Uterine clearance of non-antigenic markers (Cr51) in response to a bacterial challenge in mares potentially susceptible and resistant to chronic uterine infection. J Reprod Fertil Suppl 44:283–288.

Troedsson MHT, Concha C, Einarsson S, Holmberg OA. 1990. A preliminary study of uterine derived polymorphonuclear cell function in mares with chronic uterine infections. Acta Vet Scand 31:187–192.

Troedsson MHT, Liu IKM, Ing M, et al. 1993a. Multiple site electromyography recordings of uterine activity following an intrauterine bacterial challenge in mares susceptible and resistant to chronic uterine infection. J Reprod Fertil 99:307–313.

Troedsson MHT, Liu IKM, Thurmond MM. 1993b. Function of uterine and blood derived polymorphonuclear neutrophils (PMN) in mares susceptible and resistant to chronic uterine infection (CUI): Phagocytosis and chemotaxis. Biol Reprod 49:507–514.

Troedsson MHT, Liu IKM, Thurmond M. 1993c. Immunoglobulin (IgG and IgA) and complement (3) concentrations in uterine secretion following an intrauterine challenge of Streptococcus zooepidemicus in mares susceptible to versus resistant to chronic uterine infection. Biol Reprod 49:502–506.

Troedsson MHT, Steiger BN, Ibrahim NM, et al. 1995. Mechanism of sperm-induced endometritis in the mare. Biol Reprod 2(Suppl)52:133.

Troedsson MHT, Spensley MS, Fahning ML. 1997. Retained fetal membranes. In: Robinson NE, ed. Current Therapy in Equine Medicine, 4. Philadelphia: WB Saunders, pp 560–562.

Troedsson MHT, Liu IKM, Crabo BG. 1998. Sperm transport and survival in the mare: A review. Theriogenology 50:807–818.

Troedsson MHT, Franklin RK, Crabo BG. 1999. Suppression of PMN-chemotaxis by different molecular weight fractions of seminal plasma. Pferdheilkunde 15:568–573.

Troedsson MHT, Lee CS, Franklin RK, Crabo BG. 2000. Post-breeding uterine inflammation: The role of seminal plasma. J Reprod Fertil Suppl 56:341–349.

Troedsson MHT, Alghamdi AS, Mattisen J. 2002. Equine seminal plasma protects the fertility of spermatozoa in an inflamed uterine environment. Theriogenology 58:453–456.

Trommerhausen-Bowling A, Millon L, Hughes JP. 1987. An update on chromosomal abnormalities in mares. J Reprod Fertil Suppl 35:149–155.

Tucker HA. 2000. Hormones, mammary growth, and lactation: A 41-year perspective. J Dairy Sci 83:874–884.

Turner TI. 2001. The study of varicocele through the use of animal models. Hum Reprod Update 7:78–84.

Turner TT, Tung KSK, Tomomasa H, Wilson LW. 1997. Acute testicular ischemia results in germ cell-specific apoptosis in the rat. Biol Reprod 57:1267–1274.

Tyler JW, Cullor JS, Thurmond MC, et al. 1990. Immunologic factors related to survival and performance in neonatal swine. Am J Vet Res 51:1400–1406.

Tyler JW, Hancock DD, Thorne JG, et al. 1999. Partitioning the mortality risk associated with inadequate passive transfer of colostral immunoglobulins in dairy calves. J Vet Intern Med 13:335–337.

Van Demark NL, Moeller AN. 1950. Spermatozoan transport in the reproductive tract of estrus cows. J Dairy Sci 33:390–391.

Van Demark NL, Moeller AN. 1951. Speed of spermatozoan transport in the reproductive tract of estrus cows. Am J Physiol 165:674–679.

Vanderplassche M, Spincemaille J, Bouters R. 1971. Aetiology, pathogenesis and treatment of retained placenta in the mare. Equine Vet J 3:144–147.

Velasquez-Pereira J, Chenoweth PJ, McDowell LR, et al. 1998. Reproductive effects of feeding gossypol and vitamin E to bulls. J Anim Sci 76:2894–2904.

Von Reitzenstein M, Callahan MA, Hansen PJ, LeBlanc MM. 2002. Aberrations in uterine contractile patterns in mares with delayed uterine clearance after administration of detomidine and oxytocin. Theriogenology 58:887–898.

Waelchli RO, Winder NC. 1991. Mononuclear cell infiltration of the equine endometrium: Immunohistochemical studies. Equine J Vet 23:470–474.

Wakerley JB. 1998. Milk ejection. In: Knobil E, Neill JD, eds. Encyclopedia of Reproduction. San Diego: Academic, 3:264–275.

Wathes DC. 1984. Possible actions of gonadal oxytocin and vasopressin. J Reprod Fertil 71:315–345.

Watson ED, Thomson SRM. 1996. Immunolocalization of aromatase P-450 in ovarian tissue from pregnant and non-pregnant mares and in ovarian tumors. J Reprod Fertil 108:239–244.

Watson ED, Stokes CR, Bourne FJ. 1987a. Cellular and humoral mechanisms in mares susceptible and resistant to persistent endometritis. Vet Immunol Immunopathol 16:107–121.

Watson ED, Stokes CR, Bourne FJ. 1987b. Influence of arachidonic acid metabolites on vitro and in uterine washings on migration of equine neutrophils under agarose. Res Vet Sci 43:203–207.

Watson D. 1998. Transmission of passive immunity in the sheep In: Pastoret P-P, Griebel P, Bazin H, Govaerts A, eds. Handbook of Vertebrate Immunology. San Diego: Academic, pp 513–515.

Watson DL. 1980. Immunological functions of the mammary gland and its secretion: Comparative review. Aust J Biol Sci 33:403–442.

Weaver DM, Tyler JW, Scott MA, et al. 2000a. Passive transfer of colostral immunoglobulin G in neonatal llamas and alpacas. Am J Vet Res 61:738–741.

Weaver DM, Tyler JW, Van Metre DC, et al. 2000b. Passive transfer of colostral immunoglobulins in calves. J Vet Intern Med 14:569–577.

Weldon WC, Thulin AJ, MacDougald OA, et al. 1991. Effects of increased dietary energy and protein during late gestation on mammary development in gilts. J Anim Sci 69:194–200.

Welsh TH, Johnson BH. 1981. Stress-induced alterations in secretion of corticosteroids, progesterone, luteinizing hormone, and testosterone in bulls. Endocrinology 109:185–190.

Welsh TH, McCraw RL, Johnson BH. 1979. Influence of corticosteroids on testosterone production in the bull. Biol Reprod 21:755–763.

Wheat JD. 1966. Penile paralysis in stallions given propiopromazine. J Am Vet Med Assoc 148:405–406.

Widders PR, Stokes CR, David JSE, Bourne FJ. 1984. Quantification of the immunoglobulins in reproductive tract secretion in the mare. Res Vet Sci 37:324–330.

Widders PR, Stokes CR, David JSE, Bourne FJ. 1985. Specific antibodies in the equine genital tract following systemic and local immunization. Immunology 54:763–769.

Wilson JD. 1994. Translating gonadal sex into phenotypic sex. In: Short RV, Balaban E, eds. The Differences Between the Sexes. Cambridge: Cambridge University Press, pp 203–212.

Wilson DV, Nickels FA, Williams MA. 1991. Pharmacologic treatment of priapism in two horses. J Am Vet Med Assoc 199:1183–1184.

Winter AJ, Broome AW, McNutt SH, Casida LE. 1960. Variation in uterine response to experimental infection due to the hormonal state of the ovaries: I. The role of cervical drainage, leukocyte numbers and non-cellular factors in uterine bactericidal activity. Am J Vet Res 21:668–674.

Wong WW, Thomas CMG, Merkus JMWM, et al. 2000. Male factor subfertility: Possible causes and the impact of nutritional factors. Fertil Steril 73:435–442.

Woolveridge I, De Boer-Brouwer M, Taylor MF, et al. 1999. Apoptosis in the rat spermatogenic epithelium following androgen withdrawal: Changes in apoptosis-related genes. Biol Reprod 60:461–470.

Xu R-J. 1996. Development of the newborn GI tract and its relation to colostrum/milk intake: A review. Reprod Fertil Dev 8:35–48.

Xu ZZ, Gaverick HA, Smith GW, et al. 1995. Expression of follicle stimulating hormone and luteinizing hormone receptor messenger ribonucleic acids in bovine follicles during the first follicular wave. Biol Reprod 53:951–957.

Ying S-Y. 1989. Inhibins, activins and follistatins. J Steroid Biochem 33:705–713.

Yamamoto CM, Sinha Hikim AP, Huynh PN, et al. 2000. Redistribution of Bax is an early step in an apoptotic pathway leading to germ cell death in rats, triggered by mild testicular hyperthermia. Biol Reprod 63:1683–1690.

Yanagimachi R. 1994. Mammalian fertilization. In: Knobil E, Neill JD, eds. The Physiology of Reproduction, 2nd ed. New York: Raven, pp 189–281.

Yoshimura Y, Aoki N, Sueoka K, et al. 1996. Interactions between insulin-like growth factor-1 (IGF1) and the renin-angiotensin system in follicular growth and ovulation. J Clin Invest 98:308–316.

Young SL, Hudson RS, Walker DF. 1977. Impotence in bulls due to vascular shunts from the corpus cavernosum penis. J Am Vet Med Assoc 171:643–648.

Zachrisson U, Mikuni M, Wallin A, et al. 1966. Cell-specific localization of nitric oxide synthases (NOS) in the rat ovary during follicular development, ovulation and luteal formation. Hum Reprod 11:2667–2673.

Zavos PM, Zarmakoupis-Zavos PN. 1996. The inhibitory effects of gossypol on human sperm motility characteristics: Possible modes of reversibility of those effects. Tohoku J Exp Med 179:167–175.

Zirkin BR. 1998. Spermatogenesis, hormonal control of. In: Knobil E, Neill JD, eds. Encyclopedia of Reproduction. San Diego: Academic, 4:556–563.

PATHOPHYSIOLOGY OF MUSCLE DISEASE

Stephanie J. Valberg

SKELETAL MUSCLE STRUCTURE AND FUNCTION

Structure. Skeletal muscle fibers are long multinucleated spindle-shaped cells that have remarkable properties of conductibility and contractility. Conductile properties are conferred by the array of ion channels in the phospholipid bilayer of the muscle cell membrane (sarcolemma). Myogenic precursor cells called satellite cells lie between the sarcolemma and the myofiber's basement membrane. The basement membrane, comprised of glycoproteins and collagen, acts as structural support during contraction as well as a scaffold for muscle regeneration by satellite cells. Bundles of muscle fibers arranged in parallel form fascicles that are surrounded by connective tissue (Figure 8.1). Nerve branches and blood vessels are found within the connective tissue. Nerve branches are composed of motor neurons extending from the ventral root of the spinal cord into the muscle fascicle and communicating with muscle fibers at a specialized site in the sarcolemma called the *motor end plate* (Figure 8.2). The sarcolemma at the motor end plate has numerous folds, the crests of which contain densely packed acetylcholine receptors. A synaptic cleft exists between the motor end plate and the nerve terminal, which contains numerous synaptic vesicles containing the neurotransmitter acetylcholine.

The motor neuron and all the muscle fibers that it supplies are together termed a *motor unit*. Each time that the nerve is stimulated, all of the muscle fibers under its control will contract. The conduction velocities of motor neurons vary such that high-frequency, fast conduction velocities are found in motor units supplying fast-twitch muscle fibers and low-frequency, slow conduction velocities are found in motor units supplying slow-twitch muscle fibers. Trophic interactions between nerve and muscle

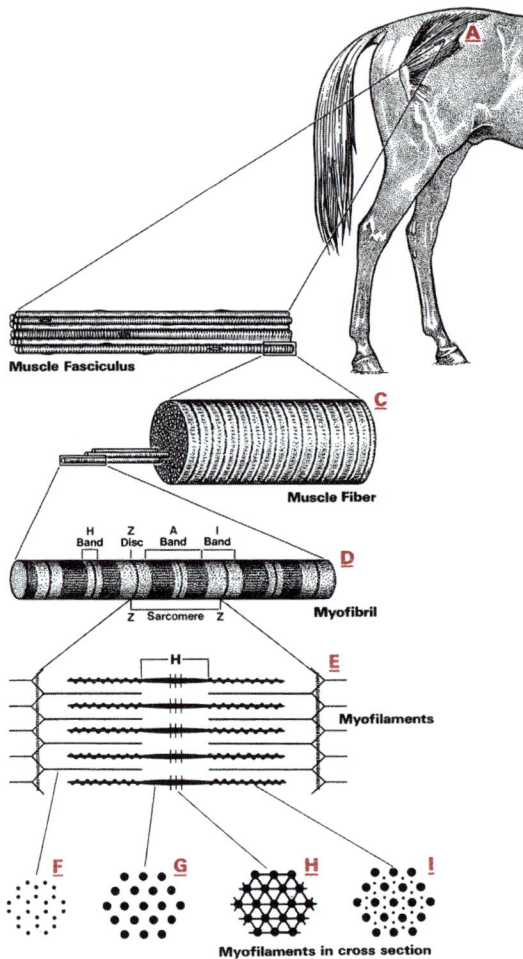

FIG 8.1—The organization of skeletal muscle cells and contractile proteins from the gross to the molecular level. (Adapted from Bloom and Fawcett 1986:282, and Hodgson and Rose 1994.)

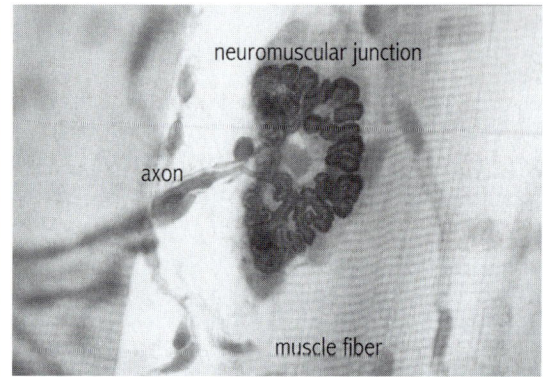

FIG. 8.2—High-power light-microscopic picture of a motor neuron and the neuromuscular junction, which is highlighted by esterase staining. Note the extensive folds of the sarcolemmal membrane at the motor end plate that contain the acetylcholine receptors. (Photo courtesy of Dr. G.H. Cardinet III.)

fibers regulate the structural, metabolic, and biochemical properties of the muscle fiber. A lack of neural firing results in atrophy of the fiber, and a change in the frequency of nerve firing decreases oxidative enzyme activities as well as the contractile speed of the muscle fiber.

A muscle's unique ability to contract is conferred by the highly organized parallel, overlapping arrangement of thick and thin filaments (Figure 8.1). These repeating contractile units or sarcomeres extend from one end of the cell to the other in the form of a myofibril. Each muscle fiber is packed with myofibrils that are arranged in register, giving skeletal muscle a striated appearance under the microscope. The proteins actin, troponin, and tropomyosin comprise the thin filaments. The main component of the thick filaments is myosin, which has many different isoforms that are differentially expressed in certain muscles and muscle fibers. In general, myosin consists of two heavy chains and four light chains. Isoforms of both light chains and heavy chains exist and characterize muscle fibers in different stages of development, different locations, and different contractile types. Nine myosin heavy-chain isoforms have been identified in adult skeletal muscle, with three types occurring most commonly (Lopez Rivero 1996a). A complex cytoskeleton comprised of actin, intermediate filaments, and microtubules maintains myofibrillar alignment and cell shape during contraction. Myofibrils are surrounded by mitochondria, glycogen particles, the sarcoplasmic reticulum, and invaginations of the sarcolemma called *T tubules* (Figure 8.3). The sarcoplasmic reticulum is an intracellular membrane system highly enriched in pumps and channels for sequestering and releasing calcium. T tubules are closely aligned with the terminal cisternae of the sarcoplasmic reticulum. A triad junction between a T tubule and two terminal cisternae occurs twice in each sarcomere.

Excitation-Contraction Coupling. When a motor unit is recruited, an action potential travels down the motor neuron. When the action potential reaches each nerve terminal, presynaptic voltage-gated calcium channels open transiently. Calcium flux into the cytosol of the nerve terminal stimulates exocytosis of synaptic vesicle containing acetylcholine. Acetylcholine crosses the synaptic cleft and binds to receptors on the postsynaptic membrane. This results in a net flux of sodium through the acetylcholine receptor channel into the muscle cells with subsequent depolarization of the sarcolemma at the motor end plate. A wave of depolarization spreads from the motor end plate in all directions, including deep into the muscle cell by way of the invaginating T tubules. The voltage-gated calcium channel (dihydropyridine receptor), also known as the

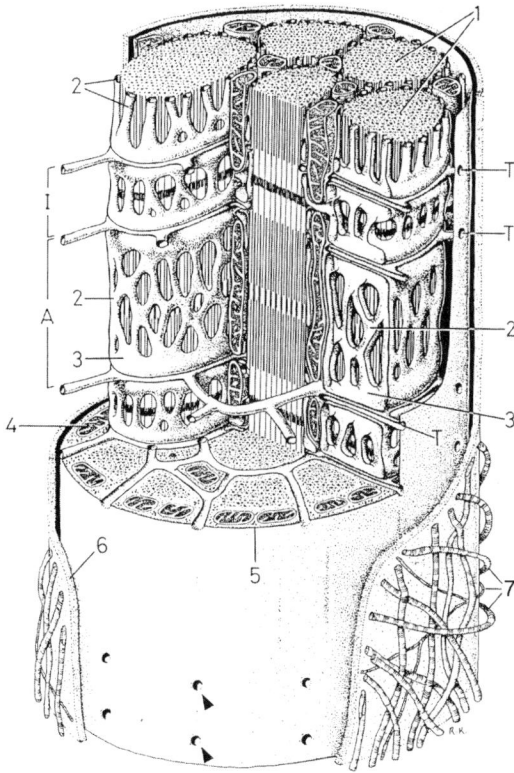

FIG. 8.3—A three-dimensional view of the internal structure of a muscle fiber. Every myofibril (1) is surrounded by a parallel arrangement of sarcoplasmic reticulum (2) that converges at the terminal cisternae (3). Between each terminal at the A–I junction is an invagination of the sarcolemma called a T tubule (T). Mitochondria (4) are present between myofibrils. The sarcolemma is surrounded by a basement membrane (6) and a network of reticular and collagen fibrils (7) surround the cell. (Adapted from Kristic 1984:265.)

TABLE 8.1—Properties of muscle fiber types in untrained horses

	Type 1	Type 2A	Type 2B
Speed of contractions	Slow	Fast	Very fast
Fatigability	Low	Intermediate	High
Oxidative capacity	High	Intermediate	Low
Glycolytic capacity	Low	High	High
Glycogen content	Low	High	High
Fat content	High	Intermediate	Low
Myoglobin	High	Intermediate	Low

(Table 8.1). Type 1 fibers contain slow myosin, contract slowly, have a high volume of mitochondria, and can hold a tetanic twitch for long durations without fatigue. Their resistance to fatigue is in part related to their ability to generate adenosine triphosphate (ATP) through mitochondria oxidation. In addition to having the highest oxidative capacity, type 1 fibers also have the highest myoglobin stores, lipid stores, and density of capillaries, as well as the lowest glycogen stores and glycolytic enzyme capacity of the three fiber types. Fast-twitch muscle fibers or type 2 fibers contract faster and fatigue earlier than do type 1 fibers. In cats, swine, horses, and ruminants, fast-twitch fibers are readily divided into type 2A and 2B fibers. Type 2B fibers contain the IIx myosin heavy-chain isoform and have the fastest contractile speed, the largest cross-sectional area, the highest glycogen stores and glycolytic capacity, and the lowest oxidative capacity (Lopez Rivero 1996b). As such, they are ideally suited to short, fast bursts of power. Type 2A fibers contain the IIa myosin heavy-chain isoform, are intermediate in contractile speed, and have metabolic properties intermediate between type 1 and type 2B fibers. Distinctive light-chain and heavy-chain myosin isoforms have been found in some fibers of the masseter muscle in dogs; these fibers have been designated as type 2M (Orvis and Cardinet III 1981).

In birds and rodents, many muscles exclusively contain fast-twitch or slow-twitch muscle fibers. Most muscles in domestic animals contain a mixture of muscle fiber types (Figure 8.4A). The muscle fiber composition, the percentage of type 1, 2A, and 2B fibers, and muscle fiber cross-sectional areas vary greatly between muscle groups, among individuals, and between breeds. These proportions are not constant, as training can alter the fiber composition and fiber size in the same muscle over time. Breed differences have been extensively studied in horses (Snow and Valberg 1994). These studies show that propulsive locomotor muscles such as the gluteus contain a predominance of fast-twitch type 2 muscle fibers, with the highest density of type 1 fibers located deeper within the muscle. In general, quarter horses and thoroughbreds have the highest percentage of fast-twitch muscle fibers (80% to 90%), standardbreds have an intermediate number (75%), and donkeys have the lowest percentage of type 2 fibers in locomotor muscles. Greyhounds have a higher proportion of fast-twitch fibers than do other dog breeds

voltage sensor, within T tubules is activated by depolarization triggering the opening of the juxtaposing terminal cisterna calcium-release channel (ryanodine receptor). The efflux of calcium from the sarcoplasmic reticulum into the myoplasm binds to troponin C on the thin filaments of the myofibrils. The activated troponin-tropomyosin complex then allows actin and myosin interaction and the generation of force through myosin crossbridge cycling and adenosine triphosphatase (ATPase) activity. Myosin slides over the thin filament in a ratchetlike fashion shortening the length of the entire sarcomere, which in turn shortens the length of the myofibril and subsequently the muscle fiber.

Muscle Fiber Types. Myosin isoforms determine the speed with which a muscle cell can contract, and the activity of enzymes involved in oxidative metabolism will determine how readily a muscle fiber fatigues

(Gunn 1978). With growth and training, there is a change in the length and breadth of a fiber, and a change in the proportion of fiber types rather than an increase in the number of muscle fibers. In young horses intensively trained at speed, the proportion of type 2A fibers increases concomitant with a decrease in type 2B fibers (Roneus et al. 1993).

Muscle Fiber Recruitment. When a muscle contracts during exercise, it does so in response to a predetermined recruitment of particular muscle fibers. This orderly recruitment of muscle fibers leads to smooth, coordinated movement. Each motor unit contains fibers of the same type. As exercise begins, a select number of motor units are recruited to provide the power to advance the limb. At slow exercise intensities, type 1 muscle fibers and a small number of type 2A muscle fibers are stimulated. The force produced by any muscle is proportional to the cross-sectional area that is active. As the speed or duration of exercise increases, more muscle fibers will be recruited, which occurs in the order of their contractile speed. Only at near-maximal exercise intensities or after several hours of submaximal exercise are type 2B fibers recruited (Valberg 1986).

Metabolic Responses to Exercise

ENERGY PATHWAYS. The basic unit of energy in the cell is *adenosine triphosphate* (ATP). This molecule stores energy in the form of high-energy phosphate bonds. During muscle contractions, ATP is utilized to shorten the contractile proteins and to power the cell-membrane ion pumps. Glycogenolysis, glycolysis, the Krebs cycle, oxidative phosphorylation by the electron-transport chain, β oxidation of free fatty acids (FFAs), and purine nucleotide deamination all serve to supply the muscle cell with ATP. A number of interdependent factors appear to influence the metabolic pathways used for energy production during exercise. These include the speed and duration of exercise, the muscle fiber composition, the metabolic properties of the muscle fibers recruited, and the availability of oxygen and different energy substrates.

ENERGY SOURCES. Creatine phosphate serves as a small store of immediate energy within the muscle fibers. Glucose is stored in the body in the form of glycogen, a long, branched polymer of glucose molecules. The largest deposits of glycogen are in the liver and muscle cells. Up to 8% of the liver's weight and up to 1% to 2% of the muscle's weight may be in the form of glycogen. Sympathetic stimulation of the nervous system, as occurs in exercise, causes an increase in the circulating levels of epinephrine and glucagon. These hormones activate the breakdown of glycogen to glucose molecules. The muscle or liver cells shift from glycogen formation to glycogenolysis to supply free glucose. When this process occurs in the liver, free glucose is released into the bloodstream. Muscle cells obtain glucose from the blood and from glycogen stored within the muscle cell. Fat serves as another energy-rich fuel source. FFAs released from adipose tissue or from the liver can be taken up by the muscle cells and burned aerobically. Small intracellular triglyceride stores are also present within type 1 and 2A muscle fibers.

METABOLIC PATHWAYS. Anaerobic pathways such as glycolysis, creatine phosphate, and the purine nucleotide cycle are found within the cell cytoplasm. This pathway, which converts glucose to pyruvate and then lactate, provides two molecules of ATP for each molecule of glucose metabolized. Aerobic pathways such as the Krebs cycle, β oxidation of FFA, and the electron-transport chain are located within the cell's mitochondria and provide the bulk of ATP for the cell as long as oxygen is plentiful. The efficiency of mitochondrial pathways is demonstrated by the ability to generate 38 molecules of ATP from oxidation of 1 molecule of glucose or the generation of up to 146 molecules of ATP from β oxidation of an FFA.

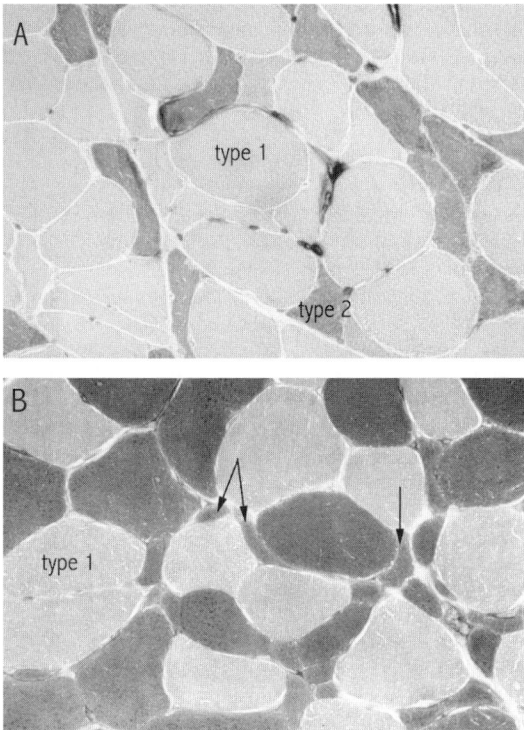

FIG. 8.4—**A:** An ATPase stain (pH 9.4) of a cross section of skeletal muscle from a dog with denervation atrophy. Note the angular shape of both lightly stained (type 1) and darkly stained (type 2) fibers. **B:** An ATPase stain (pH 9.4) of a cross section of skeletal muscle from a dog with Cushing's disease. The myogenic atrophy is characterized by small type 2 fibers (arrows). (Photo courtesy of Dr. G.H. Cardinet III.)

AEROBIC EXERCISE. At submaximal exercise speeds, oxygen is readily available, and slow-twitch fibers as well as fast-twitch fibers with a high oxidative capacity are recruited (Valberg 1986). Intramuscular supplies of ATP and creatine phosphate are quickly utilized and energy must be derived from glucose in the muscle fibers. Glucose is burned in the mitochondria to form waste products such as water and carbon dioxide. Glucose and FFA are delivered to the muscles by the bloodstream within minutes of beginning submaximal exercise. The muscle gradually begins to burn fat as aerobic exercise continues and, as such, the rate of intramuscular glycogen utilization steadily declines over time as the oxidation of FFA increases (Hodgson 1985). Oxidative metabolism is highly efficient. It provides much more ATP per molecule of substrate (glucose or FFA) than does anaerobic metabolism without altering intracellular pH. By using FFA, intramuscular glycogen stores are spared. Fatigue during prolonged submaximal exercise occurs when a combination of the following occurs: intramuscular glycogen concentrations become depleted, muscle temperatures become markedly elevated, electrolyte concentrations are altered, or neuromuscular fatigue occurs (Table 8.2). Very little lactic acid accumulates at fatigue in horses performing submaximal exercise (Hodgson 1985).

ANAEROBIC EXERCISE. With any form of exercise a small amount of anaerobic metabolism occurs, but at submaximal speeds the majority of energy is produced by aerobic metabolism. As the speed of exercise increases, so does the energy demand placed on the muscle. More muscle fibers are recruited, including type 2B fibers, and more oxygen is consumed by the horse until it reaches a speed where the delivery of oxygen or the ability to utilize oxidative processes becomes limiting. At the point of maximum oxygen consumption (VO_{2max}), any further energy must be generated by anaerobic glycolysis or deamination of ATP. With their rich supply of glycolytic enzymes and limited capacity for aerobic metabolism, type 2B fibers are uniquely suited for anaerobic glycolysis. With type 2B fiber recruitment at speeds beyond the point of maximal oxygen uptake, an exponential rise in blood lactate accumulation occurs. The advantages of anaerobic glycolysis are that oxygen is not required and that it provides a rapid supply of ATP. Depletion of glycogen

stores does not limit maximal exercise, because anaerobic glycolysis is inhibited by a lactic acidosis before muscle glycogen is markedly depleted. Low intramuscular pH caused by lactate and hydrogen-ion accumulation inhibits phosphofructokinase enzyme, the rate-limiting step in glycolysis (Table 8.2). Muscle pH can fall as low as 6.4 following maximal exercise, at which point both glycolysis and muscle contraction are inhibited (Harris et al. 1990). The ability to buffer or remove hydrogen ions becomes very important for muscle function during maximal exercise. The amount of lactic acid in the circulation following exercise is in part directly related to the percentage of low-oxidative type 2B fibers in the muscle and the duration of high-intensity exercise (Valberg et al. 1985).

At top speeds, as the intramuscular stores of ATP and energy demands outstrip its innate ability to produce ATP, the cell turns to its last venue of energy production: the purine nucleotide cycle (Harris et al. 1991). Short term, this produces ATP for muscle contraction from the excess of intramuscular ADP. However, the total nucleotide pool is depleted. For intracellular stores of ADP and ATP to be replenished, at least 30 to 60 minutes is required. Ultimately, fatigue may be related to depleted ATP stores within individual muscle fibers (Table 8.2). The levels of lactate and ATP in individual fibers during maximal exercise may be more important for the onset of fatigue than are the measured concentrations in whole-muscle samples (Essen Gustavsson et al. 1997).

Effect of Training

ENDURANCE TRAINING IN HORSES. Endurance training changes the contractile and metabolic profiles of skeletal muscles. After a short period of training, the volume density of mitochondria, and thus the oxidative enzyme capacity, both increase. Over a 6-month period, the ratio of type 2A/2B fibers increases in horses, the cross-sectional area of type 2B muscle fibers decreases, and the capillarization of all fiber types increases (Lopez Rivero et al. 1991). These adaptations favor the delivery of oxygen and blood-borne substrates, the early activation of oxidative metabolism, and the utilization of FFA in muscle fibers. By sparing muscle glycogen, endurance is enhanced, and fatigue is delayed.

SPEED TRAINING IN HORSES. With training at high intensities, the speed at which a horse begins to accumulate lactate should gradually increase, delaying the onset of lactate accumulation and ATP depletion. This is accomplished by an increase in the oxidative capacity (by increased mitochondrial volume) and capillarization of all muscle fiber types, including type 2B fibers. Training of 2- and 3-year-old standardbred and thoroughbred racehorses in Scandinavia had been shown to reduce the percentage of type 2B fibers and increase the percentage of type 2A fibers, as well as decrease the cross-sectional area of type 2B fibers

TABLE 8.2—Factors that contribute to fatigue during aerobic and anaerobic exercise intensities

Aerobic exercise	Anaerobic exercise
Glycogen depletion	Lactic acidosis
Hyperthermia	Inhibition of PFK
Electrolyte depletion	Impaired intracellular
Myalgia and motivation	calcium regulation
	Depletion of CP and ATP
	Myalgia and motivation

PFK, phosphofructokinase; CP, creatine phosphate; and ATP, adenosine triphosphate.

(Roneus et al. 1993). Although an increase in oxidative capacity may be metabolically advantageous, a decrease in the percentage of type 2B fibers and a decrease in their cross-sectional areas may deleteriously affect their speed and force of contraction. Muscle must have the ability to generate energy via anaerobic glycolysis for racehorses to be successful. Obviously, a balance is required between skeletal muscle fiber metabolic and contractile properties for optimum speed and endurance. Since the muscle fiber composition and fiber properties vary so greatly among horses, achievement of this balance may be different for each horse.

BASIC PATHOLOGICAL REACTIONS OF SKELETAL MUSCLE. A sound classification system for muscle disorders in domestic animals is difficult to design because the pathophysiological basis for many animal myopathies remains unknown. In the present chapter, muscle diseases are grouped under three characteristic reactions of muscle to congenital or acquired diseases: (a) muscle atrophy, (b) muscle necrosis and regeneration, and (c) abnormal electrical conduction in the neuromuscular junction and muscle cell membrane. Selected neuromuscular disorders of small and large animals are presented to highlight the various mechanisms that are capable of producing atrophy, muscle necrosis, or altered neuromuscular excitability.

Muscle Atrophy. Atrophy is defined as a reduction in muscle size, specifically a reduction in muscle fiber diameter or cross-sectional area. Muscle atrophy can be due to loss of trophic neural stimulation or to myopathic processes. Regardless of the cause, a reduction in muscle size results from muscle protein degradation by lysosomal and nonlysosomal pathways within the cell (Tawa and Goldberg 1994). Lysosomal degradation occurs by acid hydrolases and proteases within autophagic vacuoles. Stimuli include a lack of amino acids and lack of insulin. Calcium-dependent thiol proteases called calpain I and II also cause proteolysis, particularly when intracellular calcium concentrations increase due to a loss of cell-membrane integrity or loss of muscle tension. The bulk of cytosolic proteolysis in many cells occurs by an ATP-ubiquitin-dependent process that is particularly active with infection, inflammation, denervation, and malnutrition. This is the type of proteolysis that is capable of complete degradation of myofilaments to their amino acid components (Tawa and Goldberg 1994).

NEUROGENIC ATROPHY. Neurogenic atrophy is not specific for muscle fiber type and classically involves both fast-twitch and slow-twitch muscle fibers (Figure 8.4B). Denervation removes the normal low-level tonic neural stimulus that is necessary to maintain muscle fiber mass. Following denervation, lysosomal and cytosolic protein degradation is markedly increased without an overall change in protein synthesis (Tawa

and Goldberg 1994). Very small concave angular fibers are characteristically surrounded by compensatory hypertrophy of other fibers that have intact motor-unit activity. Complete denervation of a muscle results in more than a 50% loss of muscle mass within a 2- to 3-week period (Hulland 1985; Cumming et al. 1994). A good example of this is "sweeney" in horses, in which the suprascapular nerve is damaged by trauma to the shoulder, and muscles over the scapula atrophy. Conditions that cause generalized motor-neuron involvement, such as equine motor-neuron disease or progressive spinal muscular atrophy in Brittany spaniels, show a slower but marked progression toward generalized muscle atrophy. Electromyographic abnormalities following denervation are apparent within 5 days, and it may take 3 weeks for maximal changes to develop. Increased insertional activity, positive sharp waves, and bizarre high-frequency discharges and fibrillation potentials are seen with electromyographic examination of denervated muscle.

Following denervation, sprouts of nearby intact axons reinnervate muscle fibers. With enlargement of motor units, the random distribution of fiber type is altered, and a grouping of fibers according to type rather than a random mosaic pattern is seen. Histologically, this indicator of chronic denervation with reinnervation is termed *type grouping* (Figure 8.5).

MYOGENIC ATROPHY. Myogenic atrophy may occur at variable rates, depending on its cause. Disuse, malnutrition, cachexia, and corticosteroid excess result in a gradual loss of muscle mass. The overall response of skeletal muscle is to maintain essential postural muscle groups, whereas less essential groups undergo significant reduction in muscle mass. With malnutrition, 30% to 50% of the muscle mass may be lost in the first 1 to 2 months (Hulland 1985). Corticosteroid myopathy and Cushing's disease produce gradual

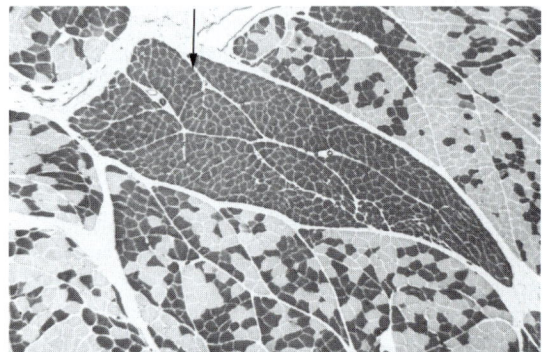

FIG. 8.5—An ATPase stain (pH 9.4) of a cross section of muscle fascicles. Note the lack of a normal mosaic pattern of type 1 and type 2 fibers with one fascicle (arrow) consisting solely of type 2 fibers. This pattern is called type grouping and is typical of denervation followed by renervation. (Photo courtesy of Dr. G.H. Cardinet III.)

marked atrophy and weakness of extremity and trunk limb muscles. With normal feed consumption, corticosteroid-induced atrophy appears primarily related to decreased protein synthesis, whereas in animals with poor appetites, atrophy may be primarily from enhanced ATP-dependent proteolysis (Tawa and Goldberg 1994). Myogenic atrophy is often distinguished from neurogenic atrophy by slow progression, normal electromyographic findings, and muscle biopsy specimens that are characterized by exclusive atrophy of type 2 muscle fibers (Figure 8.4B). Rapid myogenic atrophy may occur following severe rhabdomyolysis due to cellular breakdown. In addition, rapid atrophy of specific muscle groups can occur with immune-mediated myopathies due to cellular damage and muscle wasting (see the section *Specific Causes of Rhabdomyolysis* for more information).

Muscle Necrosis and Regeneration

NECROSIS. Muscle necrosis or rhabdomyolysis involves injury to all organelles within a muscle fiber and may affect an entire fiber or a segment of several sarcomeres within a fiber. Loss of muscle membrane integrity can occur from oxidant damage, toxicities, electrolyte imbalances, infections, immune-mediated disorders, and heritable defects in the subsarcolemmal cytoskeleton (Table 8.3). Metabolic disturbances resulting in an inability to produce ATP or inability to regulate myoplasmic calcium concentrations may also cause rhabdomyolysis. Although the inciting causes may differ, they usually share a final common pathway leading to cell death (McArdle and Jackson 1997). Under normal conditions, myoplasmic calcium concentrations are extremely low (10^{-7} M), and considerable energy is expended to pump the calcium that accumulates in the sarcoplasm during contraction back into the sarcoplasmic reticulum. If cell membrane or sarcoplasmic reticulum function is disrupted or if the energy pathways that generate ATP for the calcium pump are impaired, excessive calcium may accumulate in the sarcoplasm. Although some calcium can be sequestered by the mitochondria, eventually mitochondria become overloaded, and oxidative metabolism ceases. Oxygen free radicals are generated that damage cell membranes. Elevated myoplasmic calcium activates phospholipases, which promote inflammation via the arachidonic cascade. Calcium-dependent proteases are stimulated, resulting in proteolysis of enzymes and contractile filaments. Complement is activated, resulting in the formation of membrane-attack complexes that lyse membranous organelles. Within 16 to 48 hours of the muscle injury, macrophage infiltration occurs in order to phagocytose and remove the necrotic debris.

Histologically, acute rhabdomyolysis is characterized by a homogenized appearance of the myoplasm due to loss of the cross-striations of contractile proteins (Figure 8.6A and B). This appearance is known as *hyalinization*. Acute necrosis is easily demonstrated in frozen section with special stains that reveal mitochon-

TABLE 8.3—Causes of rhabdomyolysis

Sarcolemmal defects
    Muscular dystrophy
Nutritional
    Deficiency of vitamin E and selenium
    Electrolyte imbalances (hypokalemia)
Toxic
    Ionophores (monensin)
    Plants (white snake root)
Infectious
    Viral (influenza)
    Bacterial (*Clostridia*)
    Parasitic (*Toxoplasma* and *Sarcocystis*)
Immune mediated
    Masseter muscle myositis
    Streptococcus equi myopathy
    Polymyositis/dermatomysitis
Metabolic
    Glycogenoses (II, III, IV, V, and VII)
    Lipid storage myopathies (carnitine deficiency)
    Mitochondrial myopathies (pyruvate dehydrogenase, complex I, and cytochrome C oxidase)
    Calcium regulation (malignant hyperthermia and recurrent exertional rhabdomyolysis)

drial disruption. Within days, macrophage infiltration in the necrotic segment will be apparent and is a hallmark of myonecrosis (Figure 8.6C).

REGENERATION. Muscle has a remarkable ability to regenerate. Factors that determine the extent to which repair is possible include the extent of tissue necrosis, the preservation of nerve and blood supply, and the integrity of the architecture within the muscle. If the basement membrane of the fiber is intact, complete repair is often possible. Within hours of muscle cell damage, sarcolemmal membrane proliferation seals off muscle fiber segments (Figure 8.7). Macrophages move into the damaged segment to remove all cellular debris (Figures 8.6D and 8.7). Since myonuclei are in a postmitotic state, satellite cells are the primary source of myogenic precursor cells that migrate along the basement membrane into the damaged segment and differentiate to form myoblasts (Figure 8.7). Myoblasts fuse with the damaged fiber ends and each other to create regenerative myotubes within 3 to 4 days of injury. Myotubes appear as basophilic small myofibers with multiple large central nuclei and prominent nucleoli. As myofilaments are produced, the nuclei are pushed to a subsarcolemmal location, and mature muscle fibers develop within a month of the original damage (Cumming et al. 1994).

Extensive muscle damage that disrupts numerous cells and their blood supply prevents normal muscle regeneration by allowing fibroblast proliferation. Collagen deposition between fibers produces a major obstacle for rejoining of damaged muscle segments. Extensive connective tissue and fatty infiltration are features of end-stage muscle that signal an inability to regenerate further.

CLINICAL DETECTION. Severe muscle cell necrosis commonly produces signs of muscle pain, contracture, elevated respiratory, and excessive sweating and myo-

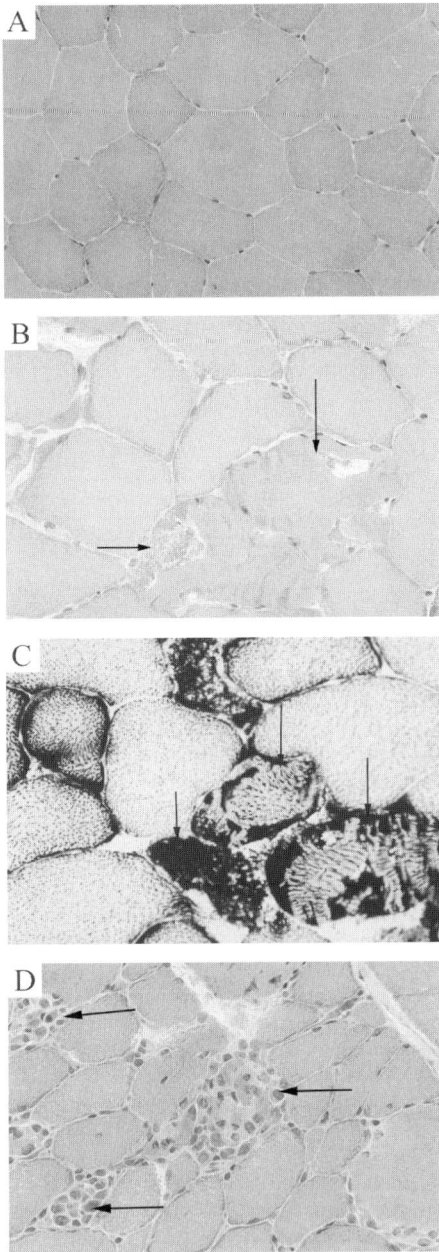

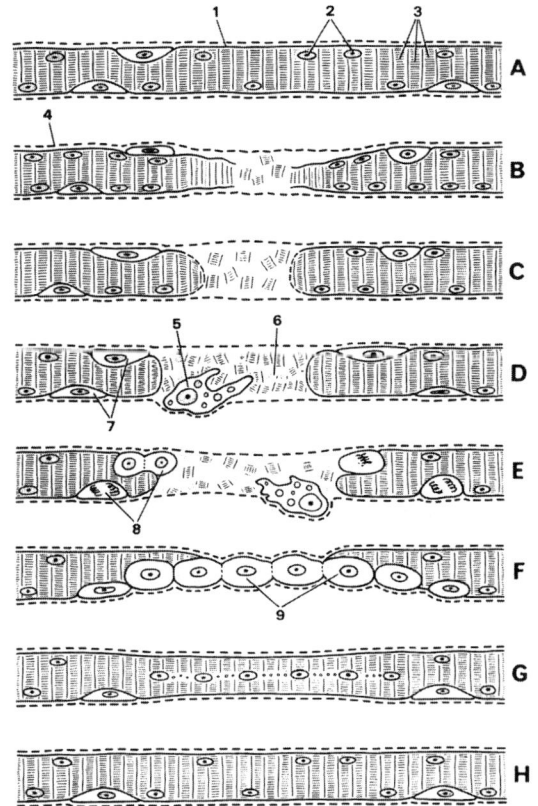

FIG. 8.7—Regeneration of a skeletal muscle fiber. **A:** A healthy fiber showing an intact sarcolemma (1), multiple subsarcolemmal nuclei (2) and myofibrils in register (3). **B:** Segmental disruption of the fiber with an intact basement membrane (4). **C:** Proliferation of the sarcolemmal membrane occurs to compartmentalize the damaged areas. **D:** Macrophages (5) infiltrate and phagocytose necrotic debris (6). **E:** Satellite cells (7) are activated and replicate to form myoblasts (8). **F:** Myoblasts fuse to form myotubes (9). **G:** Synthesis of new myofilaments and formation of myofibrils progress, and myonuclei remain in a central position. **H:** A repaired fiber with peripheral nuclei following complete myofibrillogenesis. (Adapted from Kristic 1984:273.)

FIG. 8.6—A cross section of gluteal muscle from a normal horse **(A)** and a horse with an exertional myopathy **(B)** obtained within minutes of undergoing acute necrosis. Note the loss of membrane integrity, lack of an organized contractile protein pattern (vertical arrow), and increased calcium staining darkly under the sarcolemma (horizontal arrow) in B. A nicotinamide adenine dinucleotide dehydrogenase (NADH) stain **(C)** of the same biopsy as B showing the disruption of the mitochondrial staining pattern (arrows) with acute necrosis. Hematoxylin-eosin stain of a muscle biopsy obtained 3 days after acute necrosis **(D)** shows the typical infiltration of macrophages within necrotic fibers (arrows).

globinuria. It is possible, however, to have occult myoglobinuria in animals free of pain. A clinical diagnosis of rhabdomyolysis is usually accomplished by determination of the activity or concentration of muscle proteins that leak into the serum following muscle damage. Several events may occur to cause the amount of these proteins to be elevated. Necrosis with disruption of the cell membrane results in diffusion of cellular contents, including enzymes into the lymphatic or blood circulation. Other factors may exert a modest influence upon the activities of muscle enzymes within the circulation. These include permeability of the cell membrane, rate of enzyme production, alternate sources of the enzyme, rate of enzyme excretion/

degradation, and alterations to the pathways involved in enzyme removal or inactivation (Kramer 1980).

Two enzymes are used routinely in the assessment of muscular diseases in animals: creatine kinase (CK) and aspartate transaminase (AST). Serum CK is found predominantly in skeletal and cardiac muscle and is readily liberated into the extracellular fluid when the muscle cell membrane is disrupted. Serum activity of this enzyme increases within hours in response to a significant muscle insult. A three- to fivefold increase in serum CK from normal values is believed to represent necrosis of approximately 20 g of muscle tissue (Volfinger et al. 1996). Serum AST, previously known as serum glutamic-oxaloacetic transaminase (SGOT), has high activity in skeletal and cardiac muscle and also in liver, red blood cells, and other tissues. Elevations in AST are not specific for myonecrosis, and increases could be the result of hemolysis, muscle, liver, or other organ damage. AST activity rises more slowly in response to myonecrosis than does CK, often peaking between 12 and 24 hours after the insult, and the half-life of AST is much longer than that of CK.

Elevation in serum myoglobin concentrations provides an indication of acute muscle damage, but few veterinary laboratories perform this assay. Myoglobin is a small protein that leaks into plasma immediately after muscle damage and is rapidly cleared in the urine by the kidney. Renal tubular cells attempt to resorb myoglobin from the urine. In quantities that produce urine discoloration, particularly when urine is acidic, myoglobin can cause severe renal tubular nephrosis.

Severe rhabdomyolysis can also produce fluid and electrolyte disturbances. Muscle comprises 45% of body mass and represents the largest volume of intracellular fluid. With crush injuries or severe rhabdomyolysis, intracellular electrolytes move from muscle into the bloodstream, causing hyperkalemia and hyperphosphatemia. Vascular fluid, sodium, chloride, and calcium move down a concentration gradient into damaged muscle, creating hypovolemia, hemoconcentration, hyponatremia, hypochloremia, and hypocalcemia (Perkins et al. 1998). These alterations may be life-threatening due hyperkalemic bradycardia and hypovolemic shock.

SPECIFIC CAUSES OF RHABDOMYOLYSIS

MUSCULAR DYSTROPHY. Muscular dystrophies in small animals have been defined as a group of primary myopathies that are inherited and are characterized by progressive degeneration of skeletal muscle. Muscular dystrophies have been described in a number of dog and cat breeds. As an example, an X-linked form of muscular dystrophy in golden retrievers is first seen in male puppies that are stunted, show elbow abduction, bunny hop-like gait, and possibly trismus (inability to open the jaw) (Kornegay et al. 1988). Over time, the conditions show extensive atrophy of the trunk, limb, and temporal muscles, progressing to a stiff plantigrade-like stance. Pharyngeal and esophageal muscles may be involved, and some dogs develop hypertrophy of the tongue muscles. Serum CK activity is markedly increased, with peak activity at 6 to 8 weeks of age. Muscle biopsy specimens are characterized by myofiber size variation, necrosis with prominent multifocal calcification of muscle fibers, and regeneration with perimysial and endomysial fibrosis. The form of muscular dystrophy in golden retrievers is similar to Duchenne's muscular dystrophy in humans and is the result of the lack of a large sarcolemmal protein called *dystrophin*. A splice-site mutation in the dystrophin gene results in a truncated dystrophin protein. Increased permeability of the sarcolemma to calcium occurs as a result of mechanical stress generated during contraction resulting in myonecrosis and regeneration (Schatzberg et al. 1998). Recurrent muscle damage and regeneration eventually lead to significant fibrosis.

NUTRITIONAL CAUSES OF RHABDOMYOLYSIS

Vitamin E and Selenium Deficiency [Coauthored by John Maas]. Nutritional myodegeneration (NMD) (also know as white muscle disease or nutritional muscular dystrophy) is a peracute-to-subacute myodegenerative disease of cardiac and skeletal muscle caused by a dietary deficiency of selenium and/or vitamin E (McMurray and Rice 1982; Dill and Rehbun 1985). This syndrome occurs in most farm animal species but is most commonly found in young, rapidly growing calves, lambs, kids, and foals, particularly those born to dams that consumed selenium-deficient diets during gestation. Selenium and vitamin E appear to be synergistic in preventing NMD. However, on the basis of prophylaxis and response to treatment, selenium deficiency appears to be the most important.

The effects of selenium and vitamin E deficiency have been postulated to result, at least in part, from the destruction of cell membranes and proteins, leading to a loss of cellular integrity. Selenium has been shown to be an essential component of at least five selenoproteins: three glutathione peroxidase enzymes, a deiodinase in liver and kidney that converts T_4 to T_3, and selenoprotein P (a plasma protein of unknown function) (Burk and Hill 1993). These proteins combined with vitamin E (α-tocopherol) serve as biological antioxidants. During normal cellular metabolism, highly reactive forms of oxygen (free radicals) are produced. These include hydrogen peroxide, hydroperoxides, lipoperoxides, superoxide, various hydroxy radicals, and singlet oxygen. Vitamin E is active within the cell membrane as a lipid-soluble antioxidant that scavenges free radicals that otherwise might react with unsaturated fatty acids to form lipid hydroperoxides. In contrast, glutathione peroxidase (GSH-Px) destroys hydrogen peroxide and lipoperoxides that have already been formed and converts them to water or relatively harmless alcohols. Other enzymes such as catalase and superoxide dismutase are also involved in this protective process.

Apparently, important interrelationships exist between the selenium and vitamin E status of the animal, the level of polyunsaturated fatty acids (PUFAs) in the diet and NMD, particularly in ruminants (McMurray and Rice 1982). PUFAs of dietary origin can undergo peroxidation to hydroperoxides forming toxic free radicals. During active growing periods, pasture grasses and plants contain high concentrations of linolenic acid, a PUFA. Under normal conditions, the rumen is thought to be important in saturating dietary unsaturated fatty acids. However, concentrations of PUFAs in the plasma often increase in calves recently turned out to pasture, possibly enhancing the chance of free radical formation and tissue damage. This indicates that the capacity of the various protective mechanisms can be overwhelmed by dietary factors such as high levels of PUFA. Not surprisingly, selenium or vitamin E-deficient animals may be at a greatly increased risk of tissue oxidative damage when exposed to such diets. However, the potential for induction of NMD by this process should not be overemphasized, since calves on a milk diet may be severely affected.

The precise interrelationships between selenium, vitamin E, other metabolic factors, and triggering mechanisms in NMD are not fully understood because many animals deficient in selenium and/or vitamin E have no evidence of muscle disease. In certain situations, deficiencies of both selenium and vitamin E are necessary for disease to occur. In other animals, NMD can occur when a deficiency of only one of the agents is present and the other is normal in blood and tissues.

Hypokalemia. Rhabdomyolysis in cats may occur as a result of prolonged dietary deficiency of potassium or excessive urinary potassium losses associated with chronic renal disease (Dow et al. 1989). Cats show signs of a stiff stilted gait, exercise intolerance, neck ventroflexion, and muscle pain. Serum elevations of CK and AST and hypokalemia are evident in serum biochemical profiles. Muscle biopsy samples may be normal or show a vacuolar myopathy with mild rhabdomyolysis. Weakness is likely due to hypopolarization of muscle cell membranes due to hypokalemia. The mechanisms proposed for rhabdomyolysis include ischemia due to hypokalemia-induced vasoconstriction and osmotic effects of increased membrane permeability to sodium resulting in sodium chloride, as well as free water entering the myocyte, which causes osmotic expansion (Dow and Fettman 1992). Postpartum cows treated for ketosis with repeated doses of short-acting corticosteroid also show severe muscle weakness and recumbency as a result of hypokalemia (Sattler et al. 1998). Weakness leading to prolonged recumbency may cause ischemic necrosis of the compressed muscles.

TOXIC CAUSES OF RHABDOMYOLYSIS. Toxic causes of rhabdomyolysis are rare in small animals but occur occasionally in ruminants and horses as a result of ingestion of toxic substances in feed or forage. For their growth-promotion and coccidiostat properties, ionophores are commonly added to ruminant feeds.

Accidental ingestion by dogs or horses or overdoses in ruminant feeds can produce cardiomyopathies and rhabdomyolysis (Wilson 1980; Geor and Robinson 1985). At toxic doses, ionophores form cationic complexes of calcium, sodium, and potassium ions that enhance their transport across cell membranes. This enhanced transport leads to myocardial and skeletal muscle calcium overload, mitochondrial dysfunction, and myonecrosis. Tremetone-containing plants, such as white snakeroot (*Eupatorium rugosum*) and rayless goldenrod (*Isocoma wrightii*), in hay or pasture cause severe rhabdomyolysis in horses. White snakeroot grows in shaded areas of the eastern and central United States and rayless goldenrod is common in the Southwest on open pastures (Beier et al. 1993). The precise mechanism of myonecrosis is unclear.

INFECTIOUS CAUSES OF RHABDOMYOLYSIS

Clostridial Myonecrosis. Various species of the spore-forming clostridial organisms cause acute myonecrosis in horses and ruminants. Infections are characterized by a rapid clinical course, fever, systemic toxemia, and high mortality (Rebhun et al. 1985; Erwin 1986). There is usually only one primary site of infection in a limb or trunk muscle. Areas around recent injections are common sites of myonecrosis in horses. Clostridial agents are ubiquitous to the environment and can frequently be cultured from the feces, the intestinal tract, and other internal organs of a variety of species. Development of clostridial myonecrosis following an intramuscular injection or penetrating wound may be the result of direct spore deposition into the tissue in association with penetration. If suitable conditions prevail within the muscle, the spores undergo a conversion into the vegetative, toxin-producing form of the organism. In contrast, the pathogenesis of the disease is more difficult to explain when a wound does not exist. It is postulated that clostridial agents gain access to the body through the alimentary tract, and are present in liver and muscle in the dormant spore form (Williams 1977). Subsequently, when local tissue is devitalized and conditions become appropriate for the spores to germinate, the rapid vegetative process ensues. The proliferation of clostridial agents in devitalized tissues is associated with the release of powerful exotoxins responsible for the local necrotizing myositis and systemic toxemia. The toxins vary depending on the clostridial species involved, but invariably they act to create widespread organ dysfunction.

Virus-associated Myopathies. Virus-associated myopathies are uncommon. Some viral infections of large animals—such as bovine ephemeral fever, malignant catarrhal fever, bovine virus diarrhea, and bluetongue—may produce necrosis of skeletal and cardiac muscle, in addition to clinical signs of multiple organ dysfunction. Equine influenza A2 and equine herpesvirus 1 have been reported to induce marked muscle stiffness and clinical signs resembling those seen in horses with rhabdomyolysis (Freestone and Carlson 1991).

Toxoplasmosis. Toxoplasma-related myositis is probably the most commonly reported infectious myositis in small animals, with some cases being due to *Neospora caninum* (Dubey 1977; Dubey et al. 1988). Clinical signs include pelvic limb weakness and stiffness, as well as a bunny-hopping gait. Cats serve as the definitive host for *Toxoplasma gondii*, with snails, earthworms, flies, and cockroaches serving as transport hosts for oocysts. The disease is most severe in young dogs and can be transmitted transplacentally as well as acquired by ingestion. The disease may be exacerbated by immunosuppression. Toxoplasma organisms have a predilection for skeletal muscle and can be visualized in muscle biopsy samples. Their presence induces a mononuclear granulomatous inflammation, myonecrosis, atrophy and, in chronic cases, fibrosis. In addition, nerve fiber degeneration, demyelination, and the occasional presence of endoneural cysts in peripheral nerves and nerve roots occur.

Sarcocystosis. Cysts of the sporozoan parasite *Sarcocystis* are commonly seen in routine histological sections of the heart and esophageal and skeletal muscle of cattle, sheep, goats, and horses (Dubey 1976) (Figure 8.8). More than 90% of horses over 8 years of age have sarcocysts in their esophageal muscles. Cysts may pose no problem, but multisystemic dysfunction occurs with heavy infestations (Leek et al. 1977; Fayer 1982; Traub-Dargatz et al. 1994). Acute disease is characterized by fever, mild anemia, anorexia, salivation, weight loss, weakness, muscle fasciculations, and severe depression, which may culminate in death or develop into a chronic myositis and muscle wasting. The life cycle of the parasite involves two hosts: carnivores as the definitive host and cattle or horses as the intermediate host. The most common mechanism for natural infection is by ingestion of feeds contaminated with infected carnivore feces. Laboratory analysis in the acute stages of infection may reveal elevations in serum urea nitrogen and bilirubin concentrations, sorbitol dehydrogenase, Lactate dehydrogenase (LDH), CK, and AST activities. Muscle biopsies may reveal numerous intracellular cysts and a polymorphonuclear inflammatory response that may contain eosinophils. Diagnosis of sarcocystosis requires history, clinical signs, laboratory and serological evaluation, and the demonstration of immature cysts in muscle biopsies. It is important to differentiate between the muscle cysts caused by sarcocystis and those produced by toxoplasmosis, because toxoplasmosis does not cause clinical disease in cattle (Dubey 1976).

IMMUNE-MEDIATED MYOSITIS

Masticatory Muscle Myositis. This disorder is an inflammatory myopathy of the temporal, masseter, and pterygoid muscles in dogs (Shelton et al. 1987). In the

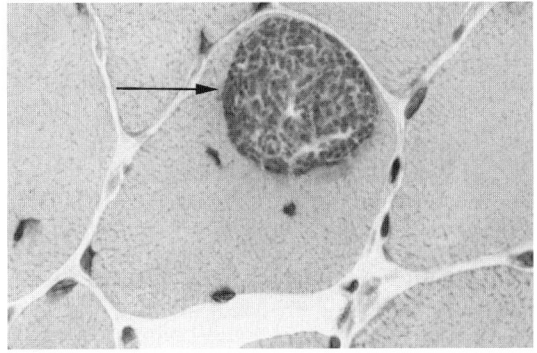

FIG. 8.8—A hematoxylin-eosin stain of equine muscle showing a sarcocyst (arrow) within a muscle fiber.

acute form, swelling and pain may be associated with these muscles. Chronically, there is marked atrophy of the temporal and masseter muscles, resulting in a skull-like appearance to the head and inability to open the jaw (trismus). Histological lesions comprise lymphocytic and plasmacytic cellular infiltrates around muscle fibers and in perivascular locations. Occasionally, eosinophils are present as the predominant infiltrate. In chronic cases, muscle atrophy and fibrosis are apparent. Masticatory muscles are comprised of type 1 and type 2M muscle fibers, which differ in myosin heavy-chain and light-chain composition from limb muscles (Orvis and Cardinet 1981). Dogs with this disorder produce circulating autoantibodies directed against type 2M muscle fibers, suggesting an immunopathogenesis (Shelton et al. 1985) (Figure 8.9).

Immune-mediated Equine Myopathy. Quarter horses have developed a myositis characterized by malaise and rapid atrophy of lumbar and gluteal muscles upon exposure to *Streptococcus equi* or unidentified respiratory infections (Valberg et al. 1996; Valberg 1999). Horses usually do not have any concurrent signs of strangles but will have persistent mild to moderate elevations in serum CK and AST. Muscle biopsies in these cases show a lymphocytic vasculitis and myofiber infiltrate, atrophy of type 2 fibers, and waves of rhabdomyolysis and regeneration (Figure 8.10). Untreated cases may show significant fibrosis around blood vessels. The myositis may reflect epitope sharing between the contractile protein myosin and the M protein of streptococcal organisms that has similar amino acid sequence. Antibody directed toward type 2 fibers has not been demonstrated, which suggests this may be a cell-mediated autoimmunity (personal observation).

Polymyositis. This disorder is a diffuse inflammatory myopathy seen most commonly in large-breed dogs that is believed to have an immune-mediated basis (Kornegay et al. 1980). Weakness, lameness, and exercise intolerance with painful musculature are fre-

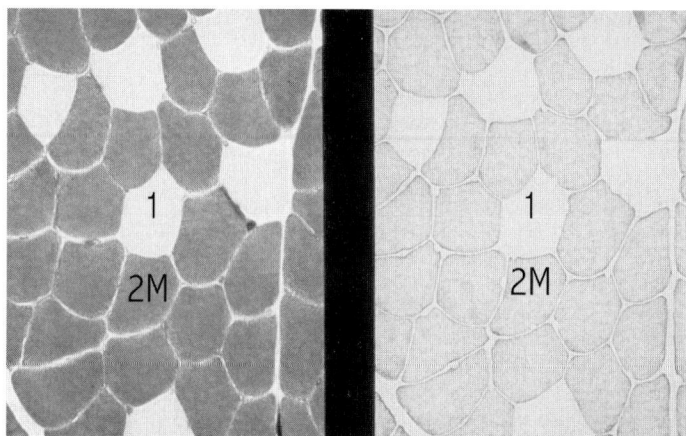

FIG. 8.9—A cross section of masseter muscle from a dog with masticatory muscle myositis stained with myosin ATPase (**left**), and a serial section (**right**) stained for canine antibodies localized by staining for peroxidase activity after incubation with the staphylococcal protein A-horseradish peroxidase conjugates. Note that darkly stained type 2M fibers have antibody staining. (Photo courtesy of Dr. G.H. Cardinet III.)

quently found. Muscle atrophy can occur and may be prominent in masticatory muscles. Occasionally, dogs will also have megaesophagus. Serum CK activity is usually high combined with hypergammaglobulinemia. Multifocal areas of necrosis and phagocytosis of type 1 and type 2 muscle fibers, and perivascular lymphocytic and plasmacytic infiltration and regeneration, are present in numerous areas of skeletal muscle. In humans with polymyositis, the predominant cell type destroying healthy muscle fibers is activated CD8+ T cells and subsequently macrophages. Polymyositis can occur as part of systemic lupus erythematosus or adverse drug

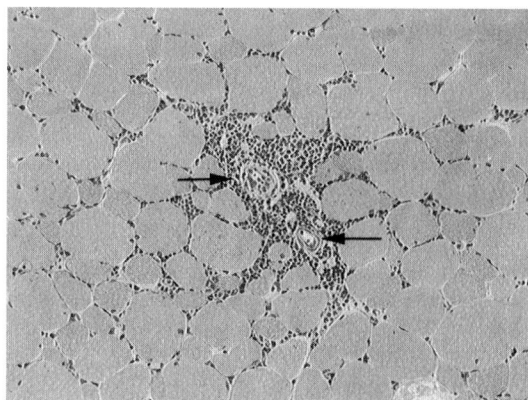

%Accumulated%=0

FIG. 8.10—A cross section of muscle from a horse with immune-mediated myositis. Note the marked mononuclear inflammatory reaction around blood vessels (arrows) and extending to surround muscle fibers.

reaction or as part of a paraneoplastic syndrome (Krum et al. 1977). An immune-mediated etiology is supported by the often rapid response to corticosteroids.

METABOLIC MYOPATHIES

GLYCOGENOSES. Numerous inherited myopathies that have been identified in animals are the result of disruption of a metabolic pathway. Such disorders affecting domestic animals are listed in Table 8.4.

Disorders of glycogen or glucose metabolism are classified as glycogenoses because they result in a characteristic accumulation of excessive amounts of glycogen or potentially abnormal polysaccharide within skeletal muscle (Figure 8.11). Clinically, glycogenoses may present as progressive muscle weakness with or without atrophy or as exertional muscle pain, contracture, and muscle necrosis. Muscle weakness most commonly occurs in Pompe's disease, debrancher, and branching enzyme deficiency (Ceh et al. 1976; Walvoort et al. 1984; Healy et al. 1995; Fyfe et al. 1992; Valberg et al. 2001). Glycogen accumulates in Pompe's disease because of the lack of the lysosomal enzyme acid maltase that degrades glycogen. Weakness has been attributed to the mechanical disruption of the contractile system by extensive accumulation of glycogen. A normal highly branched glycogen molecule provides numerous sites for glucose liberation by myophosphorylase. With branching enzyme deficiency, long straight chains of glycogen accumulate. Weakness may result from a lack of end points to liberate glucose for metabolism. With debranching enzyme deficiency, weakness may be due to the inability to liberate glucose residues from branch points within glycogen. In addition, weakness may be related to the effect of the metabolic defect on spinal motor neurons.

TABLE 8.4—Glycogen storage disorders for which a specific enzyme deficiency has been identified

Type	Species	Breed	Clinical presentation	Enzyme defect	Mode of inheritance	Ref.
II	Canine	Swedish laplands	Progressive weakness, vomiting megaesophagus, and cardiac disease	Acid maltase	AR	Walvoort et al. 1984
II	Bovine	Brahman and Shorthorn	Progressive weakness	Acid maltase	AR	Healy et al. 1995
III	Canine	German shepherd and Akita	Muscle weakness and hepatomegaly	Debrancher	AR	Ceh et al. 1976
IV	Feline	Norwegian forest	Stillbirth, muscle weakness, and atrophy	Brancher	AR	Fyfe et al. 1992
IV	Equine	Quarter horse	Stillbirth, contractures, muscle weakness, and sudden cardiac arrest	Brancher	AR	Valberg et al. 2001
V	Bovine	Charolais	Exercise intolerance and myoglobinuria	Myophosphorylase	AR	Angelos et al. 1995
V	Ovine		Exercise intolerance	Myophosphorylase	AR	Tan et al. 1997
VII	Canine	English springer spaniel	Hemolytic anemia, muscle cramping, and weakness	Phosphofructokinase (PFK-M subunit)	AR	Harvey et al. 1990

AR, autosomal recessive.

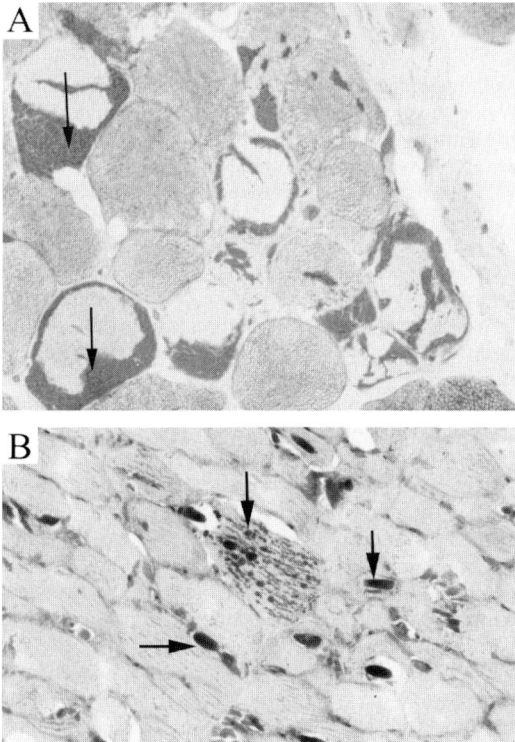

FIG. 8.11—A cross section of skeletal muscle stained with periodic acid-Schiff (PAS) from a horse with polysaccharide storage myopathy (**A**). Note that some fibers have dark myoplasmic PAS stain for glycogen, and others have very intense PAS-positive inclusions of abnormal polysaccharide (arrows). In contrast, a PAS stain from a foal with glycogen branching enzyme deficiency (**B**) shows no normal myoplasmic glycogen but numerous globular or crystalline PAS-positive inclusions (arrows).

Exertional myopathies commonly occur with myophosphorylase deficiency and phosphofructokinase deficiency (Harvey et al. 1990; Angelos et al. 1995; Tan et al. 1997). Deficiencies in glycogenolytic and glycolytic enzymes impair the muscle's ability to utilize the Embden-Myerhoff pathway and thus inhibit the muscle's ability to generate lactic acid. Exercise intolerance with aerobic exercise is believed to be due to impairment of the ability to generate pyruvate for oxidative metabolism as well as a reduction in the ability to generate the high-energy phosphate bonds in creatine phosphate and ATP (Argov et al. 2000). Whether the ATP concentrations become low enough in single muscle fibers to be the cause of muscle necrosis and muscle contractures is still a matter of debate. Draft horses and quarter horses also have a unique glycogen storage disorder that is not due to deficiencies in enzymes of glycogenolysis or glycolysis (Valberg et al. 1992, 1998, 1999). Horses with polysaccharide storage myopathy (PSSM) are reluctant to perform anaerobic exercise, but when forced, can generate normal to high concentrations of lactic acid (Valberg et al. 1999). This PSSM is characterized by the accumulation of both glycogen as well as a less highly branched polysaccharide than normal muscle glycogen. Glycogen accumulation in PSSM appears to have a novel basis related to enhanced insulin sensitivity, muscle glucose uptake, and glycogen synthesis (De la Corte et al. 1999). The connection between increased synthesis of glycogen and rhabdomyolysis has yet to be explained.

LIPID STORAGE DISORDERS. Abnormal accumulation of lipid droplets has been observed in type 1 fibers of dogs with generalized myalgia, weakness, and muscle atrophy (Shelton et al. 1998; Platt et al. 1999). In humans, lipid storage myopathies have been attributed to several different deficiencies of enzymes involved with lipid transport into mitochondria (carnitine palmitoyltransferase deficiency) or β oxidation of FFAs.

Clinical features include muscle necrosis and myoglobinuria without painful contractures. A specific enzyme deficiency remains to be defined for the lipid storage myopathies in dogs.

MITOCHONDRIAL MYOPATHIES. A deficiency of complex 1, the first step in the mitochondrial respiratory chain, was identified in a young Arabian filly that showed signs of extreme fatigue and lactic acidemia with mild exertion (Valberg et al. 1994). This horse showed no changes in serum CK activity following exercise. Histopathological evaluation of muscle biopsy specimens showed an abnormal increase in mitochondrial density with bizarre mitochondrial conformation. Pyruvate dehydrogenase deficiency is suggested to be the cause of mitochondrial myopathy in Clumber and Sussex spaniels (Herrtage and Houlton 1979; Houlton and Herrtage 1980). Old English sheepdogs have been found to have low cytochrome-c oxidase activity (Vijayasarathy et al. 1994). The dogs showed signs of extreme fatigue and lactic academia. The inability to generate ATP from the respiratory chain with mitochondrial enzyme deficiencies results in a complete reliance on anaerobic metabolism and a persistent elevation in lactic acid.

ABNORMAL INTRACELLULAR CALCIUM REGULATION. Malignant hyperthermia (MH) is a heritable disorder of skeletal muscle elicited by exposure to volatile anesthetics and depolarizing muscle relaxants (Gronert 1994). This pharmacogenetic disorder is now recognized in humans, pigs, and dogs. In the animal species and most humans, there are usually no histological or clinical signs of an underlying muscle defect in the absence of the triggering agents. However, when exposed to halogenated anesthetics or succinylcholine, genetically MH-susceptible (MHS) individuals exhibit tachycardia, hyperthermia, elevated carbon dioxide production, and die if the anesthetic is not discontinued. Metabolic acidosis and muscle rigidity are severe in both swine and humans, whereas metabolic acidosis is usually moderate and muscle rigidity is minimal in dogs (Nelson 1991). Specific interventions, including the use of the calcium-release channel antagonist dantrolene, are efficacious in reversing signs of the syndrome. In MHS swine, a hypermetabolic episode can often be initiated by various stressors, including handling, transport, mating, and slaughter. Meat from MHS pigs is typically pale, soft, and exudative (PSE) due to the deleterious effects of high muscle temperatures and low muscle pH post mortem on the water retention and pigment properties of the muscle proteins.

MH is inherited as an autosomal recessive gene in swine, but as an autosomal dominant gene in humans and dogs (Nelson 1991; MacLennan and Phillips 1992; McCarthy et al. 2000). Genetic mapping of the MH locus in pigs and humans placed it in the vicinity of the RYR1 gene, which encodes the sarcoplasmic reticulum ryanodine receptor calcium-release channel. In addition, many biochemical and physiological measurements have implicated this very large protein as the site of the defect in both pigs and humans (Mickelson and Louis 1996). In pigs, a single causative Arg to Cys RYR1 mutation at residue 615, derived from a single founder, has been found and was one of the first disorders in veterinary medicine for which a molecular basis was defined (Fujii et al. 1991). Over 20 RYR1 human mutations have now been identified (Jurkat-Rott et al. 2000; McCarthy et al. 2000). In dogs, a Val to Ala mutation at residue 547 has recently been identified, although it is not known whether this mutation is responsible for all forms of MH in this species (Roberts et al. 2001).

In all three MHS species to date, the clinical symptoms of increased muscle metabolism and muscle contracture are likely due to the effects of the RYR1 mutation on the gating properties of this channel. Many studies have shown that MHS sarcoplasmic reticulum calcium-release channels have a greater level of activity, allowing greater rates of calcium efflux from the SR terminal cisternae into the myoplasm (Mickelson 1996). This intrinsic calcium channel defect is exacerbated by the MH-triggering agents. The SR calcium ATPase is now unable to resequester the calcium back into the SR lumen fast enough, and the myoplasmic calcium concentration rises. The resulting MH episode is due to calcium stimulation of myofilament contractile activity, and the resultant stimulation of aerobic and anaerobic metabolism to fuel the contraction.

A form of dominantly inherited abnormal intramuscular calcium regulation called *recurrent exertional rhabdomyolysis* (RER) has also been proposed to exist in thoroughbred horses. Characteristically, horses have intermittent rhabdomyolysis following exercise, stress, or halothane anesthesia. The threshold for muscle contracture in response to halothane and caffeine is lower in intercostal muscles from RER horses, which suggests a defect in intramuscular calcium regulation (Lentz et al. 1999; Ward et al. 2000).

Altered Electrical Conduction. The electrical conduction system of the neuromuscular junction and muscle cell can be altered by decreased or increased release of acetylcholine at the neuromuscular junction, decreased numbers of acetylcholine receptors at the neuromuscular junction, or altered conductance of ions across the muscle cell membrane.

ALTERED MOTOR-NEURON FIRING

HYPOCALCEMIA. Electrolyte imbalances are capable of producing alterations in motor-neuron firing, which can cause muscle fasciculations, muscle cramping, or weakness. Sweat losses and alkalosis in endurance horses can produce hypocalcemia and hypomagnesemia. Lactation in dogs and horses also may cause hypocalcemia. The resultant low interstitial ionized calcium concentration increases neuronal permeability to sodium ions, allowing easy initiation of neuronal action potentials (Guyton and Hall 1996). With equine hypocalcemia, the phrenic nerve, which passes directly over the atrium, easily discharges in response to atrial depolarization, resulting in synchronous diaphragmatic flutter. Paradoxically, hypocalcemia in dairy cows results in decreased neuronal firing and flaccid paresis. The mechanism for this is unclear but may be related to decreased calcium-induced acetylcholine release from neuromuscular junctions.

ALTERED MOTOR END-PLATE DEPOLARIZATION

MYASTHENIA GRAVIS. Myasthenia gravis in dogs occurs as a congenital familial form in terriers and springer spaniels or more commonly as an acquired condition (Lennon et al. 1978, 1981; Miller et al. 1983). It manifests as postexertional muscle weakness with or without megaesophagus. The congenital form is due to a deficiency in the number of acetylcholine receptors in the postsynaptic motor end plate. The acquired condition is associated with destruction of the receptor by circulating autoantibodies directed against the acetylcholine receptor in the postsynaptic membrane (Figure 8.12). Weakness is due to complement-mediated destruction of the receptors, an accelerated rate of internalization and degradation of receptors that are crosslinked with antibody, and direct inhibition of acetylcholine receptor function by bound antibody. It is assumed that the uncontrolled production of anti-acetylcholine receptor antibodies is due to a disturbance in immunoregulation.

BOTULISM. When feeds contaminated with the *Clostridium botulinum* toxin are ingested, it leads to profound muscle weakness. Skeletal muscle paresis is caused by the toxin inhibiting release of acetylcholine from the presynaptic motor nerve terminals.

ALTERED MUSCLE CELL MEMBRANE EXCITABILITY

HYPERKALEMIC PERIODIC PARALYSIS. Hyperkalemic periodic paralysis (HyPP) is a disorder that affects quarter horses, American paint horses, Appaloosas, and quarter horse crossbred animals. Clinical signs are intermittent and include muscular fasciculations and weakness (Cox 1985; Spier et al. 1990). This disorder in horses is inherited as an autosomal dominant trait and is due to a point mutation that results in a phenylalanine/leucine substitution in a key part of the voltage-dependent skeletal muscle sodium channel α subunit (Rudolf et al. 1992). This results in a resting membrane potential that is closer to firing than in normal horses. Sodium channels are normally briefly activated during the initial phase of the muscle action potential. The HyPP mutation results in a failure of a subpopulation of sodium channels to inactivate when serum potassium concentrations are increased. As a result, an excessive inward flux of sodium and outward flux of potassium ensues, resulting in persistent depolarization of muscle cells and temporary weakness. Serum potassium concentrations during clinical manifestations of episodic weakness are increased and quickly return to normal as clinical signs recede. Electromyographic examination of affected horses may reveal abnormal fibrillation potentials, complex repetitive discharges with occasional myotonic potentials, and trains of doublets even between episodes of HyPP.

MYOTONIA. Myotonia has been described in dogs, horses, and goats (Steinberg 1962; Duncan et al. 1983; Beck et al. 1996). The pathophysiology of these disorders is likely different among different breeds of ani-

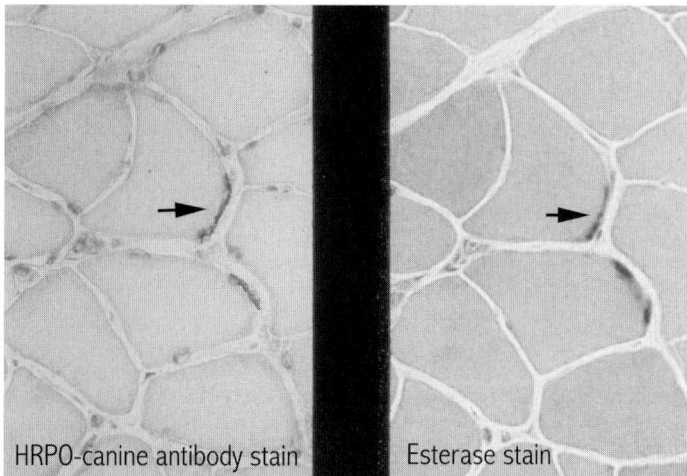

HRPO-canine antibody stain   Esterase stain

FIG. 8.12—A cross section of canine limb muscle stained for canine antibodies localized by staining for peroxidase activity after incubation with the staphylococcal protein A-horseradish peroxidase conjugates (**left**) and a serial section stained with esterase (**right**) to locate the neuromuscular junction (arrow). Note the presence of antibody at the neuromuscular junction of this dog with myasthenia gravis. (Photo courtesy of Dr. G.H. Cardinet III.)

mals. Some generally similar characteristics exist, however, including signs of gross muscle hypertrophy, muscle stiffness, rigidity, and prolonged muscle contraction with dimpling below the contraction (Figure 8.13). Muscles may remain contracted for up to a minute or more, with subsequent slow relaxation. Myotonias are best recognized by electromyography. The most characteristic finding is repetitive high-frequency discharges after needle insertion that increase and then decrease in amplitude and frequency, producing sounds similar to those produced by a dive bomber.

Following cessation of the characteristic waxing-and-waning discharges, additional discharges occur due to spontaneous repetitive discharges of single muscle fibers. In goats, the exact cause of myotonia is known to be an autosomal dominant point mutation in the skeletal muscle chloride channel. The mutation decreases the conductance of the chloride channel. This results in an accumulation of potassium in the T tubules, which in turn leads to progressive postexcitation depolarization of the muscle cell membrane and continued muscle contraction (Ptacek et al. 1993).

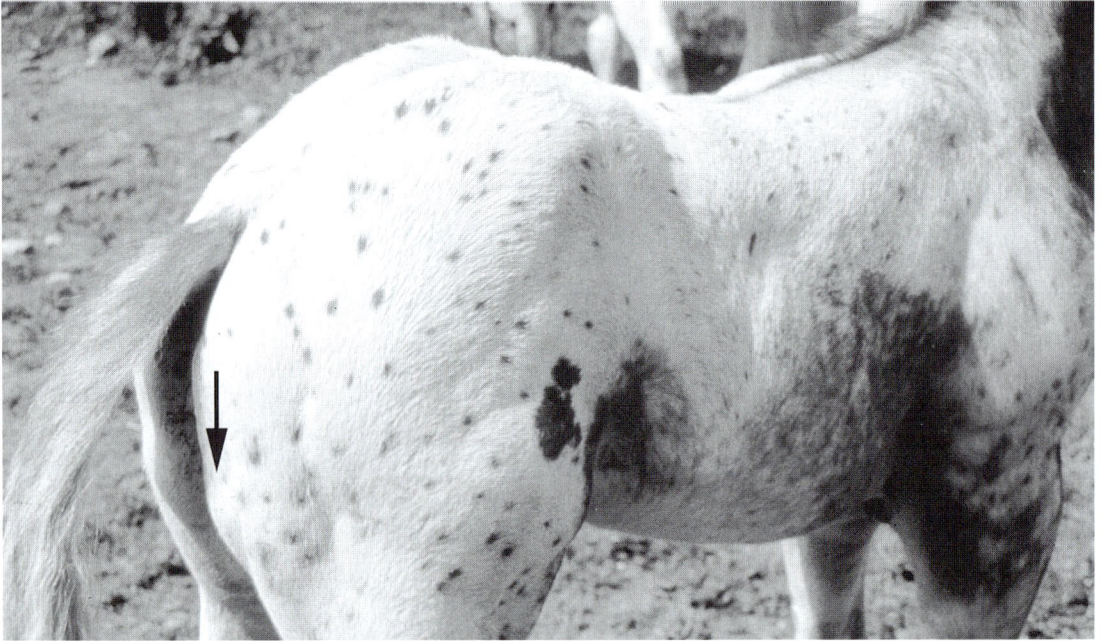

FIG. 8.13—A 2-month-old horse with myotonia. Note the large muscle mass for a foal of this age and the dimpling of areas of the semimembranosus and tendinosus muscles (arrow).

REFERENCES

Angelos S, Valberg SJ, Smith BP, et al. 1995. Myophosphorylase deficiency associated with rhabdomyolysis and exercise intolerance in six related Charolais cattle. Muscle Nerve 18:736–740.

Argov Z, Löfberg M, Arnold DL. 2000. Insights into muscle diseases gained by phosphorus magnetic resonance spectroscopy. Muscle Nerve 23:1316–1334.

Beck CL, Fahlke C, George AL Jr. 1996. Molecular basis for decreased muscle chloride conductance in the myotonic goat. Proc Natl Acad Sci USA 93:11,248–11,252.

Beier RC, Norman JO, Reagor JC, et al. 1993. Isolation of the major component in white snakeroot that is toxic after microsomal activation: Possible explanation of sporadic toxicity if white snakeroot plants and extracts. J Natural Toxins 1:286–293.

Bloom W, Fawcett DW. 1986. A Textbook of Histology. Philadelphia: WB Saunders, 282 pp.

Burk RF, Hill KE. 1993. Regulation of selenoproteins. Annu Rev Nutr 13:65–81.

Cardinet III GH, Stephens-Orvis J. 1980. Skeletal muscle function. In: Kaneko JJ, ed. Clinical Biochemistry of Domestic Animals, 3rd ed. Orlando, FL: Academic, pp 545–574.

Ceh L, Hauge JG, Svenkerud R, et al. 1976. Glycogenosis type III in the dog. Acta Vet Scand 17:212–222.

Cox JH. 1985. An episodic weakness in four horses associated with intermittent serum hyperkalemia and the similarity of the disease to hyperkalemic periodic paralysis in man. In: Proceedings of the 31st Annual Convention of the American Association of Equine Practitioners. Lexington, KY: AAEP, pp 383–391.

Cumming WJK, Fulthrop J, Hudgson P, et al. 1994. Color Atlas of Muscle Pathology. London: Mosby-Wolfe.

De la Corte FD, Valberg SJ, Williamson S, et al. 1999. Enhanced glucose uptake in horses with polysaccharide storage myopathy (PSSM). Am J Vet Res 60:458–462.

Dill SG, Rehbun WC. 1985. White muscle disease in foals. Compend Continuing Educ 7(Suppl):S627–S636.

Dow SW, Fettman MJ. 1992. Chronic renal disease and potassium depletion in cats. Semin Vet Med Surg (Small Anim) 7:198–201.

Dow SW, Fettman MJ, Curtis CR, Le Conteur RA. 1989. Hypokalemia in cats: 186 cases (1984–1987). J Am Vet Med Assoc 194:1604–1608.

Dubey JP. 1976. A review of sarcocystis of domestic animals and of other coccidia of cats and dogs. J Am Vet Med Assoc 169:1061–1078.

Dubey JP. 1977. *Toxoplasma, Hammondia, Besnotia, Sarcocystis* and other tissue cyst-forming coccidia of man and animals. In: Kreier JP, ed. Parasitic Protozoa. New York: Academic, 3:101–237.

Dubey JP, Carpenter JL, Speer CA, et al. 1988. Newly recognized fatal protozoal disease of dogs. J Am Vet Med Assoc 192:1269–1285.

Duncan ID, Griffiths IR. 1983. Myotonia in the dog. In: Kirk RW, ed. Current Veterinary Therapy, vol 8: Small Animal Practice. Philadelphia: WB Saunders, pp 686-691.

Erwin BG. 1986. Clostridial bacteria and clostridial myositis. In: Berg JN, ed. Current Veterinary Therapy 2: Food Animal Practice, 2nd ed. Philadelphia: WB Saunders, pp 567–570.

Essen Gustavsson B, Roneus N, Pösö R. 1997. Metabolic response in skeletal muscle fibers of standardbred trotters after racing. Comp Biochem Physiol [A] 117:431–436.

Fayer R. 1982. Sarcocystis: A clinical entity in bovine practice. Bovine Pract 14:117–119.

Freestone JP, Carlson GP. 1991. Muscle disorders in the horse: A retrospective study. Equine Vet J 23:86–90.

Fujii J, Otsu K, Zorzato F, et al. 1991. Identification of a mutation in porcine ryanodine receptor associated with malignant hyperthermia. Science 253:448–451.

Fyfe JC, Giger U, Van Winkle TJ, et al. 1992. Glycogen storage disease type IV: Inherited deficiency of branching enzyme in cats. Pediatr Res 32:719–725.

Geor RJ, Robinson WF. 1985. Suspected monensin toxicosis in feedlot cattle. Aus Vet J 62:130–131.

Gronert GA. 1994. Malignant hyperthermia. In: Engel AG, Franzini Armstrong C, eds. Myology. New York: McGraw-Hill, pp 1661–1668.

Gunn HM. 1978. Differences in the histochemical properties of skeletal muscle of different breeds of horses and dogs. J Anat 127:615–634.

Guyton AC, Hall JE. 1996. Parathyroid hormone, calcitonin, calcium and phosphate metabolism, vitamin D, bone, and teeth. In: Textbook of Medical Physiology, 9th ed. Philadelphia: WB Saunders, pp 985-1002.

Harris RC, Marlin DJ, Dunnett M, et al. 1990. Muscle buffering capacity and dipeptide content in the thoroughbred horse, greyhound dog and man. Comp Biochem Physiol [A] 97:249–251.

Harris RC, Marlin DJ, Snow DH, Harkness RA. 1991. Muscle ATP loss and lactate accumulation at different work intensities in the exercising thoroughbred. Eur J Appl Physiol 62:235–244.

Harvey JW, Calderwood Mays MB, Gropp KE, et al. 1990. Polysaccharide storage myopathy in canine phosphofructokinase deficiency (type VII) glycogen storage disease. Vet Pathol 27:1–8.

Healy PJ, Nicholls PJ, Martiniuk F, et al. 1995. Evidence of molecular heterogeneity for generalized glycogenoses between and within different breeds of cattle. Aus Vet J 72:309–311.

Herrtage ME, Houlton JEF. 1979. Collapsing Clumber spaniels. Vet Rec 105:334.

Hodgson DH. 1985. Energy considerations during exercise. Vet Clin North Am Equine Pract 3:447–460.

Hodgson DR, Rose RJ. 1994. The Athletic Horse. Philadelphia: WB Saunders.

Houlton JE, Herrtage ME. 1980. Mitochondrial myopathy in the Sussex spaniel. Vet Rec 106:206.

Hulland TJ. 1985. Muscle and tendons. In: Jubb KVF, Kennedy PC, Palmer N, eds. Pathology of Domestic Animals, 3rd ed. Orlando FL: Academic, 1:139–199.

Jurkat-Rott KT, McCarthy TV, Lehmann-Horn F. 2000. Genetics and pathogenesis of malignant hyperthermia. Muscle Nerve 23:4–17.

Kornegay JN, Gorgacz EJ, Dawe DL, et al. 1980. Polymyositis in dogs. J Am Vet Med Assoc 176:431–438.

Kornegay JN, Tuler SM, Miller DM, et al. 1988. Muscular dystrophy in a litter of golden retriever dogs. Muscle Nerve 11:1056–1064.

Kramer JJ. 1980. Clinical enzymology. In: Kaneko JJ, ed. Clinical Biochemistry of Domestic Animals, 3rd ed. Orlando, FL: Academic, pp 175–179.

Kristic RV. 1984. General Histology of the Mammal. New York: Springer-Verlag, pp 265–273.

Krum SH, Cardinet III GH, Anderson BC, et al. 1977. Polymyositis and polyarthritis associated with systemic lupus erythematosus in a dog. J Am Vet Med Assoc 170:61–64.

Leek RG, Fayer R, Johnson AJ. 1977. Sheep experimentally infected with sarcocystis from dogs: I. Disease in young lambs. J Parasitol 63:642–650.

Lennon VA, Palmer AC, Pflugfelder C, et al. 1978. Myasthenia gravis in dogs: Acetylcholine receptor deficiency with and without antireceptor autoantibodies. In: Rose NR, Bigazzi PE, Warner NL, eds. Genetic Control of Autoimmune Disease. New York: Elsevier North Holland, 1:295–306.

Lennon VA, Lambert EH, Palmer AC, et al. 1981. Acquired and congenital myasthenia gravis in dogs: A study of 20 cases. In: Satoyoshi E, ed. Myasthenia Gravis: Pathogenesis and Treatment. Tokyo: Tokyo University Press, pp 14–54.

Lentz LR, Valberg SJ, Balog E, et al. 1999. Abnormal regulation of contraction in equine recurrent exertional rhabdomyolysis. Am J Vet Res 60:992–999

Lopez Rivero JL. 1996a. Fast myosin heavy chain isoforms in horse skeletal muscle: An immunohistochemical and electrophoretic study. Pferdeheilkunde 12:523–527.

Lopez Rivero JL. 1996b. Immunohistochemistry versus traditional myofibrillar ATPase histochemistry for identification of muscle fiber types in the horse. Pferdeheilkunde 124:518–522.

Lopez Rivero JL, Morales-Lopez JL, Galisteo AM, Aguera E. 1991. Muscle fiber type composition in untrained and endurance trained Andalusian and Arab horses. Equine Vet J 23:91–93.

MacLennan DH, Phillips MS. 1992. Malignant hyperthermia. Science 256:789–794.

McArdle A, Jackson MJ. 1997. Intracellular mechanisms involved in skeletal muscle damage. In: Salmons S, ed. Muscle Damage. Oxford: Oxford University Press, pp 90–101.

McCarthy TV, Quane KA, Lynch PJ. 2000. Ryanodine receptor mutations in malignant hyperthermia and central core disease. Hum Mutat 15:410–417.

McMurray CH, Rice DA. 1982. Vitamin E and selenium deficiency diseases. Ir Vet J 36:57–67.

Mickelson JR, Louis CF. 1996. Malignant hyperthermia: Excitation-contraction coupling, Ca^{2+} release channel, and cell Ca^{2+} regulation defects. Physiol Rev 76:537–592.

Miller LM, Lennon VA, Lambert EH. 1983. Congenital myasthenia gravis in smooth fox terriers. J Am Vet Med Assoc 182:694–698.

Nelson TE. 1991. Malignant hyperthermia in dogs. J Am Vet Med Assoc 198:989–994.

Orvis J, Cardinet III GH. 1981. Canine muscle fiber types and susceptibility to masticatory muscle myositis. Muscle Nerve 4:354–359.

Perkins G, Valberg SJ, Madigan JE, et al. 1998. Fluid, electrolyte and renal abnormalities associated with acute rhabdomyolysis in four neonatal foals. J Vet Intern Med 12:173–177.

Platt SR, Chrisman CL, Shelton GD. 1999. Lipid storage myopathy in a cocker spaniel. J Small Anim Pract 40:31–34.

Ptacek LJ, Johnson KJ, Griggs RC. 1993. Genetics and physiology of the myotonic disorders. N Engl J Med 328:482–489.

Rebhun WC, Shin SJ, Kurg JM, et al. 1985. Malignant edema in horses. J Am Vet Med Assoc 187:732–736.

Roberts MC, Mickelson JR, Patterson EE, et al. 2001. Autosomal dominant canine malignant hyperthermia is caused by a mutation in the gene encoding the skeletal muscle calcium release channel (RYR1). Anesthesiology 95:716–725.).

Roneus M, Essen Gustavsson B, Lindholm A, Persson SGB. 1991. Muscle characteristics of thoroughbreds of different ages and sexes. Equine Vet J 23:207–210.

Roneus M, Essen Gustavsson B, Lindholm A, Persson SGB. 1993. Racing performance and longitudinal changes in muscle characteristic in standardbred racehorses. J Equine Vet Sci 13:355–361.

Rudolph JA, Spier SJ, Byrns G, et al. 1992. Periodic paralysis in quarter horses: A sodium channel mutation disseminated by selective breeding. Nature Genet 7:141–147.

Sattler N, Fecteau G, Girard C, Couture Y. 1998. Description of 14 cases of bovine hypokalaemia syndrome. Vet Rec 143(18):503–507.

Schatzberg SJ, Anderson LV, Wilton SD, et al. 1998. Alternative gene transcripts in golden retriever muscular dystrophy. Muscle Nerve 21:991–998.

Shelton GD, Cardinet III GH, Bandman E, et al. 1985. Fiber type specific autoantibodies in a dog with eosinophilic myositis. Muscle Nerve 8:783–790.

Shelton GD, Cardinet III GH, Bandman E. 1987. Canine masticatory muscle disorders: A study of 29 cases. Muscle Nerve 10:753–766.

Shelton GD, Nyhan WL, Kass PH, et al. 1998. Analysis of organic acids, amino acids, and carnitine in dogs with lipid storage myopathy. Muscle Nerve 21:1202–1205.

Snow DH, Valberg SJ. 1994. Muscle anatomy, physiology and adaptations to exercise and training. In: Rose RJ, Hodgson DH, eds. The Athletic Horse: Principles and Practice of Equine Sports Medicine. Philadelphia: WB Saunders, pp 145–179.

Steinberg S, Botelho S. 1962. Myotonia in a horse. Science 137:979–980.

Spier SJ, Carlson GP, Holliday TA, et al. 1990. Hyperkalemic periodic paralysis in horses. J Am Vet Med Assoc 197:1009–1017.

Tan P, Allen JG, Wilton SD, et al. 1997. A splice-site mutation causing ovine McArdle's disease. Neuromuscular Disord 7:336–342.

Tawa NE Jr, Goldberg AL. 1994. Protein and amino acid metabolism. In: Engel AG, Franzini-Armstrong C, eds. Myology. New York: McGraw-Hill, pp 683–707.

Traub-Dargatz JL, Schlip JW, Granstrom DE, et al. 1994. Multifocal myositis associated with *Sarcocystis* sp in a horse. J Am Vet Med Assoc 205:1574–1576.

Valberg S. 1986. Glycogen depletion patterns in the muscle of standardbred trotters after exercise of varying intensity and duration. Equine Vet J 18:479–484.

Valberg SJ. 1999. Spinal muscle pathology. Vet Clin North Am 15:87–95.

Valberg S, Essen Gustavsson B, Lindholm A, Persson SGB. 1985. Energy metabolism, in relation to skeletal muscle fibre properties, during treadmill exercise. Equine Vet J 17:439–444.

Valberg SJ, Cardinet III GH, Carlson GP, Di Mauro S. 1992. Polysaccharide storage myopathy associated with exertional rhabdomyolysis in the horse. Neuromuscular Disord 2:351–359.

Valberg S, Carlson GP, Cardinet III GH, et al. 1994. Skeletal muscle mitochondrial myopathy as a cause of exercise intolerance in a horse. Muscle Nerve 17:305–312.

Valberg SJ, Bullock P, Hogetvedt W, et al. 1996. Myopathies associated with *Streptococcus equi* infections in horses. In: Proceedings of the American Association of Equine Practitioners. Lexington, KY: AAEP, pp 292–293.

Valberg SJ, Townsend D, MacLeay JM, Mickelson JR. 1998. Glycolytic capacity and phosphofructokinase regulation in horses with polysaccharide storage myopathy. Am J Vet Res 59:782–785.

Valberg SJ, MacLeay JM, Billstrom JA, et al. 1999. Skeletal muscle metabolic response to exercise in horses with polysaccharide storage myopathy. Equine Vet J 31:43–47.

Valberg SJ, Mickelson JR, Ward TL, et al. 2001. Glycogen branching enzyme activity in quarter horse foals. J Vet Intern Med 15:572–580.

Vijayasarathy C, Giger U, Prociuk U, et al. 1994. Canine mitochondrial myopathy associated with reduced mitochondrial mRNA and altered cytochrome c oxidase activities in fibroblasts and skeletal muscle. Comp Biochem Physiol [A] 109:887–894.

Volfinger L, Lassourd V, Michaus JM, et al. 1996. Kinetic evaluation of muscle damage during exercise by calculation of amount of creatine kinase released. Am J Physiol 266:R434–R441.

Walvoort HC, Van Nes JJ, Stokhof AA, et al. 1984. Canine glycogen storage disease type II: A clinical study of 4 affected dogs. J Am Anim Hosp Assoc 20:279–286.

Ward TL, Valberg SJ, Roghair TJ, et al. 2000. Skeletal muscle membrane activities in thoroughbred horses with exertional rhabdomyolysis. Am J Vet Res 61:242–247.

Williams BM. 1977. Clostridial myositis in cattle: Bacteriology and gross pathology. Vet Rec 100:90–91.

Wilson JS. 1980. Toxic myopathy in a dog associated with the presence of monensin in dry dog food. Can Vet J 21:30–31.

9

PATHOPHYSIOLOGY OF THE CENTRAL NERVOUS SYSTEM

Marc Vandevelde, Andreas Zurbriggen, Cleta Sue Bailey, and Robert H. Dunlop

PART 1: INFECTIOUS-INFLAMMATORY DISEASES OF THE CENTRAL NERVOUS SYSTEM

MARC VANDEVELDE AND ANDREAS ZURBRIGGEN

Infectious and inflammatory diseases are a major cause of neurological dysfunction in domestic animals. Despite the widespread use of vaccination against a variety of viral infectious agents and antibiosis, veterinarians are often confronted with severe neurological problems in individual animals or in populations of animals. A range of viruses, bacteria, fungi, and parasites are known to cause central nervous system (CNS) infections. A special class of CNS infections that have caused great public health concern in recent years are the spongiform encephalopathies, such as scrapie, bovine spongiform encephalopathy (BSE), and Creutzfeldt-Jakob disease. Transmissible spongiform encephalopathies (TSEs) are a group of progressive lethal diseases with very long incubation periods (years) and spongy degeneration of the CNS. All of these diseases are transmissible at least under experimental conditions. The exact nature of the infectious agent is uncertain. TSE agents are very small and extremely resistant to physical and chemical treatment. There is no doubt that development of the disease is associated with accumulation of amyloid in the CNS, which is derived from a glycosylphatidylinositol (GPI)-anchored protein called the prion protein or PrPc. PrPc is expressed on the surface of the cell, particularly in neurons. In TSE, the normal cellular protein PrPc undergoes a posttranslational conformational change resulting in the accumulation of the protease-resistant isoform PrPsc (sc is derived from scrapie). The prion theory postulates that PrPsc is capable of initiating its own replication by acting as a template for further PrPc molecules to become abnormally folded. Thus, according to the prion theory, the infectious agent consists solely of protein. Genetics of the PrP gene and experiments with transgenic mice lend strong support to the prion theory.

The mechanisms leading to loss of the steady state in the CNS in infectious diseases are complex and only in part understood. Very generally speaking, infectious agents cause loss of steady state in the CNS as a result of direct activity of the agent in the CNS and indirectly as a result of the immune response against this agent. The latter may be compounded by the fact that infections may also induce an aberrant immune response with additional negative consequences for the host. Finally, we know of a few inflammatory diseases that arise as a result of a disturbance of the immune system without known involvement of infectious agents.

BASIC ANATOMIC AND PHYSIOLOGICAL ASPECTS. The CNS is an anatomically and histologically complex organ that consists of neurons and their processes, some of which are covered with myelin sheaths, creating the white matter. Myelin sheaths are formed by the membranes of the oligodendrocytes, a specialized type of glial cell. Another major class of glial cell is the astrocyte, which has cell processes covering most other cell elements in the nervous system. Using a considerable share of the body's energy, the nervous system is intensely vascularized with a very high concentration of capillaries. The exterior surface of the CNS is covered by the meninges, with an interior layer (pia mater and arachnoid) consisting of a mesh of chambered connective tissue and a very tough thick outer layer (dura mater) apposing the bone. The cavities of the CNS—the ventricles—are lined by ciliated ependymal cells. The CNS does not possess lymph vessels as other tissues do.

However, it has a cerebrospinal fluid (CSF) circulation. CSF is produced in the choroid plexus of the ventricles by ultrafiltration from the blood. It flows in a caudal direction and leaves the ventricles through small holes of the medullary velum at the level of the fourth ventricle, entering and filling the meningeal spaces around the CNS, where it is resorbed back into the blood. The CNS tissue itself also contributes to the CSF in that interstitial fluid is drained from the tissue toward the ventricles.

Blood-Brain Barrier. In contrast to other organs, the endothelia of the blood vessels in the nervous system are not fenestrated: the endothelial cells are connected by tight junctions creating an effective protective barrier between the blood and the nervous tissue. Lipid-mediated passive diffusion of small molecules is possible, but most traffic across the blood-brain barrier (BBB) is catalyzed carrier-mediated or receptor-mediated transport of nutrients, proteins, and electrolytes. Also involved in the BBB as a functional system are the pericytes, which, together with the endothelial cells, form a basement membrane and the astrocytic processes that cover most of the external surface of the vessels. In the normal state, little protein and hardly any cells cross the BBB. Because of this BBB, the nervous system has been considered to be an immunologically "privileged" site. As we will see, however, this barrier can be breached, rendering the CNS vulnerable to immunopathological processes. In infectious-inflammatory diseases, the BBB plays a very important role, regulating access of immune cells to the CNS (Figure 9.1). Its endothelial cells are very active when homeostasis is lost: they react by upregulating major histocompatibility complex (MHC) antigens and adhesion molecules, and can express various cytokines such as interleukin 1 (IL-1), IL-6, and IL-8.

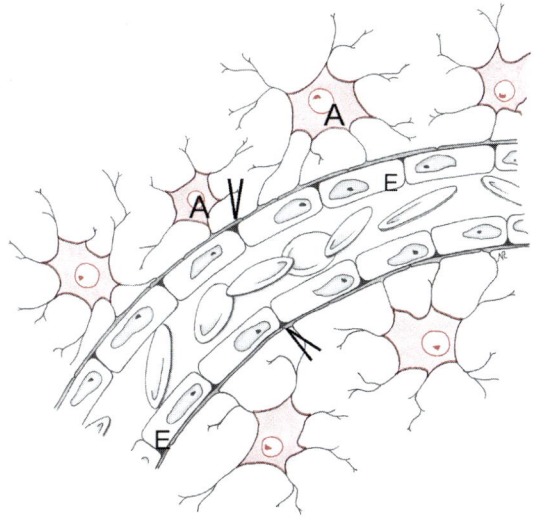

FIG. 9.1—Schematic representation of the blood-brain barrier. E, endothelial cells of the blood vessels with tight junctions between them; and A, astrocytes in the central nervous system (CNS) parenchyma with processes forming astrocytic endfeet, which envelop the basement membrane of the endothelial cells (*arrowheads*).

Entry of Infectious Agents into the Nervous System. Infectious agents can enter the nervous system in several ways. Most infections are species specific, although some, such as rabies virus and tick-borne encephalitis, have a wider species spectrum. This implies that agents use specific receptors to enter the CNS. Within a given species, susceptibility may be genetically determined. An extreme example of genetic susceptibility is found in spongiform encephalopathies in sheep, mice, and people. In this case, susceptibility or resistance is determined by certain polymorphisms of the prion gene. Certain configurations of the prion protein appear to favor the production of its pathological form and to facilitate the interaction between PrPc and PrPsc, leading to replication of prions. This interaction is also the basis of the species barrier when TSEs are transmitted from one species to another: the more compatible the PrP molecules from donor and acceptor species are, the easier the transmission is. The primary sequence of the two prion proteins is certainly important for the species barrier, but it is clear from experiments in transgenic mice that other cellular factors are also involved.

Hematogenous spread is common in bacterial infections with primary involvement of other organs and septicemia. Not much is known about how bacteria can cross the BBB. Both receptor-mediated and pinocytotic transport across the endothelial cells have been described in vitro. In bacterial septicemia in domestic animals, small thrombi riddled with bacteria may become lodged in small blood vessels in the CNS, causing microinfarcts with disruption of the blood vessel wall, and spread from there into the tissue. The rete mirabile, a very dense network of blood vessels around the pituitary at the base of the brain in ruminants, is a site where such bacterial emboli can easily become trapped: bacterial abscesses are therefore frequently found in this area. Some viruses, such as the equine herpesvirus, hog cholera virus, and canine hepatitis virus, preferably replicate in endothelial cells, including those of the CNS, and can invade CNS cells from there. Viruses are often carried to the CNS by the mononuclear cells in which they replicate. Such cells have to penetrate the BBB to get the agent into the nervous tissue. A few areas of the CNS (the choroid plexus and circumventricular organs) have fenestrated capillaries where viruses or virus containing cells may access the brain.

Agents can also use the peripheral nerves to get into the nervous system by traveling through the axons (Figure 9.2). The bacterium *Listeria monocytogenes* enters the brain through the trigeminal nerve in ruminants. This happens at the time of change of teeth, when the nerve endings of the dental branch of the trigeminal nerve are exposed. Many viruses use the peripheral nervous system as the site/route of entry. For example, herpes suis virus enters the CNS by way of the oropharyngeal nerve endings of the cranial nerves in carnivores and in pigs. In the latter species, the virus also enters the CNS through the olfactory nerves. Rabies virus is another example whereby the virus is inoculated by biting wounds. Following primary replication in the muscle cells, rabies virus travels to the CNS through the retrograde axoplasmic flow of the axons. Once inside the nervous system, the same principle of axonal spread applies whereby the agent is transported from one neuronal pool to the next. Infectious agents can also spread through the CSF. This is common in bacterial infections, once the agents have entered the spinal fluid. In canine distemper, infected mononuclear cells in the CSF fuse with the ependymal surface, from which the virus spreads in the brain. This explains why lesions are often found in subependymal and subpial locations in distemper.

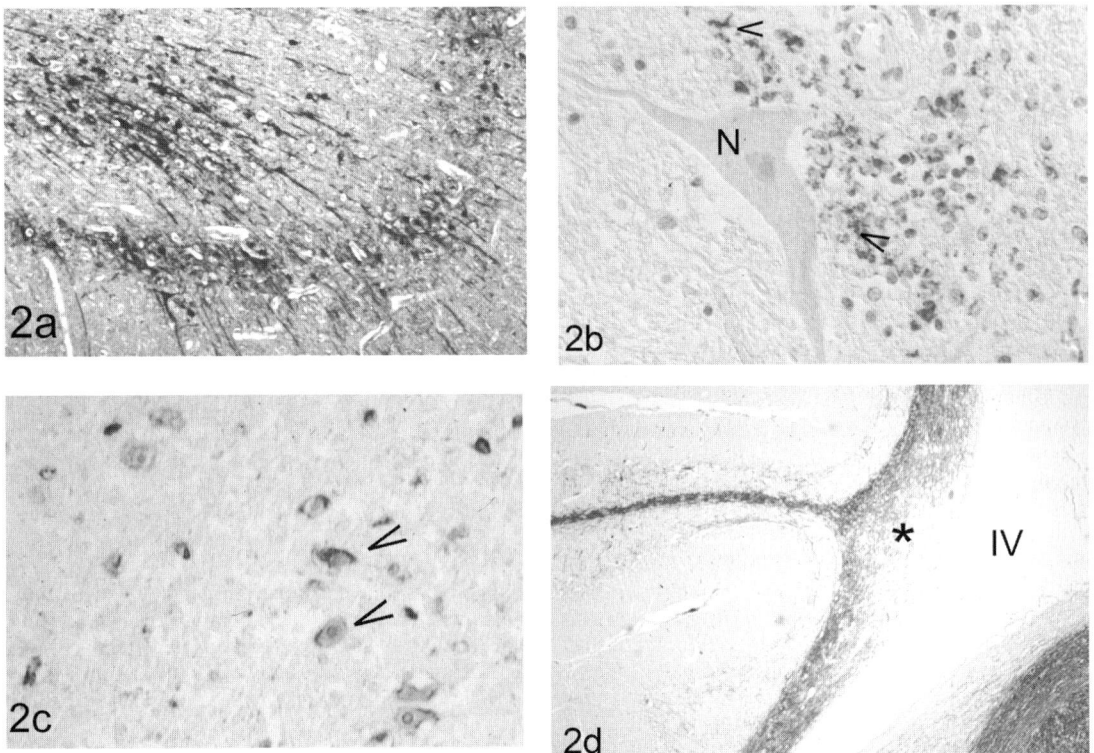

FIG. 9.2—Spread of infectious agents in the central nervous system (CNS). **a:** Cerebral cortex. Darkly labeled neurons contain canine distemper virus (CDV). Virus is also present in long-cell processes, suggesting axonal spread between cells. In situ hybridization for phosphoprotein (P) mRNA of CDV. ×100. **b:** Cerebral cortex. Several labeled neurons containing rabies virus without apparent cell damage. Immunocytochemical staining for rabies virus antigen. ×250. **c:** Brain stem. *Listeria monocytogenes* (darkly labeled grains, *arrowheads*) in the nervous parenchyma close to a neuron (N) of the trigeminal nucleus. ×400. **d:** Cerebellar white matter (darkly stained tissue). The *asterisk* depicts demyelinating lesion. Myelin sheaths have disappeared as a result of CDV infection. Immunocytochemical stain for myelin basic protein. ×25.

In spongiform encephalopathies, similar patterns of spread have been observed. In several species, TSE agents replicate in lymphatic tissues before entering the CNS very much like in many conventional viral infections. In experimental mouse scrapie, follicular dendritic cells play an important role in the transmission of the agent to the brain. In scrapie, the agent enters the lymphoid tissues in the gut, with primary replication in the lymphatic tissues such as the spleen. From there, the agent spreads by way of the splanchnic nerves to the spinal cord. Once in the CNS, further spread from neuron to neuron occurs by way of cell processes. This process is also very strain specific in that only specific neuronal populations are involved, leading to a specific distribution pattern of the lesions. In BSE, the route of entry in the CNS has not been elucidated. Replication of the BSE agent in lymphatic tissues appears to be lacking. In experimental BSE in cattle, some infectivity has been found in the wall of the distal ileum but none in any other extraneural organ. It is possible that the BSE agent can enter the CNS by way of the nerve endings in the oropharyngeal and gastrointestinal mucosa. Direct spread by way of the cranial nerves has also been observed in hamsters.

DIRECT EFFECTS OF THE AGENTS ON THE TISSUE

Damage to the Blood-Brain Barrier. Bacterial toxins damage endothelial cells with profound disturbance of the blood vessel permeability. Serum components and whole blood leak into the CNS parenchyma or into the CSF. As a result, leaked proteins increase osmotic pressure, with formation of brain edema. When larger areas of the brain are affected with brain edema, the brain swells and intracranial pressure rises with potential detrimental consequences for the host. A massive rise in intracranial pressure decreases brain perfusion, causing ischemia and compression of the brain stem with dysfunction of the vital centers.

Some bacteria such as *Haemophilus somnis* induce blood clots that obliterate blood vessels, causing focal ischemia with formation of infarcts. Several viruses such as equine herpesvirus and hog cholera virus replicate in endothelial cells, inducing permeability changes with hemorrhagic necrosis of perivascular CNS tissue.

Changes in Neurons. Many agents, especially viruses, have an affinity for neurons. Frequently, certain viruses have a specific preference for certain neuronal populations; for example, enteroviruses have an affinity for the motoneurons of the cord and the brain stem. The clinical signs reflect such particular localization and can help to establish a diagnosis.

The process of viral replication in neurons differs between agents, but, generally, penetration, uncoating, transcription, and translation lead to formation of infectious particles that are then transmitted to other neurons. The process of replication may kill the neuron by apoptosis or necrosis, evidently leading to serious loss of function. Rabies virus destroys the neurons of the hippocampus by apoptosis. Herpes suis virus destroys large numbers of the cerebral cortical neurons, leading to encephalomalacia. In other infections, the cells are not directly killed at all, but their function may be altered. Some work has been done on such functional deficits at the single-neuron level in tissue culture systems. In acute canine distemper, there is sometimes massive neuronal infection of the cerebral cortex, leading to marked changes in the electroencephalographic pattern and seizures, even though little neuronal cytolysis is detectable on pathological examination. In diseases such as scrapie and BSE, functional deficits may be pronounced at the level of the autonomic nervous system, with bradycardia and reduced rumination. A hallmark of these diseases is accumulation of the abnormal prion protein in the tissue as amyloid or so-called scrapie-associated fibrils. It is not clear whether this phenomenon has something to do with the degenerative changes in neurons. PrPsc appears to be toxic for neurons in vitro, yet experiments with infected brain grafts in transgenic PrP knockout mice did not suggest toxicity in vivo. The mechanism of vacuolation of the neuropil and neuronal somata in spongiform encephalopathies is hardly understood. In addition to these changes, there is neuronal cell loss in certain predilection areas. For example, in BSE, a significant reduction in the number of neurons in the lateral vestibular nucleus has been detected by morphometric techniques even though degenerative changes in neurons in this nucleus are not very obvious. It is thought that neurons in TSE die by apoptosis. In BSE, few apoptotic neurons have been found, but DNA fragmentation of glial cells is apparent especially in areas in which prion protein accumulation is concentrated.

Changes in the Myelin. A number of viruses have an affinity for the white matter of the CNS. Visna in sheep and canine distemper in dogs are characterized by white-matter lesions whereby the myelin sheaths are selectively damaged. The pathogenesis of demyelination has been studied in dogs with distemper. Canine distemper virus (CDV) causes severe immunosuppression and neurological disease in dogs that is associated with demyelination. In the early stage of the infection, demyelination is associated with viral replication in the white matter. Oligodendrocytes, the myelin-producing cells, support transcription of all CDV genes, although very little viral protein can be found in these cells. This restricted infection does not necessarily kill the cells but leads to a massive downregulation of myelin transcription and metabolic impairment of the myelin-producing cells. As a result, the turnover of myelin sheaths can no longer be maintained, and myelin disintegrates. Myelin sheaths greatly enhance the efficiency of transmitting impulses through saltatory conduction whereby action potentials jump from one node of Ranvier to the next one. Nerve conduction is severely slowed when the myelin sheaths are removed.

SECONDARY CHANGES

Reaction-Defense Mechanisms in the Central Nervous System. As already indicated, the CNS is, immunologically speaking, poorly equipped. Besides the lack of a lymphatic drainage system and the existence of a BBB, effectively shielding the CNS from the blood, neurons and glial cells in normal CNS do not express MHC molecules on their surface. The MHC I and II antigen-presenting molecules are important for interaction of cells with either CD8–Tc lymphocytes (cytotoxic cells) or CD4-ThTI lymphocytes (helper cells). Furthermore, there are almost no lymphocytes available in CNS tissue: only very few lymphocytes are found in the perivascular spaces and spinal fluid (Figure 9.3). Some antigen-presenting cells are available: the so-called resting microglia, which are derived from the mononuclear phagocyte system. These cells migrate into the CNS during ontogenesis: some are in a perivascular location, whereas others occur diffusely in the tissue. They are capable of expressing MHC molecules. In tissue culture, it has been shown that astrocytes can express MHC II following stimulation, but it is uncertain whether this plays a major role in vivo.

In view of all of these shortcomings, one would not expect that the CNS could effectively cope with infectious agents. This is by no means the case.

Information to the Immune System. How is the immune system informed about the presence of an infection in the CNS?

In most infections, the agent is also present in other tissues, such as respiratory and gastrointestinal systems. In this way, the immune system is already sensitized to the agent. Nevertheless, the immune system must still be informed that the infection is also present in the brain. Antigen can drain from the CSF into the blood through the arachnoid villae of the meninges or by way of the olfactory bulb through the ethmoid perforations to the cervical lymph nodes. Also, antigens can be expressed on the luminal surface of the endothelial cells in the CNS, whereby such antigens are transported through the BBB. Viruses that infect endothelial cells can be released in the blood or can induce MHC molecules on the surface, rendering these cells recognizable by T lymphocytes. Furthermore, processes of antigen-presenting cells on the brain side of the BBB may penetrate through the barrier and expose antigen on the luminal face of the blood vessels.

The replication of agents in the cells of the CNS also leads to upregulation of immune molecules in cells other than endothelial cells of the CNS, preparing these cells to participate effectively in the immune response. For example, in canine distemper, there is a diffuse upregulation of MHC II molecules into the microglial cells of the white matter.

Cytokines play an important role in the regulation of the immune response and in the induction of CNS lesions. They may derive directly from CNS cells but also from the blood. Some cytokines—such as IL-1, IL-2, IL-8, IL-12, tumor-necrosis factor α (TNF-α), and interferon-γ (IFN-γ)—have proinflammatory functions, whereas IL-4, IL-10, and transforming growth factor β are known to have anti-inflammatory functions.

TNF-α and IL-6 increase invasion of leukocytes into the CNS by an upregulation of adhesion molecules on endothelial cells and by increasing BBB permeability. In addition, cytokines may be directly involved in the demyelinating process in distemper; for example, TNF-α and IL-6 have some toxic effects on myelin.

Chemotaxis is also an important mechanism to attract certain cell populations to the CNS. For example, in viral and bacterial infections and in canine steroid-responsive meningitis arteritis, spinal fluid contains substances that are chemotactic for lymphocytes or neutrophils. In acute canine distemper, we have found high levels of IL-8 in the CSF that is chemotactic for lymphocytes. It is possible that this IL-8 is produced by the microglial cells that are activated in distemper.

Chemotaxis and upregulation of immune molecules will not lead to much activity inside the CNS per se because, as already mentioned, the main players—the leukocytes—are not available in the CNS itself. They must be recruited from the circulation. For example, in steroid-responsive meningitis arteritis in dogs, strong chemotactic signals are generated in the CSF with invasion of leukocytes in the meninges and the induction of a very painful meningitis. Glucocorticosteroid therapy effectively inhibits migration of leukocytes into the meninges, resulting in dramatic clinical improvement. However, the chemotactic signal continues to exist; when the treatment is stopped, the signs recur.

Import of Immune Cells into the Central Nervous System. The next step in the process is thus invasion of

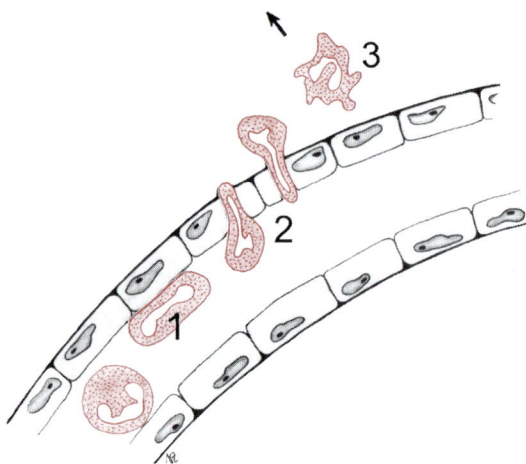

FIG. 9.3—Migration of inflammatory cells from the blood to the central nervous system (CNS): (1) adhesion of the leukocyte to the endothelial lining, (2) penetration through endothelial cell, and (3) entry into the perivascular space (Virchow-Robin space).

immune cells from the blood through the BBB into the CNS. Initially, this requires that the circulating lymphocytes that have recognized their targets stick to the endothelial cell surface. This is mediated by a range of molecules: the adhesins and integrins that are upregulated in activated endothelial cells and mononuclear cells alike. The upregulation is the result of chemokine secretion by the mononuclear cells. For example, lymphocytes express lymphocyte function-associated antigen (LFA-1), and endothelial cells express intercellular adhesion molecule (ICAM-1), which is a ligand between T cells and endothelial cells. Following adhesion to the luminal surface, lymphocytes and macrophages have to penetrate the BBB. In some infections, as we have already seen, the infection itself leads to damage of the blood vessel wall, thus facilitating entry of the cells into the CNS. The process of crossing the barrier is usually more subtle, with transport by pinocytosis through the endothelial cells. Lymphocytes also secrete enzymes to dissolve the basement membrane of the endothelial cells to get on the CNS side of the barrier.

In recent years, it has been recognized that there is also a nonspecific trafficking of lymphocytes across the BBB whereby activated lymphocytes, irrespective of their specificity, migrate into the CNS. The cells that are sensitized against antigens in the CNS remain in the CNS compartment, whereas the others return into the blood circulation. This phenomenon has been well studied in experimental allergic encephalitis in rodents. We have observed a diffuse increase in the residential lymphocyte population in the CNS in normal vaccinated dogs shortly after challenge with virulent distemper. It appears that cytotoxic lymphocytes have a tendency to migrate quickly in the tissue, whereas CD4 cells remain longer around the blood vessels, causing perivascular cuffing, the morphological hallmark of the immune response in the CNS (Figure 9.4).

Development of the Intrathecal Immune Response.
The imported specifically sensitized immune cells quickly expand upon interaction with their target, with recruitment of many additional cells from the blood into the CNS, and a fully fledged immune response is established. Initially, CD8 cells invade, followed by CD4 cells and the establishment of a mature immune response. The induction by invading T cells of

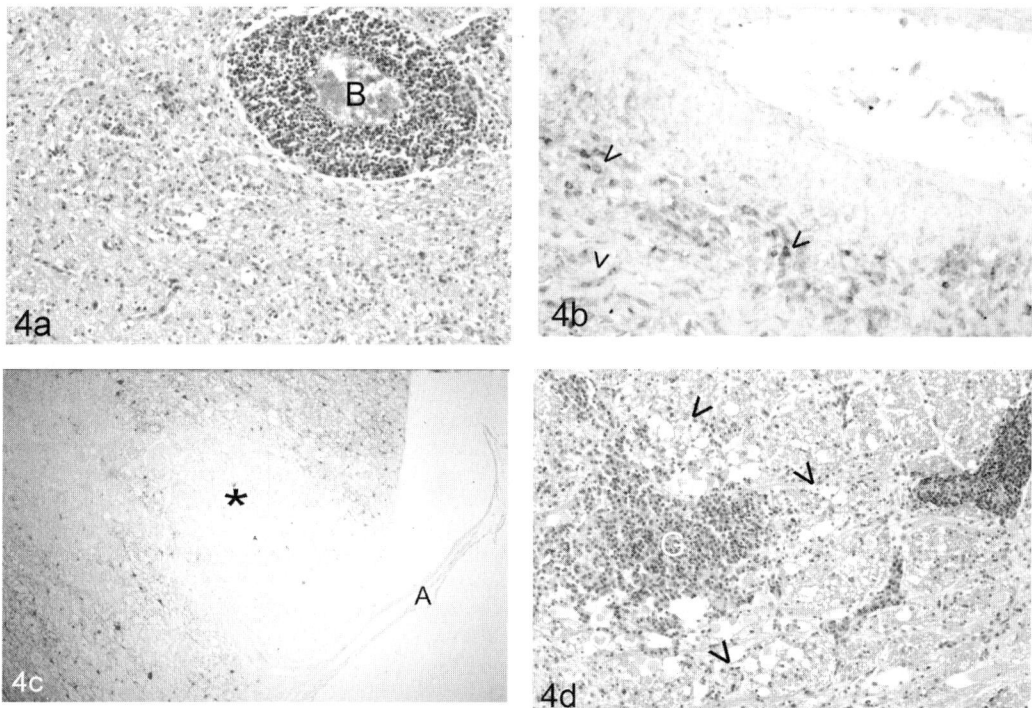

FIG. 9.4—Inflammation in the central nervous system (CNS). **a:** Hallmark of CNS inflammation: perivascular cuffing with inflammatory cells. B, Lumen of a cerebral blood vessel. Borna disease in a horse. Hematoxylin-eosin, ×100. **b:** Upregulation of cytokines in the CNS. Lymphocytes expressing interleukin 4 (IL-4) (*arrowheads*) in a periarterial infiltrate. Meninges in a case of canine steroid-responsive meningitis-arteritis. In situ hybridization for canine IL-4 mRNA. Hematoxylin-eosin, ×250. **c:** Clearance of canine distemper virus (CDV) in a spinal cord lesion. The *asterisk* depicts an inflammatory focus in which CDV has been removed. Compare with the surrounding tissue containing many darkly labeled CDV-infected cells. Immunocytochemical stain for CDV antigen. ×100. **d:** Inflammatory tissue destruction in listeriosis. The *arrowheads* depict necrosis of the brain stem around a granuloma (G). Hematoxylin-eosin, ×100.

chemokine production by microglial cells and astrocytes is an important mechanism to attract and facilitate influx of more inflammatory cells in the CNS. Next to the cellular immune response, a humoral immune response is initiated as B cells are recruited and develop into immunoglobulin-producing plasma cells.

The immune response in the CNS tissue is reflected in the composition of the CSF. The invading leukocytes are also present in the CSF, accounting for pleocytosis, an important clinical marker for inflammation. The differential cell count in the CSF may also provide information on the nature of the disease. For example, viral infections provoke a mononuclear pleocytosis, whereas bacteria cause polymorphonuclear cell infiltrates. The local production of immunoglobulin is also reflected in the composition of the CSF. The amount of intrathecally produced immunoglobulin can be measured in the CSF with immunoelectrophoretic techniques using albumin as a reference protein. The latter is necessary to estimate the contribution of leakage of immunoglobulin through the BBB, which is frequently damaged in inflammatory diseases. Whereas all albumin in the CSF is derived from the blood, immunoglobulin either can leak through the barrier or can be locally produced by infiltrated plasma cells. Based on albumin and immunoglobulin titers in blood and CSF, the so-called immunoglobulin index can be calculated, which is also a marker for an intrathecal immune response. The different immunoglobulin classes are also found in the CSF of domestic animals and measured by electrophoretic techniques or enzyme-linked immunosorbent assays (ELISAs). Isoelectric focusing of CSF reveals different immunoglobulin bands. In chronic diseases, the number of these bands may be restricted, which is called oligoclonal banding. Whereas it is very difficult to study the specificity of the intrathecal cellular immune response, the humoral immune response can be assessed by a variety of antibody assays in the CSF (e.g., by a virus-neutralization test or an ELISA). Local CNS cells also participate in the inflammatory reaction in the CNS.

HOST-PATHOGEN INTERACTION WITH ELIMINATION OF THE AGENT. The intrathecal immune response directed against an agent should ideally lead to elimination of the agent and to recovery. Generally, the humoral immune response should be able to neutralize extracellular agents, whereas CD8 cytotoxic cells should eliminate infected cells. Both together should lead to clearance of the infection. Indeed, this is frequently observed in immunocytochemical studies of viral infections of the CNS. For example, in Central European tick-borne encephalitis in dogs, the agent is cleared rapidly. However, as to how far an animal will recover is another question. This depends on the infectious load in the CNS and how many cells have been infected. When the immune response evolves very early and rapidly, spread of the agent within the CNS is limited. In experimental CDV infection in susceptible dogs,

usually a small number of dogs exhibit only mild transient clinical signs without neurological disease. However, neuropathological examination of such animals reveals the presence of small glial nodules in the CNS. Closer examination of such brains reveals that nodules contain numerous T cells, and that there is a diffuse upregulation of T lymphocytes in the CNS, but that the virus is no longer present. Thus, in these cases, the agent has been cleared effectively and rapidly from the CNS, with little impairment of structural integrity and function of the tissue. Unfortunately, in many infectious diseases, considerable primary damage has already occurred before the immune response becomes effective. When large neuronal populations are lost, permanent loss of function occurs, although a remarkable degree of compensation is possible.

Immunopathological/inflammatory damage to the tissue. The antiviral immune response directed against intracellular agents is inevitably also damaging to the tissue when, together with the agent, cells are also killed. In addition, the inflammatory process by itself generates a wide range of reactive molecules that affects not only infected cells but also adjacent tissue. The macrophages play a central effector role in this process. In chronic nervous canine distemper, there is violent inflammatory reaction in the brain, with considerable damage to the white matter. The inflammation is characterized by infiltration of lymphocytes, plasma cells, and macrophages, plus a vigorous intrathecal production of antiviral antibodies. Indeed, we observe viral clearance in inflammatory lesions but also severe destruction of the tissue. We have attempted to understand the mechanism of inflammatory destruction in dog brain cell cultures. We found that anti-CDV antibodies bound to the surface of infected cells react with the Fc receptors of neighboring macrophages, inducing a respiratory burst in these cells. These macrophages release reactive oxygen radicals, which are short-lived molecules with a highly destructive potential. This is particularly dangerous in the white matter: we found that oligodendrocytes, the myelin-producing cells, are very vulnerable to oxygen radicals, perhaps because oligodendrocytes contain iron compounds, which catalyze the production of highly destructive hydroxyl ions from the superoxide anion released by the macrophages (Fenton reaction). We also showed that macrophages stimulated in various ways, including anti-CDV antigen-antibody complexes, damage adjacent oligodendrocytes. We concluded from these experiments that the intrathecal antiviral immune response in distemper leads to clearance of the virus but also to considerable destruction of innocent bystander cells. Thus, inflammatory destruction of white matter in distemper is in fact bystander demyelination associated with an antibody-dependent cell-mediated cytotoxicity reaction.

Another example of inflammatory tissue destruction occurs in *Listeria monocytogenes* infection in ruminants. CNS listeriosis is one of the most common CNS infections in ruminants and is characterized by severe inflammation and tissue destruction in the brain stem. Macrophages appear to play an important role in tissue damage in listeriosis. We found that perivascular macrophages strongly express MHC II molecules, whereas macrophages in microabscesses and in glial nodules strongly express inductible nitrous oxide synthetase (iNOS). Calcium-binding proteins S100A8 and S100A9 were expressed in macrophages only weakly expressing iNOS. Thus, it appears that, in listeriosis, iNOS is expressed by a restricted set of macrophages. These cells produce NO, resulting in nitrite generation. This mechanism helps to eliminate bacteria but is also responsible for tissue destruction.

Immunopathological complications result in severe tissue damage in feline infectious peritonitis. The mechanism is based on the formation of circulating viral antigen-antibody complexes. Such complexes are trapped in the wall of arteries with complement fixation and subsequent induction of a suppurative inflammatory response with necrosis/obliteration of the vessel wall. Complexes are also trapped at the level of the choroid plexus, with severe pyogranulomatous chorioiditis, ependymitis, and meningitis.

Spongiform Encephalopathies: An Exception to the Rule. Generally, intrathecal immune reactions and inflammation occur in the vast majority of infectious diseases. Notable exceptions are the spongiform encephalopathies, in which bilaterally symmetrical degenerative lesions are found in the absence of inflammatory reactions such as perivascular cuffing. There are local reactions of the microglia/macrophage system, but the relentless lethal course of these diseases is evidently due to a lack of an effective intrathecal immune response. In the light of the prion theory, the lack of an intrathecal immune response seems logical. The "replication" of prions with accumulation of protease-resistant amyloid in the tissue is derived from the host's own prion protein. Thus, prions are not recognized as nonself. Apparently, the conformational change of the prion protein does not render this protein immunogenic. The best monoclonal antibodies against prions have been developed in mice with a PrP0 background. There are some indications that the immune system is somehow involved in TSE. Sheep with scrapie have increased gammaglobulin levels in the blood, and in BSE we observed a diffuse infiltration with T lymphocytes.

Space Occupation. In some infections, invasion and proliferation of inflammatory cells are so intense that large space-occupying inflammatory lesions are formed. This is the case in granulomatous encephalitis in *Lentivirus* infections in small ruminants and in canine granulomatous meningoencephalitis (GME), a relatively common disease of unknown etiology in adult dogs. Such large granulomas behave like tumors, causing compression and dislocation of brain tissue. Another form of space-occupying lesions is brain abscess arising from bacterial and fungal infections. Space-occupying lesions in the CNS cause compression of the surrounding tissues, formation of edema, and a rise in intracranial pressure similar to that seen in neoplasms.

Obstruction of Cerebrospinal Fluid Pathways. Inflammatory changes in the ventricles can cause obstruction of CSF flow. When this occurs at the level of the mesencephalic aqueduct in the midbrain, rapid accumulation of CSF in the lateral and third ventricles leads to internal hydrocephalus, with compression and atrophy of cerebral tissues, enlargement of the head, and increased intracranial pressure. Inflammation at the level of the ependymal lining also interferes with resorption of spinal fluid from the tissue to the ventricles, with similar effects. A typical example of inflammatory hydrocephalus is streptococcal infection in piglets (Figure 9.5).

Functional Impairment of the Nervous System. Inflammatory cells produce a wide range of molecules

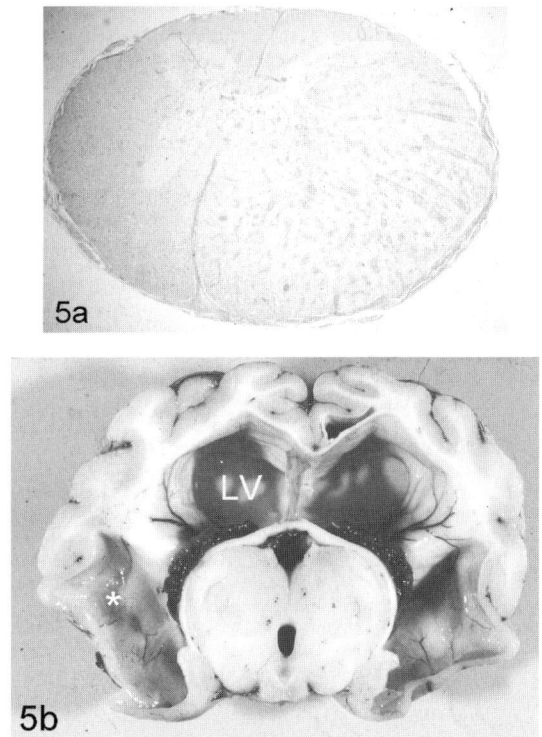

FIG. 9.5—Secondary effects of central nervous system (CNS) inflammation. **a:** Granulomatous inflammation of the spinal cord in caprine arthritis-encephalitis virus infection with massive enlargement of the cord. Hematoxylin-eosin, ×25. **b:** Hydrocephalus in porcine streptococcal infection. Marked enlargement of the lateral ventricles (LV) as a result of meningitis and ependymitis. Suppurative material visible on the surface of the ventricle (*asterisk*).

that can interfere with CNS function. Inflammation can lead to tissue destruction with loss of function. Depending on the localization of such destructive lesions, a large variety of neurological signs can occur. Direct loss of function (e g., flaccid paralysis of a limb) results from destruction of motoneurons in the corresponding spinal cord segment. Disinhibition occurs when an inhibitory center or its connection to the lower motoneurons is lost. For example, a severe thoracic spinal cord lesion causes spasticity in the hindlimbs. Other signs result from compensation for loss of function (e.g., a wide-based stance following cerebellar damage). Lesions in certain sites can have irritative effects (e.g., seizures). Since infectious-inflammatory diseases frequently cause multiple lesions in various locations, it can be expected that neurological signs occur referring to more than one area of localization. However, a multifocal clinical presentation is by no means always available: one localization may dominate the clinical picture, masking other affected sites.

SELECTED READING

Accatino A, Jaggy A, Gaillard C, Aeschbacher G. 1997. Electroencephalographic findings of encephalitis in beagle dogs experimentally infected with canine distemper virus. J Vet Med 44:39–40.

Alldinger S, Wunschmann A, Baumgartner W, et al. 1996. Upregulation of major histocompatibility complex class II antigen expression in the central nervous system of dogs with spontaneous canine distemper virus encephalitis. Acta Neuropathol (Berl) 92:273–280.

Banks WA. 1999. Physiology and pathology of the blood-brain barrier: Implications for microbial pathogenesis, drug delivery and neurodegenerative disorders. J Neurovirol 5:538–555.

Burgener I, Van Ham L, Jaggy A, et al. 1998. Chemotactic activity and IL-8 levels in the cerebrospinal fluid in canine steroid responsive meningitis-arteritis. J Neuroimmunol 89:182–190.

Collins RC, AL Pearlman. 1990. Introduction. In: Pearlman AL, Collins RA, eds. Neurobiology of Disease. New York: Oxford University Press, pp xi–xvii.

Frisk AL, Baumgärtner W, Gröne A. 1999. Dominating interleukin-10 mRNA expression induction in cerebro-spinal fluid of dogs with natural canine distemper virus induced demyelinating and non-demyelinating CNS lesions. J Neuroimmunol 97:102–109.

Graber H, Müller C, Vandevelde M, Zurbriggen A. 1995. Restricted infection with canine distemper virus leads to down-regulation of myelin gene transcription in cultured oligodendrocytes. Acta Neuropathol (Berl) 90:312-318.

Gröne A, Frisk AL, Baumgärtner W. 1998. Cytokine mRNA expression in whole blood samples from dogs with natural canine distemper virus infection. Vet Immunol Immunopathol 65:11–27.

Jungi TW, Pfister H, Sager H, et al. 1997. Comparison of inducible nitric oxide synthase expression in the brains of *Listeria monocytogenes*-infected cattle, sheep and goats and in macrophages stimulated in vitro. Infect Immun 65:5279–5288.

Kritas SK, Pensaert MB, Mettenleiter TC. 1994. Role of envelope glycoproteins gI, gp63 and gIII in the invasion and spread of Aujeszky's disease virus in the olfactory nervous pathway of the pig. J Gen Virol 75:2319–2327.

Kritas SK, Nauwynck HJ, Pensaert MB. 1995. Dissemination of wild-type and gC-, gE-and gI-deleted mutants of Aujeszky's disease virus in the maxillary nerve and trigeminal ganglion of pigs after intranasal inoculation. J Gen Virol 76:2063–2069.

Lassmann H. 1997. Basic mechanisms of brain inflammation. J Neural Transm Suppl 50:183–190.

Ledeen RW, Chakraborty G. 1998. Cytokines, signal transduction, and inflammatory demyelination: Review and hypothesis. Neurochem Res 23:277–289.

Miller DW. 1999. Immunobiology of the blood-brain barrier. J Neurovirol 5:570–578.

Müller C, Fatzer R, Beck K, et al. 1995. Studies on canine distemper virus persistence in the nervous system. Acta Neuropathol (Berl) 89:438–445.

Reams RY, Glickman LT, Harrington DD, et al. 1994. *Streptococcus suis* infection in swine: A retrospective study of 256 cases. Part II. Clinical signs, gross and microscopic lesions, and coexisting microorganisms. J Vet Diagn Invest 6:326–334.

Schobesberger M, Zurbriggen A, Summerfield A, et al. 1999. Oligodendroglial degeneration in distemper: Apoptosis or necrosis? Acta Neuropathol (Berl) 97:179–187.

Selmaj KW, Raine CS. 1988. Tumor necrosis factor mediates myelin and oligodendrocyte damage in vitro. Ann Neurol 23:339–346.

Theil D, Fatzer R, Schiller I, et al. 1998. Neuropathological and aetiological studies of sporadic non-suppurative meningoencephalomyelitis of cattle. Vet Rec 143:244–249.

Tipold A. 1995. Diagnosis of inflammatory and infectious diseases of the central nervous system in dogs: A retrospective study. J Vet Int Med 9:304–314.

Tipold A, Jaggy A. 1994. Steroid-responsive meningitis-arteritis in dogs: A long-term study of 32 cases. J Small Anim Pract 35:311–316.

Tipold A, Fatzer R, Holzmann H. 1993. Zentraleuropäische Zeckenenzephalitis beim Hund. Kleintierpraxis 38:619–628.

Tipold A, Pfister H, Zurbriggen A, Vandevelde M. 1994. Intrathecal synthesis of major immunoglobulin classes in inflammatory diseases of the canine CNS. Vet Immunol Immunopathol 42:149–159.

Tipold A, Vandevelde M, Zurbriggen A. 1995. Neuroimmunological studies in steroid-responsive meningitis-arteritis in dogs. Res Vet Sci 58:103–108.

Tipold A, Moore P, Jungi TW, et al. 1998. Lymphocyte subsets and CD45RA positive T-cells in normal canine spinal fluid. J Neuroimmunol 82:90–95.

Tipold A, Moore P, Zurbriggen A, et al. 1999. Early T-cell response in the central nervous system in canine distemper virus infection. Acta Neuropathol (Berl) 97:45–56.

Vandevelde M, Zurbriggen A. 1995. The neurobiology of canine distemper virus infection. Vet Microbiol 44:271–280.

Waxman SG. 1990. Normal and demyelinated axons. In: Pearlman AL, Collins RA, eds. Neurobiology of Disease. New York: Oxford University Press, pp 3–21.

Westmoreland BF, Benarroch EE, Daube JR, et al. 1994. Medical Neurosciences: An Approach to Anatomy, Pathology, and Physiology by Systems and Levels. Boston: Little, Brown.

Wünschmann A, Alldinger S, Vogl C, et al. 1997. Phenotypical characterization of lymphocytes in acute, subacute and chronic demyelinating brain lesions of dogs with spontaneous canine distemper encephalitis. Immunobiol Abstr 197:369.

Zurbriggen A, Graber H, Wagner A, Vandevelde M. 1995. Canine distemper persistence in the nervous system is associated with noncytolytic virus spread. J Virol 69:1678–1686.

Zurbriggen A, Schmid I, Graber HU, Vandevelde M. 1997. Oligodendroglial pathology in canine distemper. Acta Neuropathol (Berl) 95:71–77.

PART 2: PATHOPHYSIOLOGY OF NONINFECTIOUS NEUROLOGICAL DISEASES

CLETA SUE BAILEY

"In the investigation of Epilepsies, or any kind of nervous disease, we have three lines of investigation. We have:

To find the Organ damaged (Localization)
To find the Functional affection of nervous tissue.
To find the Alteration in nutrition.
There is, in brief, (1) Anatomy, (2) Physiology, (3) Pathology in each case."

JOHN HUGHLINGS JACKSON, 1873

This statement by John Hughlings Jackson, the famed British neurologist often called the Father of English Neurology, describes the essence of understanding the pathophysiology (mechanisms) of neurological disease as we see it expressed in animals or people. In other words, where is the disease, what is the functional affect of the disease, and what are the changes in the normal cellular processes that produced the abnormalities of the disease? This statement also incorporates the necessary steps in the diagnosis of neurological disease:

1. Is neurological disease present?
2. If so, where is the neurological lesion, and how many lesions are present?
3. What are the possible causes for the lesion(s)?

The term *neurological lesion* refers to a point of localized dysfunction within the nervous system. Lesions can be anatomic, with dysfunction resulting from structural damage (e.g., trauma, infection, or tumors). Lesions also can be physiological, reflecting functional abnormality in the absence of anatomic abnormality. Examples of the latter are metabolic disorders and some seizure conditions.

Detection of the presence of neurological disease requires knowledge of the normal and abnormal neurophysiological functioning of the animal (as well as the ability to perform a neurological examination). Localization of lesions requires knowledge of neuroanatomy in addition to neurophysiology. Finally, discerning the cause of the disease requires knowledge of neuropathology.

IS NEUROLOGICAL DISEASE PRESENT?
Because the nervous system is so complex and because so many different causes of neurological disease exist, these diseases may develop in a variety of ways and have a variety of clinical signs. Underlying this variety, however, are some basic themes. Recognition of these basic patterns will assist in the diagnosis of the disease.

Onset and Development of Neurological Disease. The onset of neurological disease may be either sudden or slow. For example, an animal may be traumatized and incur an immediate injury to its spinal cord. In contrast, a brain tumor may develop and grow very slowly. Having occurred, a disease may then become progressively worse over time, remain static, regress, or recur episodically. The clinical signs caused by the various types of neurological diseases tend to appear and progress in characteristic fashion (Table 9.1 and Figure 9.6). Clinical signs that are transient and rapidly reversible, such as seizures, are typical of physiological or biochemical abnormalities. Deficits that appear suddenly and either remain static or regress are suggestive of trauma or a vascular disorder. A steplike quality to the progression, or clear evidence of remissions and relapses, implies recurrent episodes of ischemia or perhaps immune-mediated disease. Signs that progress over days or weeks, with a crescendo of worsening, are typical of an expanding mass lesion, whereas steadily progressive deficits, particularly when confined to one neural system, suggest a degenerative process. Acquiring an accurate history about the appearance and progression of clinical signs is an essential and helpful initial step in the diagnostic process.

At least two noteworthy exceptions to the expected appearance and development of neurological signs occur. Trauma typically produces neurological signs

---

TABLE 9.1—Characteristic age of affected animal, speed of onset, progression, and distribution within the nervous system of the major types of neurological disease

Disease type	Age	Onset	Progression	Distribution
Degenerative	Young	Insidious	Progressive	Variable
Anomalous	Young	Birth	Nonprogressive	Focal and multifocal
Metabolic	Variable	Variable	Variable	Diffuse
Neoplastic	Adult	Insidious	Progressive	Focal and multifocal
Nutritional	Variable	Insidious	Progressive	Diffuse
Immune	Variable	Variable	Progressive	Variable
Inflammatory	Variable	Variable	Progressive	Multifocal and diffuse
Ischemic	Adult	Sudden	Nonprogressive	Focal and multifocal
Toxic	Variable	Variable	Progressive	Diffuse
Traumatic	Variable	Sudden	Nonprogressive	Focal and multifocal

Note: Exceptions to each are possible.

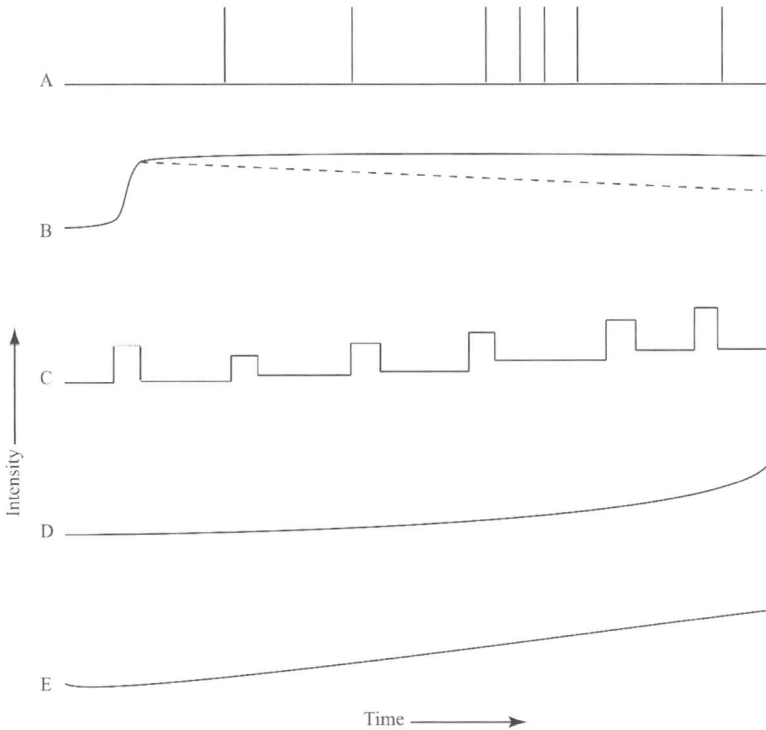

FIG. 9.6—Characteristic time courses for various types of neurological disorders. **A:** Brief episodes of neurological abnormality are typical of seizures and some biochemical disorders. **B:** A sudden onset of neurological dysfunction followed by either a static course or improvement of function is characteristic of traumatic and vascular diseases. **C:** A relapsing-remitting course is characteristic of some immune-mediated diseases. **D:** Progressively worsening dysfunction with a crescendo course is suggestive of a mass lesion. **E:** A steadily worsening course of neurological deficits is typical of degenerative disorders.

that appear immediately at the time of the injury. These signs may become more severe over the ensuing few hours, but over the next few days to weeks the abnormalities usually remain static or regress. In some instances, however, neurological signs may not be apparent at the time of the injury, but instead develop hours to days later. Two scenarios suggested by this type of history are (a) the trauma initiated some progressive process, such as hemorrhage or infection, and (b) the trauma produced a condition that is aggravated over the next few days, such as spinal instability eventually producing spinal cord trauma or compression.

The second exception is the sudden appearance of neurological signs associated with a slowly progressive disease. This often occurs in association with tumors or other mass lesions in the brain or spinal cord and suggests a vascular incident (hemorrhage or infarction) has occurred. Vascular incidents may also occur with inflammatory diseases. A sudden onset or sudden worsening of clinical signs could also be caused by a brain mass as a result of a rapid increase in intracranial pressure (ICP) and brain herniation.

Neuronal Activity and Clinical Signs Associated with Neurological Disease. The expected result of neurological disease is a loss of the normal activity of neural cells, resulting in a clinical loss of function (often called a *negative* sign, defect, or phenomenon; Table 9.2). An example of this situation is an injury to the motor-neuron axons descending from the brain to the spinal cord (axons of upper motoneurons), resulting in a loss of excitatory input to the motoneurons innervating skeletal muscles (lower motoneurons). The clinical result of such excitatory loss is weakness or absence of voluntary movement (paresis or paralysis). (See Table 9.2 for other examples.)

Neurological disease is somewhat unique, however, in that the clinical results of a loss of neuronal activity are not always a loss of function. Neurons form complex networks and circuits that produce and control neurological functions. When some of the neurons in a circuit stop functioning, the circuit itself may continue to function but in an inappropriate, unbalanced fashion. Upper motoneuron lesions provide a classic example. In contrast to the loss of voluntary movement caused by upper motor lesions, the reflex movements mediated

TABLE 9.2—Physiological basis of clinical signs

Neuronal activity	Loss of clinical function (negative sign)	Increased or abnormal clinical function (positive sign)
Decreased activity	Loss of neural facilitation or excitation Examples: paralysis, areflexia, anesthesia, and blindness	Loss of neural inhibition Examples: spasticity, rigidity, and cerebellar tremor
Increased activity	Increased inhibition Example: some types of seizures	Increased neuronal excitability Examples: spasticity, some tremors, and seizures

by the diseased or injured upper motoneurons become excessive (hyperreflexia). This is an example of a *positive* sign (defect or phenomenon). (See Table 9.2 for other examples.)

Also somewhat unique is that neurological disease may result in an increase in neural activity rather than a loss of activity. The clinical result of this increased activity depends on the normal function of the diseased structure. As with decreased neural activity, increased activity can result in either negative or positive clinical signs. Note in Table 9.2 that spasticity is given as a clinical example of decreased neuronal activity and also increased neuronal activity. Because of the multiplicity of neural functions and the complexity of neural networks, this type of situation is probably the rule rather than the exception; that is, neurological disease often results in a myriad of neurophysiological alterations that produce a number of clinical signs. For example, upper motoneuron spasticity is probably the result of loss of descending facilitation as well as descending inhibition, the development of denervation hypersensitivity, sprouting of primary afferent neurons, and a variety of changes in presynaptic and postsynaptic membranes. Some of these mechanisms take days to weeks to develop (denervation hypersensitivity and neuronal sprouting), but some occur immediately or within minutes of the development of the lesion (loss of neural input and imbalance of neuronal circuit activity).

Although individual clinical signs usually can be explained neurophysiologically, particularly when given a hypothetical lesion, the clinical situation is rarely so simple. We currently know quite a lot about the phenomenology of neurological disease, but are relatively deficient in understanding the underlying physiological mechanisms as expressed in individual patients. However, with the recent advances in the ability of diagnostic procedures to examine the nervous system at the cellular and molecular levels, this situation is rapidly changing.

WHERE IS THE NEUROLOGICAL LESION?

Just as many neurological diseases have a characteristic onset and progression, many also have typical locations within the nervous system. Therefore, identification of the disease location gives a clue to the general type of disease and often its specific cause. Aside from providing valuable clues as to the cause of a neurological disease, localization of the lesion is necessary in order to choose the appropriate diagnostic procedures.

Many of the neurodiagnostic procedures must be *aimed* at the part of the nervous system that contains the lesion. The best examples of this situation are the various radiological and imaging procedures, such as magnetic resonance imaging and computed tomography. Obviously, radiographing the vertebral column will be of little or no help in diagnosing a brain tumor. The location of a lesion can be described by

Distribution
System localization
Rostrocaudal (longitudinal) location
Transverse (segmental) location
Cellular and molecular location

Distribution. Many diseases affect the nervous system at a single site, and a patient's signs reflect dysfunction of the structures at that single site. A common example is spinal cord compression by a herniated intervertebral disc. In this situation, the disease is described as having a *focal distribution*. A disease may also affect the nervous system at several, separate sites; this is called a *multifocal distribution*. Equine protozoal encephalomyelitis is an example of this type of disease. Lastly, a disease may cause widespread neurological dysfunction, exhibiting a *diffuse distribution*. This condition is typical of metabolic or toxic disorders, in which necessary nutrients are not delivered to the nervous system or toxic waste products are not removed. As demonstrated by the examples given for each of these distributions, many neurological diseases have characteristic distributions (see Table 9.1).

In diagnosing neurological disease, the clinician must not only answer the question "Where is the lesion?" but also "How many lesions are present?" The assumption is generally made that all the signs are caused by one lesion, a focal disease. If all of the clinical and historical signs cannot be explained by a lesion at a single site, then the presence of a multifocal or diffuse disease must be assumed. Determining the distribution will aid in the construction of an appropriate list of probable diseases, which will in turn guide the diagnostic plan.

System Location. Having decided the number of lesions that are present in a patient with neurological disease, further insight into the pathophysiology of the disease, and further assistance in developing the diagnostic plan, are achieved by anatomically localizing the lesion or lesions. As a first step in this process, it is useful to consider the nervous system as several major and separate but interconnected systems (neural networks), each of which subserves a particular type of function. These systems are

Motor system
Sensory system
Visual system
Auditory system
Vestibular system
Somatosensory system
Olfactory system (difficult to assess in animals)
Gustatory system (difficult to assess in animals)
Consciousness system
Autonomic nervous system (including limbic system)
Cerebrospinal fluid system
Vascular system

Localizing lesions to particular neural systems requires knowledge of the normal functioning of these systems, and the manner in which dysfunction of them is manifested in the animal.

Rostrocaudal Location. Location along the length of the neuraxis is probably the most important localization for the purpose of directing radiographic imaging procedures and other *focal* diagnostic procedures. These diagnostic procedures include electromyography, nerve conduction-velocity studies, cerebrospinal fluid (CSF) collection, tissue biopsy, and even exploratory surgery. The major rostrocaudal loci are

1. Brain
    a. Telencephalon
    b. Diencephalon
    c. Mesencephalon
    d. Metencephalon
    e. Myelencephalon
2. Spinal cord
    a. Cervical area (C1–5)
    b. Cervicothoracic area (C6–T2)
    c. Thoracolumbar area (T3–L3)
    d. Caudal lumbar area (L4–6)
    e. Lumbosacral area (L6–S2)
    f. Sacral area (S1–3)
    g. Caudal area (Cd1–5+)
3. Cauda equina
4. Peripheral nerve: major named spinal and peripheral nerves

Using the history and specific neurological signs, rostrocaudal localization within the brain may be done even more precisely. This is particularly true if cranial nerve dysfunction is evident, as the cranial nerves and their nuclei are essentially located linearly along the length of the brain.

More precise rostrocaudal localization within the spinal cord is usually difficult unless sensory dysfunction is obvious. For example, motor deficits may indicate a lesion between T3–L3 (upper motoneuron signs

in the pelvic limbs, thoracic limb function normal), but hyperesthesia may be present at the T13–L1 area, and anesthesia may exist caudal to the midlumbar area. These abnormalities help to refine the lesion localization to the T13–L1 area. Within the thoracolumbar area, assessment of the cutaneus trunci reflex may also help localize a lesion more accurately. This reflex has bilateral projections that ascend the spinal cord from their point of entry (spinal nerves L3–4 to T2–3) to the C8 and T1 spinal cord segments. Severe unilateral or bilateral spinal cord lesions may cause the reflex to be absent to stimuli administered caudal to the lesion. Thus, an animal with a severe, bilateral T13–L1 lesion would not exhibit a cutaneous trunci reflex to stimuli applied along the back caudal to the midlumbar area.

Of particular importance in rostrocaudal localization is the knowledge of which systems cross the midline to the other side of the body, and where the decussation takes place. For example, a focal, unilateral lesion in the spinal cord produces predominantly ipsilateral motor and sensory deficits. Such a lesion in the cerebral cortex, however, would produce contralateral deficits because many of the involved neural pathways decussate in the brain stem.

Transverse Location. In the process of lesion localization, the clinician must also consider the placement of the lesion in the transverse plane, that is, within the cross section of the brain or spinal cord. Within the spinal cord, a lesion may be localized to the gray matter or white matter based on the presence of lower motoneuron or upper motoneuron signs. However, because of the limitation in our ability to examine detailed motor and sensory function in our animals, localization to fasciculi and tracts within the spinal cord is difficult. In the brain, localization within a transverse plane is often possible and often depends on observing dysfunction of several structures that are known to be adjacent at a particular site in the brain.

Localization Based on Syndromes. A *syndrome* is a constellation of signs frequently associated with each other and suggesting a common origin. Syndromes are usually produced because several structures are located close to each other and are commonly affected by a single lesion in that area. A syndrome may also be produced because a structure has several distinct functions that go awry when the structure becomes diseased. An example of the former is the cerebellomedullary angle syndrome, in which a lesion at the craniolateral aspect of the medulla produces dysfunction of cranial nerves V, VII, and VIII, ipsilateral motor and sensory deficits in the limbs, and ipsilateral cerebellar signs. An example of the latter is the cerebrocortical syndrome of circling, hemiparesis and deficits in placing reactions, disturbance of consciousness, and focal seizures. The recognition of syndromes is especially helpful in the localization of lesions and in narrowing the list of probable causes.

Specific Structural Location. The ultimate morphological localization is to a specific structure or structures, or portion thereof, such as the optic chiasm, the right side of the spinal cord at C6 and C7, or the sciatic nerve between the origins of the proximal caudal cutaneous sural nerve and the lateral cutaneous sural nerve. Although localization to this degree is the goal, this is not always possible or necessary. Many neurological diseases can be diagnosed based on a less specific localization. However, the more precisely we can locate the lesion, the better understanding we will have of the disease process itself, and the better chance we will have of devising adequate therapy.

Cellular and Molecular Localization. Recent advances in neuroscience have enabled us to localize disease processes to the cellular and molecular levels, yielding such concepts as *biochemical lesions* and *functional disorders* (Table 9.3). Understanding the mechanisms of neurological disease at this level seems to be the essence of neuropathophysiology and clinical neurology.

WHAT IS THE CAUSE OF THE LESION? The answer to this question is not simply the name of the disease or disorder affecting the animal, but the description and understanding of the cellular and biochemical mechanisms resulting in the neural dysfunction. In answering this question, we meld the basic neuroscientists with the neuroclinicians. Both contribute vitally to the goal of diagnosing and managing neurological disease. The possible variations in the mecha-

TABLE 9.3—Cellular and molecular localization of neurological lesions, with examples

1. Local neuronal circuits (focal epilepsy)
2. Neuron (amyotrophic lateral sclerosis of people, equine motor neuron disease, and rabies)
3. Axon (vitamin E deficiency, organophosphate poisoning, and progressive axonopathy of boxer dogs)
4. Schwann cell (hairy shaker lamb disease, myoclonia congenital of piglets, and hypomyelinogenesis of springer spaniels)
5. Myelin (multiple sclerosis of people, canine distemper, and acute canine idiopathic polyradiculoneuritis)
6. Synapse
   a. Presynaptic membrane (tick paralysis, botulism, and congenital myasthenia gravis of Gammel Dansk Honsehund dogs)
   b. Synaptic cleft (anti-acetylcholinesterase drugs, organophosphate toxicity, and carbamate toxicity)
   c. Postsynaptic membrane (congenital and acquired myasthenia gravis, and curariform drugs)
7. Membrane ion channels (equine hyperkalemic periodic paralysis)
8. Metabolic pathways
   a. Cofactor deficiency (vitamins B_1 and B_{12})
   b. Enzyme dysfunction (gangliosidosis, globoid cell leukodystrophy, and Niemann-Pick disease)
   c. Substrate deficiency (hypoxia and hypoglycemia)
   d. Toxins (ammonia and uremic compounds)

Sources: Oliver et al. 1997; Pearlman and Collins 1990; and Summers et al. 1995.

nistic themes are nearly as numerous as the people and animals with neurological disease, but again some basic processes exist that form the pathophysiological underpinnings.

Reactions of Neurons to Injury. A neuron may be altered in a number of ways by disease processes. These can be classified as disorders of the axolemma, the axoplasm, the neuron cell body, or the myelin sheath.

AXOLEMMAL DISORDERS. The axon membrane may undergo changes that block impulse (action potential) conduction without histological alteration or destruction of the axon. These changes are caused (a) by blockade or enhancement of neurotransmitter activity or (b) by interference with the maintenance of ion distribution across the membrane, and therefore with generation of resting or action membrane potentials. These disorders may be caused by electrical, mechanical, thermal, or chemical means. The changes are usually transient, and include the familiar phenomenon of a limb *going to sleep*. Common examples of these types of disorders include mechanical conduction block caused by pressure or distortion of a nerve, nerve block with local application of ice or local anesthetics, and inhibitory neurotransmitter blockade by strychnine.

AXOPLASMIC DISORDERS. Axons may be affected by acute or chronic disorders of the axoplasm.

WALLERIAN DEGENERATION. Cutting or crushing an axon, either in a tract within the brain or spinal cord or within a peripheral nerve, causes changes in the part of the neuron still connected to the cell body (the proximal segment) as well as in the part of the axon disconnected from the cell body (the distal segment). Physiologically, synaptic transmission fails within hours, even before morphological changes become apparent. Histologically, both segments swell, the cell body undergoes central chromatolysis, and the distal segment undergoes a dissolution called Wallerian degeneration after Augustus Waller, who first described it (Figure 9.7). Subsequently, the myelin sheath around the distal segment also degenerates. The duration of this process can range from a few days (e.g., in the peripheral nervous system) to several months [e.g., in the central nervous system (CNS)]. Additional changes include atrophy of any muscle fibers innervated by the severed axon (denervation atrophy) and retrograde and anterograde transneuronal degeneration.

AXONAL DYSTROPHY AND DYING BACK. When axons are sublethally injured, for example, by toxins or metabolic derangements, they may become narrowed (dystrophic or atrophic; Figure 9.7). In other situations, degeneration may occur in the distal portion of the axon and proceed in a retrograde direction toward the cell body. This latter process is called the *dying back* pattern of axonal degeneration. The cell body typically

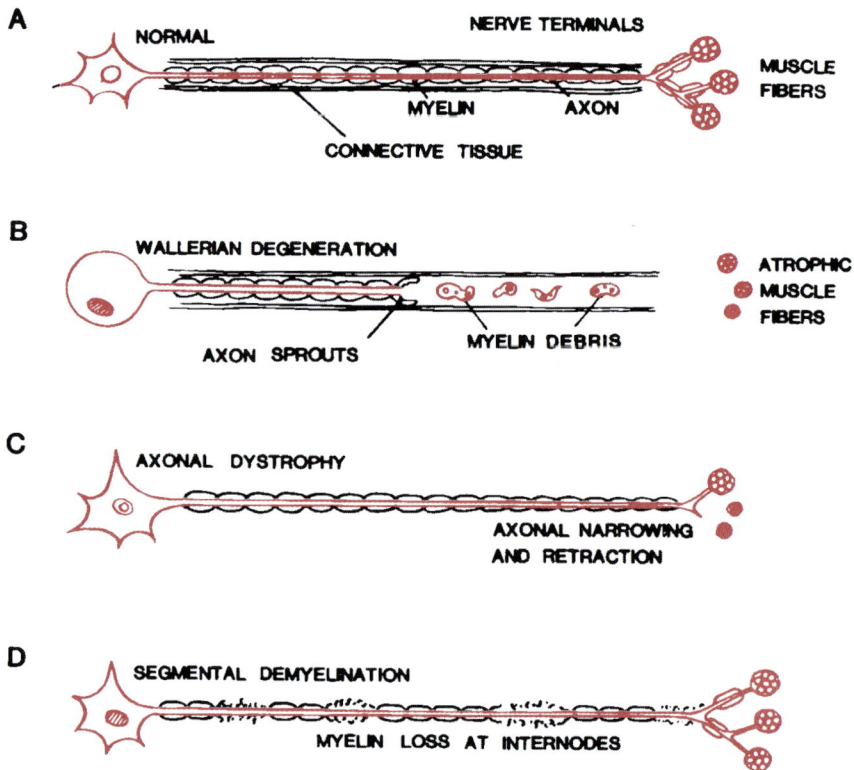

FIG. 9.7—Pathological changes in peripheral nerve fibers. **A:** Normal axon. **B:** Wallerian degeneration occurs distal to local destruction of an axon and is associated with central chromatolysis and muscle fiber atrophy. Regeneration occurs along the connective tissue path. **C:** Axonal dystrophy results in distal narrowing and dying back of nerve terminals, due to either intrinsic axon or motor-neuron disease. **D:** Segmental demyelination destroys myelin at scattered internodes along the axon without axonal damage. (By permission of Mayo Foundation for Medical Education and Research.)

survives this process, as does the more proximal portion of the axon, which maintains its ability to conduct an action potential with normal conduction velocity. These axonal diseases are classified under the general term *axonopathies*. An example is the disorder caused by chronic exposure to organophosphate chemicals.

The distal, or dying-back, axonopathies affect the longest axons first—typically those innervating the distal portions of the limbs. Because axons have no ribosomes, they have no capacity for protein synthesis. Thus, the axon and its terminal depend on the nerve cell body for their supply of structural elements, which are delivered to the terminal by axonal transport mechanisms. This arrangement has some inherent risks, particularly for the longest axons. The preference of the dying-back phenomenon for neurons with long axons is classically attributed to interference with these axonal transport mechanisms. At least two other mechanisms may also explain the preferential involvement of the distal limbs. One explanation is that the disease process may require the cooler temperatures of the distal limbs, such as is necessary for the replication of

Mycobacterium leprae in the pathogenesis of leprosy. A second explanation is that a disease may attack the axon at any point along its length, not just the distal portion, and longer axons have a higher probability of *hits* along their length.

NEURONAL CELL DEATH: NECROSIS AND APOPTOSIS. Although the oft-stated dogma that dead neurons cannot be replaced is now known to be false, it is true that neuron regeneration does not occur in a widespread, clinically useful manner. As a result, the death of neurons is problematic and often catastrophic.

The cell death and tissue degeneration that are caused by disease have long been regarded as passive events. Severe disturbance of the intracellular homeostatic control and swift cell disruption characterize the injury that leads to tissue necrosis. In contrast, an active and highly regulated form of cell death has been described within the past two decades. In this type of death, termed *apoptosis*, the cell plays an active role in its own demise and disposal, which often occur discretely without tissue necrosis. Cellular necrosis and apoptosis have different morphological and molecular features and implications for the tissue.

Cellular necrosis is characterized by cellular swelling, mitochondrial damage, rapid energy loss, and a random breakdown of the cell's nucleus. Lysis of the cell membrane quickly follows, with release of the cell's contents into the parenchyma, which often invokes an inflammatory response. The inflammatory response generally consists of cellular infiltration, vascular injury, and edema, and damages the surrounding tissue. Apoptosis literally means a "falling away." In this process, an individual cell undergoes a genetically controlled transition from an intact metabolically active state into a shrunken remnant more or less retaining its membrane integrity. Lysis of cellular organelles does not occur until late in this process, and little leakage of the contents of the dying cell can be detected. As a consequence, apoptotic cells do not induce an inflammatory response of the same type or degree as necrotic cells. Instead, the shrunken apoptotic bodies are specifically recognized and phagocytosed, leaving the tissue's structural organization essentially unaltered. Thus, apoptosis provides an organism with a safe way to turn over cells continuously in any tissue. Apoptosis also provides the capacity to remove specific, perhaps abnormal, cells during development. A surprise finding in the study of development was that the death of neurons is a normal and widespread occurrence during embryonic development. Up to half of all neurons initially generated are removed by apoptosis.

The dysregulation of apoptosis (pathological apoptosis) may be an important mechanism underlying many diseases. Increased apoptosis may be involved in the long-lasting neurodegenerative conditions such as Alzheimer's disease, AIDS-related dementia, and multiple sclerosis in people. Apoptosis may also be important in the delayed cell death following cerebral ischemia. In contrast, a suppression of apoptosis could disturb the fine balance between cell proliferation and cell death, favoring the growth of neoplastic cell clones. Also, the suppression of apoptosis in autoreactive T-cell clones may promote the onset of autoimmune diseases.

Necrosis and apoptosis seem to be distinct and different modes of cell death. However, they may actually represent the extremes of a continuum. The two processes can be initiated by the same stimuli, and whether apoptosis or necrosis occurs can be influenced by the intensity or duration of the inciting insult. Additionally, the two processes may be present in a tissue at the same time or occur sequentially.

TRIGGERS OF NEURONAL DEATH. A countless variety of signals, stimuli, and conditions can lead to neuronal death. The most comprehensive information on the mechanisms of cell death exists for acute degenerative disorders, particularly ischemia. We now know, however, that the same cellular and molecular mechanisms that lead to acute cell death also operate in chronic neurodegenerative disease.

INTRACELLULAR CA^{2+} OVERLOAD. A widely accepted theory—the calcium hypothesis of neuronal cell death—is that increased intracellular calcium and its effects represent a *final common pathway* leading to irreversible cell injury. Thus, a loss of calcium homeostasis may play a major role in causing neuronal necrosis in both acute and chronic neurodegenerative disorders. Numerous cellular functions require calcium signals or simply the maintenance of a set calcium concentration. The major requirement for the signaling function of calcium is the existence of a concentration gradient between the extracellular fluid and the interior of the cell, and cells are continuously faced with the problem of maintaining a gradient of more than 4 orders of magnitude across the plasma membrane. Within the cell, calcium is largely sequestered into different organelles, such as the endoplasmic reticulum and mitochondria. Various physiological stimuli increase the cytosolic concentration of calcium transiently, either by allowing an influx of calcium from the extracellular space or by releasing calcium from its intracellular stores, thereby inciting cellular responses. Under pathological conditions, however, changes in intracellular concentration of calcium are more pronounced and sustained. When calcium accumulates to pathophysiological levels, it can induce a number of potentially destructive reactions, including the following:

1. *Mitochondrial dysfunction:* Increased cytosolic calcium leads to a loss of the mitochondrial membrane potential and loss of mitochondrial function. Intramitochondrial stores of calcium can then be released into the cytosol, aggravating the situation. Mitochondrial failure also results in the loss of cellular energy production through loss of adenosine triphosphate (ATP) production and loss of production of reactive oxygen species that incite oxidative stress and damage.

2. *Activation of hydrolytic enzymes:* The main classes of hydrolytic enzymes include proteases, kinases, endonucleases, and phospholipases. These enzymes can attack receptor and ion-channel proteins, break down the cytoskeleton, fragment DNA, and release arachidonic acid resulting in additional generation of reactive oxygen species.

3. *Altered gene expression:* The cascade of events initiated by elevated intracellular calcium can also affect gene transcription and translation, activating the expression of several immediate early genes such as c-*fos* and c-*jun*. These genes may be important in the initiation and progression of cell death, as well as in the reparative response of sublethally injured cells.

CAUSES OF INTRACELLULAR CALCIUM OVERLOAD. A number of pathological events can result in elevated intracellular calcium. Two of the most studied, and apparently most ubiquitous, are excitotoxicity and oxidative stress. *Excitotoxicity* is a term applied to the harmful effects of excessive stimulation of excitatory, ion-channel-linked glutamate receptors, such as the *N*-methyl-D-aspartate receptor (NMDA-R), a ligand-gated Ca^{2+} channel. Excitotoxicity has been implicated in the acute neuronal death accompanying hypoxia, ischemia, hypoglycemia, brain and spinal cord trauma, and seizures. Excitotoxic mechanisms have also been implicated in chronic neurodegenerative diseases such as Alzheimer's disease, Parkinson's disease, amyotrophic lateral sclerosis (ALS, Lou Gehrig's disease), epilepsy, and chronic pain syndromes. In these latter diseases, weak or slow excitotoxicity may occur either due to abnormalities in excitatory amino acid receptors or as a consequence of defects in energy metabolism. Excitotoxicity is accompanied by increases in intracellular calcium that then leads to a number of deleterious consequences and neuronal cell death, as already noted.

Oxidative stress results from the loss of regulation of the pro-oxidant/antioxidant balance. Oxygen plays a vital role in cellular respiration as the terminal electron acceptor, yet the oxygen metabolites formed during this process include free oxygen radicals, which are potentially toxic to cells. (A *free radical* is any chemical species that contains one or more unpaired electrons and is capable of existing independently.) Because of its high metabolic activity, the brain uses large amounts of oxygen and therefore generates high levels of free oxygen radicals. Additionally, the brain has high levels of polyunsaturated fatty acids. The unsaturated bonds in these molecules render them susceptible to oxidative damage by free radicals. Considering its importance, one would assume that the nervous system would be amply endowed with defense mechanisms to counter oxidative stress. Contrary to this expectation, however, the CNS, and especially the brain, does not have an abundance of processes to neutralize oxygen radicals and is very vulnerable to attack by reactive oxygen species. A large number of physiological and pathological sources of oxygen radicals exist. Sources of exogenous agents include photochemical smog, ozone, pesticides, xenobiotics, and ionizing radiation. A number of endogenous cellular processes also generate free radicals. Free oxygen radicals can cause lipid peroxidation, oxidize proteins, and damage DNA. Thus, these radicals have a variety of deleterious effects on neuronal function, including increased blood-brain barrier permeability, altered tubulin formation, inhibition of mitochondrial respiration, and perturbations in synaptic transmitter and ion functions.

MYELIN SHEATH DISORDERS. Some nerve fibers of mammals are covered with a lipid-rich sheath, called *myelin*. Myelin is formed in the CNS by the modified processes of oligodendrocytes, and in the peripheral nervous system by Schwann cells. Myelin has a high electrical resistance and low capacitance, allowing it to function as an electrical insulator. The myelin is formed in distinct segments known as internodes separated from each other by nodes of Ranvier. As a consequence, conduction of action potentials along myelinated fibers must *jump* from uninsulated point to uninsulated point (node to node), a process termed *saltatory conduction*. In unmyelinated fibers, conduction occurs by a moving depolarization along the entire length of the fiber, a much slower process than saltatory conduction. The conduction velocity of mammalian unmyelinated fibers ranges from 0.5 to 2 meters per second; the conduction velocity of myelinated fibers ranges from 5 to 120 meters per second.

Destruction of the myelin sheath exposes the internodal axon (Figure 9.7), which is essentially electrically inexcitable due to a lack of sodium channels, and allows leakage of current across the nerve fiber membrane of the internodes. The depolarization of the next node of Ranvier is delayed, altering impulse conduction. Extensive demyelination actually blocks action-potential conduction. Abnormalities in conduction that can occur in demyelinated, or partially demyelinated, axons are

1. Decreased conduction velocity
2. Temporal dispersion of impulses, a result of unequal slowing of conduction in the fibers of a given nerve or tract, resulting in reduced or absent nerve action potentials (this could account for loss of tendon reflexes and vibration sensibility, which rely particularly on synchronous bursts of neural activity)
3. Partial blockage of high-frequency trains of action potentials
4. Total conduction block

These abnormalities result in neurological deficits that reflect the normal function of the affected nerves (i.e., paresis, paralysis, and reflex deficits if motor nerves are affected; sensory and reflex deficits if sensory nerves are involved).

Demyelination can also produce abnormalities of action potential generation, which may be responsible for *positive* signs that accompany myelin disorders. Ectopic potential generation (action potentials arising at or near the site of demyelination) may be responsible for apparent paresthesia or dysthesia. Electrical interaction (cross talk) between demyelinated axons, a process called *ephaptic transmission*, also may produce abnormal sensory phenomena. Increased sensitivity to mechanical stimuli may cause dysthesia and pain on percussion or pressure at the demyelinated site.

Not all nerve fibers are myelinated; in fact, over two-thirds of all fibers in peripheral nerves are type C fibers (or type IV fibers in the sensory nerve classification), which are unmyelinated. These fibers carry impulses from some types of pain, itch, temperature, and crude touch receptors. The function of these fibers should be preserved in strictly demyelinating, peripheral nerve diseases.

Demyelination occurs in various neurological conditions, and is the main feature in the so-called *demyelinating diseases*. These are diseases in which the pathological process selectively involves myelin sheaths and often spares the axons in a remarkable manner. This situation is termed *primary demyelination*. Only a few primary demyelinating diseases occur in animals. Canine distemper and visna maedi of sheep are two inflammatory diseases in which myelin is selectively destroyed (termed *myelinoclastic diseases*). An example of a human demyelinating disease is multiple sclerosis. In another class of diseases, the leukodystrophies, myelin sheath abnormalities are caused by enzymatic disorders of genetic origin. These disorders, which are familial, are suitably called *dysmyelinating disorders.* Nonspecific injury to myelin resulting in demyelination occurs in a number of other situations, as well, specifically following axonal damage (termed *secondary demyelination*). Demyelination is also a feature of massive white-matter lesions such as cerebral infarcts, hemorrhages, and cerebral tumors. In these latter situations, the physiological and clinical effects of demyelination are likely complicated and overridden by the neuronal damage.

Ischemia-Hypoxia. Ischemia, which is the reduction of blood flow to a level incompatible with normal function, occurs with many disease processes, including inflammatory diseases, neoplasia, trauma, and primary vascular disorders. Ischemia may be global (generalized) as with cardiac arrest or severe hemorrhage, or it may be focal as with stroke in people or fibrocartilagenous embolism of the spinal cord in animals. As the blood is the delivery system for oxygen, ischemia and hypoxia usually coexist, and the injury mechanisms of each are intertwined. Hypoglycemia is also usually involved, contributing to the cellular energy failure, which is the root of ischemic pathophysiology. Experimental and clinical evidence shows two distinct periods of neuronal loss after a reversible ischemic-hypoxic injury. Some neurons die during the initial insult—the primary phase—but approximately 2 to 12 hours after the injury, further neuronal loss occurs—the secondary phase. The processes of cell death during the two phases are similar, but differences exist (Table 9.4), which may have implications for therapy.

Restoration of blood flow after an ischemic insult is essential for recovery. However, reperfusion may lead to further tissue damage. The mechanisms of reperfusion injury are poorly understood, but are believed to include the formation of oxygen free radicals, eicosanoids, and cytokines, as well as an influx of leukocytes, initiating a cascade of damage. Leukocyte accumulation may obstruct the microcirculation, contributing to the secondary phase of neuronal loss.

Edema. This is the abnormal increase in water and sodium content in a tissue. The CNS has several

TABLE 9.4—Mechanisms of neuronal cell loss in the phases of ischemic–hypoxic injury

Mechanism	Primary phase	Secondary phase
Increased intracellular calcium	+++	±
Membrane instability	++++	+
Increased production of oxygen-free radicals	+	+
Excitotoxicity	+++	+++
Apoptosis	–	++++

anatomic attributes that protect it from edema. A lymphatic system is not present, and the interstitial space between cells, especially in the gray matter, is much less than in other tissues. Additionally, the capillaries of the CNS are designed to limit fluid transport from the circulation into the neuropil. Except for specialized structures in the nervous system that have a secretory function, the neural capillaries are not fenestrated as they are in other tissues. Instead, these capillaries have tight junctions between endothelial cells. Also, the endothelial cells have few pinocytotic vesicles for transcellular transport. Despite these protective mechanisms, though, cerebral edema probably develops to some extent in all pathological states.

Edema has been classified in a variety of ways. Current concepts describe three types of edema: cellular (old term is cytotoxic), vasogenic, and interstitial (aka hydrocephalic). Cellular edema is characterized by swelling of all the cellular elements of neural tissue (neurons, glia, and endothelial cells), due to a net shift of water from the extracellular space to the interior of the cells. Among the many causes of cellular edema are hypoxia, ischemia, metabolic disorders, drug poisoning, water intoxication, and acute hyponatremia. Vasogenic edema, the most common type of neural edema, results from increased permeability of the blood-brain barrier, which allows plasma to leak into the neuropil. White matter is particularly affected. Vasogenic edema occurs with ischemia, hemorrhage, neoplasia, trauma, and vasculitis. Interstitial edema is characterized by the accumulation of edema fluid (in this case CSF) predominately around the ventricles. This typically occurs with obstructive hydrocephalus (hydrocephalus caused by obstruction of intraventricular or extraventricular CSF pathways). Inflammation of the lining of the ventricles can also produce interstitial edema by allowing leakage of CSF across the damaged ependyma.

The clinical effects of neural edema, particularly brain edema, can be catastrophic, if not fatal. The increased volume of contents (i.e., the edema fluid) within the rigid cranial vault or vertebral canal results in increased pressure within the neural tissue, distortion of the ventricles in the brain, distortion of the subarachnoid space, decreased blood circulation, ischemia, hypoxia, and metabolic failure of the neural cells. An additional complication of brain edema and increased ICP can be brain herniation (see the *Brain Herniation* section).

Increased Intracranial Pressure. Because the bony skull is virtually incompressible, ICP rises when the volume of the intracranial contents is increased. The intracranial contents have three normal components: neural tissue (brain, meninges, and associated cellular tissue), CSF within the ventricles and the subarachnoid space, and blood in the vessels within and outside the brain (Figure 9.8A). If the volume of any of these constituents increases, the volume of the others can compensate by decreasing. This is particularly true of CSF and blood volume (Figure 9.8B and C). Brain volume

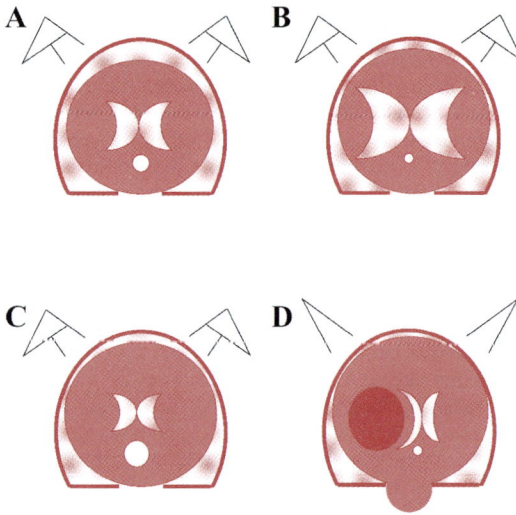

FIG. 9.8—Schematic representation of relationships among brain (*gray circle*), subarachnoid space and brain ventricles (*light grey*), and brain vasculature (*white circles*) within the rigid cranium (*heavy black line*). **A:** Normal condition. **B:** Noncommunicating (obstructive) hydrocephalus. **C:** Impaired venous drainage or global vasodilation. **D:** Mass lesion (*black oval*) with brain herniation.

can decrease, as well, by atrophy (which takes quite a bit more time) or by the escape of brain tissue from the cranial vault (brain herniation; Figure 9.8D). ICP rises when the volume increase of any of these three constituents outstrips the compensatory mechanisms. ICP can also rise if the volume capacity of the cranial vault itself is decreased, as with skull deformation associated with trauma or neoplasia. Examples of the numerous causes of increased ICP are presented in Table 9.5.

The results of increased ICP include impaired cerebral blood circulation resulting in ischemia and hypoxia, edema, neural dysfunction, brain herniation, and death. Neurons that are very active metabolically

tend to suffer first; thus, cerebral cortical signs, particularly decreased consciousness, are often the first signs noted (other than focal signs if the inciting lesion is focal). In addition to the intracranial effects of increased ICP, several systemic effects may occur, including cardiac arrhythmias, pulmonary edema, gastrointestinal ulceration, and sudden death. An interesting phenomenon has been documented in people with advanced stages of increased ICP: the occurrence of plateau waves. In this situation, the ICP elevates dramatically for 15 to 20 minutes, then returns to normal, and may recur hourly. The waves indicate a failure of the compensatory mechanisms for maintaining a normal ICP. Plateau waves may occur in patients with increased ICP due to a variety of causes. In people, these are most commonly observed with tumors, trauma, and hydrocephalus.

Brain Herniation. This is the displacement of a portion of the brain from its normal position in the cranial vault. These displacements are around the various osseous or fibrous barriers of the cranial vault, such as

1. Cerebral hemisphere under the falx cerebri
2. Occipital lobe(s) and/or diencephalon under the tentorium cerebelli
3. Cerebellum through the foramen magnum

The cause of brain herniation is an increased volume of contents within a compartment of the cranial vault, which may then lead to increased ICP. If the normal compensatory mechanisms for increased ICP (decrease in CSF and blood volume) are exceeded, the brain tissue itself will be pushed out of its normal position into an adjacent compartment of the cranial vault. The causes of increased ICP are given in the preceding *Increased Intracranial Pressure* section. The specific cause and location of the lesion determine the type of herniation that occurs. Focal lesions, such as a tumor of one cerebral hemisphere, can produce a relatively *focal* herniation, such as the herniation of the involved hemisphere under the falx cerebri. Diffuse diseases of the brain, such

TABLE 9.5—Causes of increased intracranial pressure

Increased volume of tissue components	Increased cerebrospinal fluid (CSF) volume	Increased blood volume	Decreased volume of cranial vault
Inflammation (inflammatory cells and vasogenic edema fluid)	Neoplasia (obstructive hydrocephalus, and increased CSF secretion by choroid plexus tumor)	Cardiovascular/respiratory disease (cerebral vasodilation due to hypoxia)	Neoplasia (skull tumor)
Metabolic and toxic disorders (cellular edema)	Trauma (obstructive hydrocephalus)	Inflammation (impaired hydrocephalus)	Trauma (compression skull fracture)
Neoplasia (tumor cells and vasogenic edema fluid)		Neoplasia (vascular tumors, impaired venous drainage, venous compression, and tumor thrombosis or embolism)	
		Trauma (hemorrhage, hematoma, and impaired venous drainage)	

as toxic, metabolic, and some inflammatory diseases, can produce herniation at multiple sites. The herniation may occur spontaneously as the disease process progresses, or may be precipitated by an event that suddenly lowers the pressure within the communicating spinal subarachnoid space, such as the aspiration of CSF.

As usual, the clinical signs produced by the herniation depend on the specific neurological structures affected. The clinical signs are the result of compression of the herniated tissue (e.g., the occipital lobes) and also compression of the tissue normally lying adjacent to the barrier (e.g., the midbrain under the tentorium cerebelli). Clinical signs may also be the result of obstructive hydrocephalus (e.g., compression and occlusion of the mesencephalic aqueduct in the midbrain), and impaired circulation because of compression of vascular structures in the area. Herniations can occur quite suddenly and be quickly fatal owing to compression of vital areas of the brain, such as the respiratory centers.

Hydrocephalus. This is the condition of an increased CSF volume within dilated brain ventricles. CSF is formed principally by the choroid plexuses in the lateral, third, and fourth ventricles. A smaller amount is formed extrachoroidally by the diffusion of brain interstitial fluid across the ependyma or pia mater. CSF flows from the sites of production to sites of absorption. Fluid formed in the lateral ventricles flows through the paired interventricular foramina into the third ventricle and then through the mesencephalic aqueduct into the fourth ventricle. The majority of the CSF exits the fourth ventricle into the subarachnoid space through the lateral foramina. Absorption occurs directly into the venous system through arachnoid villi that project into the cranial dural sinuses, through lymphatic channels in the dura, and through the perineural sheaths around the cranial and spinal nerves. The volume of ventricular CSF may increase as a result of increased production, obstruction to flow, or decreased absorption of the CSF. Hydrocephalus caused by increased production or impaired absorption of CSF is called *communicating hydrocephalus* (the ventricles still have unimpeded connection—communication— with the subarachnoid space). Hydrocephalus caused by an obstruction to CSF flow within the ventricular

system is called *noncommunicating hydrocephalus* (the communication of the ventricular system with subarachnoid space is impeded). Causes of the various forms of hydrocephalus are numerous (Table 9.6).

The clinical effects of hydrocephalus depend to a large extent on the cause and type of hydrocephalus. However, the accumulation of CSF and dilation of the ventricles have consequences independent of the inciting agent. One of the determinants of clinical signs of hydrocephalus is the presence of increased intraventricular or intracranial pressure. Increased pressure occurs particularly with noncommunicating hydrocephalus, and, within 3 to 4 hours of an acute, total obstruction, the periventricular white matter becomes edematous. A reduction in myelin lipids leads to actual thinning of the adjacent white-matter layer. This is especially evident around the lateral ventricles. The gray matter of the cerebral cortex and basal nuclei are relatively spared, at least initially. Eventually, even the gray matter atrophies and degenerates. The most common sites for obstruction are the narrow areas of the ventricular system: the interventricular foramina, the mesencephalic aqueduct, and the lateral apertures. Following obstruction, ventricular dilation occurs rostral to the obstruction. Typical clinical signs include enlargement of the head of neonates, inappropriate mental status (dementia, aggression, retarded learning), and visual deficits with normal pupillary reflexes due to cerebral cortical dysfunction. Gait and postural abnormalities may also be present as a result of cerebral cortical, internal capsule, basal nuclei, and even cerebellar dysfunction if the fourth ventricle is involved. If the obstruction is at the lateral apertures, the increased intraventricular pressure may also distend the central canal of the spinal cord, particularly the cervical cord, producing hydromyelia and syringomyelia and consequently a cervical myelopathy.

Interestingly, hydrocephalus is not always accompanied by increased ICP. Increased intraventricular pressure may return to normal as the inciting disorder stabilizes and an equilibrium state develops (arrested hydrocephalus). The term *normal-pressure hydrocephalus* is used to designate the syndrome of communicating hydrocephalus without clinical evidence of increased ICP. Normal-pressure hydrocephalus is associated with inadequacy of the subarachnoid space and

TABLE 9.6—Causes of hydrocephalus

Communicating hydrocephalus	Noncommunicating hydrocephalus
Increased CSF production	Congenital mesencephalic aqueduct malformation
Choroid plexus tumor	Intraventricular hemorrhage
Decreased CSF absorption	Ependymitis
Congenital arachnoid villi malformation	Neoplasia
Subarachnoid hemorrhage (arachnoid villi become congested with fibrin or protein)	
Meningitis (arachnoid villi become congested with fibrin or protein)	
Neoplasia of the meninges	

CSF, cerebrospinal fluid.

impaired CSF absorption. In contrast, ICP may undergo wavelike changes, so-called plateau waves, as described in the *Increased Intracranial Pressure* section.

Mass Effect. In thinking of focal lesions, a useful concept is that of mass versus nonmass lesions. A *nonmass lesion* is one that is altering cellular function in the area of the lesion but is not substantially interfering with neighboring cell performance. In this type of lesion, the pathological process is not, by virtue of its size or volume, compressing, damaging, or destroying nearby structures. The clinical signs are those of a focal or multifocal (if more than one mass is present) lesion. A *mass lesion* affects not only the tissue involved in the lesion, but also neighboring tissue and potentially even distant structures. The clinical signs are those of expanding focal (or multifocal) disease progressing to diffuse disease in the later stages. The specific clinical signs reflect the size, location, and the rate of lesion expansion. If located in a noncritical area and if compensatory mechanisms have time to develop, a mass can become quite large before producing noticeable clinical signs. The effects of mass lesions on neighboring tissue include compression with demyelination of white matter and vascular compromise, edema, and eventually cellular degeneration. The specific effects of a mass depend on the disease process producing the mass and the biological properties of the mass (e.g., the ability to affect the blood-brain barrier, resulting in vasogenic edema). Mass lesions can affect distant parts of the brain by means of increased ICP and ventricular obstruction leading to hydrocephalus. Causes of mass lesions include neoplasia, particularly noninfiltrative tumors, hematomas, granulomas, abscesses, and edema.

The concept of mass versus nonmass lesions is not so easily applied to the spinal cord. Because of its small cross-sectional area and linear structure, masses in the spinal cord have less opportunity to affect neighboring and distant structures. However, the concept of focal, multifocal, and diffuse lesions is very applicable to the spinal cord.

Neural Compression. This is an element of many neurological disease processes. Compression can be applied suddenly or gradually and can be brief or sustained. If applied suddenly and removed within a short period, the process is more of a traumatic nature and is pathophysiologically different from insidious or sustained compression. Hemorrhage and edema, particularly of the gray matter, are not characteristic of compressive lesions as they are for traumatic lesions. Instead, gradual or sustained compression affects primarily white matter, where demyelination as well as axonal degeneration occurs. With focal lesions, particularly in the spinal cord, wallerian degeneration occurs in the distal segments of the axons traversing the lesion. In severely compressive lesions, neurons in the gray matter degenerate. Mechanical deformation likely plays a major role in generating the lesion. Circulatory compromise, particularly impaired venous drainage,

may also have an effect. Mass lesions are compressive lesions, but not all compressive disorders are mass lesions (e.g., increased ICP and hydrocephalus). Compression is an element of many congenital and developmental disorders of the vertebral column, many neoplastic diseases, some inflammatory diseases (particularly those with sizeable granulomas or abscesses), some traumatic lesions, and sustained intervertebral disc protrusion.

Functional Disorders of Neurons. Agents that do not cause overt structural damage to the cells may alter neuronal function. Biochemical lesions that either block or augment neurotransmitter activity or interfere with normal ion distribution across the cell membranes exemplify this type of disorder. Transmitter disorders affect transmission of action potentials across synapses. Many of these disorders are toxic in nature, such as botulism, strychnine poisoning, and organophosphate poisoning. Congenital and acquired myasthenia gravis are also examples of transmitter disorders. Two other examples of functional disorders are the ion-channel disorders (termed channelopathies) and seizures.

CHANNELOPATHIES. Since 1990, a group of diseases resulting from small but critical alterations in ion channels has been recognized. These diseases, called *channelopathies*, are caused by genetic mutations or acquired alterations of ion-channel proteins. Defects have been found involving sodium, potassium, chloride, and calcium channels. Ion channels regulate the traffic of cations and anions across lipid cell membranes and are critical for most aspects of cellular function. In neural tissue and muscle, ion channels are particularly important in the generation, propagation, and transmission of electrical impulses (action potentials). Ion-channel defects have been identified in the heart, kidney, inner ear, and brain, but the best characterized of these disorders are those affecting skeletal muscle cells. Alterations in muscle ion-channel function produce either myotonia (muscle stiffness due to excessive electrical excitability) or paralysis (due to insufficient muscle excitability). A sodium channelopathy—hyperkalemic periodic paralysis—has been identified in horses. This disorder is caused by a change in a single base pair in one of the two sodium-channel genes, resulting in a single amino acid change in the protein product. This change alters the characteristics of the channel so that it cannot function correctly, and the horse suffers episodes of stiffness and paralysis. The disorder is dominantly inherited. Interestingly, this disorder also occurs in people, in whom it is also dominantly inherited.

SEIZURES. The term *seizure* refers to a transient alteration in behavior caused by the disordered, synchronous, and rhythmic firing of populations of neurons in the CNS or, more succinctly, a symptomatic paroxysmal cerebral dysrhythmia. Although the cellular and biochemical mechanisms are still incompletely understood, the cerebral cortex is considered to be the primary generator of seizures. The behavioral, or clinical, features of a seizure are determined by the functions normally served by the cerebral cortical region generating the seizure. Thus, as described by Lennox and Lennox (1960) for people, seizures are composed of any one or more of five recurrent and involuntary phenomena:

1. Loss or derangement of consciousness or remembrance
2. Excess or loss of muscle tone or movement
3. Alteration of sensation, including hallucination of special senses
4. Disturbance of the autonomic nervous system, with resulting vegetative and visceral phenomena of various sorts
5. Other psychic manifestations, abnormal thought processes, or moods

Based on experimental and clinical work in animals, this description seems applicable to seizures in animals, as well. Unfortunately in animals, several of these phenomena may be unrecognizable, or simply not noticed by an observer, making identification of an *event* as a seizure sometimes difficult.

Seizures have been classified into two major types: *partial* seizures and *generalized* seizures. Generalized seizures are characterized by widespread involvement of both cerebral hemispheres from the onset of the seizure. Partial seizures begin focally in a small region of the cerebral cortex. They may spread throughout the cerebral hemispheres to become generalized (termed partial seizures with secondary generalization). Several subtypes have been described for people in each of the two major seizure categories. In animals, the most commonly recognized seizures seem to be generalized, tonic-clonic seizures in which the animal loses consciousness and has a generalized contraction of muscles (tonus) followed by muscle jerking (clonus). However, actual recording of the electrical activity of the cerebral cortex (electroencephalography) immediately prior to and during seizures is done rarely in animals, and therefore accurate classification of seizure types is lacking. In people, identification of seizure type is the basis for deciding on appropriate therapy.

Seizures are the end result of a state of increased neuronal excitability and/or synchronization. Partial seizures are usually caused by a structural lesion that alters inherent neuronal properties and neuronal circuits, leading to recurrent hyperexcitability. Such structural lesions can be caused by inflammation, neoplasia, or trauma involving the cerebral cortex. The physiological basis of hyperexcitability is not well understood, but likely involves abnormalities of the cell membrane and alterations in ion-channel properties. Axonal sprouting, synaptic reorganization, and the development of aberrant interneuronal connections after an injury may also play a role. Primary generalized seizures may be the result of a congenital, diffuse, or multifocal hyperexcitable condition, such as an ion-channel abnormality.

Despite being a functional disorder, however, seizures, particularly continuous seizures (status epilepticus), can cause neuronal death. Neurons in cortical layers of the hippocampus and pyriform lobes are most susceptible. The mechanism of cell death is unclear, but appears to be associated with a massive release of excitatory neurotransmitters (excitotoxicity) induced by the excessive electrical discharge of the seizure, which then results in necrosis and apoptosis.

Epilepsy is the chronic condition of recurrent seizures caused by

1. Genetically determined primary brain dysfunction (inherited epilepsy)
2. Active brain disease (symptomatic epilepsy)
3. Inactive brain disease (symptomatic epilepsy)
4. Brain disorders of undetermined cause (idiopathic or cryptogenic epilepsy)

In people, genetic mechanisms have been implicated in over a dozen of the epileptic syndromes, and the mutant gene has been identified in over half of these. Most of these epilepsies are generalized-onset epilepsies. The identified patterns of inheritance include autosomal dominant, X-linked dominant, autosomal recessive, mitochondrial, and complex patterns. Having identified the mutant gene associated with an epileptic syndrome, the next task is to discern how the genotype produces the phenotype; in other words, how the mutation results in increased neuronal excitability and epilepsy. As already noted, one mechanism would be to change the functioning of ion channels. The mutant gene associated with autosomal dominant nocturnal frontal lobe epilepsy encodes a subunit of the ion-channel receptor for the neurotransmitter acetylcholine. Acetylcholine is thought to open the channel by triggering a conformational change that alters the association of amino acid residues in the channel. The amino acid residue at position 248 of the normal subunit is serine, whereas the amino acid residue at this position in this epileptic syndrome is phenylalanine, the result of a point mutation. What is the impact on channel function of this substitution? Is the permeability of ions through the channel modified? Is the sensitivity of the channel to various drugs changed? Ultimately, the questions are these: How do such changes in the channel physiology produce seizures? How can these physiological changes be therapeutically ameliorated?

PATHOPHYSIOLOGY OF NONINFECTIOUS NEUROLOGICAL DISEASES

Chronic Degenerative Diseases. Degenerative diseases are a group of heterogeneous diseases for which no cause is apparent. As causes for these diseases are determined (e.g., viral infection, metabolic error, and environmental toxin), they will be reclassified in the appropriate category. A number of animal diseases fall into this category, including the cerebellar abiotrophies seen in several animal species, degenerative encephalomyelopathies, motor-neuron diseases such as equine motor-neuron disease, and neuroaxonal dystrophies. In people, the most important diseases in this group are Parkinson's disease, Alzheimer's disease, and amyotrophic lateral sclerosis.

These disorders are characterized by a gradual decrease in neurological function, often with bilaterally symmetrical involvement of several levels of the nervous system. The mechanisms of chronic degenerative disease appear to be similar to those of acute disorders; these are defects in mitochondrial energy (ATP) production, excitotoxic neuronal damage, elevated intracellular calcium, enhanced levels of oxygen free radicals producing oxidative stress, and alterations in gene expression (e.g., the induction of immediate early genes) important in the initiation and progression of cell death. In these diseases, cell death is not massive and develops inconspicuously. Therefore, it seems reasonable to assume that pathological apoptosis is involved.

Genetic Neurological Diseases. More genes are expressed in the CNS than in any other tissue. This attests to the great complexity of the nervous system, particularly the brain. Several thousand human genes have been cloned and sequenced, but of greatest interest to basic and clinical neurologists has been the isolation of genes with mutations that cause neurological disease. To date, about 100 neurogenetic disorders have been identified in people, and at least twice that many are known or suspected in animals.

Recessive disorders typically involve loss of function of the mutated gene. Affected individuals, having two copies of the mutant gene, have no active protein product and suffer a consequent phenotype. Many recessive disorders are associated with loss of an enzyme activity, such as globoid cell leukodystrophy in Cairn and West Highland white terriers (deficiency of β-galactocerebroside) and fucosidosis in English springer spaniels (deficiency of α-L-fucosidase). The clinical features of such a recessive disorder may result either from the inability to produce a required metabolite downstream from the defect in the enzymatic pathway, or from the failure to remove a compound produced upstream in the pathway. In unaffected carriers of a recessive genetic defect, the one remaining normal allele produces sufficient activity to prevent the development of clinical symptoms.

Dominant disorders may also involve loss of function if a normal allele cannot fully compensate for the loss of activity (loss of the protein product) of its mutant allelic partner. More commonly, dominant mutations involve expression of a protein product with altered function— or *gain of function*. Alteration of normal function is typified by a number of channel disorders, such as hyperkalemic periodic paralysis, which is the result of a missense substitution mutation of the muscle sodium channel. Both normal and mutant alleles are expressed, but the mutant protein allows leakage of sodium ions that causes repetitive muscle firing, depolarization, and consequently muscle weakness. Another type of altered function that can be seen in dominant disorders is a so-called dominant negative mutation. In this situation, both normal and abnormal protein products are expressed, but the mutant protein interacts directly or indirectly with the normal protein and prevents it from performing its normal function. Such mutations are often associated with structural proteins in which a single abnormal subunit can inactivate an entire structure. Complex disorders involve multiple gene-gene interactions or gene-environment effects. In these disorders, individual genes may be inactivated or otherwise altered by mutations that predispose an individual to the disorder but are insufficient to cause symptoms on their own. In addition to the Mendelian inherited diseases, genetic mechanisms have now been implicated in a variety of other neurological disorders (particularly in people), including ischemia/stroke, epilepsy, multiple sclerosis, human immunodeficiency virus encephalopathy, prion disorders, Alzheimer's disease, amyotrophic lateral sclerosis, Parkinson's disease, and genetic mitochondrial disorders.

In the genetic diseases associated with premature neuronal death, symptoms may not appear until later in life. This delay in clinical onset has been assumed to reflect the accumulation of cellular damage over time. For example, oxidative stress may disrupt metabolism by cumulative damage of essential macromolecules. This hypothesis predicts that the probability of cell death will increase over time. An alternate hypothesis, the *one hit* model of cell death, arose from patient data analysis that indicated neurons died at a fairly constant rate regardless of the stage of the disease. This theory proposes that a mutation imposes a mutant steady state on the neuron, and a single event randomly initiates cell death. The one-hit model appears to be common to many forms of neurodegeneration and has implications for therapy. Particularly, the one-hit model suggests that the probability of therapeutically rescuing diseased neurons does not decrease with age.

Neoplasia. A wide variety of primary and metastatic tumors occur in the CNS. Even within the same tumor type, these tumors vary by degrees of malignancy. Benign tumors are slow growing and have few mitoses, no necrosis, no vascular proliferation, and no associated edema. Therefore, benign tumors may become quite large before having a noticeable effect, particularly in animals, which cannot describe abnormal sensations, don't use eating utensils, and aren't required to balance a checkbook. Malignant tumors are characterized by rapid growth, an invasive nature, many mitotic figures, vascular proliferation, endothelial hyperplasia, and necrosis. The mass effect of malignant tumors is augmented by vasogenic edema in surrounding white matter. Malignant tumors may actually produce a substance that compromises the blood-brain barrier, allowing the edema formation. CNS tumors rarely metastasize out of the CNS, but instead cause death by relentless local growth. Thus, the histological distinction between benign and malignant tumors is less important for CNS tumors than for tumors elsewhere in the body. The actual location of the tumor is just as important in determining the tumor's morbidity and mortality as is its degree of malignancy.

The specific cause of neuroectodermal tumors remains unknown, but like that of cancer in general it is thought to be related to altered genetic information, caused either directly by mutation or through epigenetic events such as defects in mitosis that produce segregational errors. During the development of a tumor, loss-of-function mutations lead to impairment in cellular activities that function physiologically to restrain cell proliferation. The genes that encode these growth-restraining activities are known as *tumor-suppressor genes*, and inactivating mutations of such genes have been recognized to contribute to the development of many different tumor types, including brain tumors. The second class of mutations known to contribute to the development of malignant tumors occurs in genes that are typically involved in cellular proliferation. These genes, known as *proto-oncogenes*, encode proteins that are growth factors or growth-factor receptors, mediators of signaling pathways, or regulators of gene expression. Activating mutations convert proto-oncogenes to oncogenes, which either encode a structurally different protein with novel biological activities or encode a normal protein that is expressed at inappropriately high levels or at inappropriate times. The result is uncontrolled, inappropriate, cellular proliferation. Inciting agents may be viruses, immune-system abnormalities, irradiation, or petrochemicals.

Central nervous system tumors produce neurological symptoms by the following mechanisms:

1. Cellular dysfunction due to ischemia, compression, and energy failure
2. Mass effect due to volume of tumor tissue, vascular proliferation, and edema
3. Hemorrhage resulting in inflammation and mass effect
4. Increased intracranial pressure and potentially brain herniation
5. Obstructive hydrocephalus
6. Seizures due to changes in the excitability of cortical neurons
7. Cell death by necrosis

The signs of CNS tumors tend to have an insidious onset and become slowly worse. However, deficits can develop suddenly or worsen quickly if hemorrhage, CSF obstruction, or brain herniation occurs.

Trauma. Trauma to neural tissue has two main effects: the primary immediate damage arising as a direct consequence of the physical forces, and secondary, delayed, reactive processes that are autodestructive. The primary damage encompasses mechanical damage such as concussion, contusion, laceration, distortion, distraction, compression, and transection. Neurological dysfunction is the result of the physiological blockage of action-potential generation or conduction in concussed or physically disrupted neurons. Immediate vascular effects such as hemorrhage, vasospasm, and vasodilatation resulting in an immediate reduction of blood flow, ischemia, and hypoxia contribute as well. These processes affect the gray matter more than the white matter and can result in cellular necrosis within minutes.

Although the initial effects clearly can be catastrophic, the delayed effects that occur over the next several hours make things much worse and can produce irreversible damage and even death. For example, nearly one-third of people who die from head trauma have spoken some time after their injury. The secondary phase results from the cumulative effects of systemic (affecting the whole body) phenomena as well as focal changes in the neural tissue. The systemic changes can include hemorrhage, hypotension, hypoxia, hyperglycemia, hyperthermia, and shock. The focal secondary changes are the result of neural ischemia-hypoxia, release of excitotoxic agents such as glutamate into the tissue, increased calcium levels in the cytosol with activation of the calcium-dependent hydrolytic processes, generation of free oxygen radicals and oxidative stress, vasogenic and cellular edema, increased ICP, compression and herniation, and cellular necrosis. Traumatic CNS injuries also incite an inflammatory response that begins within hours. The inflammatory response can also be destructive, enhancing vascular permeability and vasogenic edema, as well as inciting leukocyte and platelet infiltration, which compromises the blood flow even further.

Vascular Disorders. Vascular disease has two major forms: occlusive and hemorrhagic. In both forms, the blood supply to tissue is interrupted and ischemia occurs. If the ischemia is severe enough, death of the tissue—infarction—ensues. Neurons deprived of their metabolic support (oxygen and glucose) stop functioning in minutes. Thus, the hallmark of vascular disease is a sudden onset of a usually focal deficit. In addition to ischemia, hemorrhage can also produce a mass lesion. The specific clinical signs observed reflect the structures supplied by the affected vessel(s). Clinical signs are most likely to develop with disease of larger vessels (vessels that supply large amounts of tissue) and vessels that have few anastomoses with other vessels. Vascular disorders include vascular malformations, inflammation of vessels (vasculitis), vascular neoplasia, and various embolic disorders (e.g., feline ischemic encephalopathy, fibrocartilagenous embolic myelopathy of various species, and encephalomalacia following intracarotid injection in horses). In people, *stroke* (cerebrovascular accident—infarct or hemorrhage associated with degenerative vascular changes) is of immense medical, economic, and social importance. Cerebrovascular accidents comparable to those in people rarely occur in animals, probably because, for the most part, animals lack the predisposing factors of arteriosclerosis and hypertension.

RECOMMENDED READING

Astic L, Saucier D. 2001. Neuronal plasticity and regeneration in the olfactory system of mammals: Morphological and functional recovery following olfactory bulb deafferentiation. Cell Mol Life Sci 58:538–545.

Bailey CS, Kitchell RL, Haghighi SS, Johnson RD. 1984. Cutaneous innervation of the thorax and abdomen of the dog. Am J Vet Res 45:1689–1698.

Bartus RT. 1997. Calpain inhibition: A common therapeutic rationale for treating multiple neurodegenerative conditions? In: Bar PR, Beal MF, eds. Neuroprotection in CNS Diseases. New York: Marcel Dekker, pp 71–86.

Bast A, Bar PR. 1997. The antioxidant/prooxidant balance in neurodegeneration and neuroprotection. In: Bar PR, Beal MF, eds. Neuroprotection in CNS Diseases. New York: Marcel Dekker, pp 147–159.

Beal MF. 1997. Therapeutic effects of nitric oxide synthase inhibition in neuronal injury. In: Bar PR, Beal MF, eds. Neuroprotection in CNS Diseases. New York: Marcel Dekker, pp 131–146.

Cannon SC. 1998. Ion channel defects in the hereditary myotonias and periodic paralyses. In: Martin JB, ed. Molecular Neurology. New York: Scientific American, pp 257–277.

Ceballos-Picot I. 1997. The Role of Oxidative Stress in Neuronal Death. Austin: Landes Bioscience and Chapman and Hall.

Clarke PGH. 1999. Apoptosis versus Necrosis. In: Koliatsos VE, Ratan RR, eds. Cell Death and Diseases of the Nervous System. Totowa, NJ: Humana, pp 3–28.

Clarke G, Collins RA, Leavitt BR, et al. 2000. A one-hit model of cell death in inherited neuronal degenerations. Nature 406:195–199.

Collins RC, Pearlman AL. 1990. Introduction. In: Pearlman AL, Collins RA, eds. Neurobiology of Disease. New York: Oxford University Press, pp xi–xvii.

Eger CE, Howell JM. 1988. The nervous system. In: Robinson WF, Huxtable CRR, eds. Clinicopathologic Principles for Veterinary Medicine. Cambridge: Cambridge University Press, pp 330–377.

Faden AI. 1993. Experimental neurobiology of central nervous system trauma. Crit Rev Neurobiol 7:175–186.

Fishman RA. 1992. Cerebrospinal Fluid in Diseases of the Nervous System. Philadelphia: WB Saunders.

Fry EJ. 2001. Central nervous system regeneration: Mission impossible? Clin Exp Pharmacol Physiol 28:253–258.

Gluckman PD, Gunn AJ. 1997. Neuroprotection in hypoxic-ischemic encephalopathy. In: Bar PR, Beal MF, eds. Neuroprotection in CNS Diseases. New York: Marcel Dekker, pp 409–424.

Gusella JR, Martin JB. 1998. Principles of neurogenetics. In: Martin JB, ed. Molecular Neurology. New York: Scientific American, pp 1–18.

Hoffman EP. 1995. Voltage-gated ion channelopathies: Inherited disorders caused by abnormal sodium, chloride, and calcium regulation in skeletal muscle. Annu Rev Med 46:431–441.

Holt WF. 1997. Glutamate in health and disease: The role of inhibitors. In: Bar PR, Beal MF, eds. Neuroprotection in CNS Diseases. New York: Marcel Dekker, pp 87–119.

Israel MA. 1998. Molecular genetics of brain tumors. In: Martin JB, ed. Molecular Neurology. New York: Scientific American, pp 95–114.

Jackson JH. 1873. On the anatomical, physiological and pathological investigation of the epilepsies. In: The West Riding Lunatic Asylum Medical Reports, vol 3.

Johanson CE. 1995. Ventricles and cerebrospinal fluid. In: Conn MP, ed. Neuroscience in Medicine. Philadelphia: JB Lippincott, pp 171–196.

Kandel ER, Schwartz JH, Jessell TM, eds. 1991. Principles of Neural Science. New York: Elsevier.

Kempermann G, Gage F. 2000. Neurogenesis in the adult hippocampus. Novartis Found Symp 231:220–235.

Leist M, Nicotera P. 1999. Calcium and cell death. In: Koliatsos VE, Ratan RR, eds. Cell Death and Diseases of the Nervous System. Totowa, NJ: Humana, pp 69–90.

Lennox WG, Lennox MA. 1960. Epilepsy and Related Disorders. Boston: Little, Brown.

March PA. 1998. Seizures: Classification, etiologies, and pathophysiology. Clin Tech Small Anim Pract 13:119–131.

McNamara JO. 1998. Genetics of epilepsy. In: Martin JB, ed. Molecular Neurology. New York: Scientific American, pp 75–93.

Nicotera P, Leist M. 1997. Apoptosis and control of cell death. In: Bar PR, Beal MF, eds. Neuroprotection in CNS Diseases. New York: Marcel Dekker, pp 319–330.

Oliver JE Jr, Lorenz MD, Kornegay JN. 1997. Handbook of Veterinary Neurology. Philadelphia: WB Saunders.

Pearlman AL, Collins RC, eds. 1990. Neurobiology of Disease. New York: Oxford University Press.

Poirier J, Gray F, Escourolle R. 1990. Manual of Basic Neuropathology. Philadelphia: WB Saunders.

Purves D, Augustine GJ, Fitzpatrick D. 2001. Neuroscience. Sunderland, MA: Sinauer.

Schmidley JW, Maas EF. 1990. Cerebrospinal fluid, blood-brain barrier, and brain edema. In: Pearlman AL, Collins RA, eds. Neurobiology of Disease. New York: Oxford University Press, pp 380–397.

Shapiro WR, Shapiro JR. 1996. Malignant tumors of the nervous system. In: Guthkelch AN, Misulis KE, eds. The Scientific Foundations of Neurology. Cambridge, MA: Blackwell Science, pp 361–375.

Sharp FR, Honkaniemi J, et al. 1998. Molecular approaches to the therapy of stroke. In: Martin JB, ed. Molecular Neurology. New York: Scientific American, pp 115–133.

Shin C, Lee K-H. 1999. Epilepsy and cell death. In: Koliatsos VE, Ratan RR, eds. Cell Death and Diseases of the Nervous System. Totowa, NJ: Humana, pp 361–378.

Siesjo BK, Lindvall O. 1996. Degeneration and regeneration in the brain. In: Guthkelch AN, Misulis KE, eds. The Scientific Foundations of Neurology. Cambridge, MA: Blackwell Science, pp 3–31.

Summers BA, Cummings JF, De Lahunta A. 1995. Veterinary Neuropathology. St Louis: CV Mosby.

Takahashi M, Niki E. 1998. The effect of oxidative stress on cells by oxygen radicals and its inhibition by antioxidants. In: Montagnier L, Pasquier C, eds. Oxidative Stress in Cancer, AIDS, and Neurodegenerative Diseases. New York: Marcel Dekker, pp 9–14.

Watson JC, Bullock R. 1997. Neuroprotection in acute neurological disease: Trauma to the brain and spinal cord. In: Bar PR, Beal MF, eds. Neuroprotection in CNS Diseases. New York: Marcel Dekker, pp 387–408.

Waxman SG. 1990. Normal and demyelinated axons. In: Pearlman AL, Collins RA, eds. Neurobiology of Disease. New York: Oxford University Press, pp 3–21.

Waxman SG. 2000. Correlative Neuroanatomy. New York: Lange Medical/McGraw-Hill.

Waxman SG. 2001a. Acquired channelopathies in nerve injury and MS. Neurology 56:1621–1627.

Waxman SG. 2001b. Form and Function in the Brain and Spinal Cord: Perspectives of a Neurologist. Cambridge: MIT Press.

Westmoreland BF, Benarroch EE, Daube JR, et al. 1994. Medical Neurosciences: An Approach to Anatomy, Pathology, and Physiology by Systems and Levels. Boston: Little, Brown.

PART 3: MECHANISMS OF CENTRAL NERVOUS SYSTEM HOMEOSTASIS

ROBERT H. DUNLOP

CENTRAL NERVOUS SYSTEM OPERATIONS AND MAINTENANCE: SOME AUTONOMIC ASPECTS OF CENTRAL REGULATION

Regulation in the organism is the central problem in physiology.

W.B. CANNON

This chapter presents an overview of the mainly subconscious elements of brain function and dysfunction. Conceptual overlap with parts of the coverage of the pathophysiology of infections of the central nervous system (CNS) and of noninfectious diseases is inevitable but kept to a minimum. The primary focus will be placed on the general managerial aspects of the brain keeping itself "in good running order" or homeostasis and a look at some of the adaptive responses to physical and chemical challenges that require multisystem integration (Cotman and McGaugh 1980). The subject areas involved include the homeostatic roles of maintaining food and water intake (which have behavioral components as well as autonomous ones), and metabolism, waste disposal, temperature regulation, sleep-arousal-emergency activity, sexual arousal and other reproductive behaviors (which are covered in another section), and other neuroendocrine responses. Central control of blood circulation and breathing is obviously part of the story, but the dysfunctions are covered elsewhere in this book under the relevant body systems (Chapters 5 and 6). Similarly, numerous aspects of endocrine dysfunction are addressed under endocrinology, reproduction, and lactation.

CENTRAL NEUROTRANSMITTER FUNCTIONS.
Histofluorescence, lesioning, selective pharmacological agents, and advances in biochemical analysis, commencing in the 1950s, made possible the visualization and functional description of many of the brain's neurotransmitter (NT) systems (Nestler et al. 2001) (Table 9.7).

Catecholamines in the Central Nervous System: Dopamine, Norepinephrine, and Epinephrine

DOPAMINE. Dopamine (DA) neurons (totaling about 3500) are centered in the midbrain ahead of the norepinephrine (NE) elements that are mainly based in the pons and medulla. DA neurons occur in major cell groups A8 and A9 in the large black mass of neurons called the substantia nigra. Their fibers pass to the largest basal ganglia: the caudate nucleus and the putamen. Together, the latter two are called the striatum

TABLE 9.7—Classes of central neurotransmitters

Cholinergics
  Acetylcholine
    Nicotinic receptors—nAChR
    Muscarinic receptors—mAChR
Catecholamines
  Dopamine
  Norepinephrine
  Epinephrine
Indoleamines
  Serotonin (5-hydroxytryptamine)
Imidazoleamines
  Histamine
Amino acids
  Glutamate
  Aspartate
  GABA
  Glycine
Peptides (many)
  Purinergics
    P1 receptors—ATP and ADP
    P2 receptors—AMP and adenosine
  Enkephalins and other opioids
Nitrergics
  Nitric oxide

(appear striped). The output of A8 and A9 forms the nigrostriatal pathway and is made up of very fine fibers that contain 75% of the DA in the brain. The role of DA involves motor integration. If the nigrostriatal pathway is damaged, failure to make DA available results in severe motor disturbances. Parkinson's disease is characterized by a fine tremor of the hands at rest, rigid resistance to passive movement of the limbs, and a decrease in the frequency of voluntary movement. It involves progressive degeneration of the dopaminergic pathway from the substantia nigra to the striatum in the basal ganglia. The balance between dopaminergic and cholinergic inputs to the striatum that control fine movements is lost as dopaminergic neurons are lost. Then, the dominant cholinergic activity causes tremor. The problem can be reduced by treatment with levodopa, which is a precursor of DA and can make up for the shortfall. With time, however, the treatment loses its value and leads to dyskinesia, with uncontrollable movements of mouth, cheeks and limbs.

Five metabotropic G protein-linked DA receptors have been sequenced. DA cells in the hypothalamus control secretion of certain pituitary hormones. Veterinary applications are still in the experimental stage. However, the drug domperidone is a competitive antagonist at peripheral DA_2 receptors and has been tested with some encouraging results in mares that graze endophyte-infected tall fescue and thus have low prolactin concentrations in their plasma. Other applications of DA have included intensive care of hypotensive foals on fluid therapy to exploit its stimulation of α- and β-adrenergic receptors to achieve a pressor effect. DA has also been tried in paralytic ileus to restore intestinal motility. An excellent illustration and description of gastrointestinal ileus by G.D. Lester (2002) can be found in *Large Animal Internal*

Medicine (Smith 2002 Figure 30-44). This is an excellent schematic diagram of neural and hormonal influences on intestinal motility. Studies are needed on the central neural actions of DA and other neurotransmitters in diseases affecting domestic mammals.

NOREPINEPHRINE. NE neurons are estimated to total only about 10,000 in or around the locus coeruleus (LC), mostly in the dorsal part of the pons-medulla region. They are designated A1 to A7 plus A11 (A1 to A4 are in the medulla, and A5 to A7 are in the pons). Remarkably, these neurons send fibers to almost all major functional parts of the brain. The A6 nucleus in the LC is particularly remarkable for the elaborate branching of its axons throughout the brain, including the fanlike Purkinje cells of the cerebellum and a bundle to the cortex (forebrain). One branch, the *dorsal bundle*, innervates the hypothalamus, thalamus, hippocampus, and cerebral cortex. Other fibers pass to the septum, basal ganglia, amygdala, limbic lobe and surrounding olfactory cortex, and olfactory bulb. The fibers to the cortex go directly without a relay in the thalamus. The other cell groups feed into a major fiber cable: the *ventral bundle*. That lies deeper in the reticular formation. At the level of the hypothalamus, the dorsal and ventral bundles merge and then separate again as they head for the forebrain. The brain's NE cells comprise the *sympathetic nervous system* of the brain, serving the brain nuclei much as the peripheral sympathetic nervous system, with its network of vessels, neurons, ganglia, and fibers, integrates a wide range of functions and responses in organs peripheral to the brain. Some of the fibers from the medulla and pons send axons to the gray matter of the spinal cord, the link between central and peripheral systems.

NE is formed from DA by the enzyme β-hydroxylase. It is important in arousal via widespread release of NE, which acts mainly as a modulator of other NTs. NE is not released directly into synapses. Rather, it is liberated at a distance from its receptors. This has the effect of creating the equivalent of a generalized *neural arousal*. Within the LC, the NE neurons have a low firing rate during sleep that increases during arousal. When fully awake, their frequency of firing increases with the intensity of the focus on the task at hand.

EPINEPHRINE. A small number of the catecholamine neurons in the brain contain the enzyme, phenylethanolamine *N*-methyltransferase (PEMT), which is necessary to form epinephrine (Epi) from NE.

6-Hydroxydopamine has devastating effects on central noradrenergic neurons: when injected near them, they accumulate it, and it kills them apparently via toxic metabolites that it forms.

Acetylcholine in the Ventral Nervous System

CHOLINERGIC NEUROTRANSMISSION. Projecting from the brain stem, both somatic and autonomic preganglionic motoneurons are cholinergic, using acetylcholine (ACh) as the NT. The CNS has three main cholinergic NT systems:

1. The *pontine reticular formation* sends axons (a) back to the spinal cord or (b) forward to forebrain structures.
2. The *basal forebrain nuclei* connect widely with the cortex.
3. The *septum* projects to the *hippocampus.*

Cholinergic neurons use choline acetyltransferase (ChAT) to make ACh from acetylcoenzyme A (ACoA). Note that ACh is the *only* NT whose synaptic action is terminated in the synapse. Active neuronal uptake processes functionally inactivate other NTs. The agent responsible is the esterase enzyme AChE. After it acts, the choline moiety is recovered. Receptors (R) for ACh are either (a) *nicotinic receptors* (nAChR), which are ligand-gated, or (b) *muscarinic receptors* (mAChR), which are metabotropic and G protein linked.

NICOTINIC RECEPTORS. In the CNS, nicotinic acetylcholine receptors (nAChRs) are confined mainly to the Renshaw cells, which are glycinergic interneurons in the ventral horn of the spinal cord that are activated by collaterals of α motoneurons and produce inhibitory postsynaptic potentials (IPSPs) that suppress weakly firing motoneurons and dampen strongly firing ones, a general modulating effect. Their blockade by strychnine results in convulsions due to failure of the recurrent inhibition. Note the mechanistic connection between the nicotinic receptors of the Renshaw cells and those of the neuromuscular junction.

MUSCARINIC RECEPTORS. Central muscarinic receptors are widely distributed in the CNS. There are two types: (a) M1 receptors, which are postsynaptic, and (b) M2 receptors, which are presynaptic. Note that in their peripheral distribution muscarinic acetylcholine receptors (mAChRs) mediate fast transmission in autonomic ganglia and at the neuromuscular junctions of skeletal muscle. They are also present in smooth muscle of *hollow organs*, including blood vessels and viscera, cardiac muscle, and glands.

In the brain, their function is to mediate long-term facilitation of cortical neurons. The overall effect is to promote cortical arousal in response to rewarding stimuli. This is different from the arousing effect of noradrenergic stimulation. Sites with cholinergic neurons include

1. The medial septum, which projects to the hippocampus
2. The magnocellular forebrain nuclei of the basal forebrain, which projects to the cerebral cortex
3. Part of the pontine reticular formation in the brain stem with axons that project rostrally to the amygdala, thalamus, and basal forebrain, as well as back to the spinal cord

Central cholinergic neurons in the brain stem are involved in regulating sleep and awake states. Wakefulness requires midbrain reticular system projections to the thalamus. In non-rapid eye movement (REM) or slow-wave sleep (SWS) stage 2, thalamic neurons fire bursts called *sleep spindles*, but, in deeper sleep (stages 3 and 4), the thalamic firing ceases, disconnecting it from the cortex. This is because the excitatory drive from the hypothalamus to the thalamus stops. Cholinergic neurons that are quiet in the awake state become active in REM sleep. In REM sleep, thalamocortical neurons are excited by stimuli from the preoptic hypothalamus, and the cholinergic input from pons to thalamus becomes highly active, exciting the cortex and giving rise to the pontine-geniculate-optical (PGO) spikes of the electroencephalogram (EEG). The pontine cells that cause the REMs and autonomic irregularities trigger these. The reticular system of the medulla and pons blocks all sensory input and motor output (hence loss of muscle tone), disconnecting the brain from the external world during REM sleep. It has been postulated that the role of sleep may be to edit the load of information coming in during wakefulness, retaining a memory of only *significant* events (designated by a programmed brain?). Such a process of selective *unlearning* could account for the transient cortical arousal of dreaming that is followed by forgetting (Mallick and Inoue 1999).

Cholinergic sites are vulnerable to a wide range of toxicants: biological products of bacteria, poisonous plants, animal venoms, synthetic chemicals. The affected synapse may be central or peripheral, somatic or autonomic. Some of the targets include

1. Plasmalemmal sodium ion (Na^+)-dependent choline transport system: Hemicholinium causes neuromuscular blockade by competing with choline for the choline carrier, inhibiting its uptake. Choline mustard aziridinium analogues compete with choline for entry into cholinergic neurons.
2. Synthesis of ACh via choline acetylase: (a) Naphthoquinones (halogenated cholines) reduce ACh synthesis. (b) There are false cholinergic NTs.

Massive losses of cholinergic pathways from basal forebrain and septum to hippocampus are a major feature of the brain in Alzheimer's dementia.

INDOLEAMINES: SEROTONIN OR 5-HYDROXYTRYPTAMINE. 5-Hydroxytryptamine (5-HT or serotonin) neurons are in the Raphe nuclei along the upper edge of the midline from the lower part of the midbrain down into the medulla oblongata. 5-HT has a favorable effect on mood—almost a NT for happiness. Unlike the general stimulatory effect of glutamate and the inhibitory one of γ-aminobutyric acid (GABA), NE and 5-HT distribute their modulators over a wide network of fibers modulating their function. 5-HT stems from a cluster of neuronal foci in the raphe nuclei. Nine nuclei form a ridge through the very center of the brain stem, and these neurons send their axons to release 5-HT, virtually throughout the brain. They are most active when mammals are awake and active, and least active during

sleep. Mice genetically engineered to lack a 5-HT receptor are hyperaggressive to any new mouse placed in their cage.

Some 5-HT neurons are important in pain sensation, sending axons back to the dorsal horn of the spinal cord that inhibit nociceptor input to the spinothalamic tract. Also, some synapse with preganglionic autonomic neurons. Rostrally, 5-HT fibers run in the medial forebrain bundle supplying many forebrain structures, including the choroid plexus [which regulates cerebrospinal fluid secretion] and the cerebral blood vessels (which regulate blood flow). The amino acid tryptophan (T) is hydroxylated by T hydroxylase to form 5-HT. The transporter for 5-HT reuptake ends this NT's action. Tricyclic antidepressants and 5-HT reuptake inhibitors (e.g., fluoxetine) inhibit this. Monoamine oxidase (MAO) catabolizes 5-HT to 5-hydroxyindoleacetic acid (5-HIAA). Receptors for 5-HT are mostly metabotropic except for 5-HT itself, which is *ligand gated* (a term for many NT receptors that combine receptor and ion-channel functions in a single molecule) and nonspecific. Another large group of receptors for NTs and hormones is that of the G protein-coupled receptors (metabotropic receptors). In this case, their binding by agonists activates intracellular G proteins.

When 5-HT is acetylated and then methylated enzymatically, it is transformed to melatonin (Mt). Mt is downregulated by light. The *pineal gland* is a circumventricular organ that secretes Mt into the bloodstream from nightfall until dawn (or when some other dark-light program is imposed by animal husbandry practices). The Mt in the blood readily crosses the blood-brain barrier (BBB) and then acts on the suprachiasmatic nucleus (SCN). Only sites geographically situated on the equator have equal dark and light segments each day. Everywhere else, night and day lengths vary every 24 hours. This process codes the secretion of Mt. Longer Mt signals during the seasonal decrease in day length regulate the hypothalamic-pituitary-gonadal axis and cause some species (e.g., sheep) to activate estrous cycles in females and parallel testicular growth in males. Sleep-wake cycles are also affected.

The mechanism involves light reaching the retina and being relayed via the retinohypothalamic tract, which uses glutamate as its NT, synapsing in the SCN of the anterior hypothalamus. Specific neurons in the SCN respond to varying day length by varying their firing frequency, being circadian oscillators. The Mt secretion in the dark period is inhibited by light. Retinal stimuli go via the retinohypothalamic tract to the SCN, where associated neurons inhibit the paraventricular nucleus of the hypothalamus. From there, axons go via the brain stem to synapse with preganglionic sympathetic neurons in the intermediolateral horn of spinal cord segments T1 and T2. These neurons project to the superior cervical ganglion from which postganglionic cells innervate the pineal gland. The NE released activates the β-adrenoceptors of the pinealocytes, stimulating them to secrete Mt (in the dark hours). The Mt entrains the circadian clock in the SCN, resetting the sleep-wake cycle. Moving mammals across several time zones by air desynchronizes the rhythm, resulting in sleep disturbance. Mt (and some other drugs) can help avoid the disruption and ease the transition.

IMIDAZOLEAMINES: HISTAMINE. Long ago established as a potent vasoactive agent that causes vasodilation and increased capillary permeability, histamine was much more recently found to be an NT. Earlier it was found to stimulate gastric hydrogen chloride (HCl) secretion and be released by platelets and mast cells in allergic and immunologic reactions. Histamine occurs in high concentration in the hypothalamus, from which histaminergic neurons send projections to many parts of the CNS. A histaminergic pathway could originate in the mesencephalic reticular formation and send long neurons to telencephalic areas, possibly playing a role in arousal mechanisms. The brain has histamine receptors H_1 and H_2. The well-established sedative effect of most commercial antihistamines is support for the concept that their basic role may be related to arousal (Garbarg et al. 1980).

AMINO ACIDS: GLUTAMATE AND ASPARTATE (EXCITANT). Glutamate (Glu) receptors are classified by their signal transduction systems:

1. Several have *metabotropic* receptors that act via second messenger systems, a series of mGlus.
2. Others have *ionotropic* receptors with ligand-gated channels with much molecular and functional diversity. A few have been categorized by their susceptibility to neurodegeneration by specific toxic agonists: alpha-amino-3-hydroxy-5-methyl-4-isoxazole propionic acid (AMPA), kainic acid (KA), and *N*-methyl-D-aspartate (NMDA) (Spencer and Schumberg 2000).

It is important to note the remarkable potential of endogenous Glu to change from being the key mediator of orderly excitant communication in the CNS to an agent that is capable of triggering widespread neuronal destruction. Glu excitotoxicity can result from a variety of toxic agonists acting at Glu receptors or as antagonists at GABA receptors to induce neuronal degeneration or necrosis.

The metabotropic Glu receptors are coupled via G proteins to intracellular effectors and stimulate increases in Ca^{2+} concentration in cells. A number of poisonous plants (e.g., cycads) and fungi (fly agaric) lead to an initial state of excitement and myoclonus, followed by depression and loss of consciousness (the latter is GABA mediated).

The ionotropic receptors have been defined to some extent by pharmacological and electrophysiological studies. AMPA agonists induce degeneration of nitric oxide synthase-containing neurons and GABA-ergic cortical neurons. One of these AMPA agonists is present in the grass pea (*Lathyrus sativus*). The syndrome of lathyrism, a spastic paraparesis with pyramidal tract dysfunction, affects people who use the pea as a dietary staple.

The KA receptors have been studied because of their value as a lesioning agent in neural research. KA is a product of *Digenea* seaweed used in the Orient as a vermifuge. The related toxicant—domoic acid—has been studied for its clinical impact. People consumed the agent in mussels contaminated with this algal toxin that readily enters the brain. A series of neurological disorders resulted, and pathology studies revealed severe damage to the amygdaloid nucleus and hippocampus. The toxicant also occurs in razor clams along the West Coast of the United States.

The NMDA receptors have Glu and glycine as coagonists for a receptor channel, with modulation of its opening by the polyamines spermine and spermidine, as well as by protons, redox agents, and zinc. The divalent cations of magnesium (Mg^{2+}), cobalt (Co^{2+}), nickel (Ni^{2+}), and manganese (Mn^{2+}) block the channel, whereas that of calcium (Ca^{2+}) activates several key enzymes, including nitric acid synthase, which may increase NT release. There are several receptor antagonists at the NMDA site or the polyamine site. Exogenous blockers include ketamine (MK801) and phencyclidine (PCP). PCP, which is also known as angel dust, has profound effects on the function of the CNS. NMDA and AMPA receptors may be stimulated simultaneously, allowing entry of both sodium ions (Na^+) and potassium ions (K^+) through the plasmalemmal membrane, depolarizing the cell, which produces seizures and synaptic edema while causing the mechanisms that maintain the architecture of the cell to fail, allowing the neurons to swell (Figure 9.9).

Glu may be joined by aspartate in this function. Both are nonessential dicarboxylic amino acids that are abundant in the brain. Glu is an excitatory neurotransmitter and plays a major role in the function of the CNS.

GABA (INHIBITOR). γ-Aminobutyric Acid or GABA, which is synthesized from Glu, is released from nerve terminals and acts at two types of receptors: GABA-A and GABA-B. The A receptors mediate fast inhibitory postsynaptic potentials that are activated by chloride (Cl^-) conductance and antagonized by bicuculline. The GABA-B receptors are located at both presynaptic and postsynaptic sites and are not antagonized by bicuculline. There are binding sites for benzodiazepines, barbiturates, steroid anesthetics, and picrotoxin. Other GABA antagonists include penicillin G, pentylenetetrazole, several bicyclophosphates, and picrotoxin. Benzodiazopines enhance GABA-ergic transmission and have been used as sedatives, anticonvulsants, and anxiolytics. Examples include diazepam (Valium) and chlordiazepoxide. This class of drugs induces a spectrum of clinical signs of CNS depression plus some hyperactive and aggressive behavioral disturbances (Rang et al. 1995).

The anticonvulsant barbiturates (e.g., phenobarbital) activate GABA-A receptors at high concentrations and cause sedation. On the other hand, picrotoxin (made from an Indonesian shrub and containing picrotin and picrotoxin; the latter has been used to incapacitate fish) is a powerful CNS stimulant in mammals that causes

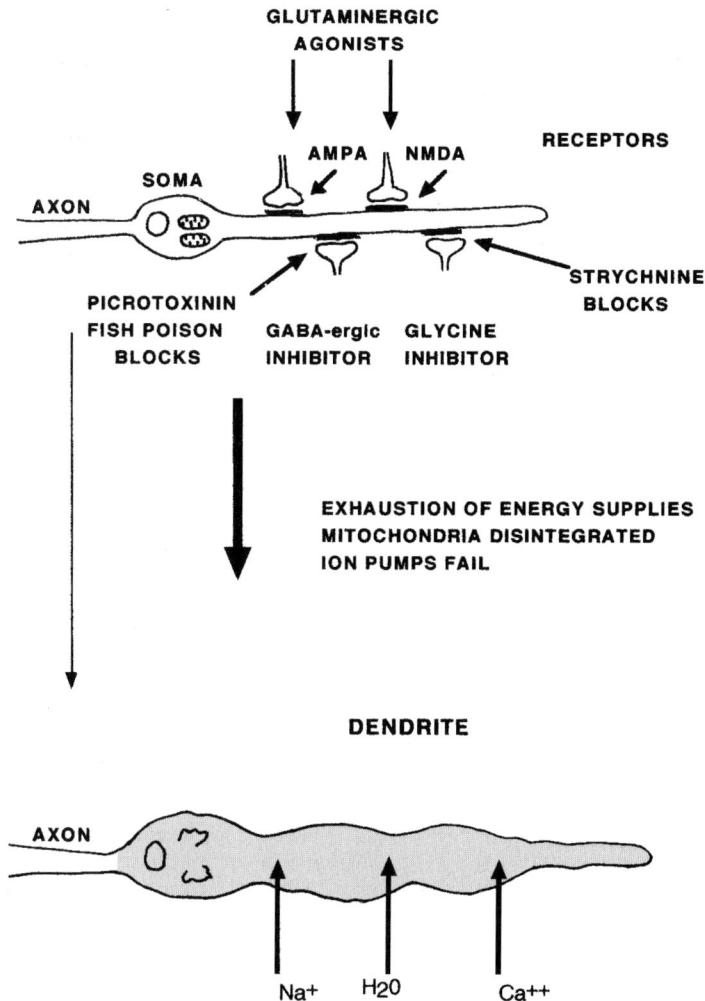

FIG. 9.9—Glutaminergic excitotoxicity in the central nervous system (CNS). An excess of the endogenous neurotransmitter glutamate (Glu) or any other agonist that stimulates the Glu receptors can cause excitotoxic damage to central neurons. Examples include aspartate, which occurs with Glu and sesquiterpenoids in the yellow star thistle, which induces extrapyramidal disease in horses; the fish poison picrotoxin; domoic acid, a Glu analogue produced by toxic mussels; and kainate extracted from *Digenea* seaweed, an algal toxin that readily crosses the blood-brain barrier.

The receptors are AMPA (alpha-amino-3-hydroxy-5-methyl-4-isoxazole propionic acid) and NMDA (*N*-methyl-D-aspartate). Mitochondria are also susceptible to damage.

Glu is the key mediator of orderly excitant communication between neurons, but it can change into a lethal agent that triggers excitotoxicity and cell death after energy stores are exhausted. The ion pumps in the membrane fail, mitochondria disintegrate, and the soma and dendrites swell.

convulsions. The convulsant effect of penicillin on the CNS is attributable to its antagonistic action on GABA-mediated neurotransmission. Several organochlorine insecticides have convulsant effects that are believed to be due to the GABA-A receptor, which responds to picrotoxin (lindane, toxaphene, aldrin, dieldrin, endrin, and endosulfan), and the toxicity induces tremor and convulsions (Hardman et al. 2001) (Figure 9.9).

Other agents that interact with GABA-A receptors with similar effects are several mycotoxins and some (type 2) pyrethroids, which also affect the Na^+ channels. Avermectin may either stimulate or inhibit GABA binding to its receptor.

The GABA-B receptors mediate late inhibitory postsynaptic potentials and release of GABA presynaptically. Their actions are coupled to K^+ channels via G proteins.

GLYCINE (INHIBITOR). Glycine (Gly) is another amino acid that acts as an inhibitory NT, mainly in the brain stem and spinal cord:

1. In interneurons, it depresses firing by motoneurons regulating antagonistic muscles and by neurons in spinal sensory, auditory. and visual pathways. It is synthesized from serine by enzymatic action.
2. Strychnine acts at the postsynaptic glycine receptor. Gly binds to the receptor in a way that opens the ion channel for chloride ion, Cl^-, hyperpolarizing the neuron.

Gly antagonists are mostly neurotoxicants that reduce the inhibitory effect of Gly, thus abnormally enhancing the activity of motor (and some other) neurons.

Strychnine binds with high affinity to the Gly receptor and blocks inhibition of glycinergic synapses, eliciting hyperreflexia, tetanic muscle contraction with opisthotonos, and changes in tactile, auditory, vestibular, and visual function.

The anthelmintic drug avermectin B inhibits noncompetitively strychnine binding to Gly receptors. Strychnine is an indole alkaloid from trees such as *Strychnos nux vomica*.

Several other plant alkaloids—notably gelsemine, a yellow jasmine convulsant—block Gly receptors.

TETANUS TOXIN. Tetanus toxin from *Clostridium tetani* inhibits Ca^{2+}-dependent release of NTs in the following order of efficacy: Gly more so than GABA more so than D-Asp more so than ACh.

The light chain of the toxin is retrogradely transported in lower motoneuron axons, crossing the synapse to bind to Gly-inhibitory terminals, and reducing presynaptic release of Gly, thereby serving to disinhibit α and γ motoneurons.

Afferent stimuli arising from the periphery trigger motor trains undamped by Gly. This causes generalized muscular rigidity and painful muscle spasms, including those of the jaw (lockjaw), face (risus sardonicus in humans), larynx, abdomen, and back along with the muscles of respiration.

METABOLIC REGULATION: BRAIN MECHANISMS

Brain Energy. The brain has a lot of neurons—perhaps 100 billion or so. *Inputs* come in from the sensory systems monitoring the external and internal environment. *Outputs* go to the muscles and other body systems to affect function consciously and unconsciously. In addition, the brain is actively engaged in internal activities—thinking and dreaming that may or may not involve or require sensory input. Ottoson (1983:192–195, 209–213) has concisely and captivatingly reviewed the key discoveries that led to the pathway to understanding the CNS. The remarkable internal architecture of the brain, which is comprised of neurons, was demonstrated by microscopy after silver-chromate staining by Golgi. Cajal then showed that neurons were separate cells, not directly continuous. They shared the Nobel Prize in 1906. Loewi showed that stimulation of the vagus nerve

liberated an active biochemical substance—acetylcholine—in the heart that slowed its rate of beating, proving that nerve impulses were chemically transmitted. The electrochemical pulse causes a transmitter to be released from the neuron's ending and then crosses the narrow synaptic gap to act on the postsynaptic neuron. Typically, one neuron releases a particular type of chemical agent to many different neurons. This effect may be modulated by other factors.

Two NTs play key roles in the brain: Glu and GABA. Glu is excitatory to the second neuron, whereas GABA is inhibitory. Each neuron receives inputs from thousands of other neurons via their synapses. Glu is a real Jekyll-and-Hyde player because it serves as a major signaling system among neurons, enhancing message sending as its major function, but when the brain becomes hypoxic, Glu reuptake fails and the transmitter accumulates at the affected synapses. The receptors on the postsynaptic neurons, if electrically excited, open and allow continuous activation that leads to the death of the neurons, for example, in a region affected by anoxia, such as is seen in a stroke.

There are many other NTs, but most serve as modulators rather than primary stimulators or inhibitors. NE has an important role as the arouser, alerting the brain to higher levels of selective attentiveness and focus. Thus, it is the central fight-or-flight activator. For example, the cat's LC becomes very active when it is confronted with a barking dog (Abercrombie and Jacobs 1987a, b). The relatively modest number of norepinephrine neurons (about 10,000 total) make contact with vast numbers of other neurons via long axons and their branches, a seemingly ideal design for an alarm system, "be prepared for the unexpected." Thus, the LC serves as a central activating system that acts in conjunction with the peripheral parts of the sympathetic nervous system and the adrenal medulla.

Sensitivity of the Central Nervous System to Failure of Energy Supply. The brain is extremely dependent on its vascular oxygen supply to be able to use the limited number of metabolic substrates that it is designed to catabolize for generation of the high-energy compounds that make its wondrous ways possible. Therefore, it is particularly sensitive to hypoxia and anoxia. For example, in less than 10 seconds without oxygen, consciousness is lost. Lose it for 10 seconds or longer and muscle control goes. Within 5 minutes, serious damage to neurons is setting in and, within 10 minutes, many may die. Two factors stand out in accounting for this dramatic vulnerability (Bager et al. 1992):

1. The low-energy storage capacity is combined with high dynamic requirements (many other organs survive severe hypoxia—some even for hours without oxygen).
2. One of the main neurotransmitters of brain—glutamate—also can be a powerful neurotoxin. In acute regional hypoxia as in stroke, the rapid decline in oxygen leads to failure to reuptake Glu that normally pumps it back into the terminus of the neuron it came

from, so it accumulates in the synapses of the brain, giving continuous stimuli to the postsynaptic receptors (R). A particular one of these Rs is only stimulated to open when two conditions are met: (a) the cell must be electrically excited (i.e., the membrane ion pumps must be active) and (b) Glu must be present. In stroke, both are in place, and the continuous activation causes neuronal death, a deadly combination. This explains why strokes and some other neurodegenerative diseases can create such catastrophic pathophysiology in regions of the brain affected by vascular occlusion.

Homeostatic Mechanisms of Brain Dysfunctions. A valuable introduction to understanding *central systems* is provided in Part 4 of *Neurobiology* by Shepherd (1994), which is illustrated with very clear diagrams.

The brain is partly insulated from the metabolic and physical stresses of the rest of the body. As the CEO, it has a lot of *underlings* whose contributions are far from obvious and must be ferreted out by assiduous research. *Energy homeostasis* involves maintaining equilibrium between the intake and expenditure of energy. The only way to regulate intake is to modulate food consumption. Obesity is a consequence of failure to balance intake and expenditure. Excess energy can be dissipated by exercise. Lack of exercise and reduced thermogenesis contribute to obesity. Changes in body weights are associated with changes in energy expenditure.

Mammals have evolved mechanisms for precise control of body temperature that operate effectively and spontaneously (Cunningham 2002). Thermoreceptors (both external and internal), hypothalamic nuclei, various nerves and neurotransmitters, biochemical pathways, and physical mechanisms are involved. If the environment is cold, *thermogenesis* is activated. If it is warm, *sweating* and panting lead to heat loss. The sympathetic nervous system and adrenal responses must be developed or newborn calves will succumb to hypothermia (Olson et al. 1981).

Central Control of Food Intake. The evolution of the brain, its homeostatic regulation, and behavior were addressed by Sarnat and Netsky in 1981. Every veterinary student should be familiar with Chapter 13 in Sarnat's book (Sarnat and Netsky 1981:379–398). Also, Allman (2000) has written a very stimulating book on evolving brains.

Suckling mammary glands is the defining characteristic of all neonatal mammals. Maternal protection, cooperation, and assistance are required as innate behavioral activities that establish the interactive sensory bonding. On the other hand, a newborn mammal must make a considerable effort to come to terms with its extrauterine situation, start to respire, and establish preliminary mastery of movement so that it can locate the mother and rise to seek the teats that are essential to its survival. Initial vigorous licking of the infant is an important stimulus to promote respiration and arouse the newborn, establishing the permanent olfactory connection and orienting her position so that the mammary glands are within reach. Car-

nivora may lick their mammary area to help puppies or kittens locate and access the teats. Neonatal herbivores, however, have to make the big effort to stand up and walk so that they reach the mammary glands. Facial and neck muscles needed for suckling are well developed at birth, even though, in some species, the eyes may be closed.

The urge to suckle is an innate motivation, and, once the teats are located, they are taken into the mouth, triggering the strong suckling reflex. The reflex oxytocin secretion in the dam triggers milk letdown, and the suckling action of the newborn squirts the milk into the pharynx for swallowing so that its homeostatic programs can be established. A crucial reflex is designed to preserve a patent airway during suckling and swallowing of milk. This involves dropping the soft palate behind the back of the tongue and being held there by the epiglottis, allowing milk to pass around the epiglottis into the esophagus, although the airway between nares and trachea stays open. Using radioactively labeled 2-deoxyglucose, studies of the importance of the olfactory sense in establishing and maintaining suckling motivation revealed that a special area at the extreme dorsomedial margin of the olfactory bulb is highly active during suckling. This is where the typical small, round glomeruli of the bulb are replaced by a "necklace" of modified glomeruli in which the cells respond to a specific odor that stimulates receptors in a subset of cells in the olfactory epithelium. A placental antigen appears to be the suckling cue, an interesting link between mother and fetus that carries through after delivery to maintain the bond.

Suckling is an intermittent act that is provided for by the hypothalamus, which regulates the letdown process. The hormone oxytocin is synthesized in neurons in the paraventricular and supraoptic nuclei. Their axons carry it to the posterior lobe of the pituitary gland to the terminals. Sensory inputs to the cells of the nuclei result in synaptic depolarization that increases impulse generation and stimuli that travel to the pituitary, triggering release of stored oxytocin into the circulation. After it reaches the mammary gland, oxytocin causes the smooth muscle of the mammary gland to contract, pushing the milk down to the cisterns and the nipples. Normally, the newborn responds with vigorous suckling. Obviously, the system is vulnerable to failure from numerous potential problems (Gardiner 1980a, b). The environment can introduce many hazards. The important ingredient is the *life force* of infants and mother in the face of thermal or man-made stresses. The arousal of the newborn is the essential variable. In species that have large litters, the latest in the line being born (e.g., piglets) tends to be most vulnerable because its reserves may be depleted. There is some evidence for autocrine feedback control of milk secretion (Linzell and Peaker 1971; Peaker 1995; Peaker and Wilde 1996).

CHALLENGES TO AFFECTIVE RESPONSES

Emotion and Expression. The term *emotion* evolved from *mental agitation* to its modern usage implying reactive feeling as distinct from memory and rational thought. It is often manifested by facial expressions, postures, and movements that communicate feelings and attitudes, including some that are instinctive or unconscious (Panksepp 1998). The common term used to encompass this phenomenon is *body language*. Working with cats in the late 1920s Hess (1969) established that the hypothalamus was the site that controlled the expressions of rage and fear. However, Bard showed that, although the program for the expression of rage is in the hypothalamus, it lacks the directed conscious component if cortex, basal ganglia, and thalamus are removed. They termed the resulting expression *sham rage*. This capacity is lost if the brain is transected below the hypothalamus. A combination of autonomic and somatic responses are needed for the rage display to be deployed as affective attack, designed to threaten and dominate, defend territory, and so on. Predation differs in having autonomic activation without the expressive warnings. It involves behavior focused on the hunt and the *quiet biting* of successful capture. These features of feline behavior are central to the life of a cat, a carnivorous predator. Herbivores, as prey species, had to focus on the flight aspect. Only understandable via a neuroevolutionary approach, anger stems from the neurodynamics of subcortical circuits that we share (homologously) with other mammals. Their locations were identified by electrical stimulation.

RAGE CIRCUITRY AND AGGRESSION. *Rage* circuitry runs

1. From medial *amygdala*
2. Through discrete zones of the *hypothalamus*
3. Down into the periaqueductal gray of the *midbrain*

Aggression is when animals threaten, bite, or kill each other. There are three distinct circuits in mammal brain for rage:

Predatory: because a mammal needs food to survive
Intermale: not enraged; just competing to be champ for sex resources
Affective attack: the only one that provokes enraged behaviors (i.e., *anger*)

The circuitry is different for each of these three, that is, three types of aggression. However, they are not fully distinct from *seeking* circuits.

Other possible circuits that are common behaviors in nature (could be some combination of the other three) include killing and injury to young. Also, could *defensive aggression* emerge from a dynamic mix of *rage* and *fear* systems? In general, is there much less aggression when mammals have known each other for a long time than when they are strangers? In stable societies, mammals usually develop acceptance of their social status, knowing their priority status in the line for resources: *hierarchy*. If they do not know each other,

physical confrontation is much more likely. Larger-scale warlike tendencies stem from the higher cortical centers and are not instinctual potentials of the old mammalian brain.

EVOLUTIONARY SOURCES OF AGGRESSION AND RAGE. James said, "Our ancestors bred pugnacity into our bone and marrow, and thousands of years of peace wont breed it out!" (*Essays on Faith and Morals*). However, there is good evidence that breeding for aggression can markedly heighten aggressiveness in both male and female rodents within half a dozen generations. It is as effective in females as in males.

Clues come from aggression induced by electrical stimulation of the brain (ESB), with evaluation of the aggressive sequences it evokes. For example, a cat with an indwelling electrode in the medial hypothalamus is sitting peacefully. After ESB is applied, in a few seconds it is transformed emotionally; claws unsheathed, fangs bared, hissing and spitting, it leaps viciously toward the researcher. Less than 1 minute after ESB is stopped, it is again relaxed and peaceful, and can be petted without retribution.

Hypothalamus and Limbic System. The hypothalamus and associated limbic structures regulate homeostasis directly via the autonomic nervous system and endocrine secretions. It also integrates input from the neocortex involving the control of arousal, emotion, and motivated behaviors. Many vital functions regulated by the hypothalamus can be affected by toxicants. Temperature regulation, heart rate and force of contraction, blood pressure, plasma osmolality, food and water intake, and circadian rhythms are significant examples. Excitatory amino acids such as glutamate and aspartate in neonatal mammals damage the arcuate hypothalamic nucleus, which leads to dysfunctional development and subnormal endocrine secretions. Regulation of the control of food intake involves

1. Internal mechanisms governing hunger and satiety (Gershon 1998)
2. External factors that regulate (a) the availability of food and (b) the desire to eat

Internal cues to coordinate/regulate mechanisms are (a) short-term modulation of meal initiation (ingestion), meal size, and meal ending; and (b) long-term modulation of energy consumption (food intake), energy expenditure, and maintenance of fuel stores.

External cues are important, too. For instance, food intake is shaped by ecological constraints, such as total amount of food available, individuals' societal status (i.e., which animals get to eat, how much, what is eaten, and the pattern of intake), ability to get food, timing of access, choices available, and quality (including possibility of distasteful or poisonous content). The effect of previous experience is important in determining whether the same type of food will be eaten again. For example, if a particular food source leads to side effects such as nausea or abdominal discomfort within a short time after starting ingestion, this may lead to stopping consumption in the short term. It may also establish an aversion to that particular food or component (Garcia and Koelling 1966; Ashe and Nackman 1980). On the other hand, if eating a certain food results in a discernibly pleasant sensation, it will be sought out again.

Internal drives exist for particular nutrients that affect selection for foods that contain them (e.g., sodium chloride, water, essential minerals, specific core nutrients such as sugars, and amino acids/proteins). Some foods contain materials that are appetite enhancers. For some species (e.g., carnivores), there are strong drives to consume body tissues, including bones, which can be hazardous. Puppies are notorious chewers of sticks, stones, natural and synthetic fibers, and even soil and fecal material, frequently with serious consequences requiring surgical intervention.

Depraved appetites (pica) occur in many species. Pica may be related to malnutrition, such as diets too low in energy and protein or sodium and potassium (sheep). Cattle on phosphorus-deficient diets develop osteophagia, a craving for bone chewing. This pathophysiology has been reproduced experimentally by exteriorizing the parotid duct and feeding a low-phosphorus diet. Because of carcass contamination with *Clostridium botulinum*, death may result from paralysis due to botulism.

AROUSAL, SOMNOLENCE, AND SLEEP. Despite the large time commitment of the mammalian life span to sleep, it was the 1970s before physiological events during sleep were researched systematically. Considering the very high incidence of individual concerns about insomnia, tiredness and fatigue, snoring, frequent awakenings, a tendency to fall asleep during the day, excessive sleepiness, and dreaming, this seems, in retrospect, to be quite remarkable. It was only with the development of sleep labs equipped to monitor events and physiological status during sleep that a genuine understanding of the normal and pathophysiological pattern was developed (Guilleminault 1976; Shepherd 1994; Smolensky 2001).

Unequivocal evidence was obtained that the basis of many problems was respiratory disorder, often associated with hypertension and obesity, and involving significant hypoxia. Gradually, the perspective emerged that sleep apnea was an important pathophysiological syndrome. Laboratory research on the stages of sleep led to the definition of paradoxical sleep or REM sleep and its probable role in dreaming. Jouvet and Michel (1958) did classical work on cats. Ponto-geniculo-occipital (PGO) waves are seen during sleep, are critical for it, and are memory dependent (Datta 1999). Sleep-deprived animals have sleep-promoting factors in their tissues. One of these factors is the cytokine, interleukin 1, that stimulates immune function and is formed in glial cells and macrophages. It appears to promote REM sleep, raising the speculation that sleep may be needed for maintenance of an effective immune response (Husband 1995; Husband and Bryden 1996).

Sleep-disordered Breathing. Hendricks makes the point that the typical initial examination of a veterinary patient cannot constitute an adequate assessment of pathophysiology. Stressors such as exercise are not conducted, and episodic dysfunctions such as seizures, arrhythmias, and behavioral aberrations are likely to be missed. Continuous monitoring of function over a 24-hour period is required. This is particularly true of sleep disorders involving sleep-disordered breathing (SDB).

Sleep with instrumentation in place is needed to record oxygen saturation (S_aO_2), respiratory efforts, electrocardiogram, and electroencephalogram (EEG). Repeated respiratory arrests accompanied by reduction in oxygen saturation enable SDB to be identified. Airflow rate measured with a nasal thermistor accompanied by monitoring changes in movements of the rib cage and abdomen may reveal factors involved in a reduction of oxygen saturation.

Brachycephalic breeds of dogs have anatomic features that predispose them to disordered respiration. As the animal falls asleep, the EEG wave pattern slows down, increases in amplitude, and assumes the SWS pattern. Respiratory rate declines with increased tidal volume, eye movements are slow, and neck muscle tone is maintained. Homeostatic regulators operate subconsciously. After an interval characteristic of the species, the wave pattern and muscular activities change dramatically. Major muscle groups relax, allowing the head and limbs to be lowered to the ground. Extraocular muscles are aroused into REM activity. Standing animals (including horses that can sleep standing) will lie down, and there are bursts of twitching activity in small distal muscles that results from rapid neuronal firing. Inspiratory diaphragmatic records show the appearance of pauses with erratic breaths in both dogs and cats.

Photoperiodic Rhythms. The study of biorhythms in veterinary medicine is as yet in its relative infancy compared with human medicine. Most attention so far has been given to *circadian* (24 hour) rhythms (CRs). There is now a growing awareness of their importance to pathophysiology in veterinary practice. By definition, CR implies variations in the patterns and levels of cellular activities affecting functional parameters and responses over the course of the 24-hour "day." Study of their phasing and amplitude in health and disease can yield perspectives that advance understanding of *normality* and *pathophysiology*. This allows a new degree of predictability regarding the expected manifestations of many medical conditions over time, aiding interpretation of clinical laboratory data and prognosis. Of particular significance is the relationship between biorhythms and pharmacokinetics that forms the basis of the new art of chronotherapeutics, which has demonstrated varying vulnerability of, for example, certain tumors over the 24-hour period. Thus, one can now conceive of purposeful varying of dose, and so on, over time to optimize therapeutic outcomes in the framework of the time course of each disease (Shepherd 1994; Smolensky 2001).

The real pioneer of circadian veterinary studies in domestic mammals was the late Yves Ruckebusch, Professor of Physiology at the National Veterinary School in Toulouse, France (Ruckebusch et al. 1981). It is an important goal of this book to extend his ideas from normal functional chronobiology to the transition to pathophysiology and the early stages of disease when intervention based on in-depth understanding is much more likely to be capable of reversing the damage than in later stages when the pathology is more severe. It will be necessary to go beyond circadian data to the entire time course of each disease, integrating the data on daily rhythms and extending it to include other time-based rhythms. Ruckebusch made his contributions by setting up 24-hour-a-day continuous physical recording and biochemical sampling systems involving tremendous dedication and investment of time, including direct observation of functional events and behaviors. The concept of rhythmicity determinants in pathophysiology needs investigation. The rhythms of each species differ and are affected by environmental factors. The milieu of living things undergoes continuous cyclical changes with time that are geared to the planet's calendar time scale—that is, circannual, circamenstrual, circadian, and shorter periods within a day. Hours of darkness and light in a day have a major effect on the activities and rhythms of mammals as they adapt to be either diurnal or nocturnal.

Thermoregulation Dysfunctions. The effects of endophyte-infected tall fescue (EITF) and environmental temperature on follicular and luteal development have been studied. Heifers grazing EITF–infested pastures had reduced prolactin levels, smaller follicles than controls, and lower estrogen levels. Impaired follicle function could explain reduced pregnancy rates. Grazing EITF and high environmental temperature both caused higher rectal temperature and respiratory rates. Consumption of EITF in summer can cause severe hyperthermia in cattle. The temperature rise of the core temperature is especially marked at night, due mainly to a reduction in cutaneous heat transfer but not other mechanisms of heat loss.

Electroencephalographic (EEG) Evidence of Dysfunction. A useful brief introduction to the EEG is available in Shepherd (1994).

Varying electrical fields on the surface of the skull that are generated by neurons of the cerebral cortex can be recorded by using suitable electrodes and leads. The changes in the resulting waveforms are attributable to changes in the membrane potential of the nerve cells. The recordings can provide clues to dysfunction that may be of clinical significance. The record registers the summated activity of the cells as it changes with time.

Projected to the brain areas affecting the recording leads, it generates a similar pattern of dipoles.

The source of the potential changes on the cortical surface arises mainly from postsynaptic potentials at dendrites of the pyramidal cells. These potentials have lower amplitude than the action potentials but last significantly longer. As the pyramidal cells are positioned at right angles to the surface of the cortex, their activity generates dipoles in the direction of the surface more efficiently than that of other cortical cell types, thereby giving them a larger impact on the surface potential. Also, since they are all oriented in parallel, their equidirectional potential changes are summated with those of their neighbors. Thus, there is opportunity for synchronous activity if simultaneous depolarization of several pyramidal cells as a group occurs.

Sodium ions enter the neurons during an excitatory postsynaptic potential (EPSP). In their wake, they leave a local negative extracellular potential that causes an efflux of potassium ions along the cell membrane, generating a local positive extracellular potential. Activation of the excitatory synapse at the apical end of a dendrite creates a dipole with a negative potential at the surface.

The frequency of the recorded waves can be diagnostically significant: If a patient is awake with eyes open, beta waves are predominant, about 14 to 30 Hz. With eyes closed, the slower alpha waves are dominant, at 8 to 13 Hz. Sleep spindles have frequencies in this range, but these have higher-amplitude sharp spikes. Sheep affected with polioencephalomalacia (PEM) induced by amprolium were found to generate sleep spindles that started at 3 Hz and rose to 6 Hz (Dunlop et al. 1981). Higher rates have been recorded in people. Other slow deflection frequencies are seen, such as the omega (4 to 7 Hz) and delta (0.5 to 3 Hz) waves, usually only in the young and adolescents. However, delta waves are seen in adults during deep sleep. Also, in diseases like dementia, slower frequencies may be present and, in bipolar disorders, accelerations may be observed. The EEG has special value in epilepsy that is characterized by massive synchronized excitation of cortical neurons. Seizure spikes or spike and wave complexes may be present. In brain death, all electrical activity ceases and the EEG is flat (i.e., isoelectric).

OVEREXCITATION OF THE CENTRAL NERVOUS SYSTEM: TICS AND EPILEPSY. The most extreme case of overexcitation of the CNS is that of epilepsy. Seizures are a result of synchronized, widespread excitation of a lot of neurons. The outcome is generalized activation of motor and sensory activity, and higher levels of cortical activity (emotional and cognitive), accompanied by less apparent autonomic functions. Depending on the cortical site affected, one or the other of these functions may be affected more. The bursts of depolarization can start locally and spread. The motor effects are the most visible and dramatic (i.e., *convulsions*). The trigger is activation of calcium-ion channels that open the nonspecific cation channels, resulting in paroxysmal depolarization of neurons. This process is restrained by the activation of K^+ and Cl^- channels by Ca^{2+}. When a certain critical number of neurons have been excited, a seizure occurs. Some strains of animals, such as the Tennessee falling goats, exhibit genetic susceptibility. Other root causes include malformation of the brain, trauma, cranial hemorrhage, hypoxia, tumor, cerebral edema, abscesses or other infections of the CNS, hyperventilation, hypomagnesemia, hypocalcemia, and several toxicants. The major component of the neuronal membrane polarity is the K^+ gradient maintained by the potassium channels that are fueled by Na-K ATPase. Inhibitory neurons reduce depolarizations in the normal brain via GABA that is made by the vitamin B_6-dependent glutamate decarboxylase. Vitamin B_6 deficiency increases susceptibility.

Blood-Brain Barrier Responses. An overview of pathways of entries of agents that cause CNS infections will be found in a brilliant illustration by A.L. Smith (1998:538) in Schaechter's text on *Mechanisms of Microbial Disease*, 3rd edition. Further coverage of CNS infections is provided in Chapter 9, Part 1, of this book by Vandevelde. The remainder of the discussion of *blood-brain barrier responses* is restricted to aspects of the BBB per se.

The blood vessels in the CNS are separated from the extracellular fluid (ECF) surrounding the neural tissues by endothelial cells connected by *tight junctions* induced by astrocytes. These tight junctions prevent passage between endothelial cells by toxicant molecules in the circulating blood unless they can traverse the capillary endothelium *and* the plasma membranes of astrocyte foot processes abutting the outer surface of the capillaries. The penetration of any substances that are ionized and/or protein bound is restricted. Only lipid-soluble agents can get through readily. Even the latter are restricted to some extent by the action of phase 1 enzymes in the walls of brain microvasculature. Overall, this BBB is absent from the choroid plexus and the circumventricular organs. The latter are discrete regions of the brain that are involved with neuroendocrine secretion. The regions include area postrema, hypophysis, pineal body, hypothalamic nuclei, subfornical organ, and the supraoptic crest.

The cerebrospinal fluid (CSF) is formed mainly in the choroid plexus of the lateral ventricles and flows via interventricular foramina to the third ventricle then to the fourth ventricle via the aqueduct. The foramina of Luschka and Magendie convey it into the subarachnoid space and arachnoid villi of the sinuses of the dura mater on its way to the venous sinuses. If CSF flow is hindered or obstructed at any of these structures, *hydrocephalus* will start as *backward congestion*. Malformations or disease can cause such obstruction (Feldman 1989).

Basal Ganglia in Physiopathology. The components of the basal ganglia are (a) the corpus striatum, which is the caudate nucleus plus putamen; (b) the globus pallidus, inner and outer; (c) the subthalamic nucleus; and (d) the substantia nigra (pars reticulata and compacta). The basal ganglia participate in movement control—in conjunction with the cerebellum, the motor cortex, the corticospinal tracts, and the motor nuclei in the brain stem.

Glutamate is the activator for striatal neurons, arising from cortical neurons.

GABA, an inhibitory transmitter, is a key agent for internal connections among the basal ganglia, which has an inhibitory effect on the thalamus via GABAergic neurons in the inner pallidum of the globus pallidus and in the subthalamic nucleus. These neurons are activated by glutamate from the neurons of the subthalamic nucleus.

DA from the subthalamic nucleus has a mixed action on striatal neurons—part activating and part inhibiting. These neurons are also activated by cholinergic neurons. Any imbalance between inhibitory and activating influencing has a detrimental effect on control of motor functions, either hypokinetic or hyperkinetic. Degeneration of dopaminergic neurons in the subthalamic nucleus was discovered in Parkinson's disease in the 1960s, the first demonstration of an NT deficiency with a neurological disease.

Cerebellum in Physiopathology. The cerebellum does not influence muscle strength or sensation other than in events relating to orientation in space, coordination of complex movements requiring precision, and maintenance of posture both at rest and during movement. Coordination of antagonistic muscles such as flexors and extensors is crucial. The cerebellum enables both the postural adjustments and the voluntary movements to be performed in a smooth and precise way. It is a key regulator of posture, gait, stereotyped movements, and fine skilled movements.

The vestibulocerebellum responds to changes in head position and movements, adjusting the tone of eye, trunk, and proximal limb muscles to coordinate eye movements and reset posture.

The spinocerebellum responds to much input from receptors, especially those in neuromuscular spindles and tendon organs, and then adjusts and corrects body position, muscle length, and tension to regulate posture and coordinate stereotyped voluntary movements.

The cerebrocerebellum regulates timing, range, force, and direction of skilled voluntary movements of distal parts of extremities and facial muscles.

The semicircular canals of the labyrinth feed information via the 8th cranial nerve to the vestibular nucleus in the brain stem, indicating the position of the head in space. The neurons in the vestibular nucleus send axons to the medial region of the spinal cord. One area and those of the proximal limb muscles target muscles of the neck and back by another. The superior colliculus, which projects to medial groups in the cervical cord and whose role in generation of eye movements is well established, has a significant role in generating orienting movements of the head.

Postural control requires some complex interactions among muscle groups. Some of these are dependent on a unique feature of the reticular activating system: *feed-*

forward mechanisms for postural control. Cats that had been trained to strike an object with a forepaw were used to demonstrate that this movement of the forepaw required feed-forward adjustments in the other legs that shift the weight distribution from its even distribution over the four feet to a diagonal pattern with the weight being borne mainly by the nonstriking forelimb and the ipsilateral hindlimb. Motor cortex neurons initiate the movement of the forelimb and the postural adjustments to maintain stability. The forelimb response involves direct connections from cortex to spinal cord while the postural adjustments are mediated over connections from motor cortex to reticular formation. Such feed-forward mechanisms may not be enough to achieve postural stability, in which case sensory inputs are deployed to correct the situation. The latter arise from the vestibular nucleus and go to the cord to correct any postural instability. Other inputs are received from muscle spindles, Golgi tendon organs, and the visual system's detection of motion.

Dysfunctions of the cerebellum include delayed onset and arrest of movements, failures in movement coordination, and erroneous judgment of many aspects of movements (dysmetria). Tremors may be present, and control of balance is defective. Common signs are standing with legs spread and nystagmus.

PAIN

Acute Pain. Acute Pain is a function of a healthy nervous system: an alarm system to protect an animal from injury or disease. It is usually in good working order for this role (Fields 1987; Day 1998; Greenstein and Greenstein 2000; Fields and Martin 2001).

Advances in Gate Theory of Pain Relevant to Laminitis. The classical paper by Melzack and Wall in 1965, "New Theory of Pain," revolutionized thinking about mechanisms involved in phenomena observed in modulation of the sensory signals coming in from the periphery. The somatosensory system is amazing in its diversity and complexity. The receptors located in the skin have their neuronal homes in dorsal root ganglia that relay the signals arising from the periphery into the spinal cord. The fibers continue into the spinal cord and then enter the dorsal horn, where they synapse with *dorsal horn cells* (DHCs). Repeated stimuli result in release of *substance P*, an excitatory peptide transmitter that causes prolonged firing of the DHCs.

The nociceptors in the skin send signals up the nerve fibers to the cord. There are two categories of such fibers. One category, the A-delta group, are fast responding, sense sharp pain, and also show sensitization to prolonged heat. The other category, the fine C fibers, are polymodal, responding to mechanical forces, heat, and certain chemical agents released when tissues are damaged. These fibers give a sensation of burning pain more slowly in onset and less localized but also distinctly more unpleasant. In this sense, they resemble

visceral pain. Such pain probably involves bradykinin and prostaglandin-E release. However, this is not the end of the story.

The DHCs, before the pain signals proceed up the spinothalamic tracts to the thalamus and other destinations, are subject to modulation. Larger-diameter A-beta fibers from mechanoreceptors send concurrent incoming signals to an inhibitory interneuron that sends its axon to the same DHCs of the spinothalamic tract. This *closes the gate* on the pain signals coming in from the nociceptors. Excitations and inhibitions are independently controlled. From the *gate theory* has come the realization that there is changeable transmission; that is, the pain-signaling and pain-modulating systems are capable of changing in different circumstances.

The typical clinical pains arise from trauma and inflammation. Damaged nerves give rise to neuropathic pain. Both types cause profound changes in spinal cord and brain. Damaged tissue releases potent mediators that alter and sensitize sensory receptors while excitability changes occur in neuropathic form within the nerve. Such peripheral changes can cause marked central changes and sometimes lead to hyperalgesia. This is the problem with pathophysiology: the potential for maladaptive compensation. Repeated C-fiber input elicits increased spinal neuron responses in animals. As the spinal neurons become more excitable, their receptive fields expand. This could explain one aspect of secondary hyperalgesia.

Glutamate is a transmitter involved in central sensitization and, in conjunction with potent peptides, a key factor in setting the level of pain transmission. In the dorsal horn, the AMPA receptors for Glu set the baseline level of activity, and, when activated, the NMDA receptors cause the windup amplification. This happens only when the scale of the pain stimuli exceeds a certain level. Peptides may participate by removing the magnesium block of the NMDA receptor. Block of nitric oxide production abolishes windup and reduces hyperalgesia.

In addition to the spinal modulation of pain, there is a descending pain-suppression system from the brain stem. The neurons arise from the hypothalamus, the periaqueductal gray, rostral ventromedial medulla, and dorsolateral pontine tegmentum. These circuits influence pain-sensitive ST cells in the dorsal horn with the periaqueductal gray as command center, having opiate receptors and enkephalins that can bind to them. The enkephalins activate the rostral ventromedial medulla, which releases 5-HT in the dorsal horn. The 5-HT activates interneurons containing enkephalins. These act on opioid receptors on pain-responsive neurons in the cord, making them less responsive to the incoming pain signals. The periaqueductal gray also activates the dorsolateral pontine tegmentum, which also sends its NE-releasing neurons to the spinal cord.

Modulation of nociceptive input (endogenous pain) has at least three source agents that have an overall analgesic effect: serotonin, enkephalin, and NE. Furthermore, β-endorphin is a pituitary hormone whose production arises, along with adrenocorticotropic hormone (ACTH), from various stresses and interventions, including pain, parturition, exercise stress, surgery, and acupuncture. It is noteworthy that the skin of pigs has heat-sensitive nociceptors (Lynn et al. 1996).

Veterinary medicine needs to deploy the new techniques and knowledge about pain in addressing unsolved problems of pathophysiology, such as laminitis in the horse.

The Elusive Search for the Pathophysiology of Itch with Nociception (Metze and Luger 2001). Neurogenic inflammation is a result of activation of a class of nociceptors that often exhibit vasodilation and protein extravasation in mammalian skin. A century ago, Bayliss (1901) described antidromic vasodilation after electrical stimulation of centrally cut dorsal nerve roots. With keen insight, he called this an efferent response from afferent nerve fibers. Recently, using dermal microdialysis, some of the specific neuropeptides and their receptors responsible for the induction of such neurogenic inflammation in mammalian skin have been identified. The pivotal agents are calcitonin gene-related peptide (CGRP) and substance P. Other neuropeptides identified in primary afferent neurons include neurokinins A and B, somatostatin, galanin, and endomorphins (Schmelz and Peterson 2001).

Activation of fine C-fiber nerve endings in the skin generates action potentials that are conducted to the spinal cord and give rise to a sensation of pain or itch in the CNS. These same action potentials will also invade retrogradely the arborizations of the primary afferent neuron and release neuropeptides from their terminals. This phenomenon is known as *axon reflex erythema*. Mechanoinsensitive but heat-sensitive and chemosensitive C receptors have been found responsible for neurogenic vasodilation in pig skin (Schmelz et al. 1997).

The evidence of neuropeptide release was obtained by using capsaicin, a potent activator of sensory nerves that induces intense pain, and also by antidromic electrical stimulation of nerves. The possibility of mast cell degranulation releasing histamine being the mechanism for such responses arising from injection of allergens or some other peptides was eliminated by using microdialysis to show that histamine was not released in the flare area induced by capsaicin (either intradermally or topically applied).

Using microdialysis to infuse substance P, the axon reflex reactions could not be antagonized by histamine H1-blocking agents. Similar results were obtained with CGRP. It was concluded that mast cell activation did not occur in neurogenic inflammation in normal skin. Further studies will explore whether the situation is different in inflammatory dermatitis.

Release of neuropeptides by capsaicin and by antidromic nerve stimulation has been demonstrated in animals (Szolcsanyi 1996). There are significant species differences in qualitative and quantitative responses to irritants and to neuropeptides, so a great deal of investigative work is needed. However, given the widespread prevalence of severe sensory discomfort of dermal origin in domestic animals, coupled with the high risk of dermal mutilation by scratching, the solution of the mysteries of the pathophysiology of dermal itch and related pain should be a very high priority for enlightened research in this field in veterinary medicine.

Chronic Pain. Chronic pain is like a broken alarm. It is in fact neuropathology. It is not just attributable to an underlying disease process (as used to be thought) that, if corrected, would result in a cure of the pain. This is *not* so. Defined as pain that persists for over 6 hours, chronic pain is estimated to affect about 40 million Americans. It outlives its original cause and develops a life of its own. It is pathology of the nervous system. The pain process unleashes a continuing cascade of negative hormones that progressively have adverse effects upon immune functions and renal function.

It has been shown that cancer pain, if treated with morphine, enables patients to live longer just because the pain is reduced, yet many such patients seldom get adequate treatment for pain relief. Pain, especially chronic pain, is poorly understood, and its therapy is still not defined in a way that the medical professions can implement dependably and effectively. Individuals and health professionals have often taken a "wait it out" approach, which is unwise and dangerous to the patient because of the pathophysiological damage that chronic pain exacts.

Chronic pain gets worse over time because physical pain changes the body in the same way as emotional loss watermarks the soul. β-Endorphin accounts for *runner's high* by providing a state like anesthesia. With prolonged injury, progressively deeper levels of pain cells in the spinal cord are activated.

Neuropathic Pain. Neuropathic pain is a kind for which opiates are least effective. The new antiseizure drug gabapentin (Neurontin) a centrally active GABA agonist, has also been found to act as a nerve stabilizer that quiets misfiring nerves that cause this kind of pain. It must be recognized that, after trauma or surgery, structures may look healed, but the nerve networks can not be imaged like the skeletal ones or be made visible by contrast media, yet they are the sites of the pain condition. Examples include backache and tubes into thorax after treatment for collapsed lung. The pain is terrible because the region has one of the richest nerve networks in the body. Postmastectomy pain can be extremely severe. Kathleen Foley at Sloan-Kettering Institute showed the pain was due to the technique that included cutting a thoracic nerve. Modifications to avoid this avoided the problem. When these types of chronic pain are extreme, patients become desperate— even crazed—because they cannot get relief.

Anxiety and Depression. Anxiety and depression can be outcomes of severe chronic pain. These are pathophysiological responses as well as cognitive consequences. They share neural circuitry using similar transmitters/pathways (serotonin and endorphins). Chronic pain uses up serotonin, like a car running out of gas. Depression and stress often enhance pain.

During pain research over 30 years of pain studies, 60 genes affecting pain were found, one at a time. Now, in the past year alone, using gene-chip technology, 1500 have been found. The information overload is getting extreme. There is an abnormal sodium-ion channel that is expressed only in sensory nerves that are damaged. It could lead to blockers for these channels that might control neuropathic pain. It is clear that there is such a thing as *cellular pain memory* of damage to the immature nervous system (e.g., circumcision without anesthesia). Children exhibit a lower pain threshold. Also there is *pathological cortical reorganization*. If a motor nerve is cut, the response is predictable: paralysis. But if sensory nerves are cut, the outcome is less predictable. They may become "dead" or numb but may start to fire spontaneously and the pain may be severe. Postsurgical chronic pain can be devastating. It can lead to pathological cortical reorganization.

PATHOPHYSIOLOGY OF AGING. Two hypotheses about the pathophysiology of aging have led the pack among many theories put forward:

1. *Programmed cell death:* "your time is up." This proposes that there is an internal, built-in clock that is programmed to trigger changes that lead to cell self-destruction.
2. *Cumulative functional errors* that lead to progressive deterioration and inability to repair the damage. Epidemiological studies have shown that almost all living species/individuals have a maximal life span that is genetically determined (i.e., set by the genes).

A major discovery was made in 1961 that human cells divide only 80 to 90 times and then stop. Even though the cells can live much longer, they gradually lose their ability to resist degeneration and most infections, as well as to repair traumatized tissue.

Also they start to produce enzymes that hydrolyze proteins and make the perpetual grind of maintaining homeostasis less well coordinated. When a cell divides, all of its chromosomes replicate completely except for their tips or *telomeres*, which lose a little bit at each cell division. The enzyme telomerase, which was discovered in 1984, enables cells to rebuild their telomeres and proliferate indefinitely. It is present in most cancer cells but not in all cells from healthy tissue. Studying this area of molecular biology is a very hot topic of current research because there is still much to be learned about the process and how it can be manipulated.

Free radicals or oxyradicals are also strong candidates for involvement in aging. These consist of reactive oxygen in the form of molecules with an additional *free electron* (e.g., O$^-$ and OH$^-$) that damage other molecules they encounter, particularly DNA. The mammalian body is equipped to protect itself from attack by free radicals. Its guardians include vitamin E, selenium-containing enzymes, glutathione peroxidase, superoxide dismutase and β carotene. Also, reducing food intake by about 30%, a regimen that lowers body temperature, spontaneous activity, and *appetites*, can lower the rate of free radical formation. It must be recognized that aging is a complex process that involves many interconnected components of body function and their adaptation to the changing needs of homeostasis in a dynamic physical, biological, and emotional environment.

Metabolism of substrates leads to ATP synthesis and energy release as heat. Mitochondria reoxidize reduced coenzymes and phosphorylate ADP. Energy released by mitochondria is a significant component of thermogenesis because coupling of cellular respiration to ATP synthesis cannot be accomplished without heat production because the overall reactions are exothermic. Regulatory thermogenesis is a special role of brown adipocytes. Their heat production is due to the synthesis of a proton transporter in the inner membrane of their M (mitochondrial proton channel)-uncoupling protein (UCP-1). Other UCPs have been discovered that may control M response to oxidants.

Neuronal Apoptosis. Unlike necrosis, where the organelles swell and the plasma membrane becomes permeable on the road to dissolution, apoptosis is an alternative mechanism for weeding out tired or surplus cells without causing ill-effects to neighboring cells. Neuronal apoptosis differs from that of other cell types in proliferative tissues (Graham and Chen 2001; Mattson 2001). To sustain the function of neuronal circuits, neurons must survive for the lifetime of the organism. This is particularly evident for neurons involved in long-term memory and nonautonomic thought processes. The mammalian organism starts out by developing a surplus number of neurons. Many of these neurons undergo apoptosis. These cell deaths occur mainly in the period dedicated to synaptogenesis. Apparently, the selection involves tuning of the circuits and prioritizing by a signaling system using neurotrophic growth factors.

Apoptosis is initiated by a *death signal* that activates a cascade of intracellular events, which include increases in the entry of oxyradicals and ionized calcium into the cell and the mitochondria that initiates a complex series of changes. One of them is a rapid increase in apoptosis response and translocation of proapoptotic Bcl-2 to the mitochondrial membrane with formation of permeability transition pores. These allow cytochrome c to escape the mitochondrion into the cytosol, where it forms a complex with Apaf-1 and caspase-9 that begins the final process of apoptosis via enzymatic degradation with blebbing of the plasma membrane and exposure of phosphatidylserine on the surface of the cell. This is a trigger for macrophages and microglia to initiate phagocytosis of the damaged cell. The nuclear chromatin clumps and fragments, and the cell is history.

NUTRITION-RELATED FAILURES INVOLVING CENTRAL NERVOUS SYSTEM HOMEOSTASIS.

A few selected syndromes are considered here. These and many others are addressed in the major encyclopedic texts dealing with CNS disorders, for example, Mayhew (1989), Oliver et al. (1997), Aiello (1998), Bagley and Gavin (1998), Radostits et al. (2000), and Smith (2002).

Laminitis in Horses. Laminitis is a most hazardous and injurious condition to which horses are uniquely susceptible because of the design of their hooves and the dynamic laminar structure with its vulnerable circulatory and neural supply. The other design feature involved is their complex digestive tract and its associated organs and circulation. As a hindgut fermenter equipped with splendid grinding molars plus effective cutting incisors, the horse is, by its evolutionary design, the result of focus on fibrous plant materials for its diet. Biting, chewing, ensalivating, and swallowing, followed by secretions and digestion in stomach and small intestine, the fibrous residue passes to cecum and colon for microbial digestion. After domestication and management, the focus became exacting physical labor, either as traction or riding (Marie 2000).

Unable to get the necessary hours grazing to meet their nutritional needs, better pastures were developed and hay was made on a large scale, supplemented by concentrated grain feeds usually in the form of oats. The high workload generated strong appetites and a need for higher energy intake. Various concentrate formulations were created, as by-products became available. These richer diets set the stage for digestive disturbances, including acidic indigestion and enteritis, often with toxic microbial products such as amines and endotoxins (Rowe et al. 1994; Moore and Allen 1996). Some of these ideas stemmed from experience with lactic acidosis in ruminants, which showed the significance of lactic fermentations in the rumen that resulted in acidosis, endotoxemia, osmotic dehydration and, sometimes, histamine absorption. Following absorption, such factors led to damage of vulnerable endothelial sites, including the vascular supply to the laminae of the bovine hoof.

A common outcome of the excessive demands made on working horses was laminitis (also known as founder or fever in the feet), the bane of horse owners, trainers, and grooms. The stress from long hard drives, rides, or transport (e.g., voyages over water) could be the trigger. Often these activities lead to mechanical stresses on the feet and thermoregulatory challenges such as overheating, heavy sweating, and chilling. The primary problem for the affected horse is anguish from the severe pain in the hooves, especially the forefeet, which typically bear 60% of the body weight. Desperate for relief, the horse tries to take more weight on its hindfeet by extending its forefeet forward, taking the weight on the heels, and *roaching* the back so that the hindfeet are further forward to take a larger share of the weight (Figure 9.10). Not infrequently, the coffin bone

drops and rotates so that its point presses down on the sole, a very serious situation. Reluctant to move, the animal becomes stiff, even boardlike.

Several classes of specific events that may trigger laminitis have been observed or studied:

1. Making horses perform excessive physical work without allowing breaks when discomfort occurs, especially on hard or rough surfaces
2. Allowing overheated, weary horses to drink excessively
3. Feeding horses high-concentrate diets (e.g., wheat or barley or other concentrated feeds), particularly if rich in readily fermentable carbohydrates
4. Turning onto lush pasture and allowing horses ad libitum ingestion when they are hungry
5. Failing to provide appropriate exercise and nursing care for horses on long sea voyages or during truck transport

The acute syndrome often affects more than one limb. Usually, the forefeet are more severely affected than the hind. The clinical signs include sweating, tachypnea and tachycardia, agitation, and repeated lifting of affected limbs. The continuous anguish results in staring and a complete loss of interest in eating or drinking. A progressive onset of depression sets in along with a desire to lie down. This proves to be difficult, but, once down, the affected horse tends to lie for a long time.

Two syndromes that are the bane of horse owners, trainers, and grooms are laminitis and colic. Both have complex etiology and pathophysiology. (Colic is covered in Chapter 4.) Laminitis occurs in ungulates generally, but, particularly in equidae, it is one of the most prevalent and devastating conditions that has defied explanation by pathophysiological research throughout the last half-century. For the horse, the primary concern is extreme pain indicating serious damage in the hooves. Most research on it has focused on the vascular responses in the hoof, with a presumption that the dysfunction involves suboptimal blood flow that causes tissue hypoxia and pain. The vulnerability stems from the unique architecture of the hoof that provides the dynamic suspensory apparatus that bears the weight and cushions the bones within the hoof that is relatively inflexible, except at the heel.

Pathophysiological Investigations into Laminitis. The central concept that has evolved is that laminitis is a metabolic and vascular disease involving the inner sensitive laminae of the feet (Riggs and Knottenbelt 1998; Linford 2002). In some cases, it may start when bacterial endotoxins and lactic acids (D and L) from the intestines enter the blood plasma, causing acidosis and endotoxemia. The agents dilate the large arteries to the feet, increasing the overall blood flow, but, because there appears to be intense constriction of many of the capillary sphincters, causing many of the laminae to be bypassed, most of the blood is shunted around the lami-

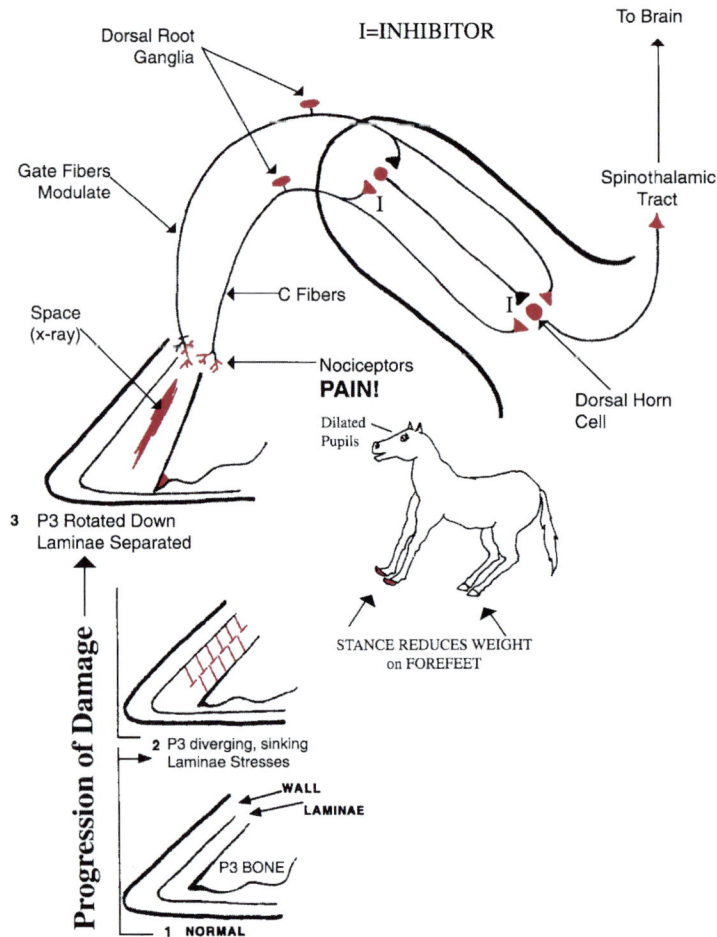

FIG. 9.10—Factors in the pathophysiology of laminitis: neural, vascular, cellular, and metabolic aspects.

1. Etiology may involve dietary readily fermentable carbohydrate (CHO) overload with microbial toxemia of intestinal origin, including epithelial damage. Several alternative stresses may be involved.

2. The vascular reactions to various toxins and cytokines lead to obstructions of capillary circulation, damage to the endothelium, and local hypoxia with severe pain, amplified by the animal's weight.

3. The vascular cushion of frog, bars, and heel vessels provide pumplike action and relief while moving is lost.

4. The sensitive and insensitive laminae are pulled apart, letting the coffin bone [third phalanx (P3)] drop toward the sole, with the widening of the space between hoof wall and P3.

5. Complete separation of the laminae lets the P3 bone rotate down, pulled by the deep digital flexor tendon. The damage in the space between wall and corium laminae is extensive and may become irreversible.

6. The excessive pain input up the C fibers overrides the modulating gate effect of the other fibers, resulting in hyperalgesia involving higher neural centers.

7. The hoof wall and laminae grow down from the coronary band, a very slow process.

nar capillaries. The resulting pathophysiology is hypoxia and restricted exposure to the capillary filtrate. At the same time, the laminae swell slightly and, being confined, as the sensitive tissues degenerate, they become extremely painful. Controversial is the finding that there may be microvascular thrombosis and venoconstriction in digital microvasculature (Weiss et al. 1995, 1996). There is evidence of changes in platelet function although other coagulation criteria are in the normal ranges. An experimental model in ponies and horses showed that platelets accumulated in the hoof area of animals overloaded on cornstarch. Glycoprotein changes in platelets enabled aggregation with fibrinogen. Platelets may be activated in the enterohepatic circulation, and intestinal permeability may be increased through mucosal damage. The platelet effect occurred within the first 12 hours although the animals did not become lame until 32 to 48 hours. A test of the peptide inhibitor, glycoprotein 2β plus 2α, eliminated platelet function for several hours. This finding seemed worthy of follow-up.

A vascular factor causes ischemia of the laminae but the precise pathogenesis has been very elusive for researchers, pathologists, and clinicians, mainly because of inconsistency of research data. There is severe metabolic dysfunction of the laminae that quickly results in mechanical crisis with extreme pain. The laminar damage can become so serious that the P may separate from the hoof capsule. Something (as yet unknown) triggers the ischemia, sometimes accompanied by coagulopathy and thrombi in the peripheral vasculature supplying the hoof support laminae. This leads to degeneration of the junction between the horny and the sensitive laminae (Pollitt 1996). As a consequence of their loss of cohesion, the pedal bone (third phalanx or P3) loses its secure attachment under the pressure of the animal's weight over time, tending to settle ventrally and, under the backward pull of the deep flexor tendon, often rotating down so that its point presses into the sole. The P3 bone is normally suspended securely by the large surface area of the interdigitating epidermal and sensitive laminae, but this suspensory system is pulled apart, creating a painful, often crippling, lesion. The obstruction to blood flow results in shunting of the arterial supply to the venous system via the many arteriovenous shunts in the area, thereby bypassing the corium.

The coronary band is hard hit, and the stagnation of its blood flow leads to failing both of capillary exchange and of essential metabolic processes needed for repair of the laminae and for keratinization. The latter requires sulfur-containing amino acids. Digestive and postpartum uterine disturbances or infections, such as Potomac fever, resulting in endotoxemia are alternative predisposing factors for laminitis. Excessive carbohydrate intake (grain overload) or turning onto lush pastures, especially if obese or unfit animals are exercised too much, can set the stage for laminitis. Using black walnut (*Juglans nigra*) shavings leads to a form of laminitis that has been proposed as an interesting model to study the pathophysiology of the condition. as it causes a drop in leukocyte level, limb edema, and laminitis. The as-yet-unknown toxin is not the naphthoquinone ingredient juglone.

The link between overfeeding of feeds/diets high in readily fermentable carbohydrates and the outcome of the laminitis (founder) syndrome in large animals is well established as one etiological avenue to the syndrome. If this is present, steps must be taken to neutralize any further absorption and promote removal of the contents of the bowel (Jeffcott 1998).

A number of systemic inflammatory and toxic conditions can also be involved in the pathogenesis. The horse is the most vulnerable to the syndrome among farm species, but a similar process affects the hooves of cloven-hoofed species such as cattle, small ruminants and, less often, swine. In these species, it is usually less severe. Cattle that gain access to feed stores of growing, ripening grain crops or immature maize may develop the condition. Also, cattle deliberately overfed

in an attempt to increase the rate of gain in the feedlot, of milk production after parturition, or in preparation for the show ring may engender rumen fermentative changes that cause osmotic dehydration, lactic acidosis, and toxic end products, resulting in vascular changes that trigger founder syndrome. Decomposition and infection of the uterine contents can lead to similar problems in the hooves. Even subclinical laminitis can predispose dairy cattle to hoof disease and founder, as can some forms of mastitis.

The syndrome of laminitis has been studied most intensely in horses (Belknap 2001). However the research focus has been almost entirely on the pathophysiology in the hoof rather than on the enormous impact of the pain it causes in the horse, other than prescribing analgesics and anti-inflammatory agents. The inflexible nature of the keratinized wall of the hoof does not allow for stretching to give relief except at the heel. The heavy weight of the animal combined with the hypoxic pathogenetic process give rise to unbearable pain. Perhaps it is time to think of new ways to relieve part of the agony. One possibility might be to devise pneumatic cushioning fittings within which the pressure could be oscillated or cycled up and down to create a pump-assisted promotion of circulation and edema removal from the hoof and lower part of the limb. If combined with subsolar support and agents to reduce vasoconstriction and the venoconstriction of small venules to help mobilize vascular flow, there might be some possibilities for using physiotherapy to help the animal through the acute nociceptive crisis stage.

Reducing tension on the laminae can have a protective effect if it allows more of the weight to be taken on the frog and sole, and less on the wall of the hoof and the tip of the P. Elevation of the heel with an 18-degree wedge reduces the pull of the digital flexor tendon, reducing tension on the laminae (Redden 1992). Sole supports as bandages or special shoes are used. Deep straw and shavings (or sand) as bedding help. Sedation to promote recumbency is desirable for weight and pain relief. The degree of rotation of the P over time is an indicator of the likely prognosis.

Further studies are needed of the specific nociceptive neural pathways and NTs involved, the nature of the stimuli that aggravate or modulate them, and the synaptic, smooth muscle and endothelial antagonists to the pathophysiological mediators that result in the ischemia, hypoxia, and pain. Such manipulative efforts might reduce the risk of the devastating degeneration of the sensitive laminae that can lead to breakdown of the bond that lets the P sink and rotate within the hoof capsule, which can progress toward irreversibility. The gate-control theory of pain has opened thinking to the various ways pain sensation can be modulated by interaction involving other sensory nerves (A-delta as well as C fibers) and a variety of interneurons (Figure 9.10).

The hoof grows continuously from the keratinocytes of the coronary corium at about 0.2 inch per month. The inward-growing leaves of the insensitive laminae grow down at the same rate matched by that of the interlocked leaves of the sensitive laminae growing out from the corium of the pedal bone. The epidermal laminae suspend the distal phalanx (P3) of each hoof, thereby bearing the fraction of body weight borne by each hoof touching the ground at a given moment during movement. Given damage to the laminae, the suspension mechanism eventually fails, allowing the P3 to drop vertically and tip toward the sole. The blood vessels perfusing the most dorsal laminae have passed through the vascular channels of the P3 bone. Detachment of the laminae with tilting downward of that bone obstructs perfusion of the damaged laminae. The pain resulting from laminar degeneration is accentuated greatly by the weight component on each foot. Bovine research has revealed that hoof cells proliferate and undergo keratinization at rates that vary with time of year (seasonal) and reproductive status (MacCallum et al. 2002).

The pain itself has a number of negative consequences, including peripheral and central release of catecholamines and vasoconstriction. The laminar degeneration is considered to be a consequence of a combination of ischemic (hypoxemic) and cytotoxic injury. In a healthy hoof cut parallel to the coronary band (i.e., close to horizontally), the length of the epidermal laminae is approximately equal to one-third of the thickness of the wall of the hoof. The distance between the dorsal cortex of the distal (P3) phalanx and the inner surface of the hoof wall is normally about 75% of that of the thickness of the hoof wall and parallel to it.

Peracute cases of laminitis, on the other hand, can have total degeneration of the secondary epidermal laminae of the hoof wall with separation from the collagen fibers of the corium. Necrotic foci may occur in those laminae or subsolar tissues. As a consequence, the distal phalanx may escape from its laminar moorings and sink toward the sole. If it rotates down at the point of the bone, it may even penetrate the sole. There is a variable degree of elongation of the epidermal laminae, depending on severity and duration. Less acute cases are more typical, but if there is any separation of the laminae with a widening angle between the hoof wall and the distal part of the P3 bone, there is always a high risk of progressive degeneration toward irreversibility. There is a need to locate and correct the cause at the earliest possible moment, restore digital circulation, reduce tension on and in the laminae (i.e., stop the forces that are pulling them apart), reduce inflammation, and ease pain (typically with nonsteroidal anti-inflammatory agents and antihistamines). It should be noted that corticosteroids decrease protein synthesis, increase vasoconstriction and promote microthrombi. Hence, they may be contraindicated. Heparin may be protective from negative coagulation-promoting events.

In recent years, the reperfusion following virtually complete shutdown of blood flow has been found to have serious consequences, with a postischemic hyperemic influx of polymorphonuclear neutrophils and cytotoxins. During this phase, nociceptors and neural circuits are overstimulated. As the basement membrane disintegrates, there is mechanical deformation of the tissues and loss of functional integrity, with inhibition of differentiation of keratinocyte repair processes. The attachment of the dense connective tissue of the coffin bone (P3) gradually gives way, leading to a high risk of its downward rotation.

Searching for a New Paradigm for Laminitis. It is time to probe a little deeper into the early stages of the genesis of the syndrome. Exciting findings and contradictory results have beset the ongoing search for critical aspects of the pathophysiology of laminitis. Despite the plethora of research data, there still seems to be no agreed distillate of analysis to allow confident decision making to guide clinicians. Some rethinking is called for in planning broader investigations.

Bowker (1999) studied the sensory neural systems of the equine foot. He noted the often overlooked fact that the hoof is a horse's *touch sense* between it and the surface environment it travels on. This sensory system enables horses to respond dramatically to environmental surface changes that are transmitted to the CNS via fast myelinated fibers. Several types of mechanical receptors are subject to activation by the physical deformation resulting from impact of hooves with the ground. The large lamellated pacinian corpuscles are an important example, as they are localized in specific areas such as the heel bulbs. As the heels are the first part of the hooves to touch the ground in a moving horse, they must play a significant role in guiding interactive reflex responses involving muscles. Another type of lamellated mechanical receptor is smaller and found around the navicular suspensory apparatus and neurovascular structures. Using immunoreactive staining for neuropeptides such as substance P and CGRP, such fibers were detected in synovial linings of the navicular bursa, within the navicular bone, and in the deep digital flexor tendon. These fibers are myelinated but slower conducting and convey pain sense in addition to the pain sense conveyed by unmyelinated nerves that conduct slowly. Thus, there are sensory fibers guiding the horse via the touch modality, the proprioceptive modality, and the pain modality.

Rethinking laminitis pathophysiology, Bowker noted that the great advance in premium athletic shoes for people was the development of the gel-filled cushioned shoes to run in. In these shoes, the fluid moves as each foot hits the ground, converting a jolt to a bounce. The movement of the gel diffuses some of the shock by dissipating energy before it can travel back up through the limb. Bowker perceives of horses' hooves being analogous to gel-filled shoes. Reviewing old ideas that the digital cushion (the wedge-shaped mass of tissue between the frog below and the deep digital flexor tendon above) was the major shock absorber, Bowker found that soundness correlated with stiffer, rather than softer, springy digital cushions. He tested the idea that, for the digital cushion to absorb shock by flexing the wall of the hoof laterally, as one theory proposed, there would have to be a major rise in hydrostatic pressure in the digital cushion when each hoof struck the ground. Measured with accelerometers in Denmark, it was shown that this did not happen and that the hydrostatic pressure actually declined and became negative at that moment.

Reexamining the issue, it was shown that those horses that had tough digital cushions had many more small blood vessels throughout the lateral or ungual cartilages that arise from the P3 or coffin bone than the ones that had springier cartilages. It was concluded that the cushion effect must be attributable to more blood being forced out through the LCs. The narrower a channel is in a moving stream, the faster the fluid moves and the lower the pressure within it. Thus, a concept emerged that hemodynamic theory required that the hydrostatic pressure would decline, transiently dissipating the shock wave that would travel up the leg on impact in a moving horse, a brilliant design feature. The only caveat is that the blood must be flowing for the theory to work.

The key feature of Bowker's biomechanical and hemodynamic hypothesis is that *transient peak impact energies are dissipated almost simultaneously by two events*:

1. The pillars of the hoof wall force the digital cushions to rotate outward as their axial projection is pushed upward, thereby creating a negative pressure within the digital cushion.
2. The impact energy is transmitted via the pillars to the digital cushions and thence to the fluid in the vascular network within the vascular channels of the digital cushions—specifically the venovenous anastomoses of the microvasculature.

These two events are highly dynamic and produce an increase in blood flow out of the vasculature of the caudal foot, creating the negative pressure on ground contact that enables it to refill rapidly after cushioning the impact by dissipating the impact energy. Horses vary in the composition of their digital cushion, with evidence suggesting that those having a stiffer fibrocartilagenous makeup have superior cushion function protecting the lower parts of the limbs. Marked differences were observed between the forefeet and hindfeet. No doubt, this evolved because of the greater stresses on the former at fast gaits and because they bear a greater fraction of the body weight.

Sound horses also tended to have three anatomic characteristics: a large frog to contact the ground, prominent bars to bear some of the weight, and a short toe. Feral horses that have not been constrained have small feet for their body mass and seem to avoid foot problems. It was concluded that a horse's hoof had evolved to bear its weight on the rear part of the sole, not on the toe or hoof wall. The optimum seemed to be to have two-thirds of the foot behind the apex of the frog and ample opportunity to exercise when very young as the structures are developing and for the next 8 months or so. Unfortunately, the practice tends to be the opposite. Because of the timing of the racing season, it is perceived to be advantageous to have mares

foal in February in North America. However, in many regions, the foals are kept in stalls at that time because of the climate.

Shoeing is another critical factor because the shoes prevent the hoof wall from being worn away, resulting in the base of the hoof moving forward and the toe becoming shaped more like an oval. Following this change, the farrier shapes the shoes to fit the new shape. Presumably, there could be compensation by filing down the growing parts of the wall and toe at each change of shoes. An elongated toe, in particular, puts leverage on the laminae, which forces them to lengthen and activates pain receptors that induce reflex contraction of the deep digital flexor tendon pulling on the P3 bone. One approach is to set the shoe to the P3 bone rather than to the hoof wall to keep the contact stress on the solar heel and off the toe and wall.

The most prominent clinical sign is *pain*. The horse is hurting. This type of acute pain is a sign that there is serious hypoxia along with the local pressure on the sensitive area due to the weight bearing down on the damaged structures in the hoof, as has been appreciated for a long time. However, most investigators have gone directly to look into the pathology of the hoof (e.g., Obel 1948) and that became the standard. Yet these structural changes were preceded by the body's early warning signal: pain. The horse stops moving around because, if it does, it hurts. So it tries to find positions that give it some relief. Usually, the forefeet are most painful, partly because they bear 60% or more of the body weight and partly because the forefeet of a horse are more sensitive than the hindfeet. This is because of their central neural design and representation within the cortex. So the horse adjusts its position to redistribute the weight, moving the rear feet forward and the forefeet as well so their stress is more on the heels than the wall. So far, all these are adjustments selected by the affected horse.

Certainly, the goals must be to help the animal achieve relief from suffering and to minimize damage by halting the pathogenetic process as rapidly as possible. First it is necessary to investigate and trace the etiological factors that triggered the onset of the syndrome. Epidemiologically, it has been estimated that 60% to 70% of cases today are attributable to ingesting an excess of readily fermentable carbohydrate grains or other concentrate feeds. Another group of cases of uncertain incidence is secondary to infections of the uterus or other organs and seems to involve endotoxins and other immunologic factors. Management errors associated with physical or nutritional stresses, such as working overfat ponies too hard or letting overheated horses drink ad libitum, have also been implicated in some cases of founder syndrome. Corrective measures can be taken to minimize damage in the case of intestinal dysfunctions.

The main research focus on the damage to the laminae and associated circulatory pathophysiology has been salutary and has advanced understanding. An excellent illustration summarizing a majority of the findings to date is to be found in Riggs and Knottenbelt (1998:4, Figure 1). However, the aspect that seems to cry out for investigation is the neurological response that leads to hyperalgesia in situations like the one in the hooves of a laminitic horse. Research on extreme pain in laboratory animals has revealed some molecular changes that occur when the modulators of the gate system in the dorsal horn and central circuits are overwhelmed by profound changes due to the intensity of the resulting hyperexcitability arriving via the dorsal root ganglia. The process involves the very rapid primary effect of excitatory amino acids (glutamate and aspartate), substance P, and CGRP that results in activation of the AMPA receptor, followed by the NMDA receptor. These events set the stage for expression of the c-*fos* and other genes after interneurons release dynorphin. Other regions of the brain broaden the pathophysiological response pattern. Obviously, major species differences must be expected, and the equine hoof is unique in having such a tightly contained structure that is vulnerable to the Velcro-like tearing apart of the sensitive laminae from their interdigitated insensitive partners projecting in from the hoof wall. However, the neural apparatus and its response systems seem to have a comparable design in principle among the major domesticated herbivores. There is evidence of long-term remodeling consequences from persistent severe pain that have detrimental effects on recovery and reparative processes. (See earlier section on Gate Theory of Pain Relevant to Laminitis)

HYPOMAGNESEMIA: TETANY

Pathophysiology of Hypomagnesemia

EFFECTS OF HYPOMAGNESEMIA. The effects of hypomagnesemia are

1. Increased neuromuscular excitability, hyperreflexia, cramping.
2. Tachycardia, arrhythmias, and hypertension.
3. Decreased release of PTH, which may cause hypercalcemia as lower Mg concentration results in increased Ca^{2+} entering cells. The activity of NMDA channels is favored by Mg deficiency. Dendrites of pyramidal cells have voltage-gated Ca^{2+} channels that open on depolarization: increased depolarization is promoted by Mg^{2+}.

Body magnesium is distributed as about 70% in bone and about 30% in intracellular fluid, with only a small proportion in extracellular fluid.

HOMEOSTATIC REGULATION OF MAGNESIUM. In the mammalian body, homeostatic regulation of magnesium (Mg) is still somewhat indistinct (Schwartz et al. 1988). Similarly, the homeostatic functions of Mg are unclear, as plasma Mg varies between hypo and hyper (i.e., the extracellular fluid concentration of Mg is not

tightly regulated). One problem is that ECF Mg is but a small fraction of body Mg. Most of the Mg is intracellular or bound in bone.

Hypothermia causes an increase in plasma Mg, which also rises quickly when hibernating species go into hibernation. This is not due to hemoconcentration. It then declines slowly and returns to normal within an hour of arousal.

The role in thermoregulation varies based on the species. Injection of Mg in nonhibernators results in a fall in body temperature. In hibernators, it may induce hibernation. Injection of Mg into hypothermic dogs reduces their tolerance to low environmental temperatures.

Evidently, homeostatic mechanisms of nonhibernators compensate for body cooling up to a point, but injection of Mg can initiate a trigger in hibernators and lower temperatures of cooled tissues may trigger release of Mg from cells with a similar effect.

Experimentally induced acidosis (respiratory or metabolic) or alkalosis may affect plasma Mg concentration quite quickly, but the direction varies with the circumstances. Plasma Mg concentration starts to decline in women early in pregnancy, becoming about 20% below normal by term.

Ultrafilterable Mg is about 70%, with protein-bound Mg being about 30%, of the total Mg. In milk, the Mg concentration is about 1 mM in humans and up to 10 mM in the cows, with about 25% protein bound in human milk but only 0.4 mM ionized in cow milk having 2.5 mM Mg, the rest being complexed with citrate, phosphate, and other ligands in cow milk. Also, processing affects the Mg concentration.

The *optimal* Mg content for an organism would be the appropriate starting point for study of tolerated ranges in Mg content, compartmentation, and the consequences of departures from these ranges for dysfunction and symptomatology.

MAGNESIUM DEPRIVATION DURING GROWTH. Mammals develop poorly on Mg-deficient diets because protein synthesis is impaired. Deficiency develops in growing mammals, not because of negative balance between intake and output but because of the demands of new tissue growth. Thus, hypomagnesemia in young animals (e.g., calves) occurs because net absorption (intake less fecal excretion) has provided insufficient Mg to meet the needs of the new tissue plus the unavoidable postabsorption losses via kidneys and secretions.

Hypomagnesemia in adult animals is usually a result of inadequate Mg intake (acute or chronic). Abnormal calcification leads to concretions in Henle's loops in the kidneys. Dogs can get atherosclerosis if kept on low-Mg diets. The Purkinje cells of the cerebellum show degenerative changes. During lactation, dietary requirements of Mg increase considerably, with depletion occurring if intake and/or absorption are low. Malabsorption and diarrhea cause increased losses of Mg in the feces.

Cell damage (as in delirium tremens in alcoholics) results in loss of Mg from cells and subsequent excretion, the result being hypomagnesemia. The CNS symptoms include confusion, delirium, convulsions, tremors, twitching, hyperirritability, and athetoid movements. *Spasmophilia* (latent tetany with electromyographic changes) occurs.

Cattle, when put out to pasture on lush grass in the spring, can develop hypomagnesemia very rapidly because of diminished Mg uptake without a large negative balance.

Plasma Mg may fall to very low levels in lactating cows and ewes (Figure 9.11). Milk content, however, does not fall. This clinical syndrome must be a deficiency in the ECF without significant depletion. Clinical signs include anorexia, restlessness, tetany, and staggers, progressing to convulsions. Tetany is more likely on switching from dry feed to lush grass. Also, use of ammonium (NH_4) fertilizer results in $MgNH_4PO_4$ complexes. Lush grass is high in ammonium also. Adult ruminants are much less able to mobilize bone Mg than are nonruminants. Even fasting causes a rapid fall in plasma Mg, indicating a unique susceptibility to the syndrome. In calves, the large intestine is most important in Mg absorption, but, as they mature into ruminants, the small intestine becomes the main site of inward transport (Hess 1969; Hatfield 2001; Radostits et al. 2000).

It has been shown that spinal cord Mg content increases in experimental rabies.

Rabbits on vitamin E-deficient diets have reduced muscle Mg concentration. Human epileptics have high CSF Mg concentration and hypomagnesemia, whereas psychotic patients have a low Mg concentration.

Hypomagnesemic Tetany in Cows. Vulnerability to grass tetany is a pathophysiological risk for ruminants—notably for bovines. Hypomagnesemia is a complex metabolic disorder featuring abnormally low levels of Mg in plasma and CSF: typically less than 1.2 mg/dL in plasma and 1.0 in CSF. This is attributable to inadequate intake of absorbable Mg to meet the demand created by growth and/or milk production. It should be noted that body reserves of Mg are not great, which is the basis of the vulnerability. Maintenance requirements are estimated to be about 3 mg/kg for maintenance and 120 mg/kg of milk. Adult lactating cows and ewes grazing lush spring pastures or young green cereal crops are at the highest risk. The risk is greater when intakes of potassium and ammonia are high and are accompanied by hypocalcemia. The lush forages predispose ruminants to metabolic acidosis and to diarrhea that reduces Mg absorption (Dua and Care 1995). Underfed beef animals exposed to cold environments are vulnerable, too.

Magnesium ion is a cofactor in many metal ion-activated enzymes facilitating the union of substrate and enzyme. Thus, it is important in many metabolic pathways (e.g., oxidative phosphorylation, pyruvate, and α-ketoglutarate oxidation) and phosphate transfers, β oxidation of fatty acids, and the pentose phosphate pathway. Low levels of Mg affect cell membrane ion function, accelerating transmission of nerve impulses, including autonomic synapses. Many body functions are affected by Mg deficiency. Growth is impaired, and peripheral vasodilation, anorexia, and a range of neural and muscular dysfunctions occur. The latter include hyperirritability, muscular stiffness, incoordination, and convulsions. Heart rate is increased, and blood pressure is reduced along with body temperature. Thiamine concentration in tissues is reduced. Minerals from the skeleton are mobilized after an initial drop in plasma Mg concentration. An illustrated summary of abnormalities of magnesium balance is presented in Silbernagl and Lang (2000:126–127).

The clinical signs of the acute form of tetany appear to be CNS related: extreme nervousness and unpredictable behavior, muscle tremors and abnormal ear movements, jaw champing with frothy salivary drooling, extreme hypersensitivity with episodes of bellowing and frenzied galloping may be observed, as well as incoordination, collapse, thrashing with tonic-clonic convulsions, and death (Smith 2002).

Subacute cases have slower onset and similar but less severe clinical signs. Chronic subclinical cases are thought to occur in herds where acute cases are seen. Ewes feeding twin lambs on lush pastures may be affected. Spring pasture grasses contain organic acids that complex Mg and reduce its nutritional availability. In particular, transaconitic acid (TAA) may chelate Mg ion. When this acid was administered orally with potassium chloride to cattle, it induced grass tetany. Studies with cattle on wheat pasture detected a sudden rise in TAA in the wheat forage when the animals developed tetany. TAA is rapidly converted in the rumen to tricarballylic acid that is absorbed and may inhibit aconitase while increasing Mg excretion (Cheeke 1998).

HYPOMAGNESEMIC TETANY IN CALVES. Hypomagnesemic tetany occurs in calves 2 to 4 months old, in calves fed milk only, or in younger calves with chronic scours fed milk replacer. The latter have reduced absorption of Mg. Clinical signs are very similar to those of adult cows.

Hypomagnesemic tetany is an important disease in lactating ewes grazing young grass pastures in spring and in any sheep grazing young wheat or other cereal grain crops. Plasma Mg undergoes an abrupt decline at lambing continuing in early lactation. This is more severe in the case of ewes with fast-growing twin lambs. The pathophysiology is basically dietary and environmental. Seasonal pasture and reproductive cycles set the stage. Wet weather in spring or fall, hormonal impact of parturition and lactation, plus use of ammonium fertilizers trigger growth of grass or grain plants rich in protein, potassium, and aconitate. The result is in high ammonia levels in rumen contents with higher pH that reduces availability of both calcium and Mg, and low carbohydrate. As plasma Mg falls, some skeletal mobilization of Mg does occur but not enough to prevent a change in neural and muscular cell membranes to a state of hyperirritability when Mg concen-

Predisposing Factors

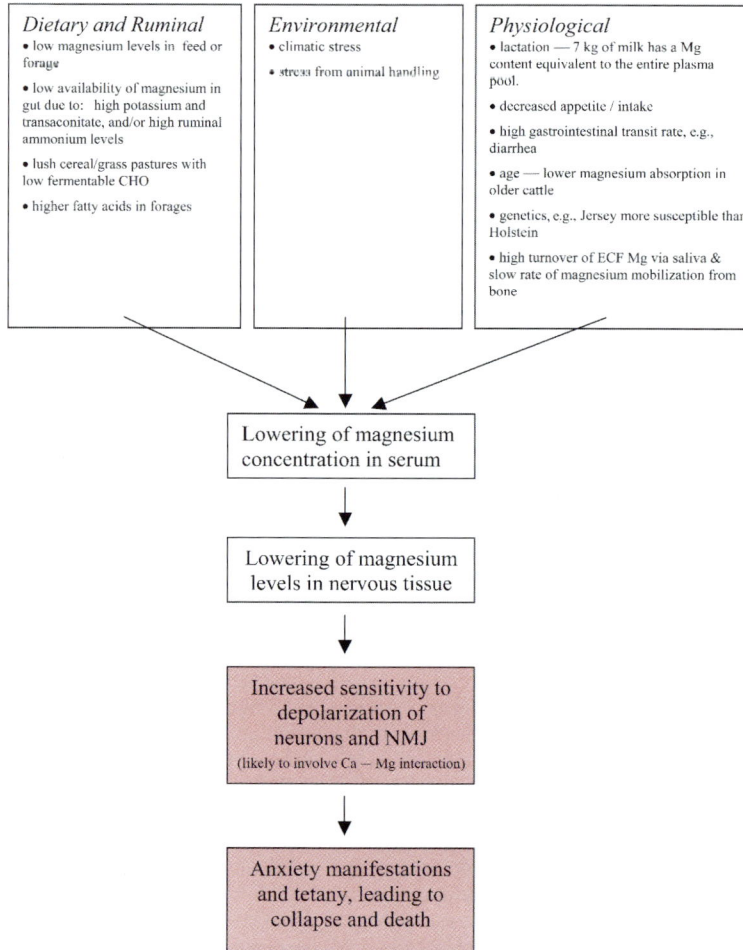

FIG. 9.11—Hypomagnesemic tetany in ruminants. The chart outlines the predisposing factors relating to the nutrition and ruminal environment that result in too little magnesium (Mg) being absorbed and the physiological factors that affect availability, such as the high turnover of extracellular fluid (ECF) magnesium via the high-volume flow of saliva. Also, the magnitude of the loss of Mg via milk in early lactation and, in young calves, the high demand of rapidly growing tissues are major factors to consider. Other stresses contribute to neural insults. The consequences are low extracellular fluid and cerebrospinal fluid (CSF) Mg levels that result in lower thresholds for depolarization of neurons and neuromuscular junctions (NMJs). The outcome is anxiety, abnormal (sometimes dangerous) belligerent behavior, and tetany. This carries a high risk of collapse and death. CHO, readily fermentable carbohydrate.

tration falls below 0.7 mg/dL. This causes behavioral dysfunction; easily startled, lambs show signs of panic with hyperventilation, head shaking, and tremors that lead to stiffness and uncoordinated movements. Affected animals may fall and develop tetany and convulsive behavior. After that stage, a high proportion will die unless the neural and muscular dysfunction is reversed promptly by appropriate therapy. It should be noted that hypomagnesemia is often accompanied by hypocalcemia (Aiello 1998).

Postmortem diagnosis can be aided by Mg assay of vitreous humor for up to 2 days after death. Before death, clinical signs are more closely correlated with CSF levels.

MANGANESE DEFICIENCY. The functions of manganese (Mn) revolve around its role in the activation of several metalloenzymes, notably pyruvate carboxylase, glucosyltransferase, and a superoxide dismutase. Activation of glucosyltransferases is essential for synthesis of the mucopolysaccharides of cartilage and participates in the synthesis of prothrombin. Mn deficiency can lead to skeletal deformities in calves and kids, resulting in leg weakness with pasterns and joints deformed by generalized weakness and ataxia (Underwood and Suttle 1999:397–420; Radostits et al. 2000:1513).

Mn toxicity has mainly been studied as an occupational disease in people. Of particular interest was the finding that the olfactory bulb has one of the largest concentrations of Mn in the human brain, raising the probability that Mn-related hyperosmia is linked to the high content of Mn there. Mn interferes with the nigrostriatal system, causing dysfunctions in the dopaminergic NT network. It concentrates in the basal ganglia, with changes in DA and 5-HT. Functional effects of Mn excess include motor-coordination dysfunctions, including unsteady gait, limb weakness, and clumsiness, with sensitivity greater during developmental stages. This is not surprising, since the dopaminergic system develops before weaning. There are also disturbances in catecholamine metabolism.

The highest levels of Mn were in the hypothalamus and cerebral cortex. There is progressive weight loss leading to neuronal degeneration and encephalopathy. In people, the signs include locomotor-activity changes and problems with movement coordination reminiscent of Parkinson's disease and of the acute syndrome evoked by methylphenyltetrahydropyridine (MPTP). This compound is related to a meperidine analogue, MPPP, a drug of abuse that was found to cause damage to neurons in the substantia nigra with neuronal loss and gliosis. MPTP is used for animal models of Parkinson's disease. Tetrahydroisoquinoline, found in some cheeses, wines, and various foods in high doses, can result in Parkinson's disease. Similar compounds have been isolated from CSF of some patients with Parkinson's disease. The antipsychotic agent haloperidol can cause Parkinson's disease as a side effect. It is a DA antagonist and depresses mitochondrial complex 1 activity, inhibiting oxidative phosphorylation. The herbicide paraquat has similar structure to MPP^+. Both it and diquat can induce Parkinson's disease. Now that Mn compounds are replacing lead compounds as antiknock in gasoline, they may have to be monitored as potential toxicants.

PATHOPHYSIOLOGY OF BOVINE KETOSIS AND OVINE PREGNANCY TOXEMIA.

Cows in early lactation and ewes in late pregnancy face enormous challenges to their capacity for metabolic adaptation that often exceed their homeostatic regulators' ability to keep crucial parameters within acceptable ranges, particularly in the cases of high-yielding dairy cows and twin-pregnant ewes. If additional stresses are encountered in these vulnerable periods, such as extremes of climate or nutritional inadequacy, the risks of a subclinical metabolic disorder proceeding to a symptomatic disease are enhanced. In the bovine situation, the huge increase in metabolic demand for glucose for milk lactose synthesis from weeks 1 to 6 of lactation evokes major changes in substrate flow among metabolic pathways in the effort to mobilize the needed molecular energy sources. If the corrective efforts fail, the clinical syndrome takes the form of decreased feed intake, reduced milk yield, and signs of neurological destabilization (Bruss 1989).

The metabolic crisis involves the accumulation of ketone bodies in the tissues that can be detected in the blood: acetoacetate, D-3-hydroxybutyrate, and acetone; increased plasma nonesterified fatty acids and hepatic triglycerides; and decreased hepatic glycogen and plasma glucose concentrations. In ewes, the huge demand for energy comes from the two lambs in utero. This condition is more threatening to the survival of dams than in the bovine case because of the approaching event of parturition as a major additional stress.

In both the bovine and ovine syndromes, the increased metabolic demand for glucose involves an increase in food intake that increases metabolic rate and the oxygen demand of the visceral tissues. The marvel of the ruminant's metabolism is that it usually handles the situation by expanding its remarkable capacity for gluconeogenesis to meet the need. However, there is a breaking point. The lack of preformed glucose reaching the intestine because of the metabolic activities of the rumen biota means that the host must take the products of microbial metabolism plus any undigested (in the reticulorumen) nutrients that escape microbial metabolism and convert them into forms that can contribute to gluconeogenesis. Once in the tissues of the host animal, there are many adaptations to the pathways and nutrient flows. In addition, there is significant proliferation of lining cells of the gut wall all the way from the rumen back. This is accompanied by alimentary ketogenesis (Rowe and Pethick 1994).

Pregnancy Toxemia of Ewes: Ovine Ketosis or Twin-lamb Disease. In late pregnancy, ewes, particularly those carrying multiple fetuses, may develop a pathophysiological syndrome involving failure of homeostatic mechanisms to keep up with the increasing metabolic demands of the twin (or more) fetuses. One factor may be an inadequate diet that is too low in energy (Caple and McLean 1986). The malaise of the ewe often leads to feed refusal, compounding the problem. Poor body condition can be another predisposing factor. Further metabolic hazards may result from inclement weather, concurrent disease, and other stresses, such as moving long distances.

The early signs are a loss of their normal competitiveness at the feed trough and a decline in awareness of their environment. Fasting, of course, is the worst thing affected ewes could do, but it is commonly seen. With less propionate being formed in the rumen and being absorbed to provide the liver with the substrate needed for gluconeogenesis, the result is hypoglycemia. This leads to a reduction of insulin secretion by the islet cells and increased glucagon secretion. One outcome is activation of hormone-sensitive lipase and catabolism of fat to fatty acids and glycerol. The fatty acids are oxidized to form ketones, but the relative lack of glucose reduces the ability of the tricarboxylic acid cycle to utilize acetylcoenzyme A (acetylCoA) [lack of oxaloacetic acid (OAA) to accept it and form citrate], so it is shunted into ketogenesis. Several body tissues can utilize ketones as an energy source. In some species, the brain can be one of these. Unfortunately, the sheep is not one that can use them as a major energy supply for its brain; hence the decline in neural function. Accumulation of ketones causes ketonemia and ketonuria. The metabolic challenge is clearly demonstrated by studies that showed that only about 3% of expired carbon dioxide was derived from ketones in fed pregnant ewes, compared with 30% in fasted ewes. To compensate, the body has to increase proteolysis to amino acids to use for gluconeogenesis. If intervention is attempted, the diagnosis must be made early after the onset of the pathophysiology. Otherwise, there fetuses will die in utero.

Ewes carrying twin lambs are trapped in a homeostatic challenge in the last 2 months of their pregnancy (Figure 9.12). In lactating bovine animals, as plasma glucose levels decline, the mammary glands slow the rate of lactose synthesis. This eases the rate of glucose utilization and allows lifesaving homeostatic adjustments to occur. Affected cows will be sick and their milk production will fall significantly, but they will survive in most cases. Twin-pregnant ewes, on the other hand, can get no relief from the burgeoning consumption of glucose and amino acids by the twin fetuses during the last 2 months before parturition. Hence, if the animals sicken, a high mortality is avoidable only by the induction of parturition or cesarean section to remove the fetuses.

A remarkable feature of ovine fetal metabolism is the very low concentration of glucose in fetal plasma—typically less than 8 to 10 mg/dL. This situation maintains a steep gradient from maternal to fetal circulation even when the ewe is hypoglycemic. All of the fetal metabolic building blocks must arrive via the placental blood. The fetal plasma compensates by developing a large *store* of plasma fructose—typically 80 to 100 mg/dL. This is synthesized from glucose by the placenta and does not pass significantly back to the maternal side. The fructose acts like a *cushion* against a major fall in glucose because fetal tissues use about twice as much glucose as fructose despite the disparity of concentrations in favor of fructose. Also remarkable is the extraordinary capacity of fetal tissues to acquire the glucose they need despite the very low concentration in the fetal plasma. By late pregnancy, the two metabolically voracious fetuses are growing rapidly, leaving less room in the abdomen for digestive organs and their venous drainage.

Gluconeogenesis from protein breakdown is less effective in ewes than in cows. Hormonal changes in late-pregnant ewes activate lipolysis, releasing long-chain fatty acids that are catabolized to form acetyl-CoA too rapidly for available supplies of OAA to feed it through the tricarboxylic acid cycle. Some is con-verted to ketone bodies, and some is reformed into triglycerides that stay in the liver; hence the source of hepatic lipidosis. It is important to note that β-hydroxybutyrate and acetoacetate are relatively strong acids and that their accumulation pushes the acid-base balance of the plasma and ECF toward acidosis. This uses up plasma buffers by formation of Na^+ and K^+ salts of these acids, which must be excreted, resulting in acidosis and dehydration.

It is important to grasp that late twin-pregnant ewes and high-yielding dairy cows are examples of biological systems pushed to their homeostatic limit. It takes minor stresses to push the system past its limit of tolerance. The rising level of ketone bodies depresses the CNS, including appetite (Sainz and Morris 2002).

Bovine Ketosis. Bovine ketosis differs from the ovine syndrome in that it occurs after a calf is born, when the cow is in rising volume lactation. Because of the very high yield of modern dairy cows, a very high metabolic demand occurs during lactation. Consequently, early lactation is the time of maximum metabolic demand, unlike in sheep, for which it comes in late pregnancy. Untreated, bovine ketosis leads to a fall in milk production. Clinical signs come on gradually and may take one of three forms: underfeeding ketosis, alimentary ketosis, or spontaneous ketosis. Some affected cows show marked behavioral disturbances, such as aggression and frenzy, kicking compulsively, head pressing, and bellowing. However, a majority of affected cows show a fall in milk production and reduced appetite resulting in weight loss and lethargy. Pica is often observed. Untreated, there can be catastrophic falls in milk production as metabolic compensation (Bruss 1989).

VITAMIN A-DEFICIENCY PATHOPHYSIOLOGY.

Ruminant species require the provitamin β carotene or preformed vitamin A. They typically make and store vitamin A in the liver if they are fed on green herbage containing β carotene. If pregnant and lactating cows are fed diets low in the vitamin or its provitamin, their calves will have inadequate hepatic reserves of the vitamin. Various metabolic defects are likely to result. Lack of vitamin A leads to slow adaptation to night vision—xerophthalmia—with drying, thickening, and clouding of the cornea and conjunctiva as early changes resulting in loss of a protective film over the ocular surfaces. Cattle deficient in vitamin A often exhibit daytime blindness with mydriasis. Such eye lesions, particularly in horses, may result in keratinization and corneal ulceration.

In the bovine CNS, the arachnoid epithelium secretes abnormal amounts of mucopolysaccharides, and the dura mater becomes thickened, leading to compression of the arachnoid villi and impaired reabsorption of CSF, increased CSF pressure, and encephalopathy with papilledema. Bouts of syncope and convulsions may occur. Pigs deficient in vitamin A develop neurological

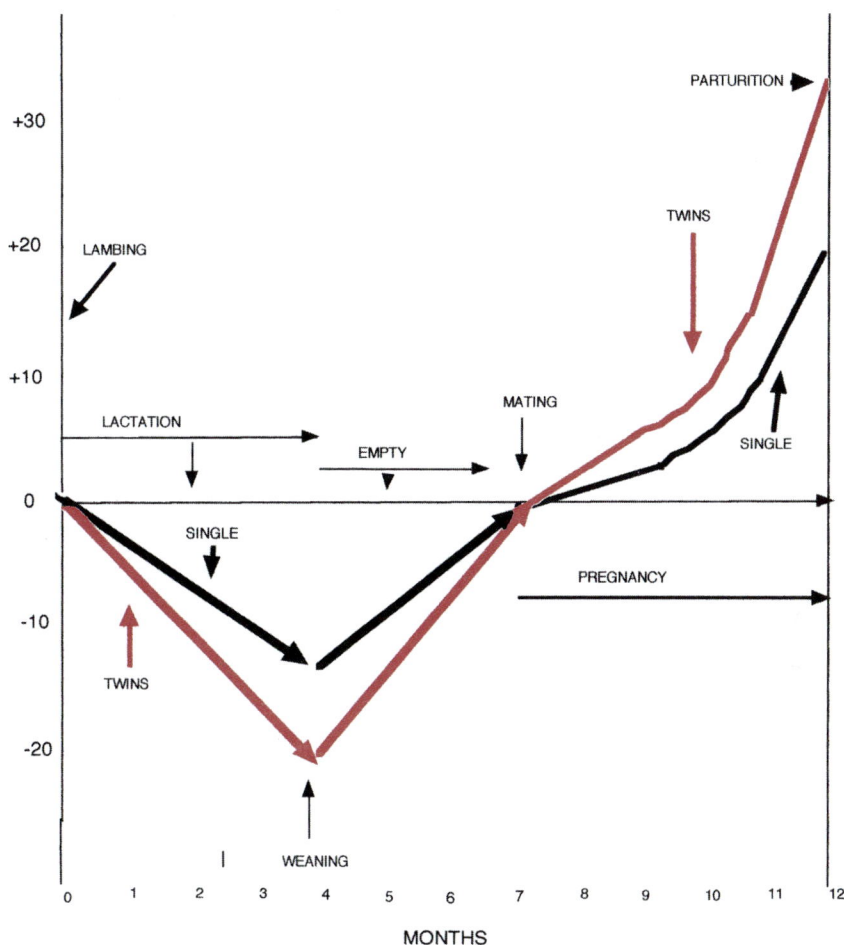

FIG. 9.12—Annual cycle of physiological consequences in a 150-pound ewe carrying one versus two (*red line*) lambs. This illustrates why pregnancy with twin fetuses is such a severe physiological stress and often results in pregnancy toxemia.

dysfunctions and myelin degeneration accompanied by osteodystrophy, high CSF pressure, and paralysis (Gorgacz et al. 1975).

Puppies from bitches deficient in vitamin A may develop degeneration of the middle ear due to stenosis of foramina. The aminosulfonic acid taurine is an essential amino acid for cats for both photoreceptor and cardiac cell function. Deficiency leads to cardiomyopathy. Dogs can utilize β carotene, unlike cats, which lack the mucosal cleavage enzyme and must ingest preformed vitamin A.

Selenium Malnutrition and Toxicity. Selenium (Se) deficiency can cause unthriftiness and white-muscle disease in calves and lambs that affects cardiac and/or skeletal muscle. The deficiency occurs particularly in areas with volcanic soils. The heat of eruptions was so great that the Se vaporized to a gas and was carried away by the wind, leaving behind a Se-deficient soil. Many mountainous areas have this type of geology. Other areas can have an excess of the element, resulting in toxic forages. This toxicity was discovered long before the potential deficiency. Several other Se-responsive syndromes impair function, growth, or reproduction. There are connections between Se and vitamin E in protective functions and antioxidant effects. Glutathione peroxidase is a selenoprotein, and a number of other selenoproteins have been identified. The amino acid selenocysteine is the primary component. The genetic code has codons for 20 amino acids that are assembled into proteins during translation. Although over 100 amino acids are found in various proteins, only one above the 20 established as *essential* is put into mammalian proteins by the translation machinery itself. This exception is selenocysteine. Its structure is the same as that of cysteine except that it has a Se atom in place of the sulfur atom. Its codon is a UGA—typically a stop codon in *Escherichia coli*, but in mammals it can also be translated directly as selenocysteine in RNA molecules. This *sec* occurs as a component of various enzymes—selenoproteins that contain the *21st essential amino acid*. It is incorporated into proteins as they are synthesized by ribosomes; hence, it needs a special transfer RNA and a stop codon (Hatfield 2000).

Some plants accumulate high levels of Se in seleniferous areas. Se toxicity can evoke a range of symptoms, depending on the chemical form of the element and the level and duration of intake. The signs of the disease vary with the level of Se ingested and interactive factors. Chronic intoxication leads to emaciation, stilted gait with incoordination, rough coat accompanied by loss of hair, lameness, and painful hoof pathology. The pathophysiology involves epidermal cellular degeneration, with tubules of the stratum medium being replaced by parakeratotic debris and disruption of the germinal layer. These signs are seen in the condition known as *alkali disease*. Some plants are notorious accumulators of Se, making the role of the element in rangeland toxicity very hard to investigate without a great deal of dietary characterization and analysis (O'Toole et al. 1996). Se has the greatest potential for toxicity among all the essential trace mineral elements, but the full picture of acute toxicity is incomplete for the condition known as *blind staggers*. The vulnerable tissues involve the integument, notably skin, hair, and hooves. The result is lameness, pain, and degeneration of the hoof wall, even ending up in sloughing of the hoof. The pain can be so severe that the animal may become immobilized, unable to reach food and water. The tubules are replaced by parakeratotic material. As Se crosses placenta, calves may develop deformed hooves. Hoof lesions may occur in cattle, sheep, and swine.

DYSFUNCTIONS ATTRIBUTABLE TO SULFUR.
Elemental sulfur is the most heavily used chemical for crop protection in California, comprising one-third of the total weight of pesticides used, mainly as a dust to combat fungal diseases of plants (rots, spots, mildews, rusts, and scabs) plus some for mites and insects as plant pests. The main crop it is used on is grapes, followed by tomatoes and sugar beets. Organic farming has led to heavy use of sulfur in *integrated pest management*.

The fate of sulfur is oxidation to sulfite and then to sulfate and sulfuric acid. Exposure of workers to sulfur causes dermatitis. Animal manure and its derivatives also increase levels of sulfur in farmlands, contributing to the resulting acidity. The combustion of coal and oil liberates sulfur dioxide (SO_2) and hydrogen sulfide to the atmosphere to return later as acid rain. Sulfur dioxide is used as a fumigant gas that hydrates to sulfurous acid, which dissociates into bisulfite (HSO_3) and sulfite (SO_3) ions. Sulfur dioxide is used as a food additive as a preservative for its antimicrobial action and enzyme inhibition, the latter to arrest discoloration. Also, in winemaking, it selectively inhibits acetic acid-forming and lactic acid-forming bacteria. The parent chemicals

are known to be hazardous, and precautions are required to protect the respiratory tract, eyes, and skin. Environmental pollution has led to heavy loss of life and severe illnesses in situations where sulfur dioxide levels reached a peak of 1.34 ppm. The effectiveness of the ciliary mucus escalator of the respiratory passages was seriously impaired.

Pet food preserved with sulfur dioxide led to thiamine deficiency in dogs and cats. Clinical signs included depression, pupillary dilation, and ataxia, with some cases progressing to seizures and sudden death caused by cardiac failure (Studdert and Labuc 1991). Pet foods containing fish-based ingredients frequently contain thiaminase-like activity. When preserved food samples had sulfur dioxide levels above 800 mg/kg, the thiamine levels were markedly reduced. In the presence of sulfiting agents such as sulfur dioxide, thiamine is cleaved into its constituent pyrimidine and thiazole moieties, rendering it inactive. It should be noted that the principal toxic effect of sulfur on the CNS of ruminants is a direct effect of sulfur and not a secondary effect resulting from thiamine deficiency. In pig feed, high-moisture barley treated with sulfur dioxide at 1%(wt/wt) had a preserving effect; that is, it was longer before mold growth became evident. However, the thiamine content of the meal was only 7.6% of that of the controls. These pigs had cardiac hypertrophy with reductions in feed intake and weight gain. The direct effects of sulfur dioxide could have been responsible for the toxicity, rather than the consequences of thiamine deficiency. The World Health Organization (WHO) recommends foods that contribute significantly to thiamine intake should not be treated with sulfur dioxide or other sulfites.

The major animal health concern of sulfur is for ruminants: the association between excessive sulfur ingestion and PEM, also known as cerebrocortical necrosis (CCN). In ruminants, microorganisms in the rumen convert sulfur to hydrogen sulfide, which is readily absorbed (Cummings et al. 1995a, b). Sulfide inhibits various enzymes involved in oxidative metabolism. It inhibits respiration by blocking the carotid body and by combining with hemoglobin to form sulfhemoglobin, thereby reducing the oxygen-carrying capacity of the blood. High ruminal concentrations of sulfur may lead to secondary thiamine deficits, but the mechanisms have not been discovered (Olkowski et al. 1992). Sulfite ion is a strong nucleophile that readily binds to thiamine (to the positively charged nitrogen in the thiazole ring), leading to secondary deficits of vitamin B_1. Veterinary problems associated with the ingestion of excessive sulfur include PEM, a severe brain disease of ruminants. Field incidents and lab data have clearly shown that dietary sulfur intake in these animals needs to be carefully regulated.

Clinical signs can occur from a few hours to several weeks after exposure to excess sulfur. These include mild excitement and restlessness, loss of appetite, and avoidance of light, progressing to head pressing, rigidity, blindness, violent convulsions, coma, and death. Young animals appear to be more susceptible. Removal of the animals from the source of sulfur leads to some improvement. Feeding sheep or cattle on elevated levels of sulfur in the diet or drinking water has given rise to PEM. Treatment of forage with elemental sulfur has led to cases. Similarly, when ammonium sulfate was added to feed (instead of the usual ammonium bicarbonate as a urinary acidifier), several cases of PEM occurred, with severe lesions present in the thalamus and striatum (Jeffry et al. 1997).

Cattle died in New Zealand after being fed on kale containing 8500 mg/kg of sulfur (0.85% of dry matter), as did sheep in Scotland fed pellets containing 0.43% sulfur. The latter showed depression, blindness, head pressing, nystagmus, and opisthotonos (dorsiflexion of the neck). The level of sulfur ingestion was calculated to have been 170 mg/kg per day. Although injected thiamine did not reverse the clinical signs, there were no further cases after treatment was started and sulfur was removed from the diet. Cattle drinking well water containing high levels of sodium sulfate (7200 ppm) suffered an outbreak of PEM in Canada. A flock of sheep grazing alfalfa stubble that had been sprayed with an aqueous suspension of 35% elemental sulfur 14 to 16 hours earlier at 53 pounds per acre had rapid onset of incoordination within 2 to 4 hours, even though they were moved to an unsprayed pasture within 2 hours. Mortality was 10%, but the rest survived and made a full recovery. On necropsy, the rumen smelled strongly of rotten eggs (i.e., hydrogen sulfide) and had a pH of 6.0 to 6.5, with no visible mucosal lesions. Necropsies of animals that died between 5 and 30 days revealed PEM lesions in their brains.

PEM has been reproduced experimentally by feeding calves a high-sulfate diet and noting that hydrogen sulfide (H_2S) accumulation in the rumen was higher in animals that developed PEM than in asymptomatic calves. Lambs dosed with sodium hydrogen sulfide (0.94 M) every 20 minutes directly into the esophagus developed clinical signs of PEM within 45 minutes of the first dosing in all lambs. PEM lesions were already present in the brains.

PEM is one of the most devastating outcomes among neurotoxicities and/or deficiencies. The toxicants may be the enzyme thiaminase or sulfur in the reduced form of hydrogen sulfide.

Over the last 10 years, the focus on probable etiology of CCN or PEM has seen a major research transition. Earlier studies had concluded that the cause was ruminal thiaminase (ingested or made by microbes) that destroys thiamine or makes a toxic antithiamine metabolite. More recently, another scenario has been explored based on evidence of high-sulfur intakes, usually as sulfates, that are reduced in the rumen milieu to hydrogen sulfide, which is a very potent neurotoxin and readily penetrates cell membranes and the BBB. There is good evidence that there may be two routes that achieve a similar terminal pathophysiology of widespread necrosis of various parts of the cerebral cortex (Gould 2000; Niles et al. 2002).

In one form of PEM, there is strong evidence of thiaminase in the rumen digesta and very low levels of thiamine pyrophosphate (TPP) in blood and brain. Thornber and colleagues (1979) produced classical PEM signs and CNS pathology in young lambs fed milk substitute with ingredients from which all thiamine had been extracted; however, it took over 5 weeks to appear. Thiaminases were present in rumen ingesta from field cases, and a TPP effect on erythrocyte transketolase was demonstrated. Also, the condition responded to high doses of parenteral thiamine as therapy, if begun early enough (Strain et al. 1990).

In the other form of PEM, there is good evidence of very high sulfur intake (usually as sulfate) but not of thiaminase in the gut or of low TPP in tissues. However, there is evidence of hydrogen sulfide presence in the rumen gas cap (Gould 1998, 2000) (Figure 9.13). This could be an indication of entry of the toxicant via the respiratory tract as well as via absorption directly into the blood, as has been shown for eructated methane. There are significant differences in the time course between the two types of PEM (Alves-de-Oliveria et al. 1993).

The thiaminase model requires a much longer lead time because it may have to establish an acute deficiency of the cofactor, TPP (Thornber et al. 1980). It has not been shown conclusively that an antithiamine compound is formed, despite a major effort to locate one, although direct toxicological studies using amprolium (Loew and Dunlop 1972) have shown the possibility exists if one were found in a clinical case. In those studies, continuously recorded EEG revealed the appearance of bursts of sleep-type spindles before clinical signs of PEM were observed (Dunlop et al. 1981; Itabisashi et al. 1990). Suzuki and colleagues (1990) made similar observations in cases of PEM/CCN in Japanese black calves. PEM occurs sporadically in ruminants grazing on wild plants that may be sulfate accumulators such as *Kochia* species on saline soils.

Hyperammonemia Pathophysiology. Cattle are often fed *urea* as a low-cost source of nitrogen. This involves depending on their reticuloruminal bacteria to incorporate it into amino acids and proteins after initial degradation to ammonia (NH_3) by urease in bacteria attached to the rumen wall. However, this does not meet the needs of microbes that need preformed amino acids. Furthermore, other risk factors exist in such forms as urea supplements offered as free-choice licking of blocks or as liquids, through incomplete mixing of feeds, leaving pockets of urea in some batches, or via errors in formulation of rations or materials. Ammonia has a pK_a of over 9. If ammonia levels in the rumen liquor exceed 20 mg/mL, the rumen pH may rise enough for absorption to occur and it to be carried via the portal venous system to the liver. The risk of toxicity rises as the concentration increases because the ammonia increases the rumen pH and the rate of absorption (Plumlee 2002; Stockham and Scott 2002).

Nitrogen is a very essential element in animal nutrition. Its metabolic currency is ammonia, which is used for biosynthesis in metabolic pathways via the ubiquitous amino group, NH_2. Moved from one organic compound to another, it is a key factor in achieving versatility in metabolism. Unfortunately, if ammonia

RISK FACTORS   H₂S

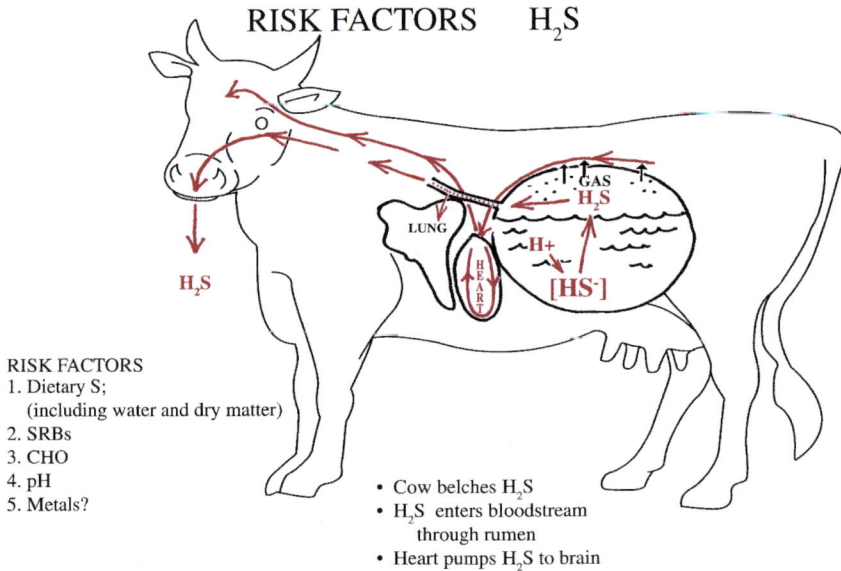

RISK FACTORS
1. Dietary S;
    (including water and dry matter)
2. SRBs
3. CHO
4. pH
5. Metals?

• Cow belches H₂S
• H₂S enters bloodstream
    through rumen
• Heart pumps H₂S to brain

FIG. 9.13—Sulfur-related polioencephalomalacia (PEM) in ruminants.

1. Excessive *sulfur* ingestion is a major factor in the incidence of PEM whenever water and/or feeds (certain plants and coproducts) are high in sulfates.
2. Once ingested, the *sulfate-reducing bacteria* (SRBs) in the rumen convert it to the sulfide form after a period of microbial adaptation of the flora.
3. Diets high in *readily fermentable carbohydrates* (CHOs) cause a buildup of acids [volatile fatty acid (VFA)and lactic acid] that may also modify microbial ecology.
4. The fall in pH increases the proportion of sulfide volatilized to hydrogen sulfide (H₂S) in the gas cap. Hydrogen sulfide is readily absorbed and crosses the blood-brain barrier.

Trace elements (e.g., copper, molybdenum, iron, and zinc) affect chemical interactions involving sulfur in the rumen, but their contribution to the incidence of PEM is not known. Hydrogen sulfide appears to be the toxicant that causes the widespread necrosis of cerebrocortical neurons.
Note: An alternative avenue to the induction of PEM is via microbial or plant thiaminase in the rumen. This causes thiamine inadequacy over a period of several weeks. The possibility of an antithiamine compound being formed in the rumen has not been confirmed, but the coccidiostat amprolium does produce a similar syndrome. (Illustration courtesy of D.H. Gould, Colarado State University modified.)

accumulates to high levels in body fluids, it becomes extremely toxic. Brain is the most sensitive organ for this. It functions almost exclusively on glucose as its primary energy source. It oxidizes glucose to acetylCoA for entry to the citric acid cycle. However, it requires a source of oxaloacetate to accept the acetate unit. The brain cells generate OAA by the carboxylation of pyruvate. Since brain pyruvate carboxylase is limiting, considerable recycling of OAA is needed to keep the cycle running. However, if much ammonia is present, the glutamate dehydrogenase activity is tilted toward glutamate, resulting in the formation of glutamine. Thus, the levels of cycle intermediates are reduced, and less OAA is regenerated. The brain is deprived of its ATP, and the pathophysiology of ammonia toxicity develops. Furthermore, glutamine and aspartate accumulate and have NT activities that can accentuate the dysfunctions.

Absorbed ammonia crosses the BBB readily, giving rise to behavioral consequences. These include restlessness, bellowing, and aggression. Physiological dysfunctions include bruxism, bloat, tremors, and convulsions. Sudden death may occur within a few hours.

Nonruminant animals are less susceptible to ammonia toxicity because the mammalian metabolism evolved to provide protection from the dangerous ammonia. In particular, the liver converts it to urea, which is uncharged and stops free ammonia from crossing the cell membranes by "mopping it up" into the urea sink, from which it can be readily eliminated via the urine or recycled by gut microbes. Ammonia is found in urine, but this is all formed via reactions in the kidneys. During starvation, after mobilizable glycogen stores are exhausted, the major source for gluconeogenesis becomes muscle protein. Decreased secretion of insulin by the pancreas and increased glucocorticoid secretion by the adrenal cortex hasten such degradation of muscle tissue to expedite glucose formation by using interconversions among amino acids to yield alanine and glutamine. Early in starvation, the liver takes alanine and makes glucose and urea. Later, glutamine is

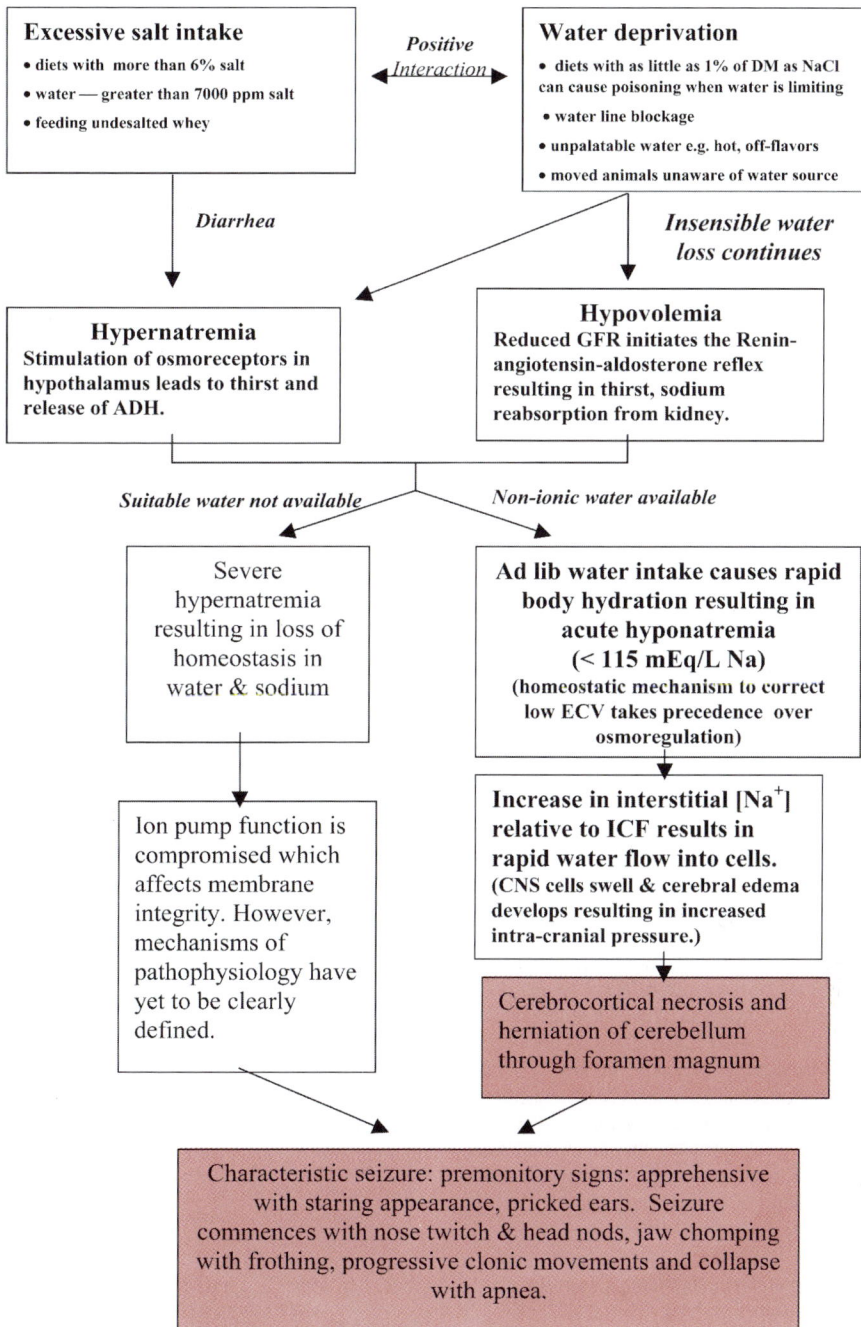

FIG. 9.14—Pathophysiology of osmotic encephalopathies in pigs that is caused by water deprivation and/or excessive salt intake. The combination of inadequate water intake with excessive ingestion of sodium chloride leads to hypovolemia and hypernatremia. Two syndromes can occur, depending on whether there is water available. A continuing lack of water causes failure of sodium and water homeostasis. The dysfunction of the ion pumps results in failure of the functional integrity of neuronal cell membranes. Alternatively, if adequate water is available ad libitum, the rapid rehydration from excess drinking results in marked hyponatremia because correction of hypovolemia takes precedence over osmoregulation. The rapid entry of water into neurons causes the cells to swell, and many die. The clinical signs are listed. CNS, central nervous system; DM, dry matter; ECV, extracellular volume; GFR, glomerular filtration rate; ICF, intracellular fluid; and ppm, parts per million.

used both to form more alanine and to serve as a favored substrate for replicating intestinal epithelial cells, which are subject to constant sloughing even in starvation and must be replaced.

Also, after a few days of fasting, the increased rate of lipid mobilization leads to a progressive buildup of ketone bodies that must be eliminated in the urine in the effort to maintain acid-base balance by avoiding ketoacidosis in body fluids. The homeostatic counter to this is to use the ammonia from glutamine in the kidney, which also frees up the carbon skeleton for use in renal gluconeogenesis along with the glycerol released during fat mobilization. During starvation, the total nitrogen excreted decreases, as there is a need to conserve nitrogen for use in metabolism, and urea loss is greatly reduced while the amount of ammonia excreted as a buffer to ketones in urine increases. In summary, the three phases of gluconeogenesis over time of fasting are (a) from hepatic glycogenolysis, (b) hepatic from liberated glycerol and amino acids from muscle, and (c) renal from glutamine residues and liberated glycerol.

Ammonia is a very toxic gas. People can smell it at 10 ppm or even less. The gas is a problem encountered in confinement facilities for livestock. It is an irritant and causes tears, shallow respiration, and nasal discharge. At levels of up to 100 ppm, it is a stressor and reduces resistance to infection and growth rate. Levels in the range of 100 to 150 ppm in ambient air cause young pigs to suffer about a 30% decrease in growth rate and also exacerbate turbinate bone lesions. In addition, it worsens the consequences of ascarid larvae infection.

Ammoniated Forage Toxicosis or "Bovine Bonkers". This is a syndrome seen when anhydrous ammonia has been added to low-quality forages to improve their nutritional value and reduce some toxic fungal metabolites (e.g., from *Acremonium*, which produces prolactin-like endophyte toxins). Overammoniation (over 3% on a dry matter basis) may result in formation of 4-methylimidazole, which also enters the milk and affects calves. Molasses treatment increases the risk. The toxins cause CNS dysfunction with hyperesthesia, ataxia, and adoption of a sawhorse stance. There may be bouts of frenzy lasting several minutes involving bellowing and running into things (blindness), progressing to recumbency sometimes accompanied by convulsions. Levels of ammonia in blood and CSF are elevated.

Osmotic Encephalopathy: Sodium Chloride (Salt) Poisoning. An acute toxic dose of sodium chloride (salt) is 2.2 g/kg, and a chronic toxic dose is 1.75 g/kg. Growth and weight are affected at 1.5 g/kg or less. Salt poisoning can be a problem where artesian bore water is used for stock and sporadic deaths may occur, especially among thirsty animals.

In pigs, the neurological syndrome consists of CNS signs: opisthotonos, nystagmus, tremors, blindness, deafness, wandering, head pressing, circling, pivoting, and epileptiform convulsions at regular intervals. The course is typically 2 to 4 days until death (Bradley and Done 1986). Ruminants often show anorexia, thirst, bawling, weight loss, hypothermia, dehydration, incoordination, and convulsions. Plasma sodium increases from 135 to 145 to 170 to 210 mEq/L, and, at the postmortem, gastritis or abomasitis can be found. To save affected animals, feed and water should be changed immediately. Adequate access to water is imperative whenever salty feeds like whey or a salted grain diet is being fed to reduce urolithiasis. Water should be less than 0.5% salt. Cerebral decompression by use of diuretics may provide relief (Stockham and Scott 2002).

Salt or sodium toxicity is a life-threatening water-deprivation sodium-ion toxicosis. It is a result of an excessive intake of sodium chloride in a situation where water access is cut off or very scarce, as when water is faulty or frozen. Although it can affect all species, it most often occurs in swine. The acute oral lethal dose for pigs is 2.2 g/kg, whereas that for sheep is 6.0 g/kg. It is unlikely to occur in the latter, provided ample water is available. Range-fed cattle may get chronic poisoning if given high-salt feed and excessive salt and mineral blocks. Affected pigs show thirst, pruritus, and constipation, and may be blind and deaf, oblivious to their environment, anorexic, unresponsive, and wander in a daze, bumping into objects, circling, or pivoting around on one limb. Intermittent seizures occur, with the animal sitting on its haunches, jerking its head upward, and then falling on its side into clonic-tonic seizures in a comatose state, accompanied by paddling (Bradley and Done 1986; Dunlop and Hugo 2002) (Figure 9.14).

At serum and CSF [Na^+] levels over 160 mEq/L (over 1800 ppm wet weight), pigs develop eosinopenia, eosinophilic cuffs around blood vessels in the cerebral cortex and adjacent meninges, and cerebral edema and necrosis. Excessive drinking will result in cerebral edema with high mortality in severe cases. Cattle get gastric inflammation, edema of skeletal muscles, and hydropericardium.

REFERENCES

Abercrombie ED, Jacobs BL. 1987a. Single-unit response of noradrenergic neurons in the locus coeruleus of freely moving cats: I. Acutely presented stressful and non-stressful stimuli. J Neurosci 7:2837–2843.

Abercrombie ED, Jacobs BL. 1987b. Single-unit response of noradrenergic neurons in the locus coeruleus of freely moving cats: II. Adaptation to chronically presented stressful stimuli. J Neurosci 7:2844–2848.

Aidley D. 1998. The Physiology of Excitable Cells, 4th ed. Cambridge: Cambridge University Press.

Aiello SE, ed. 1998. The Merck Veterinary Manual, 8th ed. Whitehouse Station, NJ: Merck.

Allman, JM. 2000. Evolving Brains. Scientific American Library, a division of HPHLP.

Alves-de-Oliveria L, Jean-Blain C, Komiscarczuk-Bony S, et al. 1993. Microbial thiamin metabolism to the rumen simulating fermenter (RUSITEC): The effects of acidogenic conditions, a high sulfur level and added thiamin. Br J Nutr 78:599–613.

Argenzio RA. 1989. Intestinal transport of electrolytes and water. In Swenson MJ, ed. Dukes' Physiology of Domestic Animals. Ithaca, N.Y., Cornell University Press.

Ashe JH, Nackman M. 1980. Neural mechanisms in taste aversion learning. Prog Psychobiol Physiol Psychol 9:223–262.

Austin AB, Pawson L, Meek S, et al. 1997. Abnormalities of heart rate and rhythm in bovine spongiform encephalopathy. Vet Record 141:352-357.

Bager F, Braggins TJ, Devine CE, et al. 1992. Onset of insensibility at slaughter in calves: Effects of electropectic seizure and exsanguination on spontaneous electro-cortical activity and indices of cerebral metabolism. Res Vet Sci 52:162–173.

Bagley RS, Gavin PR. 1998. Evaluation of the Nervous System of Domestic Animals. Sydney: Post Graduate Foundation in Veterinary Science, University of Sydney.

Baskys A, Remington G. eds. 1996. Brain Mechanisms and Psychotropic Drugs. Part I: Basic Physiology. Boca Raton, Florida: CRC Press, pp 3-54.

Bayliss WM. 1901. On the origin from the spinal cord of the vaso-dilator fibers of the hind limb, and on the nature of these fibers. J Physiol (Lond) 32:1025–1043.

Belknap J. 2001. The laminitis puzzle. Auburn Univ CVM Q 24:3.

Blakemore C. 1977. Mechanics of the Mind. Cambridge: Cambridge University Press.

Bowker RM. 1999. Insights into the Biology of the Equine Foot. In: Sixth Annual Veterinarian Farrier Conference. College of Veterinary Medicine, University of Minnesota, Agricultural Extension Service. Saint Paul, Minnesota.

Bradley R, Done JT. 1986. Nervous and muscular systems. In: Leman AD, Straw BE, Mengeling WL, Glock RD, eds. Diseases of Swine, 6th ed. Ames: Iowa State University Press, p 65.

Bruss ML. 1989. Ketogenesis and Ketosis. In: Kaneko JJ, ed. Clinical Biochemistry of Domesticated Animals, 4th ed. San Diego: Academic, pp 86–105.

Caple IW, McLean JG. 1986. Acetonemia and pregnancy toxemia. In: Howard JL, ed. Current Veterinary Therapy: Food Animal Practice 2. Philadelphia: WB Saunders.

Cheeke PR. 1998. Natural Toxicants in Feeds, Forages, and Poisonous Plants, 2nd ed. Danville, IL: Interstate.

Cotman CW, McGaugh JL. 1980. Behavioral Neuroscience: An Introduction. New York: Academic.

Crawley AC, Jones MZ, Bonning LE, et al. 1999. Alpha-mannosidosis in the guinea pig: a new animal model for lysosomal storage disorders. Pediatric Research 46:501-509.

Cummings BA, Gould DH, Caldwell DR, Hamar DW. 1995a. Identity and interactions of rumen microbes associated with dietary sulfate-induced polioencephalomalacia in cattle. Am J Vet Res 56:1384–1389.

Cummings BA, Gould DH, Caldwell DR, Hamar DW. 1995b. Ruminal microbial alteration associated with sulfide generation in steers with dietary sulfate-induced polioencephalomalacia. Am J Vet Res 56:1390–1395.

Cunningham JG, ed. 2002. Textbook of Veterinary Physiology, 3rd ed. St Louis: WB Saunders.

Dantzer R. 1994. Animal welfare methodology and criteria. Rev Sci Tech 13:277-302.

Datta S. 1999. PGO (ponto-geniculo-occipital) wave generation: Mechanism and functional significance. In: Mallick BN, Inoue S, eds. Rapid Eye Movement Sleep. New Delhi: Narosa, pp 91–106.

Day JW. 1998. Pain syndromes and pain control. In: Day JW, et al. Pathophysiology I: Year Two Curriculum, 1999–2000. Nervous System and Muscle Disorders. Minneapolis: University of Minnesota Medical School, pp 48–56.

Dua KK, Care AD. 1995. Impaired absorption of magnesium in the etiology of grass tetany. Br Vet J 151:413–426.

Dunlop R, Hugo. 2002. Osmotic encephalopathy. Personal communication.

Dunlop RH, Bueno L, Ruckebusch Y. 1981. Slow wave spindle bursts in ovine polioencephalomalacia. In: Giesecke D, Dirksen G, Stangassinger M, eds. Metabolic Disorders in Farm Animals. Munich: Munich University, pp 198.

Feldman BF. 1989. Cerebrospinal fluid in disease. In: Kaneko JJ, ed. Clinical Biochemistry of Domesticated Animals, 4th ed. New York: Academic, pp 855–860.

Fields SL. 1987. Pain. New York: McGraw-Hill.

Fields HL, Martin JB. 2001. Pain: Pathophysiology and management. In: Braunwald E, Fauci AS, Hauser SL, et al., eds. Pain: Harrison's Principles of Internal Medicine, 15th ed. New York: McGraw-Hill, pp 55–60.

Galean ML, Eng KS. 1998. Application of research findings and summary of research needs. In Britton Memorial Symposium on Metabolic Disorders of Feedlot Cattle. Journal of Animal Science 76:323-327.

Garbarg M, Barbin G, Llorens C, et al. 1980. Recent developments in brain histamine research: Pathways and receptors. In: Essman WB, Calzelli L, eds. Neurotransmitters, Receptors and Drug Action. New York: Spectrum, pp 179–202.

Garcia J, Koelling RA. 1966. Relation of cue to consequence in avoidance learning. Psychonom Sci 4:123–124.

Gardiner RM. 1980a. Cerebral blood flow and oxidative metabolism during hypoxia and asphyxia in the newborn calf and lamb. J Physiol (Lond) 305:357–376.

Gardiner RM. 1980b. Potassium transfer from brain to blood during sustained hyponatremia in the calf. J Physiol (Lond) 306:463–472.

Gershon MD. 1998. The Second Brain: The Scientific Basis of Gut Instinct. New York: Harper Collins.

Gorgacz EJ, Nielsen SW, Frier HI, et al. 1975. Morphologic alterations associated with decreased cerebrospinal fluid pressure in chronic bovine hypervitaminosis A. Am J Vet Res 36:171–180.

Gould DH. 1998. Polioencephalomalacia. J Anim Sci 76:309–314.

Gould DH. 2000. Update on sulfur-related polioencephalomalacia. Vet Clin North Am Food Anim Pract 16:481–496.

Graham SH, Chen J. 2001. Programmed cell death in cerebral ischemia. J Cereb Blood Flow Metab 21:99–109.

Greenstein B, Greenstein A. 2000. Color Atlas of Neuroscience. New York: Thieme.

Guilleminault C. 1976. Emotion-laden situations and stimuli trigger attacks extending to REM in narcolepsy. Adv Sleep Res 3:125–143.

Hardman JG, Limbird LE, Gilman AG. 2001. Goodman and Gilman's The Pharmacological Basis of Therapeutics, 10th ed. New York: McGraw-Hill.

Hatfield DL, ed. 2001. Selenium: Its Molecular Biology and Role in Human Health. Boston: Kluwer.

Hess WR. 1969. Hypothalamus and Thalamus: Experimental Documentations, 2nd ed. Stuttgart: Thieme.

Husband AJ. 1995. The immune system and integrated homeostasis. Immunol Cell Biol 73:377–382.

Husband AJ, Bryden WL. 1996. Nutrition, stress and immune activation. Proc Nutr Soc Aust 20:60–70.

Itabisashi T, Horino R, Hirano K, Maeda M. 1990. Electroencephalographic observation on sheep and cattle with experimental cerebrocortical necrosis. Nippon Juigaku Zasshi 52:551–559.

Jeffcott LB. 1998. Laminitis. In: Aiello SE, ed. The Merck Veterinary Manual, 8th ed. Whitehouse Station, NJ: Merck, pp 816–818.

Jeffry M, Duff JP, Higgins RJ, et al. 1997. Polioencephalomalacia associated with the ingestion of ammonium sulfate by sheep and cattle. Vet Rec 134:343–348.

Jouvet M, Michel F. 1958. EEG of cat during sleep. CR Soc Biol (Paris) 152:1167–1170.

Kleiber M. 1971. The Fire of Life. New York: John Wiley.

Knight AP, Lassen D, McBride T, et al. 2000. Adaptation of Pregnant Ewes to an Exclusive Onion Diet. Vet and Human Toxicol 42:1-4.

Lawrence AB, Terlorus EM, Kyriazakis I. 1993. The Behavioral effects of undernutrition in confined farm animals. Proceedings Nutritional Society 52:219-229,

Lester GD. 2002. Gastrointestinal ileus. In: Smith BP, ed. Large Animal Internal Medicine, 3rd ed. St Louis: CV Mosby, pp 674–678.

Linford RL. 2002. Laminitis (founder). In: Smith BP, ed. Large Animal Internal Medicine. St Louis: CV Mosby, pp 1116–1124.

Lingappa VR, Farey K. 2000. Physiological Medicine: A Clinical Approach to Basic Medical Physiology. New York: McGraw-Hill, Medical Publishing Division.

Linzell JL, Peaker M. 1971. The effects of oxytocin and milk removal on milk secretion in the goat. J Physiol (Lond) 216:717–734.

Livesey CT. 1997. Polioencephalomalacia associated with the ingestion of ammonium sulfate by sheep and cattle. Veterinary Record 134:343-348.

Loew FM, Dunlop RH. 1972. Induction of thiamine inadequacy and polioencephalomalacia in adult sheep with amprolium. Am J Vet Res 33:2195–2205.

Lynn B, Schutterle S, Pierau FK. 1996. The vascular component of neurogenic inflammation is caused by a special subclass of heat-sensitive nociceptors in the skin of the pig. J Physiol (Lond) 494:587–593.

MacCallum AJ, Knight CH, Hendry KAK, et al. 2002. Effects of time of year and reproductive state on the proliferation and keratinisation of bovine hoof cells. Vet Rec 151:285-289.

Mallick BN, Inoue S, eds. 1999. Rapid Eye Movement Sleep. New York: Marcel Dekker.

Marie T. 2000. Hoofs under pressure. Equus 280:42–48.

Mattson MP. 2001. Mechanisms of neuronal apoptosis and excitotoxicity. In: Mattson MP, ed. Pathogenesis of Neurodegenerative Disorders. Totowa, NJ: Humana.

Mayhew IG. 1989. Large Animal Neurology: A Handbook for Veterinary Clinicians. Philadelphia: Lea and Febiger.

Melzack R, Wall PD. 1965. Pain mechanisms: a new theory. Science 150:971–979.

Metze D, Luger T. 2001. Nervous system in the skin. In: Freinkel RKS, Woodley DT, eds. The Biology of the Skin. Boca Raton, FL: CRC.

Mims C, Nash A, Stephen J. 2001. Mim's Pathogenesis of Infectious Disease 5d ed. San Diego/London: Academic Press.

Moore JN, Allen D Jr. 1996. The pathophysiology of acute laminitis. Vet Med 91:936–939

Nestler EJ, Hyman SE, Malenka RC. 2001. Molecular Neuropharmacology: A Foundation for Clinical Neuroscience. New York: McGraw-Hill.

Niesink RJM, Jaspers RMA, Kornet LMW, et al. eds. 1999. Introduction to Neurobehavioral Toxicology: Food and Environment. Boca Raton, Florida: CRC Press pp 115-162, 231-251, 368.

Niles GA, Morgan S, Edwards WC, Lalman D. 2002. Effects of dietary sulfur concentrations on the incidence and pathology of polioencephalomalacia in weaned beef calves. Vet Hum Toxicol 44:70–72.

Obel N. 1948. Studies on the histopathology of acute laminitis [PhD diss]. Uppsala: Almqvist and Wiksells.

Oliver JE, Lorenz MD, Kornegay JN. 1997. Handbook of Veterinary Neurology, 3rd ed. Philadelphia: WB Saunders.

Olkowski AA, Gooneratne SR, Rousseaux CG, Christensen DA. 1992. Role of thiamin status in sulphur-induced polioencephalomalacia in sheep. Res Vet Sci 52:78–85.

Olson D, Ritter RC, Papasian CJ, Gutenberger S. 1981. Sympatho-adrenal and adrenal hormone responses of newborn calves to hypothermia. Can J Comp Med 45:321–326.

O'Toole D, Raisbeck M, Case JC. 1996. Selenium-induced blind staggers and related myths: A commentary on the extent of historical livestock losses attributed to selenosis on western US rangelands. Vet Pathol 33:104–116.

Ottoson D. 1983. Physiology of the Nervous System. New York: Oxford University Press.

Panksepp J. 1998. Affective Neuroscience: The Foundations of Human and Animal Emotions. New York: Oxford University Press.

Peaker M. 1995. Autocrine control of milk secretion: Development of the concept. In: Wilde CJ, Peaker M, Knight CH, eds. Intercellular Signalling in the Mammary Gland. New York: Plenum, pp 193–202

Peaker M, Wilde CJ. 1996. Feedback control of milk secretion from milk. J Mamm Gland Biol Neoplasia 1:307–315.

Plumlee KH. 2002. Feed additives. In: Smith BD, ed. Large Animal Internal Medicine, 3rd ed. St Louis: CV Mosby.

Pollitt CC. 1996. Basement membrane pathology: A feature of equine laminitis. Equine Vet J 28:38–46.

Purves D, et al., eds. 1997. Neuroscience. Sunderland, Massachusetts: Sinauer Associates.

Radostits OM, Gay CC, Blood DC, Hinchcliff KW. 2000. Veterinary Medicine, 9th ed. London: WB Saunders.

Rang HP, Dale MM, Ritter JM, Gardner P. 1995. Pharmacology. New York: Churchill Livingstone.

Redden RF. 1992. Eighteen degree elevation of the heel as an aid to treating acute and chronic laminitis in the equine. Proc Am Assoc Equine Pract 38:375–379.

Ridley RM, Baker HF. 1998. Fatal Protein. Oxford: Oxford University Press.

Riggs CM, Knottenbelt DC. 1998. Acute and subacute laminitis. In: Watson TDG, ed. Metabolic and Endocrine Problems of the Horse. London: WB Saunders, pp 1–22.

Rowe JB, Pethick DW. 1994. Starch digestion in ruminants: Problems, solutions and opportunities. Proc Nutr Soc Aust 18:40–52.

Rowe JB, Lees MJ, Pethick DW. 1994. Prevention of acidosis and laminitis associated with grain feeding in horses. J Nutr 124:2742S–2744S.

Ruckebusch Y, Phaneuf L-P, Dunlop RH. 1981. Physiology of Small and Large Animals. Philadelphia: BC Decker.

Sainz RK, Morris JG, et al. 2002. Department of Animal Science and College of Veterinary Medicine, University of California, Davis. Personal communication.

Sarnat HB, Netsky MG. 1981. Evolution of the Nervous System, 2nd ed. New York: Oxford University Press.

Schmelz M, Petersen LJ. 2001. Neurogenic inflammation in human and rodent skin. News Physiol Sc NIPS 16:33–37.

Schmelz M, Schmidt R, Bickel A, et al. 1997. Specific C-receptors for itch in human skin. J Neurosci 17:8003–8008.

Schwartz R, Topley M, Russell JB. 1988. Effect of tricarballylic acid, a non-metabolizable rumen fermentation product of trans-aconitic acid, on Mg, Ca and Zn utilization of rats. J Nutr 118:83–88.

Shepherd GM. 1994. Neurobiology, 3rd ed. New York: Oxford University Press.

Silbernagl S, Lang F. 2000. Color Atlas of Pathophysiology. New York: Thieme.

Smith AL. 1998. Central nervous system. In: Schaechter M, Engleberg NC, Eisenstein BI, Medoff G, eds. Mechanisms of Microbial Disease, 3rd ed. Baltimore: Williams and Wilkins. [See Figure 58.2: Pathways of entry of agents that cause CNS infections.]

Smith BP, ed. 2002. Large Animal Internal Medicine, 3rd ed. St Louis: CV Mosby.

Smolensky MH. 2001. Circadian rhythms in medicine. CNS Spectrums 6:467–482.

Spencer PS, Schaumberg HH, eds. 2000. Experimental and Clinical Toxicology, 2nd ed. New York: Oxford University Press.

Stockham SL, Scott MA. 2002. Fundamentals of Veterinary Clinical Pathology. Ames: Iowa State Press.

Strain GM, Claxton MS, Olcott BM, Turnquist SE. 1990. Visual-evoked potentials and electroretinograms in ruminants with thiamin-responsive polioencephalomalacia or suspected listeriosis. Am J Vet Res 51:1513–1517.

Studdert VP, Labuc RH. 1991. Thiamin deficiency in cats and dogs associated with feeding meat preserved with sulphur dioxide. Aust Vet J 68:54–57.

Suzuki M, Sitizyo E, Takeuchi J, Saito T. 1990. Electroencephalogram of Japanese black calves affected with cerebrocortical necrosis. Nippon Juigaku Zasshi 52:1077–1087.

Szolcsanyi J. 1996. Capsaicin-sensitive sensory nerve terminals with local and systemic efferent functions: Facts and scopes of an unorthodox neuroregulatory mechanism. Prog Brain Res 113:343–359.

Thornber EJ, Dunlop RH, Gawthorne JM, Huxtable CR. 1979. Polioencephalomalacia (cerebrocortical necrosis) induced by experimental thiamine deficiency in lambs. Res Vet Sci 26:378–380.

Thornber EJ, Dunlop RH, Gawthorne JM. 1980. Thiamin deficiency in the lamb: Changes in thiamin phosphate esters in the brain. J Neurochem 35:713–717.

Underwood EJ, NF Suttle. 1999. The Mineral Nutrition of Livestock, 3rd ed. New York: CABI.

Weiss DJ, Trent AM, Johnston G. 1995. Prothrombotic events associated with the prodromal stages of acute laminitis. Am J Vet Res 56:986–991.

Weiss DJ, Monreal L, Angles AM, Monasterio J. 1996. Evaluation of thrombin-antithrombin complexes and fibrin fragment D in carbohydrate-induced acute laminitis. Res Vet Sci 61:157–159.

10

WELFARE, STRESS, BEHAVIOR, AND PATHOPHYSIOLOGY

Donald M. Broom and Richard D. Kirkden

Welfare is a term that is restricted to animals, including humans. It is regarded as particularly important by many people but requires strict definition if it is to be used effectively and consistently. A clearly defined concept of welfare is needed for use in precise scientific measurements, in legal documents, and in public statements or discussion. If animal welfare is to be compared in different situations or evaluated in a specific situation, it must be assessed objectively. The assessment of welfare should be quite separate from any ethical judgment, but, once an assessment is completed, it should provide information that can be used to make decisions about the ethics of a situation.

An essential criterion for a useful definition of animal welfare is that it must refer to a characteristic of the individual animal rather than something given to the animal by humans. The welfare of an individual may well improve as a result of something given to it, but the thing given is not itself welfare. The loose use of the term welfare with reference to payments to poor people is irrelevant to the scientific or legal meaning. However, it is accurate to refer to changes in the welfare of an initially hungry person who uses a payment to obtain food and then eats the food. We can use the word welfare in relation to a person, as above, or an animal that is wild or is captive on a farm, in a zoo, in a laboratory, or in a human home. Effects on welfare that can be described include those of disease, injury, starvation, beneficial stimulation, social interactions, housing conditions, deliberate ill-treatment, human handling, transport, laboratory procedures, various mutilations, veterinary treatment, or genetic change by conventional breeding or genetic engineering.

We have to define welfare in such a way that it can be readily related to other concepts, such as needs, freedoms, happiness, coping, control, predictability, feelings, suffering, pain, anxiety, fear, boredom, stress, and health.

WELFARE DEFINITION. If, at some particular time, an individual has no problems to deal with, that individual is likely to be in a good state, including good feelings, that is indicated by body physiology, brain state, and behavior. Another individual may face problems in life that are such that it is unable to cope with them. Coping implies having control of mental and physical stability, and prolonged failure to cope results in failure to grow, failure to reproduce, or death. A third individual might face problems but, using its array of coping mechanisms, be able to cope but only with difficulty. The second and third individuals are likely to show some direct signs of their potential failure to cope or difficulty in coping, and they are also likely to have had bad feelings associated with their situations. "The welfare of an individual is its state as regards its attempts to cope with its environment" (Broom 1986). This definition refers to a characteristic of the individual at the time. The origin of the concept is how well an individual is faring or traveling through life, and the definition refers to state at a particular time [for further discussion, see Broom (1991a, b, 1993, 1996) and Broom and Johnson 1993]. The concept refers to the state of the individual on a scale from very good to very poor. This is a measurable state, and any measurement should be independent of ethical considerations. When considering how to assess the welfare of an individual, it is necessary to start with knowledge of the biology of the animal. The state may be good or poor; in either case, however, in addition to direct measures of the state, attempts should be made to measure those feelings that are a part of the state of the individual.

This definition of welfare has several implications (Broom and Johnson 1993), some of which are discussed in more detail later:

1. Welfare is a characteristic of an animal, not something given to it. In recent American usage, welfare can refer to a service or other resource given to an individual, but that is entirely different from this scientific usage. Human action may improve animal welfare, but an action or resource provided should not be referred to as welfare.

2. If welfare were viewed as an absolute state that either existed or did not exist, then the concept of welfare would be of little use when discussing the effects on individuals of various conditions in life or of potentially harmful or beneficial procedures. It is essential that the concept be defined in such a way that welfare is amenable to measurement. Once the possibility of measurement is accepted, welfare has to vary over a range. If there is a scale of welfare and the welfare of an individual might improve on this scale, it must also be possible for it to go down the scale. Many scientists assessing the welfare of animals accept that welfare can get better or can get poorer. It is therefore illogical to try to use welfare as an absolute state or to limit the term to the good end of the scale. Welfare can be poor as well as good.

Good welfare, with associated pleasure or happiness, is an essential part of the welfare concept, but the view of welfare as referring only to something good or "conducive to a good or preferable life" (Tannenbaum 1991) is not tenable if the concept is to be practically and scientifically useful. Fraser (1993), referring to well-being as the state of the animal, advocates assessing it in terms of level of biological functioning, such as injury or malnutrition, extent of suffering, and amount of positive experience. However, despite using well-being to refer to scales of how good an animal's condition is, some of his statements explaining well-being imply only a good state of the animal, a limitation that is neither logical nor desirable.

3. Welfare can be measured in a scientific way that is independent of moral considerations. Welfare measurements should be based on a knowledge of the biology of the species and, in particular, on what is known of the methods used by animals to try to cope with difficulties and of signs that coping attempts are failing. The measurement and its interpretation should be objective. Once the welfare has been described, moral decisions can be made.

4. An animal's welfare is poor when it is having difficulty in coping or is failing to cope. Failure to cope implies fitness reduction and hence stress. However, there are many circumstances in which welfare is poor without there being any effect on biological fitness. This occurs if, for example, animals are in pain, they feel fear, or they have difficulty controlling their interactions with their environment because of (a) frustration, (b) absence of some important stimulus, (c) insufficient stimulation, (d) overstimulation, or (e) too much unpredictability (Wiepkema 1987; Broom 1988).

If two situations are compared, and individuals in one situation are in slight pain but those in the other situation are in severe pain, then welfare is poorer in the second situation even if the pain or its cause does not result in any long-term consequences, such as a reduction in fitness. Pain, or the other aforementioned effects, may not affect growth, reproduction, pathology, or life expectancy, but it does mean poor welfare.

5. Fraser (1993) follows Broom (1986) and Broom and Johnson (1993) in drawing a conceptual parallel with the term *health* that is encompassed within the term welfare. Like welfare, health can refer to a range of states and can be qualified as either good or poor.

6. Animals may use a variety of methods when trying to cope, and there are various consequences of failure to cope. Any one of a variety of measurements can therefore indicate that welfare is poor, and the fact that a measure, such as growth, is normal does not mean that welfare is good.

7. Pain and suffering are important aspects of poor welfare. Pain is a sensation that is very aversive, and suffering is an array of unpleasant subjective feelings that are also aversive and avoided where possible. Even though some pain and suffering may be tolerated so that some important objective can be attained, both of these involve increased difficulty in coping with the environment and hence poorer welfare. The relationship between welfare and feelings is considered again later in this chapter.

8. Welfare is affected by what freedoms are given to individuals and by the needs of individuals, but it is not necessary to refer to these concepts when specifying welfare.

The term *well-being* is often used interchangeably with *welfare*, but well-being is often used in a looser, less precise way. Welfare is the word used in English versions of modern European legislation.

WELFARE AND FEELINGS. The feelings of an animal are an extremely important part of its welfare (Broom 1991b). Suffering is a negative, unpleasant feeling that should be recognized and prevented wherever possible. However, although we have many measures that give us some information about injury, disease, and both behavioral and physiological attempts to cope with the individual's environment, fewer studies tell us about the feelings of the animal. Information can be obtained about feelings by using preference studies, and other information giving indirect information about feelings can be obtained from studies of physiological and behavioral responses of animals.

As previously discussed, feelings are aspects of an individual's biology that must have evolved to help in survival (Broom 1998), just as aspects of anatomy, physiology, and behavior have evolved. They are used in order to maximize an individual's fitness, often by helping the individual to cope with its environment. It is also possible, as with any other aspect of the biology of an individual, that some feelings do not confer any advantage on the animal but are epiphenomena of neural activity (Broom and Johnson 1993). The coping systems used by animals operate on different time scales. Some must operate during a few seconds in order to be effectual, others take hours or months. Optimal decision making depends not only on an evaluation of energetic costs and benefits but on the urgency of action, in other words the costs associated with injury, death, or failure to find a mate (Broom 1981:80). In the fastest acting, urgent coping responses, such as avoidance of predator attack or risk of immediate injury, fear, and pain play an important role. In longer time scale coping procedures, where various risks to the fitness of an individual are involved, feelings rather than just intellectual calculations are among the causal factors affecting what decisions are made. In attempts to deal with very long term problems that may harm an individual, aspects of suffering contribute significantly to how the individual tries to cope. In the organization of behavior so as to achieve important objectives, pleasurable feelings and the expectation that these will occur have a substantial influence. The general hypothesis advanced is that whenever a situation exists where decisions are made that have a big effect on the survival or potential reproductive output of an individual, it is likely that feelings will be involved. This argument applies to all animals with complex nervous systems, such as vertebrates and cephalopods, and not just to humans. Feelings are not just a minor influence on coping systems—they are a very important part of them.

In circumstances where individuals are starting to lose control and fail to cope, feelings may exist. These feelings might have a functional role in damage limitation. However, they might also occur when an individual is not coping at all, and the feelings have no survival function then. Extreme suffering or despair are probably not adaptive feelings, but an observer of the same species might benefit, and a scientist might use indications of such feelings to deduce that an animal is not coping.

If the definition of welfare were limited to the feelings of the individual, as has been proposed by Duncan and Petherick (1991), it would not be possible to refer to the welfare of a person or an individual of another species that had no feelings because it was asleep, or anesthetized, or drugged, or suffering from a disease that affects awareness. A further problem, if only feelings were considered, is that a great deal of evidence about welfare—like the presence of neuromas, extreme physiological responses, or various abnormalities of behavior, immunosuppression, disease, inability to grow and reproduce, or reduced life expectancy—would not be taken as evidence of poor welfare unless bad feelings could be demonstrated to be associated with them. Evidence about feelings must be considered for it is important in welfare assessment, but to neglect so many other measures is illogical and harmful to the assessment of welfare and hence to attempts to improve welfare.

In some areas of animal welfare research, it is difficult to identify the subjective experiences of an animal experimentally. For example, it would be difficult to assess the effects of different stunning procedures by using preference tests. Disease effects are also difficult to assess using preference tests. There are also problems in interpreting strong preferences for harmful foods or drugs. However, research on the best housing conditions and handling procedures for animals can benefit greatly from studies of preferences that provide information about the subjective experiences of animals. Both preference studies and direct monitoring of welfare have an important role in animal welfare research. Welfare assessment should involve a combination of studies and of other factors providing information about coping.

WELFARE AND STRESS. The word *stress* should be used for that part of poor welfare that involves failure to cope. If the control systems regulating body state and responding to dangers are not able to prevent displacement of state outside the tolerable range, a situation of different biological importance is reached. The use of the term stress should be restricted to the common public use of the word to refer to a deleterious effect on an individual [see Broom and Johnson (1993) for more detailed information on this subject]. A definition of stress as just a stimulation or an event that elicits adrenal cortex activity is of no scientific or practical value. A precise criterion for what is adverse for an animal is difficult to find, but one indicator is whether there is, or is likely to be, an effect on biological fitness. *Stress can be defined as an environmental effect on an individual that overtaxes its control systems and reduces its fitness or seems likely to do so* (Broom and Johnson 1993; see also Broom 1983, 2001; Fraser and Broom 1990). Using this definition, the relationship between stress and welfare is very clear. Firstly, although welfare refers to a range in the state of an animal from very good to very poor, whenever there is stress, welfare is poor. Secondly, stress refs only to situations where there is failure to cope, but poor welfare refers to the state of an animal both when there is failure to cope and when the individual is having difficulty in coping. It is very important that this latter kind of poor welfare, as well as the occasions when an animal is stressed, is included as part of poor welfare. For instance, if a person is severely depressed or if an individual has a debilitating disease but there is complete recovery with no long-term effects on fitness, then it would still be appropriate to say that the welfare of the individuals was poor at the time of the depression or disease.

WELFARE ASSESSMENT. The general methods for assessing welfare are summarized in Table 10.1, and a list of measures of poor welfare is presented in Table 10.2. Most indicators will help to pinpoint the state of an animal wherever it is on the scale from very good to very poor. Some measures are most relevant to short-term problems, such as those associated with human handling or a brief period of adverse physical conditions, whereas others are more appropriate to long-term problems. [For a detailed discussion of measures of welfare, see Broom (1988, 1991a, b), Fraser and Broom (1990), and Broom and Johnson (1993).]

Some signs of poor welfare arise from physiological measurements. For instance, increased heart rate, adrenal activity, adrenal activity following adrenocorticotrophic hormone (ACTH) challenge, or reduced immunological response following a challenge can all indicate that welfare is poorer than in individuals that do not show such changes. Care must be taken when interpreting such results, as with many other measures described here. The impaired immune system function and some of the physiological changes can indicate what has been termed a *prepathological state* (Moberg 1985).

Behavioral measures are also of particular value in welfare assessment. The fact that an animal avoids an object or event strongly reveals information about its feelings and hence about its welfare. The stronger the avoidance is, the worse is the welfare while the object is present or the event is occurring. An individual that is completely unable to adopt a preferred lying posture despite repeated attempts will be assessed as having poorer welfare than one that can adopt the preferred posture. Other abnormal behavior, such as stereotypies,

self-mutilation, tail biting in pigs, feather pecking in hens, or excessively aggressive behavior, indicates that the perpetrator's welfare is poor.

In some of these physiological and behavioral measures, it is clear that an individual is trying to cope with adversity, and the extent of the attempts to cope can be measured. In other cases, however, some responses are solely pathological, and an individual is failing to cope. In either case, the measure indicates poor welfare.

Disease, injury, movement difficulties, and growth abnormality all indicate poor welfare. If two housing systems are compared in a carefully controlled experiment, and the incidence of any of the aforementioned is significantly increased in one of them, the welfare of the animals is worse in that system. The welfare of any diseased animal is worse than that of an animal that is not diseased, but much remains to be discovered about the magnitude of the effects of disease on welfare. Little is known about how much suffering is associated with different diseases. A specific example of an effect on housing conditions that leads to poor welfare is the consequence of severely reduced exercise for bone strength. In studies of hens (Knowles and Broom 1990; Norgaard-Nielsen 1990), those birds that could not sufficiently exercise their wings and legs because they were housed in battery cages had considerably weaker bones than did those birds in percheries that could exercise. Similarly, Marchant and Broom (1996) found that sows in stalls had leg bones only 65% as strong as sows in group-housing systems. The actual weakness of bones means that the animals are coping less well with their environment so welfare is poorer in the confined housing. If such an animal's bones are broken, there will be considerable pain and the welfare will be worse. Pain may be assessed by aversion, physiological measures, the effects of analgesics [for example, see Duncan et al. (1991)], or the existence of neuromas (Gentle 1986). Whatever the measurement, data collected in studies of animal welfare provide information about the position of the animal on a scale of welfare from very good to very poor.

The majority of indicators of good welfare that we can use are obtained by studies demonstrating positive preferences by animals. Early studies of this kind included that by Hughes and Black (1973) showing that hens given a choice of different kinds of floor to stand on did not choose what biologists had expected them to choose. As techniques of preference tests

TABLE 10.1—Summary of welfare assessment

General methods	Assessment
Direct indicators of poor welfare	How poor

Tests of   a) Avoidance
      b) Positive preference
Measures of ability to carry out normal
   behavior and other biological functions
Other direct indicators of good welfare
	a) Extent to which animals have to live with avoided situations or stimuli
	b) Extent to which that which is strongly preferred is available
	How much important normal behavior or
	   physiological or anatomic development cannot occur
	How good

Modified after Broom 1999b.

TABLE 10.2—Measures of welfare

Physiological indicators of pleasure
Behavioral indicators of pleasure
Extent to which strongly preferred behaviors can be shown
Variety of normal behaviors shown or suppressed
Extent to which normal physiological processes and
    anatomic development are possible
Extent of behavioral aversion shown
Physiological attempts to cope
Immunosuppression
Disease prevalence
Behavioral attempts to cope
Behavior pathology
Brain changes, e.g., those indicating self-narcotization
Body damage prevalence
Reduced ability to grow or breed
Reduced life expectancy

After Broom 2000.

developed, it became apparent that good measures of strength of preference were needed. Taking advantage of the fact that gilts preferred to lie in a pen adjacent to other gilts, Van Rooijen (1980) offered them the choice of different kinds of floors that were either in pens next to another gilt or in pens farther away. With the floor preference titrated against the social preference, he was able to gain better information about strength of preference. A further example of preference tests, in which operant conditioning with different fixed ratios of reinforcement were used, is the work of Arey (1992). Preparturient sows would press a panel for access to a room containing straw or one containing food. Up to 2 days before parturition, they pressed, at ratios of 50 to 300 per reinforcement, much more often for access to food than for access to straw. At this time, food was more important to the sows than was straw for manipulation or nest building. On the day before parturition, however, at which time a nest would normally be built, sows pressed just as often, at fixed ratio 50/300, for straw as for food. Another indicator of the effort that an individual is willing to use to obtain a resource is the weight of door that is lifted. Manser and colleagues (1996), studying floor preferences of laboratory rats, found that rats would lift a heavier door to reach a solid floor on which they could rest than the weight of a door they would lift to reach a grid floor.

The third general method of welfare assessment, listed in Table 10.1, involves measuring what behavior and other functions cannot be carried out in particular living conditions. Hens prefer to flap their wings at intervals but cannot in a battery cage. whereas veal calves and some caged laboratory animals try hard to groom themselves thoroughly but cannot in a small crate, cage, or restraining apparatus.

In all welfare assessment, it is necessary to take account of individual variation in attempts to cope with adversity and in the effects that adversity has on the animal. When pigs have been confined in stalls or tethers for some time, a proportion of individuals show high levels of stereotypies, whereas others are very inactive and unresponsive (Broom 1987). There may

also be a change with time spent in the condition in the amount and type of abnormal behavior shown (Cronin and Wiepkema 1984). In rats, mice, and tree shrews, it is known that different physiological and behavioral responses are shown by an individual confined with an aggressor, and these responses have been categorized as active and passive coping (Von Holst 1986; Koolhaas et al. 1983; Benus 1988). Active animals fight vigorously, whereas passive animals submit. A study of the strategies adopted by gilts in a competitive social situation showed that some sows were aggressive and successful, and a second category defended vigorously if attacked, whereas a third category avoided social confrontation, if possible. These categories of animals differed in their adrenal responses and in reproductive success (Mendl et al. 1992). As a result of differences in the extent of different physiological and behavioral responses to problems, it is necessary that any assessment of welfare should include a wide range of measures. Our knowledge of how the various measurements combine to indicate the severity of the problem must also be improved.

HEALTH, DISEASE, AND PATHOLOGY. Health may be defined as "an animal's state as regards its attempts to cope with pathology" (Broom 2000). In this statement, animals include humans.

In their veterinary dictionary, Blood and Studdert (1999) define pathology as

1. The branch of veterinary science involving treating the essential nature of disease, especially the changes in body tissues and organs which cause or are caused by disease.
2. The structural and functional manifestations of disease.

This is almost identical to the definition of pathology in Dorland's (1988) dictionary of human medicine.

Thus, pathology refers both to a scientific discipline and to the object of its study. The second definition is the relevant one in the present context, but it is not satisfactory. Although this definition is faithful to the etymology of the term *pathology*, which literally means the study of disease, it does not get us any closer to an understanding of the subject, since it begs the question of what disease is. Rather than taking the circuitous route of answering this question and deducing from it what pathology must actually mean, it is simpler to refer to several veterinary pathology textbooks that have advanced definitions without invoking disease. For example,

Pathology is the study of the derangement of molecules, cells, tissues and function that occur in living organisms in response to injurious agents or deprivations. (Jones et al. 1997)

Pathology, in the broadest sense, is abnormal biology. As a science it encompasses all abnormalities of structure and function. It involves the study of cells, tissues, organs, and body fluids.... Pathology is essentially the search for and study of lesions, the abnormal structural and functional changes which occur in the body. (Cheville 1988)

These definitions refer to the discipline of pathology, not to its object of study. Nevertheless, the object of study is made clear. The foregoing definitions suggest that pathology is "the derangement of molecules, cells, tissues and function that occur in living organisms in response to injurious agents or deprivations," or "the abnormal structural and functional changes which occur in the body."

One shortcoming of these definitions of pathology is that they imply, but do not explicitly state, that pathology is always detrimental to the organism. The terms *derangement* and *abnormal* are loaded in that, in common usage, they usually refer to undesirable changes or states, but they need not do so. In practice, pathologists study detrimental changes in structure and function, not beneficial ones, and the definition of pathology should reflect this. It is suggested that the terms derangement and abnormal be qualified by the word *detrimental*.

Cheville's use of the term *lesion* is also somewhat problematic. In veterinary medicine, lesions are generally thought of as gross abnormalities occurring at the level of the organs or tissues, not at the level of the cell. Hence, there can be pathology in the absence of lesions. Blood and Studdert's (1999) definition of a lesion, as "any pathological,... discontinuity of tissue or loss of function of a part" reflects its general usage. There is also a syntactic difference between the terms pathology and lesion, which Cheville's usage reflects. *Pathology* can be, and most frequently is, employed as a collective noun, whereas *lesion* is a particular noun. Unless there is only one lesion, pathology describes a collection of lesions. The plural, *pathologies*, is sometimes used to refer to the existence of pathology in more than one animal.

The distinction that pathologists make between structure and function is essentially one between the morphology of a cell, tissue, or organ and its operation. Functional abnormalities include physiological changes, which are the subject of a subdiscipline known as *pathophysiology*. These physiological changes are seen as departures from the normal day-to-day balance or steady state. Functional abnormalities also include more obvious changes, such as loss of appetite and diarrhea, that are often employed as clinical signs. The term *lesion* usually refers to a structural abnormality but is also applied to functional abnormalities, which may or may not have morphological counterparts. The term *pathogenesis* refers to the way in which a lesion develops over time (Slauson and Cooper 1990).

The veterinary definition of the term *disease* is in fact very similar to that of pathology. Blood and Studdert (1999) begin by stating that disease is "tradi-

tionally defined as a finite abnormality of structure or function with an identifiable pathological or clinopathological basis, and with a recognizable syndrome or constellation of clinical signs," but go on to add that "the definition has long since been widened to embrace subclinical diseases in which there is no tangible clinical syndrome but which are identifiable by chemical, hematological, biophysical, microbiological or immunological means." Slauson and Cooper's (1990) definition is "the culmination of those various defects, abnormalities, excesses, deficiencies, and injuries occurring at the cell and tissue level which ultimately result in clinically apparent dysfunction." This usage of the term disease, like the widespread veterinary usage of the term pathology, refers to injuries as well as to the effects of pathogens although, for many people, injury would not initially fall under the heading of disease. Furthermore, these definitions of disease, like the aforementioned definitions of pathology, are too inclusive, describing diseases as *abnormalities*, whereas the study of disease is exclusively concerned with changes that are detrimental to the organism.

Pathology or disease is classified in three ways: (a) according to its causes, (b) according to the type of tissue changes that are involved, and (c) according to the identity of the tissue or organ that is affected. The classification of pathology according to the type of tissue changes involved is probably the least ambiguous approach. Five types of tissue changes have been identified: cellular degeneration and death, circulatory disturbances common to all tissues, inflammation and repair, immunopathology, and disturbances of growth, including neoplasia (Cheville 1988; Slauson and Cooper 1990). However, the classification of pathology according to causes is more useful for the purposes of present review, since this approach is compatible with the classification of welfare measures already discussed. Because so many diverse causes exist, and because most pathology is multifactorial, it is not easy to devise a rigorous system of classification on this basis. In practice, most veterinarians employ a mixture of categories, relating not only to cause, but also to the identity of the affected tissue, when they make diagnoses. Nevertheless, attempts have been made to classify pathology by its causes [for example, see Cheville (1988) and Slauson and Cooper (1990)]. Slauson and Cooper's (1990) system is presented in Table 10.3.

Slauson and Cooper (1990) provide examples of the pathologies that would fall into these categories but do not offer an exhaustive list.

TABLE 10.3—Classification of pathology according to its causes

Genetic abnormalities
Physical injury
Thermal injury
Chemical injury
Infections or infestations
Metabolic abnormalities
Nutritional injury

Thermal injury should include not only direct tissue damage but also consequences of hyperthermia and hypothermia (Cheville 1988).

Infections and infestations can be subclassified, according to the pathogen, into those caused by viruses; *Mycoplasma*; *Rickettsia*; *Chlamydia*; bacteria; protozoa (e.g., coccidia); and parasitic helminths and arthropods (Jones et al. 1997). Prions should be added to this list.

The category of metabolic abnormalities is quite difficult to define, owing to the complex etiology of many metabolic disorders. Slauson and Cooper (1990) list hormonal imbalance, enzyme defects, membrane defects, and structural protein defects as examples of metabolic abnormalities. This list emphasizes pathology in which metabolic dysfunction is the sole cause. It would not include many conditions normally classed as metabolic diseases, particularly those associated with nutritional deficiency. Blood and Studdert (1999) define metabolic disease as

> diseases in which normal metabolic processes are disturbed and a resulting absence or shortfall of a normal metabolite causes disease, eg. hypocalcaemia in cows, or an accumulation of the end products of metabolism causes a clinical illness, eg. acetonaemia of dairy cows. Many diseases in this group really have their beginnings in a nutritional deficiency state.

In fact, very few disorders in domestic animals are caused solely by metabolic dysfunction (Payne 1989). Even parturient hypocalcemia and ketosis (acetonemia) in dairy cows are associated with nutrition, arising from an imbalance between nutrient intake and the excessive metabolic demands of lactation. Slauson and Cooper's (1990) perspective reflects the human medical usage of the term *metabolic disease* more than the veterinary usage. In people, the term metabolic disease implies some inherent defect, such as the congenital absence of an enzyme (e.g., storage diseases, in which metabolites slowly accumulate), or an endocrinologic failure (e.g., diabetes mellitus). The veterinary usage is looser, admitting nutritional deficiencies and more complex disorders that result from a breakdown in an animal's capacity to meet the physiological demands of high productivity (Payne 1989) (see Figure 10.1).

There is substantial overlap between metabolic disease and the so-called production diseases, defined by Blood and Studdert (1999) as

> diseases caused by systems of management, especially feeding and the breeding of high-producing strains of animals and birds, in which production exceeds dietary and thermal input. Includes the group of diseases known in the veterinary literature as 'metabolic diseases'. They differ from nutritional deficiencies in which it is the nutritional supply which falls short of normal production.

Production diseases are effectively man-made, being caused by an inability to meet the demands of high pro-

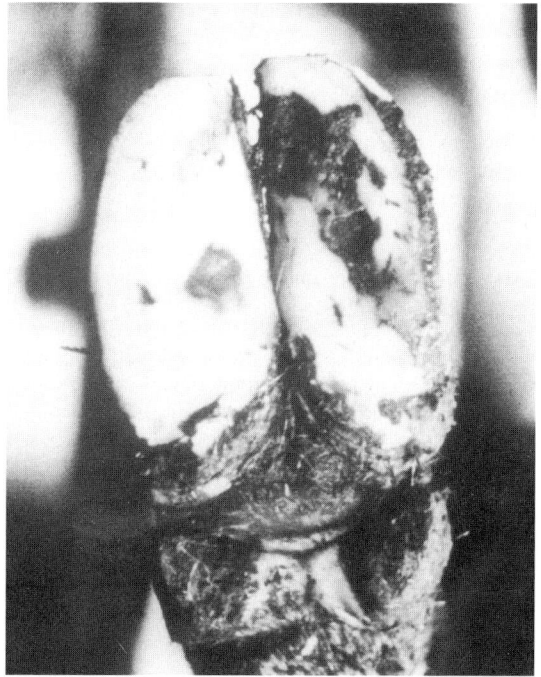

FIG. 10.1—Sole ulcer in cattle occurs more often in metabolically challenged individuals. (Photograph F.A. Galindo.)

duction (Payne 1989; Broom 1994). This category does not include nutritional deficiencies but does include many other metabolic diseases, such as parturient hypocalcemia and ketosis in dairy cattle. It is somewhat broader in general usage than Blood and Studdert's definition suggests, since it also includes acidosis and laminitis in dairy cows (Payne 1989; Webster 1993), which are diseases caused by the overfeeding of concentrates. These conditions are closely associated with high productivity, because high-yielding cows require large quantities of concentrate to meet the demands of lactation. Production diseases are discussed in more detail later.

In the category of *nutritional injury*, Slauson and Cooper (1990) include deficiency, imbalance, undernutrition, and overnutrition. This agrees with Blood and Studdert's (1999) definition of *nutritionally related disease*, as "disease caused by deficiencies or excesses of specific feed nutrients or of a total ration." The overlap between metabolic disease and nutritional disease in ordinary veterinary usage is clear from a comparison of Blood and Studdert's definitions of these terms. Also, some production diseases, including acidosis and laminitis in dairy cattle, would be classed as nutritional diseases.

In discussing the causes of pathology, the effects of environmental factors on an animal's resistance to infection is also generally acknowledged [for example, see Thomson (1984) and Slauson and Cooper (1990)]. For example, cold air and atmospheric pollutants have been shown to impair bacterial clearance from the lung in pigs by interfering with the mucociliary elevator. This may predispose them to respiratory infections. Crowding, weaning, changes of feed, and transportation are other environmental factors that are believed to reduce resistance to infection. Such factors may change subclinical or latent infection into acute or chronic disease.

It should be noted that some veterinarians would define animal health more broadly than Broom (2000). For example, Blood and Studdert's (1999) definition is "a state of physical and psychological well-being and of productivity including reproduction." This definition is inadequate, partly because *well-being* is not defined and partly because it is far too inclusive. It does not reflect the practice of veterinary medicine, which is primarily concerned with physical abnormalities. In reality, neither behavioral disturbances nor psychological stressors are considered in the classification of pathology. This review employs Broom's definition of health because it reflects the de facto meaning of the term in veterinary medicine and because it makes clear the distinction between health and welfare.

RELATIONSHIP BETWEEN WELFARE AND HEALTH. Health is a part of welfare. When an animal's health is poor, so is its welfare, but poor welfare does not always imply poor health. There are many circumstances where behavioral or physiological coping mechanisms are activated, indicating that welfare is poor, but the animal's health remains good. These include situations where the coping mechanisms are successful, such as when body temperature is maintained despite extreme ambient temperatures; circumstances where failure to cope has consequences for psychological, but not physical, stability, such as in the development of noninjurious pathological behaviors; and circumstances where detrimental effects on physical stability are compensated for by management practices, such as the routine use of antibiotics.

A comparison of Table 10.1 with Table 10.3 indicates that there are some indicators of poor welfare that are classified as pathology and, as such, will also indicate poor health. These include body damage and disease, which refers in this case to infectious disease. The prevention of normal physiological processes and anatomic development will also indicate poor health where these phenomena can be shown to be symptoms of an infectious, metabolic, or nutritional disease. Mortality rate is also an indicator of welfare in general and health in particular in many circumstances. When animals are close to death, their welfare and their health will often be very poor.

Other indicators of poor welfare, though not being signs of poor health at that time, may indicate a risk of poor health in the future. These include immunosuppression, which renders an animal susceptible to infection; the chronic activation of physiological coping mechanisms, which may cause immunosuppression; and certain behavioral pathologies and redirected behaviors, which can result in serious injury or predisposition to infection, either in the animal itself or in others. It is these measures that the review focuses on, since poor welfare precedes poor health and is instrumental in its deterioration.

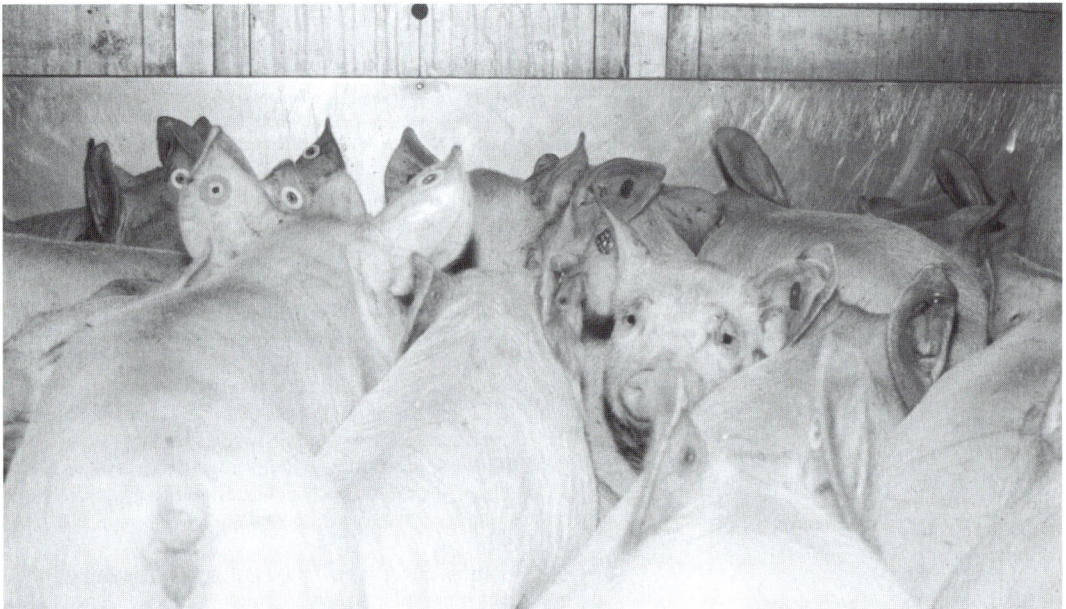

FIG. 10.2—Crowding of pigs predisposes them to various clinical conditions. (Photograph R.H. Bradshaw.)

Two pathways can be identified that link poor welfare to poor health:

1. Chronic activation of physiological coping mechanisms leads to immunosuppression that leads to infectious disease.
2. Behavioral coping mechanisms lead to injurious abnormal behavior that leads to physical injury.

This review also considers metabolic *production diseases* in which poor welfare also causes poor health. In some domestic breeds, a combination of nutrition and genetic selection for high productivity has produced a situation in which an animal is barely able to cope with the demands of its own physiology.

A third pathway, linking poor welfare to poor health, therefore corresponds to the development of metabolic production diseases:

3. Genetic selection for high productivity + nutrition leads to metabolic stress that leads to metabolic production disease.

The remainder of this review is concerned with the description of these three pathways. Examples are presented, several of which are discussed in detail.

Physiological Coping Mechanisms and Infectious Disease

GENERAL PRINCIPLES. The relationship between the chronic activation of physiological coping mechanisms, immunomodulation, and susceptibility to infectious disease has been explored in the field of psychoneuroimmunology. It is important because all environmental challenges that lead to poor welfare, whether they threaten mental or bodily stability, activate these coping mechanisms. However, the relationship is not a simple one. The response of the neuroendocrine system is not the same for all environmental challenges (Mason 1968a, b, 1975). It may also vary between species (Griffin 1989) and between individuals, depending on how they perceive the challenge. Glucocorticoids and other hormones modulate the immune system in various ways, which have been studied in vitro and are relatively well understood, at least in the case of glucocorticoids. A given change in the immune system, though, may affect an animal's susceptibility to different pathogens in different ways (Gross and Colmano 1969). These complications mean that it is often necessary to consider one challenge, one species, and one pathogen at a time.

Glucocorticoids have certain, relatively uniform, effects on the immune system (Griffin 1989). They reduce the number of circulating lymphocytes (lymphopenia) and increase the number of neutrophils (neutrophilia). In many species, they also reduce the number of eosinophils (eosinopenia). Lymphocytes, neutrophils, and eosinophils are all types of white blood cell, or leukocyte. In species with relatively high numbers of lymphocytes, such as chickens, these changes result in a reduction in the total number of circulating leukocytes (leukopenia), whereas in species with relatively low numbers of lymphocytes, including cattle, sheep, and pigs, the net result is an increased leukocyte count (leukocytosis).

Lymphocytes include B cells, T cells, and natural killer (NK) cells. B cells synthesize antibodies: the humoral immune response. These bind to circulating antigens, facilitating their ingestion by granulocytes and macrophages, neutralizing them, or otherwise assisting the host's defenses. T cells are subdivided into cytotoxic T cells, which destroy host cells presenting foreign (e.g., viral) antigens on their surface, the cell-mediated immune response, and helper T cells, which facilitate the humoral and cell-mediated immune responses. NK cells destroy host cells that do not present antigens on their surface, a characteristic of tumor cells and some cells infected by viruses. B cells and T cells are sensitive to specific antigens. In addition to performing their characteristic functions, they respond by proliferating. In the case of B cells and cytotoxic T cells, memory cells are produced that greatly increase the humoral and cell-mediated immune responses to the antigen if the host is exposed to it again: the secondary immune response. Neutrophils and eosinophils are two varieties of granulocytes, a cell population distinct from the lymphocytes, which also includes basophils. Neutrophils, which are the most numerous of the granulocytes, are attracted by chemical signals to damaged tissues, where they capture and destroy foreign material by phagocytosis. Eosinophils can also phagocytose small particles but are better suited to the destruction of large parasites by extruding enzymes into the surrounding fluid. Basophils are not phagocytic but release vasoactive amines in damaged tissues, provoking acute inflammation. A third distinct population of leukocytes is the macrophages, known as monocytes when immature, which reach damaged tissues after the neutrophils and destroy not only foreign material but also dead and dying host cells. They also assist in wound healing and secrete cytokines, which activate lymphocytes and produce feelings of illness.

The differential effects of glucocorticoids upon different leukocyte populations may explain the observation that a given stressor can increase the susceptibility of chickens to some pathogens while reducing their susceptibility to others (Gross and Siegel 1965; Gross and Colmano 1969, 1971; Gross 1972, 1976). The rapid, nonspecific immune response mediated by neutrophils is of considerable importance in dealing with certain bacterial and coccidial infections but is of little use against some agents, such as *Mycoplasma gallisepticum* and Newcastle disease virus, which can only be tackled effectively by lymphocytes (Gross 1962; Gross and Siegel 1975; Siegel 1980).

Not only do glucocorticoids reduce the number of circulating lymphocytes, they also suppress the activity of B cells and cytotoxic T cells by interacting with macrophages and helper T cells. For example, glucocorticoids decrease the synthesis of interleukin 1 (IL-1) by macrophages (MacDermott and Stacey 1981) and the synthesis of interleukin 2 (IL-2) by helper T cells (Gillis et al. 1979). These cytokines increase the activity of B cells and cytotoxic T cells, as well as that of other leukocytes, including macrophages and helper T cells.

Glucocorticoids are very important mediators of the immune system (Biondi and Zannino 1997). However, they are not the only means by which stressors influence immunocompetence (Griffin 1989; Biondi and Zannino 1997; Yang and Glaser 2000). For example, both the synthesis of β-endorphin by the anterior pituitary gland (Haynes and Timms 1987) and the release of vasopressin and oxytocin from the neurohypophysis (Wideman and Murphy 1985; Williams et al. 1985) are increased in response to environmental challenges. β-Endorphin enhances T-cell proliferation in vitro (Gilman et al. 1982), whereas vasopressin and oxytocin both stimulate helper T cells to produce more interferon-γ (Johnson and Torres 1985), a cytokine that activates macrophages and NK cells. In humans at least, catecholamines suppress the cell-mediated immune response while enhancing the humoral immune response (Yang and Glaser 2000). Furthermore, the lymphoid organs, including the bone marrow, thymus, spleen, and lymph nodes, where lymphocytes are produced and stored, are all innervated (Felten and Felten 1991; Schorr and Arnason 1999), permitting the central nervous system to influence lymphocytes directly. The situation is further complicated by the fact that vasopressin and oxytocin (Gibbs 1986a, b; Gaillard and Al-Damluji 1987) and catecholamines (Axelrod 1984) also stimulate the secretion of ACTH, while β-endorphin is secreted in parallel with ACTH, from their mutual precursor pro-opiomelanocortin (Guillemin et al. 1977; Rossier et al. 1977). With so many pathways modulating the effects that environmental challenges have on the immune system, it is not possible to make generalized predictions concerning the effects of stress upon immunocompetence.

What is clear from the study of psychoneuroimmunology is that environmental conditions that elicit physiological coping responses in animals, and that can therefore be said to cause poor welfare, alter their susceptibility to infectious agents and hence their health status (Biondi and Zannino 1997). It is also apparent that, despite the complexity of the physiological processes that mediate between the exposure of an animal to an environmental challenge and its health status, the majority of experimental studies to date have reported an increased susceptibility to pathogens (Peterson et al. 1991; Biondi and Zannino 1997). Notwithstanding this, it is essential that the effect of a given challenge upon the susceptibility of a given species to a given disease should be investigated individually.

TABLE 10.4—Effects of environmental challenges upon bacterial (including mycoplasmal) pathology

Study	Species	Challenge	Bacteria	Effects on clinical course
Gross and Siegel 1965	Chicken	Mixing	*Escherichia coli*	↓ Susceptibility
		Transportation	*Mycoplasma gallisepticum*	= Susceptibility
Gross and Colmano 1969	Chicken	Mixing	*Staphylococcus aureus*	↓ Susceptibility
			Escherichia coli	↓ Susceptibility
			Mycoplasma gallisepticum	↑ Susceptibility
Gross and Siegel 1981	Chicken	Mixing	*Escherichia coli*	↓ Susceptibility
			Mycoplasma gallisepticum	↑ Susceptibility
Gross 1984	Chicken	Various degrees of mixing stress	*Escherichia coli*	As stress increased, susceptibility ↓ then ↑
Larson et al. 1985	Chicken	Mixing	*Staphylococcus aureus*	↓ Susceptibility
Gross and Siegel 1981	Chicken	Isolation	*Mycoplasma gallisepticum*	↑ Susceptibility
Juszkiewicz et al. 1967	Chicken	Heat	*Pasteurella multocida*	↑ Speed of mortality
Juszkiewicz 1967	Chicken	Cold	*Pasteurella multocida*	↓ Speed of mortality
Moore et al. 1934	Chick	Cold	*Salmonella pullorum*	↑ Susceptibility
Ram and Hutt 1955	Chick	Cold	*Salmonella pullorum*	↑ Mortality
Bierer 1961	Chick	Cold	*Salmonella typhimurium*	↑ Mortality
Thaxton et al. 1974	Chick	Cold	*Salmonella worthington*	↑ Mortality
Soerjadi et al. 1979	Chick	Cold	*Salmonella typhimurium*	↑ Shedding
Larson et al. 1985	Pig	Isolation	*Staphylococcus aureus*	↓ Susceptibility
Armstrong and Cline 1977	Pig	Cold	*Escherichia coli*	↑ Gastroenteritis
Filion et al. 1984	Calf	Transportation + marketing	*Pasteurella haemolytica*	= Susceptibility
Binkhorst et al. 1990	Calf	Forced exercise	*Pasteurella haemolytica*	= Severity
Anderson et al. 1990	Calf	Forced exercise	*Pasteurella haemolytica*	↑ Severity
Hambdy et al. 1963	Calf	Heat + cold	*Pasteurella haemolytica* + *Pasteurella multocida* + bovine parainfluenza 3 virus	↑ Severity
Diesel et al. 1991	Calf	Cold	*Pasteurella haemolytica*	↑ Susceptibility
Owen et al. 1983	Horse	Transportation	*Salmonella typhimurium*	Reactivated

TABLE 10.5—Effects of environmental challenges upon viral pathology

Study	Species	Challenge	Virus	Effects on clinical course
Gross and Colmano 1969	Chicken	Mixing	Newcastle disease virus	↑ Susceptibility
Gross and Colmano 1971	Chicken	Mixing	Marek's disease virus	↑ Susceptibility
Gross 1972	Chicken	Mixing	Marek's disease virus	↑ Susceptibility
Mohamed and Hanson 1980	Chicken	Mixing	Newcastle disease virus	↑ Susceptibility
Lin et al. 1998	Pig	Mixing	Latent swine vesicular disease virus	Reactivated
Furuuchi and Shimizu 1976	Pig	Heat	Transmissible gastroenteritis virus	↓ Gastroenteritis
Shimizu et al. 1978	Pig	Heat	Transmissible gastroenteritis virus	↓ Gastroenteritis
Shope 1955	Pig	Cold	Latent swine influenza virus	Reactivated
Furuuchi and Shimizu 1976	Pig	Cold	Transmissible gastroenteritis virus	↑ Gastroenteritis
Shimizu et al. 1978	Pig	Cold	Transmissible gastroenteritis virus	↑ Gastroenteritis
Filion et al. 1984	Calf	Transportation + marketing	Bovine herpesvirus 1	↑ Mortality and pneumonia

EXAMPLES OF EFFECTS OF ENVIRONMENTAL CHAL-LENGES ON PATHOLOGY. In Tables 10.4 to 10.6, lists have been made of environmental challenges that have been shown to alter the susceptibility of farm animal species to specific pathogens. The studies cited are of two kinds. The majority have proceeded by inoculating experimental subjects with a pathogen, subjecting them to an environmental challenge, either before or after inoculation, and comparing the clinical course of the disease in these animals with its course in controls, which have been subjected to the environmental challenge but not inoculated. In a second, much smaller group of studies, researchers have investigated the ability of environmental challenges to reactivate pathogens whose clinical effects are either much reduced or no longer apparent, but which remain present in the body. Studies that have simply observed the effect of an environmental challenge upon the spontaneous incidence of disease have not been included, since it is often unclear which pathogen or combination of pathogens is involved.

Table 10.4 is concerned with the effects of environmental challenges on bacterial pathology; Table 10.5 with viral pathology; and Table 10.6 with parasitic pathology. It can be seen from all three tables that the number of studies that have been conducted using domestic livestock species is small. Furthermore, the majority of studies have reported an increased susceptibility to disease following environmental challenge.

It can be seen from Table 10.4 that mixing with unfamiliar animals generally reduces the susceptibility of chickens to *Escherichia coli* and *Staphylococcus*

aureus (Gross and Siegel 1965, 1981; Gross and Colmano 1969; Larson et al. 1985) although, when the mixing procedure evoked a very substantial coping response (the neutrophil/lymphocyte ratio was measured), their susceptibility to *E. coli* was increased (Gross 1984). In pigs, isolation also reduces susceptibility to *S. aureus* (Larson et al. 1985). Both mixing and isolation increase the susceptibility of chickens to *M. gallisepticum* (Gross and Siegel 1965, 1981; Gross and Colmano 1969). Exposure to low environmental temperatures increases the susceptibility of recently hatched chicks to *Salmonella* spp. (Moore et al. 1934; Ram and Hutt 1955; Bierer 1961; Thaxton et al. 1974; Soerjadi et al. 1979). However, the survival time of adult chickens inoculated with *Pasteurella multocida* is increased by low temperatures (Juszkiewicz 1967) but reduced by high temperatures (Juszkiewicz et al. 1967). In pigs, low temperatures increase susceptibility to *E. coli* (Armstrong and Cline 1977). Attempts to induce pneumonic pasteurellosis (*shipping fever*) experimentally in calves have been unsuccessful when transportation was used as a stressor (Filion et al. 1984) and have had mixed findings with forced exercise (Binkhorst et al. 1990; Anderson et al. 1990) but have been successful when using low temperatures (Diesel et al. 1991) and abrupt temperature changes (Hambdy et al. 1963). Transportation has been shown to reactivate *Salmonella typhimurium* in horses (Owen et al. 1983).

In Table 10.5, it can be seen that mixing chickens increases their susceptibility to Newcastle disease virus (Gross and Colmano 1969; Mohamed and Hanson 1980) and Marek's disease virus (Gross and Colmano

TABLE 10.6—Effects of environmental challenges upon parasitic pathology

Study	Species	Challenge	Parasite	Effects on clinical course
Hall and Gross 1972	Chicken	Mixing	*Ornithonyssus sylvarium* (northern fowl mite)	↓ Susceptibility
Gross 1976	Chicken	Mixing	*Eimeria necatrix*	↓ Susceptibility
Hall et al. 1979	Chicken	Mixing	*Ornithonyssus sylvarium*	↓ Susceptibility
Gross 1985	Chicken	Mixing	*Eimeria tenella*	↓ Susceptibility
Pierson et al. 1997	Chicken	Mixing	*Eimeria tenella*	↓ Susceptibili

1971; Gross 1972). In pigs, mixing also reactivates latent swine vesicular disease virus (Lin et al. 1998). Low temperatures increase the susceptibility of pigs to transmissible gastroenteritis virus, whereas high temperatures make them more resistant (Furuuchi and Shimizu 1976; Shimizu et al. 1978). Low temperatures also reactivate latent swine influenza virus in pigs (Shope 1955). The transportation of calves has been shown to increase the incidence of pneumonia caused by bovine herpesvirus 1 (Filion et al. 1984).

Table 10.6 indicates that mixing chickens makes them more resistant to the northern fowl mite (Hall and Gross 1972; Hall et al. 1979) and to coccidia of *Eimeria* spp. (Gross 1976, 1985; Pierson et al. 1997).

EXAMPLES IN DETAIL. Two examples are discussed in more detail below: the transportation of cattle and the transportation of sheep. An account is given of how the various environmental challenges that occur during transportation activate physiological coping mechanisms, modulate the immune system, and increase disease incidence in these species. The effects of these challenges upon the incidence of physical injury and mortality are also described.

The experimental studies that have assessed the effects of these challenges upon the immune system have employed a variety of assays, which require some explanation beforehand. These assays have been designed to measure either humoral or cell-mediated immune responsiveness following exposure to the putative stressor.

Assays of humoral immune responsiveness measure the production of specific antibodies following an experimental challenge (usually an injection) with an antigen. The antigen should be injected either during exposure to the stressor, shortly before, or shortly afterward. Sometimes, the primary antibody response is assessed by estimating the amount of antibody present in blood samples obtained 5 or more days following the injection. A common technique is agglutination, in which blood serum is added to a suspension of antigen particles, and the level of clumping or agglutination that occurs reveals the concentration of the antibody. Alternatively, the secondary antibody response may be assessed, either by administering a second antigen challenge to the animal and estimating the number of antibodies in blood samples obtained subsequently, or by means of a plaque-forming cell assay. The plaque-forming cell assay employs foreign red blood cells (erythrocytes) as the antigen. Five or more days following injection of the erythrocytes, lymphocytes are taken from the spleen and incubated, with the erythrocyte antigen and complement, between two microscope slides. *Complement* is the name given to a series of enzymes that destroy cells presenting antigen bound to antibody. A plaque, clear of erythrocytes, forms around each B cell, its diameter being proportional to the level of antibody synthesis.

Assays of cell-mediated immune responsiveness measure the activity of cytotoxic T cells. They can be classified into in vitro and in vivo techniques. In vitro techniques include measures of the proliferation of T cells, and of their production of cytokines, in response to antigen. For these tests, blood samples are obtained either during exposure to the stressor, shortly before, or shortly afterward. To measure T-cell proliferation, the cells are mixed with antigen and incubated, sometimes in the presence of a mitogen, such as phytohemagglutinin (PHA), concanavalin A (ConA) or pokeweed mitogen (PWM), which stimulates proliferation. The rate of proliferation is estimated by measuring the uptake of radiolabeled thymidine, which dividing cells incorporate into new DNA. To measure the production of cytokines, blood samples are incubated with antigen, and the resulting concentrations of cytokines are measured using a standard assay, such as the enzyme-linked immunosorbent assay (ELISA). A third in vitro technique estimates T-cell cytotoxicity following exposure to antigen. In this case, the animal is injected with the antigen around the time of exposure to the stressor, and blood samples are obtained later. T cells are then incubated with radiolabeled cells presenting the antigen. Cytotoxic action of the T cells releases the radiolabel into solution, so the final concentration of the label yields an estimate of T-cell activity. In vivo techniques are quite different. They measure a cell-mediated inflammatory response to antigen challenge on or below the skin surface, known as a *delayed hypersensitivity reaction* because it develops gradually over several days. The inflammation is caused primarily by basophils, which are attracted to the site by T cells. An inflammatory response to most antigens occurs only when an animal has had previous exposure to them; in other words, reactions of this kind are generally secondary cell-mediated immune responses. The antigen must therefore be injected intradermally on two occasions, the inflammatory response following the second injection being assessed by a measurement of skin thickness. However, certain chemical agents, including dinitrochlorobenzene (DNCB) and PHA, elicit a delayed hypersensitivity-like reaction, known as a *contact sensitivity response*, on the first exposure. This allergic cell-mediated response is peculiar in that it does not require previous sensitization to an antigen. PHA is injected intradermally, whereas DNCB is painted onto the skin surface. The inflammatory response is assessed by measuring skin thickness.

TRANSPORTATION OF CATTLE

Transport Procedures. Cattle are transported by road, rail, sea, and air for breeding, fattening, and slaughter. In Europe, the biggest trade is by road, and most research has been conducted on road transport (Tarrant and Grandin 2000).

If dairy calves are to be sold, they are normally transported to market within the first 2 weeks of life. If purchased, they are transported twice more, first to the dealer's premises and then to a beef-rearing unit (Webster 1984). Most calves exported from the United Kingdom for veal are just over 1 week old (Knowles 1999). Beef calves from suckler herds are considerably older, usually between 6 and 12 months of age, when transported for finishing (Allen and Kilkenny 1984). Beef calves are normally weaned at the same time as they are transported (MacKenzie et al. 1997), whereas dairy calves are weaned at the rearing unit, at 4 or 5 weeks of age (Allen and Kilkenny 1984). Weaning consists of removal from the dam in suckled-beef production systems or withdrawal of milk substitute in systems that rear dairy calves for beef. In the United States, journey distances for beef calves are typically much greater than in Europe: calves often travel between 1000 and 3000 km to the feedlot (Tarrant and Grandin 2000).

Most older cattle, transported to slaughter, also pass through live auction markets (Knowles 1999). In the United States, distances between feedlots and slaughterhouses are relatively short (Tarrant and Grandin 2000), but transport times are increasing in Europe, owing to a steady decline in the number of abattoirs (Knowles 1999; Tarrant and Grandin 2000).

The transportation of cattle involves exposure to a number of environmental challenges, other than the journey itself. These may include withdrawal of feed and water; mixing; introduction to a novel environment; loading and unloading; and extremes of temperature, light, noise and vibration. Some or all of these factors may contribute to the overall levels of stress and injury observed during commercial transportation. Some experimental studies have attempted to separate out these factors, while others have simulated commercial procedures.

Mortality. Young calves, less than 4 weeks of age, are not well adapted to cope with transport and marketing, often suffering very high rates of mortality (Knowles 1999). The younger the calves are, the higher is their mortality (Staples and Haugse 1974; Barnes et al. 1975; Mormède et al. 1982). Comparatively few calves actually die during transportation, but many succumb to secondary disease, mostly with symptoms of pneumonia or scouring, within 4 weeks of arrival at the rearing unit (Staples and Haugse 1974).

Mortality is very low in adult cattle transported by road (Knowles 1999). In South Africa, Henning (1993) reported a mortality rate of 0.01% in slaughter cattle in 1980 and no mortality among 22,000 cattle in the early 1990s. Mortality rates during sea journeys can be considerably higher (Hails 1978; Connell 1984).

Physical Injury. Transportation of cattle results in bruising. Jarvis and colleagues (1995) found bruising on 97% of carcasses, with a mean of 1.4 bruises per carcass (Knowles 1999). Bruising is caused by rough handling and poor road driving techniques (Grandin 1983) and exacerbated by high stocking densities, long journey times, and repeated loading and unloading.

Cattle that are handled roughly show much more bruising than those that are handled gently (Grandin 1981). In particular, the use of a stick for driving cattle increases bruising (Jarvis et al. 1995). Observations made during the journey indicate that minor losses of balance, where cattle quickly shift their footing to regain stability, are nearly all caused by driving events, including cornering, gear changes, and braking (Kenny and Tarrant 1987b, c; Tarrant et al. 1988).

Falls were rarely observed at low stocking densities (200 or 300 kg/m^2 in 600-kg steers) but were much more frequent when stocking density was high (600 kg/m^2) (Tarrant et al. 1992). They were triggered by driving events and by animals struggling to change position. Tarrant and colleagues (1992) observed that shifts of footing, to regain balance, were inhibited at the high stocking rate. After falling, cattle were unable to get up again. Fallen animals were trampled, and this caused other animals to lose their footing. The result was a high incidence of carcass bruising.

For typical commercial driving, during which accelerations causing loss of balance are frequent (Broom 1999b), there appeared to be an optimum stocking density at which bruising is minimized. Eldridge and Winfield (1988) transported 360-kg steers for 6 hours at three stocking rates. Animals transported at the intermediate density, of about 310 kg/m^2, showed the least bruising. The incidence of bruising was twice as high at a density of about 260 kg/m^2 and four times as high at a density of about 405 kg/m^2. However, when vehicles are driven well and animals are not caused to lose their balance, bruising and other indicators of poor welfare decrease in frequency as space allowance increases. The European Union Scientific Committee on Animal Health and Animal Welfare (Broom et al. 2003) recommends a space allowance for cattle standing in a transport vehicle A(in m^2) = 0.02W$^{0.67}$ where W is weight of animals in kg. This is the same as that recommended by The Farm Animal Welfare Council (1991) and similar to Randall (1993).

The extent of bruising has also been shown to increase with distance traveled and with time spent in the lairage (McNally and Warriss 1996). In lairage, mounting behavior, seen especially in groups of unfamiliar bulls, is known to cause bruising (Kenny and Tarrant 1987a). More bruising was also seen in cattle arriving for slaughter from an auction market (Jarvis et al. 1995; McNally and Warriss 1996). This may have been due either to rough handling or to social interactions such as mounting.

Physiological Measures of Welfare. Welfare problems arising during the transportation of cattle include not only the physical injury and psychological stress associated with mixing, handling, and driving, but also fatigue, hunger, dehydration, and thermal stress.

A variety of different physiological measures of welfare have been employed, some of which assess particular problems, while others are more general. Measures that are specific include the plasma concentration of creatine kinase, an enzyme released into the blood from heart and skeletal muscle after damage or vigorous exercise. High levels of this enzyme after transportation are associated with physical fatigue. Dehydration also has specific physiological correlates, including the packed-cell volume or hematocrit, defined as the percentage, by volume, of the blood that is occupied by erythrocytes, and the osmolality, a measure of the concentration of solutes in the blood. A more general measure of welfare in transit is the depletion of muscle glycogen levels, which may be a consequence either of sustained physical exertion or of chronic activation of the SAM axis sympathetic nervous system-adrenal medullary (Shackleford et al. 1994), since adrenaline mediates the conversion of stored glycogen to glucose. An allied measure is the incidence of dark, firm, dry (DFD) beef, also known as dark cutting beef. This meat has a characteristically high pH, a result of the depletion of muscle glycogen before death (Tarrant and Grandin 2000). Another relatively general measure of poor welfare during transport is plasma cortisol concentration, although this measure is not completely general, since glucocorticoid levels are not elevated by fasting or high temperatures (Mason 1968a, b).

Cattle from intensive production systems, which are accustomed to human contact, can be loaded and unloaded without poor welfare, if rough handling is avoided (Kenny and Tarrant 1987b). However, extensively raised beef cattle exhibit elevated heart rates and cortisol levels when handled (Lay et al. 1992a, b). The physiological responses of range-reared beef cattle to handling are almost as great as their responses to hot-iron branding (Lay et al. 1992a, b), and this may be the most stressful component of transport for these animals.

The effect that the process of transportation has upon plasma cortisol concentration is somewhat variable: in many studies, cortisol levels were elevated during or after transportation (Crookshank et al. 1979; Simensen et al. 1980; Kent and Ewbank 1983; 1986b; Murata et al. 1987; Kegley et al. 1997), but in several studies they were not (Blecha et al. 1984; Kegley et al. 1997). This is probably due to differences in journey time and in a wide range of factors that influence the quality of a journey. These may include stocking density, ventilation, vehicle design, the standard of driving, and the quality of the roads (Tarrant and Grandin 2000). Plasma cortisol concentration is greater at high stocking densities (Tarrant et al. 1988, 1992).

When weaning coincides with transportation, this will also make the journey more difficult for the animals. Calves that are weaned and transported simultaneously exhibit higher cortisol levels than do calves weaned 2 weeks before transportation (Crookshank et al. 1979).

The cortisol response of young calves, of less than 4 weeks of age, to transportation is reduced as compared with older cattle (Mormède et al. 1982; Fell and Shutt 1986; Kent and Ewbank 1986a; Knowles et al. 1997), but this does not indicate that they cope better with transport. On the contrary, it reflects the immaturity of their physiological coping mechanisms (Mormède et al. 1982; Knowles et al. 1997). Hartmann and colleagues (1973) have demonstrated that the reactivity of the adrenals to an ACTH challenge increases with age and is not yet fully developed in 1-week-old calves. An inability to mount an effective glucocorticoid response, which is adaptive in the short term, may be a contributing factor to the high levels of morbidity and mortality that occur in young calves. It has also been observed that young calves are unable to regulate their body temperature closely during transportation (Knowles et al. 1997).

DFD beef is generally caused by mixing and by prolonged transportation, including time spent in the lairage. Long road journeys result in a significant elevation of meat pH, between 0.1 and 0.2 pH units, and a corresponding increase in the incidence of DFD beef (Wythes et al. 1981; Tarrant et al. 1992). The prevalence of DFD meat increases substantially with time spent in the lairage (Augustini et al. 1980; Fabiansson et al. 1984; Wajda and Wichlacz 1984). The mixing of unfamiliar animals, especially bulls, is a major cause of DFD meat. Mounting behavior has been implicated (Bartos et al. 1993). Mixing also causes fighting in adult male cattle (Kenny and Tarrant 1987c) and 6-month-old calves (Trunkfield and Broom 1991), which may increase the incidence of DFD beef (Knowles 1999). DFD meat is also seen in cattle that fall during transportation (Warnock et al. 1978; Tarrant et al. 1992). In addition, sharp temperature fluctuations or temperature extremes 24 to 72 hours before slaughter have been shown to increase the incidence of DFD meat (Scanga et al. 1998).

Plasma creatine kinase has been found to be elevated after journeys of 15 hours (Warriss et al. 1995) and 24 hours (Tarrant et al. 1992), indicating physical fatigue. Cattle remain standing during short journeys (Kenny and Tarrant 1987b, c; Tarrant et al. 1988) but begin to lie down after about 16 hours of transportation, if the stocking density permits them to do so (Tarrant et al. 1992).

Weight loss and dehydration also occur during long journeys. Weight loss during the first 12 hours is primarily due to the loss of gut contents. Thereafter, weight loss continues but at a slower rate (Knowles 1999). Dehydration has been observed after 18-hour (Lambooij and Hulsegge 1988) and 24-hour (Tarrant et al. 1992; Warriss et al. 1995) journeys. On arrival, animals drank water at the first opportunity (Lambooij and Hulsegge 1988; Tarrant et al. 1992).

Immunomodulation. The transportation of calves usually produces a neutrophilia (Simensen et al. 1980; Blecha et al. 1984; Kent and Ewbank 1986b; Murata et al. 1987; Kegley et al. 1997) characteristic of a glucocorticoid response. It sometimes also results in a lymphopenia (Kent and Ewbank 1986b; Kegley et al. 1997), but this is not always the case (Simensen et al. 1980; Blecha et al. 1984; Murata et al. 1987). Some studies have also found that ACTH injection produces a neutrophilia without lymphopenia in cattle (Simensen et al. 1980; Roth et al. 1982). The reason for this apparent lack of lymphopenia is unclear, but may be due to a difficulty in distinguishing lymphocytes from monocytes under light microscopy (Hammer and Weber 1974).

Transportation generally suppresses the cell-mediated immune response. Several studies have found a reduction in the mitogen-induced proliferation of lymphocytes following transportation (Kelley et al. 1981; Blecha et al. 1984). Murata and colleagues (1987) found a reduction in the spontaneous proliferation of lymphocytes but no change in mitogen-induced proliferation. Only Murata and coworkers (1985) have observed an enhanced rate of proliferation, and this followed a very short journey of 1 hour's duration. The contact sensitivity response to agents applied to the skin has been more variable. Transportation followed by simulated marketing, in which cattle were penned and fasted for 17 hours, reduced the inflammatory response to DNCB (Kegley et al. 1997), but transportation alone had no effect upon the response to PHA (Blecha et al. 1984).

The effects of transportation upon the humoral immune response have been very variable. Transportation has been found to reduce the synthesis of antibodies to *Salmonella dublin* and to horse red blood cells (HRBCs) (Hartmann et al. 1976). However, the transportation of weaned beef calves, followed by 17 hours of simulated marketing, had no effect upon antibody responses to infectious bovine rhinotracheitis virus (IBRV) or porcine red blood cells (PRBCs) (Kegley et al. 1997), whereas the transportation of weaned and unweaned beef calves, followed by 24 hours of simulated marketing, actually increased the immunoglobulin G (IgG) antibody response to keyhole limpet hemocyanin (KLH) (MacKenzie et al. 1997).

The weaning of beef calves, which often occurs at the same time as transportation, has been shown to reduce the antibody response to PRBCs and HRBCs, compared with preweaning responses (Gwazdauskas et al. 1978). However, MacKenzie and coworkers (1997) found that weaning calves on the day of transportation had no clear effect upon the IgG response to KLH after transportation, compared with calves weaned 2 weeks before being transported, and actually increased the immunoglobulin A (IgA) response.

Several studies have investigated the effects of extreme temperatures upon immunocompetence in calves, although most have been concerned with chronic exposure, lasting for a week or more. Such studies cannot elucidate the effects of thermal stress during transportation but may have a bearing upon the development of shipping fever in an outdoor feedlot.

Kelley (1980) cited one unpublished study in which calves were exposed to a low temperature for 12 hours. The surprising result was an increased lymphocyte count and an enhanced delayed-type hypersensitivity response to *Mycobacterium tuberculosis*. However, the chronic exposure of 3-week-old calves to −5°C, for 2 weeks, reduced the delayed-type hypersensitivity response to *M. tuberculosis* and the contact sensitivity responses to 2,4-dinitro-1-fluorobenzene (DNFB or Sanger's reagent) and PHA (Kelley et al. 1982b). The mitogen-induced proliferation of lymphocytes was unaffected (Kelley et al. 1982a).

When dairy cows were exposed to very high temperatures, between 40° and 48°C, for 24 hours in an environmental chamber, the ratio of neutrophils to lymphocytes in their blood increased (Wegner et al. 1976). Chronic exposure to high temperatures during hot summers does not have this effect, because the cattle have time to acclimatize (Lee et al. 1976; Wegner et al. 1976). The exposure of 3-week-old calves to a temperature of 35°C for 2 weeks had effects upon cell mediated immunity that were similar to those of low temperatures. There were reductions in the delayed-type hypersensitivity response to *M. tuberculosis* and in the contact sensitivity responses to DNFB and PHA (Kelley et al. 1982b), whereas the mitogen-induced proliferation of lymphocytes was unaffected (Kelley et al. 1982a).

Disease Incidence. Shipping fever, also known as pneumonic pasteurellosis, is a common cause of calf morbidity and death following transportation, particularly among beef calves transported to feedlots in North America. In the United States, it has been estimated that 1% of cattle die from shipping fever (Irwin et al. 1979). It may be responsible for 50% of mortalities in feedlots and 75% of cases of sickness (Edwards 1996). Shipping fever is characterized by fever, dyspnea, and fibrous pneumonia, and less often by gastroenteritis and occasionally by internal hemorrhage (Tarrant and Grandin 2000). The disease usually occurs within 10 to 14 days after arrival at the feedlot (Radostits et al. 2000).

Shipping fever is caused primarily by the bacterium *Pasteurella haemolytica*, or occasionally *P. multocida*, but infection with this organism alone is not sufficient to produce the disease in the laboratory (Shoo 1989). It is thought that viruses, such as bovine parainfluenza-1 virus and infectious bovine rhinotracheitis virus, or mycoplasmas may act synergistically to render *Pasteurella* sp. pathogenic and that environmental stressors may also be involved (Hoerlein 1980; Radostits et al. 2000). It has often been proposed that stress caused by transportation renders calves susceptible to shipping fever (Hails 1978; Irwin et al. 1979; Yates 1982; Tarrant and Grandin 2000). The evidence for this is largely circumstantial: in the first place, outbreaks commonly follow transportation (Radostits et al. 2000), and, in the second place, transportation may cause physiological stress and immunosuppression. Frank and Smith (1983) have shown that the prevalence of *P. haemolytica* in the nasal passages of calves is increased by transportation and marketing, but the presence of *P. haemolytica* in the nasal passages is not sufficient to cause pneumonia. It must first invade the lungs, a process that is probably facilitated by a simultaneous viral infection.

Several large-scale field studies have monitored the incidence of mortality from shipping fever in beef calves arriving at North American feedlots over a 3-year (Martin et al. 1980, 1981, 1982) or a 4-year (Ribble et al. 1995b) period and related this to the distance traveled from market. Journey distances ranged from 90 km to 1326 km in Ribble and colleagues' study and from several hundred kilometers to about 3200 km in Martin and coworkers' studies. In both cases, there was no relationship between mortality and journey distance. The studies by Martin and coworkers also monitored the incidence of morbidity from shipping fever and again found no relationship with journey time. These findings demonstrate that neither long journeys per se, nor factors that increase with journey time, such as fatigue, hunger, and dehydration, play a significant role in the etiology of shipping fever.

A number of studies have identified mixing as an important factor, although it remains unclear whether this is due to the stress associated with agonistic interactions or simply to the increased risk of exposure to pathogens. Martin and colleagues (1981, 1982) and Alexander and coworkers (1989) measured the mixing of calves from various truckloads after arrival at the feedlot. They found that increased mixing at the feedlot increased the incidence of treatment for respiratory tract disease. Ribble and colleagues (1995a) traced calves arriving at the feedlot to their farms of origin in order to investigate the relationship between the level of mixing before arrival and mortality from shipping fever at the feedlot. They found that the level of mixing, given by the mean number of calves per farm in a given truckload, varied depending on the geographic origin of the animals and that feedlot mortality increased with the level of mixing.

However, mixing is not the only factor affecting the incidence of shipping fever. This was apparent in Ribble and colleagues' (1995a) study because mixing could not account for the wide variation in mortality that occurred over time, both within and between years. Ribble and colleagues (1995c) observed that the mortality rate peaked each year in November, several weeks after the number of calves passing through the markets had peaked. This could have been due to a number of factors, including crowding in the market lairage, associated with stress or exposure to pathogens; reduced efficiency in the processing of calves arriving at the feedlot; or cold and wet weather. An additional factor, which may have contributed to the downturn in mortality after November, is that many of the calves arriving in December had been weaned before leaving the farm of origin.

There is some evidence that low temperatures and high humidity, both during transportation and on the rearing unit, may increase the incidence of shipping fever (Radostits et al. 2000). Staples and Haugse (1974) observed that mortality among calves of less than 6 months of age, during the weeks following their arrival at the rearing unit, was higher in the winter months than at other times of year. The principal causes of death were pneumonia and scours. These are also the primary causes of mortality among calves of this age that are not transported (Oxender et al. 1973) The on-farm mortality of such calves is highest in the winter (Martin et al. 1975b) and is associated with cold, wet, and windy weather and with temperature fluctuations (Martin et al. 1975a, c). Jennings and Glover (1952) demonstrated that the wetting of calves to create a chill increases the severity of pneumonic lesions in animals experimentally infected with tissues taken from calves exhibiting pneumonia. Another study, by Diesel and colleagues (1991), showed that exposure to low temperatures increases the colonization of the lung by *P. haemolytica* introduced intranasally. Furthermore, Hambdy and coworkers (1963) showed that acute exposure to a high temperature followed by a low temperature increased the severity of pneumonia in calves inoculated with *Pasteurella* spp. and bovine parainfluenza-1 virus. The immunomodulation caused by exposure to extreme temperatures may play an important role in the development of shipping fever.

TRANSPORTATION OF SHEEP

Transport Procedures. Within Europe, most sheep are transported by road and are destined for slaughter, whether as meat lambs or as adults. Lambs are subjected to a series of potentially stressful events, sometimes within the space of a few days. They are weaned from the dam and transported first to market and then possibly to an exporter's premises; they are mixed with lambs from other farms, weighed, handled for assessment of conformation, ear tagged, and clipped; and finally they are transported again, either for immediate slaughter or for several weeks fattening before slaughter (Hall and Bradshaw 1998). Research has mostly been concerned with assessing the effects of road journeys. The combination of events that occur during the commercial transportation of lambs has not been investigated (Hall and Bradshaw 1998).

A number of studies have also focused on the transportation of sheep by sea from Australia and New Zealand to the Middle East. Approximately 7 million sheep are transported from Australia to the Middle East each year (Bailey and Fortune 1992). A significant proportion of these are adult Merino sheep, between 3 and 5 years of age, although the number of younger animals is increasing (Kelly 1988). In contrast, most of the sheep exported from New Zealand are lambs, less than a year old (Black et al. 1994). In both countries, sheep

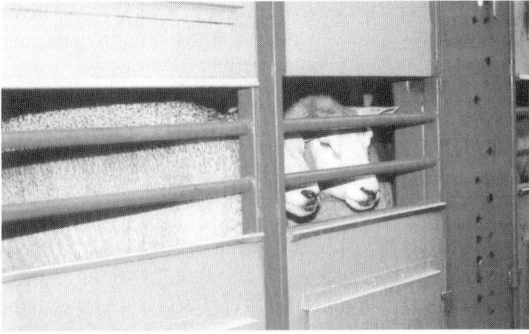

FIG. 10.3—Transport affects sheep disease incidence. (Photograph S.J.G. Hall.)

are transported by road from their farms of origin before assembly at the port feedlot.

Mortality. The mortality rate of sheep transported by road is relatively low. Within the United Kingdom, Knowles and colleagues (1994a) observed a mortality rate of 0.018% in sheep transported to slaughter.

A considerably higher rate of mortality has been estimated to occur at port feedlots in Australia, following road transportation. Feedlot managers estimated a mortality rate of around 1% for an average 7-day assembly period (Richards et al. 1989). The higher rate of mortality may be largely due to the animals not being slaughtered on arrival, giving diseases time to develop. Richards and colleagues (1989) found that the most common causes of death at the feedlot, in descending order, were salmonellosis (53.4%), miscellaneous diseases (23.8%), physical injury (12.6%), and inanition (10.2%).

Transportation by sea is also associated with a high rate of mortality. The average mortality rate on voyages from Australia to the Middle East is 2% (Kelly 1988). Richards and colleagues (1989) found that the main causes of death, in descending order, were inanition (43.4%), salmonellosis (20.2%) and physical injury (10.6%). An unpublished survey by Ryan [cited in Black et al. (1994)] indicated that the average mortality rate for voyages from New Zealand was also 2%, with the mortality on individual voyages reaching 5% to 10%. Black and colleagues (1994) observed that the most frequent causes of death, in descending order, were suffocation from smothering (31%), inanition (28%), pneumonia (25%), and dehydration (9%). Salmonellosis was not observed in this study but was seen in a subsequent study by Black (1996) and is not uncommon [Ryan, cited in Black et al. (1994)].

Physical Injury. In Richards and coworkers' (1989) study, physical injuries that caused mortality on board ship were mostly acute injuries associated with

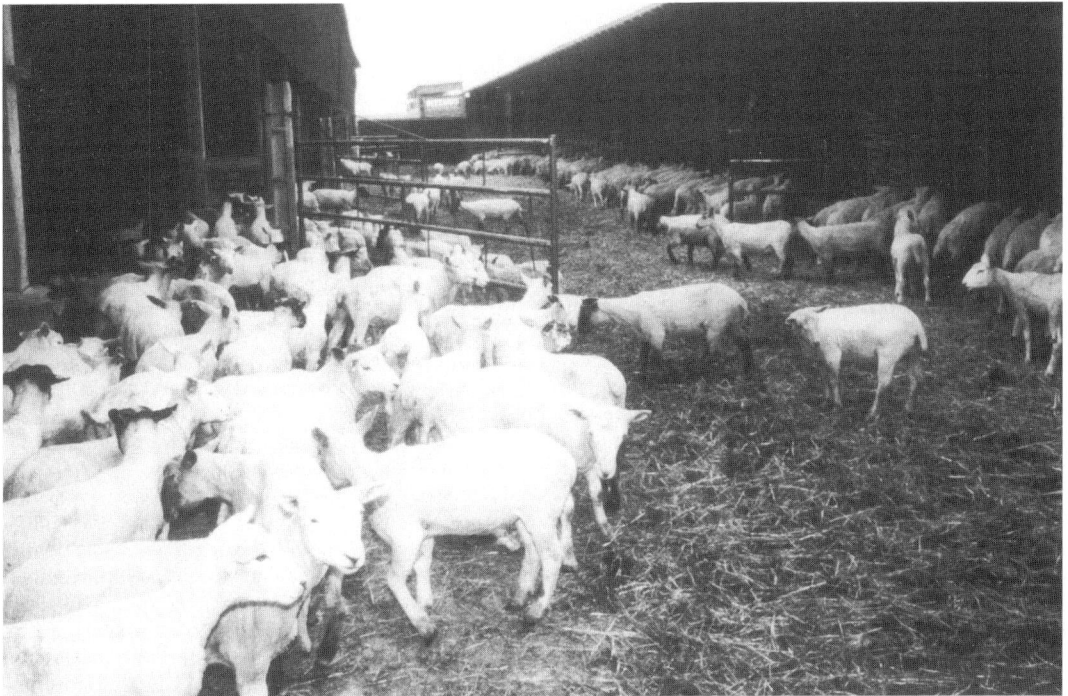

FIG. 10.4—Sheep at a transport staging point may encounter many new pathogens. (Photograph S.G.J. Hall.)

splaying of the hindlimbs on slippery floors during loading. Most of the injuries that caused mortality in the feedlot were acute or subacute and were probably sustained during transportation from the farms of origin.

"Trauma and other causes" accounted for 7% of deaths in Black and colleagues' (1994) study. However, the commonest cause of death among lambs was suffocation from smothering. This was a consequence of competition for resources, such as food and water, which were not provided ad libitum. Pushing and plunging (lifting of the forefeet from the ground and lunging forward) would sometimes cause a loss of footing, resulting in suffocation beneath other animals.

Inanition. In sheep transported long distances by sea, inanition is an important cause of mortality. Inanition occurs for different reasons in adult sheep and lambs. In lambs transported from New Zealand, it is a consequence of competition for feed (Black et al. 1994), which is not provided ad libitum during sea voyages to the Middle East. A minority of animals stop feeding altogether under these circumstances. If moved to less crowded pens, feeding normally resumes.

Among adult Merino sheep transported from Australia, deaths from inanition are instead a consequence of inappetance (Norris et al. 1990). Failure to eat is seen first in the feedlot and, in a minority of animals, persists during the voyage. The separate penning of nonfeeders on board ship makes no difference in their mortality. Furthermore, when Norris and colleagues (1990) took sheep from the port feedlot and housed them for closer observation, they found that providing groups of nonfeeders with extra trough space or ad libitum feed made no difference in their feeding, growth, or mortality. The reason for inappetance is unclear, but it has been observed that the mortality rate is much higher in sheep originating on some farms than on others. In two studies, half of all deaths aboard ship occurred among sheep from 25% (Bailey and Fortune 1992) and 14.2% (Higgs et al. 1999) of the farms of origin. Since inanition and salmonellosis are the most common causes of death on such voyages (Richards et al. 1989) and salmonellosis is generally a consequence of failure to eat, it follows that inappetance is more prevalent among sheep from some farms than others. Bailey and Fortune (1992) suggested that inappetance could be related to prior handling and feeding experience. Merinos are reared extensively, with minimal handling and usually no supplementary feeding except when young. Hence, they may find handling and transportation very stressful and may also be reluctant to eat the pelleted feed that is offered to them at the feedlot and on board ship. With respect to feeding experience, it is well established that the exposure of sheep to a particular type of feed while young is an effective method of ensuring that they will accept it later in life (Mottershead et al. 1985; Burritt and Provenza 1989). Higgs and colleagues (1999) observed that mortality rate was higher among sheep originating in zones with a longer pasture-growing season, where animals might have had less experience with supplementary feeding.

Physiological Measures of Welfare. Loading sheep onto a lorry will, to a greater or lesser extent, result in poor welfare. Several studies have found that loading caused an elevation in plasma cortisol concentration (Broom et al. 1996; Parrott et al. 1998b), although this was not observed by Cockram and colleagues (1996). Loading has also been reported to increase the plasma creatine-kinase concentration in fleeced sheep (Cockram et al. 1996; Parrott et al. 1998b) but not in shorn sheep (Parrott et al. 1998b). The release of creatine kinase into the blood is associated with tissue damage or vigorous exercise.

Mixing with unfamiliar animals leads to an increased heart rate (Baldock and Sibly 1990) but is probably not a prolonged problem for sheep during transportation (Hall and Bradshaw 1998).

Plasma cortisol concentration also increases at the onset of driving (Broom et al. 1996; Cockram et al. 1996; Parrott et al. 1998a, b) but declines during the journey (Broom et al. 1996; Cockram et al. 1996; Parrott et al. 1998a), at least when road conditions are good (Parrott et al. 1998b). Parrott and colleagues (1998a) observed an elevation for only the first 2 hours of a 3¼-hour journey, and Broom and coworkers (1996) observed an elevation for the first 3 hours of a 15-hour journey. This suggests that sheep readily adapt to motion in a carefully driven vehicle. However, when the lorry moved from major roads onto minor roads during the journey, this caused cortisol levels to increase (Parrott et al. 1998b). Bradshaw and colleagues (1996) also observed a higher plasma cortisol concentration in sheep during rough journeys compared with smooth journeys.

Extensively raised sheep have been observed to exhibit greater cortisol responses to transportation than do sheep housed indoors (Reid and Mills 1962). This may be due to the fact that extensively raised animals are less accustomed to handling. However, breed differences also exist. Hall and colleagues (1998) have shown that the plasma cortisol concentration, following 45 to 90 minutes of transportation, is greater in sheep of predominantly upland genotype, which are traditionally raised extensively, than in sheep of predominantly lowland genotype, which are normally reared with more human contact.

Sheep lose weight during road transportation, most of which is probably due to the loss of gut contents associated with feed and water deprivation. Experiments that have compared the weight loss in sheep during transportation with the weight loss caused by food and water deprivation alone have had variable findings. Knowles and colleagues (1995) found an 8% weight loss after 24 hours of transportation, mainly incurred during the first 15 hours, and the same loss in sheep held in pens for 24 hours without food and water. In contrast, Knowles and coworkers (1993) found a 6.7%

loss in sheep transported for 14 or 24 hours, but only a 1.5% loss in animals held in pens for 24 hours, suggesting that much of the weight loss that occurred during transportation could not be accounted for by feed and water deprivation. However, it is not clear what other factors might have been responsible. Catabolic activity associated with physical exertion and physiological stress could not have resulted in such a substantial difference in weight loss. Even during a 12-day period of starvation, the daily loss of body tissue through catabolism is inconsequential in relation to total body weight (Smith et al. 1938). Other studies have observed weight losses of 4% after 18 hours of transportation (Knowles et al. 1994b) and 5.7% after 14 hours confinement in a stationary vehicle (Hall et al. 1997).

Sheep do not suffer from dehydration during road journeys of up to 31 hours' duration. Packed-cell volume has been observed to decrease, not increase, during most journeys (Knowles et al. 1993; Broom et al. 1996; Parrott et al. 1998b). Similarly, plasma osmolality declines or stays the same (Knowles et al. 1993, 1994b, 1995; Broom et al. 1996; Parrott et al. 1998b). After unloading, most sheep eat before drinking (Knowles et al. 1994b, 1995; Cockram et al. 1996; Parrott et al. 1998b). In fact, Parrott and colleagues (1996) have shown that plasma osmolality is unaffected by 48 hours of food and water deprivation. This is probably because sheep have a sizable reserve of water in the rumen (Silanikove 1994).

Dehydration is an important cause of mortality among lambs transported by sea from New Zealand to the Middle East. Dehydration is associated with competition for water, which is not provided ad libitum, and with heat stress. Heat stress is exacerbated by poor air movement (reduced convective cooling); high salt content of feed and water, which increases urination, resulting in a wet floor and hence high humidity (reduced evaporative cooling); and high stocking density (increased heat production and floor wetting) (Black et al. 1994).

Immunomodulation. No experimental studies have investigated the effects of transportation upon the immune system of sheep.

Disease Incidence. Salmonellosis causes mortality among both adult sheep and lambs transported by sea but is particularly important in adult sheep. It is caused by bacteria of *Salmonella* sp. Richards and coworkers (1993) reported that the pathogen most commonly isolated at necropsy from salmonellosis mortalities on board ship was *S. typhimurium.* Other common isolates were *S. bovis-morbificans* and *S. havana.* However, epidemiological studies have revealed that *Salmonella* challenge alone is generally insufficient for the development of salmonellosis during transportation and that its development is usually caused by a combination of *Salmonella* challenge and failure to eat (Norris et al. 1990; Higgs et al. 1993). Higgs and colleagues (1993)

observed that deaths from salmonellosis were not spatially or temporally clustered on board ship, as would have been expected if pathogen challenge had been a sufficient cause. Furthermore, *Salmonella* excretion in the feces was sufficiently widespread on some journeys that most animals would have been exposed, yet only a small minority were infected with salmonellosis. In Norris and coworkers' (1990) study, mortality from salmonellosis during the voyage was very much higher in sheep that had failed to eat at the feedlot (8.8%) than in those that had eaten (0.6%), suggesting that failure to eat predisposed animals to the disease. This was confirmed by Higgs and colleagues (1993), who removed sheep from the port feedlot and housed them for closer observation. Only those animals that failed to feed developed salmonellosis.

In lambs transported by sea from New Zealand, salmonellosis also appears to be caused by a combination of *Salmonella* challenge and failure to eat. Black (1996) observed that almost all lambs exhibiting salmonellosis lesions at necropsy also exhibited signs of inanition. The incidence of primary salmonellosis was very low.

The connection between salmonellosis and failure to eat in adult sheep means that the factors responsible for inappetance in these animals are also risk factors for the development of salmonellosis. Thus, either the stress of handling road transportation or the response to a novel feedstuff or both contribute to the incidence of salmonellosis at the port feedlot and at sea.

Pneumonia in sheep often involves *P. haemolytica.* As in cattle, pneumonic pasteurellosis in sheep is an important disease worldwide and is frequently seen in ranches and feedlots in the United States (Brogden et al. 1998), not just during long sea voyages.

The etiology of pneumonic pasteurellosis in sheep is similar to that of the condition in cattle. Attempts to produce pneumonia experimentally by *P. haemolytica* challenge alone have had inconsistent results (Gilmour et al. 1980). Stress or initial infections with viral or primary bacterial agents might break down innate pulmonary immune barriers. This may release *P. haemolytica* from its usual commensal status in the nasopharynx and allow it to colonize and proliferate throughout the upper respiratory tract and induce tissue damage in the lung (Brogden et al. 1998). Various environmental challenges have been reported to predispose sheep to respiratory infections, but experimental and epidemiological investigations have not been carried out. Respiratory viral infections are known to increase the susceptibility of sheep to secondary bacterial infection, usually by interfering with mucociliary clearance mechanisms that remove organisms from the lower respiratory tract (Jakab 1982). Experimental studies infecting sheep first with virus and then with *P. haemolytica* have shown that parainfluenza-3 virus (Davies et al. 1981; Cutlip et al. 1993), bovine respiratory syncytial virus (Al-Darraji et al. 1982a-c; Sharma and Woldehiwet 1990) and an ovine adenovirus, OAV-6 (Lehmkuhl et al. 1989; Cutlip et al. 1996) can all increase the susceptibility of sheep to *P. haemolytica*. Some respiratory bacterial infections also increase the susceptibility of sheep to secondary *P. haemolytica* infection, including *Mycoplasma ovipneumoniae* (Jones et al. 1982).

Abnormal Behavior and Physical Injury

GENERAL PRINCIPLES. Abnormal behaviors that are potentially injurious include redirected behaviors, stereotypies, and heightened aggression.

REDIRECTED BEHAVIORS. Animals have evolved motivational mechanisms that govern their behavioral decisions, helping to ensure that their actions are consistent with biological priorities. The brain monitors changes in an animal's internal and external environments, interprets them in the light of experience, and generates internal variables known as causal *factors* that predispose or motivate the animal to follow various courses of action. An animal's motivational state at a given time is determined by the levels of a combination of competing causal factors. Which course of action an animal takes will depend on the relative magnitude of these factors. By influencing the weighting that the brain gives to various changes in an animal's internal and external environments when it generates causal factors, natural selection and learning both hone the animal's behavior to better meet its biological priorities (Broom 1981; Fraser and Broom 1990).

Ultimately, an animal's biological objectives are to survive and reproduce. To achieve these objectives, an animal must procure many resources, such as food, water, warmth, a mate, and a nest. The satisfaction of some motivations appears to be solely or primarily dependent on obtaining or consuming a resource. For example, preparturient sows, who show a strong motivation to build a nest from straw when housed on a bare concrete floor (Arey 1992), exhibit very little nest-building behavior when they are given a comfortable water bed on which to farrow [Baxter and Robertson, cited by Dawkins (1990)]. Another example is thermoregulation. Thermoregulatory behavior serves the objective of maintaining a constant body temperature and does not occur in thermoneutral environments.

However, species have also evolved to procure resources in specific ways to the extent that the performance of species-specific appetitive behavior patterns is often motivationally important. In fact, what is required to satisfy many motivations appears to be a combination of the behavior itself and its outcome. What an animal is motivated for in this case is best described as adequate feedback from the performance of a species-specific behavior pattern.

The evidence that animals are motivated to perform many species-specific behavior patterns includes the persistence of these activities when the resources that they would normally procure are made available for free. For example, foraging behaviors persist in many species when food is freely available, indicating that they are motivated to forage as well as to eat. Thus, growing pigs, housed in concrete pens with food pellets available ad libitum, will direct additional rooting and chewing behavior toward straw (Fraser et al. 1991) or a trough of earth (Wood-Gush and Beilharz 1983). Similarly, starlings prefer to search for mealworms than to eat them straight from a dish (Inglis and Ferguson 1986). Persistence is also seen in activities other than foraging. Unlike sows, chickens are motivated to perform nest-building behavior as well as to lie in a comfortable nest. In fact, they exhibit as much prelaying nest-building behavior in the presence of a nest that they have built on a previous day as they do when building one from scratch (Hughes et al. 1989).

The importance of adequate feedback from most of these behavior patterns is evident from the fact that few behaviors are performed in the absence of feedback of some kind. When this does occur, the behavior is said to be expressed as a vacuum activity. For example, both chickens (Martin 1975; Vestergaard 1981) and jungle fowl (Vestergaard et al. 1990), the ancestral stock of the domestic chicken, perform the movements of dust bathing when housed in wire cages, although it is possible that these birds were obtaining some limited feedback from their feed or from the feathers of other birds (Vestergaard et al. 1990).

In some cases, the motivation of animals to persist in performing such activities is very strong. Motivational strength is estimated using preference tests in which animals are required either to choose between several alternatives or to perform a task to obtain a desired outcome (Broom and Johnson 1993; Fraser and Matthews 1997). Experimental studies of this kind have revealed, for example, that caged hens are prepared to pay as much for access to a nest box before laying, in which nesting behaviors can be performed with some feedback, as they are for access to food after 20 hours of food deprivation (Duncan and Kite 1987).

The environments of captive animals are often very different from the environments in which their species evolved. They may lack suitable substrates for the performance of important behavior patterns, such as foraging and nest building. Because many motivations are tied genetically to species-specific behavior patterns, there is a limit to how much an animal's behavior can adapt such environments. Despite domestication, many species of mammals and birds remain motivated to perform activities that, although important in the wild, are biologically redundant in the captive environment. At the same time, the feedback that the captive environment provides from these activities is often inadequate. This means that, in a captive environment, animals will often be unable to obtain adequate feedback from the performance of species-specific behavior patterns, with negative consequences for their welfare (Dawkins 1990).

When the natural target or substrate of a behavior pattern is absent from the environment, the behavior will be redirected, if possible, toward a different target or substrate. The feedback that is obtained when a behavior is redirected will generally fail to fully satisfy the animal's motivation but is better than no feedback at all. For example, when growing pigs are housed in concrete pens without access to a natural foraging substrate such as earth or straw, chewing behavior is often redirected toward their penmates in the form of tail biting (Van Putten 1969). In early-weaned dairy calves fed milk replacer from a bucket, sucking behavior is redirected toward a nonnutritive teat if one is provided (Hammell et al. 1988) or toward pen fixtures and other calves if one is not (Metz 1984). Chickens housed in cages often exhibit feather pecking, which Blokhuis (1986) has argued is a redirected foraging activity, although Vestergaard (1989) has suggested that it might instead be a redirection of dust bathing.

The evidence that the feedback obtained when a behavior is redirected is generally inadequate to satisfy an animal's motivation is that most redirected behaviors are hardly ever observed when the natural substrates of these behaviors are available in the environment. Thus, although there is nothing to prevent animals from performing activities such as tail biting, cross-sucking, or feather pecking in the presence of straw, the dam, or litter, respectively, they very rarely do so. It follows that the feedback obtained from the redirected form of the behavior must be less satisfying than the natural type of feedback. Provided that the animal in the barren environment does not compensate by performing the redirected form of the behavior pattern more frequently than it would carry out the natural form in an enriched environment, its welfare can be said to be poorer in the barren environment. Where frequencies have been compared, the frequency of performing the redirected form in a barren environment has generally been found to be lower [for example, see Vestergaard et al. (1990) for jungle-fowl dust bathing] and at most no higher [see Signoret et al. (1995) for foraging in pigs] than that of the normal form in an enriched environment.

There is no a priori reason why natural substrates should be preferred to alternatives, and sometimes they are not. For example, deep litter appears to provide supernormal feedback to nesting chickens (Duncan and Kite 1989), which in feral conditions line their nests rather sparsely with vegetation (Duncan et al. 1978). Rather, a general preference for natural substrates over available alternatives is something that has been observed in practice. It arises from the fact that the available alternatives in many captive environments are very poor. In many intensive housing systems, the only substrates that can provide any kind of feedback from activities such as foraging are the pen fixtures and other animals.

As well as being associated with poor welfare, some redirected behaviors put the health of animals at risk, either that of the individual performing the behavior or that of other animals in the group. For example, tail biting among pigs and cross-sucking among calves (Sambraus 1985a; Fraser and Broom 1990).

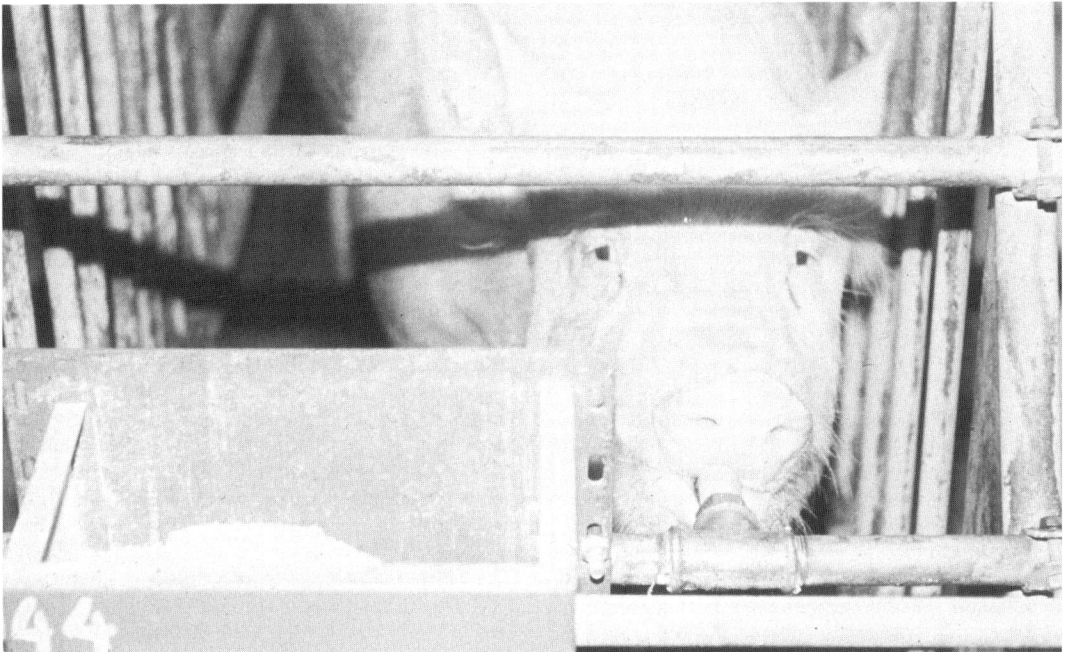

FIG. 10.5—The drinker-pressing stereotypy in a confined sow. Stereotypies are indicators of poor welfare. (Photograph D.M. Broom.)

STEREOTYPIES. Another type of behavior associated with captive environments is stereotypic behavior. A *stereotypy* is defined as "a repeated, relatively invariant sequence of movements which has no obvious function" (Broom and Johnson 1993). Despite this widely accepted definition, it is in fact unclear whether stereotypies are functional: they may or may not help animals to cope with their environments (Dantzer 1986; Mason 1991b; Rushen 1993). Like redirected behaviors, stereotypies are most often observed when animals are confined and when there are constraints on their ability to perform certain behavior patterns (Mason 1991a). Stereotypies are believed to result from the frustration of specific motivations. In restrictive environments, strongly motivated behaviors gradually become modified or "channeled" into a few simple behavioral elements, which exhibit very little variability (Lawrence and Terlouw 1993; Rushen et al. 1993).

Stereotypies sometimes arise from the redirection of an appetitive behavior pattern, such as foraging, and it may be difficult in such cases to distinguish stereotypic behavior from redirected behavior. For example, both spot picking in caged canaries, which is a redirected foraging activity (Keiper 1969), and belly nosing in weaner pigs, which is a redirection of the motivation to suckle (Van Putten and Dammers 1976), are unvarying, repetitive behavior patterns. Other stereotypies are a consequence of feed restriction and probably have more to do with hunger than with a need to perform foraging behavior. For example, postprandial stereotypies in sows, including chain manipulation, sham chewing, drinker manipulation, and excessive drinking (Terlouw et al. 1991; Lawrence and Terlouw 1993). A third group of stereotypies develop from frustrated escape attempts, such as the stereotypic pacing observed before laying in caged hens with no access to a nest box (Mills and Wood-Gush 1985).

Whether stereotypic behavior is a coping attempt or a behavior pathology, its occurrence indicates that an animal has some difficulty coping with its environment, and it is therefore an indicator of poor welfare (Broom and Johnson 1993). Some stereotypies also increase the risk of injury or other disease in that individual or in others (Sambraus 1985b; Fraser and Broom 1990).

HEIGHTENED AGGRESSION. A third type of abnormal behavior that is potentially injurious is heightened aggression. Like redirected behavior and stereotypy, heightened aggression is characteristic of intensive husbandry systems. It is either a coping mechanism or a behavioral pathology and indicates that the welfare of the aggressive individual is poor. It has a number of different causes, including inability to form a stable social group, inability to resolve conflicts, regrouping, and the frustration of specific motivations, especially feeding.

Many social species, including chickens, pigs, and cattle, normally establish a dominance order within the group, which governs access to resources and minimizes the incidence of fighting. However, when group size is large, so that individual recognition of all group members is not possible, a stable social hierarchy cannot develop. This may result in ongoing aggression, manifest as aggressive pecking (directed at the head) among laying hens (Appleby et al. 1992), as fighting among pigs (Petherick and Blackshaw 1987), and as mounting among steers (Fraser and Broom 1990). Estimates of the number of group members who can be recognized or remembered by an individual, based on observations of the point at which social disruption begins to occur, are about 80 in chickens (Guhl 1953), 50 to 70 in cattle, and 20 to 30 in pigs (Fraser and Broom 1990).

In some housing systems, it may be difficult for animals to resolve conflicts, even when group size does not prevent individual recognition. This is most apparent in pigs, in whom submission is communicated not by means of a postural signal but by fleeing. When groups of growing pigs are confined in small, bare pens, escape is not possible, and this may prolong bouts of aggression. The problem is exacerbated by a high stocking density, since crowding makes it difficult for penmates to avoid encroaching on each other's individual space, leading to more agonistic encounters (Ewbank and Bryant 1972). The incidence of aggression can be reduced by construction of partitions within the pen, which permit fleeing animals to move out of sight (Nehring 1981). The provision of *head-hides*, where an animal can place its head out of sight, also reduces aggression because the head is the focus of aggressive biting (McGlone and Curtis 1985). Unresolved conflict is also responsible for high levels of aggression between sows when they are housed individually, but in close proximity to one another, tethered or in stalls (Barnett et al. 1989).

Regrouping results in vigorous fighting among pigs (Meese and Ewbank 1973), aggressive pecking among chickens (Guhl 1953), and fighting among male adult cattle (Kenny and Tarrant 1987c) and 6-month-old calves (Trunkfield and Broom 1991). Fighting is seen less often among younger calves. The repeated regrouping of animals is a routine part of many systems of pig and cattle husbandry, so periods of intense fighting are endemic to these systems. Pigs are normally mixed first at weaning and then often again for finishing, and they are subsequently mixed both before and after transportation to the slaughterhouse. Calves from beef suckler herds that are not fattened on site are transported to a rearing unit or feedlot at older than 6 months of age. They are mixed several times during the process of transportation and marketing and again on arrival. All cattle are mixed before and after transportation to the slaughterhouse.

Aggression also occurs in response to the frustration of specific motivations, particularly the motivation to feed. Duncan and Wood-Gush (1971) observed aggressive pecking among hens when their motivation to feed was thwarted by a Perspex cover over the food container. Carlstead (1986) gave groups of growing pigs signals predicting the delivery of food and observed that the incidence of aggression was higher among groups that received unreliable signals than among groups that received reliable signals. In group-housed sows, vulva biting is associated with the use of a transponder-operated feeding station to feed animals sequentially. It develops when sows are queuing for access to the feeding station and is believed to result from the frustration of a motivation to feed when other sows are feeding. It can be reduced by the simultaneous provision of silage to all sows and by encouraging the formation of subgroups, both of which reduce competition for the feeding station (Van Putten and Van der Burgwal 1990).

EXAMPLES. In Table 10.7, a list is presented of redirected behaviors and stereotypies that can result in poor health, as well as several forms of aggressive behavior whose morphology is distinctive from normal aggression. Several other abnormal behaviors are included whose causes are as yet unclear but that are associated with indoor housing or intensive husbandry systems in which welfare is poor and that can result in poor health.

It can be seen from Table 10.7 that a large number of potentially injurious abnormal behaviors are observed in domestic animals when their welfare is poor. [Statements in this table that are not referenced come from Sambraus (1985a, b) or Fraser and Broom (1990).]

EXAMPLE IN DETAIL. One example is discussed in more detail—that of redirected sucking in calves.

SUCKING IN CALVES

Rearing Procedures. Dairy calves reared for beef or veal are removed from the dam at 1 or 2 days of age and housed individually or in groups. They are fed colostrum, and then whole milk until 6 days of age, after which they receive milk replacer. Calves reared for beef are weaned at 4 to 12 weeks of age, usually between 7 and 9 weeks. Calves raised for white veal are not weaned.

Milk replacer is most commonly fed in restricted quantities from a bucket, twice a day. In some cases, the bucket is fitted with a nipple. Bucket feeding is used

TABLE 10.7—Redirected behaviors, stereotypies, and other abnormal behaviors associated with indoor housing or intensive husbandry systems where welfare is poor, which result in poor health

Behavior	Description	Causes	Health risks
Horses			
Wind sucking and crib biting	Mouth opened, pharynx contracted, and air sucked into upper pharynx. In crib biting, sucking facilitated by clamping teeth onto some solid object.	Redirected foraging: stabled horses fed concentrates eat their feed quickly. May then gnaw objects, which leads to crib biting (Schäfer 1974). Boredom. Imitation.	Swallowing air can lead to stomach dilation, bloat, colic, and chronic intestinal catarrh. Feed intake may be reduced, leading to nutrient deficiency (Eikmeier 1970).
Litter eating	Increasingly indiscriminate consumption of litter, which may be soiled with manure or moldy.	Redirected foraging: as for wind sucking (Houpt et al. 1978). Insufficient or imbalanced feed. Worms.	Consumption of soiled or moldy litter can lead to colic (Summerhays 1973)
Polydipsia	Excessive consumption of water.	Not known. Usually seen in confined and isolated animals.	Suspected cause of gastric or intestinal volvulus (twisting), which can be fatal.
Flank biting	Biting at own sides, in the absence of any pathological skin condition, parasitism or gastrointestinal disorder.	Not known, but grazing or provision of a stall companion can ameliorate the disorder (Houpt 1981)	Usually only the hair is damaged, but occasionally results in self-mutilation.
Weaving	Head stretched forward and swayed from side to side, while body weight is shifted from one forelimb to the other.	Frustration of motivation to move forward. Commonly occurs when horse anticipates feeding or release to pasture. Boredom (Houpt 1981). Imitation.	Stereotyped motion puts great strain on tendons, joints, and hooves and can lead to pathology in these tissues. Has resulted in luxation of elbow joint (Summerhays 1973).
Pacing	Pacing or circling around a horse box.	Frustration of attempts to escape from confinement.	Considerable spinal flexion is required in circling or turning and can lead to back conditions.
Pawing	Forefoot repeatedly moved along the ground.	Not known. Usually seen in confined and isolated animals.	Continual pawing on a hard floor can result in leg injury.
Stall kicking	Head lowered, ears pulled back, back arched, and stall wall kicked forcefully with hindleg.	Not known. Possibly boredom. May be an attempt to attract attention.	Kicking can cause injury. Splintered wood may also cause injury.

(continued)

TABLE 10.7—(continued)

Behavior	Description	Causes	Health risks
Cattle			
Self-licking	Long periods spent licking own body. Licking behavior may be stereotyped in form.	Redirected activity associated with lack of straw (van Putten and Elshof 1978), social contact (Waterhouse 1978), or opportunity to explore (Webster et al. 1985). Also sodium deficiency (Phillips et al. 1999).	Hair balls may clog the rumen, leading to digestive problems (Groth 1978)
Cross-sucking	Sucking of the mouth, ears, navel, prepuce, scrotum, or udder of other calves.	Redirection of sucking at dam (Metz 1984). Also sodium deficiency (Phillips et al. 1999).	The part of the calf sucked may become inflamed, damaged, and infected (Kiley-Worthington 1977). Sucking may lead to hair balls; also to urine drinking, which can cause liver disorders. May persist in adult cows as milk sucking (Wood et al. 1967), which can cause mastitis and teat damage and udder damage.
Buller steer syndrome	Mounting in steers. The "buller" stands to be mounted by the "rider."	Redirection of sexual activity in all-male herds, also related motivationally to aggression. Exacerbated by high stocking density, large group size, and mixing; also by use of female sex hormones (Schake et al. 1979)	Weight loss in "riders." Exhaustion, injury, or collapse in "bullers."
Sheep			
Tail biting and hoof biting	Parturient sheep bite at the tails and hooves of lambs	Not known, but occurs only when animals are stabled (Hiepe 1970; Brummer 1978) and can be prevented by provision of more space and grazing. Nutritional deficiency may be a factor.	Biting can result in serious physical injury. Also, wounds may become infected. Severe biting of the tail can lead to rectal prolapse, as the affected lambs are apt to strain when defecating
Wool eating in lambs	The lamb sucks, chews, and ingests wool from the dam's stomach, udder, and tail	Not known, but occurs when animals are stabled. Possibly redirected foraging, or fiber deficiency.	Hair balls form in abomasum. Can result in severe colic and anemia. Also obstruction, which can be fatal. Flock morbidity up to 10% (Hutyra et al. 1959; Behrens 1972; Hiepe 1970)
Pigs			
Tail biting	Oral manipulation of the tails of other pigs. Gradually turns into harder biting.	Redirected foraging (van Putten 1969). Triggered by restlessness, associated with poor air quality (van Putten 1969), overstocking, thermal discomfort, and insufficient access to food or water.	Physical injury. Wounds may provoke cannibalism, which can be fatal (van Putten 1969). Bacterial infection may spread throughout the body, via the spinal cord, causing abscesses in the spinal canal, lungs, kidneys, and other organs and joint inflammation.
Anal massage	Anus of other pigs massaged with snout. When this triggers defecation, feces ingested	Not known, but may be linked motivationally with tail biting, occurring when tail biting is prevented by docking. Anal massage performed alternately with attempts to bite tails, ears, or legs, with belly nosing and with rooting and biting pen fixtures	Can lead to swelling and wounds in the area of the anus. Afflicted pigs may become weak, with reduced food intake and growth.
Belly nosing	Snout rubbed up and down against belly of other pigs and against the soft tissue between their hindlegs or forelegs.	Redirection of udder massage (Fraser 1978). Also linked with foraging, since incidence reduced by providing straw (Schouten 1986).	May cause inflammation of nipples, umbilicus, penis, or scrotum.

(continued)

TABLE 10.7—(*continued*)

Behavior	Description	Causes	Health risks
Cronism	Sows kill and eat viable piglets.	Associated with hyperexcitability. Suspected causes include lack of straw for nest building, insufficient time to acclimatize to a new environment, and pain in uterus or udder (Boothroyd 1965).	Death of piglets.
Head rubbing	Top of snout rubbed repetitively and vigorously along the underside of a bar across the front of the stall.	Not known. Seen only in sow stalls.	Rubbing may be sufficiently vigorous that the head is repeatedly bumped against the side of stall at the end of each rub. Can result in serious injury.
Vulva biting	Vulva of another sow bitten with incisors.	Frustration of a motivation to feed at the same time as other sows. Develops when sows queue for access to a feeding station (van Putten and van der Burgwal 1990).	A single bite can cause considerable damage to the vulva. Once damaged, it is likely to be bitten again. The wound usually becomes infected (van Putten and van der Burgwal 1990).
Domestic fowl			
Feather pecking	Feathers pulled out, from the back, stomach, breast, tail, and wings of other birds, and consumed.	Redirected ground pecking, which is a foraging activity (Blokhuis 1986) and a dust-bathing activity (Vestergaard 1989). Exacerbated by overstocking, insufficient space at troughs, too much light, and presence of sick birds.	Physical injury. Wounds may provoke cannibalism (body pecking), leading to death of the afflicted bird.
Toe pecking	Pecking directed at toes of other birds or occasionally at own toes.	Redirected ground pecking.	Physical injury. Infection of wounds causes weakness, reduced food intake, and reduced growth.

for both individually housed and group-housed calves. An alternative system involves feeding milk replacer ad libitum. An automatic feeder delivers the milk replacer under pressure to a series of teats. This system is used only for group-housed calves.

Calves that are suckled by the dam consume their daily milk intake in around five bouts of 10 to 15 minutes' duration each, the number of bouts declining with the age of the calf (Phillips 1993).

Welfare. Calves are motivated not only to consume milk but also to suck. This is evident from the persistence of sucking behavior when milk is available in an open bucket. For example, Hammell and colleagues (1988) observed that calves fed ad libitum from an open bucket spent 13 minutes per day on average sucking a nonnutritive teat. This was substantially more than calves fed ad libitum from a teat system: they sucked the nonnutritive teat for just 1 minute per day on average. In both cases, use of the nonnutritive teat was temporally associated with bouts of feeding. It occurred before, during, and after feeding bouts. The positive affective value of sucking is also evident from

the fact that calves that were allowed to feed ad libitum from a teat system consumed more milk than did calves that fed ad libitum from an open bucket.

The persistence of sucking behavior may have its physiological basis in the enhanced secretion of digestive hormones. De Passillé and colleagues (1993) observed greater postprandial increases in the plasma concentrations of insulin and cholecystokinin when calves were allowed to suck a nonnutritive teat after a meal than when they were not. The postprandial rise in these hormone levels has been implicated in satiety.

Calves are clearly sensitive to the quality of the feedback that a sucking substrate provides. When calves are bucket-fed a restricted quantity of milk replacer and the empty bucket is not removed after feeding, buckets fitted with nipples receive more nonnutritive sucking than do open buckets, suggesting that the shape or texture of the sucked object is important. Furthermore, removal of the bucket after feeding results in less nonnutritive sucking, in this case directed at pen fixtures and other calves, than when the empty bucket remains available, suggesting that the taste or smell of milk provides important feedback (Metz 1984).

The sucking of a nonnutritive teat, the bucket, pen fixtures, and other calves are all examples of redirected behavior. The sucking of a nonnutritive teat (Hammell et al. 1988), pen fixtures (Metz 1984), and other calves (Alexander 1954; Geddes 1954; Hoyer and Larkin 1954; Metz 1984) are all very substantially reduced in calves fed ad libitum from a teat system. The sucking of pen fixtures and other calves is also greatly reduced in calves remaining with the dam (Metz 1984).

The sucking of other calves, known as cross-sucking, is directed at various parts of the body, including the mouth, ears, navel, prepuce, scrotum, and udder. The position while sucking corresponds to that of the calf at the cow. The "bunting" movements with which a calf prepares a cow's udder are also demonstrated (Sambraus 1985a).

Health. Cross-sucking commonly results in the appearance of inflammations on the recipient animal (Sambraus 1985a). The sucked area sometimes becomes damaged and infected (Kiley-Worthington 1977). Recipients also show reduced weight gain.

Calves that cross-suck may swallow hair, leading to the formation of hair balls (Fraser and Broom 1990) that may clog the rumen, causing digestive problems (Sambraus 1985a). Sucking of the prepuce may lead to urine drinking (Stephens 1982), which can cause liver disorders (Fraser and Broom 1990).

Cross-sucking is often reduced by tethering calves for an hour following feeding (Fraser and Broom 1990). A more satisfactory solution, from the viewpoint of the calves' welfare, would be to employ an ad libitum teat-feeding system or, failing this, to fit nipples to the feeding buckets and make nonnutritive teats available.

SUMMARY. Animal welfare is the subject of rapidly increasing concern in most countries in the world, and this concern is resulting in changes in the ways in which farmers and other animal users keep and treat animals. *Welfare is defined as the state of an individual as regards its attempts to cope with its environment.* The scientific assessment of animal welfare has developed substantially, and many studies on different kinds of animals have been carried out. Information from such studies is used by legislators, food companies, and the public with the consequence that the various kinds of regulation lead to real improvements in animal welfare.

Health is defined as *an animal's state as regards its attempts to cope with pathology*, where pathology is *a detrimental derangement of molecules, cells, tissues, and functions that occur in living organisms in response to injurious agents or deprivations.* Pathology can be classified into genetic abnormalities; physical, thermal, and chemical injuries; infections and infestations; metabolic abnormalities; and nutritional disorders.

Health is a part of welfare. When an animal's health is poor, so is its welfare, but poor welfare does not always imply poor health. Some measures of poor welfare classified as pathology will therefore also be indicators of poor health, including body damage and symptoms of infectious, metabolic, and nutritional disease. Other measures of poor welfare, while not being signs of poor health at the time, indicate a risk of poor health in the future. They include immunosuppression and the occurrence of injurious abnormal behaviors. These are causal links between poor welfare and poor health. Two pathways can be identified:

1. Chronic activation of physiological coping mechanisms leads to immunosuppression that leads to infectious disease.
2. Behavioral coping mechanisms lead to injurious abnormal behavior that leads to physical injury.

The connection between physiological coping mechanisms, immune function, and susceptibility to infectious disease is complex. Different environmental challenges elicit different neuroendocrine responses; and different species and individuals may respond differently to a given challenge. Furthermore, a given neuroendocrine response has different effects on different leukocyte populations, with the consequence that susceptibility to some pathogens is enhanced, while susceptibility to others is reduced. It is therefore necessary to consider one challenge, one species, and one pathogen at a time.

Tables 10.4, 10.5, and 10.6 summarize experimental studies in which the effects of specific environmental challenges upon the susceptibility of domestic species to particular pathogens have been investigated. The number of studies that have been conducted is small. The majority of studies have reported an increased susceptibility to disease. This is in agreement with previous reviews that have included laboratory species.

The transportation of cattle and sheep has been reviewed in detail. The transportation of cattle by road usually elicits physiological coping responses and may also result in physical exhaustion, dehydration, and injury. The environmental challenges that are responsible for these welfare problems include weaning, rough handling, mixing, poor driving, high stocking density, food and water deprivation, and extreme temperatures. Transportation usually suppresses the cell-mediated immune response but has variable effects on the humoral immune response. Pneumonic pasteurellosis (shipping fever) is a common cause of mortality among calves that have undergone transportation, and it is thought, although not yet proven, that environmental challenges during transportation may play a role. The incidence of pneumonia is increased by mixing and by acute or chronic exposure to cold and wet weather.

The transportation of sheep by road elicits physiological coping responses. Extensively raised breeds exhibit greater cortisol responses than do those reared with more human contact. Australian Merino sheep held in port feedlots for 1 week after road transportation exhibit a mortality rate in the region of 1%, caused by salmonellosis and other diseases, injuries sustained during transportation, and inanition. When these animals are then transported by sea to the Middle East, the mean mortality rate is 2%, due to inanition, salmonellosis, and physical injury. Inappetance is responsible for both inanition and salmonellosis in these animals. The cause of inappetance is not known but may be a consequence either of the stress of handling and transportation or of unfamiliarity with pelleted feed. A similar level of mortality is seen in lambs transported by sea from New Zealand to the Middle East, but the causes of death are different. These animals do not show inappetance. Pneumonia is a more important cause of death than is salmonellosis. Like shipping fever in cattle, pneumonic pasteurellosis in sheep is thought to be precipitated by environmental challenges, but there is as yet no experimental evidence for this in sheep.

Abnormal behaviors include redirected behaviors, stereotypies, and heightened aggression. The redirection of behavior is a coping mechanism and hence a sign of poor welfare. Stereotypies and heightened aggression are either coping mechanisms or behavioral pathologies and also indicate that welfare is poor. Some of these behaviors are injurious, either to the animal itself or to other animals in the group. They can therefore lead to poor health.

Abnormal behaviors associated with indoor housing or intensive husbandry systems where welfare is poor, which lead to increased risk of poor health, are summarized in Table 10.7. These include redirected behaviors, stereotypies, and heightened aggression, as well as other abnormal behavior patterns whose causes are as yet unclear. A large number of potentially injurious abnormal behavior patterns have been identified.

Redirected sucking in calves has been reviewed in detail. Dairy calves reared for beef or veal are separated from the dam at 1 or 2 weeks of age and fed milk replacer from a bucket or, less frequently, from a teat system. Calves are motivated not only to consume milk but also to suck. Sucking stimulates the secretion of digestive hormones implicated in satiety. When calves are fed from a bucket, sucking is redirected toward other calves. This may lead to the formation of hair balls in the rumen, which can cause digestive problems, and to urine drinking, which can cause liver disorders. The part of the recipient that is sucked may also become inflamed, damaged, or infected.

It is concluded that there are several routes by which poor welfare results in increased disease. The pathophysiology of states typified by behavioral abnormalities and emergency physiological responses is a subject that is insufficiently investigated.

REFERENCES

Al-Darraji AM, Cutlip RC, Lehmkuhl HD. 1982a. Experimental infection of lambs with bovine respiratory syncytial virus and *Pasteurella haemolytica*: Immunofluorescent and electron microscopic studies. Am J Vet Res 43:230–235.

Al-Darraji AM, Cutlip RC, Lehmkuhl HD, Graham DL. 1982b. Experimental infection of lambs with bovine respiratory syncytial virus and *Pasteurella haemolytica*: Pathologic studies. Am J Vet Res 43: 236–241.

Al-Darraji AM, Cutlip RC, Lehmkuhl HD, et al. 1982c. Experimental infection of lambs with bovine respiratory syncytial virus and *Pasteurella haemolytica*: Clinical and microbiologic studies. Am J Vet Res 43:242–248.

Alexander GI. 1954. Rearing dairy calves. Aust Vet J 30:68–77.

Alexander BH, MacVean DW, Salman MD. 1989. Risk factors for lower respiratory tract disease in a cohort of feedlot cattle. J Am Vet Med Assoc 195:207–211.

Allen D, Kilkenny B. 1984. Planned Beef Production, 2nd ed. London: Granada.

Anderson NV, Yoanes VD, Vestweber JG, et al. 1990. The effects of stressful exercise on leukocytes in cattle with experimental pneumonic pasteurellosis. Vet Res Commun 15:189–204.

Appleby MC, Hughes BO, Elson HA. 1992. Poultry Production Systems: Behaviour, Management and Welfare. Wallingford, UK: CAB International.

Arey DS. 1992. Straw and food as reinforcers for prepartal sows. Appl Anim Behav Sci 33:217–226.

Armstrong WD, Cline TR. 1977. Effects of various nutrient levels and environmental temperatures on the incidence of colibacillary diarrhea in pigs: Intestinal fistulation and titration studies. J Anim Sci 45:1042–1050.

Augustini C, Fischer K, Schon L. 1980. Untersuchungen zum Problem des dunklen, leimigen Reindfleisches [dark cutting beef]. Fleischwirtschaft 60:1057–1062.

Axelrod J. 1984. The relationship between the stress hormones, catecholamines, ACTH and glucocorticoids. In: Usdin E, Kvetnansky R, Axelrod R, eds. Stress: The Role of Catecholamines and Other Neurotransmitters. New York: Gordon and Breach, 1:3–13.

Bailey AN, Fortune JA. 1992. The response of Merino wethers to feedlotting and subsequent sea transport. Appl Anim Behav Sci 35:167–180.

Baldock NM, Sibly RM. 1990. Effects of handling and transportation on heart rate and behaviour in sheep. Appl Anim Behav Sci 28:15–39.

Barnes MA, Carter RE, Longnecker JV, et al. 1975. Age at transport and calf survival [Abstract]. J Dairy Sci 58:1247.

Barnett JL, Hemsworth PH, Newman EA, et al. 1989. The effect of design of tether and stall housing on some behavioural and physiological responses related to the welfare of pregnant pigs. Appl Anim Behav Sci 24:1–12.

Bartos L, Franc C, Rehak D, Stipkova M. 1993. A practical method to prevent dark-cutting DFD in beef. Meat Sci 34:275–282.

Behrens H. 1972. Lehrbuch der Schafkrankheiten. Berlin: Verlag Paul Parey.

Benus I. 1988 Aggression and coping: Differences in behavioural strategies between aggressive and non-aggressive male mice [PhD thesis]. Groningen: University of Groningen.

Bierer BW. 1961. A method of inducing *Salmonella typhimurium* infection in chicks. J Am Vet Med Assoc 139:790.

Binkhorst GJ, Henricks PAJ, Van der Ingh TSGAM, et al. 1990. The effect of stress on host defense system and on lung damage in calves experimentally infected with *Pasteurella haemolytica* type A1. J Vet Med [A] 37:525–536.

Biondi M, Zannino L-G. 1997. Psychological stress, neuroimmuno-modulation, and susceptibility to infectious diseases in animals and man: A review. Psychother Psychosom 66:3–26.

Black H. 1996. Inanition, stress and immunity in the expression of salmonellosis in the live sheep export industry. NZ Vet J 44:77–78.

Black H, Matthews LR, Bremner KJ. 1994. The behaviour of male lambs transported by sea from New Zealand to Saudi Arabia. NZ Vet J 42:16–23.

Blecha F, Boyles SL, Riley JG. 1984. Shipping suppresses lymphocyte blastogenic responses in Angus and Brahman x Angus feeder calves. J Anim Sci 59:576–583.

Blokhuis HJ. 1986. Feather-pecking in poultry: Its relation with ground-pecking. Appl Anim Behav Sci 16:63–67.

Blood DC, Studdert VP. 1999. Saunders Comprehensive Veterinary Dictionary, 2nd ed. London: WB Saunders.

Boothroyd A. 1965. The control of gilts which savage their litters. Vet Rec 77:970–971.

Bradshaw RH, Hall SJG, Broom DM. 1996. Behavioural and cortisol response of pigs and sheep during transport. Vet Rec 138:233–234.

Brogden KA, Lehmkuhl HD, Cutlip RC. 1998. *Pasteurella haemolytica* complicated respiratory infections in sheep and goats. Vet Res 233–254.

Broom DM. 1981. Biology of Behaviour. Cambridge: Cambridge University Press, 325 pp.

Broom DM. 1983. The stress concept and ways of assessing the effects of stress in farm animals. Appl Anim Ethol 1:79.

Broom DM. 1986. Indicators of poor welfare. Br Vet J 142:524–526.

Broom DM. 1987. Applications of neurobiological studies to farm animal welfare. Curr Top Vet Med Anim Sci 42:101–110.

Broom DM. 1988. The scientific assessment of animal welfare. Appl Anim Behav Sci 20:5–19.

Broom DM. 1991a. Animal welfare: Concepts and measurement. J Anim Sci 69:4167–4175.

Broom DM. 1991b. Assessing welfare and suffering. Behav Proc 25:117–123.

Broom DM. 1993. A usable definition of animal welfare. J Agric Environ Ethics 6(Suppl 2):15–25.

Broom DM. 1994. The effects of production efficiency on animal welfare. In: Huisman EA, Osse JWM, Van der Heide D, et al., eds. Biological Basis of Sustainable Animal Production. Proceedings of the 4th Zodiac Symposium, EAAP Publ 67. Wageningen: Wageningen Pers, pp 201–210.

Broom DM. 1996. Animal welfare defined in terms of attempts to cope with the environment. Acta Agric Scand [A] 27(Suppl):22–28.

Broom DM. 1998. Welfare, stress and the evolution of feelings. Adv Study Behav 27:371–403.

Broom DM. 1999a. Welfare and how it is affected by regulation. In: Kunisch M, Ekkel H, eds. Regulation of Animal Production in Europe. Darmstadt: KTBL, pp 51–57.

Broom DM. 1999b. The welfare of dairy cattle. In: Aargaard K, ed. Future of Milk Farming. Proceedings of the 25th International Dairy Congress, Aarhus, 1998. Aarhus: Danish National Committee of International Dairy Federation, 3:32–39.

Broom DM. 2000. Welfare assessment and welfare problem areas during handling and transport. In: Grandin T, ed. Livestock Handling and Transport, 2nd ed. Wallingford, UK: CAB International, pp 43–61.

Broom DM. 2001. The use of the concept of animal welfare in European conventions, regulations and directives. In: Food Chain 2001. Uppsala: SLU Services, pp 148–151.

Broom DM, Barton-Gade P, Fanlazzo A, et al. 2003. Report of the Scientific Committee on Animal Health and Animal Welfare on the Welfare of Animals During Transport (details for horses, pigs, sheep and cattle). European Commission, Brussels. http://europe.eu.int/comm/food/fs/sc/scah/out 71–en.pdf.

Broom DM, Johnson KG. 1993. Stress and Animal Welfare. Dordrecht: Kluwer, 211 pp.

Broom DM, Goode JA, Hall SJG, et al. 1996. Hormonal and physiological effects of a 15 hour journey in sheep: Comparison with the responses to loading, handling and penning in the absence of transport. Br Vet J 152:593–604.

Brummer H. 1978. Verhaltensstörungen. In: Sambraus HH, ed. Nutztierethologie. Berlin: Verlag Paul Parey.

Burritt EA, Provenza FD. 1989. Food learning ability of lambs to distinguish safe from harmful foods. J Anim Sci 67:1732–1739.

Carlstead K. 1986. Predictability of feeding: Its effect on agonistic behaviour and growth in grower pigs. Appl Anim Behav Sci 16:25–38.

Cheville NF. 1988. Introduction to Veterinary Pathology. Ames: Iowa State University Press.

Cockram MS, Kent JE, Goddard PJ, et al. 1996. Effect of space allowance during transport on the behavioural and physiological responses of lambs during and after transport. Anim Sci 62:461–477.

Connell J. 1984. International Transport of Farm Animals Intended for Slaughter. Commission of the European Communities, Report EUR 9556, p 67.

Cronin GM, Wiepkema PR. 1984. An analysis of stereotyped behaviours in tethered sows. Ann Rech Vet 15:263–270.

Crookshank HR, Elissalde MH, White RG, et al. 1979. Effect of transportation and handling of calves upon blood serum composition. J Anim Sci 48:430–436.

Cutlip RC, Lehmkuhl HD, Brogden KA. 1993. Chronic effects of coinfection in lambs with parainfluenza-3 virus and *Pasteurella haemolytica*. Small Ruminant Research 11:171–178.

Cutlip RC, Lehmkuhl HD, Brogden KA, Hsu NJ. 1996. Lesions in lambs experimentally infected with ovine adenovirus serotype 6 and *Pasteurella haemolytica*. J Vet Diagn Invest 8:296–303.

Dantzer R. 1986. Behavioral, physiological and functional aspects of stereotyped behavior: A review and a reinterpretation. J Anim Sci 62:1776–1786.

Davies DH, Herceg M, Jones BAH, Thurley DC. 1981. The pathogenesis of sequential infection with parainfluenza virus type 3 and *Pasteurella haemolytica* in sheep. Vet Microbiol 6:173–182.

Dawkins MS. 1990. From an animal's point of view: Motivation, fitness and animal welfare. Behav Brain Sci 13:1–61.

De Passillé AMB, Christopherson RJ, Rushen J. 1993. Nonnutritive sucking and postprandial secretion of insulin, CCK and gastrin by the calf. Physiol Behav 54:1069–1073.

Diesel DA, Lebel JL, Tucker A. 1991. Pulmonary particle deposition and airway mucociliary clearance in cold-exposed calves. Am J Vet Res 52:1665–1671.

Dorland WAN. 1988. Dorland's Illustrated Medical Dictionary, 27th ed. Philadelphia: WB Saunders.

Duncan IJH, Kite VG. 1987. Some investigations into motivation in the domestic fowl [Abstract]. Appl Anim Behav Sci 18:387–388.

Duncan IJH, Kite VG. 1989. Nest-site selection and nest-building behaviour in domestic fowl. Anim Behav 37:215–231.

Duncan IJH, Petherick JC. 1991. The implications of cognitive processes for animal welfare. J Anim Sci 69:5017–5022.

Duncan IJH, Wood-Gush DGM. 1971. Frustration and aggression in the domestic fowl. Anim Behav 19:500–504.

Duncan IJH, Savory CJ, Wood-Gush DGM. 1978. Observations of the reproductive behaviour of domestic fowls in the wild. Appl Anim Ethol 4:29–42.

Duncan IJH, Beatty ER, Hocking PM, Duff SRI. 1991. Assessment of pain associated with degenerative hip disorders in adult male turkeys. Res Vet Sci 50:200–203.

Edwards AJ. 1996. Respiratory diseases of feedlot cattle in central USA. Bovine Pract 30:5–7.

Eikmeier H. 1970. Koppen der Pferde. In: Wamberg K, ed. Handlexikon der tierärztlichen Praxis. Copenhagen: Medical Book, 2:480–481.

Eldridge GA, Winfield CG. 1988. The behaviour and bruising of cattle during transport at different space allowances. Aust J Exp Agric 28:695–698.

Ewbank R, Bryant MJ. 1972. Aggressive behavior amongst groups of domesticated pigs kept at various stocking rates. Anim Behav 20:21–28.

Fabiansson S, Erichsen I, Reutersward AL. 1984. The incidence of dark cutting beef in Sweden. Meat Sci 10:21–33.

Farm Animal Welfare Council. 1991. Report on the European Commission Proposals on the Transport of Animals. London: MAFF.

Fell LR, Shutt DA. 1986. Adrenocortical response of calves to transport stress as measured by salivary cortisol. Can J Anim Sci 66:637–641.

Felton DL, Felton SY. 1991. Innervation of lymphoid tissue. In: Ader R, Felten DL, Cohen N, eds. Psychoneuroimmunology, 2nd ed. San Diego: Academic, pp 27–69.

Filion LG, Willson PJ, Bielefeldt-Ohmann H, et al. 1984. The possible role of stress in the induction of pneumonic pasteurellosis. Can J Comp Med 48:268–274.

Frank GH, Smith PC. 1983. Prevalence of *Pasteurella haemolytica* in transported calves. Am J Vet Res 44:981–985.

Fraser D. 1978. Observations on the behavioural development of suckling and early weaned piglets during the first six weeks after birth. Anim Behav 26:22–30.

Fraser D. 1993. Assessing animal well-being: Common sense, uncommon science. In: Lay D, ed. Food Animal Well-being. West Lafayette, IN: USDA and Purdue University, pp 37–54.

Fraser AF, Broom DM. 1990. Farm Animal Behaviour and Welfare. Wallingford, UK: CAB International, 437 pp.

Fraser D, Matthews LR. 1997. Preference and motivation testing. In: Appleby MC, Hughes BO, eds. Animal Welfare. Wallingford, UK: CAB International, pp 159–173.

Fraser D, Phillips PA, Thompson BK, Tennessen T. 1991. Effect of straw on the behaviour of growing pigs. Appl Anim Behav Sci 30:307–318.

Furuuchi S, Shimizu Y. 1976. Effect of ambient temperatures on multiplication of attenuated transmissible gastroenteritis virus in the bodies of newborn piglets. Infect Immun 13:990–992.

Gaillard R-C, Al-Damluji S. 1987. Stress and the pituitary-adrenal axis. In: Ballière's Clinical Endocrinology and Metabolism. London: Ballière Tindall, 1:319–354.

Geddes HJ. 1954. Calf rearing. Aust Vet J 30:77–79.

Gentle MJ. 1986. Neuroma formation following partial beak amputation (beak-trimming) in the chicken. Res Vet Sci 41:383–385.

Gibbs DM. 1986a. Dissociation of oxytocin, vasopressin and corticotropin secretion during different types of stress. Life Sci 35:487–491.

Gibbs DM. 1986b. Vasopressin and oxytocin: Hypothalamic modulators of the stress response—A review. Psychoneuroendocrinology 11:131–140.

Gillis S, Crabtree GR, Smith KA. 1979. Glucocorticoid-induced inhibition of T cell growth factor: I. The effect on mitogen-induced lymphocyte proliferation. J Immunol 123:1624–1631.

Gilman SC, Schwartz JM, Milner RJ, et al. 1982. β-Endorphin enhances lymphocyte proliferative responses. Proc Natl Acad Sci USA 79:4226–4230.

Gilmour NJL, Sharp JM, Donachie W, et al. 1980. Serum antibody response of ewes and their lambs to *Pasteurella haemolytica*. Vet Rec 107:505–507.

Grandin T. 1981. Bruises on Southwestern feedlot cattle [Abstract]. J Anim Sci 53(Suppl 1):213.

Grandin T. 1983. Welfare requirements of handling facilities. In: Baxter SH, Baxter MR, MacCormack JAC, eds. Farm Animal Housing and Welfare. The Hague: Martinus Nijhoff, pp 137–149.

Griffin JFT. 1989. Stress and immunity: A unifying concept. Vet Immunol Immunopathol 20:263–312.

Gröhn YT, Saloniemi HS, Syväjärvi J. 1986. An epidemiological and genetic study on registered diseases in Finnish Ayrshire cattle: III. Metabolic diseases. Acta Vet Scand 27:209–222.

Gross WB. 1962. Blood cultures, blood counts and temperature records in an experimentally produced "air sac disease" and uncomplicated *Escherichia coli* infection of chickens. Poult Sci 41:691–700.

Gross WB. 1972. Effect of social stress on occurrence of Marek's disease in chickens. Am J Vet Res 33:2275–2279.

Gross WB. 1976. Plasma steroid tendency, social environment and *Eimeria necatrix* infection. Poult Sci 55:1508–1512.

Gross WB. 1984. Effect of a range of social stress severity on *Escherichia coli* challenge infection. Am J Vet Res 45:2074–2076.

Gross WB. 1985. Effect of social environment and oocyst dose on resistance and immunity to *Eimeria tenella* challenge. Avian Dis 29:1018–1029.

Gross WB, Colmano G. 1969. The effect of social isolation on resistance to some infectious diseases. Poult Sci 48:514–520.

Gross WB, Colmano G. 1971. Effect of infectious agents on chickens selected for plasma corticosterone response to social stress. Poult Sci 50:1213–1217.

Gross WB, Siegel PB. 1965. The effect of social stress on resistance to infection with *Escherichia coli* or *Mycoplasma gallisepticum*. Poult Sci 44:998–1001.

Gross WB, Siegel PB. 1975. Immune response to *Escherichia coli*. Am J Vet Res 36:568–571.

Gross WB, Siegel PB. 1981. Long term exposure of chickens to three levels of social stress. Avian Dis 25:312–325.

Groth W. 1978. Tierschutz- und verhaltensbezogene Gesichtspunkte der Kälbermast. Tierzüchter 10:419–422.

Guhl AM. 1953. Social behavior of the domestic fowl. Tech Bull Kans Agric Exp Station, no. 73.

Guillemin R, Vargo T, Rossier J, et al. 1977. β-Endorphin and adrenocorticotropin are secreted concomitantly by the pituitary gland. Science 197:1367–1369.

Gwazdauskas FC, Gross WB, Bibb TL, McGilliard ML. 1978. Antibody titres and plasma glucocorticoid concentrations near weaning in steer and heifer calves. Can J Anim Sci 19:150–154.

Hails MR. 1978. Transport stress in animals, a review. Anim Regul Stud 1:289–343.

Hall SJG, Bradshaw RH. 1998. Welfare aspects of the transport by road of sheep and pigs. J Appl Anim Welfare Sci 1:235–254.

Hall RD, Gross WB. 1972. Effect of social stress and inherited plasma corticosterone levels in chickens on populations of northern fowl mites, *Ornithonyssus sylvarium*. J Parasitol 61:1096–1100.

Hall RD, Gross WB, Turner EC Jr. 1979. Population developments of *Ornithonyssus sylvarium* on leghorn roosters inoculated with steroids and subjected to extremes of social interactions. Vet Parasitol 5:287–297.

Hall SJG, Schmidt B, Broom DM. 1997. Feeding behaviour and the intake of food and water by sheep after a period of deprivation lasting 14 hours. Anim Sci 64:105–110.

Hall SJG, Broom DM, Kiddy GNS. 1998. Effect of transportation on plasma cortisol and packed cell volume in different genotypes of sheep. Small Ruminant Res 29:233–237.

Hambdy AH, Trapp AI, Gale C. 1963. Experimental transmission of shipping fever in calves. Am J Vet Res 24:287–294.

Hammell KL, Metz JHM, Mekking P. 1988. Sucking behaviour of dairy calves fed milk ad libitum by bucket or teat. Appl Anim Behav Sci 20:275–285.

Hammer RF, Weber AF. 1974. Ultrastructure of agranular leukocytes in peripheral blood of normal cows. Am J Vet Res 35:527–536.

Hartmann H, Meyer H, Steinbach G, et al. 1973. General adaptation syndrome (Selye) in the calf: 1. Normal behaviour of the blood picture and the content of glucose and 11-hydroxycorticosteroids. Arch Exp Vet 27:811–823.

Hartmann H, Bruer W, Herzog A, et al. 1976. [General adaptation syndrome (Selye) in cattle: 6. Influence of stress conditions on antibody levels after active and passive immunization as well as on the topographic distribution of various groups of pathogens in the gastrointestinal canal.] Arch Exp Vet 30:553–566.

Haynes LW, Timms RJ. 1987. Stress-induced release of pituitary β-endorphin may be mediated by activation of the brain stem defence areas. Int J Tissue React 9:55–59.

Henning PA. 1993. Transportation of animals by road for slaughter in South Africa. In: Proceedings of the 4th International Symposium on Livestock Environment, 6–9 July 1993. American Society of Agricultural Engineers, pp 536–541.

Hiepe T. 1970. Schafkrankheiten. Jena: VEB Gustav Fischer Verlag.

Higgs ARB, Norris RT, Richards RB. 1993. Epidemiology of salmonellosis in the live sheep export industry. Aust Vet J 70:330–335.

Higgs ARB, Norris RT, Love RA, Norman GJ. 1999. Mortality of sheep exported by sea: Evidence of similarity by farm group and of regional differences. Aust Vet J 77:729–733.

Hoerlein AB. 1980. Shipping fever. In: Amstutz HE, ed. Bovine Medicine and Surgery. Santa Barbara, CA: American Veterinary, pp 99–106.

Houpt KA. 1981. Equine behavior problems in relation to humane management. Int J Study Anim Probl 2:329–336.

Houpt KA, Wolski T, Welkovitz N. 1978. The effect of management practices on horse behavior. In: Proceedings of the First World Congress for Experimental Agricultural Ethology, vol 1. Madrid.

Hoyer N, Larkin RM. 1954. Bucket and nipple feeding of calves. Queensl Agric J 79:46–50.

Hughes B0, Black AJ. 1973. The preference of domestic hens for different types of battery cage floor. Br Poult Sci 14:615–619.

Hughes BO, Duncan IJH, Brown MF. 1989. The performance of nest-building by domestic hens: Is it more important than the construction of a nest? Anim Behav 21:10–17.

Hutyra K, Marek L, Mocsy J, Manninger R. 1959. Spezielle Pathologie und Therapie der Haustiere. Jena: VEB Gustav Fischer Verlag.

Inglis IR, Ferguson NJK. 1986. Starlings search for food rather than eat freely available, identical food. Anim Behav 34:614–617.

Irwin MR, McConnell S, Coleman JD, Wilcox GE. 1979. Bovine respiratory disease complex: A comparison of potential predisposing and etiologic factors in Australia and the United States. J Am Vet Med Assoc 175:1095–1099.

Jakab GJ. 1982. Viral-bacterial interactions in pulmonary infection. Adv Vet Sci Comp Med 26:155–171.

Jarvis AM, Selkirk L, Cockram MA. 1995. The influence of source, sex class and pre-slaughter handling on the bruising of cattle at two slaughterhouses. Livest Prod Sci 43:215–224.

Jennings AR, Glover RE. 1952. Enzootic pneumonia in calves: II. The experimental disease. J Comp Pathol 62:6–22.

Johnson HM, Torres BA. 1985. Regulation of lymphokine production by arginine vasopressin and oxytocin: Modulation of lymphocyte function by neurohypophyseal hormones. J Immunol 135(Suppl):773–775.

Jones GE, Gilmour JS, Rae AG. 1982. The effects of different strains of *Mycoplasma ovipneumoniae* on specific pathogen-free and conventionally-reared lambs. J Comp Pathol 92:267–272.

Jones TC, Hunt RD, King NW. 1997. Veterinary Pathology, 6th ed. Baltimore: Williams and Wilkins.

Juszkiewicz T. 1967. Experimental *Pasteurella multocida* infection in chickens exposed to cold: Biochemical and bacteriological investigations. Pol Arch Weter 10:615–625.

Juszkiewicz T, Cakalowa A, Stefaniakowa B, Madejski Z. 1967. Experimental pasteurella infection in normal and chlorpromazine-premedicated cockerels, subjected to heat stress. Pol Arch Weter 10:601–614.

Kegley EB, Spears JW, Brown TT Jr. 1997. Effect of shipping and chromium supplementation on performance, immune response, and disease resistance of steers. J Anim Sci 75:1956–1964.

Keiper RR. 1969. Causal factors of stereotypies in caged birds. Anim Behav 17:114–119.

Kelley KW. 1980. Stress and immune function: A bibliographic review. Ann Rech Vet 11:445–478.

Kelly AP. 1988. Review of published research in health and welfare of sheep transported by sea. In: Standing Committee on Agriculture Workshop on Livestock Export Research, February 1988, at Melbourne, Australia. Canberra: Australian Government Printing Service, pp 16–24.

Kelley KW, Osbourne CA, Evermann JF, et al. 1981. Whole blood leukocytes vs separated mononuclear cell blastogenesis in calves: Time-dependent changes after shipping. Can J Comp Med 45:249–258.

Kelley KW, Osbourne CA, Evermann JF, et al. 1982a. Effects of chronic heat and cold stressors on plasma immunoglobulin and mitogen-induced blastogenesis in calves. J Dairy Sci 65:1514–1528.

Kelley KW, Randall E, Greenfield BS, et al. 1982b. Delayed type hypersensitivity, contact sensitivity, and phytohaemagglutinin skin-test responses of heat and cold stressed calves. Am J Vet Res 43:775–779.

Kenny JF, Tarrant PV. 1987a. The behaviour of young Friesian bulls during social regrouping at the abattoir: Influence of an overhead electrified wire grid. Appl Anim Behav Sci 18:233–246.

Kenny JF, Tarrant PV. 1987b. The physiological and behavioural responses of crossbred Friesian steers to short-haul transport by road. Livest Prod Sci 17:63–75.

Kenny JF, Tarrant PV. 1987c. The reaction of young bulls to short-haul road transport. Appl Anim Behav Sci 17:209–227.

Kent JE, Ewbank R. 1983. The effect of road transportation on the blood constituents and behaviour of calves: I. Six months old. Br Vet J 139:228–235.

Kent JE, Ewbank R. 1986a. The effect of road transportation on the blood constituents and behaviour of calves: II. One to three weeks old. Br Vet J 142:131–140.

Kent JE, Ewbank R. 1986b. The effect of road transportation on the blood constituents and behaviour of calves: III. Three months old. Br Vet J 142:326–335.

Kiley-Worthington M. 1977. Behavioural Problems in Farm Animals. Stocksfield, UK: Oriel.

Knowles TG. 1999. A review of road transport of cattle. Vet Rec 144:197–201.

Knowles TG, Broom DM. 1990. Limb bone strength and movement in laying hens from different housing systems. Vet Rec 126:354–356.

Knowles TG, Warriss PD, Brown SN, et al. 1993. Long distance transport of lambs and the time needed for subsequent recovery. Vet Rec 133:286–293.

Knowles TG, Maunder DHL, Warriss PD, Jones TWH. 1994a. Factors affecting the mortality of lambs in transit to or in lairage at a slaughterhouse, and reasons for carcass condemnations. Vet Rec 135:109–111.

Knowles TG, Warriss PD, Brown SN, Kestin SC. 1994b. Long distance transport of export lambs. Vet Rec 134:107–110.

Knowles TG, Brown SN, Warriss PD, et al. 1995. Effects on sheep on transport by road for up to 24 hours. Vet Rec 136:431–438.

Knowles TG, Warriss PD, Brown SN, et al. 1997. Effects on calves less than one month old of feeding or not feeding them during road transport of up to 24 hours. Vet Rec 140:116–124.

Koolhaas JM, Schuurmann T, Fokema DS. 1983. Social behaviour of laying hens from different housing systems. Vet Rec 126:354–356.

Lambooij E, Hulsegge B. 1988. Long-distance transport of pregnant heifers by truck. Appl Anim Behav Sci 20:249–258.

Larson CT, Gross WB, Davies JW. 1985. Social stress and resistance of chickens and swine to *Staphylococcus aureus* challenge infections. Can J Comp Med 49:208–210.

Lawrence AB, Terlouw EMC. 1993. A review of behavioral factors involved in the development and continued performance of stereotypic behaviors in pigs. J Anim Sci 71:2815–2825.

Lay DC, Friend TH, Bowers CL, et al. 1992a. Behavioral and physiological effects of freeze and hot iron branding on crossbred cattle. J Anim Sci 70:330–336.

Lay DC, Friend TH, Bowers CL, et al. 1992b. A comparative physiological and behavioral study of freeze and hot-iron branding using dairy cows. J Anim Sci 70:1121–1125.

Lee JA, Roussel JD, Beatty JF. 1976. Effect of temperature-season on bovine adrenal cortical function, blood cell profile, and milk production. J Dairy Sci 59:104–108.

Lehmkuhl HD, Contreras JA, Cutlip RC, Brogden KA. 1989. Clinical and microbiologic findings in lambs inoculated with *Pasteurella haemolytica* after infection with ovine adenovirus type 6. Am J Vet Res 50:671–675.

Lin F, Mackay DKJ, Knowles NJ. 1998. The persistence of swine vesicular disease virus infection in pigs. Epidemiol Infect 121:459–472.

MacDermott RP, Stacey MC. 1981. Further characterisation of the human autologous mixed leukocyte reaction (MLR). J Immunol 126:729–734.

MacKenzie AM, Drennan M, Rowan TG, et al. 1997. Effect of transportation and weaning on humoral immune responses of calves. Res Vet Sci 63:227–230.

Manser CE, Elliott H, Morris TH, Broom DM. 1996. The use of a novel operant test to determine the strength of preference for flooring in laboratory rats. Lab Anim 30: 1–6.

Marchant JN, Broom DM. 1996. Effects of dry sow housing conditions on muscle weight and bone strength. Anim Sci 62:105–113.

Martin G. 1975. Über Verhaltensstörungen von Legehennen im Käfig. Angew Ornithol 4:145–176.

Martin SW, Schwabe CW, Franti CE. 1975a. Dairy calf mortality rate: The association of daily meteorologic factors and calf mortality. Can J Comp Med 39:377–388

Martin SW, Schwabe CW, Franti CE. 1975b. Dairy calf mortality rate: Characteristics of calf mortality rates in Tulare County, California. Am J Vet Res 36:1099–1104.

Martin SW, Schwabe CW, Franti CE. 1975c. Dairy calf mortality rate: Influence of meteorologic factors on calf mortality rate in Tulare County, California. Am J Vet Res 36:1105–1109.

Martin SW, Meek AH, Davis DG, et al. 1980. Factors associated with mortality in feedlot cattle: The Bruce County beef cattle project. Can J Comp Med 44:1–10.

Martin SW, Meek AH, Davis DG, et al. 1981. Factors associated with morbidity and mortality in feedlot calves: The Bruce County beef project, year two. Can J Comp Med 45:102–112.

Martin SW, Meek AH, Davis DG, et al. 1982. Factors associated with mortality and treatment costs in feedlot calves: The Bruce County beef project, years 1978, 1979, 1980. Can J Comp Med 46:341–349.

Mason JW. 1968a. The scope of psychoendocrine research. Psychosom Med 30:565–575.

Mason JW. 1968b. "Over-all" hormonal balance as a key to endocrine organisation. Psychosom Med 30:791–808.

Mason JW. 1975. Emotion as reflected in patterns of endocrine integrations. In: Levi L, ed. Emotions: Their Parameters and Measurements. New York: Raven, pp 233–251.

Mason GJ. 1991a. Stereotypies: A critical review. Anim Behav 41:1015–1037.

Mason GJ. 1991b. Stereotypies and suffering. Behav Proc 25:103–115.

McGlone JJ, Curtis SE. 1985. Behaviour and performance of weaning pigs in pens equipped with hide areas. J Anim Sci 60:20–24.

McNally PW, Warriss PD. 1996. Recent bruising in cattle at abattoirs. Vet Rec 138:126–128.

Meese GB, Ewbank R. 1973. The establishment and nature of the dominance hierarchy in the domestic pig. Anim Behav 21:326–334.

Mendl M, Zanella AJ, Broom DM. 1992. Physiological and reproductive correlates of behavioural strategies in female domestic pigs. Anim Behav 44:1107–1121.

Metz JHM. 1984. Regulation of sucking behaviour in calves. In: Unshelm J, Van Putten G, Zeeb K, eds. Proceedings of the International Congress on Applied Ethology in Farm Animals, Kiel, Germany 1984. Darmstadt: KTBL, pp 70–73.

Mills AD, Wood-Gush DGM. 1985. Pre-laying behaviour in battery cages. Br Poult Sci 26:247–252.

Moberg GP. 1985. Biological response to stress: Key to assessment of animal well-being? In: Moberg GP, ed. Animal Stress. Bethesda, MD: American Physiological Society, pp 27–49.

Mohamed MA, Hanson RP. 1980. Effect of social stress on Newcastle disease virus (LaSota) infection. Avian Dis 24:908–915.

Moore JM, Mallman WL, Arnold LR. 1934. Studies on pullorum disease: I. The influence of different temperatures in brooding. J Am Vet Med Assoc 84:526–536.

Mormède P, Soissons J, Bluthe R-M, et al. 1982. Effect of transportation on blood serum composition, disease incidence, and production traits in young calves: Influence of the journey duration. Ann Rech Vet 13:369–384.

Mottershead BE, Lynch JJ, Elwin RL, Green GC. 1985. A note on the acceptance of several types of cereal grain by young sheep with and without experience of wheat. Anim Prod 41:257–259.

Murata H, Takahashi H, Matsumoto H. 1985. Influence of truck transportation of calves on their cellular immune function. Jpn J Vet Sci 47:823–827.

Murata H, Takahashi H, Matsumoto H. 1987. The effects of road transportation on peripheral blood lymphocyte subpopulations, lymphocyte blastogenesis and neutrophil function in calves. Br Vet J 143:166–174.

Nehring A. 1981. One answer to the pig confinement problem. Int J Study Anim Probl 2:256–259.

Norgaard-Nielsen G. 1990. Bone strength of laying hens kept in an alternative system, compared with hens in cages and on deep litter. Br Poult Sci 31:81–89.

Norris RT, McDonald CL, Richards RB, et al. 1990. Management of inappetant sheep during export by sea. Aust Vet J 67:244–247.

Owen Rh. ap Rh., Fullerton J, Barnum DA. 1983. Effect of transportation, surgery, and antibiotic therapy in ponies infected with salmonella. Am J Vet Res 44:46–50.

Oxender WD, Newman LE, Morrow DA. 1973. Factors influencing dairy calf mortality in Michigan. J Am Vet Med Assoc 162:458–460.

Parrott RF, Hall SJG, Lloyd DM. 1998a. Heart rate and stress hormone responses of sheep to road transport following two different loading responses. Anim Welfare 7:257–267.

Parrott RF, Hall SJG, Lloyd DM, et al. 1998b. Effects of a maximum permissible journey time (31 h) on physiological responses of fleeced and shorn sheep to transport with observations on behaviour during a short (1 h) rest-stop. Anim Sci 66:197–207.

Parrott RF, Lloyd DM, Goode JA. 1996. Stress hormone responses of sheep to food and water deprivation at high and low ambient temperatures. Anim Welfare 5:45–56.

Payne JM. 1989. Metabolic and Nutritional Diseases of Cattle. Oxford: Blackwell Scientific.

Peterson PK, Chao CC, Molitor T, et al. 1991. Stress and pathogenesis of infectious disease. Rev Infect Dis 13:710–720.

Petherick JC, Blackshaw JK. 1987. A review of the factors influencing the aggressive and agonistic behaviour of the domestic pig. Aust J Exp Agric 27:605–611.

Phillips CJC. 1993. Cattle Behaviour. Ipswich, UK: Farming.

Phillips CJC, Youssef MYI, Chiy PC, Arney DR. 1999. Sodium chloride supplements increase the salt appetite and reduce stereotypies in confined cattle. Anim Sci 68:741–748.

Pierson FW, Larsen CT, Gross WB. 1997. The effect of stress on the response of chickens to coccidiosis vaccination. Vet Parasitol 73:177–180.

Radostits OM, Gay CC, Blood DC, Hinchcliff KW. 2000. Veterinary Medicine: A Textbook of the Diseases of Cattle, Sheep, Pigs, Goats and Horses, 9th ed. London: WB Saunders.

Ram T, Hutt FB. 1955. The relative importance of body temperature and lymphocytes in genetic resistance to Salmonella pullorum in fowl. Am J Vet Res 16:437–449.

Randall JM. 1993. Environmental parameters necessary to define comfort for pigs, cattle and sheep in livestock transporters. Anim Prod 57:299–307.

Reid RL, Mills SC. 1962. Studies on the carbohydrate metabolism of sheep: XIV. The adrenal response to psychological stress. Aust J Agric Res 13:282–295.

Ribble CS, Meek AH, Shewen PE, et al. 1995a. Effect of pre-transit mixing on fatal fibrinous pneumonia in calves. J Am Vet Med Assoc 207:616 619.

Ribble CS, Meek AH, Shewen PE, et al. 1995b. Effect of transportation on fatal fibrinous pneumonia and shrinkage in calves arriving at a large feedlot. J Am Vet Med Assoc 207:612–615.

Ribble CS, Meek AH, Janzen ED, et al. 1995c. Effect of time of year, weather, and the pattern of auction market sales on fatal fibrinous pneumonia (shipping fever) in calves in a large feedlot in Alberta (1985–1988). Can J Vet Res 59:167–172.

Richards RB, Norris RT, Dunlop RH, McQuade NC. 1989. Causes of death in sheep exported live by sea. Aust Vet J 66:33–38.

Richards RB, Norris RT, Higgs ARB. 1993. Distribution of lesions in ovine salmonellosis. Aust Vet J 70:326–330.

Rossier J, French ED, Rivier C, et al. 1977. Foot-shock induced stress increases β-endorphin in blood but not brain. Nature 270:618–620.

Roth JA, Kaeberle ML, Hsu WH. 1982. Effects of ACTH administration on bovine polymorphonuclear leukocyte function and lymphocyte blastogenesis. Am J Vet Res 43:412–416.

Rushen J. 1993. The 'coping' hypothesis of stereotypic behaviour. Anim Behav 45:613–615.

Rushen J, Lawrence AB, Terlouw EMC. 1993. The motivational basis of stereotypies. In: Lawrence AB, Rushen J, eds. Stereotypic Animal Behaviour: Fundamentals and Applications to Animal Welfare. Wallingford, UK: CAB International, pp 41–64.

Sambraus HH. 1985a. Mouth-based anomalous syndromes. In: Fraser AF, ed. Ethology of Farm Animals. Amsterdam: Elsevier, pp 391–422.

Sambraus HH. 1985b. Stereotypies. In: Fraser AF, ed. Ethology of Farm Animals. Amsterdam: Elsevier, pp 431–441.

Scanga JA, Belk KE, Tatum JD, et al. 1998. Factors contributing to the incidence of dark cutting beef. J Anim Sci 76:2040–2047.

Schäfer M. 1974. Die Sprache des Pferdes. Munich: Nymphenburger Verlagsbuchhandlung.

Schake LM, Dietrich RA, Thomas ML, et al. 1979. Performance of feedlot steers reimplanted with DES or Synovex-S. J Anim Sci 49:324–329.

Schorr EC, Arnason BGW. 1999. Interactions between the sympathetic nervous system and the immune system. Brain Behav Immun 13:271–278.

Schouten WGP. 1986. Rearing conditions and behaviour in pigs [PhD thesis]. Wageningen: University of Wageningen.

Sharma R, Woldehiwet Z. 1990. Increased susceptibility to Pasteurella haemolytica in lambs infected with bovine respiratory syncytial virus. J Comp Pathol 103:411–420.

Shimizu M, Shimizu Y, Kodama Y. 1978. Effects of ambient temperatures on induction of transmissible gastroenteritis in feeder pigs. Infect Immun 21:747–752.

Shoo MK. 1989. Experimental bovine pneumonic pasteurellosis: A review. Vet Rec 124:141–144.

Shope RE. 1955. The swine lungworm as a reservoir and intermediate host for swine influenza virus: V. Provocation of swine influenza by exposure of prepared swine to adverse weather. J Exp Med 102:567–572.

Siegel HS. 1980. Physiological stress in birds. Bioscience 30:529–534.

Silanikove N. 1994. The struggle to maintain hydration and osmoregulation in animals experiencing severe dehydration and rapid rehydration: The story of ruminants. Exp Physiol 79:281–300.

Simensen E, Laksesvela B, Blom AK, Sjaastad ØV. 1980. Effects of transportations, a high lactose diet and ACTH injections on the white blood cell count, serum cortisol and immunoglobulin G in young calves. Acta Vet Scand 21:278–290.

Slauson DO, Cooper BJ. 1990. Mechanisms of Disease: A Textbook of Comparative General Pathology, 2nd ed. Baltimore: Williams and Wilkins.

Smith JAB, Howat GR, Ray SC. 1938. The composition of the blood and milk of lactating cows during inanition, with a note on an unidentified constituent present in certain samples of abnormal milk. J Dairy Res 9:310–322.

Soerjadi AS, Druitt JH, Lloyd AB, Cumming RB. 1979. Effect of environmental temperature on susceptibility of young chickens to Salmonella typhimurium. Aust Vet J 55:413–417.

Staples GE, Haugse CN. 1974. Losses in young calves after transportation. Br Vet J 130:374–379.

Stephens DB. 1982. A review of some behavioural and physiological studies which are relevant to the welfare of young calves. In: Signoret JP, ed. Welfare and Husbandry of Calves. The Hague: Martinus Nijhoff, pp 47–67.

Summerhays RS. 1973. Das schwierige Pferd. Stuttgart: Frankhische Verlagsbuchhandlung.

Tannenbaum J. 1991. Ethics and animal welfare: The inextricable connection. J Am Vet Med Assoc 198:1360–1376.

Tarrant PV, Grandin T. 2000. Cattle transport. In: Grandin T, ed. Livestock Handling and Transport, 2nd ed. Wallingford, UK: CAB International, pp 151–173.

Tarrant PV, Kenny FJ, Harrington D. 1988. The effect of stocking density during 4 hour transport to slaughter, on behavior, blood constituents and carcass bruising in Friesian steers. Meat Sci 24:209–222.

Tarrant PV, Kenny FJ, Harrington D, Murphy M. 1992. Long distance transportation of steers to slaughter: Effect of stocking density on physiology, behavior and carcass quality. Livest Prod Sci 30:223–238.

Terlouw EMC, Lawrence AB, Illius AW. 1991. Influences of feeding level and physical restriction on development of stereotypies in sows. Anim Behav 42:981–992.

Thaxton P, Wyatt RD, Hamilton PB. 1974. The effect of environmental temperature on paratyphoid infection in the neonatal chicken. Poult Sci 53:88–94.

Thomson RG. 1984. General Veterinary Pathology, 2nd ed. Philadelphia: WB Saunders.

Trunkfield HR, Broom DM. 1991. The effects of the social environment on calf responses to handling and transport [Abstract]. Appl Anim Behav Sci 30:177.

van Putten G. 1969. An investigation into tail-biting among fattening pigs. Br Vet J 125:511–516.

van Putten G, Dammers J. 1976. A comparative study of the well-being of piglets reared conventionally and in cages. Appl Anim Ethol 339–356.

van Putten G, Elshof WJ. 1978. Zusatzfütterung von Stroh an Mästkälber. Aktuel Arbeit Artgemassen Tierhaltung 233:210–219.

van Putten G, Van der Burgwal JA. 1990. Vulva biting in group-housed sows: Preliminary report. Appl Anim Behav Sci 26:181–186.

van Rooijen J. 1980. Wahlversuche, eine ethologische Meth-

ode zum Sammeln von Messwerten, und Haltungseinflusse zu erfassen und zu beurteilen. Aktuel Arbeit Artgemassen Tierhaltung 264:165–185.

Vestergaard K. 1981. Behavioural and physiological studies of hens on wire floors and in deep litter pens. In: Fölsch DW, ed. Das Verhalten von Legehennen. Basel: Birkhäuser, pp 115–132.

Vestergaard K. 1989. Environmental influences on the development of behaviour and their relation to welfare. In: Faure JM, Mills AD, eds. Proceedings of the 3rd European Symposium on Poultry Welfare, Tours, France 1989, pp 109–122.

Vestergaard K, Hogan JA, Kruijt JP. 1990. The development of a behavior system: Dustbathing in the Burmese red junglefowl: I. The influence of the rearing environment on the organization of dustbathing. Behaviour 112:99–116.

Von Holst D. 1986. Vegetative and somatic components of tree shrews' behaviour. J Auton Nerv Syst Suppl, 657–670.

Wajda S, Wichlacz H. 1984. Slaughtering bulls immediately after transport. Fleischwirtschaft 64:343–345.

Warnock JP, Caple IW, Halpin CG, McQueen CS. 1978. Metabolic changes associated with the 'downer' condition in dairy cows at abattoirs. Aust Vet J 54:566–569.

Warriss PD, Brown SN, Knowles TG, et al. 1995. The effects on cattle of transport by road for up to fifteen hours. Vet Rec 136:319–323.

Waterhouse A. 1978. The effect of pen conditions on the development of calf behaviour. Appl Anim Ethol 4:286–280.

Webster J. 1984. Calf Husbandry, Health and Welfare. London: Granada.

Webster J. 1993. Understanding the Dairy Cow, 2nd ed. Oxford: Blackwell Science.

Webster AJF, Saville C, Church BM, et al. 1985. The effect of different rearing systems on the development of calf behaviour. Br Vet J 141:249–264.

Wegner TN, Schuh JD, Nelson FE, Stott GH. 1976. Effect of stress on blood leucocyte and milk somatic cell counts in dairy cows. J Dairy Sci 59:949–956.

Wideman CH, Murphy HM. 1985. Effects of vasopressin deficiency, age and stress on stomach ulcer induction in rats. Peptides 6(Suppl):63–67.

Williams AR, Carey RJ, Miller M. 1985. Altered emotionality of the vasopressin deficient Brattleboro rat. Peptides 6(Suppl):69–76.

Wood PDP, Smith GF, Lisle MF. 1967. A survey of intersucking in dairy herds in England and Wales. Vet Rec 81:396–398.

Wood-Gush DGM, Beilharz RG. 1983. The enrichment of a bare environment for animals in confined conditions. Appl Anim Ethol 10:209–217.

Wythes JR, Arthur RJ, Thompson PJM, et al. 1981. Effect of transporting cows varying distances on live weight, carcass traits and muscle pH. Aust J Exp Agric Anim Husbandry 21:557–561.

Yang EV, Glaser R. 2000. Stress-induced immunomodulation: Impact on immune defenses against infectious disease. Biomed Pharmacother 54:245–250.

Yates WDG. 1982. A review of infectious bovine rhinotracheitis, shipping fever pneumonia and viral-bacterial synergism in respiratory disease of cattle. Can J Comp Med 46:225–263.

11

PATHOPHYSIOLOGY OF THE LIVER

M. Anthony Hayes

The main objective of this chapter is to describe the normal structures and functions of the liver and to explain how these adapt or fail when the liver is diseased. Unlike the cardiovascular, respiratory, digestive, reproductive, and neuromuscular body systems, the hepatobiliary system performs its many functions in the background without much overt or dynamic evidence of what it is doing. Biochemical analyses, palpation, imaging, biopsy, and other clinical diagnostic tools reveal aspects of these processes, but we need to understand the health impact of the changes that can be observed. For example, elevated serum bilirubin (icterus) can occur when a normal liver receives too much heme to degrade or when a diseased liver underperforms the processes involved in the formation and excretion of bilirubin. The physiology and pathology of hepatic excretion therefore need to be understood before a clinical presentation of icterus can be interpreted and managed appropriately. In this chapter, we consider the major hepatic functions and use selected examples that illustrate the underlying pathophysiological principles of adaptation and dysfunction. The reader is directed to other sources for systematic consideration of liver pathology in domestic animals (Kelly 1993; Jones et al. 1997; Cullen and MacLachlan 2001); for clinical physiology and pathology of liver diseases of veterinary importance (Duncan et al. 1994; Kaneko et al. 1997), and for liver pathology and pathophysiology in the human health context (Arias et al. 1994; MacSween et al. 2002).

STRUCTURAL BASIS OF HEPATIC FUNCTION

Vasculature. The liver has multiple lobes, the number and arrangement of which vary considerably among domestic animal species (Kelly 1993; Cullen and MacLachlan 2001). It is a highly vascular multilobed parenchymal organ perfused by a variably large volume of blood, most of which is venous outflow from the gastrointestinal tract (Figure 11.1). The lobes are positioned and shaped in a manner that permits changes in size as the liver adapts to various functional demands.

The *portal vein* brings venous blood to the liver from the forestomachs, glandular stomach, intestines, spleen, and pancreas. This specialized vascular arrangement is particularly important for those liver functions regarding detoxification, nutrition, and microbial clearance. The liver has a high metabolic demand that depends on oxygenated arterial blood supplied via the aortic celiac branch. The *hepatic artery* disperses within the liver parallel with the portal veins (Figure 11.1). Most hepatic arterial blood flows through a peribiliary capillary plexus (Figure 11.2) and thence into the sinusoidal microvasculature (Ekataksin and Kaneda 1999). Some hepatic arterioles can also directly enter the sinusoids, but normally at low pressure that must not interfere with portal venous inflow. Portal and arterial blood eventually mix in the low-pressure hepatic sinusoids.

Hepatic sinusoids are cavernous microvessels lined with a combination of attached phagocytes (*Kupffer cells*) and specialized porous *sinusoidal endothelium* (Arias et al. 1994; McCuskey 2000). Kupffer cells are in direct contact with blood moving at a relatively slow velocity, and this arrangement favors their major role in phagocytic removal of particulates, especially bacteria that enter the portal blood via the lower alimentary

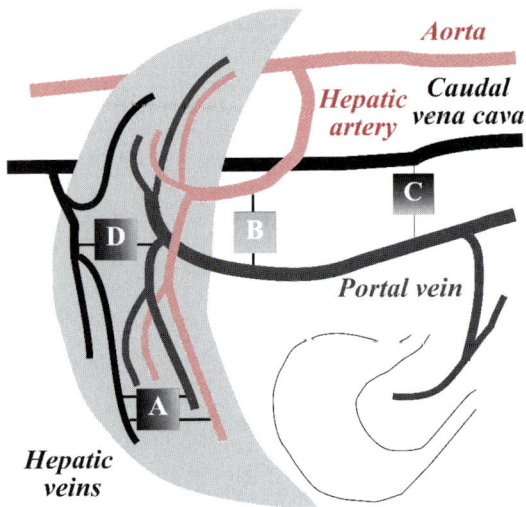

Aorta

Hepatic *Caudal*
artery *vena cava*

C

D B

Portal vein

A

Hepatic
veins

FIG. 11.1—General arrangement of normal and common
disrupted patterns of hepatic circulation. Hepatic artery from
the aorta and portal vein from the gastrointestinal tract enter
the liver and are distributed as parallel branches that mix at
low pressure at the level of the hepatic sinusoids and enter
the postsinusoidal outflow veins after interacting with
hepatocytes (**A**). Hepatic veins exit into the systemic
circulation via the caudal vena cava. Portal blood containing
waste materials from the gut can bypass the liver in various
abnormal situations. For example, anomalous anastomoses of
hepatic arteries with portal branches (**B**) or resistance to
portal flow at level A will increase portal venous pressure
and expand collateral extrahepatic (**C**) or intrahepatic (**D**)
shunts that divert portal blood into the central venous
system. Congenital shunts can also develop anomalously in
any of these locations.

tract. The sinusoids are supported by a specialized, discontinuous, or loose ECM, and the endothelial cells
have numerous small apertures or fenestrations (about
1000 angstroms) that permit the two-way exchange of
large proteins between hepatocytes and the blood
(Arias et al. 1994). This arrangement is necessary for
secretion of plasma proteins, and for hepatic uptake by
receptor-mediated endocytosis (RME) of various nutri-
ent-carrier proteins such as transferrin, bile acids,
immunoglobulin A (IgA), and growth factors that are
recycled, excreted into bile, or degraded in hepatocyte
lysosomes. Hepatocytes also have various surface
membrane transporters (Trauner et al. 1998; Ferenci et
al. 2002) by which glucose, amino acids, and many
other small molecules are taken up from or released
into the bloodstream.

Venous outflow through terminal hepatic venules
converges into larger hepatic veins that exit into the
caudal vena cava. The large and small outflow veins in
some species such as dogs and pigs are equipped with
smooth muscle walls and valve flaps that regulate the
influence of central venous pressure on the sinusoidal
blood flow (Takahashi-Iwanaga et al. 1990; Ekataksin

and Kaneda 1999; McCuskey 2000). However,
increased pressure in the vena cava during right-sided
heart failure or thrombosis (Budd-Chiari syndrome)
can impede outflow and lead to congestive distension
of the hepatic veins and sinusoids.

Anatomic Zones. Mammalian hepatocytes are organized in a relatively consistent pattern of platelike arrays
among the specialized blood vessels and bile ducts. In
two-dimensional sections, the liver parenchyma appears
as "cords" separated by microvascular channels called
sinusoids. The arrangements of inflow and outflow vasculature define the anatomic and functional subunits of
the liver parenchyma (Figure 11.2) At the sinusoidal
vascular level, the subunits are referred to as either *lobules* or *acini* (singular acinus) according to different
conventions. The more classical lobule is a six-sided
anatomic arrangement of hepatocytes centered on the
outflow venules and peripherally demarcated by connective tissue septa. In the pig and some other species
these septa form distinct lobular perimeters, but in most
species the lobular architecture is less pronounced
because connective tissue is restricted to portal tracts.
The acinus is a more physiological anatomic unit that
represents the functional domains in relation to proximity of hepatocytes to blood supply (Figure 11.2). *Zone 1*
is adjacent to the portal inflow, and *zone 3* is adjacent to
the terminal hepatic venule. *Zone 2* is a transitional
midzone that selectively involves some functions and
degenerative changes. Although the functional zone terminology is more commonly applied, the classical synonymous nomenclature relating to the classical lobule is
still widely used. Anatomic proximity to the inflow
(zone 1) is termed *periportal*, whereas proximity to outflow (zone 3) is *centrilobular*. These terms are still particularly useful in reference to the connective tissue
tracts and their vessels.

The liver has a conventional interstitial space in the
connective tissue of the surface (Glisson's capsule) and
in the vascular stroma of the portal tracts (Trutmann
and Sasse 1994; Heath and Lowden 1998). These are
supplied by fluids formed and processed in the perisinusoidal space and are drained by *lymphatics* that exit
the liver mainly via the portal hilus to the hepatic
lymph nodes and thoracic duct. Some lymphatics
around larger hepatic veins of some species such as the
dog traverse the diaphragm into the mediastinum
(Takahashi-Iwanaga et al. 1990).

There are important distinctions to be made about
how extravascular fluids are formed and processed at
the level of the hepatic sinusoid. The liver has an extensive extracellular compartment, most of which is
potential *perisinusoidal space* also referred to as the
space of Disse located between the endothelial attachment and the hepatocyte sinusoidal pole (see Figure
11.3). Unlike capillaries in most other tissues, sinusoids leak higher-protein transudate into the perisinusoidal space. This occurs in part because plasma proteins are not fully excluded by the fenestrated
sinusoidal epithelium, and because hepatocytes can

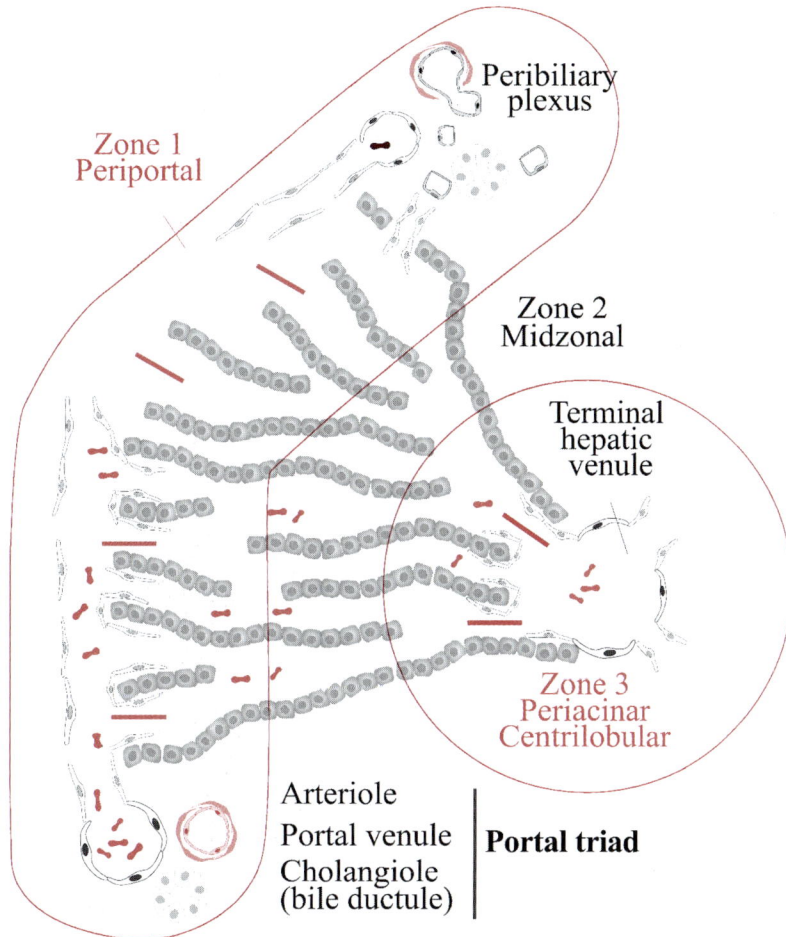

FIG. 11.2—Microanatomy of hepatic parenchyma. The illustration (not to scale) represents one-third of a classical lobule, centered on the terminal hepatic venule and demarcated by portal triads and associated connective tissue stroma. Zone 1 is the population of hepatocytes closest to the portal inflow, whereas zone 3 is the region closest to the hepatic venous outflow. These zones are illustrated by gray backgrounds separated by a midzonal region designated zone 2. Portal venules supply branches in the periphery of the lobule that open into the sinusoids, as illustrated with red arrows. Blood flows under low pressure along the hepatic sinusoids (lined by specialized endothelium; not all shown). Hepatic arterioles deliver oxygenated blood into a peribiliary capillary plexus that ultimately enters the sinusoids at low pressure, where it mixes with portal venous blood. Mixed arterial and portal blood flows along the sinusoids toward zone 3 and then out via terminal hepatic venules. Bile canalicular channels connect via small canals of Hering (not shown) into portal cholangioles that are distributed within the peribiliary plexus in the portal triad.

secrete proteins into the perisinusoidal space. When sinusoidal and perisinusoidal pressures increase, for example, in right-sided heart failure, or obstruction of hepatic venous outflow or portal hypertension due to arteriovenous fistulae, the hepatic interstitial fluid can redistribute into the peritoneal cavity as low-protein transudate known as *ascites*.

Liver Cells. While about 70% to 80% of the liver mass is composed of *hepatocytes* (referred to as *parenchymal cells*), more than 50% of liver DNA is in smaller *non-parenchymal cells* and itinerant cells (Table 11.1). The association among these various cells (Figure 11.3) is

critical to the performance of many liver functions that involve exchange of material with the blood and bile.

Hepatocytes are large cells with abundant distinctive cytoplasm that is rich in mitochondria, smooth and rough endoplasmic reticulum, lysosomes, peroxisomes, Golgi apparatus, and transport vesicles (Arias et al. 1994). The cytosolic compartment contains variable amounts of stored glycogen, triglycerides, and various proteins such as ferritin, an iron-binding protein. Hepatocyte plasma membranes have different specialized surfaces or domains that express the various cell adhesion molecules (CAMs) required to connect to each other or to neighboring cells or to the discontinuous

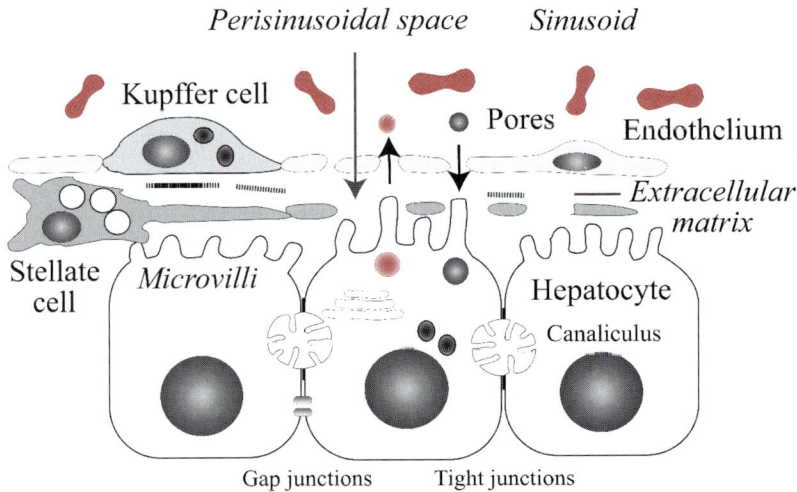

Perisinusoidal space   *Sinusoid*

FIG. 11.3—Physical relationships among major cells of the liver. In most mammals, the sinusoidal surface of the normal hepatocyte is in direct contact with proteins of the sinusoidal blood, mainly in the perisinusoidal space known as the space of Disse. Some microvilli can project through pores (fenestrations) into the sinusoidal lumen. Stellate cells (also termed perisinusoidal cells or fat-storing Ito cells) have numerous projections located in the perisinusoidal compartment between the hepatocytes and endothelial cells. There is discontinuous extracellular matrix (mainly type IV collagen) produced by perisinusoidal stellate cells, hepatocytes, and endothelial cells.

extracellular matrix (ECM) distributed along the perisinusoidal space (Figure 11.3). This ECM, composed mostly of collagen type IV, is produced cooperatively by sinusoidal endothelial cells and perisinusoidal stellate cells (Herbst et al. 1997). The canalicular domains are limited by tight adhesion between plasma membranes of adjacent hepatocytes (Figure 11.3). The intercellular surfaces or lateral domains have gap junctions through which there is regulated exchange of various small molecules between contiguous hepatocytes (Omori et al. 2001).

Kupffer cells are a specialized population of tissue macrophages located mainly at branch points in sinusoidal vessels, where they are in direct contact with slow-moving portal blood (Figure 11.4). They are proficient and eclectic phagocytes of particulates, microorganisms, and various microbial surface components,

TABLE 11.1—Cells in the normal liver

Parenchymal cells
  Hepatocytes
Nonparenchymal cells
  Biliary epithelia
  Pluripotential stem cells
  Mesothelial cells
  Endothelial cells
  Kupffer cells
  Fibroblasts
  Vascular smooth muscle cells
  Stellate (perisinusoidal) cells (Ito cells)
Blood cells
  Hematopoietic populations (mainly in fetus or neonate)
  Leukocytic infiltrates (macrophages and granulocytes)
  Lymphocytes and plasma cells

and thus serve the liver as a major "filtering organ" for clearance of bacteria from the blood. This clearance process is more effective in dogs and cats than in ruminants (Cullen and MacLachlan 2001). Kupffer cells cooperate with neutrophils in the killing of bacteria (Gregory and Wing 2002). Various pathogenic bacteria that are not efficiently killed by Kupffer cells can localize in the liver sinusoids and lead to focal necrosis and inflammation. A hematogenous pattern of multifocal necrosis and inflammation is often typical of some bacteremic forms of salmonellosis, listeriosis, Tyzzer's disease, and other infections (Kelly 1993). Kupffer cells can also sequester particulates and phagocytose apoptotic and necrotic cells. Kupffer cells are readily activated in response to biologically active materials such as bacterial lipopolysaccharides (LPS) (Bradham et al. 1998; Ring and Stremmel 2000; Ramadori and Armbrust 2001). They then secrete various inflammatory *cytokines*, especially tumor-necrosis factor, and nitric oxide that dilate vasculature of other tissues and contribute to hypotension in systemic inflammatory-response syndromes. Activated Kupffer cells also secrete cytokines such as interleukin 1 (IL-1) and IL-6 that are important in mediating the acute-phase response and some aspects of the immune and tissue regenerative responses.

Hepatic stellate cells (also termed hepatic perisinusoidal cells, fat-storing cells, lipocytes, or Ito cells) are multifunctional cells located between sinusoidal endothelium and hepatocytes (see Figure 11.3) (Geerts 2001). In their resting state, they produce and maintain ECM constituents, and store lipid droplets that are rich in *vitamin A* (Figure 11.5). Stellate cells and endothelial

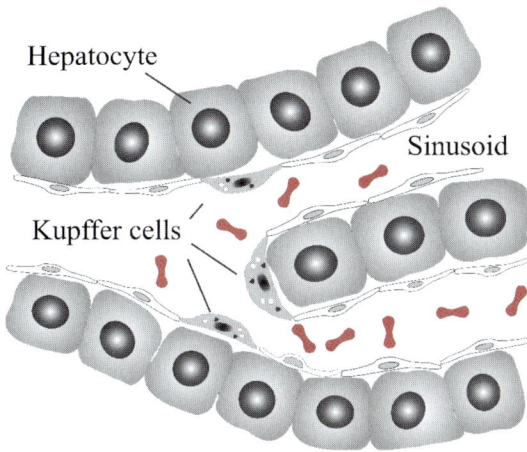

FIG. 11.4—Distribution of sinusoidal phagocytes (Kupffer cells).

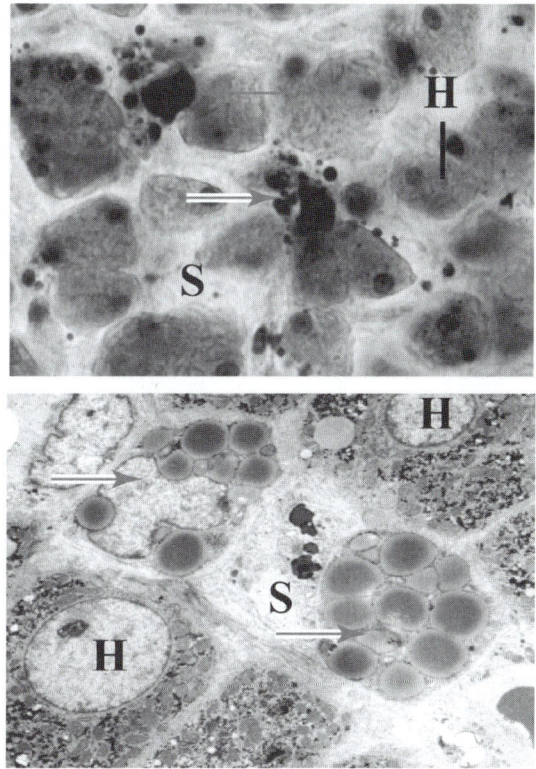

FIG. 11.5—Hepatic stellate cells in the resting state appear as large fat-storing vacuolated cells (arrows) located along the sinusoids (S) between hepatocytes (H), as illustrated by fat-stain light microscopy (**top**) or transmission electron microscopy (**bottom**). They store vitamin A and contribute to the formation of loose perisinusoidal extracellular matrix.

cells are also involved in the production of normal loose or discontinuous ECM (see Figure 11.3). The stellate cells are mainly responsible for the generation of excess ECM in pathological conditions such as cirrhosis (Geerts 2001). When activated by proinflammatory cytokines in response to tissue injuries, perisinusoidal cells alter their differentiated phenotype and secrete various factors that promote tissue repair and deposition of ECM. When reactive, they appear more like fibroblasts and produce substantially increased amounts of more densely packed ECM that transforms vessels to a less permeable capillary form (see Figure 11.6). This new substratum can then interfere locally with maintenance of the fenestrations of sinusoidal endothelium and, as a result, impede the transfer of macromolecules between the hepatocytes and the blood. In severe chronic injury leading to cirrhosis, stellate cells can become enriched with a contractile cytoskeleton that further restricts microvascular blood flow. However, stellate cells can respond to apoptosis-inducing cytokines, and this might be involved in their removal during the involution phase of hepatic fibrosis (Taimr et al. 2003). Animals with various patterns of liver injury often undergo some degree of proliferative activation of stellate cells. However, the ECM matrix deposited in the perisinusoidal space is rarely to the degree seen in severe ethanol-induced cirrhosis in humans.

Larger *bile ducts* are termed extrahepatic and intrahepatic ducts, whereas the smallest bile duct branches are called lobular ducts or, more simply, bile ductules. *Canaliculi* depend on intercellular adhesion molecules, intermediate cytokeratin filaments, and submembranous actin for secretory vesicles and for kinetic movement of bile. Canaliculi enter small bile ductules in the portal tracts (see Figure 11.2). The bile duct is a branching outflow that enters the proximal duodenum. Most species have a bile storage diverticulum (*gall-

bladder), but horses and rats are exceptions that do not. In some species, the bile duct joins the pancreatic duct before entry into the duodenum. In some fish and reptiles, the liver and pancreatic tissue is a composite organ referred to as hepatopancreas.

Mature hepatocytes are able to replicate and maintain functional liver mass, but during development and some chronic liver diseases, other precursor progenitor cells are involved in clonal regeneration. Hepatic epithelial *stem cells* are primitive undifferentiated cells that can generate new differentiated hepatocytes and bile duct cells (Forbes et al. 2002). Immature ductular cells termed *oval cells* have been considered to be hepatic stem cells because they can sometimes generate new hepatocytes, although they are more likely to become bile ducts. Hematopoietic pluripotential stem cells also appear to be able to differentiate into hepatocytes (Alison et al. 2000). Although they are likely important in the developmental formation of the liver, there is evidence that they might be induced to flourish again in some disease conditions. However, there is

Sinusoid

Dense extracellular matrix   *Capillary-type endothelium*

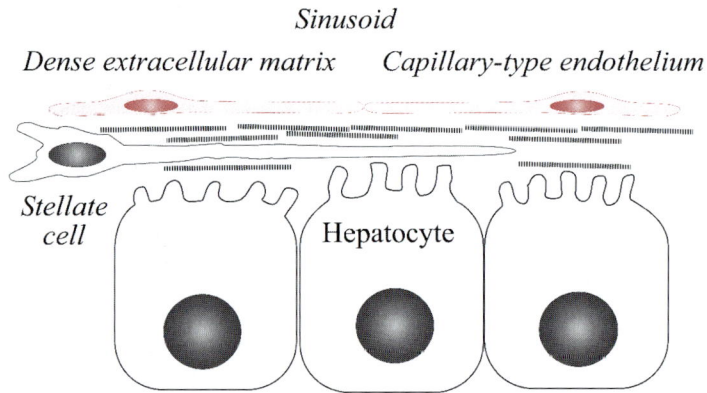

Stellate cell   Hepatocyte

FIG. 11.6—Reactive stellate cells increase deposits of extracellular matrix upon which sinusoidal endothelial cells develop in a less permeable capillary-like form.

still much to learn about the manner by which these cells contribute to liver regeneration, and how this can be stimulated when the liver is failing.

Hematopoiesis in fetal life of mammals occurs mainly in the perisinusoidal compartment of the liver sinusoids. Postnatally, hepatic hematopoietic populations regress in most species, but the perisinusoidal area retains its hospitality for extramedullary hematopoiesis (EMH). Under conditions of markedly increased demand for blood cells, EMH can resume in the liver, and the degree to which this occurs in larger species has some diagnostic significance. In rodents and other small animals, however, a small amount of hepatic EMH can be an incidental observation even in adult life.

HEPATIC FUNCTIONS. The liver is a truly versatile organ with major functions related to metabolic homeostasis (Table 11.2). Importantly, the liver is highly adaptable so metabolic resources can be efficiently allocated according to changing supply and demand. These many functions make it difficult to categorize the liver according to common tissue arrangements. It is sometimes anatomically grouped among glands accessory to the digestive tract, but based on some of its functions, it could also be considered to be a member of the excretory, circulatory, host resistance (immune), hematopoietic, and endocrine systems. As a gland, the liver is quite versatile in its ability to secrete in two directions (Figure 11.3). Secretion of bile via ducts into the intestine is exocrine, like in the adjacent exocrine pancreas, whereas proteins made in the liver are secreted into the blood, in a manner resembling that of the endocrine pancreas. As an excretory organ, production of bile seems superficially similar to excretion by the kidney, but the liver employs different ways by which it can clear substances from the blood. The liver also has an important role as a storage depot for various nutrients such as glycogen, fat, trace minerals, and

vitamins, and it sequesters some potentially harmful materials in lysosomes and phagocytes.

Functions are heterogeneously distributed across the acinus (Oinonen and Lindros 1998). Hepatocytes in zone 1 are more involved in RME and protein synthesis (Table 11.3). In zone 1, hepatocytes are more specialized for aerobic metabolism, urea cycle, fat, and cholesterol metabolism. In zone 3, the major biotransformation functions are more active, including the expression of various cytochromes P-450, glucuronyl transferases, glutathione S-transferases, and other detoxification enzymes. Zone 3 is more susceptible to injury by toxic substances that are metabolically activated by cytochromes P-450 that are more highly expressed there. By comparison, hepatocytes in zone 1 are more susceptible to direct-acting toxicants, such as metal salts. Under the influences of various inducers, the patterns of expression can extend beyond the resting limits.

Hepatocyte metabolic functions are also unevenly distributed within the cytoplasm of hepatocytes. This is particularly important in relation to the exchange of various substances across the sinusoidal and canalicular plasma

TABLE 11.2—Major functions of the liver

Micronutrient storage and supply
Lipid distribution
Protein metabolism and secretion
Carbohydrate metabolism
Plasma oncotic pressure
   Albumin
Detoxification and excretion
   Biotransformation and biliary excretion
   Ammonia removal and urea production
   Clearance of plasma proteins
Host defense
   Hemostasis (coagulation proteins)
   Antimicrobial factors (lectins, complement proteins)
   Phagocytic clearance by Kupffer cells
   Cytokines and acute-phase adaptations
Fetal and extramedullary hematopoiesis

TABLE 11.3—Zonal heterogeneity of hepatocyte functions

More in zone 1	More in zone 3
Oxidative energy metabolism	Glycolysis
Cholesterol synthesis	Lipogenesis
Fatty-acid oxidation	Most cytochromes P-450
Ureagenesis	Glutathione conjugation
Bile-acid production	Glucuronidation
Glutathione peroxidation	

membranes. Various transmembrane molecules (Table 11.4) involved in transport of bile acids, xenobiotics, and their conjugates have been characterized in the liver (Ferenci et al. 2002). Some sinusoidal transporters bring materials into hepatocytes. Excretion of conjugates and other anionic materials into the bile canaliculus depends on various adenosine triphosphate (ATP)-dependent membrane transporters located at the specialized canalicular membrane (Table 11.4) (Trauner et al. 1998).

Hepatocytes transport various substances such as transferrin, low-density lipoproteins (LDLs), and other materials within various membrane-bound cytoplasmic vesicles. Specialized membrane structures (coated pits) on hepatocytes and Kupffer cells express receptors that capture specific ligands from the blood (Table 11.5). These undergo internalization by a RME (Figure 11.7) (Arias et al. 1994; Chappell and Medh 1998; Weigel and Yik 2002). In Kupffer cells, most internalized vesicles fuse with lysosomes that degrade or sequester the contents. Within the hepatocyte, lysosomal degradation is also important, for example, in the salvage of LDLs. However, some endocytotic vesicles recycle to the sinusoidal pole, whereas others fuse with the canalicular lumen (Crawford 1996). Some vesicles transport IgA, cytokines, and other macromolecules from the blood to the bile. These vesicles are actively propelled by microtubular kinesis to the canalicular domain through which they discharge into the canaliculi. Canalicular contents are propelled directionally by peristalsis mediated by contraction cycles of pericanalicular actin filaments. These flow into bile ductules and beyond into the major bile ducts in the portal tracts.

NUTRIENT METABOLISM. The liver is the major site of exchange of various nutrients from the alimentary tract and is central to the distribution of nutritional resources that are stored or used by other tissues (Table 11.6). Hepatocytes can accumulate reserves of fat, carbohydrate, and recyclable protein for utilization in times of reduced food intake. The liver is an extraordinarily adaptive organ, in a large part because hepatocytes must perform many competing functions at varied rates under the full range of usual experiences in life. For example, the liver adjusts metabolic pathways between storage and consumption of carbohydrates, fat, and micronutrients and between anabolism and catabolism of proteins. In times of nutrient sufficiency and good health, hepatocytes are substantially committed to processes required for nutrient assimilation and distribution, in support of normal growth, pregnancy, lactation, and maintenance. They also maintain the supply of plasma proteins for host defense and the elimination of potentially noxious substances, such as ammonia and toxins, from internal or external sources. In periods of illness, anorexia, and/or starvation, the priorities shift toward host defense and/or catabolism. Under these conditions, hepatocytes can adapt to increase the supply of proteins that are more rapidly consumed from the plasma, or the cytoplasmic proteins required for detoxification, cell stress, and catabolism.

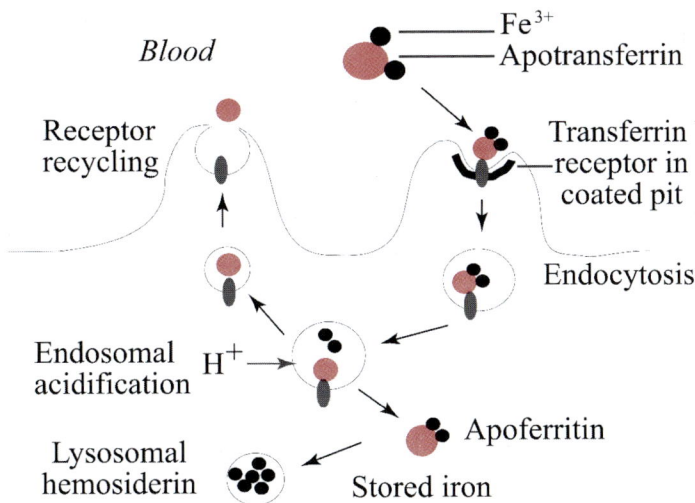

FIG. 11.7—Hepatocyte uptake of diferric transferrin by receptor-mediated endocytosis.

Table 11.4. Major small molecule transport systems of the liver

Transporter	Site[a]	Function
Na–taurocholate transporter (NTCP)	S	Bile-acid uptake
Organic anion transporting protein (OATP)	S	Uptake of bile acids and other organic anions
Multidrug-resistance protein 1 (MDR1)	C	Excretion of organic cations
Canalicular membrane organic anion transporter (cMOAT) or MDR3	C	Excretion of organic anions, bilirubin, etc.
Glucose membrane transporter 2 (GLUT2)	S	Uptake or release of glucose into plasma

[a]Location in the sinusoidal (S) and canalicular (C) plasma membranes of hepatocytes.

Micronutrients. Various *mineral* cations, including iron, copper, cobalt, and zinc, are stored in the liver and transported by proteins made by the liver. For example, the liver centrally regulates *iron* in plasma (Andrews 1999). Apotransferrin is a major liver-secreted plasma protein with an extraordinarily high affinity for ferric ions (Fe^{3+}). Fe^{3+} bound to transferrin in plasma is maintained in the oxidized state by ceruloplasmin, an acute-phase inducible plasma protein produced by hepatocytes. Because most plasma iron is transferrin bound, it is available only to cells that express surface *transferrin receptors* that mediate receptor-mediated uptake of diferric transferrin (Figure 11.7). While this restricts iron from many nonpathogenic organisms, some bacterial pathogens and parasites are equipped with various iron-binding proteins that enable them to compete for iron on transferrin. Endosomes within the liver are acidified, whereby Fe^{3+} is dissociated from apotransferrin, and the endosomes return to the sinusoidal pole and apotransferrin is recycled into plasma. Internalized Fe^{3+} is transported to various pathways in the hepatocyte, where some is used for biosynthesis of abundant liver heme proteins such as cytochromes of the respiratory transport and mixed-function oxygenase systems. Excess iron in cytosol is in the form of *ferritin* (iron bound to the protein apoferritin) or sequestered into lysosomes as an iron complex known as *hemosiderin*.

The liver rapidly removes transferrin-bound iron from circulation during the acute-phase response. This likely restricts iron available to microbial pathogens that have high-affinity iron-uptake mechanisms that

enable competitive access to transferrin-bound iron. Hepatic uptake of plasma iron is regulated by other factors. The gene mutated in some forms of hereditary hemochromatosis (*HFE*) greatly increases the ability of the liver to internalize iron (Andrews 1999; Bomford 2002). The *HFE* protein governs the rate of uptake of iron into the cell via the transferrin receptor, so the *HFE* mutations that increase efficiency of uptake can be beneficial when dietary iron is in short supply or lost to wounds or parasites. However, hemochromatosis can result when sufficient iron is available and retained by individuals with more efficient uptake. Excess iron sequestration in the liver can also occur secondarily to excessive dietary or therapeutic exposure, or accelerated turnover of hemoglobin in hemolytic diseases or multiple blood transfusions. In some arboreal bird species, iron uptake from diets designed for ground-feeding species can also be excessive, but the mechanisms are not fully explained (Crissey et al. 2000).

Stored iron is mostly present in the form of lysosomal hemosiderin in Kupffer cells and hepatocytes, particularly in older animals. Sequestered iron is not usually harmful to the host cells but can become particularly injurious if it is released and reduced. If hepatocytes die and leak iron into an acidotic milieu in which the redox state favors reduction of iron to Fe^{2+}, potently destructive reactive oxygen species (ROS) can be generated. Oxidative insults, for example, during postischemic reflow, or cytochrome P-450 generation of metabolites that undergo redox cycling (e.g., acetaminophen), can generate excess superoxide anions that

TABLE 11.5—Some receptors involved in receptor-mediated endocytosis (RME) by hepatocytes (Hs), Kupffer cells (KCs), and sinusoidal endothelial cells (ECs)

System	Cell	Plasma ligands
Transferrin receptor (Tf-R)	H	Diferric transferrin
LDL receptor (LDL-R)	H	Low-density lipoproteins (LDLs)
LDL-receptor-related protein (LRP1) or α_2-macroglobulin receptor (α_2MR)	H	Protease-modified α_2-macroglobulins, chylomicron remnants, many antiprotease complexes, etc.
Asialoglycoprotein receptor (ASGPR or GalR)	H	Galactosyl glycans on plasma proteins that lose outer sialic acids
Mannose receptors (ManRs)	EC and KC	Mannosyl glycans and glycan sulfates
Scavenger receptors (SCRs)	KC	Broad-spectrum phagocytosis
Hyaluronan receptor (HAR)	EC	Glycosaminoglycans
Mannose-6-phosphate receptor (Man6PR or IGF2R)	H	Mannose-6-phosphate modified proteins, e.g., lysosomal hydrolases and insulin-like growth factor II (IGF-II)
Epidermal growth factor receptor (EGFR)	H	Epidermal growth factor (EGF)
Polymeric immunoglobulin receptor (pIgR)	H	Immunoglobulin A for transcellular transport to bile

TABLE 11.6—Some nutrition-related metabolic functions of the liver

Micronutrients
    Vitamin A, D, E, and K storage
    Iron, copper, and zinc storage
    Cobalt and vitamin B_{12}
Lipids
    Lipoprotein biosynthesis and export
    Uptake of lipoproteins by endocytosis
    Triglyceride biosynthesis
    Peroxisomal and mitochondrial catabolism of triglycerides
    Production of cholesterol and bile acids
    Ketogenesis
Carbohydrates
    Maintenance of blood glucose
    Glycogen biosynthesis and storage
    Glycogenolysis
    Gluconeogenesis
Proteins
    Amino acid biosynthesis and transamination
    Plasma protein production
    Uptake and catabolism of plasma proteins
    Ammonia uptake and ureagenesis

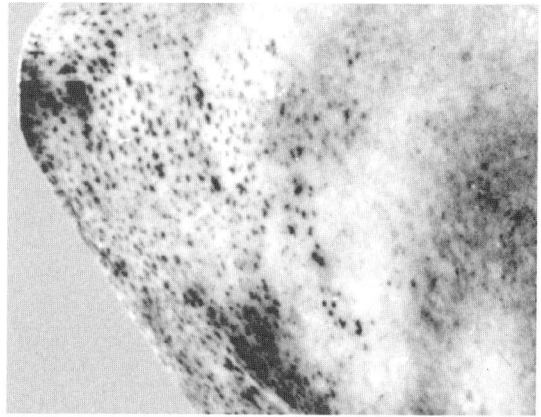

FIG. 11.8—Iron-dextran hepatotoxicity in a piglet with a centrilobular pattern of hemorrhagic hepatic parenchymal necrosis (dark areas). Normally, the liver is relatively resistant to iron while it is transferrin bound or sequestered as ferritin or hemosiderin. Free reduced iron is a potent generator of reactive oxygen species that are the injurious product of iron overload.

can reduce Fe^{3+} to Fe^{2+}. Reduced Fe^{2+} in turn favors nonenzymatic partial oxidation of hydrogen peroxide to hydroxyl radicals by the Fenton reaction.

Hydroxyl radicals and the various other ROS lead to membrane peroxidation, release of lipid-peroxidation products such as 4-hydroxynonenal, and further release of iron sequestered in those cells that die. Thus, stored iron contributes to the exacerbation of liver necrosis initiated by other insults (Eaton and Qian 2002). For this reason, antioxidants and particularly the removal of excessive stored iron by blood removal, dietary restriction, or iron chelators delay the development of cirrhosis in human patients with hereditary hemochromatosis or repeated blood transfusions. The use of iron-dextran complexes for the treatment and prevention of anemia in suckling piglets can lead to iron-catalyzed lipid peroxidation and necrosis (Figure 11.8) in animals with insufficient antioxidant defenses (e.g., marginal vitamin E levels, or selenium deficiency) (Kelly 1993).

The liver also produces several proteins involved in plasma transport and storage of *copper* in the liver. Some plasma copper is incorporated into ceruloplasmin. Copper in plasma also binds to metallothioneines from which it is internalized by an ATP-dependent Cu^{2+} transporter that is mutated in Wilson's disease, a hereditary human condition characterized by excessive copper storage in hepatocytes. A similar defect has been described in Bedlington terriers and West Highland white terriers, and is suspected in some other breeds of dogs (Figure 11.9) (Su et al. 1982; Thornburg et al. 1986; Thornburg 1998). These dogs can sequester fairly large amounts of copper in lysosomes without obvious disease. However, with time and cell turnover, sequestered levels continue to rise until there is ongoing necrosis and fibrosis leading to cirrhosis. The pathogenesis of injury appears similar to that of cirrhosis in hemochromatosis, except that the Cu^+ rather than Fe^{2+} is involved in generation of ROS and liver injury.

Sheep normally have efficient copper uptake from diet and are more susceptible to chronic copper hepatotoxicity if the amounts stored in the liver are too high. Some copper is stored in lysosomes of macrophages. Although copper can be released after liver necrosis, for example, in acute hepatic necrosis caused by some toxic plants (Howell et al. 1991), there is also a poorly understood mechanism by which the sheep liver can release copper into the blood at times of stress. Rapid release of copper after necrosis or stress can increase blood levels and cause peroxidation of erythrocyte cell membranes, leading to intravascular hemolysis. An acute fatal hemolytic crisis with icterus and hemoglobinuria is a common acute manifestation of chronic

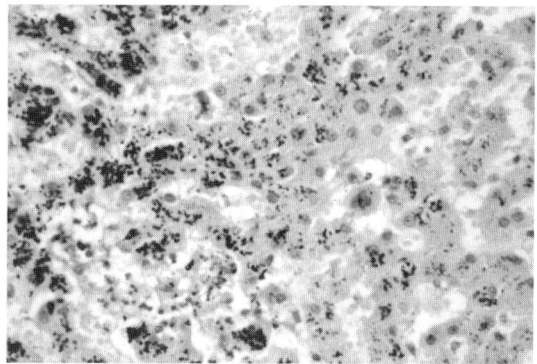

FIG. 11.9—Lysosomal storage and sequestration of copper (dark granules) in cytoplasm of hepatocytes in a section from a Doberman with cirrhosis associated with copper storage (rhodanine stain).

copper toxicosis in sheep (Kelly 1993), but rarely seen in dogs with the chronic copper storage diseases.

Vitamin A accumulates selectively in vacuoles of hepatic stellate (fat storing) cells (Figure 11.5). The liver also is involved in the first cytochrome P-450 mediated hydroxylation step in biosynthesis of 1,25-dihydroxy-cholecalciferol, the active form of *vitamin D*. The liver has various roles in the storage, transport, and metabolism of other fat-soluble vitamins (E and K), vitamin B_{12}, essential fatty acids, and trace minerals. *Vitamin K* is important in the hepatic biosynthesis of calcium-binding coagulation factors (prothrombin and factors 7, 9, and 10). It is an active cofactor for hepatic γ-glutamylcarboxylase, the enzyme that uses carbon dioxide to dicarboxylate the glutamate residues at calcium-binding sites of various coagulation factors. Toxic vitamin K analogues, such as warfarin and related coumarin anticoagulants used as rodenticides, inhibit carboxylation of coagulation factors in the liver. Without such proper posttranslational formation of calcium-binding sites on these coagulation factors, blood clotting is impaired (coagulopathy), so poisoning with these vitamin K antagonists leads to poorly controlled hemorrhage.

Deficiencies of liver *vitamin E* and/or *selenium* contribute to the severity of peroxidative liver injury in some species. For example, young pigs with these deficiencies are prone to massive liver necrosis known as hepatosis dietetica when the liver is subjected to an unusually high burden of lipid-peroxidation products (Kelly 1993; Cullen and MacLachlan 2001). Young sheep on *cobalt*-deficient pastures develop "white liver disease," a fatty liver condition resembling those described in rats with deficiencies in lipotropes such as choline, L-methionine and vitamin B_{12} (Kennedy et al. 1997). The importance of liver as a source of beneficial nutrients was known by ancient Egyptian and Greek cultures, and as a prevention of scurvy in maritime and polar explorers. The Nobel Prize in Medicine was awarded in 1934 for the discovery that uncooked liver (containing vitamin B_{12}) protects against pernicious anemia in humans. However, excessive ingestion of liver from some species can lead to hypervitaminosis A, a cause of liver cirrhosis and other problems.

The liver is the major source of plasma carrier proteins for metals, such as transferrin, metallothioneins, $α_2$-macroglobulins, and also secreted cytosolic and secreted forms of lipocalins that bind fat-soluble vitamins retinoids, fatty acids, steroids, and other hydrophobic substances.

Lipids. The liver plays a central role and highly complex physiological role in the digestion, absorption, catabolism, biosynthesis, storage, and secretion of lipids and related factors (Bruss 1997). Hepatocytes are frequently observed to have an increased content of *triglycerides* as an early sign of injury, because so much of the function of the liver is concerned with lipid metabolism. The liver is one of the main tissues that synthesize long-chain fatty acids (LCFAs) from acetyl-coenzyme A (acetyl-CoA). Hepatocytes can also per-form β oxidation, the mitochondrial utilization of LCFAs after uptake coupled to carnitine. One exclusive function of the liver is the assimilation of ingested triglycerides (TGs) and their redistribution to adipose for storage or to other tissues for β oxidation. To achieve this, the liver is involved in a complex process. First, dietary or mobilized TGs in plasma are hydrolyzed by hepatic lipase on the sinusoidal membrane. Nonesterified LCFAs are then released into the cytosol, where they are bound to carrier proteins and resynthesized to TGs that are stored in hepatocytes or exported as secreted lipoproteins.

Plasma *lipoproteins* of various classes are produced by the liver (Duncan et al. 1994; Kaneko et al. 1997). They transport various lipids as micellar structures consisting of a hydrophobic lipid core encased in an outer coat of hydrophilic apoproteins and phospholipids. Lipoproteins are distinguished by their density determined by ultracentrifugation. The major classes are chylomicrons (>80% TGs), very low density lipoproteins (VLDLs) (ca. 60% TGs), LDLs, and high-density lipoproteins (HDLs). These vary in the proportions of apoproteins, cholesterol, TGs, and phospholipids, and there are substantial species differences. Five major classes of apoproteins designated by letters A to E are found among the lipoproteins. Many more apolipoprotein forms designated by roman numerals (e.g., Apo A-III) can be distinguished by higher resolution techniques such as two-dimensional polyacrylamide gel electrophoresis.

Dietary fats are emulsified in the small intestine in the presence of bile salts secreted by the liver. TGs are then hydrolyzed by pancreatic lipases to LCFAs, monoacylglycerols, and diacylglycerols that are resynthesized in the enterocytes to TGs. The TGs are packaged with protein, cholesterol, and cholesterol esters as lipoproteins termed *chylomicrons*. These enter the blood via the lymphatics that drain the small intestine. TGs are hydrolyzed by peripheral lipoprotein lipase of endothelial cells, yielding fatty acids for β oxidation and energy. The chylomicron remnants are salvaged by endocytosis via chylomicron-remnant receptors of hepatocytes. The liver can obtain LCFAs by lipase hydrolysis of lipoprotein-associated TGs, including those on chylomicrons. Other sources include free (nonesterified) short-chain or long-chain fatty acids.

The esterified LCFAs are hydrolyzed from their ester linkages to glycerol by lipoprotein lipase and can then be used as an energy source via mitochondrial β oxidation by various cells, especially heart and skeletal muscle. In adipose tissue, fatty acids are regenerated into TGs that are stored until required. In the hepatocytes, longer-chain fatty acids are also partially oxidized by *peroxisomes*. Hypolipidemic drugs and some endogenous lipids activate the *peroxisome proliferator-activated receptor α* (PPAR-α) (Everett et al. 2000) that generally upregulates various processes involved in lipid catabolism. These include enhanced removal of TGs from the blood by induced expression of hepatocellular lipoprotein lipase. Macrophage uptake of oxidized lipids that cannot be readily catabolized leads to the formation of atheromas, cholesteomas, and xanthoma in other tissues. In the arterial vasculature, atheromas lead to atherosclerosis and thrombosis, a common pathogenesis of myocardial or cerebral infarction in humans. Domestic animals are less susceptible to atheromas, but hyperlipidemia and arterial atheromas have been associated with hypothyroidism in dogs (Liu et al. 1986).

Hepatocytes synthesize and secrete TGs as a macromolecular complex known as *very low density lipoprotein* (VLDL). TGs in VLDL can be hydrolyzed by lipoprotein lipase in endothelial cells and the LCFAs can be utilized peripherally for energy or resynthesis into stored TGs (Figure 11.10). Some TG can be stored within the cytoplasm of hepatocytes, where it coalesces into large globules, sometimes termed macrovesicles. Within the endoplasmic reticulum, TGs are assembled into VLDLs with locally synthesized apolipoproteins, phospholipids, cholesterol, and cholesterol esters. The VLDLs are packaged into secretory microvesicles in the Golgi system and then actively secreted through the sinusoidal pole into the plasma. This exocytotic process is regulated and requires microtubular cytokinetic functions.

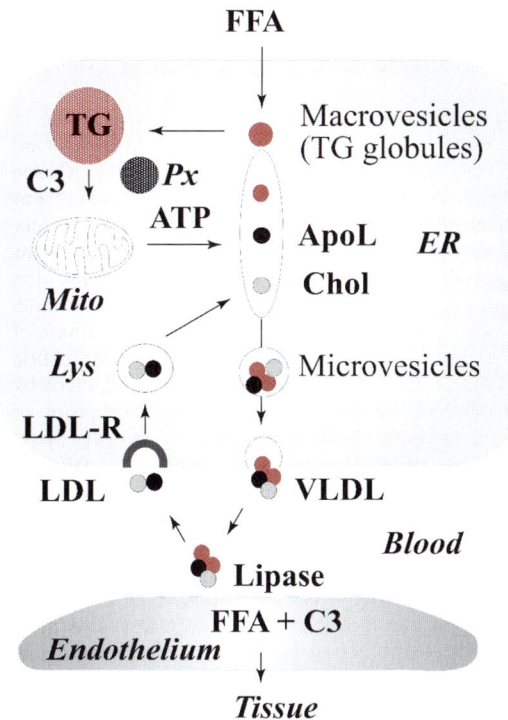

FIG. 11.10—Pathways of lipid metabolism in the normal hepatocyte: ApoL, apolipoprotein; ATP, adenosine triphosphate; C3, glycerol; Chol, cholesterol; ER, endoplasmic reticulum; FFA, nonesterified free long-chain fatty acids; LDL, low-density lipoproteins; LDL-R, LDL receptor; Lys, lysosome; Mito, mitochondria; Px, peroxisome; TG, triacylglycerol; and VLDL, very low density lipoproteins.

The liver is a major site of production of *cholesterol* that is a component of VLDL and HDL. Cholesterol is also the building block for derivatives such as steroid hormones and bile acids. Bile acids are involved in the digestion of TGs in the small intestine.

Hyperlipidemia (increased plasma lipids) occurs in various physiological and pathological conditions. Plasma normally becomes lipidemic after a fatty meal, and, depending on the amount of plasma lipid, the plasma can become transiently turbid (lipemic), but this normally clears during fasting. When it doesn't, there is usually some underlying problem such as hypothyroidism (in dogs), diabetes mellitus, cholestasis, or hyperadrenocorticism. Some breeds of dogs and cats have hereditary defects in lipoprotein clearance from the blood. For example, a hereditary deficiency of lipoprotein lipase has been described in cats. In horses, especially in obese ponies, hyperlipoproteinemia can develop after a stressful period of anorexia, parturition, or transport.

Lipidosis is a general term for any endogenous or exogenous lipid accumulation. *Steatosis* refers specifically to the accumulation of intracellular TG or "fat" to a degree above what would be normally encountered. Hepatic steatosis (also termed hepatic lipidosis, fatty liver, or fatty degeneration) is seen in many conditions, either as a physiological adaptation or as a pathological dysfunction. Healthy hepatocytes process substantial amounts of TGs as previously described (Figure 11.10). When the metabolic throughput is enhanced physiologically—for example, in pregnancy, lactation, or egg production in birds and reptiles—TG accumulates in the liver in its normal storage and export forms. In some pathological situations, such as diabetes mellitus, ketoacidosis, and fasting hyperlipidemia, the rate of mobilization of adipose TGs is substantially increased to the point that hepatic steatosis can occur. However, when hepatocytes are sublethally injured, they frequently lose some of their ability to process and secrete TG. As a result, TGs can accumulate in the cytoplasm as macrovesicles (storage globules) or microvesicles (secretory vacuoles) (Figure 11.11). These characteristic patterns represent a "backup" at different levels in the many metabolic and cytokinetic processes involved in metabolism and secretion of TGs by hepatocytes (Jaeschke et al. 2002).

Fatty liver or hepatic steatosis is readily recognized histologically and macroscopically but requires careful consideration to decide its pathophysiological significance. If it is truly a degenerative condition for which the term *fatty degeneration* is appropriate, other biochemical, functional, or morphologic evidence of liver injury and/or repair would be evident. For example, concurrent elevation of serum alanine aminotransferase (ALT), bilirubin, bile acids, or ammonia would indicate liver injury and dysfunction. Microscopic biopsy evidence of increased organelle or cell injury, or regeneration and inflammation would indicate the liver is not simply reacting physiologically to increased workload. In the absence of other evidence of hepatocyte injury or

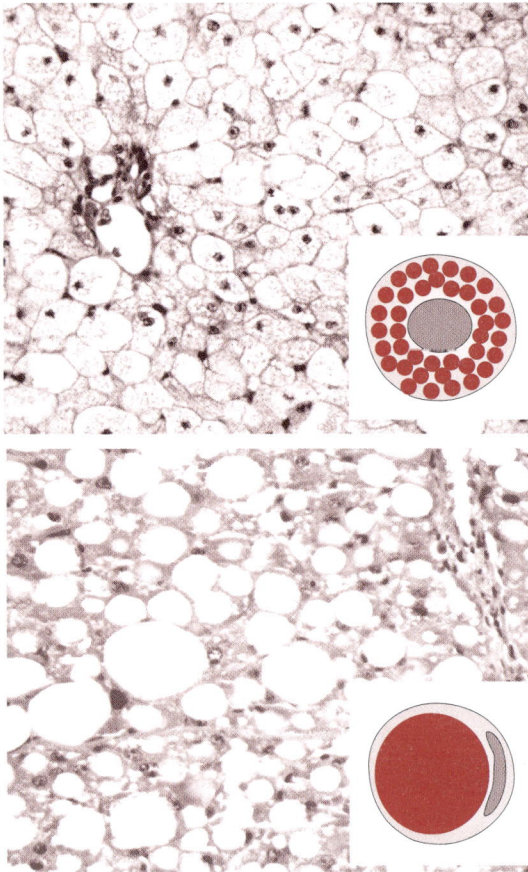

FIG. 11.11—Patterns of hepatocellular steatosis. The **top** image illustrates microvesicular steatosis in hepatocytes of a cat with fatty-liver syndrome. All hepatocytes contain small secretory vesicles containing very low density lipoproteins that do not coalesce and surround the central nucleus. In the more common forms of hepatic steatosis, free cytoplasmic triglycerides coalesce into large macrovesicles that displace the nucleus (**bottom**).

derivatives of fatty acids that can be metabolized in place of glucose in other tissues. Acetone is less available and diffuses into the respired air or urine, in which it can be recognized by its characteristic odor. Acetoacetate and β-hydroxybutyrate are acidic, so high levels of ketogenesis can lead to metabolic acidosis (ketoacidosis). This serious pathophysiological condition occurs in *pregnancy toxemia* in sheep (Figure 11.12) (Rook 2000) and sometimes in dogs with diabetes mellitus. Ketonemia and hepatic steatosis without ketoacidosis are common in high-producing lactating dairy cows. These changes occur in dairy cows if the dietary energy supply does not meet the needs of lactation, so the condition is exacerbated by conditions such as abomasal displacement.

Obese cats that experience a period of reduced food intake can develop severe fatty liver with ketosis and life-threatening anorexia, referred to as *fatty liver syndrome* or *feline hepatic lipidosis* (Pazak et al. 1998; Blanchard et al. 2002). Increased mobilization of TGs from adipose leads to the characteristic fatty liver with a mainly microvesicular pattern. Plasma concentrations of β-hydroxybutyrate and TGs are much increased. The effects of this syndrome are reduced by prior dietary supplementation with L-carnitine that is required for transport of LCFAs into the mitochondria (Blanchard et al. 2002).

Increased cell turnover can lead to excessive deposits of complex oxidized phospholipid-derived debris termed *lipofuscin* in lysosomes of hepatocytes and Kupffer cells. This is sometimes termed "wear and tear" pigment because it accumulates later in life and prematurely with chronic liver injury associated with increased cell turnover. Phospholipid debris can also accumulate in lysosomes if lysosomal hydrolases are genetically defective or if their activity is reduced by alkalinization of the lysosomal interior. Phospholipidosis can occur in rodents, dogs, and people exposed to zwitterionic drugs, such as amiodarone, that buffer lysosomal pH above the effective range for lysosomal phospholipases (Schneider 1992).

dysfunction, steatosis is likely an adaptive change of a healthy liver, responding appropriately to an energy debt by increased mobilization of TGs. However, sometimes an underlying adverse condition such as ketoacidosis is associated with an increased distribution of TGs to the liver.

Well-fed animals store substantial amounts of TG in their adipose tissue and mobilize LCFAs in times of metabolic demand. For example, during lactation, egg production, or pregnancy, demand for TGs and glucose is particularly high. Inadequate caloric intake (e.g., lack of access to feed) coupled with high demand stimulates gluconeogenesis and conversion of fatty acids to *ketones* (acetone, acetoacetate, and β-hydroxybutyrate). In ruminants, volatile fatty acids from rumenal fermentation can also be converted. The keto acids function as highly diffusible, water-soluble

Carbohydrates. The supply and control of blood glucose are major liver functions. Regulated hepatocyte membrane transporters take up dietary glucose from the blood. *Insulin* from the endocrine pancreas increases glucose uptake by other cells, whereas *glucagon* and glucocorticoids stimulate glucose uptake and the synthesis and storage of glycogen in hepatocytes. Catecholamines and other factors activate glycogenolysis or gluconeogenesis, depending on the supply of monosaccharides from the food.

Hepatic dysfunction or diseases can sometimes lead to abnormalities in glycogen and glucose metabolism (Kaneko et al. 1997). After acute diffuse hepatic necrosis with massive loss of functional mass, signs of depression of activity of the central nervous system leading to hepatic coma can be attributed in part to energy deprivation (low blood glucose) and also to neurotoxicity (high blood ammonia). Rare loss-of-function

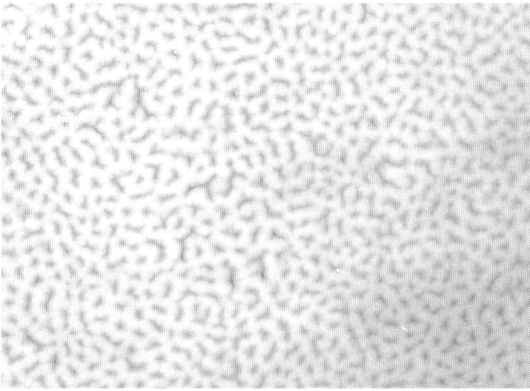

FIG. 11.12—Fatty liver from a sheep with pregnancy toxemia. Note the lobular pattern made obvious by fat accumulation in the paler area.

mutations in the liver enzyme glucose-6-phosphatase (G6Pase) have been associated with glycogen storage in hepatocytes in some families of Maltese dogs (Kishnani et al. 2001). These dogs have severely debilitating problems in maintaining their blood glucose because dephosphorylation of glucose-6-phosphate is a key step in both glycogenolysis and gluconeogenesis. The condition is typified by severe hepatocellular glycogenosis resembling G6Pase deficiency in people (von Gierke's disease or glycogen storage disease type Ia).

The liver undergoes normal daily fluctuations in the amounts of stored glycogen. In fed animals, hepatocytes contain substantial and varying amounts of glycogen that is consumed during periods of starvation or anorexia. High plasma concentrations of glucocorticoids, either as medication or endogenously generated, will induce hepatocytes to produce and store excessive amounts of glycogen, a change referred to as *glycogenosis*. Glucocorticoids also increase expression of various hepatocellular proteins, including the release of a form of inducible alkaline phosphatase (AP) into the serum in dogs. These changes are referred to as *steroid hepatopathy* (Rutgers et al. 1995). Despite the ominous name, there is only a mild influence on required hepatic functions, but some hepatocytes that are overly distended by severe glycogenosis undergo degeneration, membrane lysis, and ALT release. An observation of an increase in steroid-inducible AP in serum or marked hepatocellular glycogenosis in a liver biopsy can be diagnostically useful. For example, they might indicate the presence of a functional adrenocorticotropic hormone (ACTH)-secreting pituitary adenoma, a cortisol-secreting adrenal adenoma, or the effects of glucocorticoid treatment.

Proteins and Amino Acids. The liver plays a central role in the metabolic conversion and distribution of amino acids and in the central production and catabo-

lism of proteins. Some of the key enzymes involved in interconversion of amino acids (e.g., ALT) or management of nitrogen wastes via the urea cycle (e.g., arginase) are clinically useful indicators of liver cell necrosis because they are abundant and selectively distributed in the liver.

Hepatocytes have substantial amounts of structural and functional proteins required for their considerable metabolic repertoire. Amino acids are not stored in the liver, except as constituents of liver proteins. Accordingly, in severe malnutrition, the liver undergoes marked *atrophy* due to catabolism of hepatocellular protein after the more readily utilized glycogen and lipids are consumed. Organelles are degraded by autophagocytosis and lysosomal catabolism. Amino acids are also salvaged from apoptotic cell fragments and endocytosed plasma proteins. Cytoplasmic proteins, including those in the nucleus and cytoskeleton, are degraded by proteasomes. This involves covalent coupling of the peptide *ubiquitin* to altered cytosolic proteins that are then tagged for proteolysis. These processes evidently proceed with remarkable reliability and efficiency, because few liver problems have been related to impairments in these normal catabolic processes. Lysosomal deposits composed of lipofuscin, hemosiderin, and other matter increase with hepatocellular turnover as undegradable debris accumulates. Aggregates of undegraded cytoplasmic proteins known as *Mallory bodies* are found in hepatocytes when some hepatotoxins such as ethanol and griseofulvin interfere with protein degradation by the ubiquitin-proteasome pathway (French 2000).

The liver is a major site of production and disposal of most plasma protein except γ-globulins. Newly synthesized plasma proteins, which are formed and glycosylated in the endoplasmic reticulum (ER), acquire their mostly globular shape under the influence of various molecular chaperones, such as GRP78, calreticulin, and calnexin, in the ER of all secretory cells, including hepatocytes. Some of these ER chaperones are induced in injured hepatocytes as part of the *ER stress response* (Lee 2001), and some are binding targets for hepatotoxins that are activated in the ER (Koen and Hanzlik 2002). Newly synthesized glycoproteins are secreted through the Golgi apparatus and exported into the plasma via exocytosis of small secretory vesicles. A characteristic of many plasma proteins, both during production in the liver and in circulation, is their propensity to distribute as many differently charged forms evident as *charge trains* by two-dimensional electrophoresis (Fountoulakis et al. 2001).

Most major plasma proteins secreted by the liver are produced in ample supply, so few protein-deficiency syndromes are associated with acute liver disease. Various functions provided by *albumin*, the most abundant plasma protein, deteriorate when the liver is unable to maintain supply. Albumin is a major contributor to plasma oncotic pressure and prevents loss of fluid into the extravascular spaces. Reduced supply of albumin by the liver can lead to low plasma albumin (*hypoalbu-*

minemia), a condition that is more frequently the result of plasma protein-losing conditions, such as intestinal mucosal damage or renal glomerular leakage. Hypoalbuminemia can lead to tissue edema and in conjunction with portal hypertension contributes to the pathogenesis of ascites in some types of chronic liver disease. Because albumin is an important carrier of various substances in plasma, hypoalbuminemia can be responsible for altered hypersensitivity to some drugs and various lipophilic xenobiotics that distribute bound to albumin in the peripheral blood.

Most *coagulation proteins* in the plasma are synthesized in the liver, so some forms of liver failure are associated with coagulopathy (bleeding tendency) (Dodds 1997). Blotchy hemorrhages can develop in various tissues when the supply of fibrinogen, prothrombin, and various other clotting factors is consumed. After severe liver necrosis, hemostasis is activated within the damaged liver while regeneration of clotting factors by hepatocytes is impaired. Platelets can also be consumed in severely damaged livers. Thus, hemorrhages with increases in the prothrombin time can be observed in animals with severe hepatic necrosis of toxic or viral etiology (e.g., infectious canine hepatitis) (Dodds 1997).

Several clotting factors, including prothrombin and factors VII, IX, and X, acquire their necessary calcium-binding activity posttranslationally by a vitamin K-dependent pathway in hepatocytes. Warfarin and various other coumarin derivatives that are anticoagulants inhibit vitamin K epoxide reductase, a nicotinamide adenine dinucleotide dehydrogenase (NADH)-dependent liver enzyme that is required to maintain vitamin K in the hydroquinone form. Reduced vitamin K is a cofactor for γ-glutamylcarboxylase, the enzyme involved in adding an additional carboxyl group to glutamate residues of prothrombin. Dicarboxylated glutamate residues are the binding sites for divalent cations, especially Ca^{++}.

Thus, in warfarin toxicity and vitamin K deficiency, the calcium-binding clotting factors are secreted in an inactive form.

The liver is an important organ of the innate immune system and produces various antimicrobial factors, including complement factors, antiproteases, microbe-binding lectins, pentraxins, and many more. A large proportion of the plasma globulins consists of antiproteases, needed to neutralize proteases activated locally in hemostasis, acute inflammation, complement activation, phagocytosis, and tissue repair. Plasma antiproteases are normally present in substantial excess of what is usually required, so an unusual amount of protease activation is required to consume antiproteases before a problem with supply becomes manifest. Local inflammatory and infectious disease reactions can usually be localized by these antiproteases even when production is diminished by liver injury. Antiproteases such as α_1-proteinase inhibitor (α_1-antitrypsin), α_1-antichymotrypsin, and α_2-macroglobulin can be depleted by pancreatic trypsin, chymotrypsin, and elas-

tase released into tissues during acute pancreatitis, but the functional consequences of this are unclear.

The liver is an important site of removal of many proteins it secretes or that are released into the circulation by other tissues. However, the capacity and efficiency of these receptor-mediated clearance pathways (see Table 11.5) are such that liver disease rarely leads to a recognized problem with protein uptake and disposal. Most plasma proteins are glycosylated with attached N-linked glycans composed of complex polysaccharides covalently coupled to asparagine residues. These glycans are enriched with terminal sialic acids that shroud internal galactose, mannose or N-acetylamidosaccharide residues from endocytotic receptors expressed constitutively on hepatocytes and Kupffer cells. Thus, the liver removes "expired" plasma globulins when they lose labile sialic acids through normal wear and tear. The hepatocyte asialoglycoprotein receptor (or galactose receptor) is the most important protein clearance pathway in mammals. Other hepatocellular clearance receptors can engage mannose or sulfated polysaccharides (Weigel and Yik 2002). Some infective stages of hepatic viruses or protozoa can use endocytotic receptors as portals of entry, if they express surface glycans that mimic those on the host proteins that are cleared. Degradation of glycans can be impaired by genetic defects in lysosomal hydrolases. For example, various mucopolysaccharidoses in dogs and cats result in marked vacuolation of hepatocytes and Kupffer cells because undegraded aminoglycans accumulate in their lysosomes (Haskins et al. 1992).

Acute-phase proteins are secreted plasma proteins that change during the acute phase of inflammation (Heegaard et al. 1998, 2000). Those that change rapidly and substantially are referred to as sensitive responders. For example, serum amyloid protein A (SAA) has a short plasma half-life and is normally secreted in very low amounts, but can rapidly increase over 100-fold during the acute-phase response in most mammals. Other sensitive responders are C-reactive protein (CRP) and haptoglobin in some species, but the magnitude of the increase varies among species (Table 11.7). By comparison, fibrinogen is normally present in relatively high concentrations in plasma and has a relatively long half-life in circulation (Horadagoda et al. 1999). Concentrations decline as fibrinogen is consumed during hemostasis, but subsequently may increase two- to threefold when the liver is stimulated to produce more. Unlike the sensitive responder proteins that decline soon after the stimulus wanes, elevations in plasma fibrinogen and other slow responders can last for over a week. The kinetics of response of various plasma proteins that increase or decline during acute inflammation is diagnostically informative in several ways. Sensitive responders can be used to discover and monitor inflammatory diseases, although these responses are not necessarily specific for inflammation. The impact of subclinical inflammatory responses to infections on growth performance can be measured by elevations in some of these acute-phase proteins. Haptoglobin, major acute-

TABLE 11.7—Sensitive acute-phase proteins of different species

C-reactive protein (CRP) in humans and pigs
Serum amyloid P (SAP) in mice
Serum amyloid A (SAA) in most species
Haptoglobin in ruminants
α_2-Macroglobulin (α_2M) in rats
Major acute-phase protein (MAP) in pigs

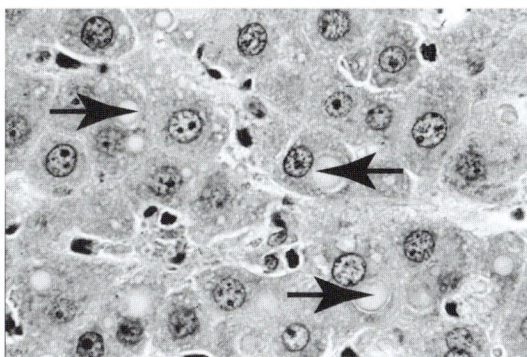

FIG. 11.13—Retained protein secretory vacuoles (arrows) caused by a microtubule poison (colcemid).

phase protein (MAP), CRP, and others have been used to monitor health status of populations of pigs and cattle (Heegaard et al. 1998; Horadagoda et al. 1999). Some acute-phase plasma proteins such as fibrinogen can be monitored to assess the status of the functions they provide (Table 11.8).

The release of plasma proteins is sometimes impaired. For example, secretory vacuoles containing proteins made in the liver can be retained if the microtubule systems involved in exocytosis are abnormal (Figure 11.13). Microtubule toxins such as colchicine have been used therapeutically to reduce the secretion of ECM proteins in canine cirrhosis (Leveille and Arias 1993).

BILE PRODUCTION AND ELIMINATION. The *bile* is a complex mixture of bile acids, waste products (bilirubin, xenobiotic conjugates, and lysosomal debris), and other functional molecules (antibodies and cytokines) that are secreted (or excreted) into the small intestine. *Bile acids* are products of cholesterol required for absorption of fat from the intestinal tract, where they dissociate TG into small micelles that are then able to complex with transport lipoproteins in the intestinal wall (Sutherland 1989; Center 1993; Thompson 1996). The resulting chylomicrons are the major form of absorbed fat in the intestinal lymph. Thus, bile duct obstructions can lead to steatorrhea (fat in the feces) and other complications associated with impaired fat absorption.

The primary *bile acids* in domestic animals are cholic acid and chenodeoxycholic acid, mostly conjugated with amino acids such as taurine and glycine (Figure 11.14). Mostly, these are absorbed in the ileum and undergo enteroportal recycling to the liver. Some are modified by microflora in the large intestine to the secondary bile acids, lithocholic acid and deoxycholic acid, respectively. These secondary bile acids can also be reabsorbed and returned to the liver. Specialized transmembrane transporter proteins (Table 11.4) move bile acid anions into the hepatocyte and across the canalicular membrane into the bile (Trauner et al. 1998, 2001).

Bilirubin is a catabolic product of heme, the major iron porphyrin of animals (Tennant 1997). Most heme comes from hemoglobin, with some from myoglobin and cytochromes. Mammals degrade heme to a yellow-brown pigment termed bilirubin and to biliverdin, a darker green precursor. Birds produce mainly biliverdin, so their bile tends to be greener. If erythrocytes are hemolyzed intravascularly, hemoglobin is bound to plasma haptoglobin and then taken up by hepatocytes, where it is degraded to bilirubin (Figure 11.15). If lysis occurs extravascularly in reticuloendothelial cells of bone marrow, spleen, or Kupffer cells, hydrophobic bilirubin is generated locally and transported bound to albumin. Bilirubin is conjugated with uridine 5′-diphosphate (UDP)-glucuronic acid by an ER enzyme, uridine diphosphoglucuronyl transferase (UDPGT) and exported into the bile via the canalicular

TABLE 11.8—Major groups of acute-phase proteins from the liver

Hemostatic and repair proteins
    Fibrinogen, fibronectin for blood coagulation, and provisional matrix
Inhibitors of proteases of microbes, thrombosis, complement, inflammation, and cell death
    α_2-Macroglobulins, α_1-proteinase inhibitor, α_1-antichymotrypsin, etc.
Anti-inflammatory factors
    C1-inhibitor, C4-binding protein, and α_2-macroglobulins
Antimicrobial proteins involved in microbial lysis and phagocytosis
    Complement factors 3, 4, and 9
    Lectins (mannan-binding lectin)
    Pentraxins (C-reactive protein, serum amyloid P)
Transport proteins for lipids, minerals, and drugs
    Serum amyloid A and other apolipoproteins
    Metallothioneins, haptoglobin, hemopexin, and ceruloplasmin
    α_1-Acid glycoprotein

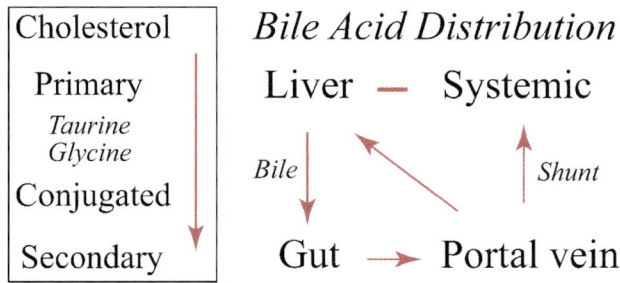

FIG. 11.14—Distribution of bile acids. Most bile acids are derived from cholesterol and conjugated with amino acids such as glycine and taurine.

multispecific organic anion transporter (cMOAT) (Trauner et al. 1998). In the intestine, bacterial β-glucuronidase can hydrolyze glucuronide conjugates, so some bilirubin can be reabsorbed into the portal vein and returned to the liver. Some bilirubin is further converted to brownish or greenish oxidation products that color the feces or are modified by enteric bacterial flora to urobilinogen that is absorbed and ultimately excreted in the urine.

Phylloerythrins are green photoactive catabolites of plant porphyrins (mainly chlorophyll) that are eliminated mostly in feces of herbivores (Kelly 1993; Tennant 1997). Some phylloerythrin is absorbed and normally excreted in the bile of herbivores. Icterus is uncommon with obstructive liver disease in ruminants, but retention of ultraviolet light-activated forms of phylloerythrin can lead to photoactive dermatitis (*hepatogenous photosensitization*).

Dysfunctions in these various bile excretion steps underlie many forms of clinical icterus (jaundice) or hepatogenous photosensitization. Icterus can result from an increased supply of heme, usually after *intravascular* or *extravascular* hemolysis. Hepatic causes of icterus are due either to impaired production of bilirubin conjugates by hepatocytes or failure of bile flow (cholestasis). Cholestatic conditions can be extrahepatic or intrahepatic, according to the level of abnormal flow (Figure 11.16).

Many hepatotoxic agents cause intracellular cholestasis by inhibiting the process of bilirubin conjugation and bile secretion into canaliculi (Crawford 1996; Tennant 1997). Various insults that damage the cytoskeleton required for canalicular kinesis cause canaliculi to become distended with retained bile. This pattern, described as intracanalicular cholestasis, can be caused by various toxicants and drugs that interfere with the polymerization or depolymerization of contractile F-actin. Other agents associated with cholestasis affect structural intermediate filaments of hepatocytes (Fickert et al. 2002). Lobular disarray as a result of toxicity by *Lantana camara*, a hepatotoxic plant that disrupts the structural integrity of hepatocyte-to-hepatocyte adhesion, can cause icterus and photosensitization in cattle (Figure 11.17) (Kelly 1993). Leaky canaliculi then allow bile pigments and phylloerythrins to leak back into the circulation.

Obstruction to outflow from major bile ducts by hepatic or pancreatic neoplasms, choleliths, and other ductal concretions, parasites, or inflammatory responses (cholangitis) causes a pattern referred to as *intraductal cholestasis*. This can also be seen after toxic injury and scarring of the biliary tracts, for example, in response to toxic doses of alsike clover, sporidesmin, and some arsenicals (Kelly 1993).

BIOTRANSFORMATION. There are numerous hepatic biotransformation systems that generate new forms of required molecules (e.g., steroid hydroxylation) or that detoxify potentially harmful chemicals of endogenous or exogenous origin (Kedderis 1996). Enzyme systems such as hepatic cytochromes P-450 are involved in the *phase I* biotransformation to reactive metabolites, most of which are intermediates in the excretion process. *Phase II conjugation* enzymes such as glutathione S-transferases, UDP-glucuronyl transferases, N-acetyltransferases, epoxide hydratases and γ-glutamyltranspeptidase (GGT) are then involved in the generation of typically less toxic but more readily excreted conjugated metabolites. For each of these classes of phase I or phase II enzymes, there are multiple genes with functionally different variably expressed products. Thus, hepatocytes with their abundant phase I and phase II systems can contend with a vast range of chemically different substrates. Some of this diversity is due to evolutionary and experiential adaptation to potentially harmful substances in the diet.

Many of these biotransformation enzymes are expressed constitutively at relatively high levels in the liver to enable efficient detoxification and elimination of a wide range of chemical substances originating in the diet or other routes of entry. Of these, some are further inducible by various chemical substances, some of which are also substrates for hepatic biotransformation.

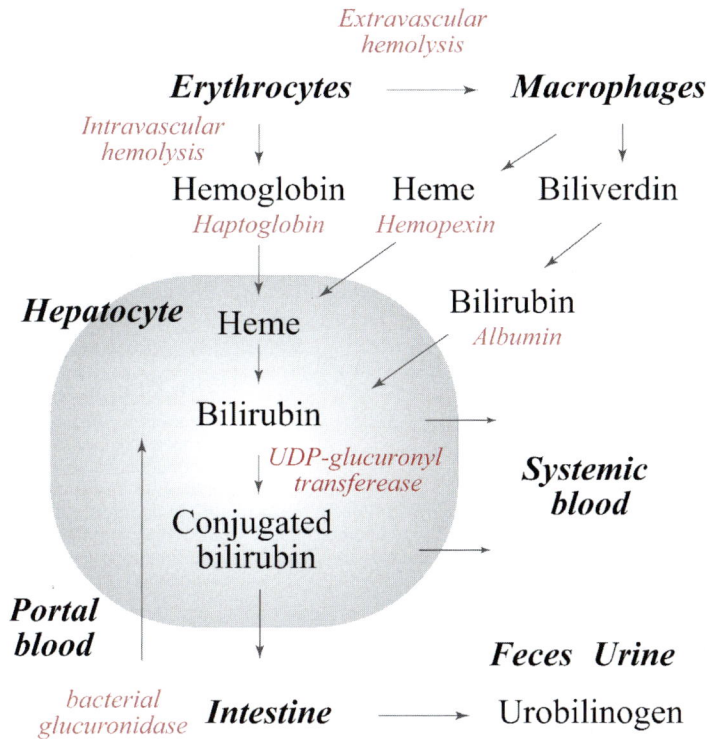

FIG. 11.15—Heme catabolism and bilirubin excretion.

Induced biotransformation activity is often a sign that the liver has been exposed to compounds or substrates capable of signaling enhanced expression of classes of biotransformation genes. Microscopically, these adaptations are often visible by an increase in smooth ER in the cytoplasm of hepatocytes in zone 3 or by increases in immunoreactive cytochrome P-450 isozymes or selected phase II enzymes. Such adaptations can have diagnostic or prognostic relevance, for example, in predicting how an individual would react to a drug or other substance that is biotransformed by the induced pathway.

Induction of microsomal biotransformation usually reduces the harmfulness of a chemical because the rates of excretion via induced phase I and phase II pathways are increased. Induction of biotransformation pathways is a frequent response of the liver to exposures to xenobiotics (De Longueville et al. 2002). Inductions are sometimes regarded as adverse outcomes in some contexts, so the potential for new medications and environmental agents to alter these functions is becoming an important aspect of safety assessment. With the advent of described genomes, DNA microarrays (De Longueville et al. 2002), mass spectrometry, and other proteomic tools (Fountoulakis et al. 2001; Galeva and Altermann 2002), the impact on expression of these and other functions can now be explored in greater detail. As an example, consider the induction of cytochrome P-450

2A1 and other microsomal enzymes in dogs on phenobarbital medication for epilepsy (Gieger et al. 2000; Muller et al. 2000). These adaptations can reduce effects of many drugs that are biotransformed and excreted by detoxification pathways that are induced by phenobarbital. This can jeopardize the benefits sought by such medications. Phenobarbital induction increases the toxicity of high doses of acetaminophen and other experimental hepatotoxins such as carbon tetrachloride and bromobenzene (Koen and Hanzlik 2002). Chronic exposure to phenobarbital leads to faster rates of hepatic removal of thyroid hormones from the plasma (Gieger et al. 2000; Muller et al. 2000) and can predispose some dogs to necroinflammatory liver disease (Dayrell-Hart et al. 1991) even though phenobarbital is not usually so toxic.

Some animals and people can lack necessary phase II functions to deal with the increased amounts of phase I metabolites. These phase II deficiencies can result from depletion of cofactors such as glutathione required for glutathione S-transferase conjugation or constitutive differences in the phase II genotypes. For example, depletion of glutathione for conjugation of acetaminophen can increase its toxicity by enabling a greater amount of phase-I-reactive metabolites to interact chemically with various functional macromolecules (Figure 11.18). Species differences in biotransformation systems can also result in differences in suscepti-

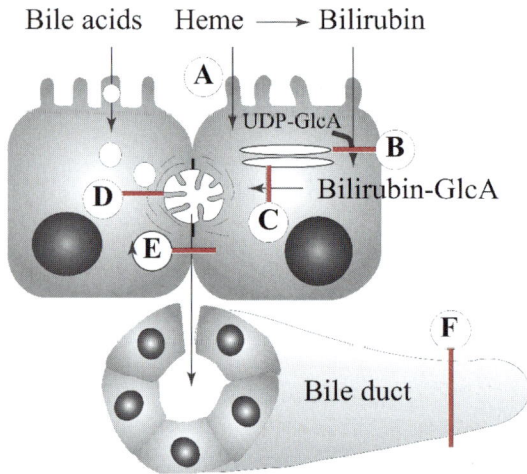

FIG. 11.16—Mechanisms of interference with bile excretion. Excess heme from breakdown of hemoglobin and myoglobin in blood is transported bound to carrier proteins (hemopexin) to the liver, where it is internalized. Most heme is catabolized to bilirubin by phagocytes. Bilirubin is then metabolically conjugated with glucuronic acid and actively transported into the bile by the canalicular membrane organic anion transporter. Bile salts in the portal blood undergo endocytosis into vesicles that move to the pericanalicular region and transport bile salts into the canalicular space. Injury to the supply of ATP for conjugation (B), secretion (C), or canalicular kinetics (D) will impede excretion. The structural integrity of the canaliculi can be disrupted by loss of cell-cell adhesion between hepatocytes and cholangiolar cells (E) such that excreted substances return to the blood. Any physical obstruction within the excretory duct system can prevent release of formed bile into the duodenum (F). A: Icterus can occur when there is an excess of these pigments (e.g., in hemolytic loss of erythrocytes).

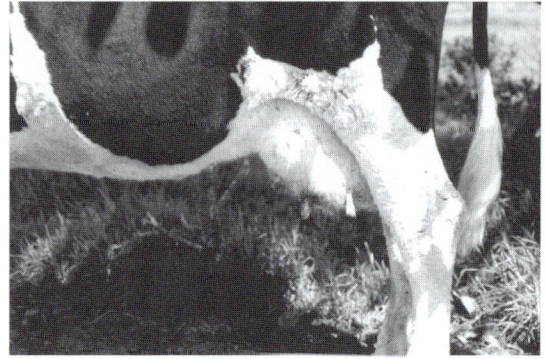

FIG. 11.17—Holstein cow with hepatogenous photosensitization due to *Lantana camara* poisoning. Phylloerythrins are heme degradation products of plant chlorophylls that can be absorbed from the intestine but excreted in the bile. Impaired biliary excretion leads to retention of phylloerythrin that causes photoactive skin injury when exposed to ultraviolet (UV) light. Note the dermatitis on the more ventral white nonpigmented skin that is most sensitive to UV exposure.

bility. Domestic cats express fewer hepatic isoforms of glucuronyl transferase compared with other species, and this difference explains in part the higher sensitivity of cats to the adverse effects of various drugs, including acetaminophen, that are detoxified by glucuronidation (Figure 11.18). The evolutionary basis for such species differences might result from the highly carnivorous makeup of the natural feline diet with minimal selection pressure from dietary phytotoxins. There is also considerable genetic diversity (polymorphism) among individual people and probably domestic animals, with associated variation in susceptibility to particular drugs and toxic substances.

ADAPTATIONS. The liver can adapt by altering expression of various genes and thereby adjust the mass and balance of its many functions. The liver of laboratory rodents undergoes a pronounced growth response after exposure to various inducers (Columbano and Shinozuka 1996). This adaptation increases the size of hepatocytes (hypertrophy) and their numbers (hyperplasia) that collectively bring a larger population of hepatocytes into service. Similar but less pronounced alterations in liver cells and total mass occur in dogs exposed to various drugs such as phenobarbital or steroids. Some of the common adaptive responses that occur in the liver are listed in Table 11.9. Conversely, the liver can undergo inverse compensation through a combination of cellular atrophy and deletion. Surplus viable hepatocytes are reduced in size by membrane blebs or eliminated by apoptosis and degradation of their fragments by neighboring hepatocytes and Kupffer cells (Columbano and Shinozuka 1996). Accordingly, hepatocytes can be lost in substantial numbers with minimal, if any, elevation in serum enzymes, such as ALT, that increase markedly when hepatocytes undergo necrosis.

Compensatory Hypertrophy and Regeneration. A healthy young liver has a remarkable ability to adapt its functional mass by regeneration and hypertrophy, but the mechanisms are not fully understood (Michalopoulos and De Frances 1997; Zimmermann 2002). Hepatic regeneration is most vigorous in young animals, but subsides with age and disease to the point where the liver can become regeneratively impaired and atrophic. Cell proliferation in the resting adult liver is low (<0.1% mitotic), but most hepatocytes can replicate after a loss of a segment of functional mass due to necrosis or resection (Michalopoulos and De Frances 1997; Laconi 2000; Zimmermann 2002). The residual tissue regenerates quickly by a transient induction of DNA synthesis and mitosis of resident cells. Many of the signaling mechanisms underlying these responses have been characterized in recent years, and the princi-

Acetaminophen *Glucuronyl transferase* → Conjugates in bile

Cyt P-450 ↓ *Sulfotransferase*

Semiquinone

Redox cycling ↓ *Glutathione S-transferase* → Glutathione conjugates

N-acetyl-benzo-quinone-imine

↓ → Oxidative damage *Glutathione depletion*

Covalent adducts

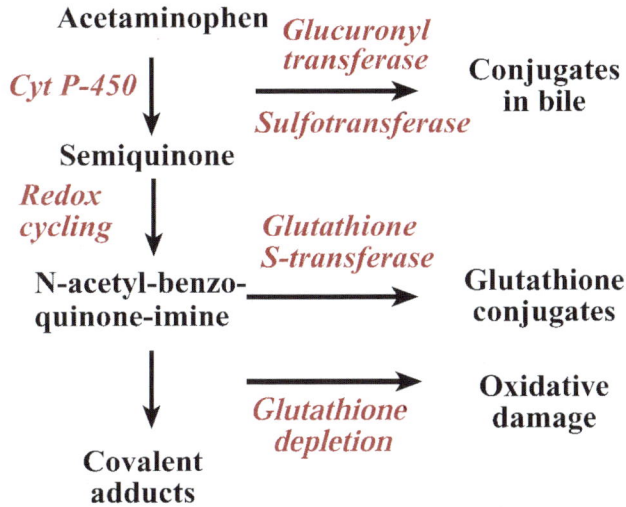

FIG. 11.18—Major biotransformation pathways for excretion and hepatotoxicity of acetaminophen. Metabolic biotransformation occurs by hepatic phase I (cytochrome P-450) and various phase II pathways [uridine-5′-diphosphate (UDP)-glucuronyl transferase, sulfotransferase, glutathione S-transferases]. Saturation of primary conjugation routes increases cytochrome P-450-mediated generation of a cytotoxic form that is detoxified by glutathione conjugation. Higher doses then lead to depletion of glutathione and so reactive acetaminophen metabolites can bind to cell proteins. Glutathione depletion increases oxidative stress, in part due to the generation of oxygen radicals during redox cycling of the metabolites, and in part because glutathione is required for glutathione peroxidase and the detoxification of organic peroxides. Some individuals or species that lack particular pathways can be more susceptible to a given dose. Other drugs that deplete cofactors potentiate toxicity. Sometimes, reactive metabolites that covalently modify proteins can be antigenic haptens.

ples behind these mechanisms serve as a paradigm for understanding the relationships between an organ function and the messages it receives from the host.

Mass of the liver is maintained within a range determined by functional requirements through a balance between multiple positive and negative signals (Michalopoulos and De Frances 1997; Laconi 2000; Zimmermann 2002). Tissue regeneration is through replication of constituent cell populations, not through reproduction of new anatomic lobules, lobes, and regeneration. Growth stimuli act rapidly by acting on preformed constituents in the target tissue. The immediate early response genes are induced and their products can be detected within minutes of partial hepatectomy. These include relocation of the urokinase receptor to the hepatocyte plasma membrane. Subsequently, urokinase activity increases, and ECM is degraded to release heparin-bound hepatocyte growth factor (HGF), also known as scatter factor. HGF then interacts with the HGF receptor expressed on hepatocytes and, in conjunction with other signals such as insulin, cortisol, and catecholamines, stimulates a wave or two of proliferation of hepatocytes and nonparenchymal cells.

Regulated Gene Expression. Hepatic adaptive mechanisms depend on physiologically regulated expression of genes involved in differentiated and proliferative functions. Some are mediated by various endogenous or exogenous *nuclear receptor* ligands. These include steroid hormone receptors, such as estrogen, androgen,

and glucocorticoid receptors, and the thyroxine receptor. Liganded receptors are transported into the nucleus, where they form dimer complexes that control gene expression by acting as gene-transcription factors that recognize specific transcriptional response elements (TREs) on various genes (Figure 11.19). Thus, activated glucocorticoid receptors engage specific glucocorticoid response elements of glucocorticoid-responsive genes, for example.

Other related nuclear receptors include the arylhydrocarbon-activated receptor (AhR), which is involved in inducing various hepatic biotransformation enzymes, particularly those induced by various halogenated polycyclic aromatic compounds that are ligands for the AhR (Hankinson 1995). PPARs are expressed abundantly in the liver, where they are a target for various lipid ligands, including unsaturated LCFAs (e.g., linoleic acid) and some eicosanoids (Leone et al. 1999; Boitier et al. 2003). Various hypolipidemic drugs and peroxisomal-proliferating xenobiotics (Cattley et al. 1995) are also activating ligands for these PPARs in the liver. Activation of PPAR-α in rodent liver is associated with peroxisome proliferation and with suppression of apoptosis and induction of hepatocyte proliferation (Boitier et al. 2003).

Many polar molecules that activate cell *surface membrane receptors*, including various endocrine peptides, cytokines, catecholamines, and others, also signal adaptive modulations of hepatocyte gene expression. The best described of many such examples are insulin and glucagon, which are important modulators

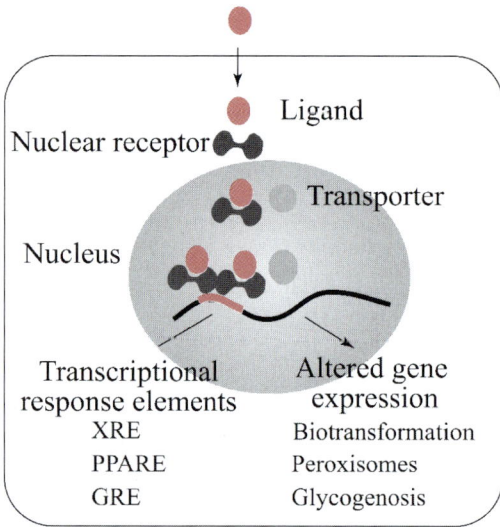

FIG. 11.19—General mechanism of nuclear receptor-mediated adaptations in hepatocytes. GRE, glucocorticoid responsive element; PPARE, peroxisomal-proliferator-activated receptor element; and XRE, xenobiotic responsive element.

TABLE 11.9—Major adaptive alterations in liver functions

Glycogen
  Glucose reserves
    e.g., Glucocorticoids of endogenous or exogenous origins
Triglyceride
  Lipid storage and transport
    e.g., Increased fat mobilization during lactation and egg production
Secreted proteins
  Acute-phase proteins
    e.g., Inflammatory cytokines and microbial components
Smooth endoplasmic reticulum
  Phase I biotransformation
    e.g., Cytochrome P-450 (CYP450s) induced by xenobiotic ligands for arylhydrocarbon receptor (AhR)
  Phase II biotransformation
    e.g., UDP-glucuronidation (conjugation) induced by xenobiotics
Pericanalicular membrane transporters
  Phase III excretion
    e.g., γ-Glutamyltranspeptidase (GGT), alkaline phosphatase (AP), and multidrug-resistance protein 1 (MDR1) induced by xenobiotics and cholestasis
Lysosomes
  Sequestration of nutrients and lipid residues
    e.g., Iron and copper storage
  Catabolism
    e.g., Increased cell or organelle turnover by apoptosis
Peroxisomes
  Long-chain fatty-acid catabolism (β oxidation)
    e.g., Induced by xenobiotics and endogenous ligands for peroxisomal-proliferator-associated receptors (PPARs)
Stress proteins
  Glucose-responsive proteins
  Some glutathione S-transferases and antioxidants
  Metallothioneins

of hepatic glucose and fat metabolism. Other growth factors—such as epidermal growth factor (EGF), HGF, and transforming growth factors α (TGF-α) induce the replicative phenotype of differentiated hepatocytes (Michalopoulos and De Frances 1997). Inflammatory cytokines such as IL-6, IL-1, and tumor-necrosis factor (TNF) participate in the induction of the acute-phase response. During the acute phase of inflammation, IL-6 and related cytokines are secreted by macrophages that are stimulated by bacterial LPS. These cytokines then induce the increased production of various acute-phase plasma proteins that are consumed during tissue injury (Table 11.8). These genes are regulated by the active form of a gene-transcription factor known as NF-κB, generated by degradation of the inhibitor I-κB (Figure 11.20). In this manner, the liver adapts to requirements for augmented host defense. Hepatocytes can also undergo apoptosis in response to TNF-α and the Fas ligand (Bradham et al. 1998).

HEPATIC DYSFUNCTIONS AND DISEASE. As the liver responds to different physiological demands, it will adjust its numerous functions according to the homeostatic responses available (Tennant 1997). However, in various disease situations, these functional adaptations may be temporarily, qualitatively, or quantitatively insufficient. Major functions of the liver, and of other tissues dependent on the liver, can deteriorate and eventually fail in irreversible ways. Hepatic dysfunctions can be characterized largely on the basis of irregularities in rates of clearance, excretion, secretion, and nutrient processing. Keep in mind however, that other phenomena will change in relation to the insults and injury involved, and the adaptive responses activated under these conditions.

Circulatory Abnormalities. Various hepatic dysfunctions are directly related to problems with circulation (Table 11.10). For example, hepatocytes normally remove ammonia and other toxic products of microbial flora of the digestive tract. Diversion of ammonia in portal blood into the systemic circulation underlies the pathogenesis of *hepatic encephalopathy* (Taboada and Dimski 1995; Howe et al. 1997). This can occur in liver cirrhosis in which the resistance to portal venous perfusion is increased.

The blood flow rate through the gut and thence to the liver is high, especially during the regular digestion and

TABLE 11.10—Some dysfunctions in liver circulation

Increased hepatic venous pressure
  Hepatic venous occlusion
  Right-sided heart failure
Increased portal venous pressure
Portal–systemic venous shunting
Abnormal plasma oncotic pressure
  Hypoalbuminemia and edema or ascites

assimilation of food. Major shifts in the distribution of blood flow occur in systemic circulatory conditions, especially congestive cardiac failure, hypovolemic shock, and peripheral vasodilatory conditions such as septic shock. In passive congestion affecting the left side of the heart, central venous pressure increases

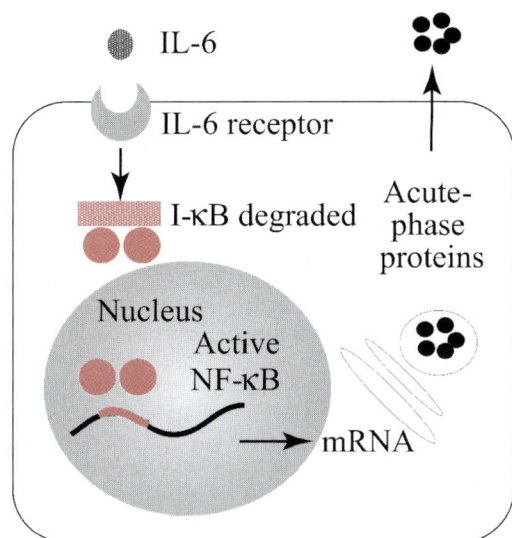

FIG. 11.20—General mechanism of cytokine-induced production of acute-phase proteins by hepatocytes. IL-6 (interleukin 6) is one cytokine that binds cell surface receptors and activates a signaling pathway that alters transcription of various acute-phase responsive genes. Those that respond have sequences that can interact with the gene transcription factor NF-κB after it becomes activated by degradation of a blocking factor, I-κB.

diffuse, venous, and sinusoidal congestion in the liver. In the short term, large volumes of blood are retained in the liver and lead to various degrees of structural alteration referred to as *chronic passive hepatic congestion* (Kelly 1993). This can lead to steatosis and interstitial edema, sinusoidal breakdown (peliosis), sinusoidal thrombosis and, ultimately, interstitial fibrosis (sometimes referred to as cardiac cirrhosis). Although the liver undoubtedly suffers from some functional compromise, few clinically important hepatic dysfunctions are more important than the extrahepatic circulatory dysfunctions associated with right-sided heart failure.

Several vascular irregularities occur in or near the liver (Kelly 1993) (see Figure 11.1 and Table 11.11). Cats and dogs sometimes are born with direct connections or *shunts* between the portal vein and major or minor branches of the hepatic outflow within the liver, or external to the liver via the azygos vein or vena cava (Boothe et al. 1996). If the shunt is a large channel, such as a persistent ductus venosus within the liver, the portal and the central venous pressures are similar, and the liver and the portal vascular bed are typically atrophic. Some breeds have a congenital hypoplasia of the portal vasculature that in turn leads to sustained elevation in portal pressure above that of the central venous system. Others have functional stenosis of outflow veins or other abnormalities in the hepatic microvasculature (Allen et al. 1999; Christiansen et al. 2000). In time, this leads to *portal venous hypertension* and increased blood flow through smaller anastomoses in the mesentery, which are more commonly present toward the esophagus, splenic mesentery, or rectum. As these dilate into many small or large bypass shunts, hepatic portal flow subsides and the liver undergoes atrophy. This pattern of *acquired shunts* can also occur secondary to inflamma-

TABLE 11.11—Vascular abnormalities in the liver

Persistent ductus venosus
    Single large intrahepatic portal-venous shunt
    Hypoplastic intrahepatic portal veins
Congenital extrahepatic shunts
    Large shunts between portal vein and vena cava, usually via the azygos vein
    Hypoplastic intrahepatic portal veins
Microvascular dysplasia
    Usually microscopic shunts within the liver
    Prominent hepatic venules
    Enlarged periacinar lymphatics and vascular smooth muscle
    Increased perivascular fibrous tissue
Aterioportal anastomoses
    Anomalous anastomosis of hepatic artery to intrahepatic portal vein
    Segment of liver with tortuous pulsatile arterialized veins
    Marked portal hypertension, and ascites
Multiple acquired shunts secondary to hepatic venous occlusion
    Small liver with cirrhosis or atrophy
    Multiple portocaval shunts along mesentery
    Fibrosis around portal and/or hepatic veins
Diffuse venous congestion (outflow resistance)
    All hepatic vessels are prominent
    Hepatic veins and sinusoids are congested
Peliosis and telangiectasis
    Cavernous hepatic sinusoids
    Vascular encroachment where parenchymal cells are lost

tory liver diseases in which there is cirrhosis along the portal or central tracts. In the latter, centrilobular veno-occlusive fibrosis initially causes sinusoidal congestion and portal hypertension until the collateral shunts develop and relieve the portal and sinusoidal pressure. If the occlusive condition is in the portal tracts, the liver undergoes more severe atrophy likely due to weaker trophic influences from the gut.

Rarely, dogs may have focal anastomoses between the hepatic arterial supply and the portal or hepatic venous branches in or near the liver (Moore and Whiting 1986). This condition is typically focal and restricted to a lobe or two of the liver. The arterial pressure elevates the portal blood and central venous pressure, and contributes to efflux of fluid into the abdominal cavity (ascites).

The pathophysiological implications of these shunting conditions vary widely. In the milder conditions, such as microvascular dysplasia, the liver mass is only mildly affected if at all (Christiansen et al. 2000). Ammonia and bile acids can bypass the liver and increase in the systemic circulation. Intermittent mild encephalopathy with seizurelike activity can occur due to ammonia toxicity. These manifestations can be more severe in cases with larger congenital or acquired shunts, and if the animal is fed a high protein diet from which more ammonia can be generated. When the shunts are the result of hepatic obstructive disease, other indicators of hepatic necroinflammatory disease may be found as well. Conditions that lead to portal hypertension are often associated with ascites.

Shunting can divert essential trophic factors, such as EGF, insulin, glucagon, and other peptides from the pancreas and intestinal Brunner's glands. Lack of trophic stimuli, coupled with diversion of portal blood, contributes to hepatic atrophy that is a common finding in dogs with portosystemic shunts. Unless the shunts are found at the end stage of fibrotic and atrophic liver disease, there is usually no serious impairment of hepatic biotransformation, excretory, secretory, clearance, or nutritional functions.

Hepatic Encephalopathy. High ammonia levels are toxic to the brain and produce hepatic encephalopathy and hepatic coma (Taboada and Dimski 1995; Howe et al. 1997). Gut microbes make ammonia and toxic thiols that are normally removed by the liver on first pass through the portal circulation. Ammonia is also generated by deamination of surplus amino acids in the liver. The resulting ammonia from these sources is then incorporated with carbon dioxide into carbamoyl phosphate and enters the *urea cycle* in the liver. Carbamoyl phosphate combines with ornithine to form citrulline and then arginine. The liver-specific enzyme arginase then splits arginine to regenerate ornithine and release *urea*, the major mammalian waste nitrogen product that is excreted by the kidney.

The major cause of high blood ammonia is insufficient removal of ammonia by the liver. Vascular shunts and insufficient hepatic mass are the usual causes, but levels can be increased when amino acid catabolism is higher. When the liver loses its ability to adequately destroy ammonia and other toxic products of gastrointestinal microflora, these products reach the brain and cause toxic injury especially to the white matter in the brain stem, which undergoes microvacuolation (Kelly 1993). Ammonia readily crosses the blood-brain barrier and interferes with neurotransmission, and also leads to local injury with vacuolation in the neuropil of the white matter of the brain stem. Hyperammonemia can result directly from liver necrosis or atrophy, or indirectly from shunting of portal blood away from the liver and into the systemic venous return. Neurological signs associated with hepatic disease are also affected by other problems, such as impaired glucose metabolism.

Necroinflammatory Diseases. Hepatocytes are often victims of insults that cause cell death. They are in the direct line of exposure to ingested infectious agents and toxic substances, and their high rates of phase I activation give them a high capacity to generate toxic levels of reactive intermediates of many xenobiotics (Kedderis 1996). Also, hepatocytes have a high requirement for oxygen and are vulnerable to ischemia in hypovolemic and passive congestive conditions.

Hepatocytes have long been used to study some of the pathogenetic pathways involved in cell death. Hepatocytes undergo classical *coagulation necrosis* in various focal and zonal patterns, or *apoptosis* in single cell patterns (Kanzler and Galle 2000; Kaplowitz 2000). Necrosis and apoptosis can be recognized by characteristic cytological details in hepatocytes. For example, necrosis is associated with catastrophic failure of cell-membrane partitions, with leakage of cytosolic contents, secondary inflammation, and relatively slow removal of cell debris by macrophages that can elicit scarring reactions. By comparison, apoptotic cell death is associated with fragmentation of hepatocytes into smaller membrane-enclosed apoptotic bodies. These undergo phosphatidylserine redistribution to the outer surface of the plasma membrane so they can be rapidly phagocytosed by adjacent hepatocytes and macrophages with minimal leakage of cytoplasmic contents. Apoptotic hepatocytes are thus rapidly removed by lysosomal degradation with some increase in accumulated lysosomal debris but otherwise minimal tissue response.

The most typical patterns of cell death of hepatocytes and the ensuing reactions give some diagnostic clues as to pathogenesis. However, it is increasingly clear that apoptosis and necrosis are reflections of the degree of cytological insult (Kaplowitz 2002). Severe alterations in membrane permeability from various causes lead to necrosis, whereas similar insults to a milder degree can result in apoptosis, the more subtle and physiological process of cell turnover in many parenchymal tissues, including the liver.

The pattern of cell death can be an important indicator of the subsequent processes that can affect the liver. For example, multifocal necroinflammatory lesions usually represent embolic infections from the alimentary tract. Zonal (or submassive) necrosis usually results from toxic or ischemic insults; however, some adverse drug reactions are multifocal for reasons that are not understood. Zone 1 necrosis is rare but can be caused by direct-acting hepatotoxic agents, particularly after they arrive via the portal blood from the alimentary tract. Direct-acting hepatotoxicants include *Amanita phalloides* (mushroom) and various metals (e.g., ferrous sulfate). Some indirect-acting hepatotoxicants such as allyl formate are activated in zone 1 by alcohol dehydrogenase. Most indirect-acting hepatotoxic agents are biotransformed to reactive cytotoxic metabolites by cytochrome P-450s located mainly in zone 3, where necrosis typically occurs in a matching zonal pattern. Indirect-acting toxicants such as carbon tetrachloride, acetaminophen, bromobenzene, halothane and many others cause zone 3 (periacinar) necrosis (Figure 11.21).

Hepatocytes can be killed by various chemical mechanisms. Microsomal activation by cytochrome P-450 can be associated with cogeneration of reactive oxygen species such as superoxide, hydrogen peroxide, lipid peroxides, peroxynitrite anions, and hydroxyl radicals. Some toxins such as carbon tetrachloride can be activated to free radical metabolites, whereas bromobenzene, acetaminophen, and halothane are converted to electrophilic metabolites that covalently bind to various essential hepatocellular macromolecules (Qiu et al. 1998; Koen and Hanzlik 2002). Those metabolites that are conjugated with glutathione, such as the semiquinone metabolites of acetaminophen, can deplete reduced glutathione levels to such a degree that further conjugation and glutathione-dependent peroxidase activity is ineffective (Figure 11.18) (Pumford et al. 1997).

When antioxidant systems are insufficient to counteract the free radical insults, peroxidative damage degrades the cell-membrane partitions and impairs the

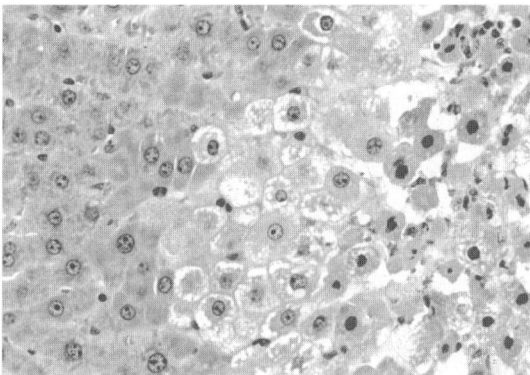

FIG. 11.21—Zone 3 hepatic necrosis due to acetaminophen toxicity.

performance of ion pumps required to maintain very low cytosolic calcium-ion concentrations. When cytosolic calcium-ion concentrations increase dramatically, hepatocytes undergo classical *coagulation necrosis*. This process is exacerbated by increased amounts of free ferrous iron, low levels of antioxidants such as vitamin E and glutathione [γ-glutamylcysteinylglycine (GSH)], and/or inadequate function of selenium-dependent glutathione peroxidase (Se-GPx) or selenium-independent glutathione peroxidase (some glutathione S-transferases). Influx of calcium ions into the cytosol activates calpains that degrade various components of hepatocytes.

Membrane leakage subsequent to hepatocyte death by necrosis can be monitored by efflux of cytosolic enzymes such as ALT, AST, LDH, and arginase. Some cytosolic proteins that leak are involved in the recruitment of phagocytes into necrotic areas in the liver, and the subsequent tissue repair processes that involve ECM secretion, perisinusoidal cell activation, and fibroblast proliferation.

Focal areas of necrosis in the parenchyma, without any particular location in the lobules, is often associated with local inflammation (hepatitis) (Kelly 1993). Many bacterial and parasitic infections cause local inflammation that may evolve into abscesses, granuloma cysts, or scars. However, focal lesions usually do not compromise the major functions of the liver until they affect a sufficient amount of functional mass or lead to thrombosis.

Chronic Hepatitis. This can result from ongoing tissue repair initiated by necrosis of hepatic parenchymal cells and/or bile ducts, or from inflammatory processes directed toward antigens located in the liver. The latter include self-antigens on hepatocytes (e.g., chronic active hepatitis) or bile ductules (primary biliary cirrhosis), or foreign antigens of liver pathogens (e.g., bacteria, viruses, protozoa, and helminths). Chronic hepatic inflammation with excessive deposition of ECM and scar tissue, often accompanied by nodular hepatocellular regeneration and ductular hyperplasia, is termed *cirrhosis*.

Necrogenic hepatotoxic chemicals elicit inflammation, fibrosis, vascular sclerosis, and nodular hepatocellular regeneration that over time give rise to the classical pattern of scarring among nodules of regenerating surviving hepatocytes (Table 11.12). The process of postnecrotic cirrhosis involves the production of specialized hepatic ECM by interstitial stellate cells (see Figure 11.6), or along the portal and central tracts by fibroblasts. Chronically activated stellate cells and fibroblasts can contract and then obstruct the flow of blood, bile, or lymphatic fluids in more severely affected regions (Geerts 2001). Secondary ischemic damage and segmental cholestasis can result, with compensatory proliferation of surviving hepatocytes and bile ducts. Some forms of cirrhosis are characterized by ongoing apoptosis with impaired hepatic regen-

Table 11.12—Patterns of hepatitis and cirrhosis

Portal
    Cholangiohepatitis
        Bile duct parasites (e.g., liver flukes)
        Bacterial cholangitis
        Duct toxins (e.g., sporidesmin)
        Duct autoantigens
Periacinar
    Ischemic necrosis
    Zone 3 necrosis
Panlobular
    Multifocal or diffuse interstitial hepatitis
        Viral hepatitis
        Embolic bacterial infections
        Chronic active hepatitis
    Various toxic insults
        Idiosyncratic drug toxicity
        Copper and iron storage
        Ethanol
        Hypervitaminosis A

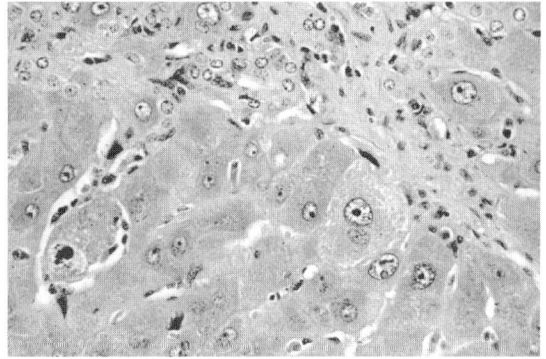

FIG. 11.22—Portal fibroplasia and bile duct proliferation with impaired regeneration of hepatocytes (megalocytosis due to pyrrolizidine alkaloid poisoning).

eration and relatively minor amounts of scarring. When the liver is reduced in functional mass, viable regions or resistant clones of hepatocytes can regenerate into nodules. These can be small (micronodular), if numerous, or large (macronodular), if there are few places from which compensatory regeneration can arise. Toxic inhibition of the ability of hepatocytes to regenerate leads to progressive reduction in the functional hepatic mass. Such injury may eventually lead to various forms of hepatic failure due to inadequate functional mass of the liver. Hepatic atrophy is more frequent in older individuals because the regenerative capacity of the liver declines with age. Atrophy is usually associated with compensatory proliferation of undifferentiated bile duct epithelial cells. Nodules of altered cells that are refractory to the inhibitory effects of the hepatotoxin may also proliferate among the proliferatively impaired hepatocytes.

Various hepatotoxins such as pyrrolizidine alkaloids (Figure 11.22) and aflatoxin cause hepatocellular apoptosis and necrosis but also impair normal liver regeneration. Most surviving hepatocytes become replicatively incompetent, but some undergo impaired nuclear division and become megalocytic (polyploid). Under these conditions, the liver mass shrinks, and the compensatory stimulus increases the replication of bile ductules (oval cells) and any populations of hepatocytes that are resistant to the inhibitory effect. The result is a small liver with regenerative nodules of hepatocytes (Figure 11.23) separated by proliferating ducts and some residual nests of replicatively impaired hepatocytes.

Idiosyncratic and other forms of hepatotoxicity are rare adverse reactions to a wide range of medications and other substances. For any one drug, problems are rare, but, collectively, hepatotoxicity is a common clinical finding. Monitoring serum ALT, GGT, and bilirubin can help in detecting early injury and hepatic dysfunction. If the exposure is ongoing, the condition can progress to cirrhosis, and impaired regeneration can lead to atrophy. Definitive implication of particular drugs as causes and predisposing dietary, genetic, and

environmental factors is difficult. However, in recent years, substantial progress has been made in informatics and in the characterization of human and other genetic polymorphisms that alter drug biotransformation. In humans, idiosyncratic hepatitis is associated with many drugs such as methyl-DOPA (3,4-dihydroxyphenylalanine), nitrofurantoin, isoniazid, phenytoin, and dapsone (MacSween et al. 2002). Similar conditions have been associated with drug therapy in dogs (Dayrell-Hart et al. 1991; Muller et al. 2000), but usually these patterns of hepatic disease are idiopathic.

Neoplasia. Major types of primary liver neoplasms arise from hepatocytes (hepatocellular adenomas and hepatocellular carcinomas), vascular endothelium (hemangiosarcomas), bile duct cells (cholangiomas

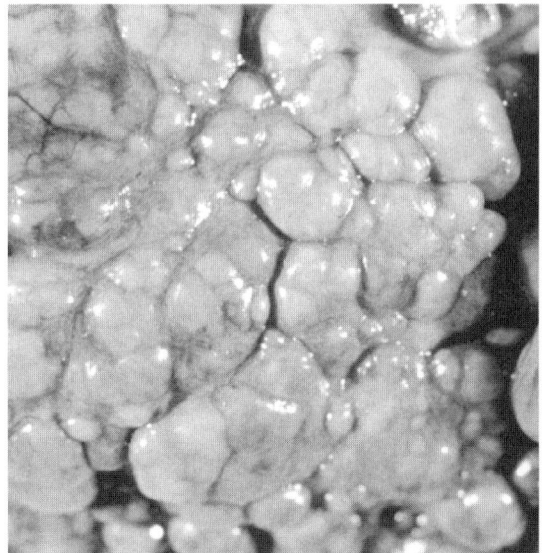

FIG. 11.23—Hepatic atrophy and macronodular

and cholangiocarcinomas), and fibroblasts (fibrosarcomas). Multicentric neoplasms that often affect the liver include sinusoidal endothelial cells (hemangiosarcomas) and hematopoietic cells (lymphomas, myeloid leukemias, etc.). The liver is a frequent site for metastatic solid neoplasms, mostly derived from stomach, intestine, and pancreas.

Hepatocellular proliferative lesions are relatively common in the liver of older dogs (Figure 11.24), but most are benign foci of atypical hyperplastic cells (Fabry et al. 1982). These arise probably as mutants, because many more such lesions develop in rodents after exposure to known mutagens. Small populations are termed altered foci, and larger expansive examples are termed hyperplastic nodules or hepatocellular adenomas. Occasionally, these lesions can become large and eventually more heterogeneous, in which case the terms hepatoma and hepatocellular carcinoma become applicable. Many of these early altered populations have induced phase II detoxification capacity and are pale because their cytochrome P-450 activity is reduced (Farber and Sarma 1987). These altered hepatocytes, together with undifferentiated ducts (oval cells) and stem cells, are sometimes more resistant to many hepatotoxins (Farber and Sarma 1987). Thus, hepatotoxins such as aflatoxin that inhibit hepatocyte proliferation and cause necrosis can selectively stimulate the enlargement of altered nodules among hyperplastic ducts.

Focal atypical hyperplasia, such as hyperplastic nodules (or nodular hyperplasia) and altered foci, are common in older rodents, fish, and dogs but are rarely seen in older horses or cats. This suggests a difference in environmental exposure of some initiating mutagen or perhaps differences in susceptibility to spontaneous mutations among species. Although some hyperplastic nodules can become clinically important by hemorrhaging or by progression to adenomas or carcinomas, the nodules are usually incidental findings when encountered by imaging, laparotomy, or necropsy. Occasionally, they can be a source of elevated alkaline phosphatase. Large focal hepatocellular adenomas can be clinically inapparent unless they are palpated or recognized by abdominal hemorrhage or pain. Typically, they permit normal hepatic function and are rarely responsible for liver dysfunction. Infiltrative neoplasms are more destructive and can destroy sufficient numbers or arrangements of hepatocytes, ducts, or vessels to result in clinical problems referable to these injuries.

ASSESSMENT OF HEPATIC FUNCTION AND DISEASE. The clinical diagnostic approaches to the investigation of liver disease are well described elsewhere (Sutherland 1989; Duncan et al. 1994; Dial 1995; Hughes and King 1995; Roth and Meyer 1995; Kaneko et al. 1997). Many aspects of these approaches have also been explained in the preceding topics, in the context of the processes they are designed to assess. Although some hepatic conditions are relatively simple problems to find and understand, some changes in the liver can be confusing even to experienced clinicians. The liver responds in various ways to physiological conditions that are changing elsewhere, so responses by the liver are often not the primary problem.

Various methods by which problems with the liver can be discovered and characterized are listed in Table 11.13. Some procedures are designed to detect some physical alteration in the liver. Others are designed to assess how well the liver is performing.

Biopsies enable targeted examination of focal liver lesions and reveal much about the pathogenic processes and causes that can be responsible for the changes in the samples that are collected. Many of the features and processes previously discussed can be discovered in well-prepared liver biopsies. Also, these can be used for biochemical and molecular biological approaches that are increasingly being developed for pharmacology and toxicological assessments.

Imaging tools (e.g., radiographs, ultrasound, magnetic resonance imaging, and laparoscopy) coupled with needle biopsy and aspirates are increasingly important in the early assessment of the liver. These approaches can reveal much about size and form of the liver, and are often the only way to access focal liver lesions that do not affect enough tissue to alter the serum biochemical indicators of liver function and disease. One of the difficulties with liver biopsies, especially those based on small samples, is that there are many background focal age-related incidental processes, some of which are not representative of the overall state of the entire organ.

Recent *necrosis* of hepatocytes can be detected by increased amounts of cytosolic hepatocellular enzymes in the serum. The utility of particular enzymes depends

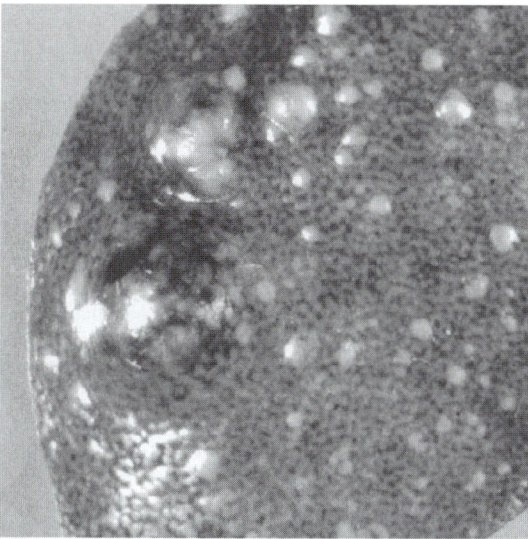

FIG. 11.24—Altered focal proliferations in the liver of an old dog. Larger nodules are referred to as *hyperplastic nodules*.

TABLE 11.13—Evaluation of liver function and disease

Focal lesions and infiltrates
  Imaging
    Laparotomy/laparosopy
    Liver biopsy
  Hepatocyte necrosis
    Serum ALT, AST, SDH, and GDH
  Cholestasis
    Serum bilirubin
    Serum GGT and H-AP
  Functional mass
    Serum albumin and globulin and ratios
    Plasma clearance rates
      BSP
  Indocyanine green
    Bile acids
    Ammonia tolerance
  Metabolic activity
    Ketonemia and ketonuria
    Cholesterol and triglycerides
    Blood urea nitrogen
    Blood glucose
  Hemostasis
    Coagulation assays
    Plasma fibrinogen
  Vascular integrity
    Blood ammonia
    Ammonia tolerance
    Serum bile acids
    Angiography
  Adaptations
    Acute-phase serum proteins
    Drug half-life
  Steroid-inducible AP

on their abundance and degree of specificity for the liver in each species of interest, and on their plasma half-life after they leak from hepatocytes. For example, ALT is liver specific and constitutively expressed but quickly cleared from serum of dogs and cats. Accordingly, the magnitude of an increase of such a "leakage" indicator correlates with severity of acute damage but not with the cumulative loss of hepatocytes during subacute and chronic injury.

Aspartate aminotransferase (AST) is similarly useful in large herbivores that have little ALT. However, AST is also released from necrotic muscle, so it is not specific for liver injury. However, muscle necrosis can be ruled out on the basis of normal serum concentrations of creatine kinase, most of which originates from skeletal muscle. Other hepatocyte-specific cytoplasmic enzymes have been useful, such as sorbitol dehydrogenase (SDH), arginase, and glutamate dehydrogenase (GDH) in ruminants.

Icterus is recognized by plasma elevations in serum bilirubin, but it is important to realize that icterus is a poor indicator of *cholestasis* unless the liver is diffusely affected. Focal canalicular or obstructive conditions can escape recognition if functional portions of the liver are available for the excretory process. For example, obstruction of the common bile duct causes marked icterus in most species, whereas obstruction of lobar ducts by a cholelith, tumor, or parasite might not be evident. In ruminants, icterus is usually the result of

hemolysis rather than primary liver disease. Similarly, in dogs, the largest elevations in serum bilirubin are generated in acute immunohemolysis.

Differentiation of conjugated and unconjugated bilirubin can provide some timely indication as to the likely pathogenesis of severe icterus. For example, hemolytic icterus is prehepatic, but most excreted bilirubin is conjugated. However, most domestic species can conjugate and eliminate some bilirubin in the kidney, so the conjugated/unconjugated ratio can sometimes be ambiguous. In some species, especially cats, icterus is a common component of anorexia due to retention of bile in canaliculi and the gallbladder.

Some serum enzymes such as GGT and hepatic alkaline phosphatase (H-AP) are useful serum indicators of *cholestasis*. Both enzymes are involved in processing bile content; GGT cleaves glutamate from glutathione and its conjugates, whereas AP hydrolyzes phosphates from various substrates for undetermined reasons. Both are expressed in the canalicular membranes and can be induced during acute and chronic cholestasis. Also, bile ductular epithelial cells that express these proliferate during obstructive cholestasis. These membrane-associated proteins are released into the bile in the presence of the detergent influences of bile salts, and some leaks back into the plasma. H-AP must be distinguished from steroid-inducible isozyme (S-AP), which is much more abundant in dogs that are exposed to glucocorticoids. GGT is also steroid responsive and is practically more useful than H-AP, especially in horses, ruminants, and pigs. Mammary GGT in colostrum can be absorbed by neonates, so it is a useful correlate of passive transfer of maternal antibodies in the neonatal calves.

Enterohepatic circulation of *bile acids* depends on an intact portal vasculature, active hepatic metabolic function, and effective uptake and secretion pathways. For these reasons, normal elevations in serum concentrations of bile acids 2 hours after feeding (postprandial) can demonstrate the integrity of hepatocellular uptake and biliary excretion. By comparison, persistent elevations in bile acids during fasting can indicate portal vascular shunts that divert more bile acids from the enterohepatic circuit into the systemic circulation (Center 1993; Thompson 1996).

High blood ammonia levels can also be measured in hepatic encephalopathy, but for more reliable diagnostic assessment of mild conditions in the context of widely fluctuating baseline levels, an ammonia tolerance test can be performed, although this is contraindicated when the ammonia levels are already elevated (Duncan et al. 1994).

Functional mass is usually first assessed by size (e.g., by palpation, ultrasound, radiographs, or magnetic resonance imaging) and then by more direct measures of function. Substantial reductions in hepatic size are usually more significant indications of functional insufficiency. Hepatomegaly (large liver) is more difficult to assess because blood, glycogen, hypertrophy, and nodules can increase the size of the liver without necessarily being detrimental to the important liver functions. Rates of clearance of endogenous substances (bile acids after a meal) and exogenous substances (such as bromosulphophthalein [BSP] and indocyanine green) are used to measure the capacity of the liver to biotransform and excrete BSP from the blood into the bile. However, the tests are difficult to perform, and various extrahepatic conditions influence pharmacokinetics. For example, expanded extracellular fluid volumes and low plasma albumin can delay clearance.

Concentrations and proportions of serum *albumin* and *globulins* (α and β) as products of the liver can sometimes be useful indicators of hepatic secretory capacity, although much liver mass needs to be lost before production deteriorates. They are also affected by other conditions, such as dehydration and renal or intestinal lesions that increase their loss. Blood clotting can be impaired in severe liver disease and in many other conditions. Clotting tests are usually performed to measure the risk of hemorrhage during biopsy or laparotomy to investigate the liver more directly.

REFERENCES

Alison MR, Poulsom R, Jeffery R, et al. 2000. Hepatocytes from non-hepatic adult stem cells. Nature 406:257.

Allen L, Stobie D, Mauldin GN, Baer KE. 1999. Clinicopathologic features of dogs with hepatic microvascular dysplasia with and without portosystemic shunts: 42 cases (1991–1996). J Am Vet Med Assoc 214:218–220.

Andrews NC. 1999. Disorders of iron metabolism. N Engl J Med 341:1986–1995.

Arias IM, Boyer JL, Fausto N. 1994. The Liver: Biology and Pathobiology. New York: Raven.

Blanchard G, Paragon BM, Milliat F, Lutton C. 2002. Dietary L-carnitine supplementation in obese cats alters carnitine metabolism and decreases ketosis during fasting and induced hepatic lipidosis. J Nutr 132:204–210.

Boitier E, Gautier JC, Roberts R. 2003. Advances in understanding the regulation of apoptosis and mitosis by peroxisome-proliferator activated receptors in pre-clinical models: Relevance for human health and disease. Comp Hepatol 2:3.

Bomford A. 2002. Genetics of haemochromatosis. Lancet 360:1673–1681.

Boothe HW, Howe LM, Edwards JF, Slater MR. 1996. Multiple extrahepatic portosystemic shunts in dogs: 30 cases (1981–1993). J Am Vet Med Assoc 208:1849–1854.

Bradham CA, Plumpe J, Manns MP, et al. 1998. Mechanisms of hepatic toxicity: I. TNF-induced liver injury. Am J Physiol 275:G387–G392.

Bruss ML. 1997. Lipids and ketones. In: Kaneko JJ, Harvey JW, Bruss M, eds. Clinical Biochemistry of Domestic Animals. San Diego: Academic, pp 83–115.

Cattley RC, Miller RT, Corton JC. 1995. Peroxisome proliferators: Potential role of altered hepatocyte growth and differentiation in tumor development. Prog Clin Biol Res 391:295–303.

Center SA. 1993. Serum bile acids in companion animal medicine. Vet Clin North Am Small Anim Pract 23:625–657.

Chappell DA, Medh JD. 1998. Receptor-mediated mechanisms of lipoprotein remnant catabolism. Prog Lipid Res 37:393–422.

Christiansen JS, Hottinger HA, Allen L, et al. 2000. Hepatic microvascular dysplasia in dogs: A retrospective study of 24 cases (1987–1995). J Am Anim Hosp Assoc 36:385–389.

Columbano A, Shinozuka H. 1996. Liver regeneration versus direct hyperplasia. FASEB J 10:1118–1128.

Crawford JM. 1996. Role of vesicle-mediated transport pathways in hepatocellular bile secretion. Semin Liver Dis 16:169–189.

Crissey SD, Ward AM, Block SE, Maslanka MT. 2000. Hepatic iron accumulation over time in European starlings (*Sturnus vulgaris*) fed two levels of iron. J Zoo Wildl Med 31:491–496.

Cullen JM, MacLachlan NJ. 2001. Liver, biliary system and exocrine pancreas. In: McGavin MD, Carlton WW, Zachary JF, eds. Thomson's Systemic Veterinary Pathology. St Louis: CV Mosby, pp 81–124.

Dayrell-Hart B, Steinberg SA, Van Winkle TJ, Farnbach GC. 1991. Hepatotoxicity of phenobarbital in dogs: 18 cases (1985–1989). J Am Vet Med Assoc 199:1060–1066.

De Longueville F, Surry D, Meneses-Lorente G, et al. 2002. Gene expression profiling of drug metabolism and toxicology markers using a low-density DNA microarray. Biochem Pharmacol 64:137–149.

Dial SM. 1995. Clinicopathologic evaluation of the liver. Vet Clin North Am Small Anim Pract 25:257–273.

Dodds WJ. 1997. Hemostasis. In: Kaneko JJ, Harvey JW, Bruss M, eds. Clinical Biochemistry of Domestic Animals. San Diego: Academic, pp 241–283.

Duncan JR, Prasse KW, Mahaffey EA. 1994. Veterinary Laboratory Medicine: Clinical Pathology. Ames, IA: Iowa State University Press.

Eaton JW, Qian M. 2002. Molecular bases of cellular iron toxicity. Free Radic Biol Med 32:833–840.

Ekataksin W, Kaneda K. 1999. Liver microvascular architecture: An insight into the pathophysiology of portal hypertension. Semin Liver Dis 19:359–382.

Everett L, Galli A, Crabb D. 2000. The role of hepatic peroxisome proliferator-activated receptors (PPARs) in health and disease. Liver 20:191–199.

Fabry A, Benjamin SA, Angleton GM. 1982. Nodular hyperplasia of the liver in the beagle dog. Vet Pathol 19:109–119.

Farber E, Sarma DS. 1987. Hepatocarcinogenesis: A dynamic cellular perspective. Lab Invest 56:4–22.

Ferenci P, Zollner G, Trauner M. 2002. Hepatic transport systems. J Gastroenterol Hepatol 17(Suppl):S105–S112.

Fickert P, Trauner M, Fuchsbichler A, et al. 2002. Cytokeratins as targets for bile acid-induced toxicity. Am J Pathol 160:491–499.

Forbes S, Vig P, Poulsom R, et al. 2002. Hepatic stem cells. J Pathol 197:510–518.

Fountoulakis M, Juranville JF, Berndt P, et al. 2001. Two-dimensional database of mouse liver proteins: An update. Electrophoresis 22:1747–1763.

French SW. 2000. Mechanisms of alcoholic liver injury. Can J Gastroenterol 14:327–332.

Galeva N, Altermann M. 2002. Comparison of one-dimensional and two-dimensional gel electrophoresis as a separation tool for proteomic analysis of rat liver microsomes: Cytochromes P450 and other membrane proteins. Proteomics 2:713–722.

Geerts A. 2001. History, heterogeneity, developmental biology, and functions of quiescent hepatic stellate cells. Semin Liver Dis 21:311–335.

Gieger TL, Hosgood G, Taboada J, et al. 2000. Thyroid function and serum hepatic enzyme activity in dogs after phenobarbital administration. J Vet Intern Med 14:277–281.

Gregory SH, Wing EJ. 2002. Neutrophil-Kupffer cell interaction: A critical component of host defenses to systemic bacterial infections. J Leukoc Biol 72:239–248.

Hankinson O. 1995. The aryl hydrocarbon receptor complex. Annu Rev Pharmacol Toxicol 35:307–340.

Haskins ME, Otis EJ, Hayden JE, et al. 1992. Hepatic storage of glycosaminoglycans in feline and canine models of mucopolysaccharidoses I, VI, and VII. Vet Pathol 29:112–119.

Heath T, Lowden S. 1998. Pathways of interstitial fluid and lymph flow in the liver acinus of the sheep and mouse. J Anat 192:351–358.

Heegaard PM, Klausen J, Nielsen JP, et al. 1998. The porcine acute phase response to infection with *Actinobacillus pleuropneumoniae*: Haptoglobin, C-reactive protein, major acute phase protein and serum amyloid A protein are sensitive indicators of infection. Comp Biochem Physiol [B] 119:365–373.

Heegaard PM, Godson DL, Toussaint MJ, et al. 2000. The acute phase response of haptoglobin and serum amyloid A (SAA) in cattle undergoing experimental infection with bovine respiratory syncytial virus. Vet Immunol Immunopathol 77:151–159.

Herbst H, Frey A, Heinrichs O, et al. 1997. Heterogeneity of liver cells expressing procollagen types I and IV in vivo. Histochem Cell Biol 107:399–409.

Horadagoda NU, Knox KM, Gibbs HA, et al. 1999. Acute phase proteins in cattle: Discrimination between acute and chronic inflammation. Vet Rec 144:437–441.

Howe LM, Boothe DM, Boothe HW. 1997. Endotoxemia associated with experimentally induced multiple portosystemic shunts in dogs. Am J Vet Res 58:83–88.

Howell JM, Deol HS, Dorling PR, Thomas JB. 1991. Experimental copper and heliotrope intoxication in sheep: Morphological changes. J Comp Pathol 105:49–74.

Hughes D, King LG. 1995. The diagnosis and management of acute liver failure in dogs and cats. Vet Clin North Am Small Anim Pract 25:437–460.

Jaeschke H, Gores GJ, Cederbaum AI, et al. 2002. Mechanisms of hepatotoxicity. Toxicol Sci 65:166–176.

Jones TC, Hunt RD, King NW. 1997. Veterinary Pathology. Baltimore: Williams and Wilkins.

Kaneko JJ, Harvey JW, Bruss M. 1997. Clinical Biochemistry of Domestic Animals. San Diego: Academic.

Kanzler S, Galle PR. 2000. Apoptosis and the liver. Semin Cancer Biol 10:173–184.

Kaplowitz N. 2000. Mechanisms of liver cell injury. J Hepatol 32:39–47.

Kaplowitz N. 2002. Biochemical and cellular mechanisms of toxic liver injury. Semin Liver Dis 22:137–144.

Kedderis GL. 1996. Biochemical basis of hepatocellular injury. Toxicol Pathol 24:77–83.

Kelly WR. 1993. The liver and biliary system. In: Jubb KVF, Kennedy PC, Palmer NG, eds. Pathology of Domestic Animals. New York: Academic, 2:239.

Kennedy S, McConnell S, Anderson H, et al. 1997. Histopathologic and ultrastructural alterations of white liver disease in sheep experimentally depleted of cobalt. Vet Pathol 34:575–584.

Kishnani PS, Faulkner E, Van Camp S, et al. 2001. Canine model and genomic structural organization of glycogen storage disease type Ia (GSD Ia). Vet Pathol 38:83–91.

Koen YM, Hanzlik RP. 2002. Identification of seven proteins in the endoplasmic reticulum as targets for reactive metabolites of bromobenzene. Chem Res Toxicol 15:699–706.

Laconi E. 2000. Differential growth: From carcinogenesis to liver repopulation. Am J Pathol 156:389–392.

Lee AS. 2001. The glucose-regulated proteins: Stress induction and clinical applications. Trends Biochem Sci 26:504–510.

Leone TC, Weinheimer CJ, Kelly DP. 1999. A critical role for the peroxisome proliferator-activated receptor alpha (PPARalpha) in the cellular fasting response: The PPAR-alpha-null mouse as a model of fatty acid oxidation disorders. Proc Natl Acad Sci USA 96:7473–7478.

Leveille CR, Arias IM. 1993. Pathophysiology and pharmacologic modulation of hepatic fibrosis. J Vet Intern Med 7:73–84.

Liu SK, Tilley LP, Tappe JP, Fox PR. 1986. Clinical and pathologic findings in dogs with atherosclerosis: 21 cases (1970–1983). J Am Vet Med Assoc 189:227–232.

Macsween RNM, Burt AD, Portmann BC, et al. 2002. Pathology of the Liver. Edinburgh: Churchill Livingstone.

McCuskey RS. 2000. Morphological mechanisms for regulating blood flow through hepatic sinusoids. Liver 20:3–7.

Michalopoulos GK, De Frances MC. 1997. Liver regeneration. Science 276:60–66.

Moore PF, Whiting PG. 1986. Hepatic lesions associated with intrahepatic arterioportal fistulae in dogs. Vet Pathol 23:57–62.

Muller PB, Taboada J, Hosgood G, et al. 2000. Effects of long-term phenobarbital treatment on the liver in dogs. J Vet Intern Med 14:165–171.

Oinonen T, Lindros KO. 1998. Zonation of hepatic cytochrome P-450 expression and regulation. Biochem J 329:17–35.

Omori Y, Zaidan-Dagli ML, Yamakage K, Yamasaki H. 2001. Involvement of gap junctions in tumor suppression: Analysis of genetically-manipulated mice. Mutat Res 477:191–196.

Pazak HE, Bartges JW, Cornelius LC, et al. 1998. Characterization of serum lipoprotein profiles of healthy, adult cats and idiopathic feline hepatic lipidosis patients. J Nutr 128:2747S–2750S.

Pumford NR, Halmes NC, Hinson JA. 1997. Covalent binding of xenobiotics to specific proteins in the liver. Drug Metab Rev 29:39–57.

Qiu Y, Benet LZ, Burlingame AL. 1998. Identification of the hepatic protein targets of reactive metabolites of acetaminophen in vivo in mice using two-dimensional gel electrophoresis and mass spectrometry. J Biol Chem 273:17,940–17,953.

Ramadori G, Armbrust T. 2001. Cytokines in the liver. Eur J Gastroenterol Hepatol 13:777–784.

Ring A, Stremmel W. 2000. The hepatic microvascular responses to sepsis. Semin Thromb Hemost 26:589–594.

Rook JS. 2000. Pregnancy toxemia of ewes, does, and beef cows. Vet Clin North Am Equine Pract 16:293–317.

Roth L, Meyer DJ. 1995. Interpretation of liver biopsies. Vet Clin North Am Small Anim Pract 25:293–303.

Rutgers HC, Batt RM, Vaillant C, Riley JE. 1995. Subcellular pathologic features of glucocorticoid-induced hepatopathy in dogs. Am J Vet Res 56:898–907.

Schneider P. 1992. Drug-induced lysosomal disorders in laboratory animals: New substances acting on lysosomes. Arch Toxicol 66:23–33.

Su LC, Ravanshad S, Owen CA Jr, et al. 1982. A comparison of copper-loading disease in Bedlington terriers and Wilson's disease in humans. Am J Physiol 243:G226–G230.

Sutherland RJ. 1989. Biochemical evaluation of the hepatobiliary system in dogs and cats. Vet Clin North Am Small Anim Pract 19:899–927.

Taboada J, Dimski DS. 1995. Hepatic encephalopathy: Clinical signs, pathogenesis, and treatment. Vet Clin North Am Small Anim Pract 25:337–355.

Taimr P, Higuchi H, Kocova E, et al. 2003. Activated stellate cells express the TRAIL receptor-2/death receptor-5 and undergo TRAIL-mediated apoptosis. Hepatology 37:87–95.

Takahashi-Iwanaga H, Fujita T, Takeda M. 1990. Canine hepatic vein branches associated with subendothelial mast cells and an adventitial lymphatic plexus. Arch Histol Cytol 53:189–197.

Tennant BC. 1997. Hepatic function. In: Kaneko JJ, Harvey JW, Bruss M, eds. Clinical Biochemistry of Domestic Animals. San Diego: Academic, pp 327–352.

Thompson MB. 1996. Bile acids in the assessment of hepatocellular function. Toxicol Pathol 24:62–71.

Thornburg LP. 1998. Histomorphological and immunohistochemical studies of chronic active hepatitis in Doberman pinschers. Vet Pathol 35:380–385.

Thornburg LP, Shaw D, Dolan M, et al. 1986. Hereditary copper toxicosis in West Highland white terriers. Vet Pathol 23:148–154.

Trauner M, Meier PJ, Boyer JL. 1998. Molecular pathogenesis of cholestasis. N Engl J Med 339:1217–1227.

Trauner M, Fickert P, Zollner G. 2001. Genetic disorders and molecular mechanisms in cholestatic liver disease: A clinical approach. Semin Gastrointest Dis 12:66–88.

Trutmann M, Sasse D. 1994. The lymphatics of the liver. Anat Embryol (Berl) 190:201–209.

Weigel PH, Yik JH. 2002. Glycans as endocytosis signals: The cases of the asialoglycoprotein and hyaluronan/chondroitin sulfate receptors. Biochim Biophys Acta 1572:341–363.

Zimmermann A. 2002. Liver regeneration: The emergence of new pathways. Med Sci Monit 8:RA53–RA63.

12

PATHOPHYSIOLOGY OF ENDOCRINE HOMEOSTASIS: EXAMPLES

Charles C. Capen, Editor, and Timothy D. O'Brien

PART 1: PATHOPHYSIOLOGY OF CALCIUM-PHOSPHORUS METABOLISM AND BONE

CHARLES C. CAPEN

PHYSIOLOGY OF CALCIUM IN THE BODY. Calcium is an essential mineral component of the skeleton and plays a central role in maintaining the homeostasis of vertebrate animals. Ionized calcium is involved in a wide variety of physiological processes, including muscular contraction, blood coagulation, enzyme activity, neural excitability, hormone secretion, and cell adhesion. The levels of calcium in the body are influenced by a variety of endocrine factors. These include parathyroid hormone (PTH) synthesized and released by the chief cells of the parathyroid glands, calcitonin secreted by the parafollicular or C cells of the thyroid gland, and calcitriol (1,25-dihydroxycholecalciferol; 1,25-dihydroxyvitamin D), the bioactive vitamin D metabolite derived from cholecalciferol (vitamin D_3). Disruption of the normal regulation of calcium balance in animals results in hypercalcemia or hypocalcemia (Chew et al. 1992) and can lead to metabolic disease and death.

Pathological effects associated with abnormal levels of calcium in the body include mineralization of vital organs and other soft tissues, rickets, osteoporosis, and metabolic disorders such as parturient hypocalcemia and paresis in dairy cattle and puerperal tetany in bitches.

Approximately 99% of the calcium of the body is present in the inorganic matrix of bone as hydroxyapatite (Figure 12.1). Most of the remaining calcium is sequestered in the plasma membrane and endoplasmic reticulum of cells. Extracellular fluid contains 0.1% of the body's calcium mass with a total calcium concentration of about 2.5 mmol/L. Approximately 50% of the

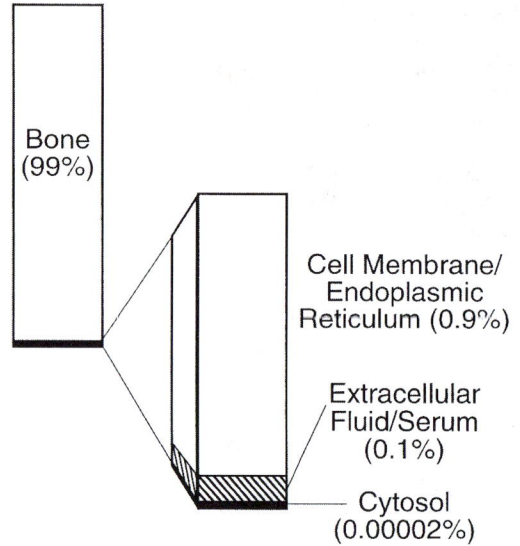

FIG. 12.1—Distribution of calcium (Ca) in the body. (From Rosol et al. 1995.)

extracellular calcium (1.2 mmol/L) is in the ionized form (Ca^{2+}), which is the biologically active form of calcium. Neonatal animals have slightly greater concentrations of extracellular calcium compared with adult animals. There is very little calcium in the cytosol, approximately 100 nM, which is predominantly in the ionized form.

Vertebrates, such as the marine fishes, originally evolved in an environment with a high concentration Ca^{2+}. Seawater contains approximately 10 mmol/L Ca^{2+}, but the extracellular fluids of marine fishes contain less than 2 mmol/L Ca^{2+}. Therefore, fishes had to limit and regulate Ca^{2+} absorption from the intestinal tract, skin, or gills and develop mechanisms to efficiently excrete Ca^{2+}. Evolutionarily, this was probably conducive to the development of hormones, such as calcitonin and stanniocalcin, that reduce the Ca^{2+} concentration in the serum. Fish lack parathyroid glands, which have the primary role of reducing the loss of body Ca^{2+} and maintaining serum Ca^{2+}. Phylogenetically, parathyroid glands first appear in amphibians, which spend most of their life cycle on land in an environment low in Ca^{2+}. In terrestrial vertebrates, both the parathyroid glands and the kidneys are important regulators of total body calcium. Because there is less need for promoting the excretion of calcium or lowering serum Ca^{2+} in terrestrial animals, hormones such as calcitonin are of less importance for the maintenance of calcium homeostasis.

Functions of Calcium. Calcium serves two primary functions in the body: (a) structural integrity of bones and teeth, and (b) as a messenger or regulatory ion. There is a 10,000-fold concentration gradient of Ca^{2+} between the extracellular fluid (1.2 mmol/L) and the cytoplasm (100 nM). This gradient permits Ca^{2+} to function as a signaling ion to activate intracellular processes. The lipid bilayer of the cell membrane has a low permeability to Ca^{2+}; therefore, influx of Ca^{2+} into the cytoplasm is controlled by a heterogeneous group of calcium channels regulated by membrane potential, cell-membrane receptors, or intracellular secondary messengers. Influx of Ca^{2+} into cells can (a) regulate cellular function by interactions with intracellular calcium-binding proteins (e.g., calmodulin) and calcium-sensitive protein kinases, and (b) stimulate biological responses such as neurotransmitter release, contraction, and secretion. Ionized calcium also plays an important role in cell adhesion and blood coagulation. In addition, Ca^{2+} may regulate cellular function by binding to a G-protein-linked Ca^{2+}-sensing receptor in the cell membrane, such as in parathyroid chief cells or renal epithelial cells (Brown et al. 1995).

Maintenance of low levels of intercellular Ca^{2+} is indispensable for cellular viability. If cellular calcium homeostasis fails due to anoxia or to an energy-deprived state or perturbed membrane integrity, cell viability is threatened due to uncontrolled entry of Ca^{2+} through the plasma membrane or from extracellular stores (Siesjö 1989).

Extracellular and serum calcium exists in three forms: (a) ionized, (b) complexed to anions such as citrate, bicarbonate, phosphate, or lactate (5% of total calcium), and (c) protein bound (Figure 12.2). The protein-bound fraction of Ca^{2+} is dependent on the pH of the serum and is principally bound to negatively charged sites on albumin, with smaller amounts bound to globulins. As the pH of serum becomes more acidic, the $[Ca^{2+}]$ will increase due to the competition of hydrogen ions $[H^+]$ for binding to the negatively charged sites on serum proteins. The ionized and complexed Ca^{2+} compose the ultrafilterable fraction of Ca^{2+} and represent the fraction that is present in the glomerular filtrate. The concentration of ionized Ca^{2+} in the serum is approximately 1.25 to 1.60 mmol/L (5.0 to 6.4 mg/dL) in most domestic animals.

Renal Handling of Calcium. The kidney normally reabsorbs 98% or more of the filtered calcium. This high degree of reabsorption is an important mechanism to maintain the balance of calcium in the body. If necessary, the kidneys excrete large amounts of calcium in the urine. Ionized and complexed calcium enters the glomerular filtrate by convection and is reabsorbed by the renal tubules. Due to the high degree of blood flow and ultrafiltration in the glomerulus, the kidneys reabsorb approximately 40-fold more calcium than is absorbed by the intestinal tract. Reduction of glomerular filtration impairs the ability of the kidneys to excrete calcium. About 70% of filtered calcium is reabsorbed in the proximal convoluted tubules by diffusion and convection with water uptake between the epithelial

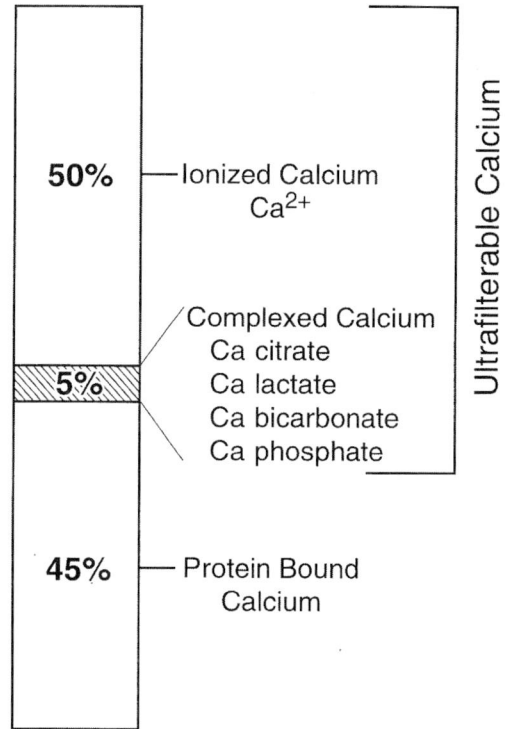

FIG. 12.2—Fractions of extracellular calcium (Ca). (From Rosol et al. 1995.)

cells (Figure 12.3). The thick ascending loop of Henle also absorbs about 20% of the filtered calcium, but the precise mechanism is unclear. Much of the calcium reabsorption appears to be passive, but an active component (Rouse and Suki 1990) may also be present in the distal convoluted tubule, which reabsorbs approximately 10% of the filtered calcium. The principal stimulator of calcium reabsorption in the distal convoluted tubule is PTH. Reabsorption of calcium in the distal convoluted tubule is an active transcellular process requiring the presence of calcium channels in the luminal cell membrane, intracellular calcium-binding proteins, such as calbindins, a Ca^{2+}-adenosine triphosphatase (ATPase), and Na^+/Ca^{2+} exchanger in the basolateral cell membranes. Renal epithelial cells express the Ca^{2+}-sensing receptor on their cell membranes, and the distribution of the receptor overlaps with the localization of PTH receptors, so the kidneys may partially autoregulate the renal reabsorption of calcium based on concentration of Ca^{2+} in the blood.

Measurements of calcium excretion in animals include calcium and calcium/creatine (Ca/Cr) ratio in the urine, fractional calcium excretion, and 24-hour calcium excretion. Urinary calcium excretion correlates with dietary absorbance in normal, adult animals. The concentration of calcium in urine is usually less

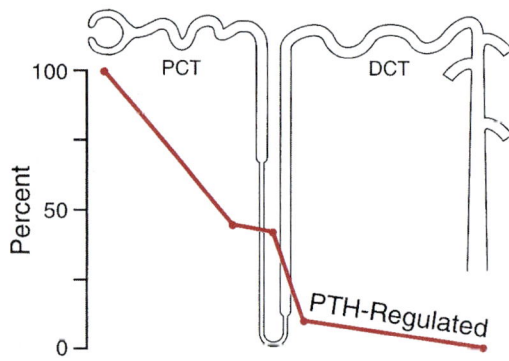

FIG. 12.3—Sites of calcium (Ca) reabsorption in the nephron. The greatest amount of filtered calcium is reabsorbed passively in the proximal convoluted tubule (PCT). The site of active regulation of calcium reabsorption by parathyroid hormone (PTH) is in the distal convoluted tubule (DCT). (From Rosol et al. 1995.)

than 4 mg/dL (1.6 mmol/L) and is of little value as a diagnostic tool due to large fluctuations in the volume of normal urine. Horses excrete larger amounts of calcium in the urine and urine [Ca] is typically much higher than 4 mg/dL (1.6 mmol/L). The Ca/Cr ratio of the urine is a better indicator of calcium excretion because it corrects for errors in timing of urine collections, urine concentration or dilution, and differences in lean body mass (Weaver 1990). Calculation of fractional calcium excretion requires measurement of urine and serum calcium and Cr concentrations and is an indication of renal calcium reabsorption at the time of analysis, as well as the degree of excretory renal function. Fractional calcium excretion is best measured in a fasting animal to eliminate the role of dietary calcium on renal calcium excretion. Measurement of calcium excretion in a fasted animal is an indirect measurement of bone resorption, since calcium released from bone and the obligate renal calcium loss are the major sources of urinary calcium when there is little gastrointestinal absorption of calcium. The 24-hour calcium excretion is a good measurement of daily calcium loss and may be used to investigate calcium balance.

Intestinal Absorption of Calcium. There are two components of calcium absorption from the intestinal tract: saturable or transcellular transport and nonsaturable or intercellular (paracellular) transport (Favus 1992). The percentage of intestinal absorption of calcium is proportional to dietary intake. Low-calcium diets are associated with absorption rates of up to 95%, whereas high-calcium diets have absorption rates of about 40%. However, high-calcium diets may increase serum calcium concentrations due to the presence of nonsaturable intestinal absorption. In contrast, diets deficient in calcium are associated with normal serum calcium con-

centrations, due to compensation by bone resorption stimulated by PTH, renal calcium reabsorption, and increased synthesis of 1,25-dihydroxyvitamin D.

Saturable transport is a carrier-mediated, vitamin D-dependent process and occurs predominantly in the duodenal segment of the small intestine and, to a lesser degree, in the cecum and colon. Saturable transport requires influx of calcium into intestinal epithelial cells via Ca^{2+} channels, movement and buffering in the cytoplasm, and basolateral exit by a Ca^{2+}-ATPase. The active form of vitamin D (1,25-dihydroxyvitamin D) stimulates transcellular transport of Ca^{2+}. One function of 1,25-dihydroxyvitamin D in the intestinal epithelial cell is to increase the expression of calbindin, an intracellular calcium-binding protein. In contrast, nonsaturable calcium transport occurs throughout the small intestine and is the main mechanism for calcium absorption in animals deficient in vitamin D. Nonsaturable Ca^{2+} transport is dependent on the luminal $[Ca^{2+}]$. As the dietary intake of calcium increases, much of the calcium in the intestinal lumen is unavailable for nonsaturable absorption, due to precipitation of calcium salts or complexes formed with other anions.

Fractional intestinal calcium absorption is approximately 20% to 40% in adult animals and can exceed 60% during increased demand for calcium. Fractional absorption is increased during pregnancy, lactation, growth, and when animals are fed low-calcium diets. The blood concentration of 1,25-dihydroxyvitamin D is the primary adaptive influence on calcium absorption. Factors that increase intestinal calcium absorption, directly or indirectly, due to stimulation of 1,25-dihydroxyvitamin D synthesis include PTH, growth hormone, testosterone, estrogen, and furosemide. Factors that reduce intestinal absorption of calcium include glucocorticoids, thyroid hormones, chronic acidosis, and luminal conditions that induce the complexation of Ca^{2+}, such as high concentrations of phosphate, phytates, oxalate, fatty acids, pH > 6.1, and other anions.

Bone and Calcium Balance. Two sources of Ca^{2+} in bone can enter the circulation: (a) readily mobilizable calcium salts in the extracellular fluid, and (b) hydroxyapatite crystals that require digestion by osteoclasts before Ca^{2+} can be released from bone. The nature and regulation of the readily mobilizable calcium in bone are poorly understood; however, readily mobilizable calcium is present in small amounts and likely plays a role in the fine regulation of serum calcium concentration. If there is a significant need for calcium from bone, the calcium must come from osteoclastic resorption of hydroxyapatite crystals. In adult animals, there is a stable balance between calcium deposition associated with bone formation and calcium release associated with osteoclastic bone resorption. In young animals, bone has a positive calcium balance due to the relative excess of bone formation. Humoral hypercalcemia of malignancy, osteolytic bone metastases, and primary hyperparathyroidism are associated with excessive bone resorption and the release of calcium from bone, which contributes to the development of persistent hypercalcemia.

Calcium Ion-sensing Receptors in the Cell Membrane. The concentration of ionized calcium in serum and extracellular fluid can regulate cellular function by interacting with a recently identified Ca^{2+}-sensing receptor in the plasma membrane of various cells (Brown and Hebert 1996; Chattopadhyay et al. 1996). The cell-membrane Ca^{2+} receptor is coupled to G protein, and the seven-transmembrane domain of this receptor is unique because the ligand for the receptor is an ion. The Ca^{2+} receptor plays an important role in the regulation of extracellular Ca^{2+} homeostasis and is present on parathyroid chief cells, thyroid C cells, renal epithelial cells, brain, and placenta, among other tissues. The Ca^{2+} receptor is responsible for sensing serum Ca^{2+} concentration and modifying PTH secretion, calcitonin secretion, and calcium transport by renal epithelial cells. Mutations in one or both of the Ca^{2+}-sensing receptor genes in humans result in familial hypocalciuric hypercalcemia or neonatal severe hypercalcemia, respectively, due to an inadequate ability to sense the extracellular Ca^{2+} concentration and coordinate the appropriate cellular response.

CALCIUM-REGULATING HORMONES

Parathyroid Hormone. Parathyroid glands are present in all air-breathing vertebrates. Phylogenetically, the parathyroids first appeared in amphibians, coincidentally with the transition of life from an aquatic to a terrestrial environment. It has been suggested that the appearance and development of parathyroid glands may have arisen from the need to protect against the development of hypocalcemia and the necessity to maintain skeletal integrity in terrestrial animals, which often are in a relatively low-calcium, high-phosphorus environment.

The parathyroid glands in domestic animal species and in most other animal species consist of two pairs of glands—the internal and the external parathyroids—usually situated in the anterior cervical region in close proximity to the thyroid gland. Embryologically, both parathyroid glands are of entodermal origin. The external parathyroid is derived from the third (III) and the internal parathyroid is derived from the fourth (IV) pharyngeal pouches, in close association with the primordia of the thymus.

FUNCTIONAL CYTOLOGY OF THE PARATHYROID GLANDS. The parathyroid glands of animals contain a single, basic type of secretory cell termed a *chief cell*, which secretes and releases PTH. Oxyphil and transitional cells, which do not have an active role in the biosynthesis of PTH, are also found in the parathyroid glands of some animal species (Figure 12.4). Chief cells have various stages of secretory activity, such as actively synthesizing, or are inactive in most animal species. Inactive chief cells are cuboidal and have

uncomplicated interdigitations between contiguous cells. The relatively electron-transparent cytoplasm contains poorly developed organelles and few secretory granules. The Golgi apparatus is small, composed of straight or curved stacks of agranular membranes, and is associated with few prosecretory granules and vesicles. Individual profiles of granular endoplasmic reticulum, ribosomes, and small mitochondria are dispersed throughout the cytoplasm. Chief cells in the active stage of the secretory cycle occur less frequently in the parathyroid glands of most species. The cytoplasm of the active chief cell has an increased electron density due to the close proximity of organelles, secretion granules, the overall density of the cytoplasmic matrix, and the loss of glycogen particles and lipid bodies.

Oxyphil cells are observed either singly or in small groups interspersed between chief cells. Oxyphil cells are larger than chief cells and their abundant cytoplasmic area is filled with numerous large, often bizarre-shaped, mitochondria. Glycogen particles and free ribosomes are interspersed between the mitochondria. Granular endoplasmic reticula, Golgi apparatuses, and secretory granules are poorly developed in oxyphil cells of normal parathyroid glands, suggesting that oxyphil cells do not have an active function in the biosynthesis of PTH. Cells with cytoplasmic characteristics intermediate between those of chief and oxyphil cells also are observed. These transitional cells also have numerous mitochondria but a few profiles of granular endoplasmic reticulum, small Golgi apparatuses, and a few secretory granules. The significance of oxyphil cells in the pathophysiology of the parathyroid glands has not been completely elucidated. Oxyphil cells are not altered in response to short-term hypocalcemia or hypercalcemia in animals, but both oxyphil and transitional cells may increase in numbers in humans in response to long-term stimulation of the parathyroid glands.

SYNTHESIS OF PARATHYROID HORMONE. The chief cells synthesize a biosynthetic precursor of PTH called preproparathyroid hormone (preproPTH) on ribosomes of the rough endoplasmic reticulum. PreproPTH (Figure 12.5) is composed of 115 amino acids and contains a hydrophobic signal or leader sequence of 25 amino acid residues that facilitate the penetration and subsequent discharge of the peptide into the cisternal space of the rough endoplasmic reticulum. Within 1 minute or less of its synthesis, preproPTH is converted to proparathyroid hormone (proPTH) by the proteolytic cleavage of the NH_2-terminal sequence of 25 amino acids (Figure 12.5). The intermediate precursor, proPTH, is composed of 90 amino acids and displaces within membranous channels of the endoplasmic reticulum to the Golgi apparatus. Enzymes with trypsinlike and carboxypeptidase B-like activity within membranes of the Golgi apparatus cleave a hexapeptide from the NH_2-terminal, biologically active end of the molecule, forming active PTH (Figure 12.5). Active PTH is packaged into membrane-limited, macromolecular aggregates in the Golgi apparatus for subsequent

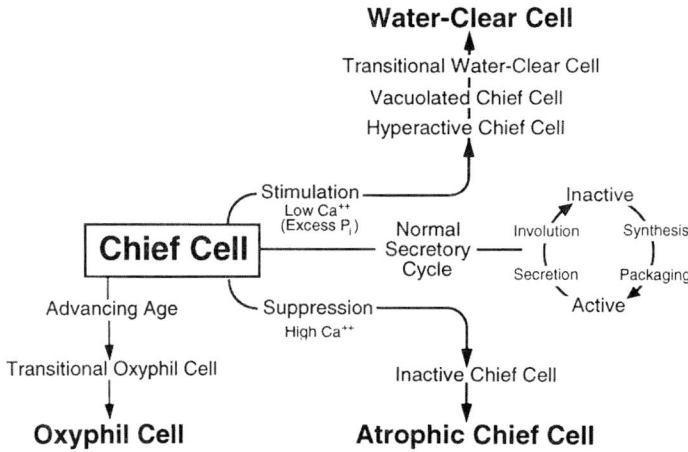

FIG. 12.4—Functional cytology of parathyroid glands under normal and pathological conditions. Ca++, ionized calcium; and P$_i$, inorganic phosphorus.

storage in chief cells (Figure 12.6). The biologically active PTH is a straight-chain polypeptide consisting of 84 amino acid residues with a molecular weight of approximately 9500 D (daltons). Molecular fragments of PTH are formed in the peripheral circulation and at the target cells of the hormone.

SECRETORY GRANULES. The secretory granules that develop by sequential accumulation and condensation of finely granular material within cisternae of the Golgi apparatus are concentrated in the vicinity of the Golgi apparatus and occasionally are observed in the process of becoming detached from the membranes of the

Golgi complex. These secretory (*storage*) granules have been demonstrated ultrastructurally within chief cells of the parathyroid glands in humans and all of the other animal species that have been examined. The secretory granules of chief cells are composed of fine, dense particles that are usually round to oval and range from 100 to 300 nm at their greatest diameter. The granules are electron dense and surrounded by a delicate, closely applied, limiting membrane. The number of granules within chief cells varies considerably between species, with bovine parathyroid cells having consistently more secretory granules than do humans and other animals.

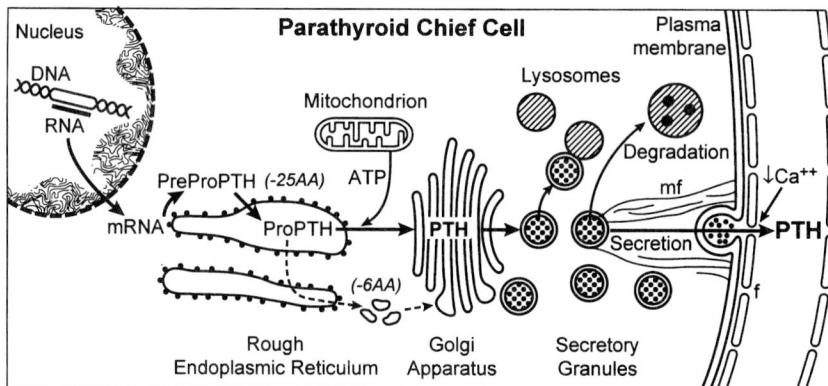

FIG. 12.5—Subcellular compartmentalization, transport, and cleavage of precursors of parathyroid hormone (PTH). The hydrophobic sequence on the amino-terminal end of preproparathyroid hormone (PreProPTH) facilitates the penetration of the leading portion of the nascent peptide into the lumen of the endoplasmic reticulum. Cleavage of a peptide fragment results in the proPTH that is transported to the Golgi apparatus and converted by carboxypeptidase to biologically active PTH. Lysosomes engulf the excess secretory granules that form in chief cells under normal conditions. Ca++, ionized calcium; and mRNA, messenger RNA, AA, amino acids; mf, microfilaments. (Adapted from Habener and Potts 1978.)

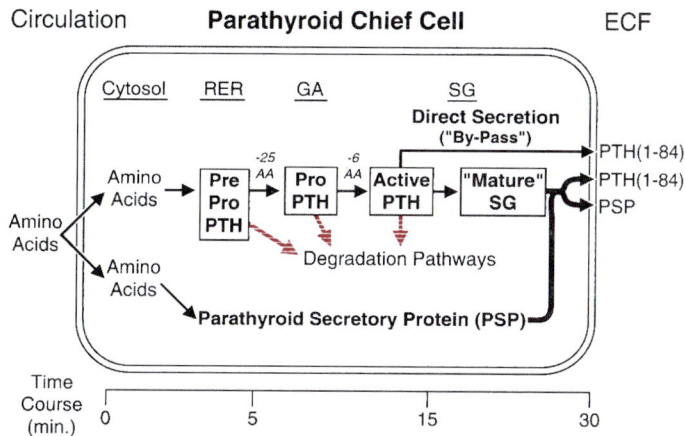

FIG. 12.6—Synthesis of parathyroid hormone (PTH) in the cytosol of the chief cell. Preproparathyroid hormone (preproPTH), the product from ribosomes of the rough endoplasmic reticulum (RER), is rapidly converted to proparathyroid hormone (proPTH) by the cleavage of a 25-amino-acid (AA) N-terminal fragment. Enzymatic removal of a 6-AA fragment from proPTH results in the biologically active PTH in the Golgi apparatus (GA). A major portion of the biosynthetic precursors and active PTH that is synthesized is degraded within the chief cell. Parathyroid secretory protein (PSP) may function as a binding protein for PTH during intracellular storage of hormone in secretory granules (SGs) and during release of PTH into the extracellular space. During periods of high demand, the active hormone PTH (1–84) may be secreted directly into the perivascular space. ECF, extracellular fluid.

Chief cells have relatively few storage granules when compared with other endocrine cells concerned with the biosynthesis of polypeptide hormones, for example, the calcitonin-secreting C cells of the thyroid gland. The secretory granules that form in the Golgi apparatus migrate peripherally in chief cells, and their limiting membrane fuses with the plasma membrane of the cell. An internal cytoskeleton composed of microtubules and contractile filaments is important in the control of the peripheral movement of secretory granules and release of secretory products from chief cells. Secretory granules are extruded from chief cells into the perivascular space and pass through fenestrae of capillary endothelial cells to gain access to the systemic circulation.

CHROMOGRANIN A. In addition to PTH, secretory granules in chief cells (Figure 12.6) also contain chromogranin A (CG-A), a parathyroid secretory peptide (molecular weight, ca. 49,000 D) that was first isolated from secretory granules of the bovine adrenal medulla. CG-A comprises up to 50% of the total protein secreted by the parathyroid gland and is a major component of secretory granules of cells of the adrenal medulla, pituitary, parathyroid, thyroid C cells, pancreatic islets, endocrine cells of the gastrointestinal tract, and sympathetic nerves. CG-A shares considerable homology between species. Immunologic cross-reactivity to mammalian proteins has been observed in reptiles, amphibians, fish, and *Drosophila* tissues. CG-A is synthesized as a preprotein and is directed to the internal cavity of the rough endoplasmic reticulum by the N-terminal preregion of the peptide and cleaved by a signal peptidase.

Although the functions of CG-A are still under investigation, several roles have been postulated. CG-A is suspected to play an important role in the maturation of secretory granules. Inside the Golgi apparatus, CG-A is involved in the packaging of the contents of newly formed vesicles. CG-A precipitates as it diffuses into the trans-Golgi network, and secretory products such as PTH become entrapped in the growing CG-A conglomerate and are subsequently packaged into secretory granules. CG-A has a large calcium-binding capacity, which may enhance the stability of secretory vesicles. As granules mature, they accumulate up to 40 mM of calcium, which also may serve as a route of Ca^{2+} secretion. CG-A–calcium complexes are important in maintaining the integrity of the secretory granules. The absence of calcium causes dissociation of protein complexes and results in osmotic lysis of the vesicle.

In summary, the intragranular functions of CG-A include hormone packaging, stabilization of the granule against osmotic gradients, and the excretion of intracellular calcium. During secretion, the contents of secretory granules are extruded into the pericapillary space. The pH and calcium concentration of the extracellular fluid promote the dissociation of CG-A complexes and solubilization of bound calcium and other contents of the granule. Once solubilized, extracellular peptidases cleave CG-A into biologically active peptides that act as paracrine or autocrine regulators of endocrine secretion (Deftos 1991).

CONTROL OF PARATHYROID HORMONE SECRETION. Secretory cells in the parathyroid gland store small amounts of preformed hormone and respond to minor fluctuations in calcium concentration by rapidly altering the rate of release of stored hormone and more slowly by altering the rate of hormonal synthesis and release. The parathyroid glands have a unique mechanism for feedback control due to the cellular response to the concentration of calcium and, to a lesser extent, of magnesium ions in the serum and perivascular space.

The influence of serum levels of ionized calcium and interaction with the Ca^{2+}-sensing receptors on chief cells results in the formation of an inverse sigmoidal type of relationship between serum Ca^{2+} and PTH concentrations (Figure 12.7). The serum $[Ca^{2+}]$ that results in half-maximal PTH secretion is defined as the serum calcium *set-point*, and this is stable for an individual animal. The sigmoidal type of relationship between serum $[Ca^{2+}]$ and PTH secretion permits the chief cells to respond rapidly to a reduction in serum $[Ca^{2+}]$. Ionized calcium binds to the Ca^{2+}-sensing receptor and results in an increase in the intracellular Ca^{2+} concentration of chief cells and a reduction in PTH secretion. This makes the parathyroid chief cells unique because increased intracellular Ca^{2+} concentrations typically serve as a stimulus for secretion in most cell types.

The major inhibitors of PTH synthesis and secretion are increased serum levels of $[Ca^{2+}]$ and 1,25-dihydroxyvitamin D. Inhibition of PTH synthesis by 1,25-dihydroxyvitamin D completes an important endocrine feedback loop between the parathyroid chief cells and the renal epithelial cells because PTH stimulates renal production of 1,25-dihydroxyvitamin D (Figure 12.8). If the blood calcium level is elevated by the intravenous infusion of calcium, there is a rapid and pronounced

reduction in circulating levels of immunoreactive PTH; however, a small percentage of the PTH secretion is nonsuppressible. Therefore, there are always low concentrations of circulating PTH in the blood, even under extreme conditions of hypercalcemia. Conversely, if the blood calcium is lowered by infusion of ethylenediaminetetraacetic acid (EDTA), there is a brisk and substantial increase in the level of immunoreactive PTH.

The concentration of blood phosphorus has no direct regulatory influence on the synthesis and secretion of PTH; however, certain disease conditions with hyperphosphatemia in animals and humans are associated clinically with hyperparathyroidism. An elevated blood phosphorus level may lead indirectly to parathyroid stimulation by virtue of its ability to lower blood levels of calcium. If the blood level of phosphorus is elevated significantly by the simultaneous infusion of phosphate and calcium in amounts sufficient to prevent the accompanying reduction of blood calcium by phosphate, plasma levels of immunoreactive PTH remain within the normal range.

Magnesium ion $[Mg^{2+}]$ has an effect on secretory rate of PTH similar to that of calcium, but the effect is not equipotent to that of calcium. The reduced potency of $[Mg^{2+}]$ compared with Ca^{2+} may be due to reducing binding affinity for $[Mg^{2+}]$ for the Ca^{2+}-sensing membrane receptors on chief cells. The more potent effects of Ca^{2+} in the control of PTH secretion, together with its preponderance over Mg^{2+} in the extracellular fluid, suggest a secondary role for magnesium in the control of the parathyroid gland.

Calcium ion not only controls the rate of synthesis and secretion of PTH, but also other metabolic and intracellular degradative processes occur within chief cells. An increase of calcium ions in extracellular fluids rapidly inhibits uptake of amino acids, synthesis of proPTH and conversion to PTH, and secretion of stored PTH by chief cells, as well as increasing the intracellular degradation of PTH. The shifting of the percentage of flow of proPTH from the degradative pathways to the secretory route represents a key adaptive response of the parathyroid gland to a low-calcium diet. During periods of long-term calcium restriction, the enhanced synthesis and secretion of PTH are accomplished by an increase in the capacity of the synthetic pathway in individual hypertrophied chief cells and through hyperplasia of active chief cells.

In response to increased demand, newly synthesized PTH may be released from the cell and bypass the storage pool of mature secretory granules in the cytoplasm of the chief cell. This bypass secretion (Figure 12.9) can only be stimulated by a low circulating concentration of calcium ion and not by the other secretagogues for PTH. Lysosomal enzymes degrade the PTH stored in secretory granules of chief cells during periods of prolonged exposure to a high-calcium environment.

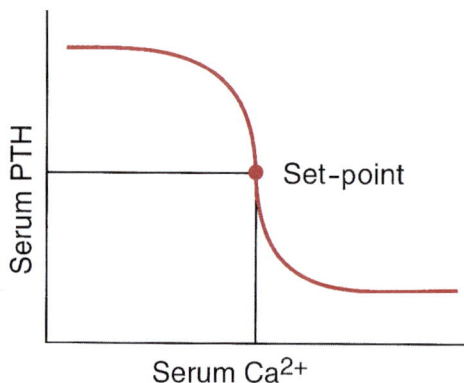

FIG. 12.7—The *set-point* for ionized calcium (Ca^{2+}) is defined as the concentration of ionized calcium at which the concentration of parathyroid hormone (PTH) in serum is half-maximal. The sigmoidal relationship between concentrations of Ca^{2+} and PTH enables the parathyroid glands to respond rapidly to a minor reduction in serum calcium and increase PTH secretion to restore the calcium concentration to normal levels in the serum. In most animals, the calcium concentration in the serum is maintained below the set-point concentration. (From Rosol et al. 1995.)

BIOLOGICAL EFFECTS OF PARATHYROID HORMONE. PTH is the principal hormone involved in the minute-to-minute, fine regulation of blood calcium in mammals. It

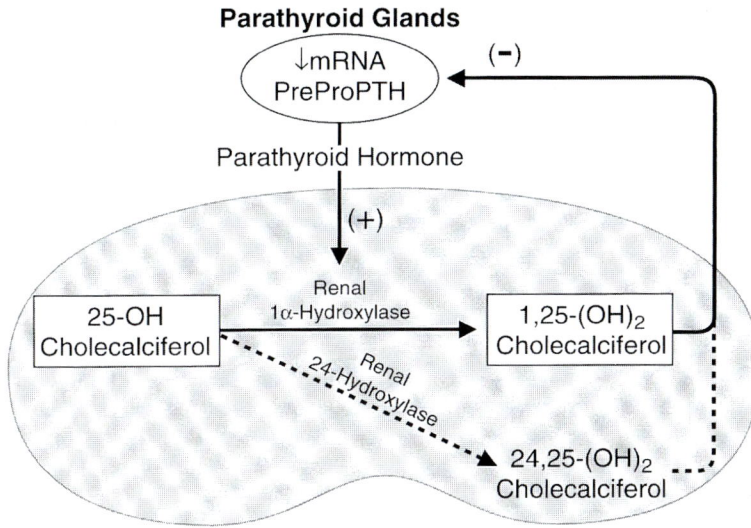

FIG. 12.8—Negative feedback exerted by vitamin D metabolites on the parathyroid chief cell to regulate the rate of parathyroid hormone secretion. 25-OH cholecalciferol is 25-hydroxycholecalciferol, and 24,25-$(OH)_2$ is 24,25-dihydroxycholecalciferol. mRNA, messenger RNA; and preproPTH, preproparathyroid hormone.

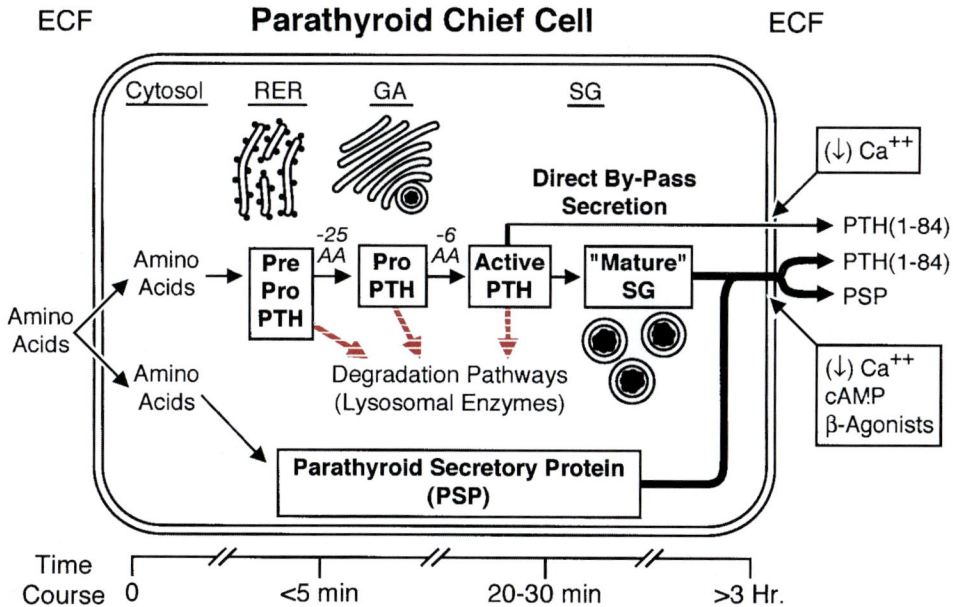

FIG. 12.9—Bypass secretion of parathyroid hormone (PTH) in response to the demand signaled by a decrease in the calcium ion (Ca^{++}) concentration in the blood. Recently synthesized and processed active PTH may be released directly from the chief cell and does not enter the storage pool of mature (*old*) secretory granules in the cytoplasm of the chief cell. Release of PTH from the storage pool is stimulated by cyclic adenosine monophosphate (cAMP) and β-agonists (e.g., epinephrine, norepinephrine, and isoproterenol) as well as by low concentrations of calcium ion in the blood. Secretion from the pool of recently synthesized PTH can be stimulated only by a decrease in the calcium-ion concentration. GA, Golgi apparatus; preproPTH, preproparathyroid hormone; proPTH, proparathyroid hormone; and RER, rough endoplasmic reticulum. (Redrawn from Cohn and MacGregor 1981.)

exerts its biological actions by directly influencing the function of target cells, primarily in the bone and kidney and secondarily in the intestine, to maintain plasma calcium at a level sufficient to ensure the optimal functioning of a wide variety of body cells. In general, the most important biological effects of PTH are to

1. Elevate the blood concentration of calcium
2. Decrease the blood concentration of phosphorus
3. Increase the urinary excretion of phosphorus by a decreased rate of tubular reabsorption
4. Increase the renal tubular reabsorption of calcium
5. Increase the rate of skeletal remodeling and the net rate of bone resorption
6. Increase the numbers of osteoclasts on bone surfaces and the rate of osteolysis
7. Increase the urinary excretion of hydroxyproline
8. Activate adenylate cyclase in target cells
9. Accelerate the formation of the principal active vitamin D metabolite (1,25-dihydroxycholecalciferol; 1,25-dihydroxyvitamin D) through a trophic effect of PTH on the 1α-hydroxylase in mitochondria of the epithelial cells lining the proximal convoluted tubules of the kidney

PTH mobilizes calcium from skeletal reserves into the extracellular fluids. The response of bone to PTH is biphasic. The immediate effects are the result of increasing the activity of existing osteocytes and osteoclasts. This rapid effect of PTH depends on the continuous presence of hormone and results in an increased flow of calcium to the bone surface through the coordinated action of osteocytes and activation of endosteal lining cells (inactive osteoblasts). The later effects of PTH on bone are of a greater magnitude of response and are not dependent on the continuous presence of PTH. Osteoclasts are primarily responsible for the long-term actions of PTH on increasing bone resorption and overall bone remodeling. This is particularly interesting in light of studies that have demonstrated the presence of receptors for PTH on osteoblasts but not on osteoclasts (Figure 12.10).

Bone resorption is a complex, multistep process that involves the activation of multiple genes and the action of multiple hormones (Teitelbaum 2000). Most hormones and cytokines that are involved in the regulation of bone resorption [e.g., PTH, calcitriol, interleukin 1β, tumor-necrosis factor (TNF), interleukin 6, and prostaglandin E_2] act via receptors on osteoblasts. Three new family members of the TNF ligand and receptor signaling system have been identified and cloned recently that play a critical role in the regulation of bone resorption [American Society for Bone and Mineral Research (ASBMR) Special Committee on Nomenclature 2000; Hofbauer 1999; Hofbauer et al. 2000]. In the presence of permissive concentrations of macrophage colony-stimulating factor (M-CSF), the new TNF superfamily molecules constitute the common pathway for regulation of osteoclast formation and function by cells of the osteoblast lineage, thereby

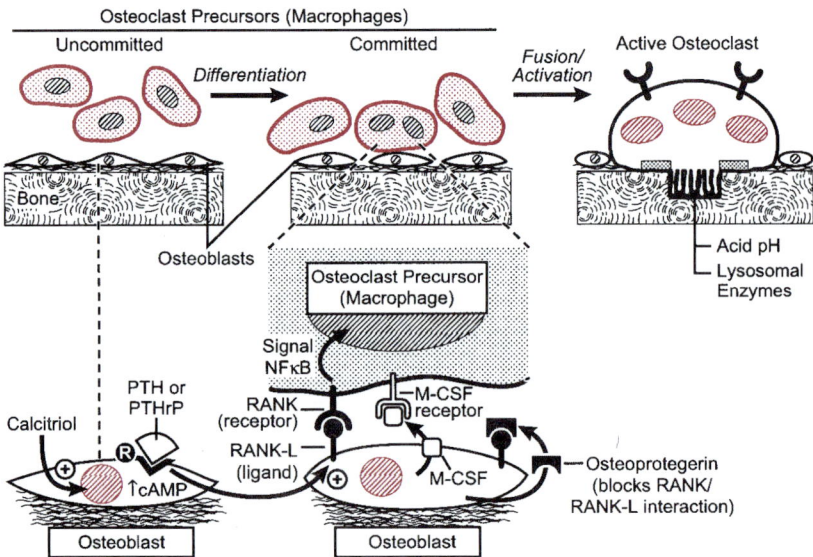

FIG. 12.10—Cellular control of bone resorption. Specific receptors for parathyroid hormone (PTH and PTH-rP) are present on osteoblasts but not on osteoclasts. RANK L) is a membrane-bound protein on osteoblasts that stimulates differentiation of cells of the osteoclast lineage. Expression of RANK L in osteoblasts is upregulated by osteotrophic factors such as PTH, calcitriol, and interleukin 11. M-CSF, macrophage colony-stimulating factor; PTH-rP, parathyroid hormone-related peptide; R, receptor for PTH or PTH-rP; R, receptor; and RANK L, receptor activator NF-κB ligand.

mediating the biological effects of many upstream hormones and cytokines (Suda et al. 1999).

The receptor ligand receptor activator NF-κB (RANK ligand or RANK L) is a membrane-bound protein on osteoblasts that serves as a common mediator for osteoclastic bone resorption (Takahashi et al. 1999; Martin and Gillespie 2001). This ligand [initially termed osteoclast differentiation factor (ODF)] and osteoprotegrin ligand (OPG L) is produced by osteoblast lineage cells and stimulates differentiation of cells of the osteoclast lineage, enhances the functional activity of mature osteoclasts, and prolongs osteoclast life by inhibiting apoptosis (ASBMR 2000; Hock et al. 2001) (Figure 12.11). Targeted deletion of the RANK L in mice leads to osteopetrosis, shortened bones, impaired tooth erup-

tion, and immunologic abnormalities. Expression of RANK L in osteoblasts/stromal cells is upregulated by osteotrophic factors such as calcitriol, PTH, and interleukin 11 (Suda et al. 1999). This molecule is identical to TNF-related activation-induced cytokine (TRANCE) or receptor activator of NF-κ B ligand (RANK L) reported in the immunology literature to stimulate T-cell growth and dendritic cell function (ASBMR 2000).

The membrane receptor (RANK) for the ligand (RANK L) on cells of the osteoclast lineage is identical with a receptor of similar name identified previously on immune cells (Suda et al. 1999; ASBMR 2000) (Figure 12.11). The receptor also has been referred to in the literature as osteoclast differentiation and activation receptor (ODAR). Binding of the ligand to this recep-

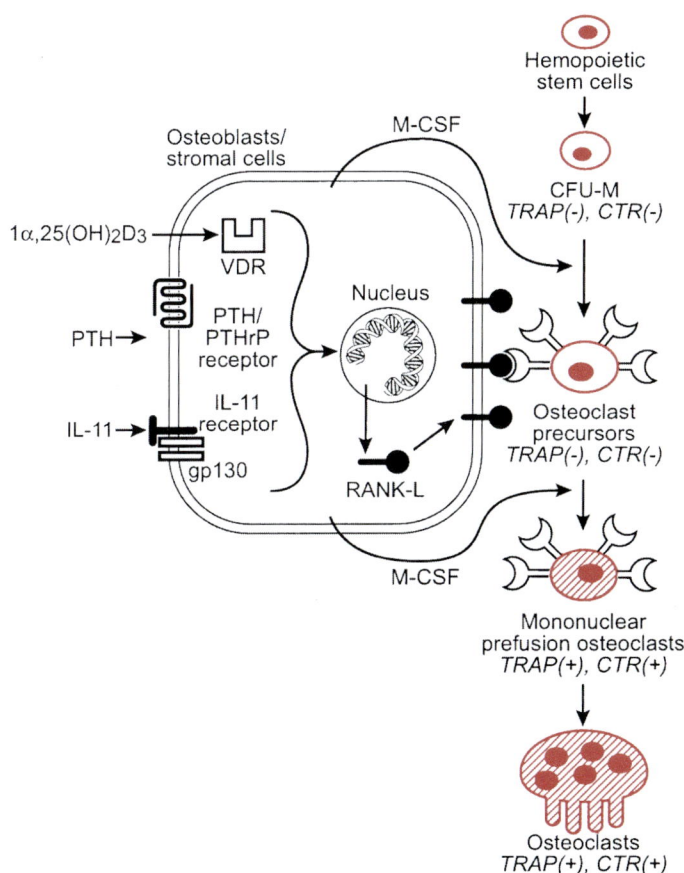

FIG. 12.11—A concept of osteoclast differentiation. Osteotropic factors such as $1\alpha,25(OH)_2D_3$ (dihydroxcholecalciferol), parathyroid hormone (PTH), and interleukin 11 (IL-11) stimulate osteoclast formation in cocultures of osteoblasts/stromal cells and hemopoietic cells. Target cells for these factors are osteoblasts/stromal cells. Three different signaling pathways mediated by the vitamin D receptor (VDR), PTH/PTH-rP receptor, and gp130 similarly induce osteoclast differentiation factor (ODF) or stromal osteoclast-forming activity (SOFA) as a membrane-associated factor in osteoblasts/stromal cells. Osteoclast progenitors of the monocyte-macrophage lineage recognize ODF/SOFA in osteoblasts/stromal cells through cell-to-cell interaction and then differentiate into osteoclasts. Macrophage colony-stimulating factor (M-CSF) produced by osteoblasts/stromal cells is a prerequisite for both proliferation and differentiation of osteoclast progenitors. CFU-M, colony-forming unit–megakaryocyte; CTR, calcitonin receptor; PTH-rP, parathyroid hormone-related peptide; RANK L, receptor activator NF-κB ligand; and TRAP, tartrate-resistant acid phosphatase. (Modified and redrawn from Suda et al. 1999.)

tor activates signaling pathways in osteoclasts that lead to increased functional activity. Osteoclast precursors express RANK, recognize RANK L through cell-to-cell interaction with osteoblasts/stromal cells, and differentiate into prefusion osteoclasts in the presence of M-CSF. Mice made deficient in RANK by targeted deletion of the gene develop severe osteopetrosis due to decreased osteoclast function and fail to develop peripheral lymph nodes (ASBMR 2000).

Osteoprotegerin (OPG) (*decoy receptor*) is a novel member of the TNF receptor superfamily produced by cells of the osteoblast lineage/stromal cells and a negative regulator of bone resorption (Hofbauer 1999; Hofbauer et al. 2000) (Figure 12.12). When this soluble decoy receptor binds to the ligand (RANK L), it prevents the ligand from binding to its biological membrane receptor (RANK), thereby resulting in its inactivation. Overexpression of this decoy receptor in transgenic mice

leads to osteopetrosis associated with decreased osteoclast formation and function. In contrast, targeted gene ablation in mice results in severe osteoporosis and arterial mineralization (ASBMR 2000).

These recent findings clearly indicate that microenvironment in bone marrow provided by osteoblast lineage/stromal cells regulates osteoclast differentiation and function. Osteoclast formation appears to be determined by the ratio of RANK L/OPG, and alterations in this ratio may be a major cause of bone loss in certain metabolic disorders such as estrogen deficiency and glucocorticoid excess (Hofbauer et al. 2000; Rodan and Martin 2000) (Figure 12.13). A long-term increase in PTH secretion also may result in the formation of greater numbers of osteoblasts and an increase in bone formation and resorption. However, because bone resorption by osteoclasts usually is greater than bone formation by osteoblasts, there is a net negative balance in skeletal mass.

The initial binding of PTH to osteoblasts lining bone surfaces causes the cells to contract, thereby exposing the underlying mineral to osteoclasts (Figure 12.10). If

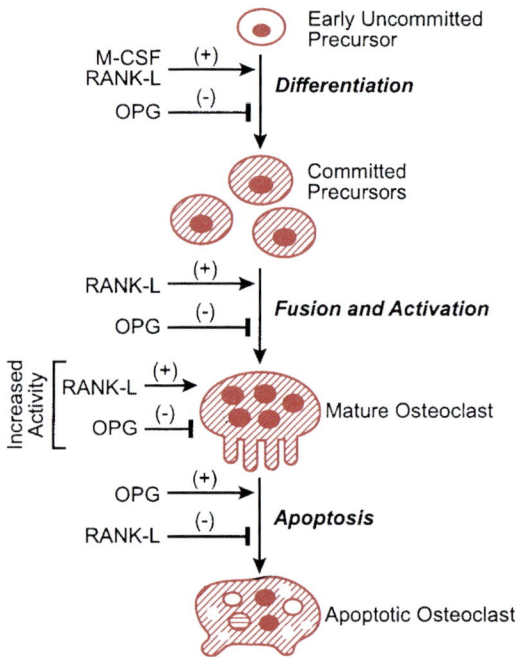

FIG. 12.12—Control of osteoclast functions by products of osteoblast cell lineage (OPG L/ODF and OPG/OCIF). Note that all steps of osteoclast formation and function are regulated by the OPG-L/OPG ratio, including initiation of differentiation, fusion of preosteoclasts to form active mature osteoclasts, regulation of osteoclast function, and osteoclast apoptosis. M-CSF is required only for the initiation of differentiation by uncommitted osteoclast precursors in bone marrow. M-CSF, macrophage colony-stimulating factor; OCIF, osteoclastogenesis inhibitory factor; ODF, osteoclast differentiation factor; OPG, osteoprotegerin; OPG L, osteoprotegerin ligand; and RANK L, receptor activator NF-κB ligand. (Modified and redrawn from Hofbauer et al. 2000.)

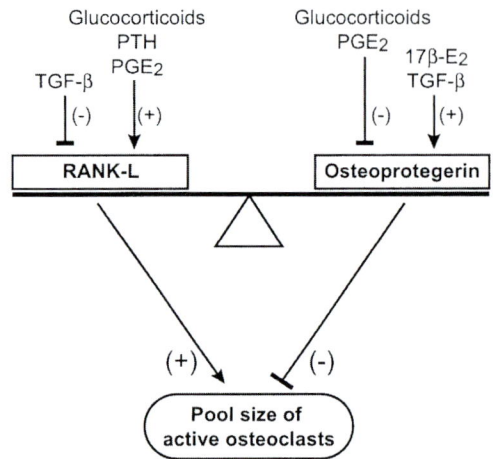

FIG. 12.13—*Convergence* hypothesis for the regulation of osteoclast functions by cytokines. This hypothesis proposes two levels of regulation of osteoclast functions. A variety of *upstream* cytokines and hormones alter the pool size of active osteoclasts by converging at the level of OPG L/ODF and OPG/OCIF. These two *downstream* factors serve as the final effectors for osteoclastogenesis and also affect osteoclast activation and osteoclast apoptosis. At steady state, there is a *balance* of levels of OPG L/ODF and OPG/OCIF that maintain a pool size of active osteoclasts that supports normal levels of bone resorption. When a change in one or more upstream factors tilts the balance toward a functional excess of OPG L/ODF, the pool size of active osteoclasts increases; when the balance tilts toward a functional excess of OPG/OCIF, the pool size decreases. 17β-E_2, 17β-estradiol; PGE_2, prostaglandin E_2; PTH, parathyroid hormone; RANK-L, receptor activator of NF-κB ligand; and TGF-β, transforming growth factor β. (Modified and redrawn from Hofbauer et al. 2000.)

the increase in PTH is sustained, the size of the active osteoclast pool in bone is increased by the activation of progenitor cells of the osteoclastic lineage. The plasma membrane of osteoclasts in intimate contact with the resorbing bone surface is modified to form a series of membranous projections referred to as the brush *ruffled* border (Figure 12.14). This area of active bone resorption is isolated from the extracellular fluids by adjacent transitional *sealing* zones, thereby localizing the lysosomal enzymes and acidic environment to the immediate area undergoing dissolution. The mineral and organic components such as hydroxyproline released from bone are phagocytosed by osteoclasts and transported across the cell in transport vesicles to be released into the extracellular fluid compartment.

PTH also has a direct and rapid effect on renal tubular function. By 5 to 10 minutes after PTH administration, the reabsorption of phosphate is decreased, causing phosphaturia. The site of action of PTH on the tubular reabsorption of phosphate has been localized by micropuncture methods to the proximal convoluted tubule of the nephron. In addition, PTH leads to the increased urinary excretion of potassium, sodium, bicarbonate, cyclic adenosine monophosphate, and amino acids. Although the effect of PTH on the tubular reabsorption of phosphate has been considered to be important, the capability of PTH to enhance the renal reabsorption of calcium is of more importance in the maintenance of calcium homeostasis. This effect of PTH upon tubular reabsorption of calcium appears to be due to a direct action on cells of the distal convoluted tubule of the kidney nephron. The other important effect of PTH on the kidney is the regulation of the conversion of 25-hydroxycholecalciferol to 1,25-dihydroxycholecalciferol and other metabolites of vitamin D (see Figure 12.8).

PTH promotes the absorption of calcium from the gastrointestinal tract in animals under a variety of experimental conditions (Nemere and Norman 1986). This effect is not as rapid as the action of PTH on the kidney and is not observed in vitamin D-deficient animals. This increased intestinal calcium transport may be due to a direct effect of PTH on the absorptive cells lining the intestine; however, the effect is more likely an indirect effect of PTH due to the stimulation of the renal synthesis of the biologically active metabolite of vitamin D.

Under normal conditions, PTH is secreted continuously from chief cells. Biologically active PTH is a linear peptide chain of 84 amino acids that is cleaved in the liver, and possibly elsewhere an amino-terminal fragment comprised of approximately one-third of the PTH molecule, and a larger carboxy-terminal fragment that is biologically inactive. PTH is secreted in two forms by chief cells: *first*, an intact PTH peptide comprised of amino acids 1 through 84 (PTH 1–84) and, *second*, a C-terminal peptide (PTH 35–84). Intact PTH (1–84) is the principal circulating biologically active form of PTH, has a half-life of less than 5 minutes, and is rapidly removed from the circulation by endopeptidases in

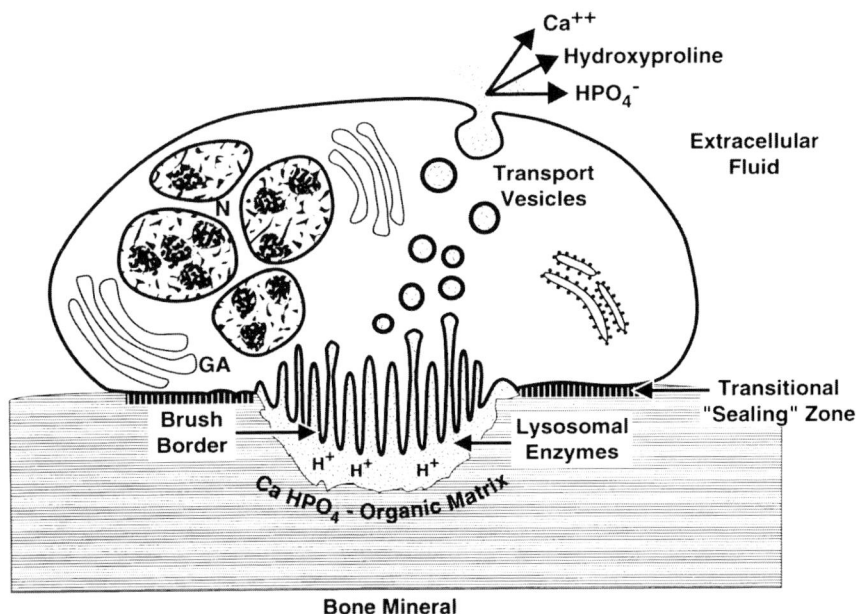

FIG. 12.14—Osteoclastic osteolysis on a bone surface with release of calcium, phosphorus, and hydroxyproline (from organic matrix of bone) into extracellular fluids. The brush border is a specialized area of the plasma membrane of osteoclasts that is in intimate contact with the underlying bone mineral. Adjacent transitional zones isolate the area undergoing active resorption and provide a mechanism for the concentration of lysosomal enzymes and acidic environment required for the dissolution of bone mineral. Ca^{2+}, ionized calcium; GA, Golgi apparatus; H+, ionized hydrogen; and HPO_4^-, phosphate ion.

hepatic Kupffer cell membranes or by glomerular filtration (Arnaud and Pun 1992). Some C-terminal peptide is released into the circulation by Kupffer cells and is then cleared by the kidney. The kidney is a major organ for the degradation of PTH. As a result, the C terminal PTH fragment has a biological half-life that is longer than that of intact PTH (1–84) and is present in the serum in higher concentrations (50% to 90% of total PTH), especially in cases of hyperparathyroidism associated with chronic renal disease.

The multiple forms of PTH and PTH fragments in the circulation made the development of specific and sensitive radioimmunoassays (RIAs) for this hormone difficult. Early assays for PTH were single-site RIAs for C-terminal peptides. These assays were suboptimal because both the biologically active and the inactive forms of PTH were measured; nevertheless, the assay was clinically useful to diagnose and monitor hyperparathyroidism in patients with normal renal function. Midregion and C-terminal RIAs measure both intact PTH (active) and C-terminal PTH (inactive), which renders them less clinically relevant. In addition, conditions that reduce the glomerular filtration rate, such as renal failure, result in a large increase in the serum concentration of C-terminal PTH. Concentrations of intact PTH in the serum of dogs, cats, and horses are best measured by a two-site immunoradiometric assay (IRMA).

PARATHYROID HORMONE RECEPTOR. The receptor for the N-terminal portion of the PTH is considered the most important region in terms of calcium regulation, and this region has been cloned and sequenced (Abou-Samra et al. 1992; Segre 1994). The receptor for N-terminal PTH is a seven-transmembrane domain receptor that is expressed in renal epithelial cells, osteoblasts, dermal fibroblasts, and also is found on cells that are not associated with the actions of PTH. Binding of PTH to the receptor results in increased levels of cytoplasmic 3′,5′-adenosine monophosphate (cAMP) and Ca^{2+} by stimulation of the adenylate cyclase and phosphatidylinositol pathways.

The calcium-mobilizing and phosphaturic activities of PTH are mediated through the intracellular accumulation of cAMP or Ca^{2+} in target cells. Binding of PTH to receptors on target cells results in activation of the receptor, binding of the receptor to stimulatory or inhibitory G proteins, and stimulation of adenyl (adenylate) cyclase or the hydrolysis of phosphatidylinositol (Figure 12.15). Receptors for PTH also bind a parathyroid-like factor, termed PTH-related protein (PTH-rP), which is an important factor in the pathogenesis of cancer-associated hypercalcemia. Stimulation of adenylyl cyclase stimulates the conversion of adenosine triphosphate (ATP) to cAMP in target cells. The accumulation of cAMP functions as an intracellular mediator or second messenger of PTH action in target cells to increase the permeability of the cell membrane for calcium ions. The cytosolic Ca^{2+} concentration may also be increased by the actions of

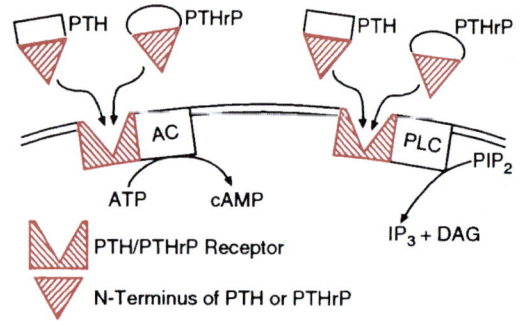

FIG. 12.15—Mechanism of action of parathyroid hormone (PTH) and parathyroid hormone-related protein (PTH-rP). The biologically active N-terminal ends of PTH and PTH-rP bind to PTH/PTH-rP receptors on the surface of the target cell. The receptor-hormone complexes are coupled to the catalytic subunit of adenylyl cyclase (AC) or to phospholipase C (PLC) by a nucleotide regulatory protein (G protein). This results in the conversion of adenosine triphosphate (ATP) to cyclic adenosine monophosphate (cAMP) by AC or phosphatidylinositol to inositol triphosphate (IP_3) and diacylglycerol (DAG) by PLC. The IP_3 that forms stimulates the release of Ca^{2+} from intracellular stores. Both cAMP and Ca^{2+} serve as second messengers for polypeptide hormones such as PTH and PTH-rP and result in the expression of the biological responses induced by these hormones. PIP_2, phosphatidyl inositol phosphate. (From Rosol and Capen 1992.)

inositol triphosphate to release Ca^{2+} from intracytoplasmic stores or by stimulation of Ca^{2+} transport through transmembrane channels. The resultant increase in cytosolic calcium, in combination with cAMP accumulation, initiates biochemical reactions in bone cells and renal epithelial cells to activate the intracellular functions of PTH.

Calcitonin. Although the appearance of calcitonin in primitive elasmobranch fish precedes the first appearance of PTH in amphibians, calcitonin or thyrocalcitonin in mammals was discovered after PTH (early 1960s compared with 1925 for PTH). Early experiments to test the McLean-Urist hypothesis of a negative-feedback control of blood calcium by PTH involved the perfusion of the parathyroid-thyroid complex of dogs with alternating low and high concentrations of calcium. However, the results were difficult to explain based on the concept that a single hormone controlled the concentration of calcium in the blood. *First*, the fall in systemic calcium following perfusion of the thyroid-parathyroid complex was more rapid and of greater magnitude than would be expected due only to the inhibition of PTH secretion. *Second*, thyroparathyroidectomy performed following the last low-calcium perfusion resulted in a continued progressive rise in blood calcium rather than the expected fall in levels of blood calcium following the removal of the source of PTH. Conflicting views on the source and role of calcitonin in mammals were resolved by definitive studies in goats, whose parathyroid glands, unlike those of dogs, can be perfused independently of the thyroid gland. The presence of a calcium-lowering hormone within the mammalian thyroid gland was further confirmed by the demonstration that a thyroid extract would produce a similar fall in plasma calcium. It is now well established that calcitonin is of thyroidal origin in mammals and that calcitonin and thyrocalcitonin are one and the same hormone.

C (PARAFOLLICULAR) CELLS IN THYROID OR ULTIMOBRANCHIAL GLANDS. Calcitonin is secreted by a second population of endocrine cells in the mammalian thyroid gland called C or parafollicular cells. These cells are distinct from the follicular cells of the thyroid gland that are responsible for the secretion of thyroxine (T_4) and triiodothyronine (T_3). The C cells of the mammalian thyroid gland are situated within the follicular wall immediately beneath the basement membrane or between follicular cells as well as in an interfollicular location. C cells do not border the follicular colloid directly, and their secretory polarity is oriented toward the interfollicular capillaries. The distinctive feature of the C cell in the thyroid gland is the presence of numerous small membrane-limited secretory granules in the cytoplasm that contain biologically active calcitonin.

Calcitonin-secreting cells are derived from cells of the neural crest. Primordial C cells migrate ventrally from the neural crest and become incorporated within the last pharyngeal (branchial) pouch of the developing embryo. The C cells are displaced caudally in the ultimobranchial body to the point of fusion with the midline primordia that gives rise to the thyroid gland. The ultimobranchial body fuses with, and is incorporated into, the thyroid hilus in mammals, and the C cells subsequently are distributed throughout the gland. Although C cells are found throughout the thyroid gland in humans and most other adult mammals, they often remain more numerous near the hilus and the point of fusion with the ultimobranchial body along major branches of the thyroid vessels. This is particularly true in the canine thyroid, where large nodules of C cells are present in the hilar region and elsewhere, and should not be misinterpreted as focal C-cell hyperplasia. In submammalian species, the C cells and calcitonin activity remain segregated in the ultimobranchial glands (bodies), which are anatomically distinct from the thyroid and the parathyroid glands. The avian ultimobranchial gland also contains a network of stellate cells with long cytoplasmic processes that support the C cells (Youshak and Capen 1971).

SYNTHESIS OF CALCITONIN. Calcitonin is a polypeptide hormone composed of 32 amino acid residues arranged in a straight chain with a 1–7 disulfide linkage. The amino acid sequence of porcine, canine, bovine, ovine, salmon, and human calcitonin, as well as for other animal species, has been determined. Calcitonin is synthesized as part of a larger biosynthetic precursor molecule (Wolfe 1982) called preprocalcitonin (Figure 12.16). It is transported to the Golgi apparatus, where it is converted to procalcitonin and then to calcitonin prior to packaging in membrane-limited secretory granules. Depending on the need for calcitonin, a proportion of the precursors and active hormone undergoes degradation prior to release from C cells. Under certain pathological conditions, C cells derived from the neural crest may secrete other humoral factors, including serotonin, bradykinin, ACTH, and prostaglandins.

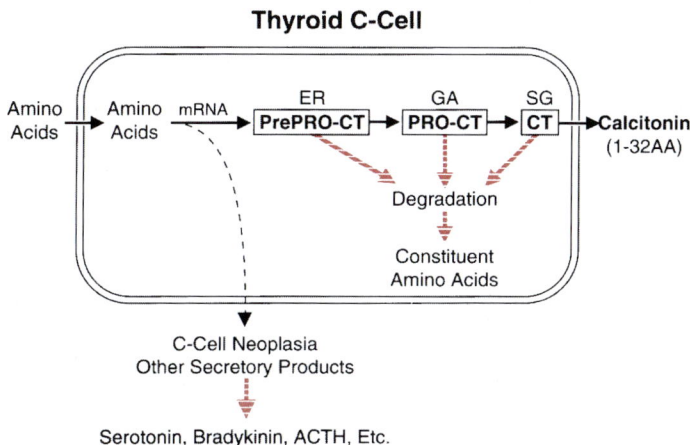

FIG. 12.16—Biosynthesis of calcitonin in C cells of the thyroid gland. Preprocalcitonin (prePRO-CT) and procalcitonin (PRO-CT) are biosynthetic precursors that undergo posttranslational processing to form biologically active calcitonin (CT). Some of these precursor molecules and biologically active calcitonin may undergo enzymatic degradation to the constituent amino acids (AAs) prior to secretion from the C cell. Under certain disease conditions, C cells may secrete other neuroendocrine products, including serotonin, bradykinin, and adrenocorticotropic hormone (ACTH). ER, endoplasmic reticulum; GA, Golgi apparatus; mRNA, messenger ribonucleic acid; and SG, secretory granule.

The calcitonin gene is expressed differently in thyroid (C cells) and than in neural tissues (Steenbergh et al. 1984; Jacobs 1985). In C cells of the mammalian thyroid the messenger RNA (mRNA) encodes primarily for pre-procalcitonin with a molecular weight of 17,400 D, whereas in neural tissues there is alternative RNA processing and encoding for calcitonin gene-related peptide (CGRP). This CGRP is a neuropeptide composed of 37 amino acids with a molecular weight of 15,900 D and participates in nociception, ingestive behavior, and modulation of the nervous and endocrine systems.

The structure of calcitonin differs considerably between species. The molecular structure of calcitonin for five selected species shares only 9 of the 32 amino acid residues. However, the amino-terminal portion of the calcitonin molecule is similar in all species. It consists of a seven-member ring enclosed by an intrachain (1–7) disulfide bridge. The complete sequence of 32 amino acids and the disulfide bond are essential for full biological activity. It is surprising that, on a weight basis, salmon calcitonin is more potent in lowering blood calcium than are any of the other calcitonins when administered to mammals, including humans. The reason for the greater biological potency of salmon calcitonin in mammals is uncertain but probably is related to an increased resistance to metabolic degradation and longer half-life or to a greater affinity for receptor sites in bone and other target tissues (Habener et al. 1972).

Serum levels of calcitonin are best measured by RIA. Because of the low degree of homology of calcitonin between species, there is poor cross-reactivity of RIAs for calcitonin. There is comparatively limited need to measure calcitonin in clinical veterinary medicine, due to the low incidence of calcitonin-secreting neoplasms and metabolic disorders resulting from abnormal levels of calcitonin. Since the sequencing of canine calcitonin, a canine-specific RIA has been developed to measure serum calcitonin in dogs (Hazewinkel 1991).

REGULATION OF CALCITONIN SECRETION. The concentration of ionized calcium in plasma and extracellular fluids is the principal physiological stimulus for the secretion of calcitonin by C cells. Calcitonin is secreted continuously under conditions of normocalcemia, but the rate of calcitonin secretion increases greatly in response to an elevation in blood calcium. Magnesium ion has a similar effect on calcitonin secretion, but this effect has been observed only under experimental conditions and for nonphysiological levels of magnesium. Under normal conditions, C cells store substantial amounts of calcitonin in their cytoplasm in the form of membrane-limited secretory granules.

The C-cell response to hypercalcemia is rapid release of stored hormone discharged into interfollicular capillaries. If the hypercalcemic stimulus is sustained, this is followed by the increased development of cytoplasmic organelles involved with the synthesis and secretion of calcitonin. The endoplasmic reticulum with attached ribosomes is hypertrophied, and the Golgi apparatus is enlarged and associated with prosecretory granules in the process of synthesis of calcitonin. Hyperplasia of C cells occurs in response to long-term hypercalcemia. When the blood calcium is lowered, the stimulus for calcitonin secretion is diminished and numerous secretory granules accumulate in the C-cell cytoplasm. The storage of large amounts of preformed hormone in C cells, and the rapid release of calcitonin in response to moderate elevations in blood calcium, probably are a reflection of the physiological role of calcitonin as an emergency hormone to protect against the development of hypercalcemia. Gastrointestinal hormones also may be important in triggering the early release of calcitonin following the ingestion of a high-calcium meal to prevent the development of hypercalcemia.

BIOLOGICAL EFFECTS AND PHYSIOLOGICAL SIGNIFICANCE OF CALCITONIN. The administration of calcitonin or stimulation of endogenous secretion results in the development of varying degrees of hypocalcemia and hypophosphatemia in animals. The effects of calcitonin on plasma calcium and phosphorus are most evident in young or older animals with increased rates of skeletal turnover. Calcitonin exerts its function by interacting with target cells located in bone, in kidney and, to a lesser extent, in intestinal cells. The actions of PTH and calcitonin on bone resorption are antagonistic (Figure 12.17), but they act synergistically to decrease the renal tubular reabsorption of phosphorus. The hypocalcemic effects of calcitonin are primarily the result of the decreased entry of calcium from the skeleton into plasma due to a temporary inhibition of PTH-stimulated resorption of bone. Hypophosphatemia develops from a direct action of calcitonin on increasing the rate of movement of phosphate out of plasma into soft tissue and bone, as well as from the inhibition of bone resorption by blockage of osteoclastic osteolysis (Figure 12.17). Osteoclasts have specific receptors for calcitonin in contrast to a lack of receptors for PTH.

Calcitonin and PTH act in concert to provide a negative-feedback mechanism to maintain the concentration of calcium in extracellular fluids within narrow limits. Under normal conditions, PTH is the major factor concerned with the minute-to-minute regulation of blood levels of calcium and protects against the development of hypocalcemia. Calcitonin functions more as an emergency hormone to (a) prevent the development of *physiological* hypercalcemia during the rapid, postprandial absorption of calcium, and (b) protect against excessive losses of calcium and phosphorus from the maternal skeleton during pregnancy. In hibernating vertebrates, the alternating secretion of calcitonin and PTH permits the cyclic withdrawal of calcium from the skeleton to maintain plasma calcium homeostasis during hibernation and ensure adequate bone structure after arousal.

Cholecalciferol (Vitamin D₃). Another major group of hormones involved in the regulation of calcium metab-

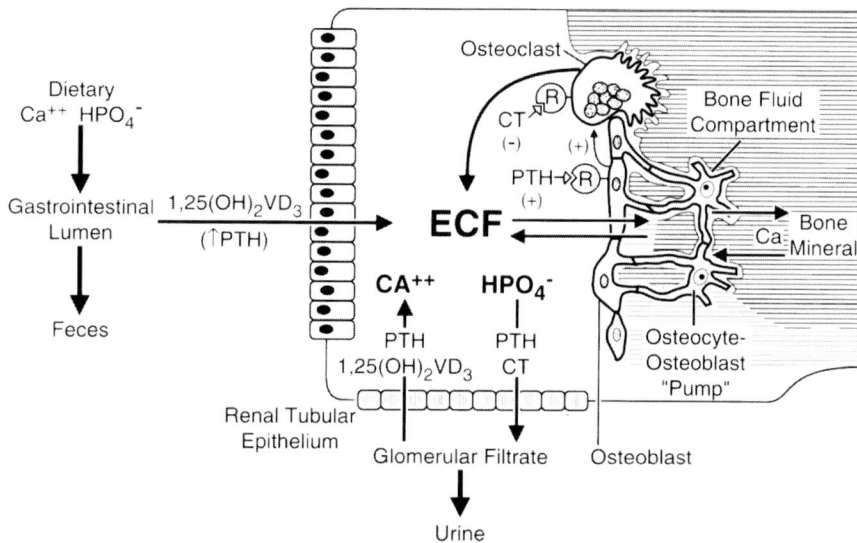

FIG. 12.17—Interrelationship of parathyroid hormone (PTH), calcitonin (CT), and 1,25-dihydroxycholecalciferol vitamin D_3 [1,25-$(OH)_2VD_3$] on the regulation of calcium (Ca) and phosphorus in extracellular fluids. CA^{++}, ionized calcium; ECF, extracellular fluid; HPO$_4^-$, phosphateion; and encircled R, PTH receptor.

olism and skeletal remodeling encompasses the various metabolites of vitamin D. The vitamin D family includes vitamin D_3 or cholecalciferol, vitamin D_2, also referred to as ergocalciferol or irradiated ergosterol, and 1,25 dihydroxycholecalciferol (calcitriol; 1,25 dihydroxyvitamin D). Due to their biological actions, these compounds, which have long been considered to be vitamins, can equally be considered hormones. Cholecalciferol is ingested in small amounts in the diet and can be synthesized in the epidermis from precursor molecules (Figure 12.18). This reaction is catalyzed by ultraviolet irradiation from the sun. A high-affinity vitamin D-binding protein in the serum transports cholecalciferol from its site of synthesis in the skin to the liver. In response to prolonged exposure to sunlight, previtamin D_3 is converted to lumisterol and tachysterol. Because the vitamin D-binding protein has no affinity for lumisterol and minimal affinity for tachysterol, the translocation of these photoisomers into the circulation is negligible, and they are sloughed with the natural turnover of the skin.

METABOLIC ACTIVATION OF VITAMIN D_3. Vitamin D_3 must be metabolically activated into a physiologically active hormonal form. The first step in the metabolic activation of vitamin D is the conversion of cholecalciferol to 25-hydroxycholecalciferol (25-OH-CC) in the liver under the enzymatic control of a hepatic microsomal enzyme referred to as calciferol 25-hydroxylase (Figure 12.18). Although 25-OH-CC may exert biological effects when substantial amounts are present, it primarily serves as a precursor for the formation of the more active metabolites of vitamin D.

High circulating levels of 25-OH-CC serve as a reservoir of vitamin D for the synthesis of the active forms of vitamin D by the kidney.

The 25-OH-CC synthesized in the liver is metabolized in the kidney to 1,25-dihydroxycholecalciferol or 1,25-$(OH)_2$-CC (Figure 12.19). The rate of formation of 1,25-$(OH)_2$-CC in mitochondria of renal epithelial cells of the proximal convoluted tubules is catalyzed by 25-hydroxycholecalciferol 1α-hydroxylase. The conversion of 25-OH-CC to 1,25-$(OH)_2$-CC is the rate-limiting step in vitamin D metabolism and is the primary reason for the time elapsed between the administration of vitamin D and the expression of biological effects. The control of this final step in the metabolic activation of vitamin D is complex and appears to be regulated by the concentration of calcium in the plasma, which influences the rate of secretion of PTH (Figure 12.19). PTH increases the conversion of 25-OH-CC to 1,25-$(OH)_2$-CC, whereas calcitonin is inhibitory under certain conditions.

A low concentration of phosphorus in the blood increases the rate of formation of 1,25-$(OH)_2$-CC, whereas a high phosphorus concentration suppresses the formation of active hormone (Figure 12.19). 1,25-Dihydroxyvitamin D_3 [1,25-$(OH)_2$-CC] is the major biologically active metabolite of cholecalciferol that interacts with target cells in the intestine and bone to enhance the rates of existing reactions and increase calcium mobilization under physiological conditions (Figure 12.20). Therefore, the onset of action is more rapid and the degree of potency is much greater than with either cholecalciferol or 25-OH-CC. A similar two-step process of metabolic activation occurs with the irradia-

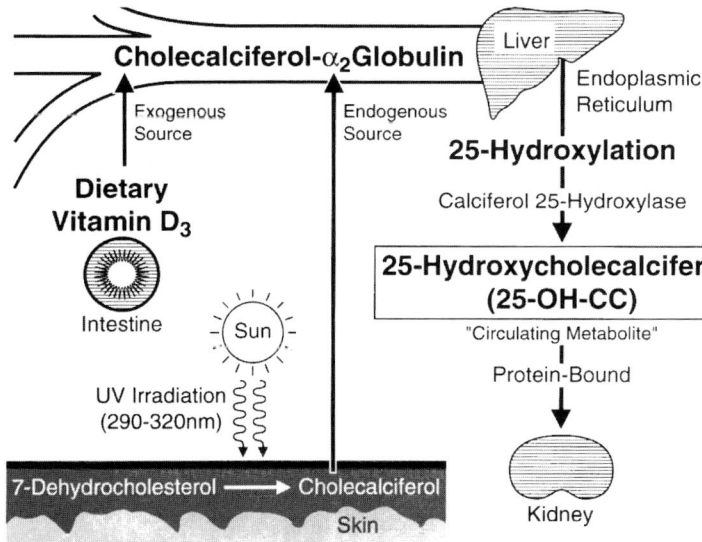

FIG. 12.18—Photochemical conversion of 7-dehydrocholesterol to previtamin D_3 in the epidermis after exposure to ultraviolet radiation from sunlight. Previtamin D_3 subsequently undergoes thermal conversion to vitamin D_3 (cholecalciferol), which enters dermal capillaries and binds to a specific binding protein (DBP, vitamin D-binding protein) for vitamin D_3. Protein-bound vitamin D_3 is transported to the liver for the initial step of metabolic activation.

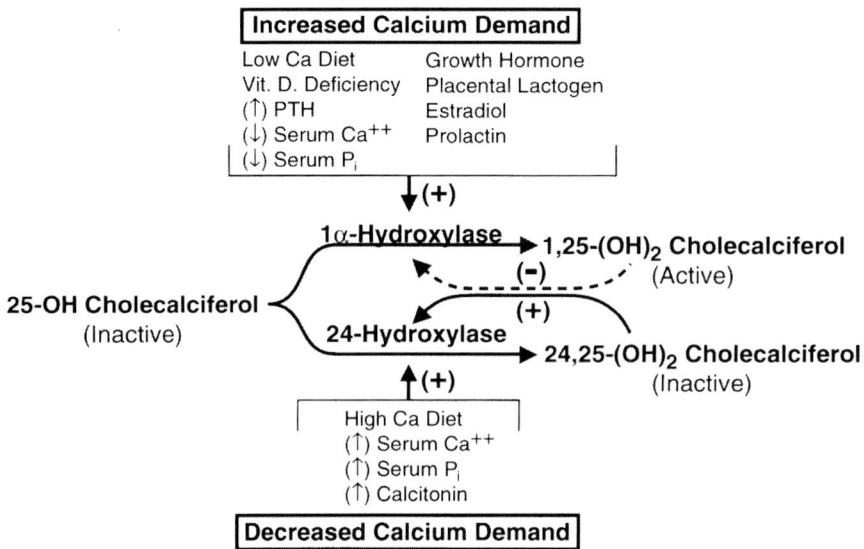

FIG. 12.19—Multifactorial control of the final step of metabolic activation of vitamin D in the kidney. Conditions associated with increased calcium demand result in the stimulation of the production of 1,25-dihydroxycholecalciferol [1,25-$(OH)_2$] from 25-OH cholecalciferol by increasing the activity of 1α-hydroxylase in the mitochondria of renal cells. Under conditions of decreased calcium demand, the production of 1,25-$(OH)_2$ cholecalciferol is diminished and 24,25-dihydroxycholecalciferol [24,25-$(OH)_2$] (an inactive metabolite) is formed by the enzymatic action of a 24-hydroxylase. CA^{++}, ionized calcium; P_i, inorganic phosphorus; and PTH, parathyroid hormone.

tion of ergosterol to form vitamin D_2. Hormones such as prolactin, estradiol, placental lactogen, and possibly growth hormone enhance the activity of renal 1α-hydroxylase and the formation of $1,25\text{-}(OH)_2\text{-}CC$. Participation of these hormones appears to be adaptive to meet the major calcium demands of the body.

BIOLOGICAL EFFECTS AND MECHANISM OF ACTION OF VITAMIN D METABOLITES. Vitamin D and its active metabolites function to increase the absorption of calcium and phosphorus from the intestine, thereby maintaining adequate levels of these electrolytes in the extracellular fluids in order to enable the appropriate mineralization of bone matrix (Figure 12.20). From a functional aspect, vitamin D can be thought to act in such a way as to cause the retention of sufficient mineral ions to ensure that the mineralization of bone matrix is adequate, whereas PTH with the "permissive effect" of vitamin D maintains the proper ratio of calcium to phosphate in the extracellular fluids.

The major target for $1,25\text{-}(OH)_2\text{-}CC$ is the absorptive cells of the mucosa of the small intestine. In the proximal part of the small intestine, $1,25\text{-}(OH)_2\text{-}CC$ increases the active transcellular transport of calcium and, in the distal intestine, the transport of phosphorus. Following synthesis in the kidney, $1,25\text{-}(OH)_2\text{-}CC$ is bound to a protein and transported to specific target cells in the intestine and bone. Circulating levels of the protein-bound $1,25\text{-}(OH)_2\text{-}CC$ are low compared with levels of 25-OH-CC. Free $1,25\text{-}(OH)_2\text{-}CC$ penetrates the plasma membrane of target cells, the hormone-receptor complex is transferred to the nucleus, and $1,25\text{-}(OH)_2\text{-}CC$ binds to specific receptors in the nuclear chromatin and stimulates gene expression, leading to the increased synthesis of vitamin D-dependent proteins such as the calcium-binding protein (CaBP) (calbindin) produced by intestinal cells (Figure 12.20). The luminal surface (brush border) of the intestinal absorptive cell is highly specialized and has numerous microvilli, which further increases the surface area of the intestine.

In response to $1,25\text{-}(OH)_2\text{-}CC$, the absorptive cells of the intestine synthesize a specific calcium-binding protein. This protein (CaBP or calbindin) has been isolated from several tissues, including the small intestine, kidney, parathyroid gland, bone, mammary gland, and the shell gland of laying hens. A vitamin D-dependent calcium-binding protein also has been demonstrated in bone, particularly in the spongiosa and cartilaginous growth plate. The absorptive capacity of the intestine for calcium is a direct function of the amount of calcium-binding protein that is present. The administration of vitamin D or feeding low-calcium and low-phosphorus diets to animals has been shown to

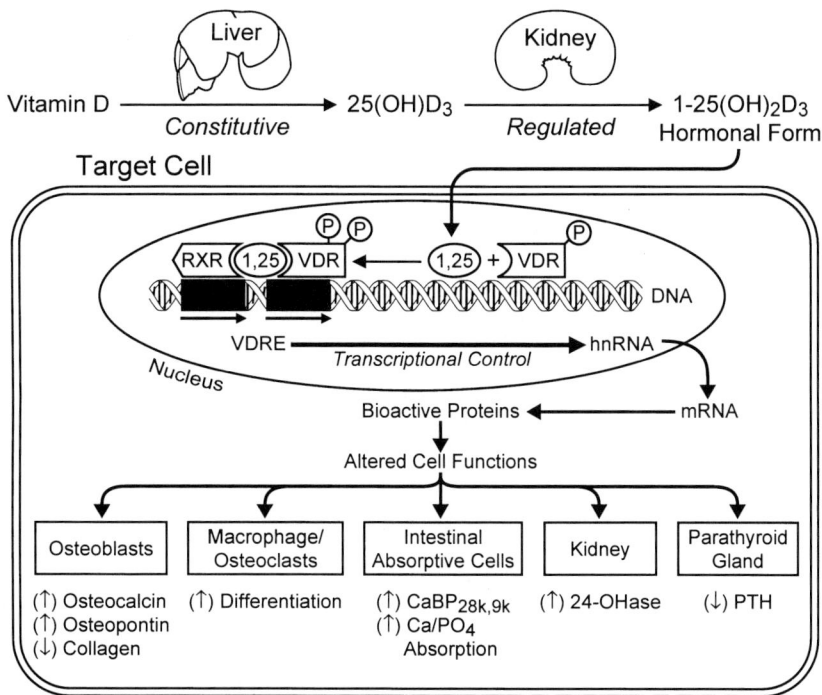

FIG. 12.20—Vitamin D metabolism and cellular actions, mediated by the vitamin D receptor (VDR)-retinoid X receptor (RXR). CaBP, calcium-binding protein (calbindin); IL-2, interleukin 2; mRNA, messenger RNA; 24-OHase, 24-hydroxylase; PO_4, phosphate ion; PTH, parathyroid hormone; and VDRE, vitamin D receptor element.

stimulate the synthesis of calcium-binding protein, which contributes to the increased absorption of calcium by intestine. The physiological functions of this binding protein are related to the transcellular transport of calcium from the luminal to basilar border of intestinal absorptive cells and in the regulation of intracellular calcium concentration to prevent injury to the cells from a high cytosolic calcium content. Calcium is exchanged for sodium at the basilar aspect of intestinal absorptive cells and enters the extracellular fluids. The active metabolites of cholecalciferol also act on bone. In young animals, vitamin D is required for the orderly growth of bone and mineralization of cartilage in the growth plate. Evidence in the literature suggests that the active metabolites of vitamin D also have a direct effect on the parathyroid gland, in addition to their well-characterized actions on intestine and bone. The parathyroid glands selectively localize 1,25-(OH)$_2$-CC and contain specific cytoplasmic and nuclear receptors for the active metabolites of vitamin D. Either alone or in combination, vitamin D metabolites directly interact with parathyroid cells to regulate transcription of preproPTH mRNA and to diminish the secretion of PTH, which in turn decreases the formation of 1,25-(OH)$_2$-CC (Figure 12.8). The active metabolites of vitamin D, in particular 1,25-(OH)$_2$-CC, have many roles in health and disease beyond the regulation of calcium metabolism (Walters 1992) (Figure 12.20). Vitamin D functions to regulate cell growth and differentiation, and the vitamin D receptor is widespread in tissues, including hematopoietic, muscle, skin, and lung cells; and cells of endocrine glands, the gastrointestinal and urinary tracts, and the reproductive and nervous systems.

PHOSPHATE METABOLISM. Phosphate in the mammalian body is present predominantly (90%) as hydroxyapatite [Ca$_{10}$(PO$_4$)$_6$(OH)$_2$] in the mineralized matrix of bone, with most of the remaining 10% occurring intracellularly in soft tissues. Phosphate is the major intracellular anion existing in organic forms (e.g., phospholipids, nucleic acids, phosphoproteins, and ATP) or inorganic forms and plays an integral role in many metabolic processes (e.g., energy metabolism, delivery of oxygen to tissues, muscle contraction, and skeletal integrity). Rapid translocations can occur between intracellular and serum phosphate pools, which can dramatically change serum phosphate concentrations. In nonruminant animals on normal diets with adequate amounts of vitamin D, the kidneys are the major regulators of serum phosphate concentration.

Serum phosphate is measured as orthophosphate (i.e., inorganic phosphate or P$_i$), since the organic forms are not routinely evaluated. Although inorganic phosphate is measured, it is often expressed as elemental phosphorus (P$_i$). Serum P$_i$ ranges from 2.5 to 6.0 mg/dL (0.8 to 1.9 mmol/L) in adult animals; however, serum P$_i$ concentrations are greater in young animals (especially giant-breed dogs) and may be outside the normal range for adult animals. Most serum inorganic phosphate (80%) is in the dibasic form, HPO$_4^{2-}$ and the remaining 20% is primarily in the monobasic form, H$_2$PO$_4^-$.

It is important to prevent hemolysis of blood samples, which will artificially increase the measurement of serum phosphate due to the release of intracellular stores. Phosphate circulates as a free anion; bound to Na$^+$, Mg^{2+}, or Ca^{2+}; or bound to protein (10% to 20% of total serum phosphate). Serum phosphate is an unreliable indicator of body stores, and its level may be higher in younger animals, since growth hormone increases renal phosphate reabsorption. High-carbohydrate diets or glucose infusions will decrease serum phosphate due to a shift of phosphate intracellularly in response to increased glycolysis and the need for phosphorylated intermediates. High-meat diets may increase serum phosphate due to their high phosphate content.

Absorption of dietary phosphate is approximately 60% to 70% and occurs by active transport using a sodium-phosphate cotransporter and by passive diffusion. In ruminants, the transporter may be coupled to H$^+$ rather than Na$^+$ (Shirazi-Beechey et al. 1996). Absorption takes place principally in the forestomachs (ruminants) and duodenum and jejunum (monogastric animals and ruminants). Horses may absorb some phosphate from the large intestine. The active form of vitamin D (1,25-dihydroxyvitamin D) increases intestinal phosphate absorption. Low dietary levels of phosphate result in adaptive changes in the intestine that result in increased net phosphate absorption.

The source of dietary phosphorus affects its availability. Inorganic sources of phosphate and bone and meat meals have high bioavailability (95%). Some diets contain substances or nutrients that can antagonize phosphate absorption, including aluminum and magnesium. Diets high in calcium and fat raise the requirement for phosphorus. Most phosphorus in concentrate sources is in the organic form of phytate, which is poorly utilized in nonruminants. Ruminants have phytases to release the phosphate from the sugar skeleton, but nonruminants do not.

In ruminants, large amounts of endogenous phosphate enter the gastrointestinal tract from salivary secretions (Care 1994; Barlet et al. 1995). Parotid saliva in ruminants is 16 to 40 mmol/L phosphate, and total phosphate secretion by the salivary glands is significantly greater than the dietary supply of phosphate. The endogenous salivary secretion of phosphate is complimented by intestinal phosphate absorption and massive recycling of phosphate resulting in greater phosphate absorption in the gastrointestinal tract in ruminants compared with monogastric animals. Increased endogenous salivary secretion of phosphate will lead to increased intestinal absorption but also increased endogenous fecal loss resulting in a net loss of phosphate. Ruminants fed a high-roughage diet use endogenous fecal loss of phosphate as the principal mechanism to regulate phosphate excretion. In contrast, ruminants on concentrate diets excrete more phosphate in the urine due to reduced saliva flow and a reduction in endogenous fecal loss. Therefore, the quantity of saliva and regulation of phosphate concentration in salivary secretions are important determinants of phosphate excretion in ruminants.

Renal excretion of phosphate is determined by the glomerular filtration rate (GFR) and the maximum tubular reabsorption rate (TmP) (Yanagawa and Lee 1992). The majority of renal phosphate reabsorption occurs in the proximal convoluted tubule, with small amounts in the distal nephron. Reabsorption is sodium dependent since phosphate transport is performed by a brush border sodium-phosphate cotransporter (Biber et al. 1996). The sodium gradient is maintained by a Na-K ATPase, and therefore phosphate reabsorption is indirectly energy dependent. The regulation of renal phosphate reabsorption can adapt to the body's need for phosphate. Reabsorption is increased with growth, lactation, pregnancy, and low-phosphate diets and is decreased during slow growth, renal failure, or excess dietary phosphorus (Lötscher et al. 1996). The major hormonal regulator is PTH, which decreases the TmP and increases renal phosphate excretion (Murer et al. 1996). Other hormones that inhibit Na-P_i cotransport include calcitonin, atrial natriuretic peptide, epidermal growth factor, transforming growth factors α and β, and PTH-related protein. In contrast, insulin, growth hormone, and insulin-like growth factor I stimulate Na-P_i cotransport by renal epithelial cells (Kempson 1996).

REFERENCES

Abou-Samra A-B, Jüppner H, Force T, et al. 1992. Expression cloning of a common receptor for parathyroid hormone and parathyroid hormone-related peptide from rat osteoblast-like cells: A single receptor stimulates intracellular accumulation of both cAMP and inositol triphosphates and increases intracellular calcium. Proc Natl Acad Sci USA 89:2732–2736.

American Society of Bone and Mineral Research (ASBMR) Special Committee on Nomenclature. 2000. Proposed standard nomenclature for new tumor necrosis factor members involved in the regulation of bone resorption. Bone 27:761-764.

Arnaud CD, Pun K-K. 1992. Metabolism and assay of parathyroid hormone. In: Coe FL, Favus MJ, eds. Disorders of Bone and Mineral Metabolism. New York: Raven, p 107–122.

Barlet JP, Davicco MJ, Coxam V. 1995. Physiologie de l'absorption intestinale du phosphore chez l'animal. Reprod Nutr Dev 35:475–489.

Biber J, Custer M, Magagnin S, et al. 1996. Renal Na/Pi-cotransporters. Kidney Int 49:981–985.

Brown EM, Hebert SC. 1996. A cloned extracellular Ca^{2+}-sensing receptor: Molecular mediator of the actions of extracellular Ca^{2+} on parathyroid and kidney cells? Kidney Int 49:1042–1046.

Brown EM, Pollak M, Seidman CE, et al. 1995. Calcium-ion-sensing cell-surface receptors. N Engl J Med 333:234–240.

Care AD. 1994. The absorption of phosphate from the digestive tract of ruminant animals. Br Vet J 150:197–205.

Chattopadhyay N, Mithal A, Brown EM. 1996. The calcium-sensing receptor: A window into the physiology and pathophysiology of mineral ion metabolism. Endocr Rev 17:289–307.

Chew DJ, Nagode LA, Carothers M. 1992. Disorders of calcium: Hypercalcemia and hypocalcemia. In: Di Bartola SP, ed. Fluid Therapy in Small Animal Practice. Philadelphia: WB Saunders, p 116–176.

Cohn DV, MacGregor RR. 1981. The biosynthesis, intracellular processing, and secretion of parathormone. Endocr Rev 2:1–26.

Deftos L. 1991. Chromogranin A: Its role in endocrine function and as an endocrine and neuroendocrine tumor marker. Endocr Rev 12:181–187.

Favus MJ. 1992. Intestinal absorption of calcium, magnesium, and phosphorus. In: Coe FL, Favus MJ, eds. Disorders of Bone and Mineral Metabolism. New York: Raven, p 57–82.

Habener JF, Potts JT Jr. 1978. Biosynthesis of parathyroid hormone. N Engl J Med 299:580–585.

Habener JF, Singer FR, Neer RM, et al. 1972. Metabolism of salmon and porcine calcitonin: An explanation for the increased potency of salmon calcitonin. In: Talmage RV, Munson PL, eds. Calcium, Parathyroid Hormone and the Calcitonins. Amsterdam: Excerpta Medica, p 152–163.

Haussler MR, Haussler CA, Jurutka PW, et al. 1997. The vitamin D hormone and its nuclear receptor: Molecular actions and disease states. J Endocrinol 154(Suppl):S57–S73.

Hazewinkel HAW. 1991. Dietary influences on calcium homeostasis and the skeleton. In Proceedings of the First Purina International Nutrition Symposium. Orlando, FL: Eastern States Veterinary Conference, pp 51–61.

Hock JM, Krishnan V, Onyia JE, et al. 2001. Osteoblast apoptosis and bone turnover. J Bone Miner Res 16:975–984.

Hofbauer LC. 1999. Osteoprotegerin ligand and osteoprotegerin: Novel implications for osteoclast biology and bone metabolism. Eur J Endocrinol 141:195–210.

Hofbauer LC, Khosla S, Dunstan CR, et al. 2000. The roles of osteoprotegerin and osteoprotegerin ligand in the paracrine regulation of bone resorption. J Bone Miner Res 15:2–12.

Holick MF. 1981. The cutaneous photosynthesis of previtamin D$_3$: A unique photoendocrine system. J Invest Dermatol 77:51–58.

Jacobs JW. 1985. Calcitonin gene expression. J Bone Miner Res 3:151.

Kempson SA. 1996. Peptide hormone action on renal phosphate handling. Kidney Int 49:1005–1009.

Lötscher M, Wilson P, Nguyen S, et al. 1996. New aspects of adaptation of rat renal Na-Pi cotransporter to alterations in dietary phosphate. Kidney Int 49:1012–1018.

Martin TJ, Gillespie MT. 2001. Receptor activator of nuclear factor kappa B ligand (RANK L): Another link between breast and bone. Trends Endocrinol Metab 12:2–4.

Murer H, Lötscher M, Kaissling B, et al. 1996. Renal brush border membrane Na/Pi-cotransport: Molecular aspects in PTH-dependent and dietary regulation. Kidney Int 49:1769–1773.

Nemere I, Norman AW. 1986. Parathyroid hormone stimulates calcium transport in perfused duodena from normal chicks: Comparison with the rapid (transcaltachic) effect of 1,25-dihydroxyvitamin D$_3$. Endocrinology 119:1406–1408.

Rodan GA, Martin TJ. 2000. Therapeutic approaches to bone diseases. Science 289:1508–1514.

Rosol TJ, Capen CC. 1992. Biology of disease: Mechanisms of cancer-induced hypercalcemia. Lab Invest 67:680–702.

Rosol TJ, Chew DJ, Nagode LA, Capen CC. 1995. Pathophysiology of calcium metabolism. Vet Clin Pathol 24:49–63.

Rouse D, Suki WN. 1990. Renal control of extracellular calcium. Kidney Int 38:700–708.

Segre GV. 1994. Receptors for parathyroid hormone and parathyroid hormone-related protein. In: Bilezikian JP, Marcus R, Levine MA, eds. The Parathyroids. New York: Raven, pp 213–229.

Shirazi-Beechey SP, Penny JI, Dyer J, et al. 1996. Epithelial phosphate transport in ruminants, mechanisms and regulation. Kidney Int 49:992–996.

Siesjö BK. 1989. Calcium and cell death. Magnesium 8:223–237.

Steenbergh PH, Hoppener JWM, Zandberg J, et al. 1984. Calcitonin gene related peptide coding sequence is conserved in the human genome and is expressed in medullary thyroid carcinoma. J Clin Endocrinol Metab 59:358–360.

Suda T, Takahashi N, Udagawa N, et al. 1999. Modulation of osteoclast differentiation and function by the new members of the tumor necrosis factor receptor and ligand families. Endocr Rev 20:345–357.

Takahashi N, Udagawa N, Suda T. 1999. A new member of tumor necrosis factor ligand family, ODF/OPGL/TRANCE/RANKL, regulates osteoclast differentiation and function. Biochem Biophys Res Commun 256:449–455.

Teitelbaum SL. 2000. Bone resorption by osteoclasts. Science 289:1504–1508.

Walters MR. 1992. Newly identified actions of the vitamin D endocrine system. Endocr Rev 13:719–764.

Weaver CM. 1990. Assessing calcium status and metabolism. J Nutr 120:1470–1473.

Wolfe HJ. 1982. Calcitonin: Perspectives and current concepts. J Endocrinol Invest 5:423–432.

Yanagawa N, Lee DBN. 1992. Renal handling of calcium and phosphorus. In: Coe FL, Favus MJ, eds. Disorders of Bone and Mineral Metabolism. New York: Raven, pp 3–40.

Youshak MS, Capen CC. 1971. Ultrastructural evaluation of ultimobranchial glands from normal and osteopetrotic chickens. Gen Comp Endocrinol 16:430–442.

PART 2: METABOLIC DISORDERS OF CALCIUM-PHOSPHORUS HOMEOSTASIS

CHARLES C. CAPEN

HYPERPARATHYROIDISM. This is a metabolic disorder in which excessive amounts of PTH secreted by pathological parathyroid glands disturb mineral and/or skeletal homeostasis. The predominant clinical features are the result of disturbances of serum calcium and bone metabolism, due to prolonged hypersecretion of parathyroid hormone (PTH) (Capen 2001b). The skeletal lesion of generalized fibrous osteodystrophy (osteitis fibrosa) is characterized by increased bone resorption, decreased radiographic density, and incomplete fractures.

Primary Hyperparathyroidism. PTH is produced in excess of normal in primary hyperparathyroidism by a functional lesion in the parathyroid gland for no useful purpose. This disease is encountered less frequently in older dogs than is the relatively common secondary hyperparathyroidism.

The normal control mechanisms for PTH secretion by the concentration of blood calcium ion are lost in primary hyperparathyroidism. Hormone secretion is autonomous, and the parathyroid gland produces excessive amounts of hormone despite a sustained increase of blood calcium. Cells of the renal tubules are particularly sensitive to alterations in the amount of circulating PTH. The hormone acts on these cells initially to promote the excretion of phosphorus and the retention of calcium (Figure 12.21). A prolonged increased secretion of PTH results in accelerated osteocytic and osteoclastic bone resorption. Mineral is removed from the skeleton and replaced by immature fibrous connective tissue. The bone lesion of fibrous osteodystrophy is generalized throughout the skeleton but is accentuated in local areas.

The lesion responsible for the excessive secretion of PTH in dogs usually is an adenoma composed of active chief cells with interspersed oxyphil and water-clear cells (Capen 2001a). Chief cell adenomas usually are single and result in considerable enlargement of the parathyroid gland. They can be located either in the cervical region near the thyroid or infrequently within the thoracic cavity near the base of the heart. Other lesions occasionally associated with primary hyperparathyroidism are chief cell hyperplasia and chief cell carcinoma. C cells in the thyroid gland are usually hyperplastic but are unable to return the blood calcium to normal.

The pathophysiological disturbances observed are the result of weakening of bones by excessive resorption. Lameness due to fractures of long bones may occur after relatively minor physical trauma. Compression fractures of vertebral bodies can exert pressure on the spinal cord and nerves, resulting in motor and/or sensory dysfunction. Excessive resorption of cancellous bone of the skull, resulting in a loosening or loss of teeth from alveolar sockets, and hyperostosis of the mandible and maxilla, due to proliferation of woven bone, have been observed in dogs with primary hyperparathyroidism. Radiographic evaluation reveals areas of subperiosteal cortical resorption, loss of lamina dura around the teeth, soft-tissue mineralization, bone cysts, and a generalized decrease in bone density with multiple fractures. Mineralization of renal tubules and formation of multiple calculi may occur in advanced cases of primary hyperparathyroidism in dogs with substantial elevations of blood calcium. Hypercalcemia results in anorexia, vomiting, constipation, depression, and generalized muscular weakness due to decreased neuromuscular excitability.

The most important and practical laboratory tests to aid in establishing the diagnosis of primary hyperparathyroidism are quantitation of total and ionized blood calcium and intact PTH immunoassay. Hypercalcemia is a consistent finding and results from accelerated release of calcium from bone and increased renal calcium reabsorption (although total urine calcium excretion is increased because of the increased filtered calcium) (Figure 12.21). The blood calcium of normal

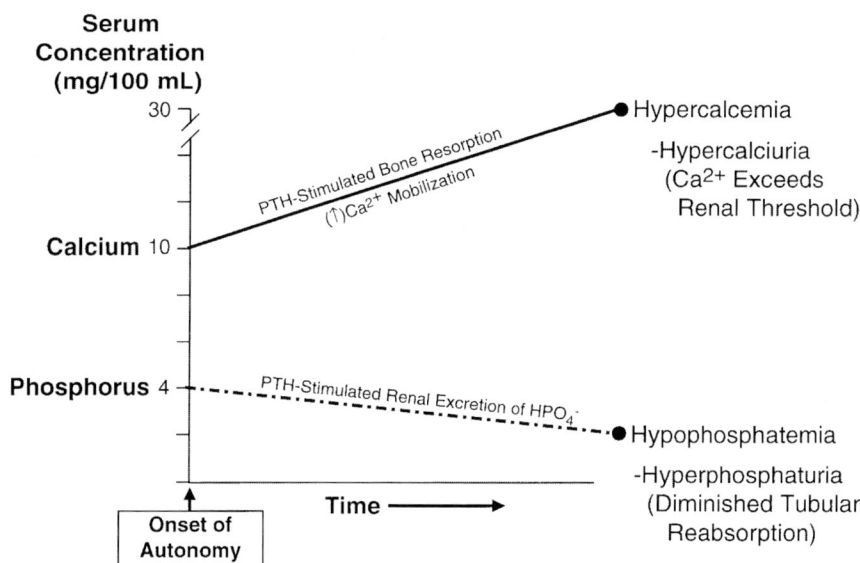

FIG. 12.21—Primary hyperparathyroidism. Alterations in serum calcium and phosphorus in response to an autonomous secretion of parathyroid hormone (PTH) in primary hyperparathyroidism. Ca^{2+}, ionized calcium; and HPO_4^-, phosphate ion.

animals is near 10 mg/dL, with some variation, depending on the analytic method employed as well as the age and diet of the animal. Calcium values consistently above 12 mg/dL should be considered to be in the hypercalcemic range. The blood phosphorus is low (4 mg/dL or less) or in the low-normal range due to inhibition of renal tubular reabsorption of phosphorus by the excess PTH. Activity of alkaline phosphatase (an enzyme involved in both apposition and resorption of bone) may be elevated in the serum of animals with overt bone disease. The increased activity of this enzyme is thought to result from a compensatory increase in osteoblastic activity along trabeculae as a response to mechanical stress in bones weakened by excessive resorption. Serum intact PTH determined by immunoradiometric assay is consistently increased outside of the normal range.

Successful removal of the functional parathyroid lesion results in a rapid decrease in circulating PTH levels because the half-life of active PTH in plasma is short (measured in minutes). It should be emphasized that plasma calcium levels in patients with overt bone disease may decrease rapidly and be subnormal within 12 to 24 hours after operation, resulting in severe hypocalcemic tetany. Serum calcium levels should be monitored frequently following surgical removal of a parathyroid neoplasm. Postoperative hypocalcemia (5 mg/dL and lower) can be the result of (a) depressed secretory activity of chief cells due to long-term suppression by the chronic hypercalcemia or injury to the remaining parathyroid tissue during surgery, (b) abruptly decreased bone resorption due to lowered PTH levels, and (c) accelerated mineralization of

osteoid matrix formed by the hyperplastic osteoblasts but previously prevented from undergoing mineralization by the elevated PTH levels. In some dogs with hypercalcemia and parathyroid adenoma, acute hypocalcemia may occur due to spontaneous infarction and necrosis of the adenoma. Infusions of calcium gluconate to maintain the serum calcium between 7.5 and 9.0 mg/dL, feeding high-calcium diets, and supplemental vitamin D therapy will correct this serious postoperative complication.

In young German shepherds, primary hyperparathyroidism also has been described as being associated with autonomous chief cell parathyroid hyperplasia. The pups develop hypercalcemia, hypophosphatemia, increased immunoreactive PTH, and increased fractional clearance of inorganic phosphate in the urine (Thompson et al. 1984). Clinical signs include stunted growth, muscular weakness, polyuria, polydipsia, and a diffuse reduction in bone density. Intravenous infusion of calcium failed to suppress the autonomous secretion of PTH by the diffuse hyperplasia of chief cells in all parathyroids. Other lesions include nodular hyperplasia of thyroid C cells and widespread mineralization of lungs, kidney, and gastric mucosa. The disease appears to be inherited as an autosomal recessive trait in dogs.

Secondary Hyperparathyroidism

RENAL FORM. Secondary hyperparathyroidism as a complication of chronic renal failure is a metabolic disease characterized by an excessive, but not autonomous, rate of PTH secretion. This disorder is encountered most frequently in dogs but also occurs in cats and other animal species. The secretion of hormone by the hyperplastic parathyroid glands in this disorder usually remains responsive to fluctuations in blood calcium.

The primary etiologic mechanism in renal hyperparathyroidism is a long-standing, progressive renal disease resulting in severely impaired function. Chronic renal insufficiency and failure (CRF) in older dogs result from interstitial nephritis, glomerulonephritis, nephrosclerosis, or amyloidosis. Several congenital anomalies, such as cortical hypoplasia, polycystic kidneys, and bilateral hydronephrosis, cause renal insufficiency in younger dogs. When the renal disease progresses to the point where there is significant reduction in glomerular filtration rate, phosphorus is retained and progressive hyperphosphatemia develops (Figure 12.22). Although the concentration of blood phosphorus has no direct regulatory influence on the synthesis and secretion of PTH, it may, when elevated, contribute to parathyroid stimulation by virtue of its ability to lower blood calcium.

The pathogenesis of secondary renal hyperparathyroidism is complex, but it has been recently recognized that 1,25-dihydroxyvitamin D (calcitriol) plays an important role in this disease (Figure 12.22) (Nagode and Chew 1992; Felsenfeld and Llach 1993). Animals with advanced CRF have decreased circulating concentrations of 1,25-dihydroxyvitamin D caused by decreased renal synthesis. Initially, the elevated blood phosphorus depresses the activity of the 1α-hydroxylase in the kidney. In the later stage of chronic renal dis-

ease, there are decreased numbers of tubular epithelial cells with 1α-hydroxylase activity to form the active form of vitamin D. Early stages of CRF are often associated with normal concentrations of circulating 1,25-dihydroxyvitamin D (even with the loss of nephrons) due to the correcting effects of increased PTH on renal 1α-hydroxylase that enhance renal tubular synthesis of 1,25-dihydroxyvitamin D (Figure 12.23).

1,25-Dihydroxyvitamin D is an important regulator of parathyroid chief cell function and acts to decrease PTH mRNA expression, increase expression of the vitamin D receptor, and control the set-point of chief cell responsiveness to negative feedback by the serum calcium concentration. The function of 1,25-dihydroxyvitamin D serves to complete the endocrine feedback loop with the parathyroid gland to control serum calcium concentration (see Figure 12.8). Decreased circulating levels of 1,25-dihydroxyvitamin D in animals with CRF results in chief cell hyperplasia and increased secretion of intact PTH. The increased circulating PTH correlates with the degree of uremia and has been suggested to play a role in both the clinical signs and progression of CRF (Nagode and Chew 1992) (Figure 12.24).

The use of dietary phosphorus restriction and intestinal phosphate binders in animals with mild uremia can reduce serum phosphate. Reduced serum phosphate results in decreased serum PTH concentrations due to the removal of phosphate inhibition of 1,25-dihydroxyvitamin D production by the kidneys, but may not return PTH levels to normal. The oral admin-

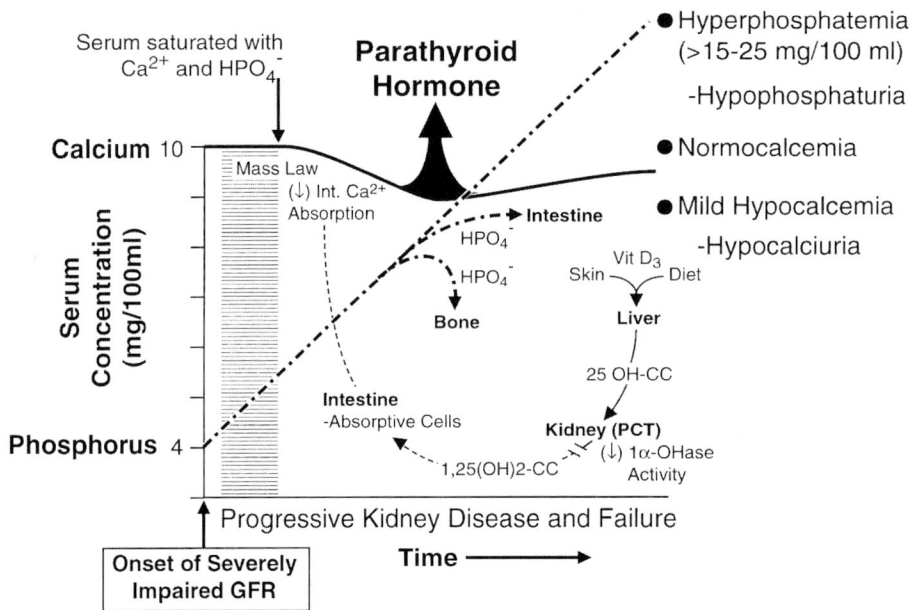

FIG. 12.22—Alterations in serum calcium and phosphorus during the pathogenesis of secondary hyperparathyroidism associated with progressive renal failure. Ca^{2+}, ionized calcium; GFR, glomerular filtration rate; HPO$_4^-$, phosphate ion; Int. Ca^{2+}, intestinal calcium absorption; 1OHase, 24-hydroxylase; PCT, proximal convoluted tubule; and Vit D$_3$, vitamin D$_3$.

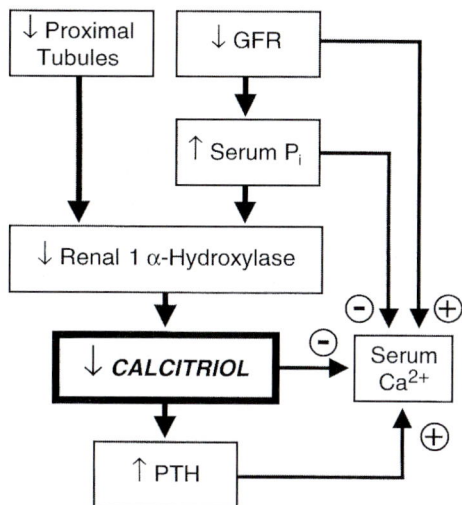

FIG. 12.23—Hyperparathyroidism and chronic renal failure. Role of 1,25-dihydroxyvitamin D (calcitriol) in the pathogenesis of renal secondary hyperparathyroidism. GFR, glomerular filtration rate; Ca^{2+}, ionized calcium; P_i, inorganic phosphorus; and PTH, parathyroid hormone. (From Rosol et al. 1995.)

istration of low doses (1.7 to 3.4 ng/kg) of 1,25-dihydroxyvitamin D has been shown to normalize serum PTH in dogs and cats with naturally occurring CRF and may reduce the progression of disease (Nagode et al. 1996). Removal of the parathyroid glands does not reduce the progression of experimentally induced renal failure in dogs; however, serum PTH levels were not as high in the experimental animals as in dogs with spontaneous, advanced renal disease (Finco et al. 1994).

Parathyroid stimulation in patients with chronic renal disease can be attributed directly to the hypocalcemia that develops during the pathogenesis of the disease. As the phosphorus concentration increases, blood calcium decreases reciprocally. Impaired intestinal absorption of calcium due to an acquired defect in vitamin D metabolism also plays a significant role in the development of hypocalcemia in chronic renal insufficiency and uremia. Chronic renal disease impairs the production of 1,25-dihydroxycholecalciferol (the biologically active metabolite of vitamin D) by the kidney, thereby diminishing intestinal calcium transport and leading to the development of hypocalcemia. Initially, the elevated blood phosphorus depresses the activity of the 1α-hydroxylase in the kidney. In the later stage of chronic renal disease, there are decreased numbers of tubular epithelial cells with 1α-hydroxylase activity to form the active metabolite of vitamin D.

All four parathyroid glands are enlarged due to organellar hypertrophy initially and cellular hyperplasia later as compensatory mechanisms to increase hormonal synthesis and secretion in response to the hypocalcemic stimulus. Since the parathyroid gland stores comparatively little preformed hormone, the rate of peptide synthesis appears to be rate limiting for hormonal secretion. Although the parathyroids are not autonomous, the PTH concentration in the peripheral blood in patients with chronic renal failure may exceed that of primary hyperparathyroidism, due to a decreased rate of degradation by the kidney. A greatly increased number and size of chief cells are required, therefore, to

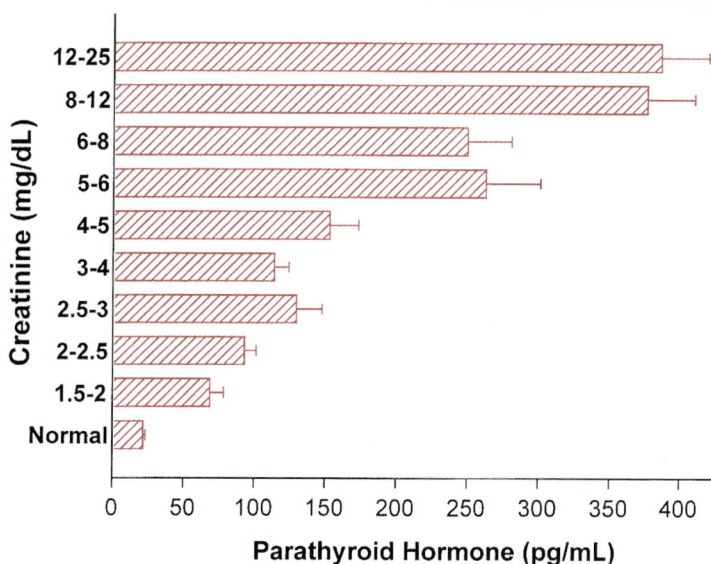

FIG. 12.24—Relationship of serum N-terminal parathyroid hormone to levels of serum creatinine in 35 normal dogs and 333 canine patients with uremia (mean ± SEM). (From Nagode and Chew 1992.)

sustain the vastly increased rates of hormonal secretion in patients with long-standing renal disease.

PTH accelerates osteocytic and osteoclastic resorption, results in release of stored calcium from bone, and returns the blood calcium toward normal (Figure 12.22). The long-standing increase in bone resorption eventually results in the metabolic bone disease associated with chronic renal insufficiency. Progressive glomerular and tubular dysfunction with loss of target cells interferes with expression of the phosphaturic response by the increased circulating PTH in renal disease. Phosphorus is retained and the blood concentration continues to rise despite the secondary hyperparathyroidism.

Although skeletal involvement is generalized with hyperparathyroidism, it does not affect all parts uniformly. Bone lesions become apparent earlier and reach a more advanced degree in certain areas. Resorption of alveolar socket bone and loss of lamina dura dentes occur early in the course of the disease. This results in loose teeth that may be dislodged easily and interfere with mastication. Cancellous bones of the maxilla and mandible also are sites of predilection in hyperparathroidism. Due to the accelerated resorption, the bones become softened and readily pliable (i.e., *rubber-jaw disease*), and the jaws fail to close properly. Long bones of the abaxial skeleton are less dramatically affected. Lameness, stiff gait, and fractures after relatively minor trauma may result from the increased bone resorption. Areas of subperiosteal resorption by numerous osteoclasts may disrupt the osseous attachment of tendons, leading to elevation and stretching of the periosteum, bone pain, and an inability to support the body's weight.

A small percentage of dogs with chronic kidney disease will have moderate hypercalcemia. Although the exact mechanism for the development of hypercalcemia with renal disease is uncertain, it may be the result of diminished PTH degradation by the damaged kidney, decreased urinary calcium excretion, or hypercitricemia with the increased formation of calcium-citrate complexes. When hypocalcemia occurs, it is largely the result of decreased intestinal absorption of calcium due to decreased serum 1,25-dihydroxyvitamin D. An additional effect can occur due to mass-law interactions of calcium with very high serum concentrations of phosphate as calcium-phosphate salts are deposited in soft tissues. Consequently, hypocalcemia usually reflects advanced loss of nephron mass.

NUTRITIONAL FORM. The increased secretion of PTH with this metabolic disorder is a compensatory mechanism directed against a disturbance in mineral homeostasis induced by nutritional imbalances. The disease occurs commonly in cats (Rowland et al. 1968), dogs, certain nonhuman primates (Hunt et al. 1967), and laboratory animals, as well as in many farm animal species (Capen 1982; Gilka and Sugden 1984).

Dietary mineral imbalances of etiologic importance in the pathogenesis of nutritional secondary hyperparathyroidism are (a) low content of calcium, (b) excessive phosphorus with normal or low calcium, and (c) inadequate amounts of vitamin D_3. The significant end result is hypocalcemia that results in parathyroid stimulation. A diet low in calcium fails to supply the daily requirement even though a greater proportion of ingested calcium is absorbed and hypocalcemia develops (Figure 12.25). Ingestion of excessive phosphorus results in increased intestinal absorption and elevation of blood phosphorus. Hyperphosphatemia does not stimulate the parathyroid gland directly but does so indirectly by virtue of its ability to lower blood calcium when the serum becomes saturated with respect to these two ions. Diets containing inadequate amounts of vitamin D_3 (even with normal levels of vitamin D_2) cause diminished intestinal calcium absorption and hypocalcemia in certain New World monkeys.

In response to the nutritionally induced hypocalcemia, all parathyroid glands undergo cellular hypertrophy and hyperplasia. Active chief cells stimulated by diet-induced hypocalcemia become larger and more tightly arranged together compared with those in parathyroids of normal animals. Since kidney function is normal, the increased levels of PTH result in diminished renal tubular reabsorption of phosphorus and increased reabsorption of calcium, and blood levels return toward normal (Figure 12.25). In addition, bone resorption is accelerated, and release of calcium elevates blood calcium levels to the low-normal range. Continued ingestion of the imbalanced diet sustains the state of compensatory hyperparathyroidism, which leads to progressive development of the metabolic bone disease.

Nutritional secondary hyperparathyroidism develops in young cats fed a predominantly meat diet (Rowland et al. 1968). For example, beef heart or liver contains minimal amounts of calcium (7 to 9 mg/100 g) and has a markedly imbalanced calcium to phosphorus (Ca/P) ratio (1:20 to 1:50). An adequate diet for kittens up to 6 months of age should supply 200 to 400 mg calcium and approximately 200 μm iodine daily, and from 10,000 to 15,000 IU of vitamin A weekly.

Kittens fed beef heart or liver develop functional disturbances within approximately 4 weeks. Clinical signs are dominated by disturbances in locomotion manifested by a reluctance to move, posterior lameness, and an uncoordinated gait. The cortex of long bones is progressively thinned due to increased reabsorption, and the medullary cavity is widened. Affected kittens become quiet, are reluctant to play, and assume a sitting position or are in sternal recumbency. Normal activities may result in sudden onset of severe lameness due to incomplete or folding fractures of one or more bones. The high content of digestible protein (over 50% on a wet basis) and fat promotes rapid growth in kittens fed beef heart. They appear well nourished, and their hair coat maintains a good luster. In general, kittens are more susceptible and develop more severe skeletal lesions than do adult cats fed a similar diet. The disease develops rapidly because the dietary imbalance is wide and the skeletal metabolic rate of kittens is high. Vertebral fractures with compression of

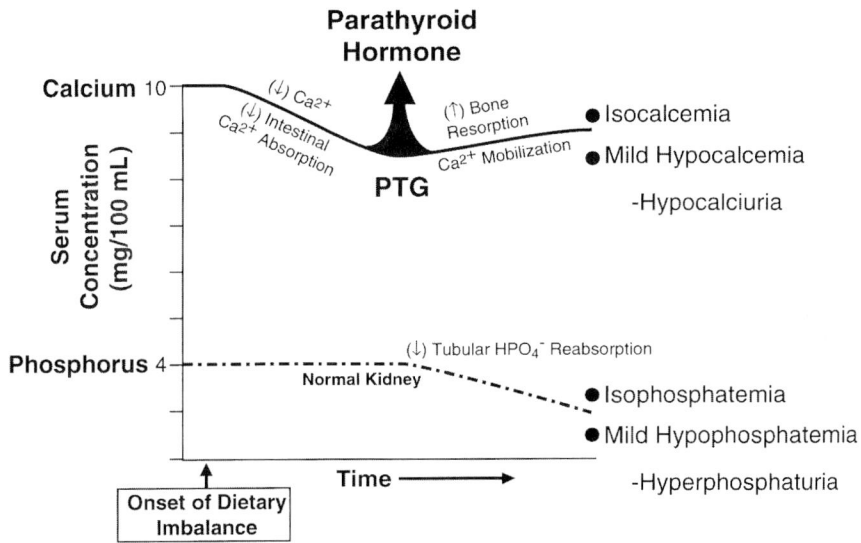

FIG. 12.25—Nutritional secondary hyperparathyroidism. Alterations in serum calcium and phosphorus in the pathogenesis of nutritional secondary hyperparathyroidism caused by feeding a diet low in calcium (Ca^{2+}) or deficient in cholecalciferol but with a normal amount of phosphorus. HPO_4^-, phosphate ion; and PTG, parathyroid gland.

the spinal cord and paralysis are common complications in kittens but are infrequent in adult cats.

Secondary hyperparathyroidism of nutritional origin also occurs in collections of aviculturists (domestic and captive birds) (Long et al. 1983), zoological parks (caged lions and tigers, green iguanas, crocodiles, etc.) (Anderson and Capen 1976), and laboratory animals used for research (ground squirrels, nonhuman primates, etc.) (Lehner et al. 1967).

In horses, the most frequent nutritional imbalance involves the ingestion of excessive phosphorus. This results in an increased intestinal absorption of phosphorus and elevation of the blood phosphorus concentration. Hyperphosphatemia does not stimulate the parathyroid gland directly but does so indirectly by virtue of its ability to lower blood calcium. Horses that develop the disease usually have been fed high-grain diets with below-average-quality roughage. Evidence of high phosphorus intake may be difficult to establish inasmuch as the excess phosphorus may be fed by the owner in the form of a bran supplement added to a grain diet to improve the health of the horse. The diet usually is palatable and nutritious except for the unbalanced phosphorus (excessive amounts) and calcium (marginal or deficient) content. A calcium-deficient diet fails to supply the daily requirement even though a greater proportion of ingested calcium is absorbed, and hypocalcemia develops. Occasionally, horses may develop nutritional hyperparathyroidism after pasturing on grasses with a high oxalate content. This results in intestinal malabsorption of calcium (Walthall and McKenzie 1976). The oxalates appear to form insoluble complexes with calcium in the intestine, resulting

in an elevated fecal calcium/phosphorus ratio (2.35:1) compared with horses on a similar calcium and phosphorus intake but without the oxalate-rich plants (fecal calcium/phosphorus ratio 1.2:1). The interference in intestinal calcium absorption results in the development of progressive hypocalcemia that leads to parathyroid stimulation and development of the metabolic bone disease.

Initial clinical signs in horses with nutritional secondary hyperparathyroidism usually include a transitory shifting lameness in one or more limbs, generalized tenderness of joints, and a stilted gait. The lameness develops as a result of increased osteoclastic resorption of outer circumferential lamellae, with disruption of tendinous insertions and bone trabeculae supporting the articular cartilage, resulting in disruption of joint cartilage on weight-bearing. Resorption of alveolar socket bone and loss of lamina dura dentes occur early and may result in loose teeth. Later in the course of the disease, severe lesions develop in bones of the skull, especially the maxilla and mandible, resulting in bilateral firm enlargements of the facial bones immediately above and anterior to the facial crests. The horizontal rami of the mandibles are irregularly thickened by a progressive hyperostotic fibrous osteodystrophy (*big head*) that develops in horses with nutritional secondary hyperparathyroidism. The hyperostosis of skull bones results from osteoid and fibrous connective tissue deposition in excess of the volume of bone resorbed. The chronic excess intake of phosphorus and increased secretion of PTH result in stimulation of osteoblasts to form osteoid in excess of the amount of bone resorbed by osteoclasts and progressive enlargement of skeletal bones. The hyperostotic fibrous osteodystrophy may impinge upon the nasal cavity, resulting in dyspnea, especially after exertion.

Changes in urine calcium and phosphorus levels are more consistent and useful in the clinical diagnosis of nutritional secondary hyperparathyroidism in horses. The increased secretion of PTH acts on the normal kidneys to increase urinary phosphorus excretion markedly but decrease calcium loss in the urine compared with normal horses. Blood urea nitrogen, serum creatinine, and other parameters used to assess renal function are within normal limits in horses with nutritional hyperparathyroidism. Serum alkaline-phosphatase levels often are in the high normal range or are elevated in horses with overt bone disease, reflecting the increased osteoblastic and osteoclastic activity in hyperparathyroidism. Under experimental conditions, horses fed a high phosphorus diet (phosphorus, 1.4%; calcium 0.7%) are able to more rapidly normalize their blood calcium following an ethylenediaminetetraacetic acid (EDTA)-induced hypocalcemia than controls fed a balanced diet (phosphorus, 0.6%; calcium 0.7%) owing to the increased parathyroid activity (Argenzio et al. 1974).

A metabolic disorder has been recognized in primates for many years and has received numerous appellations, including cage paralysis, simian bone disease, and osteomalacia. Hypocalcemia resulting from either inadequate dietary vitamin D_3 intake in New World laboratory primates housed indoors or excessive phosphorus in the diet of pet monkeys leads to long-term stimulation of the parathyroid glands. The monkeys become inactive, offer less resistance to handling, and have difficulty masticating their food. In the more advanced stages there is maxillary hyperostosis due to osteoid deposition and proliferation of fibrous connective tissue, joint pain, and distortion of limbs by palpable fractures without mineralized calluses. There is radiographic evidence of generalized skeletal demineralization, loss of lamina dura dentes, subperiosteal cortical bone resorption, bowing deformities, and multiple folding fractures of long bones. Cortical bone is thinned due to the activity of increased numbers of osteoclasts. The resorbed bone is partially replaced by the proliferation of immature fibroblasts and neocapillaries.

HYPOPARATHYROIDISM. In hypoparathyroidism either subnormal amounts of PTH are secreted by pathological parathyroid glands or the hormone secreted is unable to interact normally with target cells. Hypoparathyroidism has been recognized occasionally in dogs, particularly in the smaller breeds such as schnauzers and terriers (Jones and Alley 1985). However, the incidence of occurrence is much less than hyperparathyroidism in both dogs and cats. Several pathogenic mechanisms can result in an inadequate secretion of PTH. The parathyroid glands may be damaged or inadvertently removed during the course of operation on the thyroid gland. If the glands or their vascular supply have only been damaged but not removed, functional parenchyma often regenerates and clinical manifestations subsequently disappear.

Agenesis of both pairs of parathyroids is a rare cause of congenital hypoparathyroidism in pups. Idiopathic hypoparathyroidism in adult dogs usually is associated with diffuse lymphocytic parathyroiditis resulting in extensive degeneration of chief cells with partial replacement by fibrous connective tissue. In the early stages of lymphocytic parathyroiditis, there is extensive infiltration of the gland with lymphocytes and plasma cells, and nodular regenerative hyperplasia of the remaining chief cells. Later, the parathyroid gland is completely replaced by lymphocytes, fibroblasts, and neocapillaries with only an occasional viable chief cell. The lymphocytic parathyroiditis most likely develops by means of an immune-mediated mechanism, since a similar destruction of secretory parenchyma and lymphocytic infiltration has been produced experimentally in dogs by repeated injections of parathyroid tissue emulsions. Other possible causes of hypoparathyroidism include invasion and destruction of parathyroids by primary (thyroid, salivary, etc.) or metastatic neoplasms in the anterior cervical area.

The pathophysiological disturbances of hypoparathyroidism primarily are the result of increased neuromuscular excitability and tetany. Bone resorption is decreased and blood calcium levels diminish progressively (4 to 6 mg/dL) due to the lack of PTH (Figure 12.26). Affected dogs are restless, nervous, and ataxic with intermittent tremors of individual muscle groups that progress to generalized tetany and convulsive seizures. Concurrently, blood phosphorus levels are substantially elevated due to increased renal tubular reabsorption.

HYPOCALCEMIC SYNDROMES IN ANIMALS. A number of metabolic disorders characterized primarily by the development of hypocalcemia and associated manifestations occur in several different animal species. Many of these hypocalcemic syndromes develop near the time of the increased calcium demand associated with parturition and are a reflection of a temporary failure of calcium homeostatic mechanisms. A comparable hypocalcemic syndrome associated with parturition does not occur in human beings. The eclampsia that develops in women is related to a toxemia of pregnancy with degenerative changes in the liver, kidney, and placenta rather than disturbances in mineral homeostasis. Parturient hypocalcemia in dairy cows and puerperal tetany of bitches are examples of hypocalcemic syndromes of major economic significance and will be discussed in greater detail.

Parturient Hypocalcemia in Dairy Cows. Parturient hypocalcemia is a metabolic disease of high-producing dairy cows characterized by the development of severe hypocalcemia, hypophosphatemia, and paresis near the

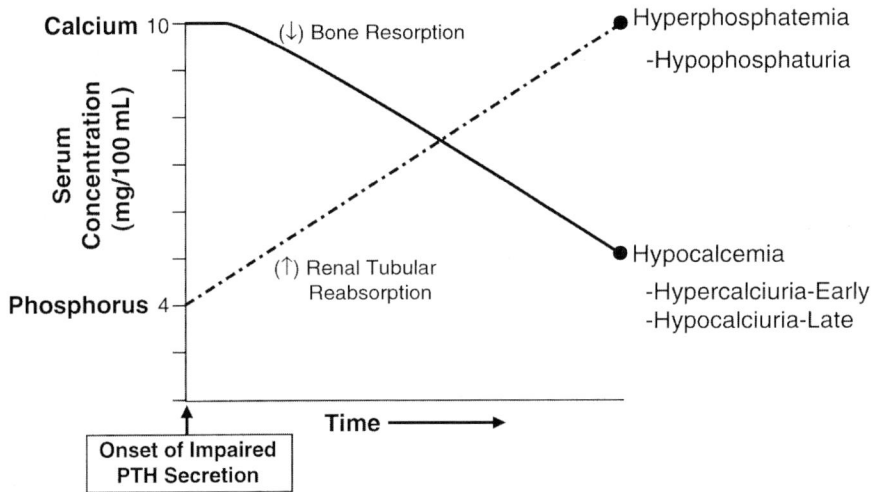

FIG. 12.26—Hypoparathyroidism. Alterations in serum calcium and phosphorus in response to an inadequate secretion of parathyroid hormone. Progressive increases in serum phosphorus levels and a marked decline in serum calcium levels that result in a neuromuscular tetany.

time of parturition. The pathogenic mechanisms responsible for the rapid and precipitous decrease in calcium and phosphorus levels in the blood are complex and involve several interrelated factors. Total and ionized calcium levels decrease progressively beginning several days before parturition. Serum magnesium may increase reciprocally as calcium declines. The blood glucose concentration often is increased in response to hypocalcemia due to an interference with the secretion of insulin from β cells. An adequate amount of calcium ion in extracellular fluids is required for insulin secretion in response to glucose and other secretagogues for insulin. The uptake of calcium by β cells appears to stimulate the contraction of microfilaments which triggers the peripheral migration of storage granules and release of insulin. Infusion of glucose in a cow with severe hypocalcemia fails to increase blood levels of insulin; however, if calcium is administered before the injection of glucose, there is a rapid and substantial increase in insulin secretion.

The development of parturient hypocalcemia in dairy cows for a number of years was considered to be the result of an inadequate response of the parathyroid glands to the substantial demands for calcium imposed by the mineralization of fetal bones and the initiation of lactation. Ultrastructural and endocrinologic studies have demonstrated that parathyroid chief cells in cows with parturient hypocalcemia were capable of responding to the increased demands for calcium by the secretion of stored hormone, hypertrophy of secretory organelles concerned with the synthesis of new hormone, and elevation of blood levels of PTH. Chief cells were primarily in the active stage of their secretory cycle and were depleted of storage granules or the

secretory granules had migrated peripherally and were fused with the plasma membrane. These structural findings suggested an active secretory response by parathyroid glands in cows with parturient hypocalcemia and were in agreement with biochemical studies. The ability of parathyroid glands to respond to the challenge for extra calcium mobilization with increased hormonal synthesis and secretion has been shown not to be defective in cows that develop parturient hypocalcemia.

Target cells in bone and skeletal calcium reserves of cows with parturient hypocalcemia are temporarily refractive to the action of the elevated levels of PTH. Investigations have shown that the elevation of serum calcium in response to exogenous parathyroid extract is less when administered prepartum than postpartum. Bone turnover, particularly resorption, is low in cows with parturient hypocalcemia and only a few osteoclasts are present on smooth inactive trabecular bone surfaces. The urinary excretion of hydroxyproline, derived from the breakdown of bone matrix, does not increase significantly during late gestation in cows that develop the disease, as occurs in cows that maintain their serum calcium near normal through parturition and early lactation. A secretion of calcitonin prepartum in cows fed high calcium diets is one factor that contributes to the inability of increased PTH levels to mobilize calcium rapidly from skeletal reserves and maintain blood levels during the critical period near parturition. The thyroid content of calcitonin is reduced (14% of control cows) and many C (parafollicular) cells are degranulated.

The decline in blood calcium may be rapid in certain high-producing dairy cows near parturition and the initiation of lactation. Since bone resorption during the prepartal period is relatively low due to a substantial intake of dietary calcium, there is a relatively small pool of active bone-resorbing cells capable of responding to PTH. Therefore, when PTH secretion increases because of the rapidly developing hypocalcemia, the increase in activity of the few active osteoclasts present is insufficient to restore the plasma calcium concentration to normal. The activation of osteoprogenitor cells and the subsequent conversion of preosteoclasts to osteoclasts under the influence of increased PTH with expansion of the pool of active bone-resorbing cells require time (as long as 48 to 72 hours in an adult cow) and an adequate concentration of calcium in extracellular fluids. If the extracellular fluid calcium falls below a critical level, the increased circulating concentration of PTH may be ineffective in causing an elevation of cytosol calcium in target cells to activate new bone-resorbing cells. Neither an increased endogenous secretion of PTH nor the exogenous administration of parathyroid extract to cows will restore homeostasis once the hypocalcemia is profound. Only the administration of calcium and elevation of calcium in extracellular fluids will restore the responsiveness to PTH, trigger bone resorption, and correct the hypocalcemia.

The composition of the prepartal diet fed to dairy cows has been shown to be a significant factor in the pathogenesis of parturient hypocalcemia. High calcium diets have been incriminated in significantly increasing the incidence of the disease, whereas low calcium diets or prepartal diets supplemented with pharmacological doses of vitamin D have been reported to reduce the incidence of the disease (Black et al. 1973b). Although cows fed a high calcium diet have higher blood calcium levels prepartum, they are less able to maintain serum calcium near the critical time of parturition. Plasma immunoreactive PTH levels are lower prepartum than in cows fed a balanced diet and decline further at 48 hours postpartum. Chief cells in the inactive stage of the secretory cycle predominate in cows fed high calcium diets, whereas actively synthesizing chief cells are most numerous in parathyroids of cows fed balanced prepartal diets (Black et al. 1973a). In response to the elevated blood calcium in cows fed high calcium prepartal diets, thyroid stores of calcitonin were diminished and C cells were partially degranulated and appeared to be actively synthesizing more hormone (Black et al. 1973b). This stimulation of C cells was accompanied by a decrease in bone turnover near parturition. Trabecular bone surfaces were inactive and few osteoclasts are resorbing bone.

A test of the immediately available calcium reserves by ethylenediaminetetraacetic acid (EDTA)-induced hypocalcemia compares the long-term effects of high calcium and balanced prepartal diets on the function of parathyroid glands and bone. Cows fed balanced diets responded to the experimental hypocalcemic challenge with a more rapid and greater increase in plasma PTH levels and the return of blood calcium to preinfusion levels was faster than in cows fed a high calcium diet (Figure 12.27). This was accompanied by a marked increase in urinary hydroxyproline excretion, suggesting increased bone matrix catabolism in response to the PTH secretion. These findings suggested that the long-term feeding of a high calcium diet prepartum partially suppressed chief cells in the parathyroid glands, so that they were less able to respond rapidly by increased PTH synthesis and secretion to a hypocalcemic challenge either induced by EDTA infusion or associated with parturition and the initiation of lactation.

Calcium homeostasis in pregnant cows fed a high calcium diet appears to be maintained principally by intestinal calcium absorption (Figure 12.28). This greater reliance on intestinal absorption rather than on PTH-stimulated bone resorption is a significant factor in the more frequent development of profound hypocalcemia near parturition in cows fed high calcium prepartal diets. These cows are more susceptible to the decreased calcium available for absorption as a result of the anorexia often associated with the high blood estrogen levels at parturition. Calcium homeostasis in cows fed balanced or relatively low calcium diets prepartum has been shown to be more under the fine control of PTH secretion with the approach of parturition. The higher levels of PTH secreted during the prepartal period by an expanded population of actively synthesizing chief cells results in a larger pool of active bone-resorbing cells to fulfill the increased needs for calcium mobilization at the critical time near parturition and the initiation of lactation. Cows fed balanced or relatively low calcium diets are less susceptible to the influence of decreased calcium absorption and flow of calcium into the extracellular calcium pool resulting from the anorexia and intestinal stasis associated with parturition (Figure 12.29).

A syndrome biochemically and pathophysiologically resembling naturally occurring parturient paresis has been produced experimentally in cows by the prepartal administration of diphosphonates (Yarrington et al. 1976). These compounds are synthetic analogues of pyrophosphate and are proven inhibitors of bone resorption. When cows with no known history of parturient paresis were fed a low calcium diet and administered dichloromethane diphosphonate (CL_2MDP) postpartum, they consistently developed hypocalcemia and hypophosphatemia with muscular weakness, incoordination, and eventually sternal or lateral recumbency (Yarrington et al. 1977a). These studies suggest an important role for the skeleton in the maintenance of calcium homeostasis at parturition in dairy cows (Yarrington et al. 1977b). Following an intravenous EDTA infusion given 10 days prepartum, CL_2MDP-treated cows developed a severe and prolonged hypocalcemia despite elevated levels of PTH. Urinary excretion of hydroxyproline was low and remained relatively unchanged during the 24 hours of the EDTA study. The rapid mobilization of calcium reserves in cows administered CL_2MDP prepartum was impaired because of diminished resorption of bone even though secretion of PTH increased in response to severe hypocalcemia induced by parturition or EDTA. These

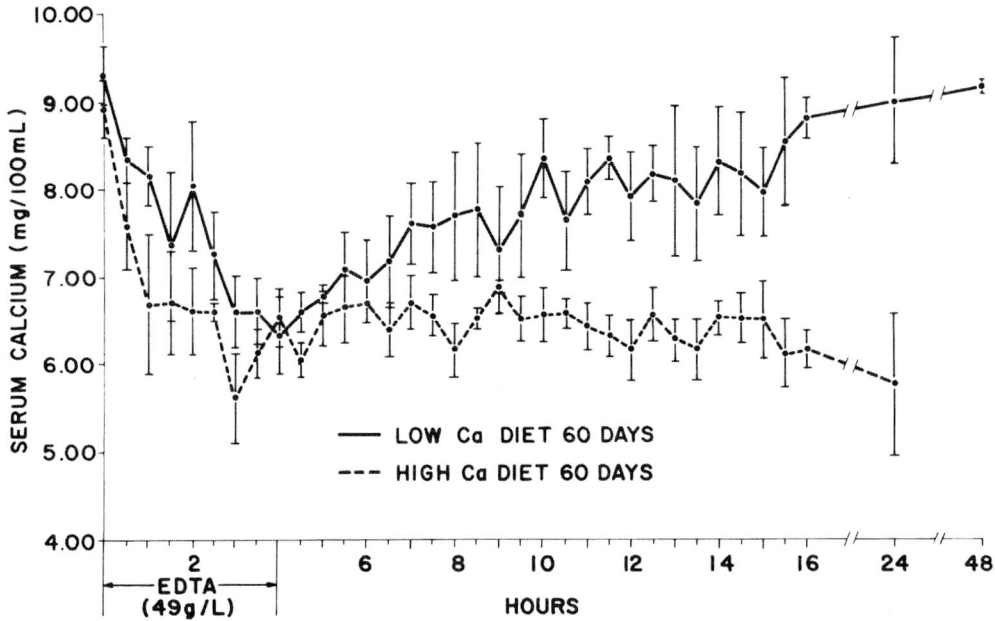

FIG. 12.27—Immediately available calcium (Ca) reserves in pregnant cows fed a low-calcium diet compared with those in pregnant cows fed a high-calcium diet prior to parturition. In response to a hypocalcemic challenge provided by EDTA infusion, cows fed the low-calcium diet are able to mobilize calcium from skeletal reserves and return the blood calcium level to the normal range more rapidly than cows fed a high-calcium diet, thereby preventing the development of hypocalcemia. In cows fed the high-calcium diet, chief cells in the parathyroid gland are inactive, and there are few osteoclasts on bone surfaces. Cows fed the low-calcium diet have predominantly actively secreting chief cells in the parathyroids and frequent osteoclasts on bone surfaces. (From Capen 1989.)

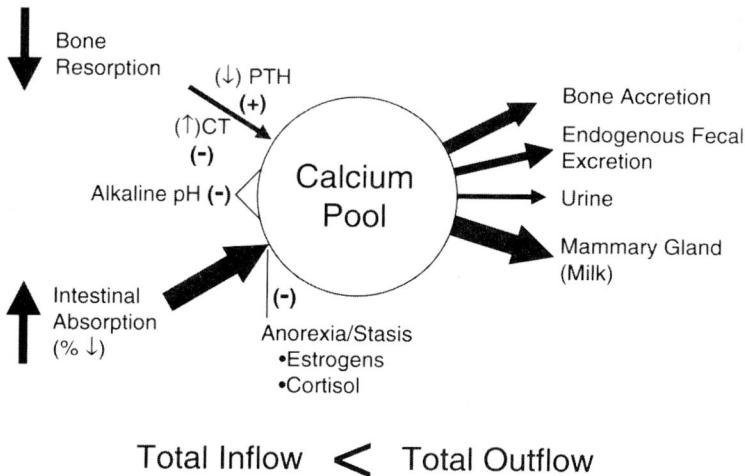

FIG. 12.28—Calcium homeostasis in cows fed a high-calcium prepartal diet primarily depends on intestinal calcium absorption. The rate of bone resorption is low, and the parathyroid glands are inactive. Anorexia and gastrointestinal stasis that can often occur near parturition interrupt the major inflow into the extracellular fluid calcium pool. Outflow of calcium with the onset of lactation exceeds the rate of inflow into the calcium pool, and the cows develop a progressive hypocalcemia and paresis. CT, calcitonin; and PTH, parathyroid hormone. (From Capen 1989.)

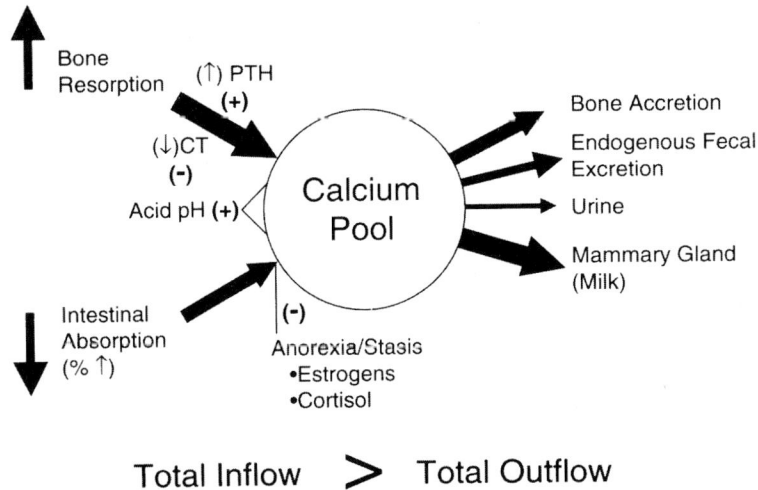

FIG. 12.29—Calcium homeostasis in cows fed a low-calcium prepartal diet. Bone resorption and intestinal absorption both contribute substantially to the inflow of calcium to the pool in extracellular fluids. The anorexia and gastrointestinal stasis that often occur near parturition may temporarily interrupt one inflow pathway. However, there is more likely to be an adequate pool of active bone-resorbing cells capable of responding to the increased PTH secretion under these dietary conditions to maintain an approximate balance between calcium inflow and outflow, thereby preventing the development of progressive hypocalcemia. Total inflow > total outflow. CT, calcitonin; and PTH, parathyroid hormone. (From Capen 1989.)

results suggest that the CL_2MDP-treated cows that developed parturient hypocalcemia were similar to cows fed a high calcium diet in that they were more dependent on calcium absorption from the gastrointestinal tract than upon skeletal calcium mobilization for the maintenance of calcium homeostasis.

Pharmacological doses of vitamin D_2 have been administered to dairy cows prepartum to develop an effective method for the prevention of parturient hypocalcemia and paresis. High levels of the parent vitamin D compound are known to increase the rate and quantity of calcium and phosphorus absorbed from the intestinal tract in cattle, to progressively elevate the blood calcium and phosphorus levels after 3 to 5 days, and to increase the net calcium deposition and retention in areas of new bone growth. The calcium mobilization rate and the immediately available calcium reserves increase in cattle after vitamin D injection. Vitamin D_2 (20 to 30 million IU) fed daily for at least 3 but not more than 7 days before parturition prevented approximately 80% of the cases of parturient hypocalcemia. However, due to the inherent difficulty in accurately predicting the date of parturition, clinical and pathological evidences of toxicity have been observed in cattle given vitamin D in large doses for an extended period. These included gastrointestinal stasis, diuresis and anorexia, abnormal cardiac function, reduced rumination, weight loss, and extensive mineralization of the cardiovascular system. Cardiovascular mineralization was not present after 7 days of administration of the parent vitamin D compound but was observed after 10 days and became extensive and widespread after 21

days. The 3- to 5-day delay preceding a significant elevation in blood calcium and phosphorus and the cardiovascular toxicity following administration for extended periods have limited the usefulness of the parent vitamin D compound in preventing the development of hypocalcemia in susceptible cows.

Active vitamin D metabolites have several advantages in the prevention of parturient hypocalcemia and paresis in susceptible cows. The more rapid onset of action (6 to 8 hours), greater potency (up to several hundredfold), and ability to regulate more precisely the magnitude of elevation in blood calcium, thereby minimizing potential toxic effects, are distinct advantages of the principal active metabolite of vitamin D_3 (1,25-dihydroxycholecalciferol) over the parent vitamin D compound in the development of an effective prophylactic regimen for parturient paresis-susceptible dairy cows.

There is a substantial body of literature that suggests that the anion-cation balance of the prepartal diet fed to dairy cows is an important factor in influencing the cow's ability to maintain the blood calcium concentration at parturition and initiation of the substantial loss of calcium and phosphorus into the milk (Block 1984; Oetzel et al. 1988; Gaynor et al. 1989; Tucker et al. 1991; Constable 1999). On the day of parturition, dairy cows commonly produce 10 L or more colostrum containing 23 gm or more of calcium, approximately 6 times the amount of calcium in the extracellular pool (Goff et al. 1991). Cows fed diets with excess anions [e.g., NH_4Cl, $(NH_4)_2 SO_4$] compared with cations (Na^+, K^+) were better able to maintain the circulating ionized and total calcium concentrations through parturition and were less likely to develop parturient hypocalcemia with paresis. The feeding of an acidic prepartal diet to dairy cows enhances bone resorption (as measured by increased plasma levels of hydroxyproline), results in a greater magnitude of 1,25-dihydroxyvitamin D produced by the kidney per unit increase in serum PTH (Goff et al. 1991) a lesser magnitude of decrease in total serum calcium near parturition (Joyce et al. 1997), increased fractional excretion of urinary calcium (Oetzel et al. 1991; Wang and Beede 1992); and improves the rate of return of the blood calcium to normal following EDTA-induced hypocalcemia.

In vitro studies have shown that metabolic acidosis increases the uptake of PTH by bone resulting in increased cyclic AMP production (Martin et al. 1980). By comparison, metabolic alkalosis decreases net calcium efflux from bone by suppressing osteoclasts and stimulating osteoblasts (Bushinsky 1996). Osteoclastic β-glucuronidase release was decreased by alkalosis whereas osteoblastic collagen synthesis was enhanced by an increased pH in the culture medium.

Dairy cows fed high cationic prepartal diets (e.g., high cation [Na + K]-anion [Cl + S] difference are less able to maintain their blood calcium (total and ionic) concentration near parturition and initiation of the lactational calcium drain, and developed a higher incidence of parturient hypocalcemia with paresis (Block 1984; Oetzel et al. 1988; Goff et al. 1991; Goff and Horst 1997). The elevated pH (alkalosis) in extracellular fluids decreased the response of bone (lower plasma hydroxyproline levels) to the calcium-mobilizing action of PTH and suppressed the magnitude of 1,25-dihydroxyvitamin D production by the kidney per unit increase in serum PTH (Goff et al. 1991; Goff and Horst 1997). These adverse effects of alkalosis on bone and kidney suppress the rate of movement of calcium ions into the extracellular fluids to counteract the rapid and substantial loss of calcium into the colostrum. Therefore, the rate of outflow of calcium from the extracellular pool exceeds the rate of inflow from bone and kidney in cows fed strong cationic diets resulting in progressive lowering in blood levels; similar to that observed in dairy cows fed prepartal diets high in calcium (Yarrington et al. 1976, 1977a).

Puerperal Tetany in Dogs. Less is known about the development of hypocalcemic syndromes in other animal species than in the cow. Puerperal tetany is most frequently encountered in the small, hyperexcitable breeds of dogs. The clinical course is rapid and the bitch may proceed from premonitory signs of restlessness, panting, and nervousness to ataxia, trembling, muscular tetany, and convulsive seizures in 8 to 12 hours.

Functional disturbances associated with hypocalcemia in the bitch are primarily the result of neuromuscular tetany, whereas in cows the clinical signs are related to paresis (Figure 12.31).

The occurrence of either tetany or paresis in response to hypocalcemia appears to be the result of basic physiological differences in the function of the

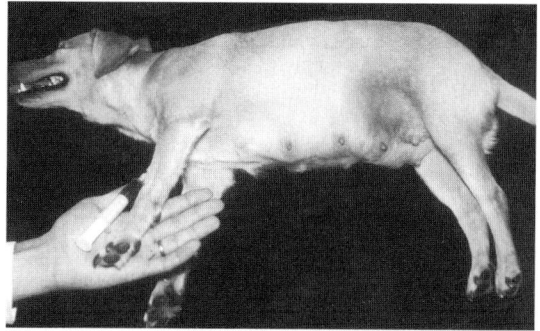

FIG. 12.30—Puerperal tetany in a bitch with hypocalcemia. Increased neuromuscular excitability occurs in the bitch with hypocalcemia, since excitation-secretion coupling is maintained at the motor endplate. (From Capen 1989.)

neuromuscular junction of the cow and the bitch. The release of acetylcholine and transmission of nerve impulses across neuromuscular junctions are blocked by hypocalcemia in cows (but not in bitches) leading to muscle paresis. The dog appears to have a higher margin of safety in neuromuscular transmission in that the degree the endplate potential exceeds the firing threshold is greater in the dog than in the cow. Excitation-secretion coupling is maintained at the neuromuscular junction in the bitch with hypocalcemia. Tetany occurs in the bitch as a result of spontaneous repetitive firing of motor nerve fibers (Figure 12.30). Due to the loss of stabilizing membrane-bound calcium, nerve membranes become more permeable to ions and require a stimulus of lesser magnitude to depolarize.

There is no evidence to suggest that puerperal tetany (eclampsia) in heavily lactating bitches is the result of an interference in PTH secretion. Severe hypocalcemia and often hypophosphatemia develop near the time of peak lactation (approximately 1 to 3 weeks postpartum), most likely the result of temporary failure in homeostasis resulting in an imbalance between the

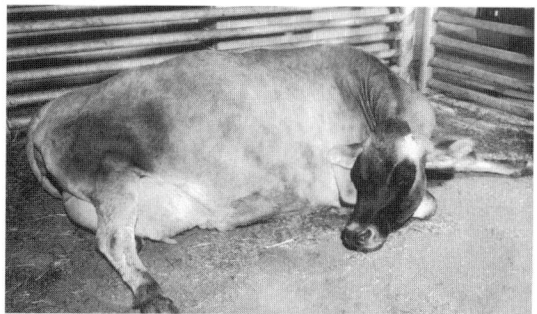

FIG. 12.31—Paresis in a Jersey cow with parturient hypocalcemia owing to a blockage in neuromuscular transmission. (From Capen 1989.)

rates of inflow to and outflow from the extracellular fluid calcium pool. The administration of intravenous calcium to stop the tetany combined with temporarily decreasing the lactational drain of calcium by removing the pups usually corrects the disruption of calcium homeostasis in the majority of bitches. Supplemental dietary calcium and vitamin D have proven useful in preventing relapses.

Hypocalcemic Syndromes in Other Species. A number of metabolic disorders characterized primarily by the development of hypocalcemia and associated pathophysiological alterations occur in several other animal species including the queen, ewe, goat, mare, sow, and chinchilla. Many of these hypocalcemic syndromes develop near the time of the increased calcium demand associated with parturition and probably are a reflection of a temporary failure of calcium homeostatic mechanisms resulting from an imbalance between outflow and inflow to the extracellular pool of calcium. A comparable hypocalcemic syndrome associated with parturition does not occur in human beings. The eclampsia that develops in women is related to a toxemia of pregnancy with degenerative changes in the liver, kidney, and placenta rather than disturbances in mineral homeostasis.

HYPOVITAMINOSIS D

Dietary Deficiency or Inadequate Exposure to Sunlight. Young animals fed diets deficient in vitamin D and housed indoors without exposure to ultraviolet irradiation develop rickets. Mineralization of the cartilaginous matrix fails to occur in affected animals and the formation of woven bone on spicules of cartilage and subsequent remodeling to lamellar bone are blocked in this disease. The epiphyseal plate is irregularly thickened as progressively more primordial cartilaginous matrix accumulates and fails to mineralize. The administration of either cholecalciferol, 25-OH-CC or 1,25-(OH)$_2$-CC to animals leads to the reestablishment of a normal calcification front in the osteoid on bone surfaces and at the growth plate. Phosphorus deficiency will also result in rickets because of the failure to maintain an adequate ion product of serum calcium and phosphorus at the zones of mineralization in bone. However, phosphorus deficiency does not result in hypocalcemia and serum levels of 1,25-dihydroxyvitamin D are normal or increased. Rickets seldom occurs in suckling animals unless the dam provides too little milk.

Vitamin D-dependent Rickets. Deficiency of vitamin D results not only from simple dietary lack or inadequate exposure to sunlight but also from a deficiency of the hydroxylase enzymes essential for metabolic activation of precursor molecules. Vitamin D-dependent rickets, Type I, in both pigs and human beings is a familial disease inherited by an autosomal recessive gene. Newborn pigs appear healthy and have normal blood calcium and phosphorus concentrations. At 4 to 6 weeks of age blood calcium and phosphate decrease, serum alkaline-phosphatase activity increases, and clinically detectable rickets develops during the following 3 to 4 weeks. The pigs develop deformities of bone in the axial and abaxial skeleton, severe pain, and classic lesions of rickets. Serum 25-hydroxycholecalciferol levels are markedly increased compared with those of control pigs, whereas serum 1,25-dihydroxyvitamin D levels are depressed in rachitic pigs compared with normal pigs. Homozygous, rachitic animals have no renal 25-hydroxycholecalciferol-1-hydroxylase in kidney homogenates or mitochondrial preparations, which is responsible for the insufficient renal production of 1,25-dihydroxyvitamin D.

Vitamin D-dependent rickets, type II, is a group of disorders characterized by target-organ resistance to 1,25-dihydroxyvitamin D. The disease is characterized by increased serum 1,25-dihydroxyvitamin D levels, hypocalcemia, secondary hyperparathyroidism, and clinically by rickets or osteomalacia. New World primates have a relative end-organ resistance to 1,25-dihydroxyvitamin D and require high levels of vitamin D$_3$ in their diet. The common marmoset has been shown to represent a model of vitamin D-dependent rickets, type II. Marmosets have increased serum 1,25-dihydroxyvitamin D concentrations compared with rhesus monkeys, and some marmosets have developed osteomalacia even when on high vitamin D$_3$ diets. The resistance to 1,25-dihydroxyvitamin D is likely due to low-affinity binding of 1,25-dihydroxyvitamin D to its nuclear receptor.

HYPERVITAMINOSIS D

Intoxication by Calcinogenic Plants: Large Animals. Livestock grazing on various calcinogenic plants develop a progressive debilitating disease with widespread soft-tissue mineralization. *Cestrum diurnum* (day-blooming jessamine) in Florida and elsewhere in the Southern United States and *Trisetum flavescens* in the Bavarian and Austrian Alps cause calcinosis in horses, cattle, and sheep. *Solanum malacoxylon* in Argentina and Brazil produces the disease *enteque seco* or *espichamento* in cattle, which is characterized by the development of hypercalcemia, hyperphosphatemia, and severe soft-tissue mineralization. Morphologically similar diseases occur in Jamaica (Manchester wasting disease) and Hawaii (*Naalehu* disease). Sporadic cases of extensive mineralization occur in cattle throughout the world.

The leaves of these calcinogenic plants contain a substance(s) possessing vitamin D-like biological activity. The dried leaves of *S. malacoxylon* contain a steroid-glycoside conjugate in which the steroidal component is identical to 1,25-dihydroxycholecalciferol. The leaves are not palatable when green but are eaten readily when dry. The calcinogenic plants appear to produce disease only in herbivores after ingestion of leaves. Intoxication produces rapid wasting and

·marked elevations in the calcium and phosphorus levels in the blood. The patterns of these elevations in blood electrolytes as well as the soft-tissue mineralization are comparable to those produced by intoxication by vitamin D. The leaves of *S. malacoxylon* are remarkably potent, with as little as 2 g being capable of producing elevations in calcium and phosphorus in the blood of adult cattle. The typical wasting syndrome is seen clinically when animals are forced to eat large quantities of the leaves. The animals develop kyphosis, with contraction of the tendons and ligaments resulting in an inability to completely straighten their front limbs. Contraction of the abdominal aponeurosis gives a unique tucked-up line to the abdomen, resulting in affected animals having a racehorse-like appearance. Many animals develop severe vascular and pulmonary disease as a result of irregular or occasional exposure to the plant, due to mineralization and ossification of interalveolar septa in the lung.

These diseases associated with the ingestion of calcinogenic plants are not restricted to cattle but occur also in goats, sheep, and horses, although with lesser frequency and severity. Mature animals are most commonly affected, with the diseases usually producing progressive debility. The earliest signs are those of stiffness and wasting. There is a subtle progression to permanent lameness due to contraction of the tendons. At this stage, affected animals often are excitable, tire easily if made to exercise, and may show signs of acute cardiac insufficiency. If they are removed from affected areas, the stiffness and deformity are not lessened, but the wasting is stopped and the animals gain weight if good pasture is available.

Necropsy reveals widespread mineralization of the tissues, particularly the aorta, heart, and lungs often with areas of ossification. Small mineralized blood vessels are encountered in the subcutaneous tissues, and mineralized plaques are present on the parietal and visceral pleura. Portions of the lungs fail to collapse, and these represent areas of mineralization in which the parenchyma is disrupted and emphysematous. Areas of mineralization are present microscopically in the mucosa of the abomasal fundus, as well as in other fibroelastic tissues. Mineralization of ligaments and of the fibrocartilagenous portions of the tendons is responsible for the stiffness along with the degenerative arthropathy that usually is present in affected animals. In chronic cases, the bones become extremely dense as new trabeculae are formed in the marrow spaces. These trabeculae appear to develop in an atypical basophilic matrix similar to that deposited in vitamin D poisoning. Parathyroid chief cells appear initially to accumulate secretory granules after the feeding of *S. malacoxylon* leaves and later to undergo involution and atrophy.

Intoxication by Cholecalciferol-containing Rodenticides: Small Animals. The incidence of hypercalcemia due to vitamin D intoxication in small animals has increased due to use of vitamin D (cholecalciferol) as a pesticide and rodenticide. The ingested vitamin D is converted to 25-hydroxyvitamin D in the liver and is the major toxic metabolite. 25-Hydroxyvitamin D has a much reduced binding affinity for the vitamin D receptor (500- to 1000-fold) than does 1,25-dihydroxyvitamin D (the active form of vitamin D), but is present at such high concentrations that it stimulates hypercalcemia by increasing intestinal absorption of calcium. Only small amounts of the 25-hydroxyvitamin D are converted to the active form of vitamin D, 1,25-dihydroxyvitamin D, which often is present in the circulation at normal to subnormal levels. This is due to inhibition of renal 1α-hydroxylase by low serum PTH levels, hypercalcemia, hyperphosphatemia, and negative feedback from 25-hydroxyvitamin D that binds to the vitamin D receptor. The hypercalcemia of hypervitaminosis D is usually accompanied by hyperphosphatemia (since vitamin D also increases intestinal absorption of phosphorus in addition to calcium) and normal serum alkaline-phosphatase activity. Skeletal disease is not a consistent feature, since the increased concentrations of blood calcium and phosphorus are derived principally from augmented intestinal absorption; however, widespread mineralization of soft tissue occurs similar to animals ingesting calcinogenic plants.

CANCER-ASSOCIATED HYPERCALCEMIA. Hypercalcemia is a common disorder that affects animals and has many causes. The most common cause of hypercalcemia in animals and people is cancer-associated hypercalcemia (Rosol and Capen 1992; Capen and Rosol 1993). There are three mechanisms of increased serum calcium induced by neoplasms: (a) humoral hypercalcemia of malignancy (HHM), (b) hypercalcemia induced by metastases of solid tumors to bone, and (c) hematologic malignancies. Hypercalcemia results from an imbalance of calcium released from bones, calcium excretion by the kidney, and/or calcium absorption from the intestinal tract (Rosol and Capen 1992).

The clinical signs of hypercalcemia are similar regardless of underlying cause and depend on the rapidity of onset of increased serum ionized calcium levels (Rosol et al. 1995). Animals with serum calcium values in excess of 16.0 mg/dL (4.0 mmol/L) generally have the most severe clinical signs. Exceptions to this rule occur, and occasionally animals with severe hypercalcemia have mild clinical signs. Horses and rabbits have normal total serum calcium concentrations greater than those of other domestic animals, which should be considered before hypercalcemia is diagnosed in these species. Metabolic acidosis will enhance the severity of clinical signs since it will result in an increase in the ionized fraction of serum calcium.

Increased serum ionized calcium will induce clinical signs relating to the gastrointestinal, neuromuscular, cardiovascular, and renal systems (Rosol et al. 1995). Decreased contractility of the gastrointestinal smooth muscle may be associated with anorexia, vomiting, or constipation. There may be generalized locomotive weakness due to decreased neuromuscular excitability. Behavioral changes, depression, stupor, coma, seizures, and muscle twitching have been observed in dogs with hypercalcemia. Lameness and bone pain from demineralization of bone or pathological fractures may be clinical signs with long-standing hypercalcemia. Hypercalcemia results in increased myocardial excitability and diminished ventricular systole that may result in weakness and syncope associated with cardiac dysrhythmia. There is shortening of the Q-T interval and prolongation of the P-R interval (first-degree heart block). Ventricular fibrillation may develop in severe hypercalcemia. Hypercalcemia can predispose some animals to develop pancreatitis. The pathogenesis of pancreatitis associated with hypercalcemia is unknown but may be related to degeneration of pancreatic acinar cells and leakage of cytoplasmic enzymes (Frick et al. 1995).

Polyuria and polydipsia are commonly encountered and may be the reason for an animal owner to seek medical attention. Initially, polyuria and polydipsia are due to impaired renal concentrating ability. The mechanism of this defect is not completely understood, but it appears that hypercalcemia inhibits the antidiuretic hormone-dependent resorption of ammonium chloride in the diluting segment of the nephron by decreasing adenylate-cyclase activity. Urine specific gravity often is low (<1.020) and may be hyposthenuric (1.001 to 1.007). Sodium excretion usually remains unchanged due to the vasoconstrictor effect of hypercalcemia, which results in a reduction in the glomerular filtration rate.

Hypercalcemia also has a toxic effect on renal tubules either directly or from ischemia induced by vasoconstriction. Renal failure is an important consequence of severe or long-standing hypercalcemia (Kruger et al. 1996). Tubular epithelial cells undergo degeneration, with the collecting system most severely affected. There is mineralization of epithelial cells and basement membranes of tubules. Glycosuria may occur due to failure of tubular reabsorption and granular cast formation from degenerate tubular epithelial cells. Azotemia will occur when renal injury is severe, and the polyuria and polydipsia are secondary to renal failure. The magnitude of mineralization and tubular damage can be reduced by phosphate restriction.

Humoral Hypercalcemia of Malignancy (*Pseudohyperparathyroidism*). HHM is a syndrome associated with diverse malignant neoplasms in animal and human patients (Rosol and Capen 1992, 1997). Characteristic clinical findings in patients with HHM include hypercalcemia, hypophosphatemia, hypercalciuria (often with decreased fractional calcium excretion), increased fractional excretion of phosphorus, increased nephrogenous cAMP, and increased osteoclastic bone resorption. Hypercalcemia is induced by humoral effects on bone, kidney, and possibly the intestine (Figure 12.32). Increased osteoclastic bone resorption is a consistent finding in HHM with increased calcium release from bone. The kidney plays a critical role in the pathogenesis of hypercalcemia and hypophos-

phatemia, since renal calcium reabsorption is stimulated by PTH-related peptide (PTH-rP), and phosphorus reabsorption is inhibited due to binding to and activation of the renal PTH/PTH-rP receptors. In some forms of HHM, there are increased serum 1,25-dihydroxyvitamin D levels, which may increase calcium absorption from the intestine (Rosol et al. 1992). Malignant neoplasms that are commonly associated with HHM in animals include the adenocarcinoma derived from apocrine glands of the anal sac in dogs, some T-cell lymphomas of dogs, myelomas, and miscellaneous carcinomas that sporadically induce HHM in various species, such as cats and horses (gastric squamous cell carcinoma) (Rosol and Capen 1992; Rosol et al. 1994).

Excessive secretion of biologically active PTH-rP plays a central role in the pathogenesis of hypercalcemia in most forms of HHM; however, cytokines such as interleukin 1 (IL-1), tumor-necrosis factor α (TNF-α), or transforming growth factor α (TGF-α) and TGF-β or 1,25-dihydroxyvitamin D may have synergistic or cooperative actions with PTH-rP (Figure 12.33) (Merryman et al. 1993, 1994; Gröne et al. 1996). Before PTH-rP was identified, it was thought that nonparathyroid tumors associated with humoral hypercalcemia of malignancy induced a syndrome that mimicked primary hyperparathyroidism due to secretion of a PTH-like factor that was antigenically unrelated to PTH. Purification of the PTH-like activity from the adenocarcinoma derived from apocrine glands of the anal sac in dogs and multiple human tumors associated with HHM resulted in the discovery of PTH-rP (Moseley and Gillespie 1995). PTH-related protein also can be demonstrated in a number of normal tissues by immunohistochemical and biochemical analyses, where it appears to function primarily as a paracrine factor (Gröne et al. 1994).

PTH-rP binds to the N-terminal PTH/PTH-rP receptor in bone and kidney but does not cross-react immunologically with native PTH. PTH-rP stimulates adenylate cyclase and increases intracellular calcium ion in bone and kidney cells by binding to and activating the cell-membrane PTH/PTH-rP receptors. This results in a stimulation of osteoclastic bone resorption, increased renal tubular calcium reabsorption, and decreased renal tubular phosphorus reabsorption. IL-1 also stimulates bone resorption in vivo and in vitro and is synergistic with PTH-rP (Rosol and Capen 1992). TGF-α and TGF-β can stimulate bone resorption in vitro and have been identified in tumors associated with HHM, including adenocarcinomas derived from apocrine glands of the anal sac in dogs (Rosol et al. 1991; Merryman et al. 1989, 1993, 1994).

The clinical syndrome of pseudohyperparathyroidism has been well characterized in elderly female dogs associated with a perirectal adenocarcinoma (Rijnberk et al. 1978). The dogs had persistent hypercalcemia and hypophosphatemia that returned to normal following surgical excision of the neoplasm in the perirectal area. The hypercalcemia persisted following

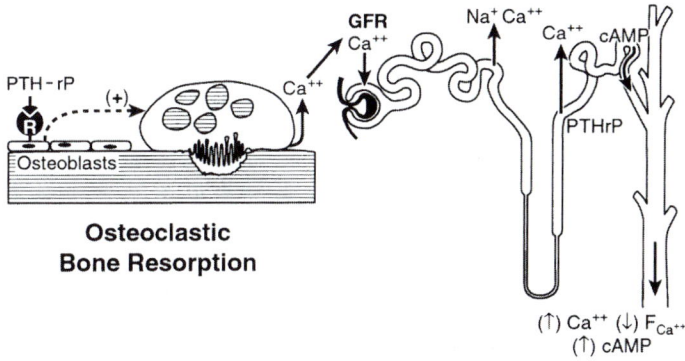

FIG. 12.32—Humoral hypercalcemia of malignancy develops in animal and human patients when neoplasms constitutively secrete parathyroid hormone-related protein (PTH-rP). PTH-rP binds to receptors on osteoblasts, which subsequently signal osteoclasts to increase bone resorption, and renal epithelial cells in the distal nephron to enhance calcium reabsorption [decreasing fractional (F) and calcium (Ca^{++}) excretion], resulting in persistent hypercalcemia. cAMP, cyclic adenosine monophosphate; $F_{Ca^{++}}$, fractional calcium; GFR, glomerular filtration rate; Na^+, ionized sodium; and encircled R, receptor. (From Rosol and Capen 1992.)

removal of the parathyroid glands. Immunoreactive PTH (iPTH) levels were within range of normal for dogs but were inappropriately high for the degree of hypercalcemia. Detailed clinical, macroscopic, and histopathological features of the adenocarcinomas arising from the apocrine gland of the anal sac have been reported in dogs (Meuten et al. 1981). This unique clinical syndrome occurred in aged, predominantly female dogs, and was characterized by persistent hypercalcemia and hypophosphatemia. Serum calcium values ranged from 11.4 to 24.0 mg/dL, with a mean of 16.2 mg/dL. Tumor ablation resulted in a prompt return to normocalcemia, but the hypercalcemia recurred with tumor regrowth, suggesting that the neoplastic cells were producing a humoral substance that increased calcium mobilization. All tumors had histopathological features of malignancy, and most had metastasized to iliac and sublumbar lymph nodes.

Skeletal demineralization in dogs with pseudohyperparathyroidism is mild in comparison with primary hyperparathyroidism and usually undetectable by conventional roentgenographic methods. Neoplastic cells from the perirectal adenocarcinomas rarely metastasize to bone and cause osteolysis (Meuten et al. 1981). Variable numbers of osteoclasts have been detected on bone surfaces in dogs with marked hypercalcemia, possibly reflecting different states in the course of the disease and phases of bone-remodeling activity. Histomorphometric analyses indicate that dogs with adenocarcinomas and hypercalcemia have significantly decreased trabecular bone volume as compared with age-matched control dogs. Total resorptive surface (Howship's lacunae with and without osteoclasts) is increased significantly, as are the number of osteoclasts per millimeter of trabecular bone. By comparison, dogs with primary hyperparathyroidism also have a significantly increased total resorptive surface and number of osteoclasts (Meuten et al. 1983b).

Renal mineralization is detected histologically in approximately 90% of dogs with pseudohyperparathyroidism associated with apocrine adenocarcinomas of the anal sac, particularly when the calcium-times-phosphorus product is 50 mg/dL or greater (Meuten et al. 1981). Tubular mineralization is most pronounced near the corticomedullary junction but also is present in cortical and deep medullary tubules, Bowman's capsule, and the glomerular tuft. Mineralization is present less frequently in the fundic mucosa of the stomach and endocardium.

The parathyroid glands are small and difficult to locate or not visible macroscopically in dogs with a cancer-associated hypercalcemia (Meuten et al. 1981). Atrophic parathyroid glands are characterized by nar-

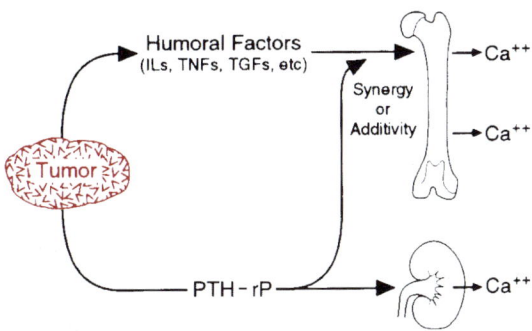

FIG. 12.33—Humoral factors, such as parathyroid hormone-related protein (PTH-rP), interleukin-1 (IL-1), tumor necrosis factors (TNFs), or transforming growth factors (TGFs), produced by tumors induce humoral hypercalcemia of malignancy (HHM) by acting as systemic hormones and stimulating osteoclastic bone resorption or increasing tubular reabsorption of calcium (Ca^{2+}). (From Rosol and Capen 1992.)

row cords of inactive chief cells with an abundant fibrous connective tissue stroma and widened perivascular spaces. The inactive chief cells have a markedly reduced cytoplasmic area, prominent hyperchromatic nuclei, relatively straight cell membranes with uncomplicated interdigitations, and are closely packed together. These findings indicate that the cancer cells are not producing a substance that stimulates PTH secretion by chief cells, but rather that the parathyroid glands are responding to persistent hypercalcemia by undergoing trophic atrophy. Thyroid parafollicular cells (C cells) often respond to the persistent elevation in blood calcium by undergoing diffuse or nodular hyperplasia (Meuten et al. 1981).

Hypercalcemic dogs with carcinomas have a significantly greater urine calcium excretion [0.35 ± 0.11 mg/dL glomerular filtrate (GF)] than either control dogs (0.02 ± 0.01 mg/dL GF) or normocalcemic tumor control dogs (0.04 ± 0.01 mg/dL GF), and have increased urine calcium compared with dogs with primary hyperparathyroidism (0.12 ± 0.06 mg/dL GF) (Meuten et al. 1983b). In addition, the results for fractional excretion of calcium indicate that the urinary excretion of calcium in dogs with cancer-associated hypercalcemia is significantly increased compared with that of clinically normal dogs. Urinary cAMP concentrations are significantly higher in hypercalcemic dogs (mean, 3.37 ± 0.44 nM) compared with clinically normal dogs (mean, 1.94 ± 0.16 nM) but not compared with tumor control dogs (mean, 2.70 ± 0.57 nM).

Most dogs with HHM have increased circulating concentrations of PTH-rP (Figure 12.34).

Plasma concentrations of PTH-rP are greatest (10 to 100 pM) in dogs with adenocarcinomas derived from apocrine glands of the anal sac and sporadic carcinomas associated with HHM (Rosol et al. 1990, 1992). The serum calcium concentrations in these dogs correlate well with circulating PTH-rP concentrations and are consistent with the concept that PTH-rP plays a primary role in the pathogenesis of HHM in these dogs (Figure 12.35).

Some dogs with cancer-associated hypercalcemia have inappropriate levels of 1,25-dihydroxyvitamin D (maintenance of normal range or increased) for the degree of hypercalcemia (Rosol et al. 1992). This suggests that the humoral factors produced by the neoplastic cells from some neoplasms are capable of stimulating renal 1α-hydroxylase and increasing the formation of 1,25-dihydroxyvitamin D even in the presence of increased blood calcium. Plasma immunoreactive PTH was not increased in hypercalcemic dogs and was significantly less in dogs with primary hyperparathyroidism (Figure 12.36). Surgical removal or radiation therapy of the adenocarcinoma results in a rapid return to normal of serum calcium and phosphorus levels, increased serum PTH, and decreased 1,25-dihydroxyvitamin D (Rosol et al. 1992).

Physiological Role of Parathyroid Hormone-related Protein. PTH-rP was first identified in 1982 as an important PTH-like factor that plays a central role in the pathogenesis of humoral hypercalcemia of malignancy. PTH-rP is a 139-, 141-, or 173-amino-acid peptide, originally isolated from human and animal tumors associated with humoral hypercalcemia of malignancy. The PTH-rP peptide shares 70% sequence homology with the first 13 amino acids of intact PTH. The N-terminal region of PTH-rP (amino acids 1 to 34) binds to and activates PTH receptors in bone and kidney cells with equal affinity as PTH. However, PTH-rP is not strictly a calcium-regulating hormone, and it has been determined that PTH-rP is widely produced in the body and acts as a paracrine factor in the tissues in which it is produced.

ROLE IN THE FETUS. The fetus maintains higher concentrations of serum calcium compared with the dam. Because the fetal parathyroid glands produce low levels of PTH, the mechanism of maintaining increased serum concentrations of calcium was unknown until the finding that PTH-rP maintains calcium balance in the fetus (Care 1991) and is the major hormone secreted by the chief cells of the fetal parathyroid glands. The PTH-rP produced by the placenta also stimulates the uptake of calcium by the fetus. PTH-related peptide plays a role in the differentiation of many tissues during gestation and is especially important in the growth and development of bone. Cartilage growth at the epiphyseal plate is regulated by the actions or PTH-rP, which stimulates chondrocyte proliferation, inhibits apoptosis, and inhibits the maturation of chondrocytes from the proliferative zone to the hypertrophic zone (Vortkamp et al. 1996), responses that are dependent on the translocation of PTH-rP to the nucleus and nucleolus (Henderson et al. 1995).

ROLE IN ADULT ANIMALS. In adult animals, PTH-rP is produced by many tissues, including endocrine glands; smooth, skeletal, and cardiac muscles; brain; lymphocytes; lactating mammary gland; kidney; prostate gland; lung; skin; and bone. The function of PTH-rP in most of these tissues is incompletely understood but is likely an autocrine or paracrine regulatory factor. Circulating concentrations of PTH-rP in normal animals and people are low (<1 pM) (Burtis 1992; Rosol et al. 1995), and the PTH/PTH-rP receptor is often expressed on the same or adjacent cells in tissues that synthesize PTH-rP.

Epidermal keratinocytes produce PTH-rP, which plays a role in their proliferation or differentiation. However, keratinocytes do not contain the classic PTH/PTH-rP receptor, which suggests that keratinocytes have an alternate PTH-rP receptor (Orloff et al. 1992). The greatest concentration of PTH-rP is found in milk (10 to 100 nmol/L), where it is 10,000- to 100,000-fold greater than in the serum (Ratcliffe 1992; Riond et al. 1995). The function of PTH-rP in the mammary gland and in milk is poorly understood at present. However, overexpression of PTH-rP in the mammary gland during glandular development prior to lactation results in glandular hypoplasia due to a reduction in the morphogenesis and branching of the mammary ducts.

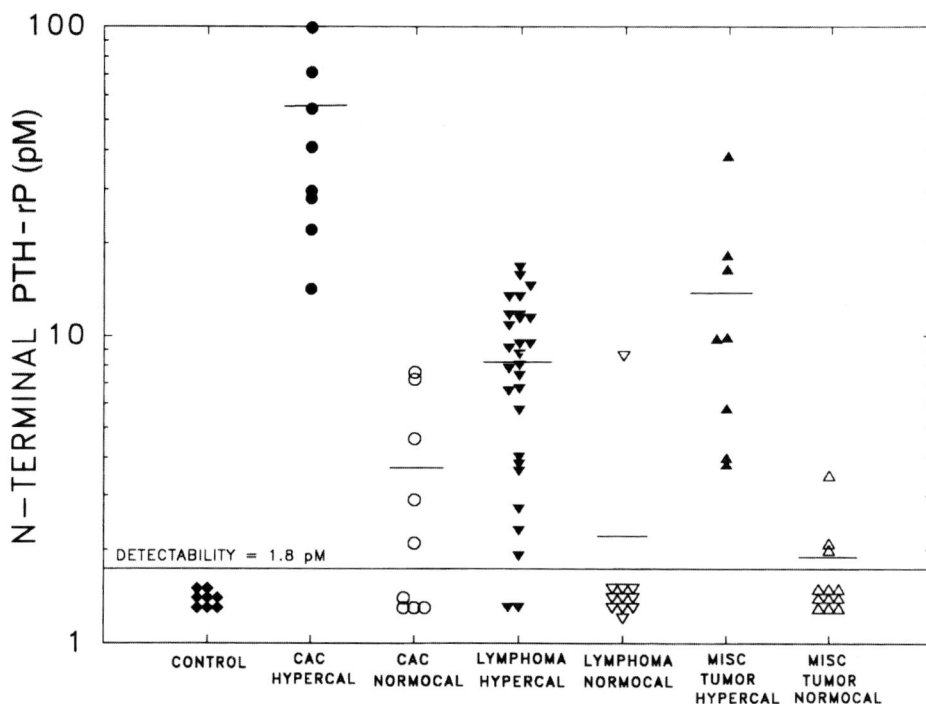

FIG. 12.34—Circulating N-terminal parathyroid hormone-related protein (PTH-rP) concentrations in normal dogs (control); dogs with hypercalcemia (>12 mg/dL) and anal-sac adenocarcinomas (CAC, canine apocrine carcinoma), lymphoma, or miscellaneous tumors (misc tumor); and dogs with normocalcemia (<12 mg/dL) and anal-sac adenocarcinomas, lymphoma, or miscellaneous tumors. (From Rosol et al. 1992.)

Biologically active PTH-rP produced by alveolar epithelial cells during lactation results in the high concentration of PTH-rP in milk, and this PTH-rP may play a role in stimulating the transport of calcium by alveolar epithelial cells from serum to milk (Parfitt 1987; Barlet et al. 1992). PTH-rP synthesis by the mammary gland abruptly ceases when suckling stops and the gland undergoes involution. The PTH-rP peptide is enzymatically cleaved in milk, but the N-terminal PTH-rP fragment retains biological activity. Although circulating concentrations of PTH-rP may be minimally increased in lactating dams, no significant relationship has been demonstrated between PTH-rP and the pathogenesis of parturient hypocalcemia and paresis in lactating dairy cattle (Riond et al. 1996). Hence, PTH-rP from the mammary gland likely plays a minor role in the systemic calcium balance of lactating animals but may have physiological functions, such as regulation of growth or differentiation of the gastrointestinal tract, in suckling neonates.

PTH-rP in hens is produced by smooth muscle, including blood vessels, uterus, urinary bladder, gastrointestinal tract, and the oviduct. In general, PTH-rP expression is increased when smooth muscle is stretched, and PTH-rP induces relaxation of smooth muscle and attenuation of contraction. With progres-

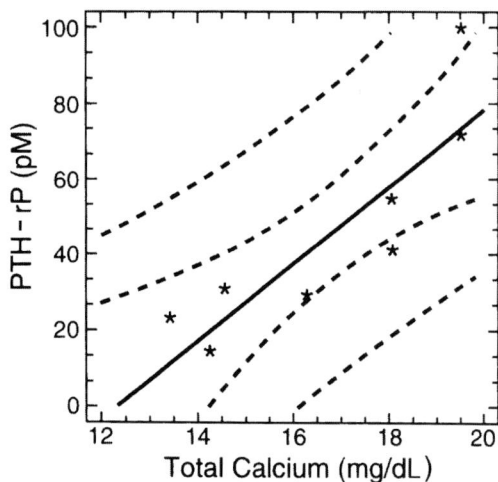

FIG. 12.35—Regression of parathyroid hormone-related protein (PTH-rP) and total calcium in dogs with anal-sac carcinoma (Ca). There was a significant linear correlation (0.87, P < 0.01) between serum calcium and N-terminal PTH-rP concentrations in dogs with humoral hypercalcemia of malignancy and adenocarcinomas derived from apocrine glands of the anal sac. (From Rosol et al. 1992.)

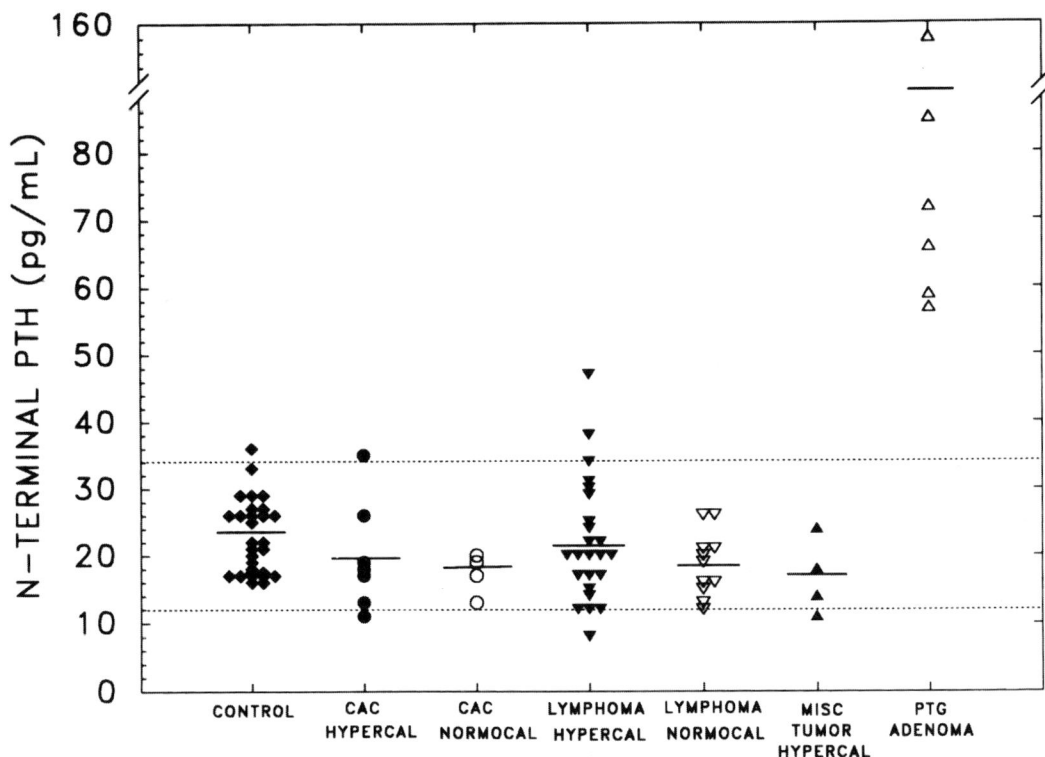

FIG. 12.36—Serum N-terminal parathyroid hormone (PTH) concentrations in normal dogs (control); dogs with hypercalcemia (>12 mg/dL) and anal-sac adenocarcinomas (CAC, canine apocrine carcinoma), lymphoma, miscellaneous tumors (misc tumor), or parathyroid adenomas [parathyroid gland (PTG) adenoma]; and dogs with normocalcemia (<12 mg/dL) and anal-sac adenocarcinomas or lymphoma. The normal range was 12 to 34 pg/mL (*dashed lines*). Bar = mean. (From Rosol et al. 1992.)

sive distension of the uterus during pregnancy or during descent of the ovum in the hen's oviduct, PTH-rP likely functions as a paracrine regulator of vascular tone, causing vasodilation and modulating vasoconstriction by other vasoactive compounds.

Two-site immunoradiometric and the N-terminal radioimmunoassays (RIAs) are available for the measurement of human PTH-rP. These assays can be used to measure PTH-rP in dogs, due to the high degree of sequence homology in PTH-rP between species. However, an N-terminal RIA for human PTH-rP has not proven useful to measure circulating PTH-rP in a small number of horses (Rosol et al. 1994). The PTH-rP concentrations are best measured in fresh or frozen plasma by using EDTA as an anticoagulant and with the addition of protease inhibitors, such as aprotinin and leupeptin (Pandian et al. 1992).

Differential Diagnosis of Hypercalcemia. Lymphoma is the most common neoplasm associated with hypercalcemia in dogs and cats (Osborne and Stevens 1973; Zenoble and Rowland 1979). Peripheral lymph node enlargement may or may not be detected, but evidence usually exists for anterior mediastinal or visceral involvement. Serum immunoreactive PTH levels have been found to be subnormal in hypercalcemic dogs with lymphoma, and plasma immunoreactive prostaglandin E_2 levels did not differ from levels in control dogs (Heath et al. 1980). Culture media from normal lymphoid tissue and control media had no effect on release of calcium 45 from prelabeled fetal mouse forelimb bones; however, media from tumor tissue increased calcium-45 release. These early findings suggested that the local production of bone-resorbing factors (e.g., osteoclast-activating factor) was important in stimulating calcium release from bone in certain dogs with lymphoma and hypercalcemia.

Malignant lymphoma is associated with hypercalcemia in 20% to 40% of the cases in dogs. Some dogs with lymphoma and hypercalcemia have HHM. Hypercalcemic lymphomas associated with HHM usually are of the T-cell subset. The affected dogs have increased fasting and 24-hour calcium excretion, increased fractional phosphorus excretion, and increased nephrogenous cAMP. Increased osteoclastic resorption was present in bones without evidence of tumor metastasis. Dogs with HHM and lymphoma may have a similar pathogenesis of hypercalcemia as occurs in people with human T-cell leukemia/lymphoma virus type I (HTLV-I)-induced lymphoma or leukemia. Human neoplastic cells with HTLV-I-induced lymphoma have increased PTH-rP production due to stimulation of PTH-rP transcription by the virally encoded Tax transcription factor (Prager et al. 1994).

Most dogs with lymphoma and HHM have significantly increased circulating PTH-rP concentrations, but levels are lower (2 to 15 pM) than in dogs with carcinomas and HHM (Figure 12.34), but there is no correlation with serum calcium concentration (Rosol et al. 1992). This indicates that PTH-rP is an important marker of dogs with HHM and lymphoma but is not the sole humoral factor responsible for the stimulation of osteoclasts and development of hypercalcemia. It is likely that cytokines such as IL-1 or TNF may function synergistically with PTH-rP to induce HHM in dogs with lymphoma (Rosol and Capen 1992). Some dogs and human patients with lymphoma and hypercalcemia have increased serum 1,25-dihydroxyvitamin D levels that may be responsible for or contribute to the induction of hypercalcemia (Rosol et al. 1992; Seymour and Gagel 1993). PTH (N-terminal) levels in dogs with lymphoma and hypercalcemia usually are in the normal range; however, an occasional dog may have levels elevated slightly out of the normal range (Figure 12.36).

Some forms of hematologic malignancies present in the bone marrow induce hypercalcemia by the local induction of bone resorption (Rosol and Capen 1992). This occurs most commonly with multiple myeloma and lymphoma. A number of paracrine factors or cytokines may be responsible for the stimulation of bone resorption. The cytokines most often implicated in the pathogenesis of local bone resorption include IL-1 and TNF-α, and tumor-necrosis β (lymphotoxin) (Martin and Grill 1992). Other cytokines or factors that may play a role include IL-6, TGF-α and TGF-β, and PTH-rP (Black and Mundy 1994). Due to increased circulating concentrations of PTH-rP, production of low levels of PTH-rP by a tumor in bone may stimulate local bone resorption without inducing a systemic response. Prostaglandins (especially prostaglandin E_2) also may be responsible for the local stimulation of bone resorption.

Some dogs with lymphoma and hypercalcemia have localized bone resorption associated with metastases to medullary cavities without evidence of increased bone resorption at sites distant from the tumor metastases (Meuten et al. 1983a). Hypercalcemic dogs with lymphoma and bone metastases had decreased serum PTH and 1,25-dihydroxyvitamin D levels; increased excretion of calcium, phosphate, and hydroxyproline; and increased serum levels of the prostaglandin E_2 metabolite (13,14-dihydro-15-keto-prostaglandin E_2). The mediator of local bone resorption has not been identified, but prostaglandin E_2 may be an important primary or secondary local mediator of bone resorption in these dogs. Other potential mediators include the cytokines, IL-1, or TNF.

Dogs with lymphoma and hypercalcemia have lower trabecular bone volume with more frequent osteoclastic osteolysis than do control dogs and dogs with normocalcemia and lymphoma (Meuten et al. 1983a). Only dogs with neoplastic cells in bone marrow have increased osteoclastic bone resorption. Dogs with hypercalcemic lymphoma often have osteoclasts on trabecular bone surfaces opposite a surface lined by osteoid and large columnar osteoblasts. Bone surfaces in normocalcemic control dogs are smooth and lined by flattened osteoblasts and rare osteoclasts. Dogs with lymphoma that are normocalcemic do not have increased bone resorption. Urine excretion of calcium, phosphorus, and hydroxyproline is higher in hypercalcemic dogs with lymphoma. Light-microscopic and electron-microscopic examination of parathyroid glands reveals inactive or atrophic chief cells and evidence of secretory inactivity in dogs with lymphoma and hypercalcemia. Ultrastructurally, lymphomas are composed of tumor cells with large nuclei and a paucity of cytoplasmic organelles.

Solid tumors that metastasize widely to bone can produce hypercalcemia by the induction of local bone resorption associated with tumor growth. This is not common in animals but is an important cause of cancer-associated hypercalcemia in people (Rosol and Capen 1992). Tumors that often metastasize to bone and induce hypercalcemia in human patients include breast and lung carcinomas. The pathogenesis of enhanced bone resorption is not well understood, but the two primary mechanisms include (a) secretion of cytokines or factors that stimulate local bone resorption, and (b) indirect stimulation of bone resorption by tumor-induced cytokine secretion from local immune or bone cells (Garrett 1993). Cytokines or factors that may be secreted by tumor cells and stimulate local bone resorption include PTH-rP (Powell et al. 1991), TGF-α and TGF-β, and prostaglandins (especially prostaglandin E_2). In some cases, bone-resorbing activity can be inhibited by indomethacin, which suggests that prostaglandins are either directly or indirectly associated with the stimulation of bone resorption. The cytokines most often implicated in indirect stimulation of bone resorption by local immune cells include IL-1 and TNF.

Malignant neoplasms with osseous metastases may cause moderate to severe hypercalcemia and hypercalciuria, but the serum alkaline-phosphatase activity and phosphorus usually are normal or only moderately elevated. These changes are believed to be due to release of calcium and phosphorus into the blood from areas of bone destruction at rates greater than can be cleared by the kidney and intestine. Bone involvement can be multifocal but usually is sharply demarcated and localized to the area of metastasis.

HYPERCALCITONINISM. Clinical syndromes associated with abnormalities in secretion of calcitonin are recognized much less frequently than are disorders of PTH secretion in both animals and people. The syndromes identified so far have been the result of excess secretion of calcitonin rather than a lack of secretion.

Calcitonin hypersecretion has been reported in humans (Hazard 1977) and bulls (Capen and Black 1974) with thyroid C-cell neoplasms (medullary or ultimobranchial). In human patients, the syndrome often is familial and affects many individuals in a kindred. Calcitonin-secreting C-cell neoplasms occur frequently in populations of adult to aged bulls. The chronic stimulation of ultimobranchial derivatives in the thyroid by the high-calcium diets fed to bulls may be related to the pathogenesis of the neoplasm (Krook et al 1971). Cows do not develop proliferative C-cell lesions under similar dietary conditions, probably because of the high physiological requirements for calcium imposed by pregnancy and lactation. The higher plasma immunoreactive calcitonin levels in bulls than in cows may be related to the bulls' greater intake of dietary calcium relative to physiological requirements.

C-cell (medullary) thyroid carcinomas also occur in dogs and horses sporadically as a firm mass in the anterior cervical region. Calcitonin activity can be localized to the cytoplasm of tumor cells by immunoenzymatic techniques. In addition to calcitonin, medullary (C cell) carcinomas in people may secrete other humoral substances, such as prostaglandins, serotonin, and bradykinin, that result in a wide spectrum of clinical manifestations. The incidence of occurrence of C-cell tumors in dogs is uncertain, but Zarrin (1977) reported that 7 of 200 thyroid tumors in dogs were derived from C cells. Due to the presence of large amounts of amyloid in the stroma, the tumors often are firm on palpation. Thyroid neoplasms of C-cell origin can be readily differentiated ultrastructurally by the presence of numerous membrane-limited secretory granules in the cytoplasm. Small granules of this type are not present in thyroid tumors derived from follicular cells.

C-cell tumors in both people and bulls can be associated with the simultaneous occurrence of pheochromocytomas in the adrenal medulla and neoplasms in other endocrine organs of neural crest origin (Sipple 1961; Capen and Black 1974). Serum calcium and phosphorus levels in adults with a chronic excessive secretion of calcitonin usually remain in the low-normal range due to the relatively slow turnover rate of bone. Osteosclerotic changes with thickening of trabeculae in vertebral bodies have been reported in bulls with this syndrome of long-term and excessive calcitonin secretion.

HYPOCALCITONINISM. Specific disease syndromes resulting from a lack of calcitonin secretion have not been recognized in either people or animals. However, experimentally thyroidectomized animals are less able than normal to handle a calcium load and may develop hypercalcemia (Swaminathan et al. 1972).

HYPOPHOSPHATEMIA. This may impair red and white blood cell function and lead to muscle weakness, recumbency, intestinal ileus, anorexia, or vomition (Hodgson and Hurley 1993; Gerloff and Swenson 1996). Red blood cell fragility and hemolysis can be increased by the lack of ATP in the erythrocyte, due to the necessity of phosphate for the erythrocytic glycolytic pathway. Intravascular hemolysis is uncommon, but the occurrence of hypophosphatemia in cattle with postparturient hemoglobinuria may predispose erythrocytes to hemolysis when the animals are exposed to hemolytic agents in plants.

The production of 2,3-diphosphoglycerate (2,3-DPG) is dependent on phosphate. Erythrocytes with low 2,3-DPG concentrations have increased binding affinity for oxygen and reduced delivery of oxygen to peripheral tissues. This may be responsible for muscle weakness in patients with hypophosphatemia. White blood cells may have decreased chemotaxis and phagocytosis also due to a lack of ATP during hypophosphatemia. The causes of hypophosphatemia include maldistribution secondary to a large carbohydrate load, respiratory alkalosis, metabolic acidosis, catecholamine release, or insulin treatment of an animal with diabetes mellitus. Hypophosphatemia also can be caused by reduced renal reabsorption in animals with primary hyperparathyroidism or renal tubular defects and reduced intestinal absorption during vitamin D deficiency.

HYPERPHOSPHATEMIA. This leads to a reciprocal reduction in serum ionized calcium concentration due to the mass-law interactions between phosphate and calcium ions and to decreased renal 1,25-hydroxyvitamin D synthesis by the kidney. The clinical signs of acute hyperphosphatemia may be due to hypocalcemia and consist of tetany and soft-tissue mineralization (especially when the serum calcium-times-phosphorus product is greater than 70 mg/dL). The principal causes of hyperphosphatemia include massive cellular lysis (e.g., during chemotherapy, rhabdomyolysis, or hemolysis), vitamin D intoxication, chronic renal failure, hypoparathyroidism, hypersomatotropism, and hyperthyroidism (Chew and Meuten 1982; Yanagawa and Lee 1992).

REFERENCES

Anderson MP, Capen CC. 1976. Nutritional osteodystrophy in captive green iguanas (*Iguana iguana*). Virchows Arch [B] 21:229–247.

Argenzio RA, Lowe JE, Hintz HF, Schryver HF. 1974. Calcium and phosphorus homeostasis in horses. J Nutr 104:18–27.

Barlet JP, Champredon C, Coxam V, et al. 1992. Parathyroid hormone-related peptide might stimulate calcium secretion into the milk of goats. J Endocrinol 132:353–359.

Black KS, Mundy GR. 1994. Other causes of hypercalcemia: Local and ectopic secretion syndromes. In: Bilezikian JP, Levine MA, Marcus R, eds. The Parathyroids. New York: Raven, pp 341–457.

Black HE, Capen CC, Arnaud CD. 1973a. Ultrastructure of parathyroid glands and plasma immunoreactive parathyroid hormone in pregnant cows fed normal and high calcium diets. Lab Invest 29:173–185.

Black HE, Capen CC, Yarrington JT, et al. 1973b. Effect of a high calcium prepartal diet on calcium homeostatic mechanisms in thyroid glands, bone, and intestine of cows. Lab Invest 29:437–448.

Block E. 1984. Manipulating dietary anions and cations for prepartum dairy cows to reduce incidence of milk fever. J Dairy Sci 67:2939–2948.

Burtis WJ. 1992. Parathyroid hormone-related protein: Structure, function, and measurement. Clin Chem 38:2171–2183.

Bushinsky DA. 1996. Metabolic alkalosis decreases bone calcium efflux by suppressing osteoclasts and stimulating osteoblasts. Am J Physiol 271:F216–F222.

Capen CC. 1982. Nutritional secondary hyperparathyroidism in horses. In: Robinson NE, ed. Current Therapy in Equine Medicine. Philadelphia: WB Saunders, pp 160–163.

Capen CC. 1989. The calcium regulating hormones: Parathyroid hormone, calcitonin, and cholecalciferol. In: McDonald LE, ed. Veterinary Endocrinology and Reproduction, 4th ed. Philadelphia: Lea and Febiger, pp 92–185.

Capen CC, Black HE. 1974. Calcitonin-secreting ultimobranchial neoplasms of the thyroid gland in bulls: An animal model for medullary thyroid carcinoma in man (Sipple's syndrome). Am J Pathol 74:377–380.

Capen CC. 2001a. Endocrine system. In: McGavin D, Carlton WW, Zachary JF, eds. Thomson's Special Veterinary Pathology, 3rd ed. St Louis: CV Mosby, pp 279–323.

Capen CC. 2001b. Overview of structural and functional lesions in endocrine organs of animals. Toxicol Pathol 29:8–33.

Capen CC, Rosol TJ. 1993. Pathobiology of parathyroid hormone and parathyroid hormone-related protein: Introduction and evolving concepts. In: Li Volsi VA, De Lellis RA, eds. Pathology of the Thyroid and Parathyroid Gland: An Update. Philadelphia: Williams and Wilkins, pp 1–33.

Care AD. 1991. The placental transfer of calcium. J Dev Physiol 15:253–257.

Chew DJ, Meuten DJ. 1982. Disorders of calcium and phosphorus metabolism. Vet Clin North Am Small Anim Pract 12:411–438.

Constable PD. 1999. Clinical assessment of acid-base status: Strong ion difference theory. Vet Clin North Am Food Anim Pract 15:447–471.

Felsenfeld AJ, Llach F. 1993. Parathyroid gland function in chronic renal failure. Kidney Int 43:771–789.

Finco DR, Brown SA, Cooper T, et al. 1994. Effects of parathyroid hormone depletion in dogs with induced renal failure. Am J Vet Res 55:867–873.

Frick TW, Mithöfer K, Fernandez-del Castillo C, et al. 1995. Hypercalcemia causes acute pancreatitis by pancreatic secretory block, intracellular zymogen accumulation, and acinar cell injury. Am J Surg 169:167–172.

Garrett IR. 1993. Bone destruction in cancer. Semin Oncol 20:4–9.

Gaynor PJ, Mueller FJ, Miller JK, et al. 1989. Parturient hypocalcemia in Jersey cows fed alfalfa haylage-based diets with different cation to anion ratios. J Dairy Sci 72:2525–2531.

Gerloff BJ, Swenson EP. 1996. Acute recumbency and marginal phosphorus deficiency in dairy cattle. J Am Vet Med Assoc 208:716–720.

Gilka F, Sugden EA. 1984. Ectopic mineralization and nutritional hyperparathyroidism in boars. Can J Comp Med 48:102–107.

Goff JP, Horst RL. 1997. Effects of the addition of potassium or sodium, but not calcium, to prepartum rations on milk fever in dairy cows. J Dairy Sci 80:176–186.

Goff JP, Horst RL, Mueller FJ, et al. 1991. Addition of chloride to a prepartal diet high in cations increases 1,25-dihydroxyvitamin D response to hypocalcemia preventing milk fever. J Dairy Sci 74:3863–3871.

Gröne A, Werkmeister JR, Steinmeyer CL, et al. 1994. Parathyroid hormone-related protein in normal and neoplastic canine tissues: Immunohistochemical localization and biochemical extraction. Vet Pathol 31:308–315.

Gröne A, Weckmann MT, Steinmeyer CL, et al. 1996. Altered parathyroid hormone-related protein secretion and mRNA expression in squamous cell carcinoma cells in vitro. Eur J Endocrinol 135:498–505.

Hazard JB. 1977. The C cells (parafollicular cells) of the thyroid gland and medullary thyroid carcinoma: A review. Am J Pathol 88:213–250.

Heath H, Weller RE, Mundy GR. 1980. Canine lymphosarcoma: A model for study of the hypercalcemia of cancer. Calcif Tissue Int 30:127–133.

Henderson JE, Amizuka N, Warshawsky H, et al. 1995. Nucleolar localization of parathyroid hormone-related peptide enhances survival of chondrocytes under conditions that promote apoptotic cell death. Mol Cell Biol 15:4064–4075.

Hodgson SF, Hurley DL. 1993. Acquired hypophosphatemia. Endocrinol Metab Clin North Am 22:397–409.

Hunt RD, Garcia FG, Hegsted DM. 1967. A comparison of vitamin D_2 and D_3 in New World primates: I. Production and regression of osteodystrophia fibrosa. Lab Anim Care 17:222–234.

Jones BR, Alley MR. 1985. Primary idiopathic hypoparathyroidism in St. Bernard dogs. NZ Vet J 33:94–97.

Joyce PW, Sanchez WK, Goff JP. 1997. Effect of anionic salts in prepartum diets based on alfalfa. J Dairy Sci 80:2866–2875.

Krook L, Lutwak L, McEntee K, et al. 1971. Nutritional hypercalcitoninism in bulls. Cornell Vet 61:625–639.

Kruger JM, Osborne CA, Nachreiner RF, Refsal KR. 1996. Hypercalcemia and renal failure: Etiology, pathophysiology, diagnosis, and treatment. Vet Clin North Am Small Anim Pract 26:1417–1445.

Lehner NDM, Bullock BC, Clarkson TB, et al. 1967. Biological activities of vitamin D_2 and D_3 for growing squirrel monkeys. Lab Anim Care 17:483–493.

Long P, Choi G, Rehmel R. 1983. Oxyphil cells in a red-tailed hawk (*Buteo jamaicensis*) with nutritional secondary hyperparathyroidism. Avian Dis 27:839–843.

Martin TJ, Grill V. 1992. Hypercalcemia and Cancer. J Steroid Biochem Mol Biol 43:123–129.

Martin KJ, Freitag JJ, Bellorin-Font E, et al. 1980. The effect of acute acidosis on the uptake of parathyroid hormone and the production of adenosine 3′,5′-monophosphate by isolated perfused bone. Endocrinology 106:1607–1611.

Merryman JI, Rosol TJ, Brooks CL, Capen CC. 1989. Separation of parathyroid hormone-like activity from transforming growth factor-α and -β in the canine adenocarcinoma (CAC-8) model of humoral hypercalcemia of malignancy. Endocrinology 124:2456–2463.

Merryman JI, Capen CC, McCauley LK, et al. 1993. Regulation of parathyroid hormone-related protein production by a squamous carcinoma cell line in vitro. Lab Invest 69:347–354.

Merryman JI, De Wille J, Werkmeister JR, et al. 1994. Effects of transforming growth factor-beta on PTRrP production and RNA expression by a squamous carcinoma cell line in vitro. Endocrinology 134:2424–2430.

Meuten DJ, Cooper BJ, Capen CC, et al. 1981. Hypercalcemia associated with an adenocarcinoma derived from the apocrine glands of the anal sac. Vet Pathol 18:454–471.

Meuten DJ, Kociba GJ, Capen CC, et al. 1983a. Hypercalcemia in dogs with lymphosarcoma: Biochemical, ultrastructural and histomorphometric investigations. Lab Invest 49:553–562.

Meuten DJ, Segre GV, Capen CC, et al. 1983b. Hypercalcemia in dogs with adenocarcinoma derived from apocrine glands of anal sac: Biochemical and histomorphometric investigations. Lab Invest 48:428–435.

Moseley JM, Gillespie MT. 1995. Parathyroid hormone-related protein. Crit Rev Clin Lab Sci 32:299–343.

Nagode LA, Chew DJ. 1992. Nephrocalcinosis caused by hyperparathyroidism in progression of renal failure: Treatment with calcitriol. Semin Vet Med Surg Small Anim 7:202–220.

Nagode LA, Chew DJ, Podell M. 1996. Benefits of calcitriol therapy and serum phosphorus control in dogs and cats with chronic renal failure. Vet Clin North Am Small Anim Pract 26:1293–1330.

Oetzel GR, Olson JD, Curtis CR, Fettman MJ. 1988. Ammonium chloride and ammonium sulfate for prevention of parturient paresis in dairy cows. J Dairy Sci 71:3302–3309.

Oetzel GR, Fettman MJ, Hamar DW, Olson JD. 1991. Screening of anionic salts for palatability, effects on acid-base status, and urinary calcium excretion in dairy cows. J Dairy Sci 74:965–971.

Orloff JJ, Ganz MB, Ribaudo AE, et al. 1992. Analysis of PTHRP binding and signal transduction mechanisms in benign and malignant squamous cells. Am J Physiol 262:E599–E607.

Osborne CA, Stevens JB. 1973. Pseudohyperparathyroidism in the dog. J Am Vet Med Assoc 16:125–135.

Pandian MR, Morgan CH, Carlton E, Segre GV. 1992. Modified immunoradiometric assay of parathyroid hormone-related protein: Clinical application in the differential diagnosis of hypercalcemia. Clin Chem 38:282–288.

Parfitt AM. 1987. Bone and plasma calcium homeostasis. Bone 8(Suppl 1):S1–S8.

Powell GJ, Southby J, Danks JA, et al. 1991. Localization of parathyroid hormone-related protein in breast cancer metastases: Increased incidence in bone compared to other sites. Cancer Res 51:3059–3061.

Prager D, Rosenblatt JD, Ejima E. 1994. Hypercalcemia, parathyroid hormone-related protein expression and human T-cell leukemia virus infection. Leuk Lymphoma 14:395–400.

Ratcliffe WA. 1992. Role of parathyroid hormone-related protein in lactation. Clin Endocrinol 37:402–404.

Rijnberk A, Elsinhorst ThAM, Kolman JP, et al. 1978. Pseudohyperparathyroidism associated with perirectal adenocarcinomas in elderly female dogs. Tijdschr Diergeneeskd 103:1069–1075.

Riond J-L, Kocabagli N, Forrer R, et al. 1995. Repeated day-time measurements of the concentrations of PTHrP and other components of bovine milk. J Anim Physiol Anim Nutr 74:194–204.

Riond J-L, Kocabagli N, Cloux F, Wanner M. 1996. Parathyroid hormone-related protein in the colostrum of paretic post parturient dairy cows. Vet Rec 138:333–334.

Rosol TJ, Capen CC. 1992. Biology of disease: Mechanisms of cancer-induced hypercalcemia. Lab Invest 67:680–702.

Rosol TJ, Capen CC. 1997. Calcium-regulating hormones and diseases of abnormal mineral (calcium, phosphorus, magnesium) metabolism. In: Kaneko JJ, Harvey JW, Bruss ML, eds. Clinical Biochemistry of Domestic Animals, 5th ed. New York: Academic, pp 619–702.

Rosol TJ, Capen CC, Danks JA. 1990. Identification of parathyroid hormone-related protein in canine apocrine adenocarcinoma of the anal sac. Vet Pathol 27:89–95.

Rosol TJ, Merryman JI, Nohutcu RM, et al. 1991. Effects of transforming growth factor-α on parathyroid hormone- and parathyroid hormone-related protein-mediated bone resorption and adenylate cyclase stimulation in vitro. Domest Anim Endocrinol 8:499–507.

Rosol TJ, Nagode LA, Couto CG, et al. 1992. Parathyroid hormone (PTH)-related protein, PTH, and 1,25-dihydroxyvitamin D in dogs with cancer-associated hypercalcemia. Endocrinology 131:1157–1164.

Rosol TJ, Nagode LA, Robertson JT, et al. 1994. Humoral hypercalcemia of malignancy associated with ameloblastoma in a horse. J Am Vet Med Assoc 204:1930–1933.

Rosol TJ, Chew DJ, Nagode LA, Capen CC. 1995. Pathophysiology of calcium metabolism. Vet Clin Pathol 24:49–63.

Rowland GN, Capen CC, Nagode LN. 1968. Experimental hyperparathyroidism in young cats. Pathol Vet 5:504–519.

Seymour JF, Gagel RF. 1993. Calcitriol: The major humoral mediator of hypercalcemia in Hodgkin's and non-Hodgkin's lymphomas. Blood 82:1383–1394.

Sipple JF. 1961. Association of pheochromocytoma with carcinoma of the thyroid gland. Am J Med 31:163–175.

Swaminathan R, Bates RFL, Care AD. 1972. Fresh evidence for a physiological role of calcitonin in calcium homeostasis. J Endocrinol 54:525–526.

Thompson KG, Jones LP, Smylie WA, et al. 1984. Primary hyperparathyroidism in German shepherd dogs: A disorder of probable genetic origin. Vet Pathol 21:370–376.

Tucker WB, Hogue JF, Waterman DF, et al. 1991. Role of sulfur and chloride in the dietary cation-anion balance equation for lactating dairy cattle. J Anim Sci 69:1205–1213.

Vortkamp A, Lee K, Lanske B, et al. 1996. Regulation of rate of cartilage differentiation by Indian hedgehog and PTH-related protein. Science 273:613–622.

Walthall JC, McKenzie RA. 1976. Osteodystrophia fibrosa in horses at pasture in Queensland: Field and laboratory observations. Aust Vet J 52:11–16.

Wang C, Beede DK. 1992. Effects of ammonium chloride and sulfate on acid-base status and calcium metabolism of dry Jersey cows. J Dairy Sci 75:820–828.

Yanagawa N, Lee DBN. 1992. Renal handling of calcium and phosphorus. In: Coe FL, Favus MJ, eds. Disorders of Bone and Mineral Metabolism. New York Raven, pp 3–40.

Yarrington JT, Capen CC, Black HE, et al. 1976. Experimental parturient hypocalcemia in cows following prepartal chemical inhibition of bone resorption. Am J Pathol 83:569–588.

Yarrington JT, Capen CC, Black HE, et al. 1977a. Effect of dichloromethane diphosphonate on calcium homeostatic mechanisms in pregnant cows. Am J Pathol 87:615–632.

Yarrington JT, Capen CC, Black HE, Re R. 1977b. Effects of a low calcium prepartal diet on calcium homeostatic mechanisms in the cow: Morphological and biochemical studies. J Nutr 107:2244–2256.

Zarrin K. 1977. Naturally occurring parafollicular cell carcinoma of the thyroid in dogs: A histological and ultrastructural study. Vet Pathol 14:556–566.

Zenoble RD, Rowland GN. 1979. Hypercalcemia and proliferative, myelosclerotic bone reaction associated with feline leukovirus infection in a cat. J Am Vet Med Assoc 175:591–595.

PART 3: PATHOPHYSIOLOGY OF THE THYROID GLAND

CHARLES C. CAPEN

PHYSIOLOGY OF THE THYROID

Unique Developmental, Structural, and Functional Aspects of the Thyroid Gland. The thyroid gland originates as a thickened plate of epithelium in the floor of the pharynx. It is intimately related to the aortic sac in its development, and this association leads to the frequent finding of accessory thyroid parenchyma in mediastinal structures, especially in dogs. This accessory thyroid tissue may undergo neoplastic transformation. Branched cell cords develop from the pharyngeal plate and migrate dorsolaterally but remain attached to the pharyngeal area by the narrow thyroglossal duct. The entodermal bud that forms the thyroid gland arises on the midline at the level of the first pharyngeal pouch. This gives rise to the thyroglossal duct, which migrates caudally. The proliferation of cell cords at the distal end of the thyroglossal duct forms the follicles of each thyroid lobe. The area at the base of the tongue marking the origin on the thyroid gland is referred to as the foramen cecum linguae in postnatal life. Calcitonin-secreting C cells of neural crest origin reach the postnatal thyroid gland by migrating into the ultimobranchial body. This last pharyngeal pouch moves caudally in mammals to fuse with the primordia of the thyroid gland and distribute C cells into each thyroid lobe.

Folliculogenesis, a complex process in the thyroid, begins by the proliferation of irregularly arranged cell cords derived from the entoderm of the thyroglossal duct on the midline of the developing pharyngeal gut. The solid cell clusters extend caudally in to the primitive mesenchyme and develop complex interdigitations of plasma membranes of adjacent cells (Takizawa et al. 1993). Primitive follicles develop either by invagination of the plasma membrane of individual follicular cells to form intracytoplasmic colloid-containing microfollicles that subsequently coalesce to form larger follicles or by the secretion of colloid in the narrow intercellular spaces limited by zonulae adherens and desmosomes. In rats with a normal 21-day gestation period, thyroid follicles begin to form between days 15 and 18 of gestation. Thyroid-stimulating hormone (TSH or thyrotropin) may not be required for the formation of the initial primitive follicles, but follicles formed on day 17 and subsequent days of gestation are responsive to TSH for their final development in rats.

A portion of the thyroglossal duct may persist postnatally and form a cyst. Thyroglossal duct cysts are present in the ventral aspect of the anterior cervical region in dogs. Their lining epithelium may undergo neoplastic transformation (see earlier the discussion of cervical cysts in parathyroid-thyroid area).

Accessory thyroid tissue is common in dogs and may be located anywhere from the larynx to the diaphragm. About 50% of adult dogs have accessory thyroid tissue embedded in the fat on the intrapericardial aorta. These nodules are usually 2 to 5 mm in dimension and may be multiple. They lack C (parafollicular) cells, which secrete calcitonin, but their follicular structure and function (ability to concentrate iodine and iodinate tyrosyl residues) are the same as that of the main thyroid lobes. Attempts to induce hypothyroidism in dogs by a surgical thyroidectomy are not consistently successful because the follicular cells in the accessory thyroids readily respond to the prompt increase in endogenous

TSH and undergo hyperplasia sufficient to sustain adequate hormone production.

The two thyroid lobes in most species are located on the lateral surfaces of the trachea. In pigs, the main lobe of the thyroid is in the midline in the caudal cervical region, with dorsolateral projections from each side. The principal blood supply to each lobe in dogs is from the cranial thyroid artery (a branch of common carotid), and the major venous drainage is via the caudal thyroid vein that enters the internal jugular vein. Lymph drainage from the cranial pole of the thyroid lobes in dogs is to the retropharyngeal lymph nodes. Lymph flow from the caudal aspect of each thyroid lobe is variable, but it often bypasses any lymph nodes before entering the brachiocephalic trunk. Efferent lymphatics usually enter directly into the cervical lymphatic trunk or internal jugular vein. This explains the frequent occurrence of pulmonary metastases from thyroid carcinoma in dogs prior to development of secondary foci in regional lymph nodes. Small efferent lymphatics may pass through the caudal cervical lymph nodes along the ventral surface of the trachea before entering the cranial mediastinum. These vascular arrangements are significant for the spread of thyroid carcinomas.

The thyroid gland is the largest of the endocrine organs that functions exclusively as an endocrine gland (Capen 2000). The basic histological structure of the thyroid is unique for endocrine glands, consisting of follicles of varying size (20 to 250 μm) that contain colloid produced by the follicular cells (thyrocytes). The follicular cells are cuboidal to low columnar (under conditions of normal iodine intake), and their secretory polarity is directed toward the lumen of the follicles. An extensive network of interfollicular capillaries provides the follicular cells with an abundant blood supply. Follicular cells have extensive profiles of rough endoplasmic reticulum and a large Golgi apparatus in their cytoplasm synthesizing and packaging substantial amounts of protein (e.g., thyroglobulin) that are then transported into the follicular lumen. The interface between the luminal side of follicular cells and the colloid is modified by numerous microvillous projections.

Varying numbers of lysosomes, histochemically stainable for enzymes such as acid phosphatase, are found in the apical portion of follicular cells. Soon after stimulation by TSH of follicular cells, intracellular droplets of ingested colloid (phagosomes), corresponding to those demonstrated light microscopically by the periodic acid-Schiff (PAS) reaction, are more numerous than in the resting state (Wetzel et al. 1965). Some of these form phagolysosomes in follicular cells by fusion with lysosomes.

Biosynthesis of Thyroid Hormones. The synthesis of thyroid hormones is unique among endocrine glands because the final assembly of hormone occurs extracellularly within the follicular lumen. Essential raw materials, such as iodide ion (I⁻), are trapped by follicular cells from plasma, transported rapidly against a concentration gradient to the lumen of the follicle, and oxidized by a peroxidase enzyme in the microvillar membranes to iodine (I_2).

The assembly of thyroid hormones within the follicular lumen is made possible by a unique protein, thyroglobulin, synthesized by follicular cells (Figure 12.37). Thyroglobulin is a high molecular weight glycoprotein synthesized in successive subunits on the ribosomes of the endoplasmic reticulum in follicular cells. The constituent amino acids (tyrosine and others) and carbohydrates (mannose, fructose, and galactose) are derived from the circulation. Recently synthesized thyroglobulin leaving the Golgi apparatus is packaged into apical vesicles that are extruded into the follicular lumen. The amino acid tyrosine, an essential component of thyroid hormones, is incorporated within the molecular structure of thyroglobulin. Iodine is bound to the tyrosyl residues in thyroglobulin at the apical surface of follicular cells to form successively monoiodotyrosine (MIT) and diiodotyrosine (DIT) (Öfverholm and Ericson 1984). These biologically inactive iodothyronines subsequently are coupled together under the influence of the thyroperoxidase to form the two biologically active iodothyronines [thyroxine (T_4) and triiodothyronine (T_3)] secreted by the thyroid gland.

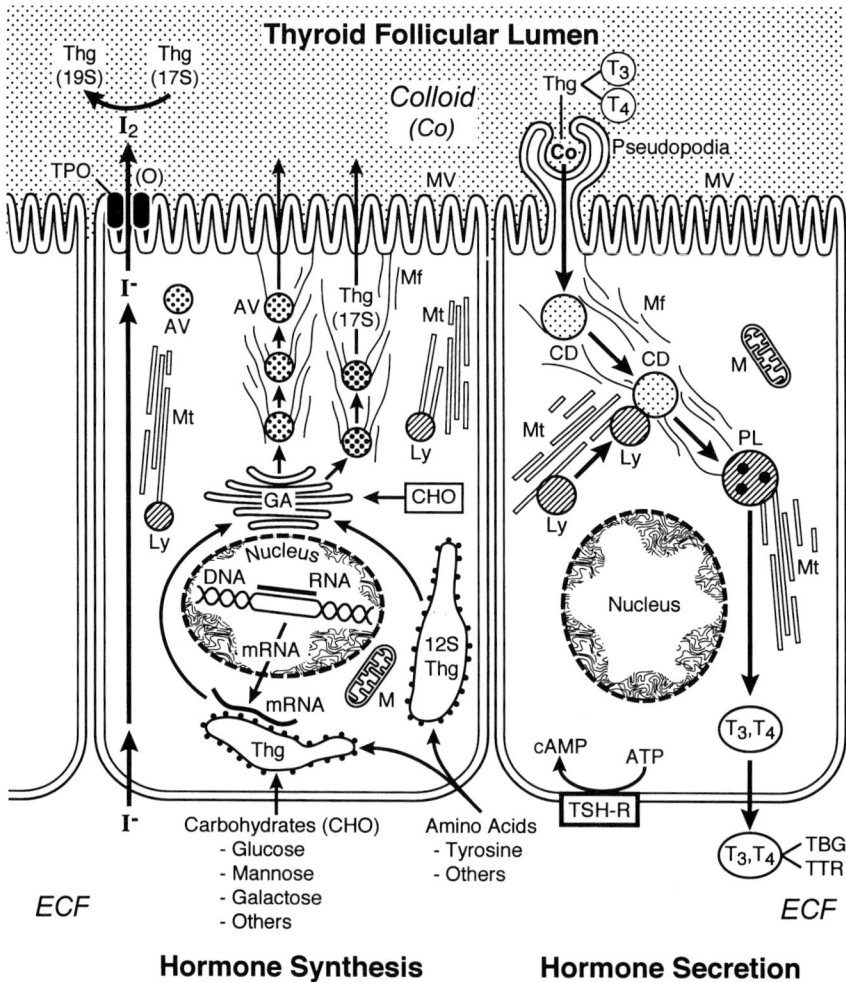

FIG. 12.37—Normal thyroid follicular cells illustrating two-way traffic of materials from capillaries into the follicular lumen and from lumen back into interfollicular capillaries. Raw materials, such as iodine, are concentrated by follicular cells and rapidly transported into the lumen **(left)**. Amino acids (tyrosine and others) and sugars are assembled by follicular cells into thyroglobulin (thg), packaged into apical vesicles (AV) and released into the lumen. The iodination of tyrosyl residues occurs within the thyroglobulin molecule to form thyroid hormones in the follicular lumen. Elongation of microvilli and endocytosis of colloid by follicular cells occurs in response to thyroid-stimulating hormone (TSH) stimulation **(right)**. The intracellular colloid droplets (Co) fuse with lysosomal bodies (Ly), active thyroid hormone is enzymatically cleaved from thyroglobulin, and free tetraiodothyronine (T_4) and triiodothyronine (T_3) are released into circulation. M, mitochondria; N, nucleus; CHO, carbohydrates; GA, Golgi Apparatus; R, receptor; TgB, thyroid binding globulin; PL, phagolysosome; TTR, transthyretin; ECF, extra cellular fluids; Mf, microfilaments; and Mt, microtubules.

The functionally important thyroperoxidase enzyme in the thyroid hormone synthetic pathway is present in the apical plasma membrane and microvilli as well as in other membranous structures of the follicular cells (Tice and Wollman 1972, 1974). Thyroperoxidase is a membrane-bound, heme-containing glycoprotein composed of 933 amino acids with a transmembrane domain. This important enzyme oxidizes (in the presence of hydrogen peroxidase) iodide ion (I⁻) taken up by follicular cells through the function of the sodium-iodide symporter into reactive iodine (I_2), which binds to the tyrosine residues in the thyroglobulin. Iodine is incorporated not only into newly synthesized thyroglobulin recently delivered to the follicular lumen but also into molecules already stored in the lumen. Thyroperoxidase also functions as a coupling enzyme to combine MIT and DIT to form triiodothyronine (T_3) or two DITs to form thyroxine (T_4).

The mechanism of active transport of iodide has been shown to be associated with a sodium-iodide (Na⁺-I⁻) symporter (NIS) present in the basolateral membrane of thyroid follicular cells (Figure 12.38) (La Perle and Jhiang 2003). Transport of iodide ion across the thyroid cell membrane is linked to the transport of Na⁺. The ion gradient generated by the Na⁺-K⁺ ATPase appears to be the driving force for the active cotransport of iodide. The transporter protein is present in the basolateral membrane of thyroid follicular cells and is a large protein containing 643 amino acids with 13 transmembrane domains.

Other tissues, such as the salivary gland, gastric mucosa, choroid plexus, ciliary body of the eye, and lactating mammary gland, also can actively transport iodide, albeit at a much lower level than the thyroid can (Lacroix et al. 2001). In the salivary glands, the NIS protein has been detected in ductal cells but not in acinar cells. Only the thyroid follicular cells accumulate iodide in a TSH-dependent manner.

The NIS gene is complex (15 exons and 14 introns), and its expression in the thyroid is upregulated by TSH. The functionally active iodine-transport system in the thyroid gland has important pathophysiological applications in the evaluation, diagnosis, and treatment of several thyroid disorders, including cancer. The NIS and active transport of iodide can be selectively inhibited by competitive anion inhibitors (e.g., perchlorate

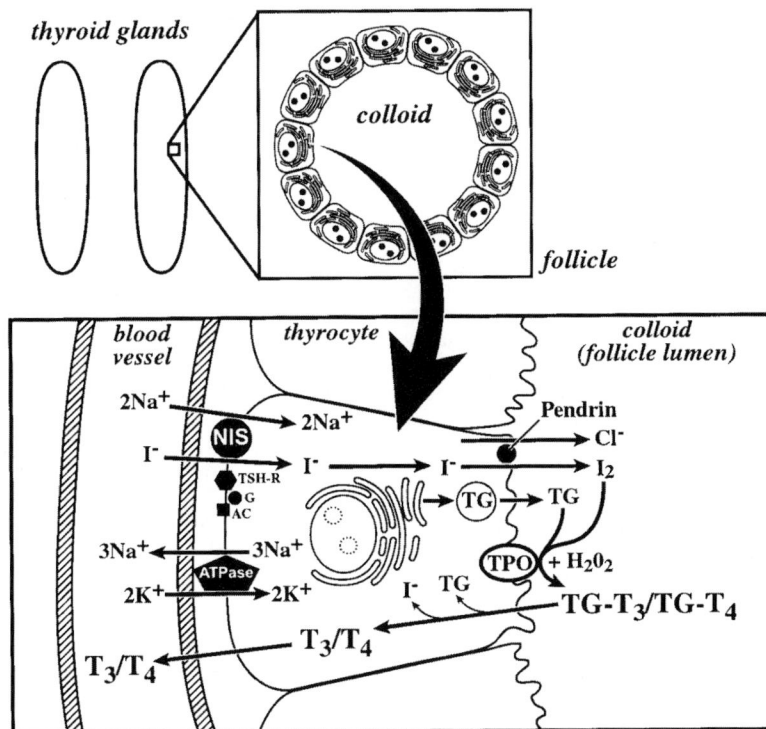

FIG. 12.38—The sodium-iodide (Na⁺-I⁻) symporter (NIS) and thyroid hormone biosynthesis. The NIS located in the basolateral membrane of thyroid follicular cells is responsible for the rapid uptake and concentration of iodide ion (I⁻) from the circulation. The enzyme thyroperoxidase (TPO) in microvilli on the lumenal surface oxidizes I⁻ in the presence of hydrogen peroxide (H_2O_2) to reactive iodine (I_2) that subsequently binds to tyrosyl residues in the thyroglobulin (TG) molecule of the colloid. Pendrin is a Cl⁻/I⁻ transport protein on the apical surface of thyrocytes. AC, adenylate cyclase; CD, colloid droplet; Cl⁻, chloride ion; G, G protein; I⁻, iodide ion; R, receptor; T_3, triiodothyronine; T_4, tetraiodothyronine (thyroxine); and TSH, thyroid-stimulating hormone. (From La Perle et al. 2003.)

or thiocyanate), thereby effectively blocking the ability of the gland to iodinate tyrosine residues in thyroglobulin and synthesize thyroid hormones.

The ability of the NIS to concentrate iodide holds clinical relevance, in addition to its physiological importance, by providing the basis for using radioactive iodine in the treatment and management of various thyroid diseases. Radioactive iodine is commonly used to destroy hyperactive thyrocytes in patients with thyrotoxicosis, to ablate normal and malignant thyroid tissues in patients who have undergone total thyroidectomy for thyroid carcinoma, and to perform whole-body scans for the detection of recurrent and metastatic thyroid cancer.

Iodide ion once within the thyrocyte is passively transported via pendrin into the follicular lumen (Royaux et al. 2000; Kohn et al. 2001). Pendrin is a ca. 86-kD chloride/iodide transport protein that is located at the apical membrane of thyrocytes and is responsible for the transport of iodide ion into the follicular lumen (Figure 12.38) (Scott et al. 1999). It is the product of the gene responsible for Pendred syndrome, a genetic disorder in human patients characterized clinically by sensorineural hearing loss and goiter (Everett et al. 1999, 2001; Kopp 1999; Bidart et al. 2000a, b). Pendrin is characterized by 11 or 12 putative transmembrane domains and is closely related to a family of sulfate-transport proteins; however, pendrin does not transport sulfate and, unlike the NIS, does not require sodium for its transport of iodide.

Thyroid Hormone Secretion. The secretion of thyroid hormones from stores within luminal colloid is initiated by elongation of microvilli on follicular cells and formation of pseudopodia. These elongated cytoplasmic projections are increased by pituitary TSH, extend into the follicular lumen, and indiscriminatingly phagocytose a portion of adjacent colloid (Figure 12.37). Colloid droplets within follicular cells subsequently fuse with numerous lysosomal bodies that contain proteolytic enzymes (Wollman et al. 1964). T_3 and T_4 are released from the thyroglobulin molecule and, because of their hydrophobic nature, diffuse out of follicular cells into the adjacent capillaries. The biologically inactive iodotyrosines (MIT and DIT) simultaneously released from the colloid droplets are deiodinated enzymatically, and the iodide generated is either recycled to the follicular lumen to iodinate new tyrosyl residues or released into the circulation under normal conditions. Thyroxine is rapidly bound in plasma to albumin and several globulin fractions [especially high-affinity thyroxine-binding globulin (TBG)] produced by the liver, and triiodothyronine is bound to albumin (transthyretin) and one globulin fraction in dogs.

Negative-feedback control of thyroid hormone secretion is accomplished by the coordinated response of the adenohypophysis and specific hypothalamic nuclei to circulating levels of thyroid hormones (especially T_3). A decrease in thyroid hormone concentration

in plasma is sensed by groups of neurosecretory neurons in the hypothalamus that synthesize and secrete a small peptide (3 amino acids), thyrotropin-releasing hormone (TRH), into the hypophyseal portal circulation. TSH or thyrotropin (TTH or thyrotropic hormone) is conveyed to thyroid follicular cells, where it binds to the basilar aspect of the cell, activates adenyl cyclase, and increases the rate of biochemical reactions involved with the synthesis and secretion of thyroid hormones (Figure 12.39).

One of the initial responses by follicular cells to TSH is the formation of numerous cytoplasmic pseudopodia, resulting in increased endocytosis of colloid and release of preformed thyroid hormones stored within the follicular lumen (Collins and Capen 1980b). If the secretion of TSH is sustained (for hours or days), thyroid follicular cells become more columnar, and follicular lumina become smaller due to increased endocyto-

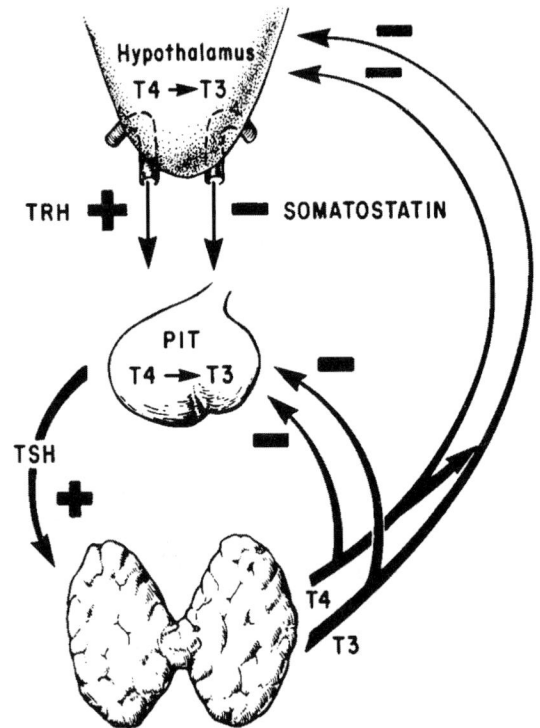

FIG. 12.39—Hypothalamic-pituitary-thyroid axis. Thyroid-stimulating hormone (TSH) from the pituitary stimulates the secretion of both tetraiodothyronine (T_4) and triiodothyronine (T_3). These act at the pituitary (PIT) level to control secretion of TSH by a negative-feedback mechanism. In addition, T_4 is converted to T_3 within the pituitary by a monodeiodinase. TSH secretion is stimulated by thyrotropin-releasing hormone (TRH) from the hypothalamus and inhibited by somatostatin and, to a lesser extent, by dopamine. Thyroid hormones act at the hypothalamus to stimulate the secretion of somatostatin. T_4 also is deiodinated to T_3 within the hypothalamus, and this conversion may play a role in feedback regulation. (From Reichlin 1998.)

sis of colloid. Numerous PAS-positive colloid droplets are present in the luminal aspect of the hypertrophied follicular cells. The converse of what has been just described occurs in response to an increase in circulating thyroid hormones and a corresponding decrease in circulating pituitary TSH. Thyroid follicles become enlarged and distended with colloid due to decreased TSH-mediated endocytosis of colloid. Follicular cells lining the involuted follicles are cuboidal and there are few endocytotic vacuoles at the interface between the colloid and follicular cells.

There are differences in thyroid morphology and function between canine breeds of European origin and the basenji, which originated in Africa (Nunez et al. 1970). At the same level of iodine intake, thyroidal turnover of iodine is two to three times faster in the basenji than in European breeds. The corresponding differences in thyroid morphology in the basenji include smaller follicles, more widespread and uniform vacuolation of the colloid, more columnar follicular epithelium, and ultrastructural features of follicular cells that more closely resemble those of the TSH-stimulated thyroid in European breeds, such as the beagle (Nunez et al. 1972).

Biological Effects of Thyroid Hormones. T_4 and T_3 once released into the circulation act on many different target cells in the body. The overall functions of the hormones are similar though much of the biological activity is the result of monodeiodination by 5′-deiodinase to 3,5,3′-triiodothyronine (active T_3) prior to interacting with target cells. Under certain conditions (protein starvation, neonatal animals, liver and kidney disease, febrile illness, etc.) or exposure to xenobiotic chemicals, thyroxine is preferentially monodeiodinated by 5′-deiodinase to 3,3′,5′-triiodothyronine (*reverse*

T3) (Figure 12.40) (Laurberg 1978). Since this form of T_3 is biologically inactive, monodeiodination to form reverse T_3 provides a mechanism to attenuate the metabolic effects of thyroid hormones in peripheral tissues.

The overall physiological effects of thyroid hormones are to increase the basal metabolic rate; make more glucose available to meet the elevated metabolic demands by increasing glycolysis, gluconeogenesis, and glucose absorption from the intestine; stimulate new protein synthesis; increase lipid metabolism and conversion of cholesterol into bile acids and other substances; activate lipoprotein lipase and increase sensitivity of adipose tissue to lipolysis by other hormones; stimulate the heart rate, cardiac output, and blood flow; and increase neural transmission, cerebration, and neuronal development in young animals (Lima et al. 2001).

The subcellular mechanism of action of thyroid hormones resembles that for steroid hormones in that free hormone enters target cells and binds loosely to cytosol-binding proteins (Figure 12.41). Free triiodothyronine initially binds to receptors on the inner mitochondrial membrane to activate mitochondrial energy metabolism and subsequently binds to high-affinity nuclear receptors and increases transcription of the genetic message (mRNA) to facilitate new protein synthesis (e.g., structural, enzymatic, and binding proteins) (Oppenheimer 1979).

Thyroid hormone functions in target cells are mediated by three nuclear receptors—T_3R α_1, T_3R β_1, and T_3R β_2—that are encoded by two genes—T_3R α and T_3R β. Thyroid hormones are essential for numerous postnatal developmental processes, including growth and neurogenesis. The T_3R α gene is widely expressed from early development, whereas the T_3R β gene is highly restricted and expressed later in development (Fraichard et al. 1997). Mice with targeted disruption of the T_3R α

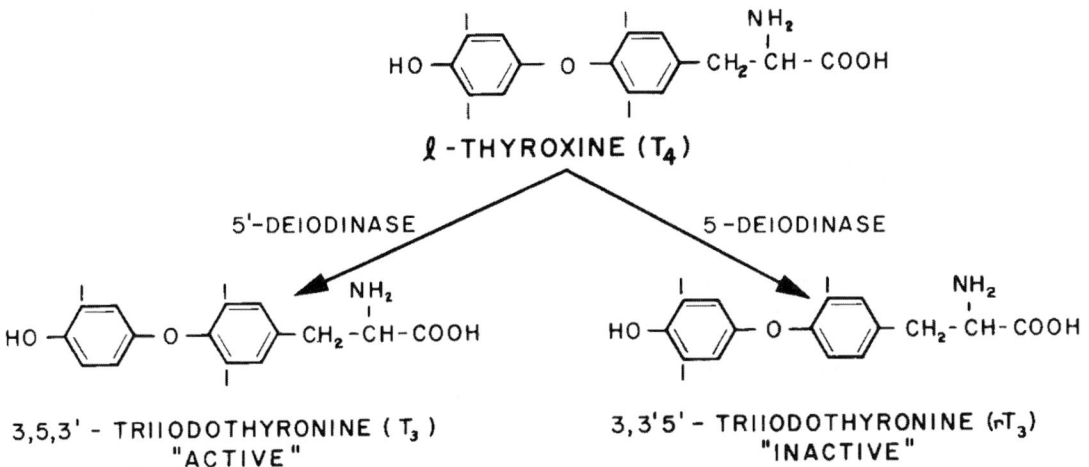

FIG. 12.40—Monodeiodination of thyroxine to form either active triiodothyronine T_3 (**left**) or inactive (reverse) rT_3 (**right**), depending upon the need for the metabolic actions of thyroid hormone. (From Capen and Martin 1989.)

THYROID HORMONE-RESPONSIVE CELL

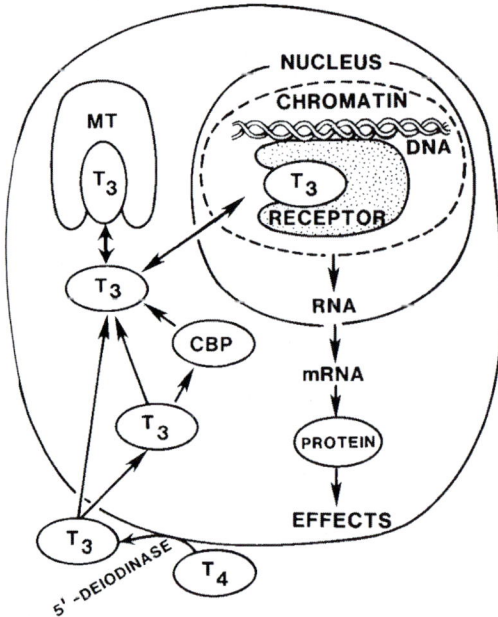

FIG. 12.41—Subcellular mechanism of action of thyroid hormones in target cells. Free triiodothyronine (T_3) primarily enters target cells because most of the tetraiodothyronine (T_4) undergoes monodeiodination in the liver or elsewhere in the periphery to form T_3. Free T_3 in the cell binds either to cytosolic binding proteins (CBPs) to high-affinity receptors on the inner mitochondrial (MT) membrane and activates oxidative phosphorylation, or to nuclear receptors in target cells. In the nucleus, T_3 increases transcription of messenger RNA, which returns to the cytoplasm to direct the synthesis of new proteins. The increased synthesis of new proteins (structural or enzyme) carries out the multiple biological effects of the thyroid hormones.

gene have markedly reduced production of both T_4 and T_3 associated with growth arrest and delayed development of bones and small intestine. By comparison, mice with targeted disruption of the T_3R β gene have an overproduction of thyroid hormones and impairment of auditory function but no developmental defects.

HYPERTHYROIDISM ASSOCIATED WITH FUNCTIONAL THYROID TUMORS. There has been a dramatic increase in the incidence of thyroid neoplasms and other focal proliferative lesions in cats resulting in hyperthyroidism since the late 1970s, and at present it is one of the two most common endocrine diseases in adult-age cats (diabetes mellitus being the other). Prior to 1980, clinical hyperthyroidism was diagnosed infrequently in cats (Holzworth et al. 1980). The reason(s) for the apparent increased incidence is (are) uncertain but appears to be related, in part, to (a) a larger

population of older cats seeking veterinary medical care since 1980, (b) improved assays for thyroid hormones, and (c) detailed characterization of the clinical syndrome and increased awareness of its common occurrence in adult to aged cats by veterinary medical clinicians (Scarlett 1994). In addition, there does appear to be a real increase in the incidence of feline hyperthyroidism over the last 30 years. Potential risk factors have been reported to include a predominantly indoor environment, regular treatment with flea powders, exposures to herbicides and fertilizers, a diet primarily of canned food, and non-Siamese breeds (10-fold greater occurrence). It has been suggested that wide variations (excessive to inadequate) in dietary iodine intake over prolonged periods may play a role in the pathogenesis of thyroid disorders in cats (Johnson et al. 1992).

Pathogenic Mechanisms. The disease in cats is mechanistically different from the clinically important Grave's disease in human patients because hyperthyroid cats do not have elevated circulating levels of thyroid-stimulating immunoglobulins comparable to long-acting thyroid stimulator (LATS) (an autoantibody that binds to the TSH receptor and activates follicular cells). Purified immunoglobulin G (IgG) preparations from hyperthyroid cats significantly increased [³H]thymidine into DNA and stimulated cell proliferation 15-fold but did not stimulate intracellular cAMP. The former could be inhibited completely by a specific TSH receptor-blocking antibody. These data suggest that elevated titers of thyroid-growth IgGs are present in cats with hyperthyroidism and most likely act by the TSH receptor. This important thyroid disease in cats most closely resembles toxic nodular goiter in human patients (Hoenig et al. 1982; Gerber et al. 1994). Hyperplastic and neoplastic thyroid tissue from cats is transplantable into athymic (nude) mice and continues to over produce T_4 and T_3 in a subcuticular location.

Studies using primary cultures of enzymatically dissociated follicles from thyroid proliferative lesions from cats with hyperthyroidism have reported that organification and [³H]thymidine labeling continue in the absence of TSH, in contrast to follicles from normal cat thyroids (Peter et al. 1991). These findings suggest that an intrinsic alteration in follicular cell function occurs in thyroids of cats with multinodular goiter leading to autonomy of cell growth and persistent overproduction of thyroid hormones (Tognella et al. 1999). A recent study reported an overexpression of the c-ras oncogene in areas of nodular hyperplasia and adenomas derived from follicular cells in cats with hyperthyroidism, suggesting that mutations in this oncogene may play a role in the pathogenesis of these proliferative lesions (Merryman et al. 1999).

Point mutations in the thyrotropin receptor (TSHR) gene cause two forms of thyrotoxicosis in humans: autonomously functioning toxic follicular adenomas and hereditary (autosomal dominant) toxic thyroid hyperplasia (Derwahl et al. 1998). The normal feline TSHR sequence between codons 480 and 640 is highly homologous to that of other mammalian TSHRs, with 95%, 92%, and 90% amino acid identity between the feline, canine, human, and bovine TSHRs, respectively. Analysis of single-stranded conformational polymorphisms in thyroid DNA from sporadic cases of feline thyrotoxicosis and leukocyte DNA from two cases of familial hyperthyroidism in cats failed to identify mutations between codons 480 and 640 of the *TSHR* gene (Pearce et al. 1997). These interesting findings suggest that *TSHR* gene mutations are not a common cause of the focal proliferative lesions of thyroid follicular cells that result in feline thyrotoxicosis.

The syndrome of hyperthyroidism in adult to aged cats can be associated either with multinodular (*adenomatous*) hyperplasia, adenomas, or adenocarcinomas derived from follicular cells. Follicular cell adenomas, often developing in a thyroid with multinodular hyperplasia, are encountered more commonly than thyroid carcinomas. Adenomas and carcinomas are most likely to be encountered in aged cats, whereas nodular hyperplasia can occur at any age. The mean age of cats with benign tumors has been reported to be 12.4 years and the mean age of cats with thyroid carcinomas as 15.8 years.

Thyroid adenomas in cats usually appear as solitary, soft, often lobulated nodules that enlarge and distort the contour of the affected lobe. Functional follicular adenomas often develop in thyroids that have multinodular hyperplasia of follicular cells in both lobes. A thin, partial fibrous capsule separates the adenoma from the adjacent, often compressed, thyroid parenchyma. Follicles in the surrounding rim of suppressed thyroid are markedly enlarged and distended by an accumulation of colloid, a lesion referred to as colloid *involution*. The follicular cells are low cuboidal and atrophied, with little evidence of endocytotic activity in response to the elevated levels of thyroid hormones produced by the adenoma, resulting in suppressed levels of TSH. Focal areas of necrosis, mineralization, and cystic degeneration are present in larger adenomas. Functional thyroid adenomas are composed of cuboidal to columnar follicular cells with occasional papillary infoldings that form follicles containing variable amounts of colloid. The follicles usually are partially collapsed and contain little colloid, due to the intense uncontrolled endocytotic activity of neoplastic follicular cells. Long cytoplasmic projections extend from the follicular cells into the lumen to phagocytose colloid.

Functional Disturbances and Evaluation of Thyroid Function. The most common clinical sign is weight loss despite a normal or increased appetite. Polydipsia and polyuria, increased frequency of defecation, increased volume of stools, and increased activity occur. A common functional disturbance is tachycardia accompanied by premature beats and/or a systolic murmur. Cardiomegaly due to left-ventricular hypertrophy may be evident on radiographs or at necropsy.

Cats with hyperthyroidism usually have markedly elevated serum thyroxine and triiodothyronine levels. Normal feline serum levels of T_4 measured by RIA are about 1.5 to 5.0 µg/dL, and serum T_3 levels are 60 to 200 ng/dL. The serum T_4 levels in cats with hyperthyroidism range from 5.0 to >50 µg/dL, and serum T_3 levels range from 100 to 1000 ng/dL (Figure 12.42) (Peterson et al. 1983). Moderately increased liver-derived serum enzyme levels, including aspartate transaminase (AST), alanine aminotransferase (ALT), serum glutamate-pyruvate transaminase (SGPT), serum glutamic-oxaloacetic transaminase (SGOT), and especially alkaline phosphatase, occur in hyperthyroid cats.

The likelihood of developing clinical hyperthyroidism associated with thyroid neoplasms in animals depends on (a) the capability of tumor cells to synthesize T_4 and T_3 (e.g., well-differentiated thyroid tumors that form follicles and produce colloid are more likely to synthesize thyroid hormones than are poorly differentiated solid neoplasms), and (b) the degree of elevation of circulating levels of T_4 and T_3, which depends on a balance between the rate of secretion of thyroid hormones by the tumor and the rate of degradation of thyroid hormones. For example, dogs have a much more efficient enterohepatic excretory mechanism for

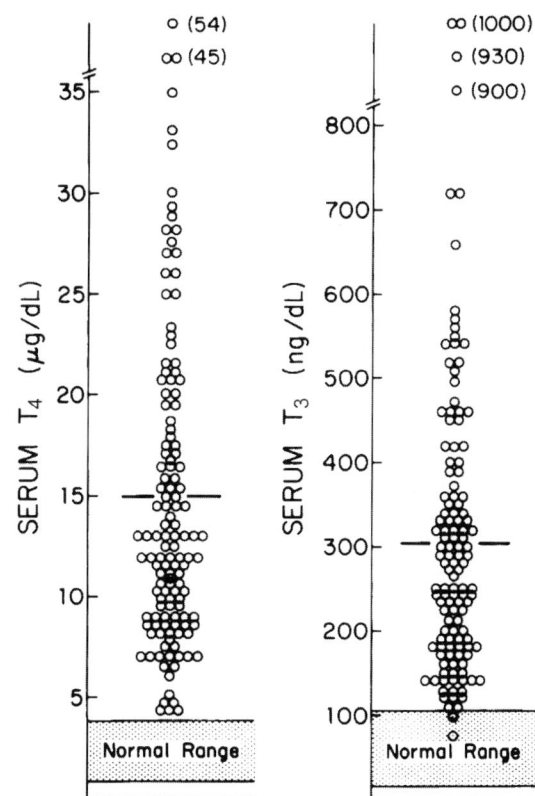

FIG. 12.42—Serum thyroid hormone levels in cats with hyperthyroidism. There is a marked elevation of serum thyroxine (mean, 15 µg/dL) and triiodothyronine (mean, 300 µg/dL) in cats with hyperthyroidism. (From Peterson et al. 1988.)

thyroid hormones than do cats and infrequently have pathophysiological changes associated with functional thyroid tumors. Cats are very sensitive to phenol and its derivatives and have a poor capability to conjugate phenolic compounds (such as T_4) with glucuronic acid and excrete the T_4-glucuronide into the bile (Jernigan 1989). The capacity of conjugation of T_3 with sulfate is limited and easily overloaded. Therefore, cats with relatively small functional proliferative lesions of thyroid follicular cells often have marked elevations in circulating levels of T_4 and T_3 with clinical signs of hyperthyroidism, whereas dogs with functional thyroid tumors have only slight elevations in serum T_4 and T_3 and less frequently develop clinical hyperthyroidism (Rijnberk and Der Kinderen 1969).

A small percentage of hyperthyroid cats when first evaluated have T_4 concentrations within the upper limits of the reference range. This most likely is due to early detection of the disease attributable to clinician awareness and readily available screening tests. Hyperthyroidism usually can be confirmed in these cats by repeating the thyroid hormone assays or performing a T_3-suppression test. In addition, a wide variety of nonthyroidal illnesses (kidney or liver diseases, diabetes mellitus, and protein malnutrition, among others) in hyperthyroid cats also may suppress the serum T_4 concentration into the normal range (Peterson and Gamble 1990).

Disturbances of Calcium Homeostasis. Hyperthyroid cats often have disturbances in calcium homeostasis and diffuse chief cell hyperplasia in the parathyroid glands (Barber and Elliott 1996). Blood ionized (not total) calcium and plasma creatinine concentrations often are significantly decreased and plasma phosphate and intact parathyroid hormone levels are increased compared with reference ranges. Hyperparathyroidism occurred in 77% of hyperthyroid cats with PTH levels elevated up to 19 times the upper limit of the reference range. Hyperphosphatemia was present in approximately 40% of hyperthyroid cats. The mechanisms for the development of hyperphosphatemia in feline hyperthyroidism are uncertain, but it appears to be related, in part, to polyphagia with increased intestinal phosphate absorption, increased catabolism of muscle proteins, and release of phosphate, due to the gluconeogenic effects of the elevated thyroid hormone levels and increased bone resorption with release of phosphate into the blood. The hyperparathyroidism and chief cell hyperplasia appear to be related to the reciprocal decline in circulating levels of ionized calcium in response to the hyperphosphatemia. An elevated blood phosphate also could inhibit the renal 1α-hydroxylase and decrease the production of the active form of vitamin D, thereby reducing intestinal calcium absorption; however, circulating levels of 1,25-$(OH)_2$-dihydroxycholecalciferol were not decreased in the limited number of hyperthyroid cats evaluated.

Serum levels of alkaline phosphatase (bone isozyme) are elevated consistently in cats with hyperthyroidism; however, there is no correlation between the magnitude of increase in alkaline-phosphatase, osteocalcin, and serum T_4 concentrations (Archer and Taylor 1996). Although the total calcium usually is in the reference range, the serum ionized calcium often (approximately 50% of cases) is reduced. These findings suggest that hyperthyroid cats have altered bone metabolism; however, the bone disease usually is not clinically significant in adult to aged cats with hyperthyroidism.

Therapeutic Approaches. Either surgical excision of affected thyroid lobe(s), medical management by thyroid-blocking drugs (e.g., methimazole and propylthiouracil), or radioactive iodine are effective treatments available for cats with hyperthyroidism. Bilateral thyroidectomy is necessary if both glands are abnormal in appearance at surgery. At least one parathyroid gland should be left with an intact blood supply if bilateral thyroidectomy is performed. A thyroid-blocking agent, such as methimazole or propylthiouracil, can be used before surgery to alleviate some of the severe clinical effects (e.g., tachycardia and cardiomegaly) of hyperthyroidism.

HYPOFUNCTION OF THE THYROID GLAND.
Hypothyroidism of adult onset is a well-recognized clinical disease in dogs but is encountered only occasionally in other animals. Although hypothyroidism may occur in many adult purebred and mixed-breed dogs, certain breeds (golden retrievers, Doberman pinschers, dachshunds, Shetland sheep dogs, Irish setters, miniature schnauzers, cocker spaniels, and Airedales) have been reported to be more commonly affected (Milne and Hayes 1981). Hypothyroidism in dogs usually is the result of primary lesions in the thyroid gland, particularly lymphocytic thyroiditis and idiopathic follicular collapse. Less common causes of hypothyroidism in dogs are bilateral nonfunctional thyroid tumors or severe iodine-deficient hyperplastic goiter. Hypothyroidism associated with long-standing pituitary or hypothalamic lesions that prevent the release of either TSH (secondary) or TRH (tertiary) is much less common in dogs. The thyroid gland in secondary hypothyroidism is moderately reduced in size and composed of colloid-distended *involuted* follicles lined by flattened follicular cells.

Pathogenic Mechanisms. In idiopathic follicular atrophy (*collapse*), there is a progressive loss of follicular epithelium and replacement by adipose tissue with a minimal inflammatory response. The gland usually is smaller and lighter in color than normal. The early lesion of follicular atrophy that is seen in dogs with mild clinical signs of hypothyroidism appears to be confined to one part of the thyroid. The affected part of the thyroid gland contains small follicles lined by tall columnar follicular cells, often with little colloid. Immediately adjacent thyroid follicles are normal. The earliest lesion of idiopathic follicular atrophy is degeneration of individual follicular cells lining thyroid follicles. Individual or small groups of degenerate follicular cells with eosinophilic cytoplasm and pyknotic nuclei are present in the follicular wall, colloid, and interstitium.

A more advanced form of follicular atrophy is seen in dogs with clinical hypothyroidism and low circulating concentrations of thyroid hormones. The thyroid gland is composed predominantly of adipose tissue with only occasional clusters of small follicles containing vacuolated colloid. When the thyroid is reduced markedly in size, it consists primarily of small follicles and individual follicular cells with PAS-positive colloid in a microfollicle in the cytoplasm. The advanced stage of follicular atrophy is characterized by a lack of normal thyroid follicles and the presence of microfollicles in the cytoplasm of individual follicular cells. The remaining hypertrophic follicular cells form small nests and are arranged closely along capillaries. The microfollicles appear to form by invagination of the apical surface of the follicular cells. Long microvilli extend into the colloid, and membrane-limited colloid droplets are present in the cytoplasm near the microfollicle, suggesting increased endocytotic activity. Small foci of lymphocytes and plasma cells may be associated with disruption of thyroid follicles and release of colloid. The mild increase in connective tissue in the interstitium appears to be the result of condensation of the normal stroma. Focal aggregations of C cells appear relatively more prominent due to progressive loss of follicular cells.

Idiopathic follicular atrophy (collapse) appears to be a primary degenerative disease of the thyroid and differs distinctly from the trophic atrophy of follicular cells secondary to diminished secretion of TSH. Under the latter conditions, thyroid follicles undergo involution, are lined by a low cuboidal epithelium, and distended by uniformly dense PAS-positive colloid with little evidence of endocytosis. Hypertrophy and hyperplasia of thyrotrophic basophils occur in the pars distalis of dogs with idiopathic follicular collapse and hypothyroidism.

Lymphocytic thyroiditis in dogs (Gosselin et al. 1982; Benjamin et al. 1996), an obese strain of chickens, nonhuman primates, and Buffalo rats closely resembles Hashimoto's disease in humans (Bigazzi and Rose 1975). Though the exact mechanism in dogs is not well established, evidence suggests a polygenic pattern of inheritance similar to that observed in the human disease (Mizejewski et al. 1971). The immunologic basis for the development of chronic lymphocytic thyroiditis in both people and dogs appears to be through production of autoantibodies directed against either thyroglobulin, thyroperoxidase (a microsomal antigen), or the TSH receptor (Foti and Rapoport 1990). Thyroglobulin autoantibodies have been found in a high percent of dogs with hypothyroidism and may be related to the development of the thyroiditis (Gosselin et al. 1980, 1981). Laboratory beagles with spontaneous lymphocytic thyroiditis also have circulating thyroid autoantibodies, but the focal thyroiditis usually is not associated with clinical hypothyroidism. Thy-

roiditis in laboratory beagles is similar serologically to human thyroiditis in that antibodies are present against thyroglobulin and thyroperoxidase; however, there is not a positive correlation between the occurrence or magnitude of the thyroglobulin antibody titers and the occurrence or severity of thyroiditis.

Thyroid glands of dogs with lymphocytic thyroiditis may be slightly enlarged and tan-white, normal, or reduced in size. Histological alterations consist of multifocal to diffuse infiltrates of lymphocytes, plasma cells, and macrophages. Lymphoid nodules are present occasionally between follicles. The remaining follicles are small and lined by columnar epithelial cells. Lymphocytes, macrophages, and degenerate follicular cells often are present in the vacuolated colloid. Either the basement membrane around thyroid follicles is thick or discrete electron-dense deposits are present between the follicular cells and the basement membrane. These electron-dense deposits are similar to those reported to represent immune complexes in people with Hashimoto's thyroiditis (Matsuta 1982). Thyroid C (parafollicular) cells are seen in small nests or nodules between follicles and often are relatively more prominent than in normal dogs. The thyroid lesion of lymphocytic thyroiditis progresses to replacement of the thyroid gland by mature fibrous connective tissue with only a few remaining scattered foci of inflammatory cells. Thyroid follicles are small and widely separated in the end stage of thyroiditis and contain only a small amount of vacuolated colloid. There is a marked increase in collagen fibers surrounding small follicles or groups of follicular cells (Benjamin et al. 1997).

Functional Disturbances. Many functional disturbances associated with hypothyroidism are due to a reduction in basal metabolic rate. A gain in body weight without an associated change in appetite occurs in some hypothyroid dogs (Nesbitt et al. 1980). The weight gain varies from slight to striking, and hypothyroid dogs usually are less active than normal. Lesions in the skin and in the hair coat occur in the majority of hypothyroid dogs. Thyroxine stimulates the anagen or active phase of hair growth, whereas a reduction in blood levels of thyroid hormones favors the telogen or resting phase. Telogen hairs are more easily dislodged from the hair follicles, resulting in thinning of the hair coat and often a bilaterally symmetrical alopecia. Areas affected initially by hair loss are those receiving frictional wear, such as the tail and cervical area. The tail may become almost completely bare in dogs with long-standing hypothyroidism.

Hyperkeratosis is a consistent finding in hypothyroidism and results in an increased scaliness of the skin. It may become severe and occur in circular scaling patches resulting in skin lesions suggestive of seborrhea. Microscopic examination consistently reveals marked hyperkeratosis that includes the external root sheath. The excessive keratin formation and accumulation within hair follicles often result in follicular keratosis that may cause a clinically observable distension of follicles. Hyperpigmentation occurs in many dogs with hypothyroidism, especially in localized areas of alopecia, such as the dorsal aspect of the nose and distal portion of the tail. Increased numbers of melanocytes are present in the basal layer of the epidermis. Changes in the thickness of the epidermis are variable in dogs with hypothyroidism. Epidermal atrophy is reported in about 50% of hypothyroid dogs, normal thickness in about 20%, and a mild to moderate epidermal thickening due to a prominent stratum granulosum with an atrophic stratum spinosum in the remaining 30%.

Myxedema may develop and produce a characteristic clinical appearance in long-standing or severe hypothyroidism. There is accumulation of mucin (neutral and acid glycosaminoglycans combined with protein) in the dermis and subcutis. This material binds considerable amounts of water and produces marked thickening of the skin. This is most obvious around the face and head, where accentuation of the normal skin folds causes a "tragic" appearance. The eyelids appear thick and drooping, thus contributing to the sad facial expression. The skin feels thick and doughy, but the characteristic pitting observed with other types of edema does not occur with myxedema. Mucin appears as a blue-purple, granular or fibrillar material that disrupts the normal collagen and elastin fibers on a skin biopsy.

Abnormalities in reproduction are common in hypothyroidism. Lack of libido and reduction in sperm count may occur in males, whereas abnormal or absent estrous cycles with reduced conception rates may result in females. The spermatogenic epithelium in the testis often is markedly atrophic in long-standing cases of hypothyroidism. Impaired joint function with evidence of pain and joint effusion also can result from severe or prolonged hypothyroidism.

The elevated serum cholesterol is responsible for many of the extrathyroidal lesions of hypothyroidism. The marked hypercholesterolemia with long-standing and severe hypothyroidism results in a variety of secondary lesions, including atherosclerosis, hepatomegaly and renal glomerular and corneal lipidosis. The decreased rate of lipid metabolism with diminished intestinal excretion of cholesterol and conversion of lipids into bile acids and other compounds in hypothyroidism results in the hypercholesterolemia. Atherosclerosis of coronary, cerebral, and other vessels may develop in dogs with severe hypothyroidism and long-standing hyperlipidemia. This occasionally results in hemorrhage and ischemic necrosis of the myocardium due to impingement of the vessel lumina by numerous lipid-laden macrophages in the tunica media and adventitia. In dogs with markedly elevated plasma lipids, renal glomeruli may become plugged with lipid, resulting in progressive renal failure. The lipid-filled glomeruli can be seen macroscopically as small yellow-white foci throughout the kidney cortex. The accumulation of excessive lipid in the liver often results in varying degrees of hepatomegaly with abdominal distension and hepatic failure. Corneal lipidosis is observed occasionally in hypothyroid dogs with hypercholesterolemia. This lesion often is unilateral because the lipid is deposited in corneas that have been previously injured and have a network of "ghost" vessels from which the lipid diffuses into the connective tissue stroma.

Evaluation of Thyroid Function. Serum cholesterol concentration is an indirect and valuable index of the peripheral action of thyroid hormone. Two-thirds of dogs with spontaneous hypothyroidism have a fasting serum cholesterol concentration above 300 mg/100 mL. However, hypercholesterolemia is as dependent on the composition of the dog's diet as on the severity and duration of hypothyroidism. Cholesterol values tend to be higher in the general population of pet dogs fed table scraps or home diets than in dogs maintained exclusively on commercially manufactured dry dog foods (e.g., housed under laboratory conditions) (Schiller et al. 1964). Hypercholesterolemia also occurs in some dogs with cortisol excess, a disease that must be considered in the differential diagnosis of hypothyroidism. Therefore, the measurement of serum cholesterol is not a specific or dependable test of thyroid function, but fasting cholesterol values greater than 600 mg/100 mL, which are often observed in hypothyroidism, infrequently occur in any other disease of dogs.

A moderate normocytic normochromic anemia often is associated with subnormal function of the thyroid in dogs. This anemia also has been observed in people as well as in experimental animals and is of a nonregenerative type. The stained blood smear characteristically has little or no evidence of active erythrogenesis, such as anisocytosis, polychromasia, or nucleated red cells. Leptocytosis may be especially prominent.

The most sensitive and accurate method for evaluation of thyroid function is measurement of total blood T_4 and T_3 levels by RIA. The normal blood level of T_4 for dogs is 1.5 to 3.6 µg/dL (mean, 2.48 µg/dL), and for T_3 it is 48 to 154 ng/dL (mean, 95 ng/dL). In dogs with primary hypothyroidism, the T_4 level usually is less than 1.0 µg/dL, and the T_3 is less than 50 ng/dL. When levels are borderline, clearer separation of dogs with hypothyroidism from euthyroid dogs can be made by injecting TSH (Sauvé and Paradis 2000). In euthyroid dogs, the T_4 level will at least double by 8 hours after intravenous or intramuscular administration of TSH. In dogs with primary hypothyroidism, T_4 and T_3 levels do not change significantly after injection of TSH. Plasma T_4 levels are no more than 0.2 µg/dL above control values at 8 hours after TSH administration, and plasma T_3 is increased by no more than 10 ng/dL after TSH administration. The increase in serum T_3 after TSH is more variable in normal dogs than for T_4, but in dogs with primary hypothyroidism there usually is little (10 ng/mL or less) change in serum T_3 at 8 hours after TSH administration (Figure 12.43).

Free thyroxine can be measured by equilibrium dialysis with tracer. Other methods of measuring free T_4 are technically less difficult but are much less accurate. The serum free T_4 in normal dogs ranges from 0.2 to

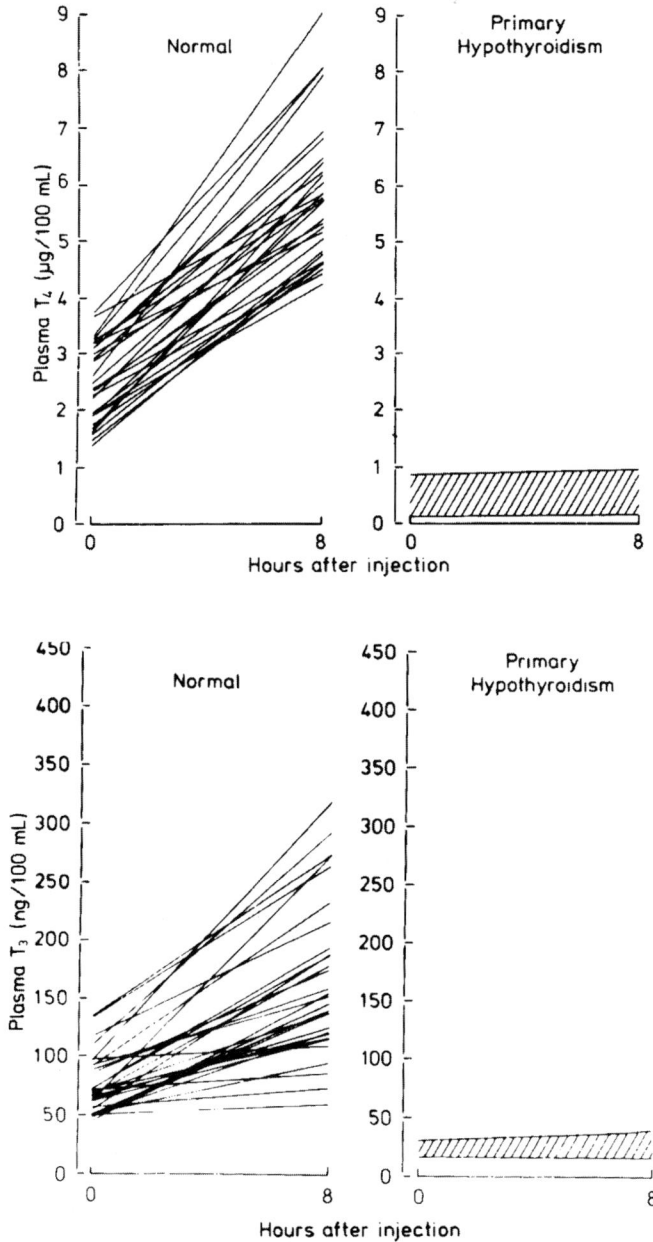

FIG. 12.43—Plasma tetraiodothyronine (T_4) **(top)** responses to thyroid-stimulating hormone (TSH) stimulation in 30 normal dogs and 28 dogs with primary hypothyroidism determined by radioimmunoassay. Only the highest and lowest response lines are shown for the hypothyroid dogs. Plasma triiodothyronine (T_3) **(bottom)** responses to TSH stimulation in 30 normal dogs and 28 dogs with primary hypothyroidism determined by radioimmunoassay. Only the highest and lowest response lines are shown for the hypothyroid dogs. (From Belshaw and Rijnberk 1979.)

1.0 µg/dL. The advantages of measuring free T_4 over total T_4 include (a) higher correlation with thyroid secretory function, (b) less overlap of hypothyroid and euthyroid levels, and (c) slower decrease with nonthyroidal illness.

In the evaluation of clinically important thyroid disease problems, an accurate quantitation of circulating levels of TSH or thyrotropin is important in the critical assessment of thyroid hormone economy (Ramsey et al. 1997; Kooistra et al. 2000). TSH is the major regulator of the synthetic and secretory processes of thyroid follicular cells. However, the immunoassay for TSH is highly species specific, with considerable interanimal and interassay variations. TSH is a glycoprotein synthesized by thyrotrophic basophils in the adenohypophysis and is composed of α and β subunits. The α subunit is similar to that of several pituitary hormones of the same family, but the β subunit is specific for TSH. The hormone circulates primarily in the free (unbound) form and has a short (ca. 15-minute) plasma half-life. Serum plasma samples for TSH assay should be collected in the morning before noon to minimize the effects of diurnal variation on hormone levels. A serum TSH procedure has been recently introduced to measure canine TSH and is available either as an immunoradiometric, luminescence, or enzyme-linked immunosorbent assay (ELISA). The β subunit of canine TSH has an 89% homology with the human subunit, and circulating TSH levels in dogs are 10- to 20-fold lower than those in people. Although the first-generation canine TSH assay is considerably less sensitive than the rat and human TSH assays, in dogs with primary hypothyroidism an increased TSH level has been demonstrated that returned to normal 24 hours after once daily T_4 therapy. A peak increase in serum TSH occurred at 30 minutes after injection of TRH and subsequently rapidly returned to baseline values.

PATHOPHYSIOLOGY OF GOITER. Nonneoplastic and noninflammatory clinical enlargements (*goiter*) of the thyroid develop in all domestic mammals, birds, and submammalian vertebrates. The major pathogenetic mechanisms responsible for the development of thyroid hyperplasia include iodine-deficient diets, goitrogenic compounds that interfere with thyroid hormone synthesis, dietary iodide excess, and genetic enzyme defects in the biosynthesis of thyroid hormones (Figure 12.44). All of these factors result in inadequate thyroid hormone synthesis and decreased blood levels of T_4 and T_3. The low blood levels are detected by the hypothalamus and pituitary to increase the secretion of TSH, which results in hypertrophy and hyperplasia of follicular cells.

Diffuse Hyperplastic and Colloid Goiter. Iodine deficiency that resulted in diffuse thyroid hyperplasia was common in many goitrogenic areas throughout the world before the widespread addition of iodized salt to animal diets. Although iodine-deficient goiter still occurs in domestic animals in large areas of the world, the outbreaks are sporadic and fewer animals are affected. Marginal iodine-deficient diets containing certain goitrogenic compounds may result in severe thyroid hyperplasia and clinical evidence of goiter. These substances include thiouracil, sulfonamides, anions of the Hofmeister series, and a number of plants from the family Brassicaceae. Young animals born to females on iodine-deficient diets are more likely to develop severe thyroid hyperplasia and have clinical signs of hypothyroidism.

Although seemingly paradoxical, an excess of iodide in the diet also can result in thyroid hyperplasia in animals and people (Figure 12.44). Foals of mares fed dry seaweed containing excessive iodide may develop thyroid hyperplasia and clinically evident goiter (Baker and Lindsey 1968). The thyroid glands of the young are exposed to higher blood iodide levels than the dam because of concentration of iodide, *first* by the placenta and *second* by the mammary gland. A high blood iodide level interferes with one or more steps of thyroid hormone synthesis and secretion, leading to lowered blood T_4 and T_3 levels, and a compensatory increase in pituitary TSH secretion. Excess iodine appears to primarily block the release of thyroid hormones by interfering with the fusion of colloid droplets and lysosomal bodies, thereby disrupting the proteolysis of colloid and release of T_4 and T_3 (Collins and Capen 1980b).

Iodine deficiency may be conditioned by other antithyroid compounds in animal feeds and be responsible, in particular situations, for a high incidence of goiter (Figure 12.44). Prolonged low-level exposure to thiocyanates, which are produced by ruminal degradation of cyanogenetic glucosides from plants such as white clover (*Trifolium*), couch grass (*Cynoden*), and linseed meal, and by degradation of glucosinolates of the *Brassica* crops, is associated with congenital goiter in ruminants. Goitrin (5-vinyl-oxazolidine-2-thione) derived from the glucosinolates of *Brassica* spp. inhibits organification of iodine.

Goiter in adult animals usually is of little clinical significance, and their general health is not impaired, except for occasional local pressure influences. However, it does continue to be of significance as a disease of newborn animals, although the previous serious losses in endemic areas are now controlled by the prophylactic use of iodized salt. Congenital hypothyroidism in domestic animals usually is associated with hyperplastic goiter, even though the dam may show no evidence of thyroid dysfunction. Gestation often is prolonged, the larger goiters may cause dystocia, and there is a tendency to retain the fetal placenta. Affected foals show extreme weakness and die within a few days after birth. Enlarged thyroid glands are readily palpable or visible in kids and lambs, but are not readily apparent in piglets because of the combination of a short neck and the development of myxedema.

Colloid goiter represents the involutionary phase of diffuse hyperplastic goiter and is usually seen in young adult and adult animals. The markedly hyperplastic follicular cells continue to produce colloid, but endocytosis of colloid is decreased due to diminished pituitary TSH levels in response to the return of blood thyroxine and triiodothyronine levels to normal. Both thyroid lobes are diffusely enlarged but are more translucent and lighter in color than with hyperplastic goiter. The differences in macroscopic appearance are the result of reduced vascularity in colloid goiter and development of macrofollicles distended with colloid.

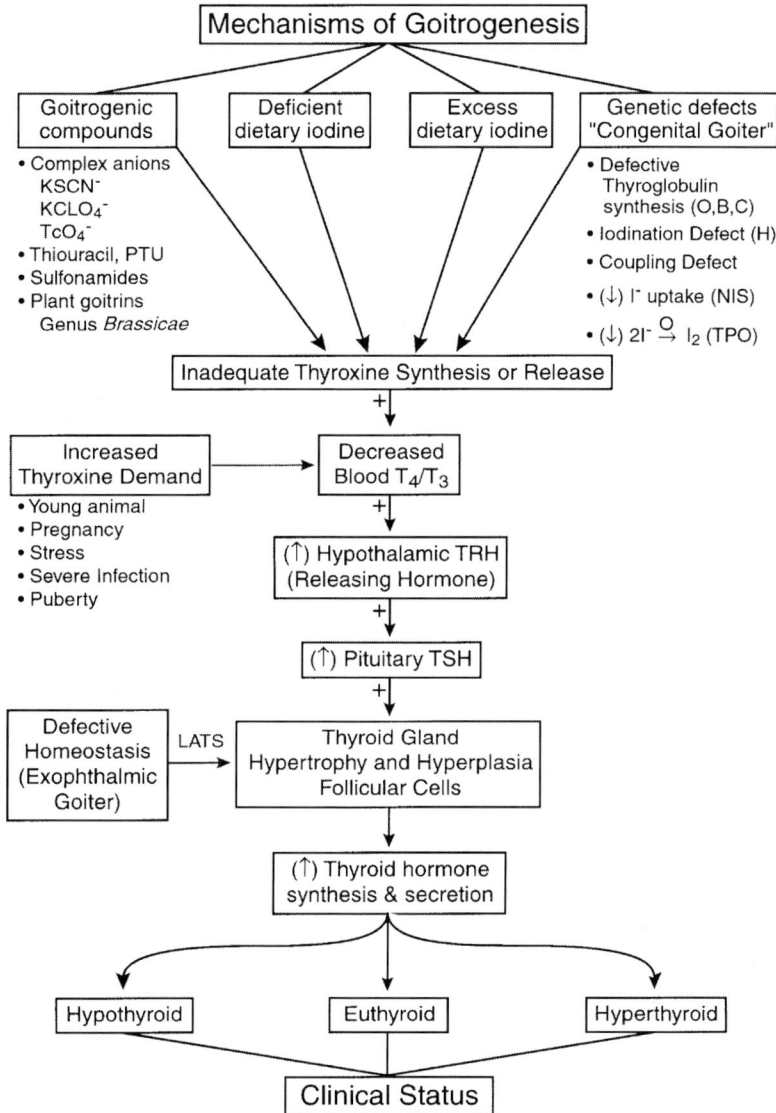

FIG. 12.44—Mechanisms of goitrogenesis. Multiple pathogenic factors (goitrogenic compounds, deficient and excess dietary iodine intake, and genetic enzyme defects) result in inadequate tetraiodothyronine (T_4)/triiodothyronine (T_3) synthesis and lead to long-term stimulation of thyroid follicular cells by an increased secretion of pituitary thyroid-stimulating hormone (TSH). Long-acting thyroid stimulator (LATS) is an autoantibody that directly stimulates follicular cells by binding to the TSH receptor on follicular cells in human beings. I_2, reactive iodine; $KCLO_4^-$, potassium perchlorate; $KSCN^-$, potassium thiocyanate; NIS, sodium-iodide (Na^+-I^-) symporter; PTU, propylthiouracil; TcO_4^-, pertechnetate; TPO, thyroperoxidase; and TRH, thyrotropin-releasing hormone.

The changes in diffuse hyperplastic and colloid goiters are consistent throughout the diffusely enlarged thyroid lobes. The follicles are irregular in size and shape in hyperplastic goiter because of varying amounts of lightly eosinophilic and vacuolated colloid in the lumen. Some follicles are collapsed due to lack of colloid. The follicles are lined by single or multiple layers of hyperplastic columnar follicular cells that in some follicles may form papillary projections into the lumen.

Colloid goiter may develop either after sufficient amounts of iodide have been added to the diet of animals with iodine-deficient hyperplastic goiter or after the requirements for thyroid hormones have diminished in an older animal. Blood thyroid hormone levels return toward normal, and the secretion of TSH by the pituitary gland is correspondingly decreased. Follicles are progressively distended with densely eosinophilic colloid due to diminished TSH-induced endocytosis. The follicular cells lining the macrofollicles are flattened and atrophic. The interface between the colloid and luminal surfaces of follicular cells is smooth and lacks the characteristic endocytotic vacuoles of actively secreting follicular cells. As a result of the lower TSH levels, interfollicular capillaries are less well developed than those with diffuse hyperplastic goiter.

Multinodular Goiter. Nodular hyperplasia (goiter) in thyroid glands of old horses, cats, and dogs appears as multiple white to tan nodules of varying size. The affected lobes are moderately enlarged and irregular in contour. Nodular goiter in most animals (except cats) is endocrinologically inactive and encountered as an incidental lesion at necropsy; however, functional thyroid adenomas often develop in glands with multinodular follicular cell hyperplasia in old cats. In contrast to thyroid adenomas, nodules of hyperplasia are multiple, not encapsulated, and result in minimal compression of adjacent parenchyma. Nodular goiter consists of multiple foci of hyperplastic follicular cells that are sharply demarcated but not encapsulated from the adjacent thyroid parenchyma. The areas of nodular hyperplasia may be microscopic, as in old cats, or grossly visible, causing enlargement of the thyroid as in old horses.

Inherited Dyshormonogenetic (Congenital) Goiter. An inability to synthesize and secrete adequate amounts of thyroid hormones beginning before or at birth has been documented in human infants and in several animal species. Congenital dyshormonogenetic goiter is inherited as an autosomal recessive trait in sheep of the Corriedale, Dorset Horn, Merino, and Romney breeds; Afrikander cattle; and Saanen dwarf goats (Falconer 1966; Rac et al. 1968; De Vijlder et al. 1978; Pammenter et al. 1978; Van Zyl et al. 1979). The subnormal growth rate, absence of normal wool development or presence of a rough sparse hair coat, myxedematous swellings of the subcutis, weakness, and sluggish behavior suggest that the affected young are clinically hypothyroid. Most lambs with congenital goiter either die shortly after birth or are highly sensitive to the effects of adverse environmental conditions.

Due to an intense diffuse hyperplasia of follicular cells, thyroid glands are symmetrically enlarged at birth. Thyroid follicles are lined by tall columnar cells but often are collapsed because of a lack of colloid resulting from the markedly increased endocytotic activity and diminished ability to synthesize thyroglobulin. The tall columnar follicular cells lining thyroid follicles have extensively dilated profiles of rough endoplasmic reticulum, but there are relatively few dense granules associated with the Golgi apparatus and few apical vesicles near the luminal plasma membrane. Numerous long microvilli extend into the follicular lumen.

Although thyroidal uptake and turnover of iodine 131 are greatly increased compared with euthyroid controls, circulating T_4 and T_3 levels are consistently low. The absence of a defect in the iodide-transport mechanism and organification or dehalogenation, together with an absence of normal 19-S thyroglobulin in goitrous thyroids, suggests an impairment in thyroglobulin biosynthesis in animals with inherited congenital goiter (Figure 12.44) (Lissitzky et al. 1973). A closely related or similar defect appears responsible in the examples of congenital goiter in sheep, cattle, and goats. The protein-bound iodine levels in sheep, cattle, and goats with inherited congenital goiter are markedly elevated (Rijnberk et al. 1977). This appears to be the result of iodination of albumin and other plasma proteins by the thyroid gland under long-term TSH stimulation, since hormonal iodide levels (T_4 and T_3) are significantly lower than in controls.

The presence of messenger ribonucleic acid (mRNA) coding for thyroglobulin has been investigated to elucidate further the molecular basis for the impairment of thyroid hormone biosynthesis in congenital goiter. Although thyroglobulin mRNA sequences are present in the goitrous tissue, their concentration is reduced to one-tenth to one-fortieth of normal, and the intracellular distribution is abnormal (nuclear fraction, 42% of normal; cytoplasmic fraction, 7%; and membrane fraction, 1% to 2%) (Van Herle et al. 1979). The lack of thyroglobulin in these examples of congenital goiter in animals appears to be due to a defect in thyroglobulin mRNA, leading to aberrant processing of primary transcripts or transport of the thyroglobulin mRNA from the nucleus to the ribosomes of the endoplasmic reticulum (Van Voorthuizen et al. 1978).

THYROTOXIC EFFECTS OF DRUGS AND XENOBIOTIC CHEMICALS. Much of the significant physiological and pathological data in the literature on thyroid function and structure have come from studies in animals. Although the basic hypothalamic-pituitary-thyroid axis functions in a similar manner in animals and people, there are differences between species that are important when extrapolating animal data from chronic toxicity and carcinogenicity studies for human risk assessment (Capen 1996). For example, long-term perturbations of the pituitary-thyroid axis by various xenobiotics or physiological alterations (e.g., iodine deficiency and partial thyroidectomy) are more likely to predispose laboratory animals to a higher incidence of proliferative lesions (e.g., hyperplasia and adenomas of follicular cells) than is the case in the human thyroid gland (Capen 1997, 1999). This appears to be particularly true in male rats, in which there usually are higher circulating levels of TSH than in females. The greater sensitivity of the animal thyroid to derangement by drugs, chemicals, and physiological perturbations also is related to the shorter plasma half-life of T_4 (12 to 24 hours) than in humans (5 to 9 days), due, in part, to the considerable differences between species in the transport proteins for T_4.

There also are marked species differences in the sensitivity of the functionally important thyroperoxidase enzyme to inhibition by xenobiotics. Thioamides (e.g., sulfonamides) and other chemicals can selectively inhibit the thyroperoxidase and significantly interfere with the iodination of tyrosyl residues incorporated in the thyroglobulin molecule, thereby disrupting the orderly synthesis of T_4 and T_3. Long-term administration of sulfonamides results in the development of thyroid *nodules* (e.g., focal hyperplasias and adenomas) frequently in the sensitive species (such as rats, dogs, and mice) but not in species resistant (e.g., monkeys, guinea pigs, chickens, and humans) to the inhibition of peroxidase in follicular cells.

The goitrogenic effects of sulfonamides have been known for many years, since the reports of the action of sulfaguanidine on the rat thyroid. Sulfamethoxazole and trimethoprim exert a potent goitrogenic effect in rats, resulting in marked decreases in circulating T_3 and T_4 levels, a substantial compensatory increase in TSH, and increased thyroid weights, due to follicular cell hypertrophy and hyperplasia. The dog also is a species sensitive to the effects of sulfonamides, resulting in markedly decreased serum T_4 and T_3 levels, hyperplasia of thyrotrophic basophils in the pituitary gland, and increased thyroid weights. By comparison, the thyroids of monkeys and people are resistant to the development of changes that sulfonamides produce in rodents (rats and mice) and dogs. Rhesus monkeys treated for 52 weeks with sulfamethoxazole with and without trimethoprim had no changes in thyroid weights, and the thyroid histology was normal.

Studies comparing the effects of propylthiouracil (PTU) and a goitrogenic sulfonamide (sulfamonomethoxine) on the activity of thyroperoxidase in rats and monkeys (using the guaiacol peroxidation assay) demonstrated the concentration required for a 50% inhibition of the peroxidase enzyme [inhibition constant 50% (IC_{50})] was 50 times greater in monkeys compared with rats. Sulfamonomethoxine was almost as potent as PTU in inhibiting the thyroperoxidase in rats; however, it required 500 times the concentration to inhibit the enzyme in monkeys compared with rats. Studies such as these with sulfonamides demonstrate distinct species differences between rodents and primates in the response of the thyroid to chemical inhibition of hormone synthesis; therefore, it is not surprising that the sensitive species (e.g., rats, mice, and dogs) are much more likely to develop follicular cell hyperplasia and thyroid tumors after long-term exposure to sulfonamides than are the resistant species (e.g., subhuman primates, humans, guinea pigs, and chickens).

The plasma thyroxine half-life in rats is considerably shorter (12 to 24 hours) than in humans (5 to 9 days). This is related in part to considerable differences between species in the transport proteins for T_4 and T_3. In humans and monkeys, circulating T_4 is bound with high avidity primarily to TBG; however, this high-affinity binding protein is not present in rodents, birds, amphibians, or fish. T_3 is transported bound to TBG

and albumin (transthyretin) in people, monkeys, and dogs but only to albumin in mice, rats, and chickens. In general, T_3 is bound less avidly to transport proteins than is T_4, resulting in a faster turnover and shorter plasma half-life in most species.

In the evaluation of potential thyroid toxicity of various xenobiotics in animals, an accurate quantitation of circulating levels of TSH is essential in order to determine whether proliferative lesions of follicular cells are mediated by a chronic hypersecretion of TSH (Capen 2001). The immunoassay for TSH is highly species specific, with considerable interanimal and interassay variations. Xenobiotics that disrupt either thyroid hormone synthesis, secretion, or peripheral metabolism often cause prompt increases in circulating TSH levels. TSH levels are higher in male than female rats, and castration decreases both the baseline serum TSH and response to TRH injection. In response to the greater circulating TSH levels, follicular cell height often is greater in male than female rats. The administration of exogenous testosterone to castrated male rats restores the TSH level to that of intact rats.

Chemical disruption of thyroid hormone synthesis and secretion in animals may occur at a number of different steps in thyroid hormone synthesis and secretion. These include blockage of iodine uptake, organification defects, blockage of hormone release, drug-induced thyroid pigmentation, inhibition of 5′-deiodinase, and induction of hepatic microsomal enzymes (Figure 12.45).

Blockage Of Iodide Uptake. The initial step in the biosynthesis of thyroid hormones is the uptake of iodide from the circulation and transport against a gradient across follicular cells to the lumen of the follicle. A number of anions act as competitive inhibitors of iodide transport in the thyroid, including perchlorate (ClO_4^-), thiocyanate (SCN^-), and pertechnetate (Figure 12.46). Thiocyanate is a potent inhibitor of iodide transport and is a competitive substrate for thyroperoxidase, but it does not appear to be concentrated in the thyroid. Blockage of the iodide-trapping mechanism has a similar disruptive effect on the thyroid-pituitary axis as iodine deficiency. The blood levels of T_4 and T_3 decrease, resulting in a compensatory increase in the secretion of TSH by the pituitary gland (Figure 12.46). The hypertrophy and hyperplasia of follicular cells following sustained exposure result in increased thyroid weight and the development of thyroid enlargement or goiter.

Organification Defect. A wide variety of chemicals, drugs, and other xenobiotics affect the second step in thyroid hormone biosynthesis. The stepwise binding of iodide to the tyrosyl residues in thyroglobulin requires oxidation of inorganic iodide (I^-) to molecular (reactive) iodine (I_2) by the thyroperoxidase present in the luminal aspect (microvillar membranes and apical cytoplasm) of follicular cells and adjacent colloid. Classes of chemicals that inhibit the organification of

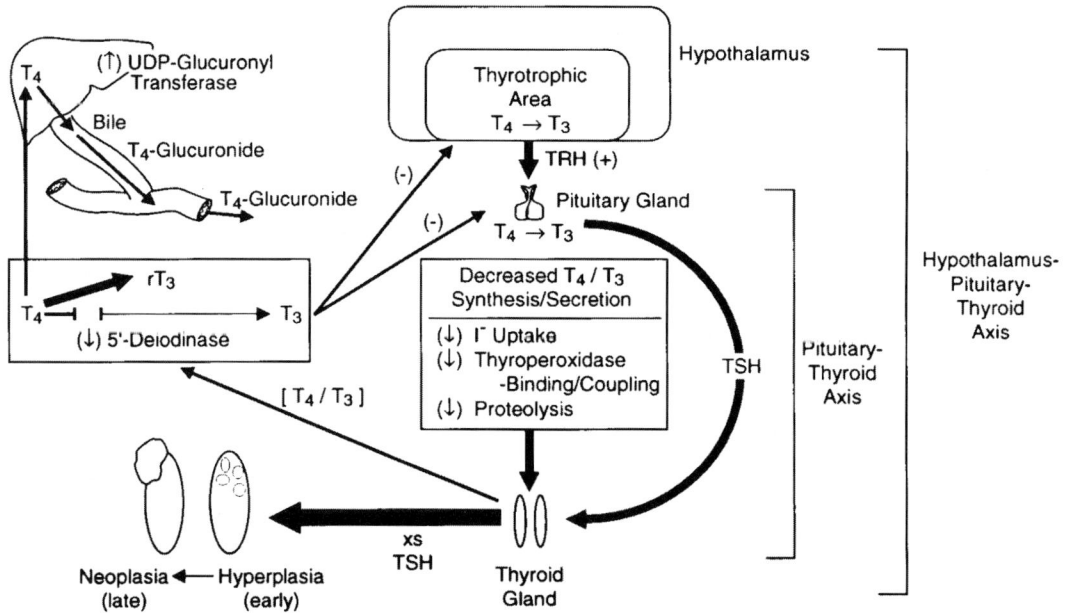

FIG. 12.45—Multiple sites of disruption of the hypothalamic-pituitary-thyroid triad by xenobiotic chemicals. Chemicals can exert direct effects by disrupting thyroid hormone synthesis or secretion and indirectly influence the thyroid through an inhibition of 5'-deiodinase or by inducing hepatic microsomal enzymes (e.g., T_4-UDP glucuronyl transferase). All of these mechanisms can lower circulating levels of thyroid hormones (T_4 and T_3), resulting in a release from negative-feedback inhibition and a compensatory increased secretion of thyroid-stimulating hormone (TSH) by the pituitary gland. The chronic hypersecretion of TSH predisposes the sensitive rodent thyroid gland to develop an increased incidence of focal hyperplastic and neoplastic (adenoma) lesions by a secondary (epigenetic) mechanism. T_3, triiodothyronine; T_4, tetraiodothyronine; TRH, thyrotropin-releasing hormone; and UDP, uridine 5'-diphosphate.

thyroglobulin include (a) thionamides (such as thiourea, thiouracil, propylthiouracil, methimazole, carbimazole, and goitrin); (b) aniline derivatives and related compounds (e.g., sulfonamides, para-aminobenzoic acid, para-aminosalicylic acid, and amphenone); and (c) substituted phenols (such as resorcinol, phloroglucinol, and 2,4-dihydroxybenzoic acid), and miscellaneous inhibitors [e.g., aminotriazole, tricyanoaminopropene, antipyrine, and its iodinated derivative (iodopyrine)].

These chemicals exert their action by inhibiting the thyroperoxidase, which causes a disruption both of the iodination of tyrosyl residues in thyroglobulin but also the coupling reaction of inactive iodotyrosines (e.g., MIT and DIT) to form active iodothyronines (T_3 and T_4) (Figure 12.46). PTU has been shown in rats to affect each step in thyroid hormone synthesis beyond iodide transport.

Blockage of Thyroid Hormone Release. Relatively few chemicals selectively inhibit the secretion of thyroid hormone from the thyroid gland (Figure 12.46). An excess of iodine inhibits secretion of thyroid hormone and occasionally can result in goiter and hypothyroidism in animals and human patients. Several mecha-

nisms have been suggested for this effect of high iodide levels on the thyroid hormone secretion, including a decrease in lysosomal protease activity (human glands), inhibition of colloid droplet formation (mice and rats), and inhibition of TSH-mediated increase in cAMP (dog thyroid slices). Rats fed an iodide-excess diet have hypertrophy of the cytoplasmic area of follicular cells, with an accumulation of numerous colloid droplets and lysosomal bodies. There is limited evidence ultrastructurally of fusion of the membranes of these organelles and degradation of the colloid necessary for the release of T_4 and T_3 from the thyroglobulin.

Lithium also has a striking inhibitory effect on thyroid hormone release. The widespread use of lithium carbonate in the treatment of manic states occasionally results in the development of thyroid enlargement, with either euthyroidism or occasionally hypothyroidism in human patients.

Drug-induced Thyroid Pigmentation. The antibiotic minocycline produces a striking black discoloration of the thyroid lobes in laboratory animals and in people, with the formation of brown pigment granules within follicular cells. The pigment granules stain similarly to melanin and are best visualized on thyroid sections

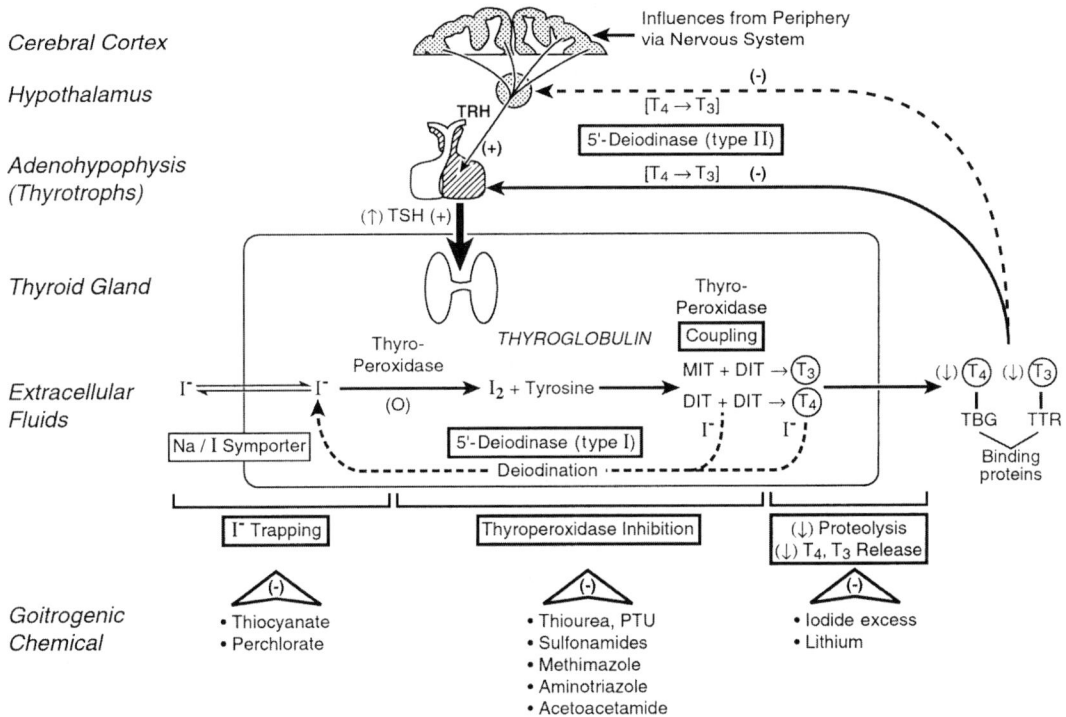

FIG. 12.46—Mechanism of action of goitrogenic chemicals on thyroid hormone synthesis and secretion. Chemicals can interfere with thyroid function either by (a) blocking iodide ion trapping, (b) inhibiting organic binding-coupling, or (c) disrupting proteolysis and release of T_4 and T_3 from colloid. DIT, diiodotyrosine; I_2, reactive iodine; MIT, monoiodotyrosine; PTU, propylthiouracil; T_3, triiodothyronine; T_4, tetraiodothyronine; TBG, thyroxine-binding globulin; TRH, thyrotropin-releasing hormone; and TSH, thyroid-stimulating hormone.

stained with the Fontana-Masson procedure. Electron-dense material first accumulates in lysosome-like granules and in the rough endoplasmic reticulum. The pigment appears to be a metabolic derivative of minocycline, and administration of the antibiotic at high dose to rats for extended periods may disrupt thyroid function and result in the development of goiter. The release of T_4 from perfused thyroids of minocycline-treated rats is significantly decreased, but the follicular cells retain the ability to phagocytose colloid in response to TSH and have numerous colloid droplets in their cytoplasm.

Other chemicals (or their metabolites) selectively localize in the thyroid colloid, resulting in abnormal clumping and increased basophilia to the colloid. Brown-to-black pigment granules may be present in follicular cells, colloid, and macrophages in the interthyroidal tissues, resulting in a macroscopic darkening of both thyroid lobes. The physicochemically altered colloid in the lumina of thyroid follicles appears to be less capable than normal colloid either of reacting with organic iodine in a stepwise manner to result in the orderly synthesis of iodothyronines or of being phagocytosed by follicular cells and enzymatically processed to release active thyroid hormones into the circulation.

Serum T_4 and T_3 are decreased, serum TSH levels are increased by an expanded population of pituitary thyrotrophs, and thyroid follicular cells undergo hypertrophy and hyperplasia and eventually develop tumors.

Inhibition of 5'-Deiodinase. The best-characterized chemical that acts as a 5'-deiodinase inhibitor and perturbs thyroid function is FD&C Red No. 3 (erythrosine). It is a tetraiodinated derivative of fluorescein with iodine accounting for about 58% of the molecular weight of the color. FD&C Red No. 3 is a red dye widely used as a color additive in foods, cosmetics, and pharmaceuticals. Amiodarone is another organic iodinated antiarrhythmic compound that disrupts thyroid hormone economy by inhibiting 5'-deiodinase. Iopanoic acid and flavonoids also inhibit the enzyme in hepatocytes.

FD&C Red No. 3 is an example of a xenobiotic that causes changes in circulating levels of thyroid hormones and morphological evidence of follicular cell stimulation by producing alterations in the peripheral metabolism of T_4 (Borzelleca et al. 1987). Inhibition of 5'-deiodinase in the liver and kidney by Red No. 3 explains the lower circulating T_3 levels. The monodeiodination of T_4 by another enzyme (5-deiodinase) to reverse T_3 and inhibition of the 5′-deiodinase [which is necessary to further degrade this inactive iodothyronine to 3,3′-diiodothyronine (T_2)] results in the striking accumulation of serum reverse T_3 (Figure 12.47). The pituitary sensing the lowered circulating levels of T_3 compensates by increasing the secretion of TSH, which results in the morphological evidence of follicular cell stimulation. FD&C Red No. 3 does not appear to be a direct-acting thyroid oncogene (Figure 12.48). Rather, in massive doses (4% of diet over lifetime beginning in utero), it acts through a secondary mechanism to promote the development of benign thyroid tumors in laboratory animals.

Induction of Hepatic Microsomal Enzymes. Hepatic microsomal enzymes play an important role in thyroid hormone economy, since glucuronidation is the rate-limiting step in the biliary excretion of T_4, and sulfation is the rate-limiting step in the excretion of T_3 by phenol sulfotransferase (Figure 12.49). Long-term exposure to many chemicals may induce these enzyme pathways and result in chronic stimulation of the thyroid by disrupting the hypothalamic-pituitary-thyroid axis (Figure 12.45) (Curran and De Groot 1991; Gaskill et al. 2000). The resulting chronic stimulation of the thyroid by increased circulating levels of TSH often increases the risk of developing tumors derived from follicular cells in chronic studies with these compounds in certain species. Xenobiotics that induce liver microsomal enzymes and disrupt thyroid function include central nervous system drugs (e.g., phenobarbital and benzodiazepines), calcium channel blockers (e.g., nicardipine and bepridil), steroids (spironolactone), retinoids, chlorinated hydrocarbons [chlordane, dichlorodiphenyl-trichloroethane (DDT), and tetrachlorodibenzodioxin (TCDD)], and polyhalogenated biphenyls [polychlorinated biphenyls (PCBs) polybrominated biphenyls (and PBBs)]. Most of the hepatic microsomal enzyme induc-

ers have no apparent intrinsic carcinogenic activity and produce little or no mutagenicity or DNA damage.

Phenobarbital has been studied extensively as the prototype for hepatic microsomal inducers that increases a similar spectrum of cytochrome P-450 isozymes. McClain (1989) reported that the activity of thyroxine-uridine (UDP) glucuronyl transferase, the rate-limiting enzyme in T_4 metabolism, is increased in purified hepatic microsomes of male rats when expressed as picamole per minute per milligram of microsomal protein (twofold) or as total hepatic activity (threefold) (Figure 12.50) (McClain et al. 1988). This resulted in a significantly higher cumulative biliary excretion of [^{125}I]thyroxine and bile flow than in controls. Most of the increase in biliary excretion was accounted for by an increase in T_4-glucuronide, due to an increased metabolism of thyroxine in phenobarbital-treated rats (Figure 12.51). Phenobarbital-treated rats develop a characteristic pattern of changes in circulating thyroid hormone levels. Plasma T_3 and T_4 are markedly decreased after 1 week and remain decreased for 4 weeks. By 8 weeks, T_3 levels return to near normal due to compensation by the hypothalamic-pituitary-thyroid axis. Serum TSH values are significantly elevated throughout the first month but often decline somewhat after a new steady state is attained (McClain et al. 1989). Thyroid weights increase significantly after 2 to 4 weeks of phenobarbital, reach a maximum increase of 40% to 50% by 8 weeks, and remain elevated throughout the treatment period. Results from these studies are consistent with the hypothesis that the promotion of thyroid tumors in rats was not a direct effect of phenobarbital on the thyroid gland but rather an indirect effect mediated by TSH secretion from the pituitary secondary to the hepatic microsomal enzyme-induced increase of T_4 excretion in the bile.

The activation of the thyroid gland during the treatment of rodents with substances that stimulate thyroxine catabolism is a well-known phenomenon that has

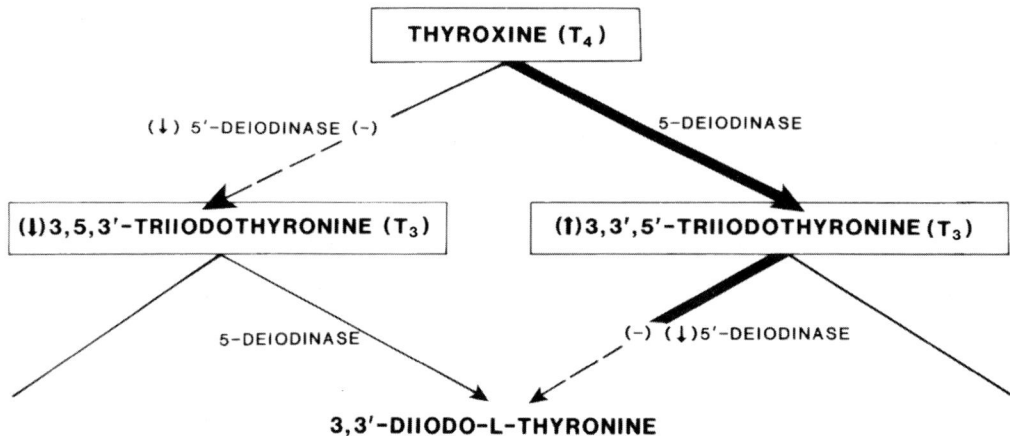

THYROXINE (T$_4$)

($\downarrow$) 5′-DEIODINASE (−)   5-DEIODINASE

($\uparrow$)3,5,3′-TRIIODOTHYRONINE (T$_3$)   **($\uparrow$)3,3′,5′-TRIIODOTHYRONINE (T$_3$)**

5-DEIODINASE   (−) ($\downarrow$)5′-DEIODINASE

3,3′-DIIODO-L-THYRONINE

FIG. 12.47—Effects of FD&C Red No. 3 (erythrosine) on in vivo metabolism of thyroxine by inhibiting the 5′-deiodinase that normally converts tetraiodothyronine (T_4) to triiodothyronine (T_3). (From Capen and Martin 1989.)

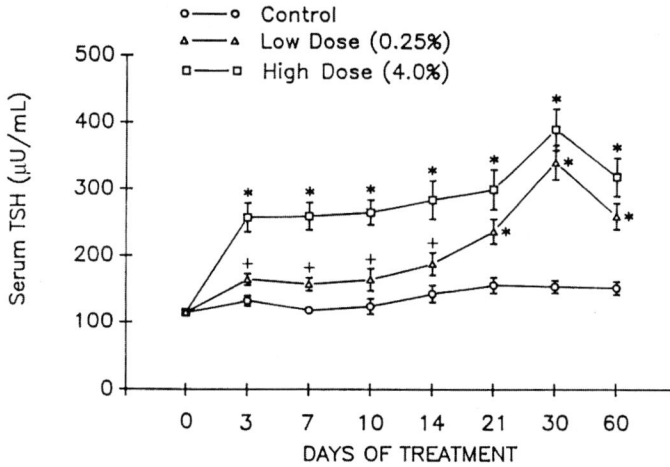

FIG. 12.48—Rapid significant increase in serum thyroid-stimulating hormone (TSH) in Sprague-Dawley rats ($N = 20$ rats/group and interval) administered a mild goitrogen (FD&C Red No. 3 that inhibits the 5'-deiodinase in peripheral tissues) in their feed. Blood for the TSH assay was collected terminally from the abdominal aorta. The significant increase in serum TSH persisted for the 60 days of the experiment in the high-dose (4%) group. (Courtesy of L.E. Braverman and W.J. De Vito, University of Massachusetts Medical School and Certified Color Manufacturers Association.)

been extensively investigated with phenobarbital and many other compounds (Clemmesen and Hjalgrim-Jensen 1981; Olsen et al. 1989; Curran and De Groot 1991). It occurs particularly with rodents, *first* because UDP-glucuronyl transferase can easily be induced in rodent species, and *second* because thyroxine metabolism takes place very rapidly in rats in the absence of thyroxine-binding globulin. In humans, a lowering of the circulating thyroxine level but no change in TSH and T_3 concentrations has been observed only with high doses of very powerful enzyme-inducing compounds, such as rifampicin with and without antipyrine.

There is no convincing evidence that people treated with drugs or exposed to chemicals that induce hepatic microsomal enzymes are at increased risk for the development of thyroid cancer (Curran and De Groot 1991). In a study of the effects of microsomal enzyme-inducing compounds on thyroid hormone metabolism in normal healthy adults, phenobarbital (100 mg daily for 14 days) did not affect the serum T_4, T_3, or TSH levels (Ohnhaus et al. 1981). Serum T_4 levels decreased after treatment with either a combination of phenobarbital plus rifampicin or a combination of phenobarbital plus antipyrine; however, these treatments had no effect on serum T_3 or TSH levels (Ohnhaus and Studer 1983). Epidemiological studies of patients treated with therapeutic doses of phenobarbital have reported no increase in risk for the development of thyroid neoplasia (Clemmesen and Hjalgrim-Jensen 1977, 1978, 1981; White et al. 1979; Shirts et al. 1986). Highly sensitive assays for thyroid and pituitary hormones are readily available clinically to monitor circulating hormone levels in patients who are exposed to chemicals that could potentially disrupt homeostasis of the pituitary-thyroid axis.

Likewise, there is no substantive evidence that people treated with drugs or exposed to chemicals that induce hepatic microsomal enzymes are at increased risk for the development of liver cancer. This is best exemplified by the extensive epidemiological information on the clinical use of phenobarbital. Phenobarbital has been used clinically as an anticonvulsant for more than 80 years. Relatively high microsomal enzyme-inducing doses have been used chronically, sometimes for lifetime exposures, to control seizure activity in human patients. A study of over 8000 patients admitted to a Danish epilepsy center from 1933 to 1962 revealed no evidence for an increased incidence of hepatic tumors in phenobarbital-treated patients when patients receiving Thorotrast (a colloidal suspension of radioactive thorium dioxide), a known human liver carcinogen, were excluded from the analysis (Clemmesen and Hjalgrim-Jensen 1978). A more recent follow-up report on this patient population confirmed and extended this observation (Clemmesen and Hjalgrim-Jensen 1981; Olsen et al. 1989). The results of two other smaller studies (2099 epileptics and 959 epileptics) also revealed no hepatic tumors in patients treated with phenobarbital (White et al. 1979).

Another classic example of a chemical that induces hepatic microsomal enzymes and disrupts thyroid function is PCB. PCBs are commonly used industrial compounds that have been released into the environment and have caused widespread contamination. The disease-producing capability of these compounds includes alterations in reproduction, growth, and development. PCBs cause a significant reduction in serum levels of thyroid hormones due to alterations in thyroid structure, in addition to the well-known induction of hepatic UDP-glucuronyl transferase and

Thyroxine Metabolism

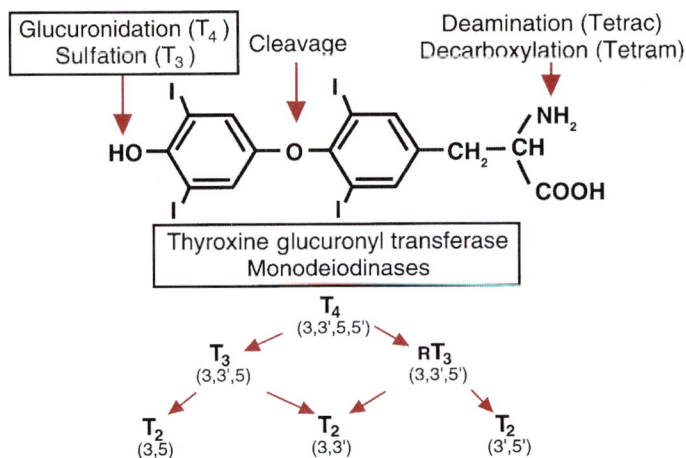

FIG. 12.49—Degradation of thyroid hormones. Thyroxine is conjugated with glucuronic acid in a reaction catalyzed by UDP-glucuronyl transferase and tetraiodothyronine (T_4)-glucuronide excreted in the bile. Triiodothyronine (T_3) is conjugated with sulfate, and T_3-sulfate is excreted in the bile. UDP, uridine 5'-diphosphate. Modified and redrawn from McClain RM (unpublished).

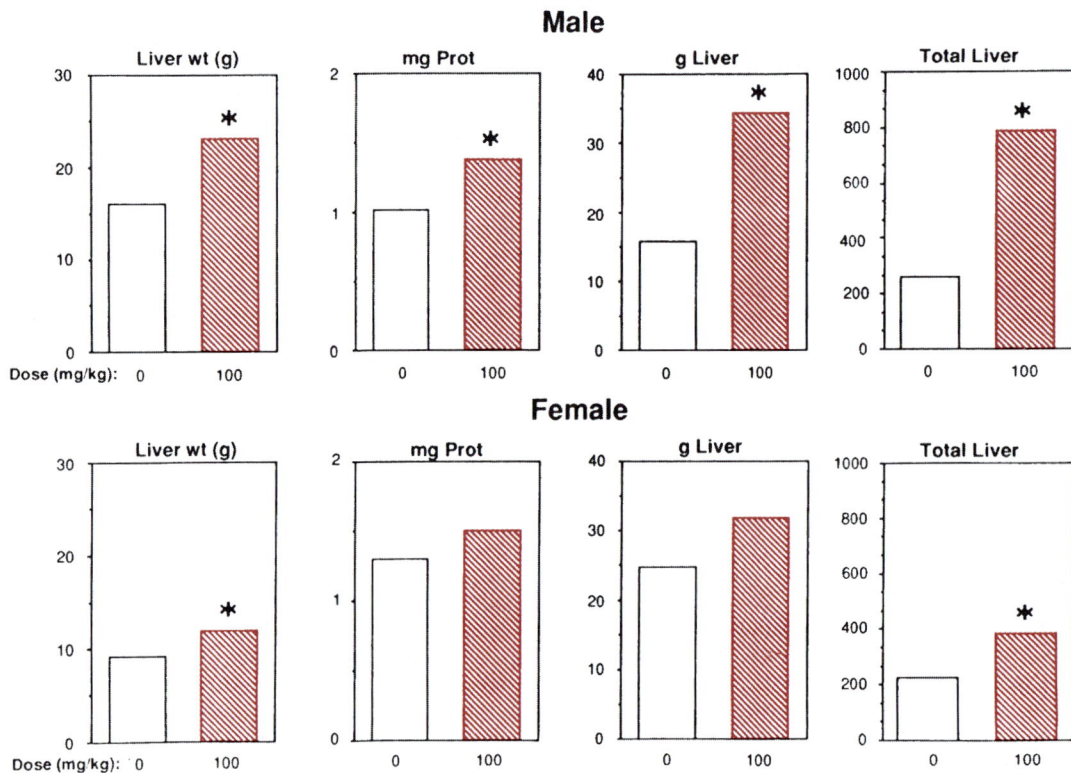

FIG. 12.50—Hepatic thyroxine UDP-glucuronyl transferase activity (pM/min) in control and phenobarbital-treated rats (100 mg/kg/day in the diet for 4 weeks). Glucuronyl-transferase activity was measured in hepatic microsomes by using thyroxine as a substrate. Phenobarbital treatment induced thyroxine-glucuronyl transferase in male and female rats; however, the effect in male rats was quantitatively larger. UDP, uridine 5'-diphosphate. (From McClain 1989.)

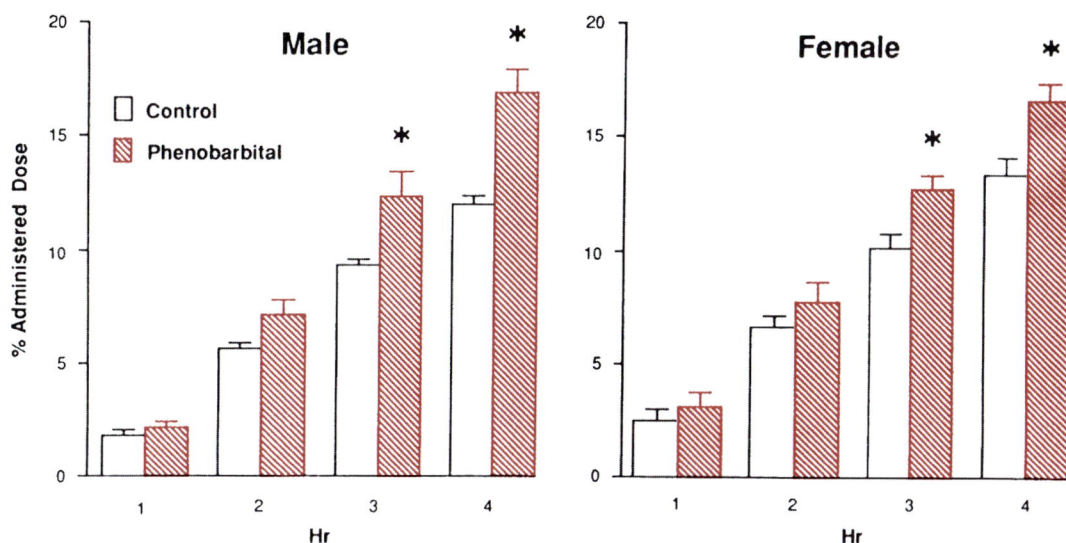

FIG. 12.51—Cumulative biliary excretion of [^{125}I]thyroxine in control and phenobarbital-treated rats (100 mg/kg/day in the diet for 4 to 6 weeks). Phenobarbital treatment resulted in increased cumulative excretion of thyroxine over a 4-hour period. Thin-layer chromatography of bile samples indicated that most of the increase in biliary excretion was accounted for by an increase in the fraction corresponding to thyroxine-glucuronide. (From McClain 1989.)

increased secretion of thyroxine-glucuronide in the bile (Collins and Capen 1980a).

Feeding of PCB produced a dose-dependent significant reduction in serum T_4 levels in rats. Following withdrawal of PCB from the diet, blood T_4 levels return to the normal range at 35 weeks but not at 12 weeks. These changes in circulating levels of T_4 were accompanied by a striking hypertrophy and hyperplasia of thyroid follicular cells compared with controls. The most consistent lesions in follicular cells following the feeding of PCB were the accumulation of numerous large colloid droplets and irregularly shaped lysosomal bodies in the expanded cytoplasmic area. Microvilli on the lumenal surface were shortened, with abnormal branchings. The chronic administration (12 weeks) of PCB resulted in a striking distension of many follicular cells, with large lysosomal bodies that were strongly acid phosphatase positive and with colloid droplets, blunt and abnormally branched microvilli, and mitochondrial vacuolation. The principal lesion produced by PCB in follicular cells that contributed to the altered thyroid function appeared to be an interference in the interaction between the numerous colloid droplets and lysosomal bodies that is necessary for the enzymatic release of thyroid hormones.

Subsequent studies have investigated whether this direct effect on follicular cells interfering with hormone secretion contributes to the lowering of thyroid hormone levels produced by PCB. These investigations have used Gunn rats, which have an impaired capability to conjugate T_4 with glucuronic acid (Collins and Capen 1980a). The serum T_4 concentration was significantly

reduced to a similar degree in both homozygous and heterozygous Gunn rats fed 500 ppm PCB daily for 6 weeks. The bile/plasma ratio of [^{125}I]T_4 was increased more than fivefold in heterozygous Gunn rats ingesting 500 ppm PCB (Figure 12.52). This was a reflection of the capability of heterozygous Gunn rats to respond to PCB with induction of hepatic T_4-UDP-glucuronyl transferase and increased conjugation and excretion of T_4-glucuronide into the bile. The bile/plasma ratio of homozygous control Gunn rats was only one-half that of heterozygous Gunn rats, reflecting their reduced biliary clearance of conjugated T_4. Biliary clearance of exogenous radiolabeled T_4 after the feeding of PCB was elevated only to that of control heterozygous Gunn rats.

Initiating Chemicals in Thyroid Carcinogenesis. In contrast to the previous categories of indirect-acting thyrotoxic compounds, certain chemicals and irradiation appear to have a direct effect on the thyroid gland, causing genetic damage that leads to cell transformation and tumor formation in animals (Doniach 1963; Lee et al. 1982; Capen et al. 1999). Examples of thyroid initiators include 2-acetylaminofluorine (2-AAF), N-methyl-N-nitrosourea (MNU), N-bis(2-hydroxypropyl) nitrosamine (DHPN), methylcholanthrene, dichlorobenzidine, and polycyclic hydrocarbons. Chemicals in this group often increase the incidence of both benign and malignant thyroid tumors. Iodine deficiency is a strong promoter of MNU-initiated thyroid tumors in rats.

Secondary Mechanism of Thyroid Oncogenesis. Understanding the mechanism of action of a new xeno-

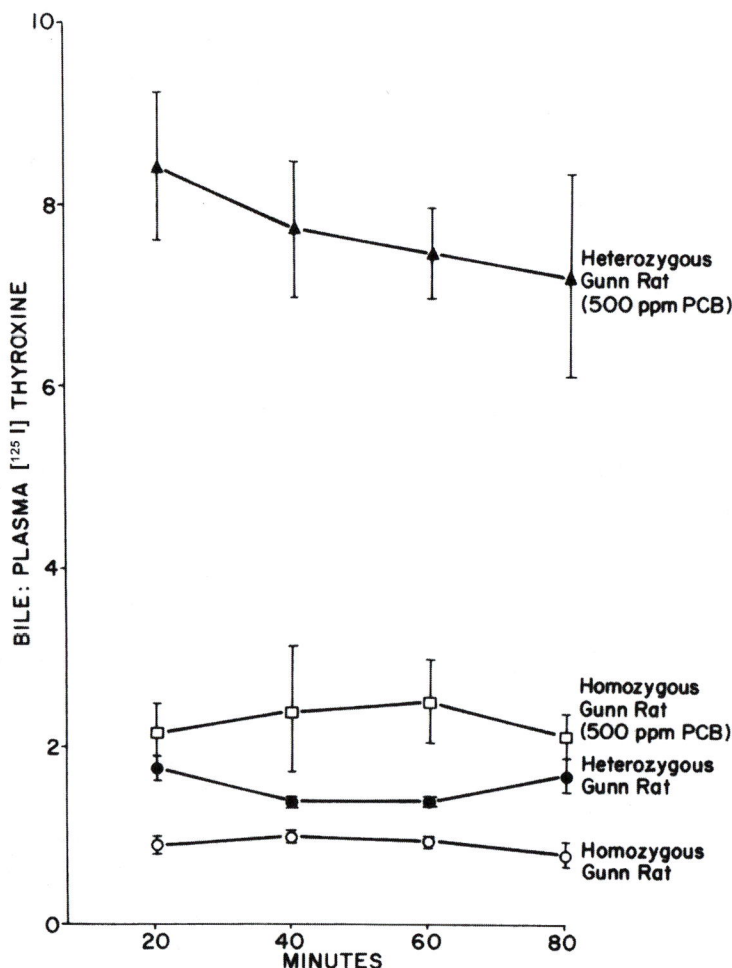

FIG. 12.52—Bile plasma [^{125}I]thyroxine in heterozygous and homozygous Gunn rats fed 0 or 500 ppm of polychlorinated biphenyl (PCB). Rats were injected with [^{125}I] tetraiodothyronine (T$_4$) 18 hours previously. (From Collins and Capen 1980b.)

biotic chemical under development on the thyroid gland provides a rational basis for extrapolation findings from long-term rodent studies to the assessment of a particular compound's safety for humans. Many chemicals and drugs disrupt one or more steps in the synthesis and secretion of thyroid hormones, resulting in subnormal levels of T$_4$ and T$_3$, associated with a compensatory increased secretion of pituitary TSH (Figure 12.45). When tested in highly sensitive species, such as rats and mice, early on these compounds resulted in follicular cell hypertrophy/hyperplasia and increased thyroid weights, and in long-term studies they produced an increased incidence of thyroid tumors by a secondary (indirect) mechanism associated with hormonal imbalances. In the secondary mechanism of thyroid oncogenesis in rodents, the specific xenobiotic chemical or physiological perturbation evokes another stimulus (e.g., chronic hypersecretion of TSH) that pro-

motes the development of nodular proliferative lesions (initially hypertrophy, followed by hyperplasia, subsequently adenomas, or infrequently carcinomas) derived from follicular cells. Compounds acting by this indirect (secondary) mechanism with hormonal imbalances usually show little or no evidence for mutagenicity or for producing DNA damage. The literature suggests that prolonged stimulation of the human thyroid by TSH will induce neoplasia only in exceptional circumstances, possibly by acting together with some other metabolic or immunologic abnormality.

REFERENCES

Archer FJ, Taylor SM. 1996. Alkaline phosphatase bone isoenzyme and osteocalcin in the serum of hyperthyroid cats. Can Vet J 37:735–739.

Baker HJ, Lindsey JR. 1968. Equine goiter due to excess dietary iodide. J Am Vet Med Assoc 153:616–630.

Barber PJ, Elliott J. 1996. Study of calcium homeostasis in feline hyperthyroidism. J Small Anim Pract 37:575–582.

Bastenie PA, Ermans AM, Bonnyns M, et al. 1975. Thyroid autoimmunity disease. In: Good RA, ed. Molecular Pathology. Springfield, IL: Charles C Thomas, pp 234–261.

Belshaw BE, Rijnberk A. 1979. Radioimmunoassay of plasma T_4 and T_3 in the diagnosis of primary hypothyroidism in dogs. J Am Anim Hosp Assoc 15:15–23.

Benjamin SA, Stephens LC, Hamilton BF, et al. 1996. Associations between lymphocytic thyroiditis, hypothyroidism, and thyroid neoplasia in beagles. Vet Pathol 33:486–494.

Benjamin SA, Saunders WJ, Lee AC, et al. 1997. Non-neoplastic and neoplastic thyroid disease in beagles irradiated during prenatal and postnatal development. Radiat Res 147:422–430.

Bidart J-M, Lacroix L, Evain-Brion D, et al. 2000a. Expression of Na^+/I^- symporter and Pendred syndrome genes in trophoblast cells. J Clin Endocrinol Metab 85:4367–4372.

Bidart J-M, Mian C, Lazar V, et al. 2000b. Expression of pendrin and the Pendred syndrome (*PDS*) gene in human thyroid tissues. J Clin Endocrinol Metab 85:2028–2033.

Bigazzi PE, Rose NR. 1975. Spontaneous autoimmune thyroiditis in animals as a model of human disease. Prog Allergy 19:245–274.

Borzelleca JF, Capen CC, Hallagan JB. 1987. Lifetime toxicity carcinogenicity study of FC&C Red No. 3 (erythrosine) in rats. Food Chem Toxicol 25:723–733.

Capen CC. 1996. Hormonal imbalances and mechanisms of chemical injury of thyroid gland. In: Jones TC, Capen CC, Mohr U, eds. Endocrine System, ser 2. Monographs on the Pathology of Laboratory Animals, 2nd ed. International Life Sciences Institute Series. Berlin: Springer-Verlag, pp 217–238.

Capen CC. 1997. Mechanistic data and risk assessment of selected toxic end points of the thyroid gland. Toxicol Pathol 25:39–48.

Capen CC. 1999. Thyroid and parathyroid toxicology. In: Harvey PW, Rush K, Cockburn A, eds. Endocrine and Hormonal Toxicology. Chichester, UK: John Wiley and Sons, pp 33–66.

Capen CC. 2000. Comparative anatomy and physiology of the thyroid. In: Braverman LE, Utiger RD, eds. Werner and Ingbar's The Thyroid: A Fundamental and Clinical Text, 8th ed. Philadelphia: Lippincott-Raven, pp 20–44.

Capen CC. 2001. Toxic responses of the endocrine system. In: Klaassen CD, ed. Casarett and Doull's Toxicology: The Basic Science of Poisons, 6th ed. New York: McGraw-Hill, pp 711–759.

Capen CC, Martin SL. 1989. The effects of xenobiotics on the structure and function of thyroid follicular and C-cells. Toxicol Pathol 17:266–293.

Capen CC, De Lellis RA, Williams ED. 1999. Experimental thyroid carcinogenesis: Role of radiation and xenobiotic chemicals. In: Thomas G, Karaoglou A, Williams ED, eds. Radiation and Thyroid Cancer. Singapore: World Scientific, pp 167–176.

Clemmesen J, Hjalgrim-Jensen S. 1977. On the absence of carcinogenicity to man of phenobarbital. Acta Pathol Microbiol Scand Suppl 261:38–50.

Clemmesen J, Hjalgrim-Jensen S. 1978. Is phenobarbital carcinogenic? A follow-up of 8078 epileptics. Ecotoxicol Environ Safety 1:255–260.

Clemmesen J, Hjalgrim-Jensen S. 1981. Does phenobarbital cause intracranial tumors? A follow-up through 35 years. Ecotoxicol Environ Safety 5:255–260.

Collins WT Jr, Capen CC. 1980a. Biliary excretion of ^{125}I-thyroxine and fine structural alterations in the thyroid glands of Gunn rats fed polychlorinated biphenyls. Lab Invest 43:158–164.

Collins WT Jr, Capen CC. 1980b. Ultrastructural and functional alterations in thyroid glands of rats produced by polychlorinated biphenyls compared with the effects of iodide excess and deficiency, and thyrotropin and thyroxine administration. Virchows Archiv [B] 33:213–231.

Curran PG, De Groot LJ. 1991. The effect of hepatic enzyme-inducing drugs on thyroid hormones and the thyroid gland. Endocr Rev 12:135–150.

Derwahl M, Manole D, Sobke A, Broecker M. 1998. Pathogenesis of toxic thyroid adenomas and nodules: Relevance of activating mutations in the TSH-receptor and *Gs-alpha* gene, the possible role of iodine deficiency and secondary and TSH-independent molecular mechanisms. Exp Clin Endocrinol Diabetes 106(Suppl 4):S6–S9.

De Vijlder JJM, Van Voorthuizen WF, Van Dijk JE, et al. 1978. Hereditary congenital goiter with thyroglobulin deficiency in a breed of goats. Endocrinology 102:1214–1222.

Doniach I. 1963. Effects including carcinogenesis of ^{131}I and X ray on the thyroid of experimental animals: A review. Health Phys 9:1357–1362.

Everett LA, Morsli H, Wu DK, Green ED. 1999. Expression pattern of the mouse ortholog of the Pendred's syndrome gene (*Pds*) suggests a key role for pendrin in the inner ear. Proc Natl Acad Sci USA 96:9727–9732.

Everett LA, Belyantseva IA, Noben-Trauth K, et al. 2001. Targeted disruption of mouse *Pds* provides insight about the inner-ear defects encountered in Pendred syndrome. Hum Mol Genet 10:153–161.

Falconer IR. 1966. Studies of the congenitally goitrous sheep: The iodinated compounds of serum and circulating thyroid-stimulating hormone. Biochem J 100:190–196.

Foti D, Rapoport B. 1990. Carbohydrate moieties in recombinant human thyroid peroxidase: Role in recognition by antithyroid peroxidase antibodies in Hashimoto's thyroiditis. Endocrinology 126:2983–2992.

Fraichard A, Chassande O, Plateroti M, et al. 1997. The T_3R gene encoding a thyroid hormone receptor is essential for post-natal development and thyroid hormone production. EMBO J 16:4412–4420.

Gaskill CL, Burton SA, Gelens HC, et al. 2000. Changes in serum thyroxine and thyroid-stimulating hormone concentrations in epileptic dogs receiving phenobarbital for one year. J Vet Pharmacol Ther 23:243–249.

Gerber H, Peter H, Ferguson DC, Peterson ME. 1994. Etiopathology of feline toxic nodular goiter. Vet Clin North Am Small Anim Pract 24:541–565.

Gosselin SJ, Martin SL, Capen CC, Targowski SP. 1980. Biochemical and immunological investigations of hypothyroidism in dogs. Can J Comp Med 44:158–168.

Gosselin SJ, Capen CC, Martin SL. 1981. Histopathologic and ultrastructural evaluation of thyroid lesions associated with hypothyroidism in dogs. Vet Pathol 18:299–309.

Gosselin SJ, Capen CC, Martin SL, Krakowka S. 1982. Autoimmune lymphocytic thyroiditis in dogs. Vet Immunol Immunopathol 3:185–201.

Hoenig M, Goldschmidt MH, Ferguson DC, et al. 1982. Toxic nodular goitre in the cat. J Small Anim Pract 23:1–12.

Holzworth J, Theran P, Carpenter JL, et al. 1980. Hyperthyroidism in the cat: Ten cases. J Am Vet Med Assoc 176:345–353.

Jernigan AD. 1989. Idiosyncrasies of feline drug metabolism. In: Proceedings of the 12th Annual Kal Kan Symposium for Treatment of Small Animal Diseases. Vernon, CA: Veterinary Learning Systems, pp 65–74.

Johnson LA, Ford HC, Tarttelin MF, Feek CM. 1992. Iodine content of commercially-prepared cat foods. NZ Vet J 40:18–20.

Kohn LD, Suzuki K, Nakazato M, et al. 2001. Effects of thyroglobulin and pendrin on iodide flux through the thyrocyte. Trends Endocrinol Metab 12:10–16.

Kooistra HS, Diaz-Espineira M, Mol JA, et al. 2000. Secretion pattern of thyroid-stimulating hormone in dogs during euthyroidism and hypothyroidism. Domest Anim Endocrinol 18:19–29.

Kopp P. 1999. Pendred's syndrome: Identification of the genetic defect a century after its recognition. Thyroid 9:65–69.

Lacroix L, Mian C, Caillou B, et al. 2001. Na+/I− symporter and Pendred syndrome gene and protein expressions in human extra-thyroidal tissues, Eur J Endocrinol 144:297-302.

La Perle KMD, Jhiang SM. 2003. Iodine: Symporter and Oxidation, thyroid hormone biosynthesis. In: Henry HL, Norman AW, eds. Encyclopedia of Hormones. Amsterdam: Academic, 2:519–522.

Laurberg P. 1978. Non-parallel variations in the preferential secretion of 3,5,3′-triiodothyronine (T$_4$) and 3,3′,5′-triiodothyronine (rT$_3$) from dog thyroid. Endocrinology 102:757–766.

Lee W, Chiacchierini RP, Shleien B, Telles NC. 1982. Thyroid tumors following ^{131}I or localized X irradiation to the thyroid and pituitary glands in rats. Radiat Res 92:307–319.

Lima FRS, Gervais A, Colin C, et al. 2001. Regulation of microglial development: A novel role for thyroid hormone. J Neurosci 21:2028–2038.

Lissitzky S, Bismuth J, Jaquet P, et al. 1973. Congenital goiter with impaired thyroglobulin synthesis. J Clin Endocrinol Metab 36:17–29.

Matsuta M. 1982. Immunohistochemical and electron microscopic studies on Hashimoto's thyroiditis. Acta Pathol Jpn 32:41–56.

McClain RM. 1989. The significance of hepatic microsomal enzyme induction and altered thyroid function in rats: Implications for thyroid gland neoplasia. Toxicol Pathol 17:294–306.

McClain RM, Posch RC, Bosakowski T, Armstrong JM. 1988. Studies on the mode of action for thyroid gland tumor promotion in rats by phenobarbital. Toxicol Appl Pharmacol 94:254–265.

McClain RM, Levin AA, Posch R, Downing JC. 1989. The effects of phenobarbital on the metabolism and excretion of thyroxine in rats. Toxicol Appl Pharmacol 99:216–228.

Merryman JI, Buckles EL, Bowers G, Neilsen NR. 1999. Overexpression of c-Ras in hyperplasia and adenomas of the feline thyroid gland: An immunohistochemical analysis of 34 cases. Vet Pathol 36:117–124.

Milne KL, Hayes HM. 1981. Epidemiologic features of canine hypothyroidism. Cornell Vet 71:3–14.

Mizejewski GJ, Baron J, Poissant G. 1971. Immunologic investigations of naturally occurring canine thyroiditis. J Immunol 107:1152–1160.

Nesbitt GH, Izzo J, Peterson L, Wilkins RJ. 1980. Canine hypothyroidism: A retrospective study of 108 cases. J Am Vet Med Assoc 177:1117–1122.

Nunez EA, Becker DV, Furth ED, et al. 1970. Breed differences and similarities in thyroid function in purebred dogs. Am J Physiol 218:1337–1341.

Nunez EA, Belshaw BE, Gershon MD. 1972. A fine structural study of the highly active thyroid follicular cell of the African Basenji dog. Am J Anat 133:463–482.

Öfverholm T, Ericson LE. 1984. Intraluminal iodination of thyroglobulin. Endocrinology 114:827–835.

Ohnhaus EE, Studer H. 1983. A link between liver microsomal enzyme activity and thyroid hormone metabolism in man. Br J Clin Pharmacol 15:71–76.

Ohnhaus EE, Burgi H, Burger A, Studer H. 1981. The effect of antipyrine, phenobarbital, and rifampicin on the thyroid hormone metabolism in man. Eur J Clin Invest 11:381–387.

Olsen JH, Boice JD, Jensen JP, Fraumeni JF Jr. 1989. Cancer among epileptic patients exposed to anticonvulsant drugs. J Natl Cancer Inst 81:803–808.

Oppenheimer JH. 1979. Thyroid hormone action at the cellular level. Science 203:971–979.

Pammenter M, Albrecht C, Liebenberg W, Van Jaarsveld P. 1978. Afrikander cattle congenital goiter: Characteristics of its morphology and iodoprotein pattern. Endocrinology 102:954–965.

Pearce SHS, Foster DJ, Imrie H, et al. 1997. Mutational analysis of the thyrotropin receptor gene in sporadic and familial feline thyrotoxicosis. Thyroid 7:923–927.

Peter HJ, Gerber H, Studer H, et al. 1991. Autonomous growth and function of cultured thyroid follicles from cats with spontaneous hyperthyroidism. Thyroid 1:331–338.

Peterson ME, Gamble DA. 1990. Effect of nonthyroidal illness on serum thyroxine concentration in cats: 494 cases. J Am Vet Med Assoc 197:1203–1208.

Peterson ME, Kintzer PP, Cavanagh PG, et al. 1983. Feline hyperthyroidism: Pretreatment clinical and laboratory evaluation of 131 cases. J Am Vet Med Assoc 183:103–110.

Peterson ME, Kintzer PP, Hurvitz AI. 1988. Methimazole treatment of 262 cats with hyperthyroidism. Vet Intern Med 2:150–159.

Rac R, Hill GN, Pain RW, Wulhearn CJ. 1968. Congenital goitre in Merino sheep due to an inherited defect in the biosynthesis of thyroid hormone. Res Vet Sci 9:209–223.

Ramsey IK, Evans H, Herrtage ME. 1997. Thyroid-stimulating hormone and total thyroxine concentrations in euthyroid, sick euthyroid and hypothyroid dogs. J Small Anim Pract 38:540–545.

Reichlin S. 1998. Neuroendocrinology. In: Wilson JD, Foster DW, Kronenberg HM, Larsen PR, eds. Williams Textbook of Endocrinology, 9th ed. Philadelphia: WB Saunders, pp 165–248.

Rijnberk A, Der Kinderen PJ. 1969. Toxic thyroid carcinoma in the dog. Acta Endocrinol Suppl (Copenh) 138:177.

Rijnberk A, De Vijlder JJ, Van Dijk JE, et al. 1977. Congenital defect in iodothyronine synthesis: Clinical aspects of iodine metabolism in goats with congenital goitre and hypothyroidism. Br Vet J 133:495–503.

Royaux IE, Suzuki K, Mori A, et al. 2000. Pendrin, the protein encoded by the Pendred syndrome gene (PDS), is an apical porter of iodide in the thyroid and is regulated by thyroglobulin in FRTL-5 cells. Endocrinology 141:839–845.

Sauvé F, Paradis M. 2000. Use of recombinant human thyroid-stimulating hormone for thyrotropin stimulation test in euthyroid dogs. Can Vet J 41:215–219.

Scarlett JM. 1994. Epidemiology of thyroid diseases of dogs and cats. Vet Clin North Am Small Anim Pract 24:477–486.

Schiller I, Berglund NE, Terry JR, et al. 1964. Hypercholesteremia in pet dogs. Arch Pathol 77:389–392.

Scott DA, Wang R, Kreman TM, et al. 1999. The Pendred syndrome gene encodes a chloride-iodide transport protein. Nat Genet 21:440–443.

Shirts SB, Annegers JF, Hauser WA, Kurland LT. 1986. Cancer incidence in a cohort of patients with seizure disorders. J Natl Cancer Inst 77:83–87.

Takizawa T, Yamamoto M, Arishima K, et al. 1993. An electron microscopic study on follicular formation and TSH sensitivity of the fetal rat thyroid gland in organ culture. J Vet Med Sci 55:157–160.

Tice LW, Wollman SH. 1972. Ultrastructural localization of peroxidase activity on some membranes of the typical thyroid epithelial cell. Lab Invest 26:23–34.

Tice LW, Wollman SH. 1974. Ultrastructural localization of peroxidase on pseudopods and other structures of the typical thyroid epithelial cell. Endocrinology 94:1555–1567.

Tognella C, Marti U, Peter HJ, et al. 1999. Follicle-forming cat thyroid cell lines synthesizing extracellular matrix and basal membrane components: A new tool for the study of thyroidal morphogenesis. J Endocrinol 163:505–514.

Van Herle AJ, Vassart G, Dunmont JE. 1979. Control of thyroglobulin synthesis and secretion. N Engl J Med 301:239–249 and 307–314.

Van Voorthuizen WF, Dinsart C, Flavell RA, et al. 1978. Abnormal cellular localization of thyroglobulin mRNA associated with hereditary congenital goiter and thyroglobulin deficiency. Proc atl Acad Sci USA 75:74–78.

Van Zyl A, Andrews EJ, Ward BC, et al. 1979. Congenital goiter in Afrikander cattle. In: Andrews EJ, Ward B, Altman N, eds. Spontaneous Animal Models of Human Disease. New York: Academic, 1:108–115.

Wetzel BK, Spicer SS, Wollman SH. 1965. Changes in fine structure and acid phosphatase localization in rat thyroid cells following thyrotropin administration. J Cell Biol 25:593–618.

White SJ, McLean AEM, Howland C. 1979. Anticonvulsant drugs and cancer: A cohort study in patients with severe epilepsy. Lancet 2:458–461.

Wollman SH, Spicer SS, Burstone MS. 1964. Localization of esterase and acid phosphatase in granules and colloid droplets in rat thyroid epithelium. J Cell Biol 21:191–201.

PART 4: PATHOPHYSIOLOGY OF THE ENDOCRINE PANCREAS

TIMOTHY D. O'BRIEN

The endocrine pancreas is a complex organ both anatomically and physiologically as befits its role as a central integrator and regulator of carbohydrate, lipid and, to a lesser extent, protein metabolism. Alterations in function may involve hypersecretion of one or more of the several hormones produced, usually in association with endocrine neoplasia, or may involve hyposecretion (mainly insulin) due to either primary or secondary disease conditions. This section presents an overview of the microscopic anatomy of the endocrine pancreas and then discusses the pathophysiology of the more common pathological entities causing either hypersecretion or hyposecretion of the hormones of the endocrine pancreas.

MICROSCOPIC ANATOMY OF THE ENDOCRINE PANCREAS. Although there is much similarity in the types and proportions of pancreatic endocrine cells occurring in mammalian species, there are also prominent differences in the topographical arrangement of these cells within the pancreas among animal species (Thomas 1937; Orci 1982). Additionally, there are regional variations in islet structure and cell content within the pancreas, and anatomic changes and quantitative changes in pancreatic endocrine cell content associated with embryogenesis and postnatal development (Bencosome and Liepa 1955; Wellman et al. 1971; Saladino and Getty 1972; Baetens et al.

1979; Saito et al. 1979; Rahier et al. 1981, 1983; Stefan et al. 1982). Because of these variations in normal pancreatic endocrine cell distribution and islet architecture, a thorough knowledge of the endocrine pancreas of each species is necessary to evaluate pathological changes correctly.

The greatest proportion of endocrine cell mass is found in the pancreatic islets (of Langerhans). These consist of more or less compact masses of endocrine cells permeated by many capillaries and autonomic nerves (Goldstein and Davis 1968). Two major types of pancreatic islets are found in adult animals, and these are derived from either the dorsal or ventral pancreatic anlage (Bencosome and Liepa 1955; Baetens et al. 1979; Orci 1982; Orci et al. 1978). Islets derived from the dorsal pancreatic anlage account for most of the pancreatic endocrine cell mass. These islets contain in decreasing proportions β cells, α cells, and δ cells, with only rare PP cells (or F cells) (Saito et al. 1979; Erlandsen 1980; Klöppel and Drenck 1983; Rahier et al. 1983). In contrast, islets derived from the ventral pancreatic anlage contain, in addition to β cells and δ cells, many PP cells, and only rare α cells. Young ruminants have, in addition to typical dorsal and ventral anlage-type islets, large islets (100 to 1600 μm in diameter) located in the interlobular connective tissue that are composed almost entirely of β cells (Bonner-Weir and Like 1980). These islets decrease in relative volume with increasing age, and are seldom seen in adults.

It is now well recognized that the endocrine pancreas of adult mammalian species is comprised principally of α cells (glucagon), β cells [insulin and islet amyloid polypeptide (IAPP)], δ cells (somatostatin), and PP cells (pancreatic polypeptide). Other cell types that may also occur within the pancreatic islets include the enterochromaffin (EC) cell (only found in islets of some species), the P cell (bombesin-like immunoreactivity; fetal islets), and G cells (gastrin; fetal islets of some species).

β Cells have been shown in numerous studies to be the most populous endocrine cell type of the mammalian pancreas (Saito et al. 1979; Klöppel and Drenck 1983; Rahier et al. 1983; O'Brien et al. 1986) and have been shown, by immunohistochemical techniques, to contain insulin and islet amyloid polypeptide (IAPP or amylin) in their secretory vesicles (Johnson et al. 1988). α Cells are the second most populous endocrine cell type of the mammalian pancreas and have been shown to contain glucagon in their secretory granules. δ Cells are the third most populous pancreatic endocrine cell type and have been firmly established to contain somatostatin.

SYNDROMES OF HYPERSECRETION. Pancreatic endocrine hypersecretion in domestic animals is principally associated with either benign or malignant neoplasms of the endocrine pancreas. Pancreatic endocrine neoplasms (PENs), while uncommon in all species, are most prevalent in dogs and ferrets and are rare in other species. The majority of these tumors are clinically associated with secretion of insulin (insulinomas), although the majority of canine pancreatic endocrine tumors are multihormonal when examined by immunohistochemical techniques. In addition, syndromes associated with excessive glucagon and excessive gastrin secretion have been described in dogs with pancreatic endocrine tumors. Hormone secretion from PENs is typically inappropriate and generally not under normal physiological control.

Despite the frequent presence of more than one hormone in the majority of PENs in dogs and ferrets, in the majority of cases the animals present with a clinical syndrome primarily related to the overproduction or inappropriate secretion of one hormone. This feature gives rise to the clinical designations of insulinoma, glucagonoma, gastrinoma, etc.

Insulinomas. Insulinomas are typically associated with complaints attributable to hypoglycemia due to inappropriate insulin secretion. Clinical signs include episodes of muscle tremors and fasciculation, seizures, and coma (Caywood et al. 1987). In dogs exhibiting the insulinoma syndrome, their PENs are composed predominantly of tumor cells containing insulin, but they may also contain islet amyloid polypeptide (IAPP, also a product of the β cell), as well as minority populations of tumor cells having glucagon, somatostatin, PP, or gastrin immunoreactivity (Hawkins et al. 1987; O'Brien et al. 1987, 1990).

Glucagonomas. Glucagonomas in dogs are associated with the clinical syndrome of superficial necrolytic dermatitis (SND) (Gross et al. 1990). Little is known about the hormonal composition of pancreatic endocrine tumors associated with SND, due to the rarity of these tumors. However, the reported cases (three) have been shown to contain a preponderance of glucagon-immunoreactive cells as well as large numbers of PP and/or insulin-immunoreactive cells (Gross et al. 1990; Torres et al. 1997). Interestingly, dogs with tumors that did contain large numbers of insulin-immunoreactive cells were not reported to have had signs of insulin hypersecretion. This may be due to either insufficient oversecretion of insulin to be clinically apparent or due to the counterinsulin effects of glucagon or both.

Gastrinomas. Gastrinomas are rare in dogs. Gastrin oversecretion (Zollinger-Ellison syndrome) is characterized by diarrhea; vomiting; esophageal, gastric, and/or duodenal ulceration; and hypertrophic gastritis. In four published cases of canine Zollinger-Ellison syndrome in which immunohistochemical analysis of the endocrine tumor was done, all of the tumors stained exclusively for gastrin (Happe et al. 1980; Hayden and Henson 1997). Thus, gastrinomas appear to be unique among canine pancreatic endocrine tumors in that they appear to be monohormonal.

Zollinger-Ellison-like Syndrome. A syndrome similar to Zollinger-Ellison syndrome may rarely occur in dogs with PENs containing pancreatic polypeptide and insulin (Boosinger et al. 1988; Zerbe et al. 1989). In one reported case, the PEN consisted mainly of PP immunoreactive cells and fewer (25%) insulin-immunoreactive cells. This tumor was negative for gastrin, glucagon, somatostatin, calcitonin, serotonin, chromogranin, L-enkephalin, and adrenocorticotropic hormone (ACTH). It is unclear as to whether the clinical syndrome was caused by oversecretion of PP (which has been reported in humans) or by some other undetected secretory product.

No clinical syndromes have as yet been attributed to the hypersecretion of IAPP, somatostatin, vasoactive intestinal polypeptide (VIP), or ACTH in domestic animals.

SYNDROMES OF HYPOSECRETION: DIABETES MELLITUS. Spontaneous diabetes mellitus (DM) among domestic species is most frequently encountered in dogs and cats, whereas it is rare in cattle, pigs, and horses.

Canine Diabetes Mellitus. Little work has been done in the area of canine DM in terms of understanding the basic mechanisms of this disease. Therefore, the precise etiopathogenesis of a large portion of canine DM cases is uncertain. Many cases are apparently attributable to indiscriminant islet destruction secondary to chronic pancreatitis. In some breeds, inherited forms of DM have been described, but these latter forms are rare. A few studies have provided evidence for the occurrence of autoimmune destruction of the pancreatic β cells in dogs by demonstration of anti-islet antibodies in affected dogs (Hoenig and Dawe 1992; Elie and Hoenig 1995; Hoenig 1995). In addition, examination of the canine endocrine pancreas in dogs with DM, but without chronic pancreatitis, reveals a paucity or complete extermination of β cells (T.D. O'Brien, unpublished results). These findings are consistent with, but do not conclusively prove, the occurrence of type I-like DM in dogs. It should also be noted that there have also been rare occurrences of type I-like DM reported in cats and cattle.

Although there has been little research into type I DM in domestic species, extensive research has been done on this condition in people and in rodents, particularly the nonobese diabetic (NOD) mouse. Recognition that human DM is heterogeneous first came clearly into view with the development of the insulin radioimmunoassay, at which time it was evident that some diabetic patients had no measurable insulin, especially those with onset of DM early in life (juvenile-onset DM), whereas others had measurable insulin, particularly those with onset in midlife or later (adult or maturity-onset DM) (Gale 2001). Since these early observations, the paradigm that juvenile-onset or type I DM is an autoimmune disease has become well established.

The principal target of the autoimmune process in type I DM is the pancreatic β cell. No definite cause or initiating factor has as yet been identified, but it is well established that type I DM is associated with dysregulated humoral and cellular immunity (Almawi et al. 1999). Evidence supports the involvement of altered production of, and response to, macrophage and T-lymphocyte-derived cytokines (Falcone and Sarvetnick 1999). Furthermore, there is a shift to a preponderance of T-helper-lymphocyte differentiation into the Th1 (helper T-lymphocyte type 1) pathway in which cytokines such as interleukin 2 and interferon-γ are produced and play a role in induction of programmed cell death (apoptosis) of β cells. In the NOD mouse, perforin, which is secreted by CD8+ T lymphocytes, has been shown to be involved in β-cell death. In addition, factors such as Fas ligand, interferon-γ, interleukin 1, and tumor-necrosis factor α have been implicated in β-cell destruction either directly or indirectly by induction of toxic molecules such as nitric oxide (Signore et al. 1998; Thomas and Kay 2000). Th1 cytokines can also promote homing of autoreactive lymphocytes to the pancreas thereby promoting destruction of β cells. More recently it has also become evident that the Th2 pathway may also be involved in β-cell destruction. In particular, it has been shown that Th2 cytokines, principally interleukin 10, play an important role by effects on the local release of other cytokines and by effects upon the microvasculature, all of which tend to increase the infiltration of the islets by autoreactive leukocytes. This exquisitely complex network of cells and signaling factors involved in the destruction of β cells continues to be revealed by ongoing research.

Feline Diabetes Mellitus. The most common form of DM in the domestic cat bears close clinical and pathological resemblance to human type II DM (T2DM) (Johnson et al. 1986). This section focuses on this form of feline DM (FDM) and does not consider other less common forms of diabetes in cats, such as type I-like diabetes, or secondary forms of diabetes, such as may occur with pancreatitis.

Despite intense research over the past 25 years, the precise pathogenesis of human T2DM and the similar forms of diabetes in cats and nonhuman primates is incompletely understood. Much of the past research concentrated on the pathophysiology of insulin resistance in T2DM, but it has become increasingly clear that β-cell dysfunction and failure are central features of this disease process. This concept is highlighted by the observation that virtually all obese people and cats are insulin resistant, but only a small proportion of these individuals become diabetic. In people, as in cats, the development of this form of DM is characterized by progressive loss of β-cell function, which corresponds to the progressive loss of β cells in the pancreatic islets. The mechanisms underlying the loss of β cells are not fully understood but may involve one or more of the following mechanisms: glucose toxicity, lipid toxicity, and islet amyloidosis. Each of these mechanisms has been linked in one or more models of diabetes to the

loss of β cells, predominantly through apoptosis. Mounting evidence now implicates the development of islet amyloidosis (IA) as an important factor in both FDM and human T2DM, and it is the focus of the remainder of this discussion.

FDM occurs mainly in middle-aged and older cats and is characterized by obesity, resistance to ketoacidosis, low but measurable fasting serum insulin concentration, absent or attenuated first-phase insulin secretion, and exaggerated or absent second-phase insulin secretion (Johnson et al. 1986; Johnson et al. 1989b; O'Brien et al. 1985, 1993). The most notable pathological feature of the endocrine pancreas of diabetic cats is the occurrence of IA and partial loss of β cells (Johnson et al. 1986, 1989b; O'Brien et al. 1993) (see Figure 12.53). These clinical and pathological features closely resemble those of human T2DM.

The precursor protein of islet amyloid is the islet hormone called islet amyloid polypeptide (IAPP, also known as amylin), which is a 37-amino-acid polypeptide (Cooper et al. 1987; Westermark et al. 1987a, b). The pancreatic islets are the main site of IAPP production, and, within the pancreatic islets of all species thus far studied, IAPP immunoreactivity is located in the pancreatic β cells and, in some species, also in the δ cells (Johnson et al. 1988; Lukinius et al. 1989). As the morphological studies predicted, IAPP and insulin are cosecreted, although the relative amounts of each hormone secreted vary with the prevailing metabolic milieu (Butler et al. 1990; Fehmann et al. 1990; Inoue et al. 1991; O'Brien et al. 1991).

IA occurs in only a limited number of species (e.g., humans, macaques, and cats), usually in conjunction with diabetic syndromes associated with aging, and does not occur in rats or mice (Johnson et al. 1989b; O'Brien et al. 1993). This observation prompted the comparison of IAPP structures in these species, which revealed highly conserved regions in the amino-terminal region (residues 1 to 19) and in the carboxy-terminal region (residues 30 to 37) while the intervening region (residues 20 to 29) showed notable sequence variations (Betsholtz et al. 1989a). Secondary structural predictions of this latter region indicated a propensity for β-pleated sheet configuration for human IAPP, whereas this was not present in mice or rats (Betsholtz et al. 1989b). This latter finding is significant since β-sheet secondary structure is critical to amyloid fibril formation. Furthermore, in vitro, peptides corresponding to human IAPP 20 to 29 readily form amyloid fibrils, whereas mouse and rat sequences will not (Westermark et al. 1990). Evidence gathered so far indicates that no mutation in the IAPP coding region is required for the development of IA in FDM or in human T2DM (Westermark et al. 1987a, b; Sanke et al. 1988; Betsholtz et al. 1989b, 1990; Nakazato et al. 1990). However, it has recently been shown that a mutant form of human IAPP, the *S20G* mutant, is associated with early-onset T2DM (Sakagashira et al. 1996; Lee et al. 2001). Significantly, this mutant IAPP shows a greater propensity to form amyloid fibrils in vitro,

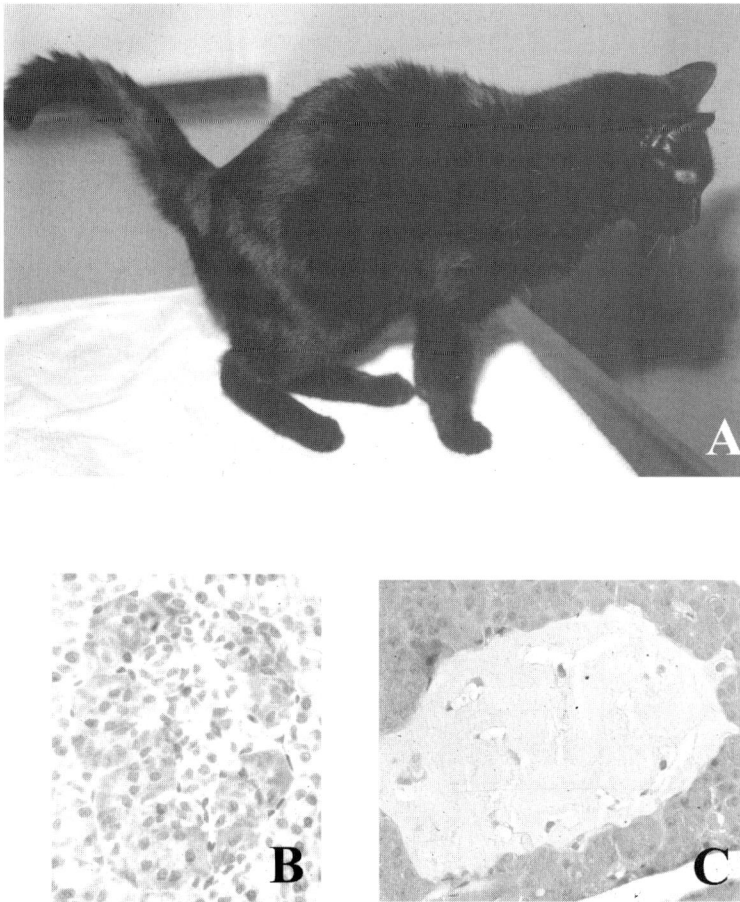

FIG. 12.53—Feline diabetes mellitus. **A:** A diabetic cat exhibiting moderate obesity. Note also the plantigrade stance in the hindlimbs that is characteristic of the peripheral polyneuropathy seen in some diabetic cats. **B:** A normal feline pancreatic islet that has been immunohistochemically stained for the presence of islet amyloid polypeptide (IAPP). IAPP occurs principally in the pancreatic β cells and is cosecreted with insulin. **C:** A pancreatic islet from a cat with diabetes mellitus. Note the extensive amyloid deposits that replace most of the normal islet tissues.

thus providing a potential link between amyloidogenicity and development of T2DM.

Simply having an IAPP sequence capable of forming amyloid fibrils is obviously insufficient for IA to develop, since not all people, cats, and macaques develop IA. It therefore appears likely that abnormalities in IAPP synthesis, processing, trafficking, secretion, or degradation by β cells must play a role in the pathogenesis of IA. One mechanism thought to be involved is increased secretion of IAPP (see Figure 12.54). Supporting this potential mechanism are studies in which increased IAPP secretion has been associated with obesity, which is an important predisposing factor for the development of FDM and human T2DM. Furthermore, it has been shown that the β cells of cats with impaired glucose tolerance have increased IAPP immunoreactivity (versus normal controls) and also

have an increased incidence of IA versus normal controls (Johnson et al. 1989a; Ma et al. 1998). Additional evidence in support of this hypothesis was recently demonstrated in an experimental cat model in which diabetes was induced by 50% pancreatectomy and treatment with drugs that produce insulin resistance (Hoenig et al. 2000). Diabetic cats were then treated with either insulin (reduces endogenous insulin and IAPP secretion) or glipizide (a sulfonyluria drug that increases endogenous insulin and IAPP secretion). In this study, glipizide-treated cats had significantly increased basal and glucose-stimulated serum IAPP concentrations (versus insulin-treated cats), and all developed IA, whereas IA formation in insulin-treated cats was almost completely prevented.

Another potentially important mechanism may involve an increase in the relative amounts of IAPP:

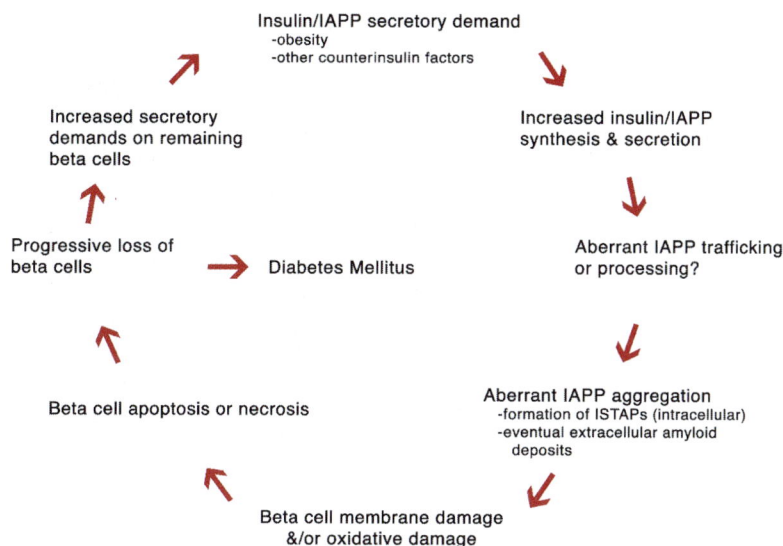

FIG. 12.54—Proposed pathogenesis for feline diabetes mellitus. IAPP, islet amyloid polypeptide; and ISTAPs, intermediate-sized toxic amyloid particles.

insulin produced and secreted by the β cells. Several in vitro studies have shown that islets in culture under varying conditions exhibit an increase in the relative amounts of IAPP secreted relative to insulin. For example, perfused pancreas from rats treated with dexamethasone or intraperitoneally administered glucose (hyperglycemic) show a significantly increased IAPP/insulin ratio in the perfusate when stimulated by 16.7 mM glucose, whereas pancreas from fasted rats showed a significantly reduced IAPP/insulin ratio (O'Brien et al. 1991). A recent study has also shown that when human islets in culture are exposed to 24.4 mM glucose, there is an increase in the cellular IAPP/insulin ratio and a similar increase in the mRNA ratios of these hormones. Under these conditions, the human islets also showed an increase in the amount of IAPP secreted through the constitutive pathway (Gasa et al. 2001). Recently, it has also been shown in a mouse model of insulin resistance that a high-fat diet was associated with maintenance of IAPP mRNA levels relative to low-fat controls, whereas insulin mRNA expression was decreased (Mulder et al. 2000). The aforementioned findings taken together show that conditions present in the diabetic state (hyperglycemia and corticosteroid excess) and in the prediabetic state (insulin resistance and hypertriglyceridemia) may increase the absolute amount of IAPP synthesized and secreted and, furthermore, may increase the IAPP/insulin ratio. In addition, experiments showing that insulin inhibits IAPP amyloidogenesis suggest a possible role for increased IAPP/insulin ratio expression in the development of IA (Kudva et al. 1998).

Evidence gathered from several human IAPP (hIAPP)-transgenic mouse models indicates that IAPP fibrillogenesis is involved in the destruction of β cells and the development of DM (De Koning et al. 1994; Couce et al. 1996; Jansen et al. 1996; Verchere et al. 1996; Soeller et al. 1998; Höppener et al. 2000). In these models, there was development of DM associated with IA. β Cells frequently contained abnormal IAPP-immunoreactive deposits within their cytoplasm, and in many instances there were actual amyloid fibrils within their cytoplasm or in the interstitium surrounding the β cells. Frequently, affected β cells had ultrastructural degenerative changes and alterations consistent with apoptosis. In each of these transgenic models, the production of high levels of hIAPP by the β cells was associated with the formation of abnormal IAPP aggregates, selective β-cell loss, and the development of DM, changes that closely recapitulate the islet lesions in FDM and human T2DM.

Several studies have demonstrated that IAPP-derived amyloid fibrils are cytotoxic and associated with apoptotic cell death and/or necrosis. COS-1 cells (mammalian cell line) that were transfected with hIAPP and expressed it at high levels developed intracellular IAPP-derived amyloid fibrils, and by 96 hours these cells were undergoing marked degenerative changes and apoptosis (O'Brien et al. 1995; Hiddinga and Eberhardt 1999). In contrast, COS-1 cells transfected with nonamyloidogenic rat IAPP (with similar high expression of IAPP) exhibited no adverse effects. hIAPP-derived fibrils have also been shown to be toxic to isolated islets in culture and to induce apoptosis (Lorenzo et al. 1994). Likewise, hIAPP-derived fibrils are toxic to neurons and PC12 cells (rat pheochromocytoma cell line) with effects that are identical to those of Aβ (the fibrillogenic protein that forms amyloid deposits in Alzheimer's disease), whereas rodent IAPP is nontoxic (May et al. 1993; Mattson and Goodman 1995; Dore et al. 1997). For both IAPP and Aβ, it is the fibrillar polymers that are cytotoxic, whereas monomers and related nonamyloidogenic polypeptides are not cytotoxic (Lorenzo and Yanker 1994, 1996; Howlett et al. 1995; Schubert et al. 1995). Furthermore, it was recently demonstrated that fibrillar assemblies of IAPP in the range of 50,000 to 200,000 D are cytotoxic and disrupt cellular membranes (Janson et al. 1999). Interestingly, the toxicity of both hIAPP and Aβ fibrils can be counteracted in cultured neurons by insulin-like growth factor I (Dore et al. 1997) and Congo red (Burgevin et al. 1994), whereas rifampicin and its analogues inhibit the toxicity of fibrillar IAPP and Aβ on PC12 cells (Mattson and Goodman 1995). These similarities in cytotoxicity by IAPP and Aβ fibrils support the concept that similar mechanisms are involved in neuronal cell death in Alzheimer's disease and β-cell death in type II DM.

The demonstrated similarities of IAPP and Aβ fibril cytotoxicity suggest that the mechanisms of Aβ toxicity in neurons are similar to the mechanisms by which IAPP-derived amyloid fibrils damage β cells and therefore may illuminate cytotoxic mechanisms involved in β-cell damage by IAPP fibrils. Mechanisms involved in Aβ cytotoxicity include oxidative damage by reactive oxygen species, lipid peroxidation, reduced mitochondrial transmembrane potential, and destabilization of intracellular calcium homeostasis (Hensley et al. 1994; Mark et al. 1997a, b). Membrane lipid peroxidation initiated by Aβ induces apoptosis in PC12 cells and cultured hippocampal neurons. This process is mediated by 4-hydroxynonenal and is prevented by Bcl-2 and antioxidants (Kruman et al. 1997). Furthermore, the neuroprotective actions of cycloheximide against Aβ induction of apoptosis are mediated by increased expression of the bcl-2 gene product (Furukawa et al. 1997). Aβ toxicity on hippocampal neurons is also prevented by EUK-8, a synthetic catalytic free radical scavenger (Bruce et al. 1996). Of special interest is the finding that membrane lipid peroxidation initiated by Aβ is also associated with impaired glucose transport into cultured rat hippocampal neurons (Mark et al. 1997b). If similar alterations are induced in β cells by IAPP fibrillogenesis, this may be of critical importance in impairing normal β-cell function.

In summary, the body of evidence for an important role for IAPP-derived IA in the pathogenesis of FDM and T2DM is growing progressively larger. However, a great deal of work still needs to done to elucidate the mechanisms underlying the initiation and toxicity of IAPP fibrillogenesis and the apoptotic pathways involved in β-cell death. Furthermore, these mechanisms need to be unequivocally demonstrated to be operational in the feline (and human) β cell during the development and progression of FDM and T2DM.

REFERENCES

Almawi WY, Tamim H, Azar ST. 1999. Clinical review 103: T helper type 1 and 2 cytokines mediate the onset and progression of type 1 (insulin-dependent) diabetes. J Clin Endocrinol Metab 84:1497–1502.

Baetens D, Malaisse-Lagae F, Perrelet A, Orci L. 1979. Endocrine pancreas: Three-dimensional reconstruction shows two types of islets of Langerhans. Science 206:1323–1325.

Bencosome SA, Liepa E. 1955. Regional differences of the pancreatic islet. Endocrinology 57:588–593.

Betsholtz C, Christmanson L, Engstrom U, et al. 1989a. Sequence divergence in a specific region of islet amyloid polypeptide (IAPP) explains differences in islet amyloid formation between species. FEBS Lett 251:261–264.

Betsholtz C, Svensson V, Rorsman F, et al. 1989b. Islet amyloid polypeptide (IAPP): cDNA cloning and identification of an amyloidogenic region associated with the species-specific occurrence of age-related diabetes mellitus. Exp Cell Res 183:484–493.

Betsholtz C, Christmanson L, Engstrom U, et al. 1990. Structure of cat islet amyloid polypeptide and identification of amino acid residues of potential significance for islet amyloid formation. Diabetes 39:118–122.

Bonner-Weir S, Like AA. 1980. A dual population of islets of Langerhans in bovine pancreas. Cell Tissue Res 206:157.

Boosinger TR, Zerbe CA, Grabau JH, Pletcher JM. 1988. Multihormonal pancreatic endocrine neoplasm in a dog with duodenal ulcers and hypertrophic gastropathy. Vet Pathol 25:237–239.

Bruce AJ, Malfroy B, Baudry M. 1996. Beta-amyloid toxicity in organotypic hippocampal cultures: Protection by EUK-8, a synthetic catalytic free radical scavenger. Proc Natl Acad Sci USA 93:2312–2316.

Burgevin MC, Passat M, Daniel N, et al. 1994. Congo red protects against toxicity of beta-amyloid peptides on rat hippocampal neurones. Neuroreport 5:2429–2432.

Butler PC, Chou J, Carter WB, et al. 1990. Effects of meal ingestion on plasma amylin concentration in NIDDM and nondiabetic humans. Diabetes 39:752–756.

Caywood DD, Klausner JS, O'Leary TP. 1987. Pancreatic insulin-secreting neoplasms: Clinical, diagnostic, and prognostic features in 73 dogs. J Am Anim Hosp Assoc 24:578–584.

Cooper GJS, Willis AC, Clark A, et al. 1987. Purification and characterization of a peptide from amyloid-rich pancreases of type 2 diabetic patients. Proc Natl Acad Sci USA 84:8628–8632.

Couce M, Kane LA, O'Brien TD, et al. 1996. Treatment with growth hormone and dexamethasone in mice transgenic for human islet amyloid polypeptide causes islet amyloidosis and β-cell dysfunction. Diabetes 45:1094–1101.

De Koning EJ, Morris ER, Hofhuis FM, et al. 1994. Intra- and extracellular amyloid fibrils are formed in cultured pancreatic islets of transgenic mice expressing human islet amyloid polypeptide. Proc Natl Acad Sci USA 91:8467–8471.

Dore S, Kar S, Quirion R. 1997. Insulin-like growth factor I protects and rescues hippocampal neurons against beta-amyloid- and human amylin-induced toxicity. Proc Natl Acad Sci USA 94:4772–4777.

Elie M, Hoenig M. 1995. Canine immune-mediated diabetes mellitus: A case report. J Am Anim Hosp Assoc 31:295–299.

Erlandsen SL. 1980 Types of pancreatic islet cells and their immunocytochemical identification. Int Acad Pathol Monogr, 21:140–155.

Falcone M, Sarvetnick N. 1999. The effect of local production of cytokines in the pathogenesis of insulin-dependent diabetes mellitus. Clin Immunol 90:2–9.

Fehmann HC, Weber V, Goke R, et al. 1990. Cosecretion of amylin and insulin from isolated rat pancreas. FEBS Lett 262:279–281.

Furukawa K, Estus S, Fu W, et al. 1997. Neuroprotective action of cycloheximide involves induction of bcl-2 and antioxidant pathways. J Cell Biol 136:1137–1149.

Gale EA. 2001. The discovery of type 1 diabetes. Diabetes 50:217–226.

Gasa A, Gomis R, Casamitjana R, Novials A. 2001. High glucose concentration favors the selective secretion of islet amyloid polypeptide through a constitutive secretory pathway in human pancreatic islets. Pancreas 22:307–310.

Goldstein MB, Davis EA. 1968. The three dimensional architecture of the islets of Langerhans. Acta Anat (Basel) 71:161–171.

Gross TL, O'Brien TD, Davies AP, Long RE. 1990. Glucagon-producing pancreatic endocrine neoplasms in two dogs with superficial necrolytic dermatitis. J Am Vet Med Assoc 197:1619–1622.

Happe RP, Van der Gaag I, Lamers CBHW, et al. 1980. Zollinger-Ellison syndrome in three dogs. Vet Pathol 17:177–186.

Hawkins KL, Summers BA, Kuhajda FP, Smith CA. 1987. Immunocytochemistry of normal pancreatic islets and spontaneous islet cell neoplasms in dogs. Vet Pathol 24:170–179.

Hayden DW, Henson MS. 1997. Gastrin-secreting pancreatic endocrine neoplasm in a dog (putative Zollinger-Ellison syndrome). J Vet Diagn Invest 9:100–103.

Hensley K, Carney JM, Mattson MP, et al. 1994. A model for beta-amyloid aggregation and neurotoxicity based on free radical generation by the peptide: Relevance to Alzheimer disease. Proc Natl Acad Sci USA 91:3270–3274.

Hiddinga HJ, Eberhardt NL. 1999. Intracellular amyloidogenesis by human islet amyloid polypeptide induces apoptosis in COS-1 cells. Am J Pathol 154:1077–1088.

Hoenig M. 1995. Pathophysiology of canine diabetes. Vet Clin North Am 25:553–561.

Hoenig M, Dawe DL. 1992. A qualitative assay for beta cell antibodies. J Vet Immunol Immunopathol 32:195–203.

Hoenig M, Hall G, Ferguson D, Jordan K, et al. 2000. A feline model of experimentally induced islet amyloidosis. Am J Pathol 157:2143–2150.

Höppener JWM, Ahrén B, Lips CJM. 2000. Islet amyloid and type 2 diabetes mellitus. N Engl J Med 343:411–419.

Howlett DR, Jennings KH, Lee DC, et al. 1995. Aggregation state and neurotoxic properties of Alzheimer beta-amyloid peptide. Neurodegeneration 4:23–32.

Inoue K, Hisatomi A, Umeda F, Nawata H. 1991. Release of amylin from perfused rat pancreas in response to glucose, arginine, β-hydroxybutyrate, and gliclazide. Diabetes 40:1005–1009.

Janson J, Soeller WC, Roche PC, et al. 1996. Spontaneous diabetes mellitus in transgenic mice expressing human islet amyloid polypeptide. Proc Natl Acad Sci USA 93:7283–7288.

Janson J, Ashley RH, Harrison D, et al. 1999. The mechanism of islet amyloid polypeptide toxicity is membrane disruption by intermediate-sized toxic amyloid particles. Diabetes 48:491–498.

Johnson KH, Hayden DW, O'Brien TD, Westermark P. 1986. Animal model of human disease: Spontaneous diabetes mellitus-islet amyloid complex in adult cats. Am J Pathol 125:416–419.

Johnson KH, O'Brien TD, Hayden DW, et al. 1988. Immunolocalization of islet amyloid polypeptide (IAPP) in pancreatic beta cells by means of peroxidase-antiperoxidase (PAP) and protein A-gold techniques. Am J Pathol 130:1–8.

Johnson KH, O'Brien TD, Jordan K, Westermark P. 1989a. Impaired glucose tolerance is associated with increased islet amyloid polypeptide (IAPP) immunoreactivity in pancreatic beta cells. Am J Pathol 135:245–250.

Johnson KH, O'Brien TD, Westermark P. 1989b. Medical intelligence: Islet amyloid, islet amyloid polypeptide and diabetes mellitus. N Engl J Med 321:513–518.

Klöppel G, Drenck CR. 1983. Immunzytochemische Morphometrie beim Typ-I- und Typ-II-Diabetes Mellitus. Dtsch Med Wochenschr 108:188–189.

Kruman I, Bruce-Keller AJ, Bredesen D, et al. 1997. Evidence that 4-hydroxynonenal mediates oxidative stress-induced neuronal apoptosis. J Neurosci 17:5089–5100.

Kudva YC, Mueske C, Butler PC, Eberhardt NL. 1998. A novel assay in vitro of human IAPP amyloidogenesis and effects of insulin secretory vesicle proteins on amyloid formation. Biochem J 331:809–813.

LaPerle KMD, Bloome EAG, Capen CC, et al. 2003. Effect of Exogenous Human Sodium/Iodide Symporter Expression on Growth of MATLyLu Cells. Thyroid 13:133–140.

Lee SC, Hashim Y, Li JKY, et al. 2001. The islet amyloid polypeptide (amylin) gene *S20G* mutation in Chinese subjects: Evidence for associations with type 2 diabetes and cholesterol levels. Clin Endocrinol 54:541–546.

Lorenzo A, Yankner BA. 1994. Beta-amyloid neurotoxicity requires fibril formation and is inhibited by Congo red. Proc Natl Acad Sci USA 91:12,243–12,247.

Lorenzo A, Yankner BA. 1996. Amyloid fibril toxicity in Alzheimer's disease and diabetes. Ann NY Acad Sci 777:89–95.

Lorenzo A, Razzaboni R, Weir GC, Yankner BA. 1994. Pancreatic islet cell toxicity of amylin associated with type-2 diabetes mellitus. Nature 368:756–760.

Lukinius A, Wilander E, Westermark GT, et al. 1989. Co-localization of islet amyloid polypeptide and insulin in the B cell secretory granules of the human pancreatic islets. Diabetologia 32:240–244.

Ma Z, Westermark GT, Johnson KH, et al. 1998. Quantitative immunohistochemical analysis of islet amyloid polypeptide (IAPP) in normal, impaired glucose tolerant, and diabetic cats. Amyloid. Int J Exp Clin Invest 5:255–261.

Mark RJ, Keller JN, Kruman I, Mattson MP. 1997a. Basic FGF attenuates amyloid beta-peptide-induced oxidative stress, mitochondrial dysfunction, and impairment of Na+/K+-ATPase activity in hippocampal neurons. Brain Res 756:205–214.

Mark RJ, Pang Z, Geddes JW, et al. 1997b. Amyloid beta-peptide impairs glucose transport in hippocampal and cortical neurons: Involvement of membrane lipid peroxidation. J Neurosci 17:1046–1054.

Mattson MP, Goodman Y. 1995. Different amyloidogenic peptides share a similar mechanism of neurotoxicity involving reactive oxygen species and calcium. Brain Res 676:219–224.

May PC, Boggs LN, Fuson KS. 1993. Neurotoxicity of human amylin in rat primary hippocampal cultures: Similarity to Alzheimer's disease amyloid-β neurotoxicity. J Neurochem 61:2330–2333.

Mulder C, Martensson A, Sundler F, Ahren B. 2000. Differential changes in islet amyloid polypeptide (amylin) and insulin mRNA expression after high-fat diet-induced insulin resistance in C57BL/6J mice. Metab Clin Exp 49:1518–1522.

Nakazato M, Asai J, Miyazato M, et al. 1990. Isolation and identification of islet amyloid polypeptide in normal human pancreas. Regul Pept 31:179–186.

O'Brien TD, Hayden DW, Johnson KH, Stevens JB. 1985. High dose intravenous glucose tolerance test and serum insulin and glucagon levels in diabetic and non-diabetic cats: Relationships to insular amyloidosis. Vet Pathol 22:250–261

O'Brien TD, Hayden DW, Johnson KH, Fletcher TF. 1986. Immunohistochemical morphometry of pancreatic endocrine cells in diabetic, normoglycemic glucose-intolerant and normal cats. J Comp Pathol 96:357–369.

O'Brien TD, Hayden DW, O'Leary TP, et al. 1987. Canine pancreatic endocrine tumors: Immunohistochemical analysis of hormone content and amyloid. Vet Pathol 24:308–314.

O'Brien TD, Westermark P, Johnson KH. 1990. Islet amyloid polypeptide and calcitonin gene-related peptide immunoreactivity in amyloid and neoplastic cells of canine pancreatic endocrine neoplasms. Vet Pathol 27:194–198.

O'Brien TD, Westermark P, Johnson KH. 1991. Islet amyloid polypeptide (IAPP) and insulin secretion from isolated perfused pancreas of fed, fasted, glucose-treated and dexamethasone-treated rats. Diabetes 40:1701–1706.

O'Brien TD, Butler PC, Westermark P, Johnson KH. 1993. Islet amyloid polypeptide: A review of its biology and potential roles in the pathogenesis of diabetes mellitus. Vet Pathol 30:317–332.

O'Brien TD, Butler PC, Kreutter DK, et al. 1995. Intracellular amyloid associated with cytotoxicity in COS-1 cells expressing human islet amyloid polypeptide. Am J Pathol 147:609–616.

Orci L. 1982. Macro- and micro-domains in the endocrine pancreas. Diabetes 31:538–565.

Orci L, Malaisse-Lagae F, Baetens D, Perrelet A. 1978. Pancreatic-polypeptide-rich regions in human pancreas. Lancet 2:1200–1201.

Rahier J, Wallon J, Henquin J-C. 1981. Cell populations in the endocrine pancreas of human neonates and infants. Diabetologia 20:540–546.

Rahier J, Goebbels RM, Henquin JC. 1983. Cellular composition of the human diabetic pancreas. Diabetologia 24:366–371.

Saito K, Yaginuma N, Takahashi T. 1979. Differential volumetry of A, B, and D cells in the pancreatic islets of diabetic and nondiabetic subjects. Tohoku J Exp Med 129:273–283.

Sakagashira S, Sanke T, Hanabusa T, et al. 1996. Missense mutation of amylin gene (*S20G*) in Japanese NIDDM patients. Diabetes 45:1279–1281.

Saladino CF, Getty R. 1972. Quantitative study on the islets of Langerhans of the beagle as a function of age. Exp Gerontol 7:91–97.

Sanke T, Bell GI, Sample C, et al. 1988. An islet amyloid peptide is derived from and 89-amino acid precursor by proteolytic processing. J Biol Chem 263:17,243–17,246.

Signore A, Annovazzi A, Gradini R, et al. 1998. Fas and Fas ligand-mediated apoptosis and its role in autoimmune diabetes. Diabetes Metab Res Rev 14:197–206.

Schubert D, Behl C, Lesley R, et al. 1995. Amyloid peptides are toxic via a common oxidative mechanism. Proc Natl Acad Sci USA 92:1989–1993.

Soeller WC, Janson J, Hart SE, et al. 1998. Islet amyloid-associated diabetes in obese A^{vy}/a mice expressing human islet amyloid polypeptide. Diabetes 47:743–750.

Stefan Y, Orci L, Malaisse-Lagae F, et al. 1982. Quantitation of endocrine cell content in the pancreas of non-diabetic and diabetic humans. Diabetes 31:694–700.

Thomas TB. 1937. Cellular components of the mammalian islets of Langerhans. Am J Anat 62:31–57.

Thomas HE, Kay TW. 2000. Beta cell destruction in the development of autoimmune diabetes in the non-obese diabetic (NOD) mouse. Diabetes Metab Res Rev 16:251–261.

Torres S, Caywood DD, O'Brien TD, et al. 1997. Resolution of superficial necrolytic dermatitis signs after surgical resection of a glucagons-secreting endocrine neoplasm in a dog. J Am Anim Hosp Assoc 33:313–318.

Verchere CB, D'Alessio DA, Palmiter RD, et al. 1996. Islet amyloid formation associated with hyperglycemia in transgenic mice with pancreatic beta cell expression of human islet amyloid polypeptide. Proc Natl Acad Sci USA 93:3492–3496.

Wellman KF, Volk BW, Brancato P. 1971. Ultrastructure and insulin content of the endocrine pancreas in the human fetus. Lab Invest 25:97–103.

Westermark P, Wernstedt C, O'Brien TD, et al. 1987a. Islet amyloid in type 2 human diabetes mellitus and adult diabetic cats is composed of a novel putative polypeptide hormone. Am J Pathol 127:414–417.

Westermark P, Wernstedt C, Wilander E, et al. 1987b. Amyloid fibrils in human insulinoma and islets of Langerhans of the diabetic cat are derived from a neuropeptide-like protein also present in normal islet cells. Proc Natl Acad Sci USA 84:3881–3885.

Westermark P, Engström U, Johnson KH, et al. 1990. Islet amyloid polypeptide: Pinpointing amino acid residues linked to amyloid fibril formation. Proc Natl Acad Sci USA 87:5036–5040.

Zerbe CA, Boosinger TR, Grabau JH, et al. 1989. Pancreatic polypeptide and insulin-secreting neoplasm in a dog with duodenal ulcers and hypertrophic gastritis. J Vet Intern Med 3:178–182.

13

PATHOPHYSIOLOGY OF HOMEOSTATIC AND TOXIC DISORDERS

Robert H. Dunlop

Acquiring an understanding of pathophysiology involves an initial consideration of the physiological limits to adaptation to extremes of the environment and the challenges these present to, in our case, the range of domesticated mammalian species. This involves reviewing the factors responsible for setting the limits of the geographic distribution of these species. Reductionist biomedical science suffers from the absence of a context within which to examine the variability of the multitude of interacting physiological and pathophysiological responses and mechanisms. Only very late was the realization arrived at that *evolution of physiological systems* would become an important researchable area relevant to pathophysiology. Thus, there has been an inadequate research effort and focus on the potential of comparative contributions involving analysis of dysfunctions attributable to ecological, behavioral, and phylogenetic constraints. Although the core of this approach is the pathophysiology of the individual animal, the nature of animal production and molecular advances in genetic research mandates consideration of the population-based aspects, as well. This chapter deals with these aspects that have a particular focus involving the nervous system that are attributable to or involve nutritional, metabolic, or toxic factors. Often these types of condition involve multiple organ systems and their interactions.

PART 1: PATHOPHYSIOLOGY OF THE METABOLIC BALANCE

THE HYPOTHALAMUS: THE BODY'S METABOLIC EXECUTIVE. The hypothalamus, sited in the lower midbrain immediately above the stalk to the pituitary gland is the central autonomic "intelligence" unit that monitors and directs adjustments to metabolic programs throughout the mammalian body. As such, it is the executive center whose departments ensure hour-by-hour, day-to-day function, survival, and adaptation of the organism: "Assignment Homeostasis" It monitors the performance of bodily organ systems and their responses to internal defects and challenges brought about by stressful events. It is the central conductor of many facets of autonomic, endocrine, and somatomotor functions, as well as a myriad of influences on behavioral responses. Many of its regulatory functions, particularly those relating to sensory systems and skeletal muscle operation, can be overridden by conscious behaviors. However, the core ones dealing with so-called vegetative functions are largely autonomous, making the body a self-correcting machine designed for survival in the face of adversity. Only the inexorable and unforgiving march of biological evolution adapting through selection against those individuals found to be unable to withstand the physical and biological hazards of their current environment (or meet the expectations of the breeders) has endured.

The range of functions subject to regulatory coordination by the hypothalamus is remarkable. It includes many aspects of food-intake regulation, electrolyte and water metabolism, temperature regulation, circadian rhythms, and arousal. The autonomous contribution of the hypothalamus to maintaining and restoring homeostasis at the physiological level is closely meshed with functions that rise to the level of consciousness and are subject to complex behavioral programming, such as

1. Mental arousal, awareness and survival responses (including the primitive *fight or flight*).

2. Foraging perception, motivation, and behavior from the neonatal seeking the nipple to the growing awareness of food to replace milk, using the special senses as well as the subconscious metabolic drives, learning the arts of biting, chewing, swallowing, eructation, drinking water, and competing.

3. An element of learning can be added to the autonomous responses involved in the elimination of wastes via urine and feces. At later stages, reproductive arousal and performance must also be learned, to some extent aided by autonomous olfactory, visual, and other stimuli. The importance of memory has not been given the attention it deserves in studies of mammalian function and behavior.

The vital functions of the circulatory and respiratory systems are based in the medulla oblongata, but they too have hypothalamic and higher cortical connections.

Overall, the basal needs of mammals are preprogrammed into neuronal and effector systems so that they are instinctive from birth. However, newborns have a great deal of learning to do. They come equipped with a metabolic platform for survival with maternal nourishment and protection plus the reflexes to ensure respiratory and circulatory function. The former involves the neurons of the hypothalamus and limbic system, and the latter involves the medulla. Progressively imposed on this platform are the learned behaviors necessary for individual autonomy after weaning. This includes everything from learning how to get up and walk to perceiving the environment as a potential source of food, water, and hazards.

Aspects of memory in domestic mammals received a significant boost from a team at the Laboratory of Cognitive and Developmental Neuroscience at Babraham Institute at Cambridge, U.K., led by Keith Kendrick (*Nature*, November 8, 2001). Their sheep were able to remember 50 other sheep faces for over 2 years. A small population of cells in the temporal and prefrontal cortices in the sheep's brains encoded faces, just as in humans. They even vocalized in response to face pictures just as they did to actual faces.

Metabolism in Hibernation. The extraordinary potential of evolved metabolic adaptations to deal with extreme environmental conditions is well exemplified by the pattern of metabolism in the North American black bear during its winter hibernation. Retreating into a den that provides shelter from extremes of cold and of gas exchange (oxygen in and carbon dioxide out) a typical bear passes up to 5 months without eating, drinking, urinating, or defecating even though its body temperature does not drop more than a few degrees Fahrenheit. The secret of its survival is mobilizing and oxidizing its fat stores. Remarkably, this yields enough water to compensate for the unavoidable insensible water loss from the skin and respiratory tract. Perhaps more surprising is the complete cessation of the need to excrete nitrogen-containing "waste" products that require water in the excreta; hence, the lack of need to pass urine or drink. Starving nonhibernators mobilize proteins and excrete extra nitrogen. So what magic switch enables a bear to pull off its metabolic marvel in which its blood urea nitrogen concentration actually falls during hibernation? It must convert N_2 by combining it internally with products that do not need to be excreted, allowing a much slower rate of urea formation. Also, the urea that is produced is reabsorbed from the bladder and returned to the gastrointestinal tract, where bacteria convert it into forms of N_2 the bear can use in metabolism, an example of natural recycling. The bear mobilizes lipids for energy, a process that yields glycerol as a basis for synthesis of amino acids, glucose, and lactate, but not urea. This allows "wasteless" maintenance, a sort of "survival anabolism." Bears give birth and suckle their young initially in the den while their independent thermoregulation is developing.

Brain Energy Homeostasis. Lab rats have a remarkable ability to balance their body's energy equation, matching output changes due to exercise and changes in metabolic activities with input changes by modifying their feeding behavior. The overall ability to sustain energy metabolism is based on adjustment of food intake to match need: an ergostatic system. The brain senses concentrations and/or whole-body content of circulating nutrients as a basis for making adjustments. It has an ongoing energy-dependent integrative process that parallels bodily processes, adjusts feeding responses, and is based on its own mechanisms and correlated processes (Panksepp 1998). This regulatory process operates throughout the day rather than responding to short-term signals.

Panksepp's studies with parabiotic (i.e., shared circulation surgically joined via a skin flap) man-made Siamese-type twins were fascinating. Each ate less until each had half the fat content of a normal rat; that is, each brain perceived its metabolic status as if it had a single rather than double fat content. Seemingly, the circulating metabolic signals of the two brains and bodies were integrated with each rat contributing half of a critical signal. The receiving station would be in the *ventromedial hypothalamus* (VMH). Lesions of this area were known to result in overeating progressing to obesity. Joining a VMH-lesioned rat to a normal partner had no effect on the lesioned rat, but the brain of the normal rat detected too strong a repletion signal from the lesioned one, lost its appetite completely, and became emaciated. Direct administration of glucose into the VMH does not make a short-term satiety signal but, instead, a longer-term one of body energy integration. Thus, injecting glucose into the brain reduced daily food intake but not the size of the meal that followed.

Feeding control areas are found in several sites in the brain from (a) the frontal cortical and temporal areas that register the value of specific foods to (b) brainstem areas that govern chewing, swallowing, gustatory acceptance, and so forth.

Lateral hypothalamus (LH) areas, if damaged, lead to severe feeding deficits. The LH handles complex integration of sensory and motor activities required as psychobehavioral routines (programs). Many of these are governed by interactions with the basal ganglia, especially ventral striatal areas such as the nucleus accumbens and ventromedial zones of the caudate nucleus (of the dorsal striatum). Massive LH lesions result in parkinsonian near paralysis with a very high metabolic rate and rapid deterioration.

Hormonal Roles in Metabolic Homeostasis in Mammals. All mammalian functions require *energy*. Specific hormones regulate its availability and use within the animal. Integrated with these subconscious biochemical signaling agents are neural programs and conscious behavioral activities that influence homeostasis. Extracorporeal factors also play major roles in defining the adaptations that are required to cope with the mammal's physical and biological environment.

Tissues and cells vary in their requirements for material and energy supply and waste disposal.

One group of hormones participates actively in energy homeostatic regulation. These can be considered to be the *metabolic hormones* that have been identified as such to date. They are *insulin, glucocorticoids, glucagon,* and *epinephrine*. In addition, more specialized general metabolic effects are attributable to *thyroid hormones* and *growth hormone* (GH). The metabolic function of T3 is primarily to ensure that core body *temperature* can be maintained while that of GH is to link the energy needed for growth to *actual* growth. On the other hand insulin, glucocorticoids, glucagon, and epinephrine direct the flows of the major metabolic fuels within the body (carbohydrate, lipid, and protein). The newcomer, *leptin*, is a signal that may dictate food intake.

A perspective on energy in homeostasis: Mammals require energy continuously to survive and function. However, they ingest food intermittently either as an occasional large meal, as in wild carnivores, or at feeding time, in human-managed production or maintenance systems. Alternatively, they may get their nourishment via grazing by pasture-fed or range-fed domestic ruminants, other herbivores, and even some omnivores such as outdoor-housed pigs. Given intermittent ingestion, mammals must have some capacity for storage to bridge the intervals between fuel intakes when they will have to be mobilized. The individual organ systems are interdependent, some focusing on storage of energy, while others focus on its functional use.

Neuroendocrine orchestration of a very complex system is the key, using modulation of the activities of regulatory enzymes that manipulate the fluxes of materials and energy, aided by feedback loops to maintain the necessary balance. Some fuels are essential for survival; for example, the plasma glucose level must be kept in a tight range if dysfunction is to be avoided. The rapidly available reserve is in the form of glycogen that is capped and kept close to that level by converting any excess to fat. Proteins can be used for gluconeogenesis to replenish plasma glucose if needed. Proteins have many other functions, but the overall level is kept near a ceiling above which they too are converted to fat stores. However, fats cannot be converted to proteins or carbohydrates directly.

Use of any metabolic fuel for energy occurs *only if it is needed*. If it overeats on carbohydrates, lipids, or proteins, a mammal lacks a mechanism to use the excess by simply converting it to carbon dioxide and water and then eliminating these products.

Thus, the excess intake mainly goes to fat. Oxidation of the metabolic fuels is tightly coupled to the production and use of energy. The citric acid cycle and β-oxidation are geared to electron transport. The electron pairs are transferred to the coenzymes isocitrate dehydrogenase [the oxidized form of nicotinamide adenine dinucleotide (NAD^+)] and flavin adenine dinucleotide (FAD) during the glycolytic and citric acid cycle enzyme catalysis. They pass to the mitochondrial electron-transport chain of linked electron carriers. This remarkably conservative process allows for reoxidation of the coenzymes so they can keep metabolic pathways operating. The electrons participate in a very dynamic sequential series of redox steps during which electrons are expelled from the mitochondria, creating an electrochemical *proton gradient* across the mitochondrial membrane that drives the synthesis of adenosine triphosphate (ATP) from adenosine diphosphate (ADP) and inorganic phosphate (*oxidative phosphorylation*).

Because electron transport is so tightly coupled to oxidative phosphorylation and the supply and demand for ADP and ATP, the citric acid cycle functions only when ADP is available. This is only the case when ATP is being utilized, because the amount of adenine nucleotides is limited. As a consequence, the oxidation of primary food fuels cannot occur at a rate needed to handle an excessive influx and eliminate it as waste. The important nutritional concept is that *regulation of body weight* is accomplished by regulation of food intake, aided by the effects of *heat loss and physical exercise*.

Another major concept is that almost all oxygen used by mammals is used for mitochondrial production of ATP. A resting mammal's brain accounts for 20% of its oxygen use, yet is only about 2% of body mass. The situation changes when the animal engages in muscular work. At rest, skeletal muscle, about 40% or so of body weight, uses only about 30% of the oxygen being used. In hard muscular work, total oxygen used by muscle can rise by up to 10-fold. Brain use does not change much. There is a large increase in use of metabolic fuels to the sites at need while maintaining brain at its vital level, along with other adjustments to maintain homeostasis and the function of other vital organs.

Homeostatic regulatory processes deploy *organ interdependency* to achieve the adaptations necessary to cope with change in the most "rational" way. For example, skeletal muscle has the highest glycolytic capacity because it must be able to generate ATP rapidly for contraction, an evolutionary priority. The brain must have glucose available as its primary source of energy, so it gets priority of this fuel. Even the heart can use various metabolic fuels and thus is less dependent on glucose than is the brain. Liver and kidney are not major users of glucose but rely mainly on fatty-acid oxidation enzymes that catalyze rate-limiting steps of glycolysis (phosphofructokinase and pyruvate kinase), reflecting their glycolytic capacity. Similarly, for the rate-limiting steps of gluconeogenesis, liver and kidney are high in the relevant enzymes enabling them to make rather than use glucose. Other tissues use glucose and cannot make it.

HYPOTHALAMIC-HYPOPHYSEAL-ADRENAL METABOLIC REGULATION. Each adrenal is comprised of a cortex (90%) and a medulla (10%). Some of the arterial blood supplying the adrenal passes through the cortex, picking up some cortical steroids en route. The cortisol reaching the medulla facilitates the synthesis of catecholamines by phenylethanolamine-*N*-methyltransferase (PNMT) that converts norepinephrine to epinephrine. Without it, only norepinephrine would be produced. The outer layer of the cortex—the zona glomerulosa—produces mineralocorticoids, notably aldosterone but also some corticosterone, under the influence of the renin-angiotensin system. It should be noted that adrenocorticotropic hormone (ACTH) has little effect on aldosterone secretion. The middle layer or zona fasciculata produces mainly cortisol and androgens. The inner zona reticularis makes mostly androgens plus some cortisol. The main adrenal form of androgen is dehydroepiandrosterone (DHEA) in the sulfate form. The latter two layers are linked and both are ACTH dependent. During gestation, there is an innermost fetal layer that degenerates soon after birth. It makes DHEA that is convertible to estrogens by the placenta. The chromaffin cells of the adrenal medulla are derived from the neural crest, making them equivalent to postsynaptic cells of a sympathetic ganglion except that they release their catecholamine transmitters into the blood to stimulate adrenergic receptors at a distance.

The regulation of glucocorticoid (i.e., cortisol) secretion is controlled by the 41-amino-acid peptide *corticotropin-releasing hormone* (CRH) that is *made in the hypothalamus*. Then CRH is conveyed by the hypothalamic-hypophyseal portal system (HHPS) vessels to the anterior pituitary, where it stimulates the secretion of ACTH into the blood for transport to the adrenal cortex. There it evokes the secretion of cortisol and some androgen. The CRH stimulates release of all agents derived from propiomelanocortin (POMC), including vasopressin, which has some additional capacity to evoke ACTH release. The isolation of CRH was an extraordinary research achievement because it is released as a complex. On arrival at the pituitary, CRH stimulates only the corticotropic cells, which hypertrophy and produce more ACTH. Many stresses stimulate CRH secretion, including cold exposure, burns, trauma, anesthesia, surgery, postoperative recovery procedures, and psychological distress.

In humans, it has been shown that there is a marked *circadian rhythm in ACTH secretion*. Its secretion is pulsatile, with about 8 pulses every 3 hours. The diurnal rhythm shows a peak of secretion on arousal and early morning, which tapers off gradually with low plasma levels during the night. ACTH is a peptide of 39 amino acids, of which the first 23 are needed for full activity and appear to be conserved in all mammalian species. The half-life of the hormone in plasma is about 5 minutes. Both ACTH and cortisol are negative-feedback inhibitors of CRH synthesis, as are exogenous glucocorticoids. Flying across time zones distorts the diurnal rhythm for a week or more. Plasma cortisol is bound mainly to cortisol-binding globulin, where it is inactive but serves as a reservoir to dampen the pulsatile secretory changes. The half-life of cortisol in plasma is quite long (over 1 hour).

METABOLIC EFFECTS OF CORTISOL. Cortisol is essential but is a double-edged sword. Required for responses to stressful situations, in excess it can give rise to severe pathophysiology. It is classed as a permissive agent because it permits a number of metabolic processes to be influenced by other agents without interference, while not having initiated them. It enters its target cell by diffusion, binds to its receptor, and moves to the nucleus, where it initiates transcription, splicing, and export of messenger RNA (mRNA) and the encoded proteins that are the actual effectors of the response to the hormone.

The metabolic impacts are complex. *Cortisol increases glucose production in liver by increasing gluconeogenesis,* by hastening release of substrate from other tissues, and by increasing protein breakdown while decreasing protein synthesis. It is also permissive to the gluconeogenetic effect of other hormones: glucagon and epinephrine. It increases glycerol release from triglycerides by promoting lipolysis. It expedites glycogenolysis in muscle, resulting in lactate formation. Insulin-mediated glucose uptake by muscle is inhibited by the effects of cortisol, which reduces glucose utilization at the cost of muscle. It also inhibits uptake and metabolism of glucose in adipose tissues, fat cells, fibroblasts, and lymphoid tissues by decreasing the transporter, mRNA. The interesting consequence is that *the hyperglycemia resulting from increases in glucocorticoids evokes an increase in insulin secretion that fails to lower plasma glucose because the cortisol causes insulin resistance.* This is a glucose intolerance not unlike that seen in type 2 diabetes mellitus, in which excess cortisol effects can lead to extreme hyperglycemia. In cortisol deficiency, hypoglycemia may occur. Note that, in Cushing's syndrome (unregulated overproduction of CRH or ACTH due to a hypothalamic or pituitary tumor), muscle wasting becomes extreme. The appearance of Cushing's syndrome in people is characterized by an abnormal pattern of fat deposition, with a puffy face and heavy trunk coupled with wasting of limb musculature. Cortisol increases appetite that can upset metabolic regulation of body mass.

ANTI-INFLAMMATORY EFFECTS OF GLUCOCORTICOIDS. The interactive actions among metabolic and immunologic effects of hormones are complex and a valuable resource text is Griffin and Ojeda (2000). Not to be overlooked is the close interaction between the hypothalamic-pituitary-adrenal (HPA) axis and the immune system. This can be a useful consequence in autoimmune diseases and allergies. On the other hand, chronic infectious lesions, like those of tuberculosis and others in which the infectious agent has not been eliminated, may be reactivated and overwhelm the host. Administration of cortisol results in a drop in peripheral lymphocyte and monocyte counts within a few hours (T cells being affected more than B cells) by virtue of redistribution from the vascular compartment to spleen, lymphatic system, and bone marrow, whereas neutrophils do the opposite and increase in peripheral count. The immune-suppressing effect of glucocorticoids is often exploited in chronic inflammatory conditions such as arthritis. Interleukin 1 (IL-1) stimulates the release of CRH that stimulates the HPA axis and vice versa. This is suggestive of interregulatory coordination between the adrenal cortex and the immune response. The pathophysiology of stress and viral infections stimulates this system. Effects of many viral infections include a phase of immune suppression involving cell-mediated immune responses. An example is presented in Figure 13.1.

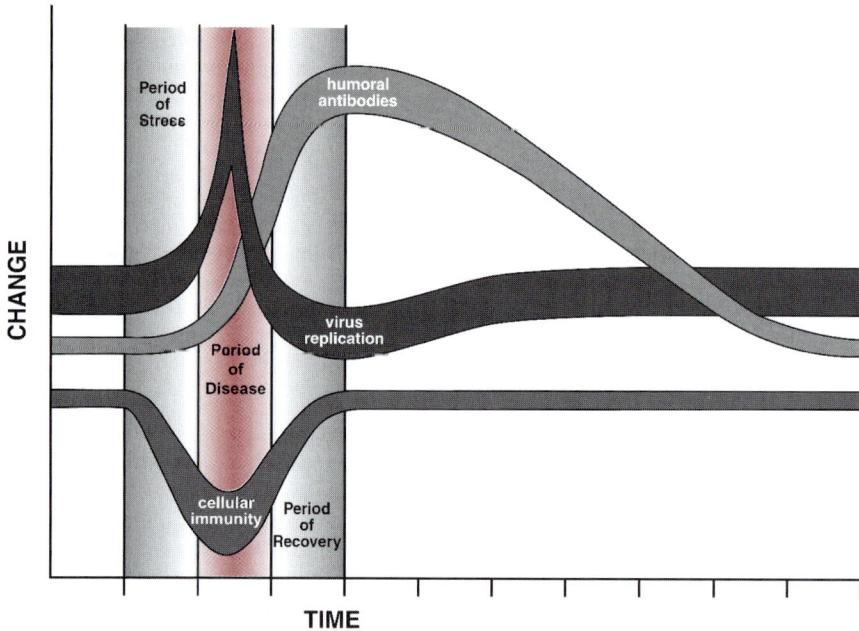

FIG. 13.1—Immune suppression in viral infection. Viral infections have profound pathophysiological effects, including, as in this case, a phase of immune suppression involving cell-mediated immune responses. The inflammatory reactions involve interleukin 2 (IL-2) and may be inhibited by glucocorticoids, prostaglandin E_2 (PGE_2) and cyclosporine. (Courtesy of Al Smith, Oregon State University.)

Elevated levels of glucocorticoids, as in pathophysiological and pharmacological situations, suppress the immune system, blocking cellular immunity more than humoral responses. Cytokines such as IL-1 stimulate hypothalamic CRH and pituitary ACTH secretion, resulting in a burst of adrenal cortisol secretion that kills mature immune cells and inhibits IL-1 production. It is interesting to note that CRH is also secreted by subpopulations of immune cells. This local effect is also suppressed by low-dose cortisol. Immature immune cells are more resistant to these effects. Glucocorticoids also have a much stronger anti-inflammatory effect than do nonsteroid anti-inflammatory drugs (NSAIDs) because glucocorticoids block production of arachidonic acid. They may do this via lipocortin, a calcium-binding protein that is a phospholipase A_2 inhibitor. Glucocorticoids have anti-inflammatory and immunosuppressive actions that can be exploited for their clinical potential in various forms of stress on the mammalian organism. Their use in therapy does not cure an underlying cause of disease but can reduce damage arising from harmful immunologic reactions, whether attributable to humoral immunity (e.g., urticaria) or from cellular responses (e.g., transplant rejection). Both the anti-inflammatory and immunosuppressive effects of glucocorticoids are linked—both involve inhibition of leukocyte functions.

Anti-inflammatory inhibition involves inhibition of several cell types involved in generating inflammation, decreasing the release of vasoactive and chemoattractive factors, secretion of lipolytic and proteolytic enzymes, extravasation of leukocytes in injured areas, and fibrosis. Glucocorticoids are modulators of the immune system, protecting the host from life-threatening consequences of inflammatory responses. The stress of infectious disease results in production of cytokines (a network of signaling molecules that integrate cellular responses): (a) macrophages/monocytes and (b) T and B lymphocytes in mounting immune responses. Among them are IL-1, IL-6, and tumor-necrosis factor α (TNF-α), which stimulate the HPA axis.

IL-1 in particular has the broadest range of actions. It leads to increased secretion of ACTH and cortisol that inhibits the immune system at multiple sites, including interferon γ (IFN-γ), granulocyte-macrophage colony-stimulating factor (GM-CSF), TNF-α, and ILs 1,2,3, 6, 8, and 12. Overall, the bidirectional actions are significant in homeostasis. The glucocorticoids (a) may upregulate the humoral arm (i.e., antibody production) of the immune response while (b) suppressing cellular immunity that involves T helper cell inhibition and thymidine (Th-2) cell activation. The HPA axis involves the regulation of ACTH secretion. Pituitary corticotropes release ACTH in fluctuating pulses that are regulated by CRH neurons in the hypothalamus (Figure 13.2). The HPA axis-immune-system interaction is manifested by

1. A basic diurnal rhythm of ACTH and cortisol
2. Marked increases in secretion during stress
3. Negative feedback that maintains levels in appropriate ranges but is overridden in stress so that much higher levels can occur

Arginine vasopressin (AVP) is a potent secretagogue for corticotropes.

Cortisol depresses osteoblast activity (i.e., new bone formation), while the activity of osteoclasts increases and calcium absorption from gut is inhibited. The overall effect on bone and connective tissue is catabolism. Renal loss of calcium is also increased. The cortisol may be of therapeutic value in the less common pathophysiology of hypercalcemia. Cortisol crosses the blood-brain barrier and affects its permeability in ways that may be beneficial in alleviating some of the pathophysiology of brain edema. It also has marked effects on moods and emotions in some patients, with elation or even psychosis if in excess and depression if cortisol is deficient. Cortisol is an effective direct inhibitor of linear growth while accelerating developmental events

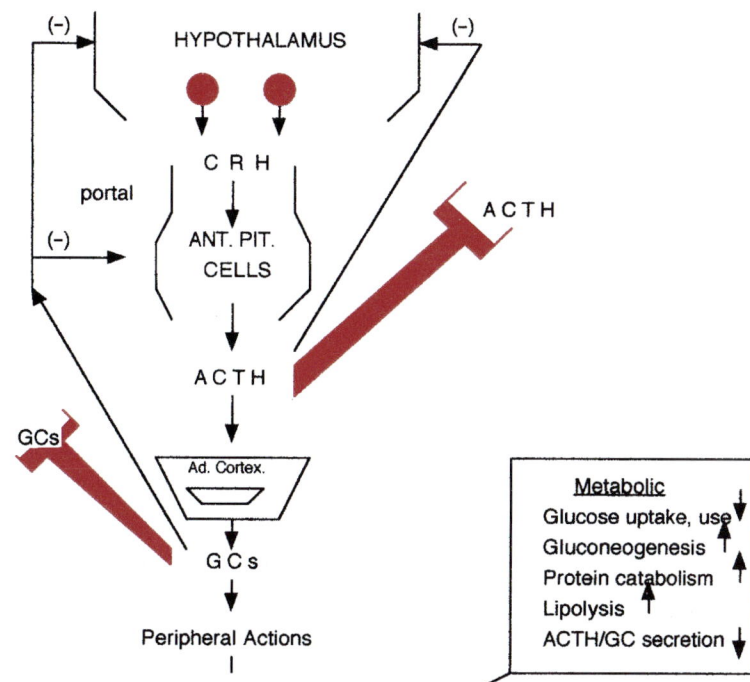

FIG. 13.2—Anti-inflammatory and immunosuppressive effects of glucocorticoids (GCs):

A. Unstressed, GC levels prevent overshoot of defense reactions seen in AdX (adrenalectomized).
B. Due to being severely stressed or receiving high pharmacological doses, elevated GCs cause marked anti-inflammatory and immunosuppressive responses:
    1. Vasodilation and fluid exudation are arrested; cellular repair processes are interrupted.
    2. Leukocyte numbers and activity decrease.
C. Cellular immune response:
    1. The number of mononuclear cells decreases.
    2. The levels of cytokines interleukin 1 (IL-1) to IL-6, IL-8, tumor-necrosis factor α, and granulocyte-macrophage colony-stimulating factor GM-CSF are lower.
    3. Eicosanoids, platelet-activating factor, and complement components in blood decline.

Consequences: Cellular immunity and activity of macrophages are suppressed.
Overall effect of high GC levels: Chronic inflammation is suppressed, along with autoimmune reactions. Protective effects and healing cells are less active.
Conclusions:

1. GCs are valuable against hypersensitivity.
2. GCs are hazardous in infections, even if dormant, without appropriate antibiotic cover. They are detrimental to healing and lead to wasting of muscle, to bone resorption, and to cartilage degradation.

ACTH, adrenocorticotropic hormone; and CRH, corticotropin-releasing hormone.

by multiple mechanisms. However, fetal tissue growth and differentiation are stimulated, particularly in the pulmonary and gastrointestinal systems. This effect gives an opportunity to treat premature neonates that may be lacking pulmonary surfactant.

THE HYPOTHALAMUS IN NEUROENDOCRINE REGULATION OF GROWTH. Broader coverage of neuroendocrine regulation of growth requires review of appropriate sections of books such as Griffin and Ojeda (2000). A brief overview is provided here. Growth hormone, or somatotropin, is a large molecule of 191 amino acids. Its roles and regulation proved to be one of the most complex and elusive to characterize. Its secretion has both stimulating and inhibiting agents. These are growth hormone-releasing hormone (GHRH) and growth hormone release-inhibiting factor, known as somatostatin (SS). The cell bodies that make GHRH are in the arcuate, ventromedial, and dorsomedial nuclei of the basal hypothalamus. Their axons terminate on the capillaries of the hypothalamic-hypophyseal portal circulation at the median eminence via which the hormone is carried to the anterior pituitary. The GHRH is released episodically, causing episodic release of GH from the anterior pituitary. The GHRH interacts with its receptor to activate the stimulatory G (G_s) protein that triggers generation of cAMP and influx of free cytosolic Ca^{2+}. This leads to release of GH from its secretory granules. Negative-feedback control of the pituitary is exerted by insulin-like growth factor 1 (IGF-1) at the pituitary level. It also acts on the hypothalamus to stimulate secretion of SS (Figure 13.3). Release of GHRH is stimulated by acetylcholine (ACh), α-adrenergic agonists, and dopaminergic agents and is inhibited by β-adrenergic agonists.

GH release is also stimulated by prostaglandin E_2 (PGE_2) and GH-releasing peptides. Recently, an endogenous ligand named *ghrelin* was identified that originates in the stomach and has potent effects on appetite plus playing a role in energy balance. SS is widespread in the central nervous system (CNS) and gut. In the CNS, it occurs mainly in the anterior periventricular nucleus, with nerve endings in the median eminence. SS inhibits release of GH and secretion of thyroid-stimulating hormone (TSH), insulin, and glucagon. GH is the most plentiful of the anterior pituitary (AP) hormones, and somatotrophs make up about 50% of anterior pituitary cells.

Plasma concentrations of GH are below 1 ng/mL through most of the day except for episodic secretion every 3 to 4 hours, with peaks up to 20 to 40 ng/mL. GH levels are very high in the mammalian fetus and then drop quickly after birth. In adolescence, peak GH is higher than in younger children. It decreases considerably in the elderly. Its half-life in plasma is about 10 to 30 minutes. The endogenous 24-hour production rate is 0.25 to 0.5 mg/m^2 surface area. Most of this is removed by the liver plus a little by the kidneys. The GH level rises with onset of stage 3 and 4 sleep. Estrogen increases GH secretion; hence, the increase in GH

in puberty. Note that both GH and SS regulate their own secretion.

IMPORTANT EFFECTS OF GROWTH HORMONE

1. Growth in stature of children
2. Stimulation of growth and calcification of cartilage, partly by IGFs
3. Positive N_2 balance

Growth effects of GH are in large part indirect. The actual mediators of growth are now called IGFs because they resemble proinsulin. Previously called somatomedins, IGFs are made in mesenchymal cells, of which most are in the liver. GH enhances growth by stimulating IGF-1 production locally by prechondrocytes in the epiphyseal growth plate.

EAT OR BE EATEN: ENERGY INTAKE

"The evolution of the animal kingdom has been a pageant of predator and prey—cat or be eaten."
HOMER W. SMITH

A mammal survives by maintaining a relative constancy of the body complex, that is, *homeostasis* (really heterostasis because the regulatory processes need to vary as a function of environmental conditions and of internal rhythms). Diverse mechanisms are involved: some like O_2-CO_2 exchange by adjustment of respiratory rate and pattern that is rapid and reflexive. Others are instinctive behavioral drives on a longer-term basis, such as the need for food and water, a learned process of arousal, hunger, thirst, and thermal discomfort. Brain mechanisms mediate appetite and distaste.

Regulation needs a framework such as set-point mechanisms that are used by autonomic systems to make the necessary adjustments physiologically to restore the desired balance. Major departures from the homeostatic balance can break through the autonomic regulatory systems into desperate cravings for water and food. At the other end of the scale is a need for a feeling of satiety when enough has been ingested to satisfy metabolic demands, not a very precise set-point judging from the behaviors of many mammals and people and their resulting obesity or indigestion. Appetite is stimulated by competition, and animals will frequently overeat to engorgement and pathophysiology only when competitors are vying for the same feed. Respiratory regulation on land is extremely well regulated by autonomic systems except when rhythmic breathing is compromised by physical obstruction of the airway or by other pathophysiology of the respiratory system. Failing respiratory homeostasis causes panic feelings. The cardiovascular system can get intimately involved in cardiopulmonary distress syndromes.

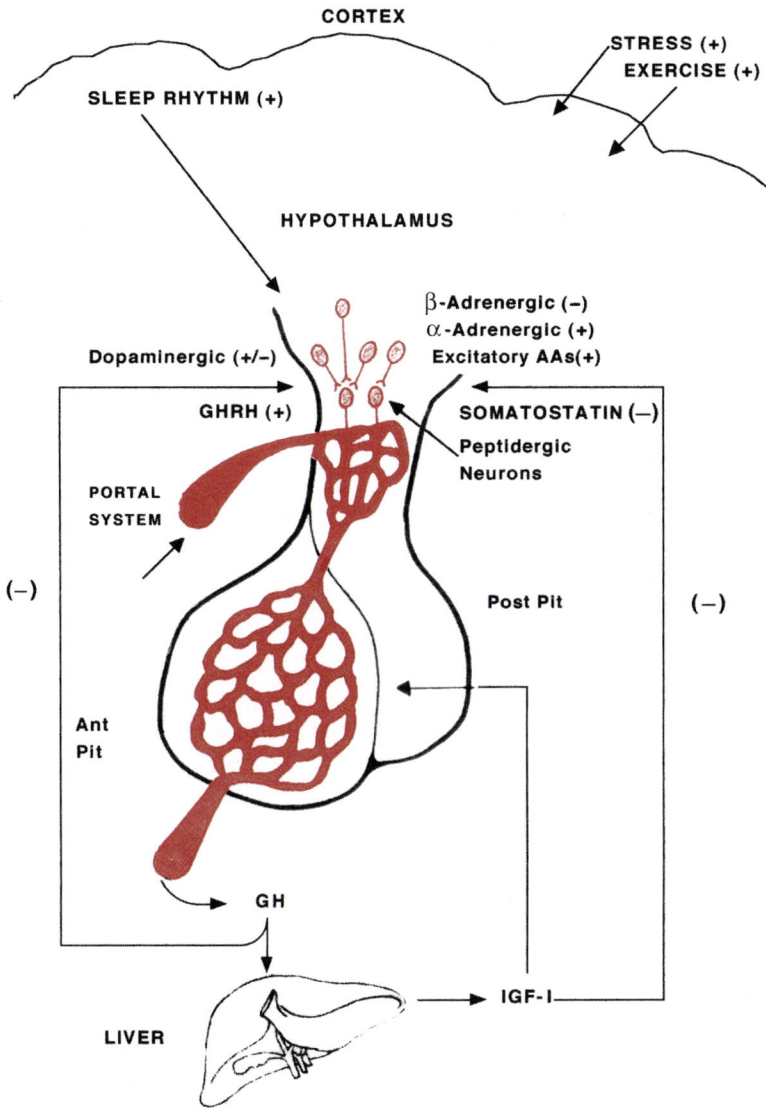

FIG. 13.3—Central regulation of growth hormone (GH) and somatostatin (SS, growth hormone-inhibiting hormone) secretion.
The basal hypothalamus has cells that synthesize three types of peptides: GHRH, growth hormone-releasing hormone; growth hormone release-inhibiting factor or SS; and growth hormone-releasing peptides (not well understood).
Cell bodies making GHRH and SS have axons ending on capillaries in the hypothalamic-pituitary portal circulation (HPPC) at the medial eminence. The GHRH is released episodically and carried via the HPPC to the anterior lobe of the pituitary gland, where its receptors on somatotroph cells activate a G protein that causes release of GH into the second capillary bed to enter the venous circulation. Insulin-like growth factor (IGF-I), which is a somatomedin produced by the liver under the influence of GH, exerts negative-feedback control of the secretion of GH while increasing SS secretion from the hypothalamus. SS also occurs in other organs, including the islet cells of the pancreas.
GH and IGF-I are important for growth of young mammals, calcification of cartilage, and achievement of a positive balance for nitrogen metabolism by promoting uptake of amino acids (AAs) by cells. GH secretion increases during the night and in deep sleep. Several neurotoxicants affect GH secretion as shown in the figure. The thyroid is also involved in growth regulation, and cortisol inhibits longitudinal growth.

Motivation in homeostatic regulation is handled through a remarkable *seeking* system that guides mammals to pursue a range of rewards from their environment. Appetitive searching for suitable nutrients is a major built-in drive. It is apparent that there is a need for a double-barreled approach: (a) a generalized, relatively nonspecific, appetitive arousal system, and (b) a need-specific, resource-finding system. A lot of behavioral learning goes into such a setup. In the case of our domestic livestock, a lot of conditioning has gone into defining the dietary options especially for food- and fiber-producing species and into providing food sources adequate to meet the production demands made on the individual species. Only in the free-ranging systems such as range-fed cattle and small ruminants is dietary selection left up to the animal itself. It should not be overlooked that gastrointestinal parasitism affects central satiety mechanisms and leads to inappetance, e.g., in *Ostertagia* infections in ruminants accompanied by a rise in abomasal pH and hypergastrinemia (Fox 1997).

TEMPERATURE REGULATION

Features of Desert Environment. There may be long, heavy, solar exposure often with little or no access to shade or cloud cover.

Air temperature may be up to 50°C by day down to about 0°C by night even in summer.

Cold deserts occur in winter, where llamas, Bactrian camels, goats, sheep, yaks, and some equidae range. Insulating hair/wool coats are essential.

In summer, hot dry air is inescapable for ungulates in warm-temperate and tropical zones at some times of the year. Vegetation is restricted to xerophytes unless irrigation is available. Such plants have bursts of growth after rain, and then later there are only dry herbage seeds and leaves to ingest. Droughts and famines are frequent. Persistent winds are hazards that increase convection. When the air temperature exceeds 39°C, it adds to the heat load. Wind also raises dust storms that make matters worse by irritating eyes, reducing respiratory cooling, and impeding foraging. Insects are a chronic source of irritation for eyes and skin.

Systems Involved in Temperature Regulation

ANATOMIC PROTECTION FROM HEAT. Fibers of the hair coat provide insulation and may be smooth in summer to reflect some solar radiation. In the tropics, short coarse hairs are most common in wild ungulates and appear to be the most effective protective covering. Seasonal shedding with regrowth adapted to the next season is seen in the dromedary and tropical cattle that seem to be regulated by photoperiod-responsive physiology. Sheep that have heavy fleece are not well adapted to hot desert conditions. However, the Merino breed is unique with its fine wool growing vertically to the skin as a compact insulating layer. In winter, this provides protection against heat loss, easily maintaining a thermal gradient of 40° to 50°C between skin and environment. A similar gradient in the opposite direction prevails in summer between the hot exposed surface and the cool skin. The insulating barrier is about 10% wool and 90% air. Tropical hair coats tend to be light in color with a dark skin beneath; for example, zebu cattle have dark skin and pale hair, with black pig-

ment on the eyelids that protects them from epitheliomas. They are better protected against ultraviolet radiation than are European breeds that are prone to get tumors of the eyelids and the pale skin around the eyes.

WATER AND ELECTROLYTE HOMEOSTASIS (SEE CHAPTER 1). The constancy of the internal environment, or at least of its core, is maintained by a combination of physiological regulatory mechanisms and behavioral actions. For example, in the case of body water, an excess is readily compensated for by increased urine production, whereas a deficiency may require a voluntary behavior, ingesting more water in response to a sense of thirst, aided by secretion of ADH (antidiuretic hormone or vasopressin). Studies in dogs have shown that 72% of a dog's drinking is related to depletion of the intracellular compartment as a result of increased extracellular sodium-ion concentration. Simply injecting hypertonic saline will lead to thirst and drinking, whereas injecting water abolishes thirst as the water "recharges" the cells. The other 28% of drinking is attributable to reduction of extracellular fluid (ECF) volume, as can be shown by infusing isotonic sodium chloride solution.

EVAPORATIVE COOLING. Evaporative cooling can minimize hyperthermia (McCutcheon and Geor 1998).

Mammalian species vary greatly in their homeostatic approaches to achieving a need to lower a hyperthermic situation. Horses use sweating by apocrine glands as a primary mechanism to exploit the cooling effect of evaporation. Dogs, on the other hand, mainly resort to panting and oronasal air movement to lower vascular temperature. Although thermal loading from exercise is the major feature limiting capacity for running in both these species, the equidae are somewhat unique in depending on dermal evaporation from sweat secretion. The efficiency of this process is compromised by the high volumes of perspiration, as it results in some of the liquid running off the body surface before it evaporates. Also, the dermal insulating effects of hair and skin impede the cooling effect on the blood vessels.

The thermoregulatory role of sweating and evaporation is the primary role of sweat glands in horses and people. Other species lack this dramatic capacity for fluid loss via the dermal sweat glands, although they have it to a lesser extent. Some animals achieve the evaporative cooling objective mainly by panting (e.g., dogs and cats). Men in the savannas and nonforested climatic zones hunted mainly small and midsized game animals and birds. Catching the former required endurance stalking and running, which demanded sweating for cooling but also had to avoid losing precious body water and electrolytes to the point of dehydration while being sufficient to ensure some evaporative cooling compatible with homeostasis.

Sweat secretion includes a surfactant compound, latherin, that lowers surface tension and causes the drops of secretion to disperse and thereby stay on the skin, reducing runoff loss of the evaporative cooling effect. Also, as sweat contains electrolytes, it carries with it considerable amounts of sodium, chloride, bicarbonate, and potassium in the longer term, invoking a serious risk of dehydration. Equine sweat is high in potassium.

Horses increase sweat secretion progressively with time of exposure to increased metabolic heat production and environmental contributions to heat load. Cattle differ in showing stepwise, rather than progressive, increases in rate of sweat secretion, whereas, in small ruminants, the increases are phasic.

It should be noted that the impact of sweat evaporation from body surfaces varies with the relative humidity and temperature of the ambient air. Evaporation of 1 L of sweated water from the surface of vascularized tissue can reduce the thermal load by up to 2428 kJ (580 kcal). The speed of running affects the rate of evaporation and cooling. Also, considerable thermal exchange involves the air movement in and out of the respiratory tract.

Dry coat or *anhidrosis* is a pathophysiological condition in horses that are unable to invoke an adequate sweating response to thermal stress (Evans et al. 1957; Warner and Mayhew 1983; McCutcheon and Geor 1998). Although particularly prevalent in nonacclimated horses subjected to heavy exercise in hot humid environments, it is a risk factor for horses generally for which the dysfunction is poorly understood. Preganglionic sympathectomy of donkeys abolished the ability to sweat, although adrenal medullary denervation did not, implicating adrenergic sympathetic neural involvement. The β_2-adrenergic antagonist propranolol blocks equine sweating (Bijman and Quinton 1984). Elevated plasma epinephrine levels could possibly lead to downregulation of the β_2-adrenergic receptors of the sweat glands. Also, the nitric oxide inhibitor L-NAME (*N*-nitro-L-arginine methyl ester) has been shown to reduce sweating significantly in exercised horses (Mills et al. 1997). Failure to sweat when raising body temperature during severe exercise results in hyperthermia, the core temperature exceeding the normal threshold, leading to incapacitation for such exercise. The loss of the normal ability to sweat and the resulting hyperthermia are accompanied by a respiratory rate that is dramatically increased and a hair coat that appears dry and thin and may have patches of hair loss.

Ruminant sweating involves α-adrenergic sympathetic systems. Dogs have both α-adrenergic and β-adrenergic receptors for sweating. Human perspiration is primarily eccrine and cholinergic and contains sebum, which has been shown to have a remarkable temperature-dependent lability of its physical properties, repelling water at lower temperatures while, at higher ones, emulsifying the sweat so that it spreads as a film over the skin and is retained on the surface for evaporative cooling.

Heat Prostration. When cooling systems fail to contain core temperature, it may rise to dangerous levels that only behavioral strategies and cooling equipment can rectify. When environmental temperature rises above 88°F (31°C), vasodilation of dermal vessels can no longer increase heat dissipation rate, as it does at temperatures up to this point. Body temperature increases unless sweating stimulates heat receptors in the skin or there is an increase in hypothalamic temperature. For the former to be fully effective, the latter must be present. The apocrine sweat glands of sheep and goats are under direct nervous control but are less important in sheep than in cattle (Robertshaw 1968). Thus, small ruminants depend more on the respiratory evaporation of water. In bovines, sweating increases with increases in body temperature. Panting is important in both cattle and sheep. It occurs at rectal temperatures above 104°F in cattle, sometimes lower. This often involves increases in salivary secretion. The evaporation occurs in the upper respiratory and oropharyngeal passages, not in the lungs. Effects of relative humidity are not too great but can start before the blood-to-brain temperature gradient increases. In sheep, body temperature rises above normal at environmental temperatures above 90°F (32°C), while open-mouthed panting cuts in at about 106°F (41°C) or above. They can survive at 110°F for hours if humidity is not too high. Zebu cattle can dissipate heat faster than European breeds. Cattle have no special water-conserving mechanisms, but zebus can dissipate more heat by evaporation from their surface and because they have more and larger sweat glands, but need water.

The clinical signs of overheating in cattle start between 107° and 115°F (41.5° to 46°C). Respiratory rate increases initially, and this may be followed by a fall. This situation can result in convulsions and death. If rectal temperature exceeds 106°F (41°C), the situation is becoming dangerous. It is often accompanied by dehydration and hemoconcentration; for example, hematocrit in excess of 60. Other signs include water seeking, decreased urine formation, and loss of 5% of body weight as water. A deficit that reaches 10% is severe. The initial fluid loss comes from the ECF. If the rate of loss is very rapid, the ECF volume decreases significantly and water shifts from the cells to the ECF. In the early stages of dehydration, there are increases in Na^+ and Cl^- in the urine, accompanied by a K^+ leak from cells. There is an increase in plasma K^+ concentration, indicating depletion of H_2O, Na^+, Cl^-, and K^+.

In people and dogs, disseminated intravascular coagulation may be seen, as well as cerebral edema. The condition is called *heat stroke*. In pigs, rectal temperature starts to climb at environmental temperatures above 86° to 90°F (30° to 32°C). If relative humidity exceeds 65, pigs cannot tolerate ambient temperatures above 95°F (35°C). At temperatures above 104°F (40°C), pigs cannot withstand any humidity in the air and may collapse quickly. Pigs in the tropics learn that mud is a better cooling medium than water, so they take every opportunity to wallow.

The temperature control of heat dissipation is associated with regions around the preoptic and supraoptic nuclei of the hypothalamus above the optic chiasm (OC) and between the OC and the anterior commissure.

Control of heat generation and conservation is regulated by the caudal hypothalamic area. This role is superimposed on the primary heat-conserving areas. Lesions of the anterior hypothalamus result in very high body temperatures.

Hyperthermia can occur from

1. The thermal effect of the physical environment on the mammalian body
2. Vigorous physical exercise
3. Fever, which is not "simple hyperthermia"

Note that in situations 1 and 2, the higher body temperature is not defended at that level by homeostatic mechanisms. In situation 3, however, it is defended at the new set-point. Further heating of the body during the plateau phase of fever is met with shivering and increased heat production.

Hypothermia. This occurs in mammals exposed to very cold environments involving very low temperatures and high winds (wind chill), and if there is precipitation such as sleet, snow, or hail (a blizzard) or if a significant part of the body is submerged in water at low temperature. The result is heat extraction from the body faster than the body can compensate for by generating extra heat and a drop in core temperature. Neonatal animals are more susceptible than adults because of a high surface area to weight ratio and because their metabolic responses may not be well developed. As tissue temperatures fall, basal heat production falls, nerve conduction becomes slower and reflexes more sluggish, heart rate slows, and arrhythmias may arise. Many homeostatic responses are impaired, resulting in cardiopulmonary and acid-base dysfunctions that become life-threatening.

Adaptation to Excessively Hot or Cold Environments. Adaptation to excessively hot or cold environments is very important for domestic mammals. Ruminants and equidae often have to endure harsh extremes of heat or cold exposure with seasonal changes and storms. For cold, some species have deposits of brown adipose tissue at certain stages of their life cycle that can develop metabolic heat when given time to adapt. A variety of physiological and behavioral adaptations are used by the different species to cope with the natural and man-made conditions imposed on them. Swine are often protected by being housed, but use of outdoor hog farming is increasing in some regions. Small carnivorous pet species, in the majority today, live much of their lives indoors, particularly cats. Hardy adapted working dogs, on the other hand, may live mainly outdoors or in unheated sheds when not working. Some breeds have been selected for certain features that make them less tolerant of thermal stresses, such as the rex-mutation breeds of cat that lack an outer hair coat. Their body temperature tends to be set a couple of degrees higher than that of their better-insulated conspecifics.

Fever and Hyperthermia. *"Physiologic" fever* may help the body overcome some of the causative factors in the response to infection, by helping to neutralize infectious agents or even other etiologic factors. This type of fever is usually not life-threatening if the core temperature does not rise more than 4°C (7°F) above the normal set-point.

In severe hyperthermia due to the loss of the balance between heat gain and heat loss, the homeostatic responses have been overwhelmed and *heatstroke* results that can be lethal. As the increase over normal core temperature rises rapidly to dangerous levels exceeding 6° or 7°F above the normal set-point, physical damage starts to occur in major organ systems such as brain, heart, liver, and kidneys. The thermostatic system of the hypothalamus brings corrective processes into play, which include anorexia, sweating, thirst, and reduced physical activity. However, if high environmental temperature and humidity plus exposure to solar radiation increase heat gain considerably faster than increased rate of heat loss can compensate, the pattern of metabolic compensation may well fail to offset the increased rate of thermogenesis.

Groups of cells lining the brain's fluid ventricles called the *circumventricular organs* have local capillaries that lack the tight junctions typical of the blood-brain-barrier system, thereby allowing monitoring of endogenous pyrogens in the systemic blood by these cells. They respond by making signaling peptides and proteins that trigger the hypothalamic nuclei to coordinate their thermostatic adjustments to reset their set-point by triggering autonomic, endocrine, and behavioral changes to achieve the goal of fever. When the level of hyperthermia exceeds 4° or 5°F, the body experiences *malaise* and starts to lose its ability to adapt. Behavioral changes include malaise and confusion, with increasing weakness.

The following is an example of behavioral adaptation by pigs to promote heat loss: In tropical environments, pigs *wallow* in mud or muddy water holes. Mud is a very efficient medium for evaporative thermolysis. In fact, heat loss is more rapid from mud-smeared skin surfaces than that of skin just wetted with water. Thus, pigs can tolerate a wider temperature gradient if they has access to a wallow.

The following is an example of hindrance to heat loss in sheep in a hot environment: Water vapor forms at skin level and passes outward through the fleece via its vapor gradient. Some is absorbed by the wool, which is hygroscopic. The fleece is a hindrance for heat loss, particularly during hot, rainy weather. The hair sheep, such as the Wiltshire horn breed, adapt better thermally to humid tropical environments than do the wool breeds.

INHERITED METABOLIC DISORDERS. Certain inherited disorders in calves cause spongiform encephalopathies that may be a result of impaired function of a specific lysosomal enzyme. The abnormal structures are filled with the products of the disordered metabolism. The problem genes, which are inherited typically as autosomal recessives, arise in lines that have been highly inbred to achieve goals such as higher milk or meat production (or desired appearance traits). Typically, the inbreeding of carrier animals leads to the expression of such genes. The calves, for example, may be born with neurodegenerative disorders and die soon after birth. Examples include (Dodd et al. 1992) the following:

1. Citrullinemia in Holstein calves, which involves a deficiency in the urea cycle enzyme, arginosuccinate synthetase. The concentration of citrulline in the brain is greatly increased, accompanied by reduced levels of neurotransmitter amino acids. Neurological signs include vocalization, ataxia, and head pressing, followed by stupor, coma, and death.

2. Branched-chain keto acid decarboxylase deficiency in polled Hereford calves. This results in maple syrup urine disease (MSUD), so called because the urine has an odor of MS. These calves have congenital myoclonus and spongiform encephalopathy.

3. Shaker calf syndrome in Hereford calves. This is associated with neurofilament accumulation in neurons and dying back of axons. In addition to cell groups in the CNS, ganglion cells of the peripheral and autonomic nervous systems may be affected. The affected calves typically remain recumbent, with tremors of the neck and hindlegs, followed by death within a few days. The most severe lesions are in the spinal cord.

Overall inborn errors of metabolism causing accumulation of indigestible metabolites within neurons because of a lack of normal capacity to metabolize them are a life-threatening hazard. The overloaded lysosomes produce marked neuronal dysfunctions. The list of examples encompasses the mannosidoses (α and β), the glycogenoses (including Pompe's disease), and the leukodystrophies, in addition to the acute neonatal ones that have been already described briefly. The lesions vary, as does the severity of the dysfunction.

Healy and Dennis (1993) noted the risk of this category of lethal recessive diseases to livestock populations. They pointed out the need to prepare for diagnosis of the very considerable potential that exists for inborn errors of metabolism to arise, given the computerized monitoring that guides selection of sires with proven potential to pass on enhanced productivity to their offspring.

RECOMMENDED READING

Annison EF, Bryden WL. 1998a. Perspective in ruminant nutrition and metabolism: I. Metabolism in the rumen. Nutr Res Rev 11:173–198.

Annison EF, Bryden WL. 1998b. Perspective in ruminant nutrition and metabolism: II. Metabolism in ruminant tissues. Nutr Res Rev 12:147–177.

Bergman EN. 1975. Production and utilization of metabolites by the alimentary tract as measured in portal and hepatic blood. In: McDonald JW, Warner ACI, eds. Digestion and Metabolism in the Ruminant. Armidale, Australia: University of New England Publishing Unit, pp 292–305.

Bergman EN. 1975. Production and utilization of metabolites by the alimentary tract as measured in portal and hepatic blood. In: McDonald JW, Warner ACI, eds. Digestion and Metabolism in the Ruminant. Armidale, Australia: University of New England Publishing Unit, pp 292–305.

Bergman EN. 1990. Energy contributions of volatile fatty acids from the gastrointestinal tract in various species. Physiol Rev 70:567–590.

Bijman J, Quinton PM. 1984. Predominantly beta-adrenergic control of equine sweating. J Am Physiol Soc 246:R349–R353.

Costa ND, McIntosh GH, Snoswell AM. 1976. Production of endogenous acetate by the liver in lactating ewes. Aust J Biol Sci 29:33–42.

Crawley AC, Jones MZ, Bonning LE, et al. 1999. Alpha-mannosidosis in the guinea pig: A new animal model for lysosomal storage disorders. Pediatr Res 46:501–509.

Dodd PR, Williams SH, Gundlach AL, et al. 1992. Glutamate and gamma-aminobutyric acid neurotransmitter systems in the acute phase of maple syrup urine disease and citrullinemia in newborn calves. J Neurochem 59:582–590.

Dove H. 1996. Rumen and the Pasture Resource: Nutrient Interactions in the Grazing Animal. Canberra: CSIRO.

Evans CL. 1966. Physiological mechanisms that underlie sweating in the horse. Br Vet J 122:117–123.

Evans CL, Smith DFG, Ross KA. 1957. Physiological factors in the condition of "dry-coat" in horses. Vet Rec 69:1.

Fox MT. 1997. Pathophysiology of infection with gastrointestinal nematodes in domestic ruminants: Recent developments. Vet Parasitol 72:285–297.

Griffin JE, Ojeda SR, eds. 2000. Textbook of Endocrine Physiology, 4th ed. New York: Oxford University Press.

Husband AJ. 1995. The immune system and integrated homeostasis. Immunol Cell Biol 73:377–382.

Husband AJ, Bryden WL. 1996. Nutrition, stress and immune activation. Proc Nutr Soc Aust 20:60–70.

Kendrick KM, Da Costa AP, Leigh AE, et al. 2001. Sheep don't forget a face. Nature 414:165–166.

Lawrence AB, Terlorus EM, Kyriazakis I. 1993. The behavioral effects of undernutrition in confined farm animals. Proc Nutr Soc 52:219–229.

McCutcheon J, Geor RI. 1998. Fluids and electrolytes in athletic horses. Vet Clin North Am 14:75–95.

Miles CO, Erasmuson AF, Wilkins AL. 1996. Ovine metabolism of zearalenone to alpha-zearalanol (zeranol). J Agric Food Chem 44:3244–3250.

Mills PC, Martin DJ, Scott SM. 1997. Nitric oxide and thermoregulation during exercise in the horse. J Appl Physiol 75:994.

Niesink RJM, Jaspers RMA, Kornet LMW, et al., eds. 1999. Introduction to Neurobehavioral Toxicology. Boca Raton, FL: CRC.

Olson D, Ritter RC, Papasian CJ, Gutenberger S. 1981. Sympatho-adrenal and adrenal hormone responses of newborn calves to hypothermia. Can J Comp Med 45:321–326.

Robertshaw D. 1968. The pattern and control of sweating in the sheep and goat. J Physiol (Lond) 198:531.

Vernon RG. 1998. Homeorhesis. In: Taylor E, ed. Hannah Research Institute Yearbook. Ayr, Scotland: Hannah Research Institute, pp 64–73.

Warner AE, Mayhew IG. 1983. Equine anhidrosis: A review of pathophysiological mechanisms. Vet Res Commun 6:249–264.

Webster AJF. 1970. Influencing resistance to infectious disease. In: Dunlop RH, Moon HW, eds. Resistance to Infectious Disease. Saskatoon, Canada: Modern.

PART 2: PATHOPHYSIOLOGY OF PLANT TOXICANTS

PLANT-BASED TOXICANTS

Origins. Thousands of species of plants have been shown to be toxic for mammals. About 4% of these have been found to be toxic for the nervous system. Presumably, the toxic species were the result of evolutionary survival achieved by natural selection aimed at the plants' main enemies: their insect predators. Foraging herbivores came along later, added to the evolutionary pressure, and had to be dealt with, too.

Mammalian nervous systems have underlying physiological vulnerabilities, many of which mirror those of insects. Many of the neurotoxicological effects of phytochemicals have been known in various human societies for hundreds, in some cases even for thousands, of years. Some have been exploited for their pharmacological effects. The terminology of neuroscience owes much to the plant-derived neurotoxins. Examples include the terms *nicotinic*, *muscarinic*, and *opiate* receptors. The subject is so vast that the focus of this chapter must be restricted to addressing the modes of action of selected families of bioactive constituents (Dorling et al. 1995). Fortunately, some wonderful texts are now available, for example, Spencer and Schaumberg and the encyclopedic Burrows and Tyrl, for those who need to delve deeper.

Narcotics from plants may have hallucinogenic, stimulant, inebriant, or hypnotic effects on mammals. Mostly studied in people, this range of effects is classed as *psychoactivity*; hence, its greater importance in human rather than veterinary medicine. Only humans (at present) can deploy the elements of knowledge, choice, and capability to obtain the products.

The tropane alkaloids, including atropine, hyoscyamine, and mandrake, were the "hexing" tools of witches in Europe, who exploited their hallucinogenic properties long before the era of modern pharmacology led to their isolation, purification, and pharmacodynamic and toxicological studies. From this research came effective drugs, like atropine and scopolamine, that could be used safely to achieve certain desirable medical effects. Scopolamine, found in the thorn apple (*Datura* species), was used in ancient Chinese and Arabic lore long before being spread to South Asia, Africa, and the Americas. These agents act by blocking the muscarinic receptors for acetylcholine (Ach) at the postsynaptic membrane. This action can be attenuated or even negated by compounds having anticholinesterase activity. Such an antidotal effect was known empirically in ancient times to be present in plants that contained galanthamine, even though its action was not understood. Physostigmine is an agent with a similar, but much briefer, action.

Marijuana or hemp from *Cannabis sativa* contains a mixture of cannabinoids obtained from alcoholic extracts of the plant known by the name *hashish*. The products tend to be variable in potency. The most pharmacologically active ingredients are tetrahydrocannabinols (THCs). The plant was originally grown for hemp fiber. Discovery of the neuroactivity probably was a result of trying the edible seeds and, later, learning to make extracts. *Marijuana* has had an interesting history in veterinary medicine. Before its hallucinogenic properties had received much attention, it became popular as a veterinary medicine for treatment of colic and pain in livestock, particularly horses (Dunlop 1997).

Opium has been known since well back into B.C., its name being derived from the old Greek word for juice, that is, the juice of the opium poppy, *Papaver somniferum*. Several potent agents were isolated from the raw juice, among which morphine was the type compound of about 20 alkaloids in the original material. Serturner isolated it in 1806 and named it after the god of dreams, Morpheus. The Middle East was where much of the poppy plant was grown and exploited by Arabian traders. It spread through Oriental and Western cultures. Initially, a major application was to relieve those afflicted with dysentery. Other effects were also discovered and used: as an analgesic and for mood enhancement and euphoria (often while inhaling the smoke from the burning product). The downside of addiction and physical dependence became apparent. The nucleus accumbens and dopaminergic pathways are involved in the emotional and motivational effects of drug-induced "reward" and its devastating consequences for degradation.

Overview of Plant Toxicity. A vast range of chemical agents, ranging from pure elements to extremely complex organic molecules, is encompassed by the term *toxicant*. Also, many interactions among chemicals affect toxicity, and many metabolic effects (by organisms from microbes to mammals) influence the intensity of the potential hazard. This huge spectrum covers microbial toxins, plant poisons, and animal venoms, among the naturally occurring agents. There is also a huge and steadily growing list of chemicals made by human purification and isolation as well as by de novo synthesis in the quest to advance technology and its application, including new drug development to combat diseases such as parasitic infections and infestations. Nowadays, there are significant concerns that some members of the medical professions are overprescribing therapeutic agents, because this increases the risks of harmful drug interactions and undesirable side effects. The goal of this chapter is to enhance the process of "thinking straight" about the contributions of toxicants to dysfunction and the progressive pathophysiology that may follow. The primary focus next is on neurotoxic aspects, but it is necessary to broaden this to include aspects of other body systems, where appropriate. As a majority of the agents gain entry to the mammal via the gastrointestinal tract and the liver, these organs affect the outcome and are often affected in some detrimental way.

The Nature of Risk of Intoxication by Plants. A plant can be considered poisonous when by consumption (or occasionally by contact), either in its natural state or after incorporation into a processed feed (e.g., hay, silage, or concentrate), it causes pathophysiological changes in the function of a host animal. Secondary factors must always be considered, such as

1. Fodder deterioration or toxicant activation due to exposure: water, radiation, or sprays
2. Infection or infestation by fungi, bacteria, viruses, or parasitic insects
3. Contamination with pathogens from human or animal sources

Vulnerability to Toxic Plants. Particularly in herbivores, vulnerability to plant toxicants is related to metabolism by ruminal and other gut flora, as well as to the detoxifying capacity of the mammal's own metabolism. The impact of the environment and seasonal conditions must also be taken into account. Many factors influence risk:

1. Appetite and motivation
2. Availability of forage, considering extreme conditions such as drought or flood that may limit access to normal pastures and force use of more isolated areas where toxic plants are present or are all that is left because they are not palatable
3. Dietary factors or crops imposed by the animals' "manager"
4. Mineral and vitamin factors as they relate to geology (both land and water) and climate
5. Interactions among dietary plants in the herbage available that may be selected and ingested by the mammal

Local knowledge with a historical perspective can be an invaluable basis for decision making about management to minimize risk of exposure to hazardous plants. The ecological factors become understandable with application and awareness of regional developments, including the political and economic pressures on livestock production. Grazing intensity and animal preferences can be learned by careful observation and the occasional opportunity afforded by an autopsy allowing inspection of rumen and other gut contents. The age, class, and condition of animals should always be kept in mind.

Special Senses and Detection of Toxicants. The neural pathways serving the special senses (a) *originate* in peripheral receptors (eye, inner ear, mouth, and nose) and (b) *terminate* in the cerebral cortex or in the brain stem/spinal cord.

Toxicants that affect these systems most commonly do so via actions on peripheral sensory receptors. Some may be damaged secondarily by edema because they are housed in inelastic structures (e.g., cochlear hair cells or optic nerve axons). Note also that afferent pathways for taste, smell, audition, and balance employ sensory neurons housed in ganglia lacking a blood-brain barrier.

Pigs and dogs stand out among domesticated mammals for their remarkable sense of smell, especially of objects on or in the ground. Pigs are supreme for their capacity to locate truffles, the delicious odoriferous subterranean fungi. Pigs have the advantage of a sensitive tactile snout that doubles as an executive functional organ used with great effect for rooting and digging. They are more particular than are dogs in terms of what they will take into the mouth and eat. Thus, dogs are more likely to suffer gastrointestinal disturbances by ingesting physically or chemically damaging material. On the other hand, some breeds of scent dogs are outstanding ground trackers. Sniffing the perianal area is an identity test for canines that is based on glandular secretions. All mammalian species use pheromone detection via the olfactory system to influence arousal and sexual behavior, including the flehmen reaction of the organ of Jacobson. Cats are famous for marking objects with the scent glands in their cheeks. Male cats in particular like to mark territory by spraying urine, a somewhat less attractive maneuver to their owners.

The caudodorsal part of the nasal mucosa contains the olfactory mucosa, which has the olfactory receptor organs that have an extraordinary range of sensitivities to the spectrum of biochemical agents sampled from the air and that dissolve in the mucosal surface fluids. As such, *the olfactory mucosa is a safety screen, an early warning system to detect other creatures, as well as toxicants in the environment and potential foods with the option of rejecting them before ingesting or swallowing.*

TASTE. Taste is a special sense that is aroused by chemicals contacting specialized receptors in the oral cavity, epiglottis, and upper anterior part of the alimentary canal. Concentrations of receptors are present in taste buds clustered in papillae (elevations) on the dorsal surface of the tongue. Each taste bud diameter is about 50 μm at the base and about 80 μm high. A single bud carries between 30 and 100 receptors. There are three types: (a) fungiform in papillae on the anterior of the tongue (these get the first taste of food being ingested); (b) behind them, at the rear of the tongue, are the vallate kind often recessed in a trench; and (c) foliate, at the posterior sides of the tongue, with numerous buds in the walls of a series of ridges. Types 2 and 3 are well situated to detect molecules in the juices of the forage and the saliva. In total, there are a few thousand taste buds, each having from several up to about 100 receptor cells. Each bud is made up of a number of cells leading up to a taste pore containing microvilli. Behind the tongue are scattered buds in the palate, pharynx, and upper esophagus. Those in the epiglottis and upper esophagus are innervated by the superior laryngeal branch of the vagus nerve. Those at the back of the tongue connect to the glossopharyngeal (9th) nerve, whereas those on the front part feed to the chorda tympani branch of the facial (7th) nerve.

There are also nociceptive axons for chemoreception in the trigeminal (5th) nerve. Some of the array of receptors in the oropharyngeal cavity are activated by irritants, including sulfur dioxide, ammonia, ethanol, acetic acid, and capsaicin. These may serve to alert an animal to potentially harmful vapors ingested or inhaled. Taste receptor cells have a short life span of about 2 weeks, after which they are regenerated. The gustatory sensory input travels via these nerves to the solitary nucleus in the brain stem and thence to the hypothalamus, amygdala, and the ventral posterior nucleus of the thalamus on its way to the insula and the postcentral gyrus of the parietal cortex.

TASTE STIMULI. Most taste stimuli are hydrophilic nonvolatile molecules soluble in saliva. The bud receptors mainly sense chemicals that would be desirable nutrients, such as sodium chloride, glucose and other sugars, organic acids, amino acids, and some lipids. Bitter-tasting molecules include many that are poisonous. These tend to deter many animal consumers, at least until they have acquired a taste for them and have learned how much they can eat without side effects. The term *dysgeusia* means an "unpleasant taste sensation." As mammals evolved, they developed dietary patterns and learned what was and was not safe. The most vulnerable times in modern agriculture were the periods of exploration and colonization when domestic mammals were introduced into unfamiliar environments containing toxic plants for which they had not yet developed taste aversions.

HOW DID/DO ANIMALS LEARN TO ASSOCIATE TASTES WITH SICKNESS? AVERSION LEARNING. A key experiment to study this issue cited by Shepherd (1994) was to pair a very tasty solution with strong X-irradiation to damage the intestine and produce sickness in rats. After recovering from the sickness, the rats refused to drink the tasty solution. It appeared that they had made the presumption of an association between ingesting the tasty treat and getting sick even though there was an interval of several hours between the two events. As only one episode of sickness was needed, such a response is called *one-trial learning*. This is typical of aversion learning as opposed to classical conditioning, which requires many trials to establish a conditioned response, and the timing of the unconditional and the conditional responses must be very precise usually within 1 or 2 seconds. Many substances can serve as the unconditional aversive stimuli, including many toxicants. However some very toxic molecules, including strychnine, are remarkably ineffective. What is so relevant to animal toxicology is that *one-trial aversive learning can only be shown by using stimulation of the tongue*. Such learning is strongest when the contact inputs come from the taste buds (tactile stimulation of the tongue can also give an aversion response).

The taste part of the learning process stems from the suspect molecule stimulating the taste bud receptors that directly stimulate endings of the afferent nerves that convey it to the CNS. This incoming message must meet the fibers coming in from the aversive pathway to make the connection between them. It is thought that the visceral afferent fibers of the vagus nerve carry the sensory input to the brain stem. The meeting point between the taste factor and the dysfunction factor appears to be the nucleus of the solitary tract, which is believed to be the convergence point for the taste and visceral inputs. The most fascinating feature is the capacity of the animal to learn from an ingestive event linked to a supposed outcome hours later. The hypothalamus and amygdala are intimately involved. It also demonstrates the important protective role of the sense of taste for the survival of the animal and emphasizes the importance of trying to understand the whole animal while thinking through the diagnostic value of associative events. The special sense of taste is often overlooked in clinical assessment of animal well-being, illness, and behavior. Because foraging is such a vital motivation and daily time commitment of the routine pattern of a mammal's waking activity, especially for herbivores, the priority assigned to it in the nature of the animal is not surprising. *The linkage of the cue with the consequence becomes an essential capacity to avoid repeat intoxication.*

COMING TO TERMS WITH THE RUNAWAY TRAIN OF RESEARCH IN BIOSCIENCE AND THE UNPREDICTABLE FUTURE. There is a need for a broader view than *toxicity* in dealing with ingested biological agents. D'Mello (2000) has broadened perspectives of this fascinating area. Three aspects of nutritional pathophysiology have been identified as a guide to thinking:

1. *Antinutritional factors* (ANFs), by definition, are those biological compounds in feeds that reduce nutrient utilization or feed intake, thereby contributing to impaired gastrointestinal and metabolic performance.
2. *Antiphysiological compounds* cause interference with regulatory systems such as reproductive function and immunocompetence.
3. *Toxic secondary metabolites* can be intrinsic phytotoxins or toxicants arising from contaminating organisms such as fungi (mycotoxins). There is considerable biochemical overlap among these three groups. When a food crop or its processed product is infested with another organism, the metabolism of both may affect the toxicity.

In this era of genetic manipulation, there will be decreasing fidelity between original genetic identity and the biological agents in circulation. The consequence of this huge change in the nature of things must be incorporated into educational and administrative thinking, if research advances and their commercialization are to be understood and managed.

ANTINUTRITIONAL FACTORS THAT HAVE SUBTLE TOXIC EFFECTS. Many are found in forages (legumes, grasses, and cruciferae), browse (legumes and pine) and grain (i.e., seeds and mainly of legumes). A great variety of plant species are represented and an even greater variety of ANFs. The tropical environments have more agents having ANF activity than the temperate ones. An interesting feature is the low nutritional value of seeds of some leguminous plants. This is cause for concern because much of the cultivated land area today is given over to production of the vigorous soybean plant. Soybeans have proteinase inhibitors and also contain antigenic proteins, which have been shown to be involved in postweaning hypersensitivity reactions in piglets and calves.

Lectins are proteins that bind carbohydrates and have affinity for cell surface membranes. Hemagglutinins are lectins that are the basis of blood cell groups. The combination of protein and carbohydrate imparts a capacity for remarkable specificity of binding. Concanavalin A occurs in jack beans and is an ANF that binds to lower parts of the villi with crypt cells having polymannose side chains.

Some storage proteins in legume seeds can cross the epithelial barrier of the intestines with adverse results for the immune system. Soybean antigens have been identified as glycinin and conglycinin. They resist denaturation by heat in thermal processing and digestive attack in the gut.

Condensed tannins in leguminous seeds and forages are also present in some grains, notably sorghum. They are combinations of flavan-3-ols and are proanthocyanidins that impede rumen fermentation and reduce the rate of gain and wool growth.

Lupins contain alkaloids that are various derivatives of quinolizidine (e.g., lupinine, augustifoline, sparteine, and lupanine).

Brassica forage crops and vegetables contain glucosinolates that are thioglucosides. Plant and microbial thioglucosidases (myrosinase) lead to release of various aglycons that may be degraded further to toxic metabolites. These include isothiocyanates and nitriles that are goitrogenic and reduce appetite.

S-methylcysteine sulfoxide (SMCO) is present in Brassica crops used for roots and forages and causes hemolytic anemia. The tropical legume, *Leucaena leucocephala*, contains mimosine, an analog of tyrosine and related central neurotransmitters, dopamine and norepinephrine.

Isoflavonoids are often endowed with estrogenic activity. Many are found in legumes. Subterranean clover and red clover contain the important toxicant isoflavone, formononetin, that is metabolized in the rumen to equol that is more estrogenic than its dietary precursor. Others such as genistein, glycitein, and daidzein occur as glycosides in soybeans. They may become less potent in the rumen.

Other toxic effects may be encountered in pasture plants (*Brachiaria* and *Panicum*). These include steroidal saponins as glycosides that are activated to become photosensitizing agents in the liver, gossypols in the cotton plant, vasoactive lipids in Western yellow pine, and cyanide as glycosides in a variety of plants (e.g., linseed, cassava, and sorghum).

PRINCIPAL FEATURES OF PLANT TOXICANTS. The two principal actions of toxic plant secondary compounds are

1. *Toxicity*, for example, alkaloids, cyanogenetic compounds, and nonprotein amino acids
2. *Binding of proteins*, including digestive enzymes of the gut, notably by tannins, phenols, etc.

Toxic molecules are usually fairly small and mobile, whereas the digestion-impairing agents are bigger and immobile. Tannins may also be hydrolyzed, in which case they become absorbable and toxic, too. Some condensed tannins (e.g., quelbracho) are toxic in ruminants. Microbes in foregut fermenters of plant fibers detoxify oxalates, alkaloids, cyanogenic glycosides, and nonprotein amino acids before they reach the intestine, where they would be absorbed.

Plant Toxicants Affecting Reproductive Function. Some plants cause *fetal deformity and abortion in ewes* if ingested early in gestation period. The timing of ingestion is usually very critical:

1. *Astragalus* genus (e.g., milk vetches)
2. *Veratrum californicum* (skunk cabbage)
3. *Gutierrezia* species (broomweed and snakeweed)

Veratrum ingested on days 13 and 14 of gestation results in cyclopian (one-eye) deformities; if eaten around day 30, collapsed trachea and limb deformities are the likely outcomes. Such tragic events cannot be reversed, so one must avoid the risk of sheep grazing these plants during the first 6 weeks of pregnancy.

Several of the species in the foregoing list cause abortions and infertility.

Clover disease of ewes is attributed to formononetin that is metabolized in the rumen to equol, resulting in inhibition of binding of estradiol to estrogen receptors. This may result in temporary infertility, with low ovulation and conception rates. The cervix fails to transport spermatozoa after insemination, and histological changes in the cervix occur that can lead to continuing dysfunction. Spermatogenesis in the ram may also be impaired. Ingestion of needles and buds of Western yellow pine can cause late-term abortion in beef cattle that is associated with a progressive decline in blood flow to the gravid uterus. The consequential decline in flow to the caruncular arterial bed leads to premature fetal-induced abortive parturition.

Reproductive function in ewes can be impaired in lupinosis as phomopsins depress ovulation rate, resulting in lower conception rates.

Plants Causing Disorders More Specifically of the Nervous System. Many range plants are *neurotoxic for sheep* in some seasons. Clinical signs include muscle tremors, compulsive chewing with salivation, incoordination, bizarre behavior, respiratory difficulty, convulsions, and even death. One problem is the large number (literally hundreds) of toxicant-producing species in some genera of plants. These include major players such as lupins and locoweeds. Unfortunately, some are quite addictive to livestock. Also, there can be considerable variability in types and content of toxic agents within genera, so evasion of risk requires considerable knowledge both of the plants and of local experience of epidemiology. The types of toxicant may be alkaloid, nitro-containing glycoside, and the like, and also may be affected by other factors, such as climate, mineral content, availability of alternative feeds/plants, management practices, and stress.

TOXIC ACCUMULATOR PLANTS. Chenopodiaceae—goosefoot family: This family includes beet plants such as sugar beet. Ten genera have been associated with toxic episodes, and two general toxic syndromes have been demarcated:

1. *Oxalate and nitrate* accumulators; some store sulfate as well. Also high levels of nitrate in runoff water increase the tendency to accumulate oxalates.
2. If fed a variety or species that has a *high sulfur content* for over a week, there may be an incidence of polioencephalomalacia (PEM).

Bassia is very similar to *Kochia*. It is palatable to sheep. If it is the only feed available to them for over 2 weeks, it causes diarrhea. This is probably attributable to potassium oxalate in the plant tissues. Sheep fed 6.1% oxalate in *B. hyssofolia* all died, having had an abrupt onset of weakness, incoordination, tetany, and coma.

Halogeton glomeratus (*halos* means "salt" and *geiton* means "neighbor"), imported in 1930s into North America, spread from Nevada in 1934 to Utah, Indiana, and Northern California in desert saltbush and sagebrush and in pinyon-juniper woodlands to over 6000 feet altitude, spread by sheep droppings along trails, in sheep holding areas, and on bare knolls. It is an annual, aggressive, adventitious, spreading species. The first losses were reported in the early 1940s, when hundreds of sheep died while being moved to winter grazing, having been let to rest while feeding on large stands of *H. glomeratus*. Hungry, thirsty animals are particularly vulnerable when water is made available in areas where tall stands of *Halogeton* are present, especially on salty soils (sodium chloride). Vigorous growths are high in soluble oxalates (up to 28% in leaves and 8% in seeds). A similar clinical syndrome has been induced by intravenous infusion of sodium oxalate. Affected sheep lose interest in the remainder of the flock and become dull within a few hours as the incoordination and weakness progress to jerky rigidity accompanied by irregular shallow breathing, coughing, and foamy drooling. Recumbency, coma, and death may ensue after periods of agitation with repeated bouts of lying down. Cattle may show similar signs plus stiffness and belligerent behavior.

Continuous intake at lower levels can lead to adaptation by elements of the ruminal microflora that degrade oxalate to carbonate. Oxalate crystals form in renal tubules, and calculi may develop. Abrupt exposure causes intestinal irritation, and steep falls in plasma calcium may occur but rarely leading to tetany. Also, calcium borogluconate IV is of little value in treating poisoned sheep, although it may be beneficial in affected cattle. Enzyme inhibition can be significant (lactate dehydrogenase and succinate dehydrogenase). Adults may rally if they survive for a few days, but affected calves get sicker, with seizures and hypersensitivity to stimuli. The rumen epithelium may be hemorrhagic and edematous.

CONTACT POISONS. *Toxicodendron:* There are five species in North America (including poison oaks, poison ivies, and poison sumac), all of which are problems for people.

Signs: Red skin, watery blisters; extremely itchy and allergic contact dermatitis.

Toxic agents: Oily resins containing a mix of catechol derivatives.

3-Alk(en)yl catechols: The general term used is urushiol. All parts of the plant contain the toxicants, and it is present in material that adheres to pets and anything it comes in contact with. Sensitization requires exposure to urushiol-containing resin. The pathophysiological response occurs within a few days. The catechol compounds penetrate the epidermal layers and undergo oxidation to a quinone form before binding to proteins and causing a cell-mediated immune reaction that results in skin damage. Exudation from the vesicles leads to crusting and scaling, with new lesions surfacing for several days. One period of exposure peaks within 1 week and resolves in 2 to 3 weeks. Treatment involves early and thorough washing of exposed areas and application of a drying agent, such as calamine lotion.

Some Examples of Major Plant Toxicants, Including Some Neural Effects: North America [for greater detail, see Burrows and Tyrl (2001)]

APIACCAE—FORMERLY UMBELLIFERAE (CARROT-PARSLEY-CELERY FAMILY). This is a very large family of plant species, including many used as foods, condiments and ornamentals. Some very important poisonous species are also included, two of which—water hemlock and poison hemlock—rank among the most hazardous to humankind among all plants. Native Americans have long been well aware of their toxicity. All major domestic mammalian species are susceptible. Several species of Apiaccae cause photosensitization, whereas others cause neurotoxicosis or teratogenic effects. Many of these species contain acetylenic compounds, including falcarinol and falcarinone, that are potent irritants. Although seldom lethal, they may cause high morbidity, with severe economic losses. Phytophotodermatitis may be a primary effect following ingestion of the plant material or topical contact. After absorption, the furanocoumarins (psoralens) and furanochromones are activated by long-wavelength ultraviolet light. Following ingestion in plant material by domestic ruminants, the furanocoumarins are orthodemethylated by ruminal microbes, followed by absorption and passage to the liver, where they are oxidized with ring cleavage and transformed to glucuronide and sulfate derivatives. The toxic effects include erythema and edema of the skin of the muzzle, ears, udder, teats, and exposed genitalia. Blisters may form. The eyes are commonly affected, showing sensitivity to light and reddening of the cornea and conjunctiva.

ASTERACEAE: *SENECIO*. This very large genus includes groundsels, ragworts, and butterweeds. Many are toxic, particularly as causes of liver disease in livestock. Widespread use in herbal teas and dietary supplements for supposed medicinal value has led to severe human intoxications. Internationally, use of related species of *Senecio* have caused veno-occlusive hepatic disease when used for treatment of chronic cough or cancer.

Livestock are vulnerable in climatic zones with long growing seasons, both as fresh herbage and in conserved forage. Because a large dose is required for toxicity in most cases, the continuous productive growth and opportunist expansion into cultivated areas increase the risk of exposure. The most common form involves long-term intake resulting in chronic liver disease. Horses and cattle are the main species affected, even though they may be reluctant to eat the plants. Sheep and goats are susceptible but much less sensitive, even though they are more willing to eat them. The tansy ragwort of the damp coastal areas, the groundsels of the Western ranges, and the widespread common groundsel have been the biggest problems for cattle and horses. Biological control by insects has helped.

The toxicants responsible for disease are variants of the group pyrrolizidine alkaloids (PAs) that occur as free base or N-oxide that are hepatotoxins. These compounds also occur in other genera. For hepatic toxicity, the necine nucleus must be unsaturated at the 1–2 position and esterified at the CH_2OH group at the C-9 position. The PAs are detoxified in the liver by ester hydrolysis and/or N-oxidation by cytochrome P-450 mixed-function oxidase (MFO), followed by dehydrogenation. Biotransformation of PAs by dehydrogenation to short-lived toxic reactive pyrroles that can act as alkylating agents is an alternative pathway that may correlate with toxicity in some situations. Because sheep are less sensitive to PA intoxication than are cattle and are more willing to eat the plants, they are used to clear areas of them. This raises the concern that the PAs in *Senecio* might predispose sheep to accumulate copper in the liver, leading to hemolytic crises, as this has been found when they ingest plants of other genera (e.g., Boraginaceae) that contain PAs.

The chronic nature of the exposure to PAs in *Senecio* poisoning results in progressive failure of hepatic metabolism and ability to clear toxic metabolites. This includes the buildup of ammonia that is carried to the CNS, where it contributes to the pathophysiology of hepatoencephalopathy. Other toxic dysfunctions occur, some involving interference with neurotransmitters and regulatory homeostasis. Liver damage leads to depression of vitamin A levels. PAs pass the placenta and enter the milk. Depression and loss of appetite are early signs. As the toxicity progresses, the level of serum hepatic enzymes elevates markedly, and other tests for hepatic dysfunction are manifested. The time course, however, can be very long. Horses express signs of hepatoencephalopathy very abruptly with head pressing, incessant aimless walking, pica such as persistent chewing of fences, yawning, drowsiness, incoordination, rectal straining with diarrhea or constipation, and ascites. Vernacular names catch the image of this clinical syndrome: Walla Walla walking disease, sleepy staggers, and walk-about disease. Cattle have similar but milder signs because the disease is subacute. Typically, there is loss of appetite and milk production, followed by weight loss and emaciation leading to rectal straining, weakness, and recumbency. Neurological signs and even mania may be present.

Four types of hepatic changes are representative of exposure to PAs:

1. Centrilobular necrosis
2. Bile duct proliferation and portal fibrosis
3. Megalocytosis/karyomegaly up to 20 times normal size
4. Fibrosis within and around central veins

Megalocytosis is very noticeable in horses. Cattle have prominent intranuclear inclusions. Similar changes are also seen in aflatoxicosis.

BRASSICACEAE OR CRUCIFERAE: MUSTARD FAMILY. Among these plants are many important food and ornamental plants, but also some responsible for disease syndrome:

1. *General problems:* Acute respiratory distress syndrome (ARDS); nitrate accumulation, photosensitization, digestive disturbances and bloat, and polioencephalomalacia
2. *Problem specific to the plant family:* Thyroid enlargement/goiter, antinutritional effects, liver hemorrhage, blindness, hemolytic anemia, reproductive problems, and tainting of milk and meats

The genus *Brassica* includes feed crops that are consumed in large amounts. Thus, the ones that contain toxicants are likely to result in high dosages of them.

Mustards include some that contain anticarcinogens and others that have neoplastic promoter activity. Many of the genera have an irritant effect on the digestive tract. Most of the Brassicae plants can cause digestive disturbances. One of the commonest causes of digestive upsets is *Sinapsis arvense*. Often, digestive dysfunctions are accompanied by neurological involvement.

There are two types of sulfur-containing *toxicants* in Brassicaceae: *glucosinolates* (formerly called thioglucosides or mustard oil glucosides), an enzyme in plant tissues; and ruminal microbes—myrosinase hydrolyzes glucosinolates to form an irritant toxic radical.

BRACKEN FAMILY: DENNSTAEDTIACEAE AND *PTERIDIUM*. Only one of these families has species of interest toxicologically: *Pteridium* is now recognized to comprise a single, albeit polymorphic, species: *P. aquilinum*, bracken fern. Bracken grows from black woody rhizomes with erect fronds. Along with the water-tolerant nardoo fern (*Marsilea drummondii*) that can dominate plant growth after flooding, ferns can contain thiaminase that can destroy all thiamine in the rumen and intestinal contents, rendering a ruminant acutely deficient in thiamine. This puts it at risk of developing PEM if repeated grazing of the ferns is continued long enough. An alternative hypothesis that thiaminase 1 causes formation of antithiamine metabolites in rumen contents has not been substantiated. However, the antithiamine coccidiostat amprolium has been used experimentally to reproduce the neuropathophysiology of PEM based on electroencephalographic studies. Note that recent work has identified a form of PEM that results from high levels of sulfur ingestion and resultant hydrogen sulfide intoxication (see Section 3 of Chapter 9).

Toxicology of Plant Secondary Compounds. Many plants contain distinctive compounds in amounts far beyond their metabolic requirements for them; hence, the term *secondary*. The list even of major categories of the compounds is long. It includes

Phenols and tannins
Terpenes
Alkaloids
Cyanogenic glycosides
Protease inhibitors
Lectins
Nonprotein amino acids
Cardiac glycosides
Oxalates etc.

Some of the specific toxicants are familiar: strychnine; reserpine, caffeine, cocaine, nicotine, colchicine, mescaline, morphine, cyanide, and urushiols (in poison ivy, oak, and sumac). Their toxicity is relative to the affected mammalian species. It is interesting to note that no foregut fermenters live in temperate forests and that the few folivores that do are hindgut fermenters.

Temperate species mainly encounter tannins in evergreen species, whereas they are not very prevalent in deciduous woody browse. Alkaloids are more highly developed in tropical lowlands, where herbivory is highly developed. In tropical forests, the polyphenols and fiber content of leaves increase with age. Plants that live in fertile soils with disturbed environments and that are fast growing are usually carbon limited and

less likely to invest much energy in chemical defenses. The defenses that are used are usually nitrogen-based (alkaloids, cyanogenetic glycosides, etc.). Nevertheless, long-term, intense browsing induces even the fast growers like willows to invest heavily in chemical defense of their adventitious shoots. Trees and shrubs adapted to infertile soils in low-disturbance areas would have low growth rates, and their parts would be long-lasting, valuable, and slow to replace, so a chemical defense would be expected. Carbon would not be limiting, so carbon-based defenses would be anticipated (phenols, tannins, and terpenes). Crop plants have a high yield in part by selection bringing a low level of protective compounds compared with their wild forebears. This works only because people protect them from predation.

MAMMALIAN RESPONSES TO SECONDARY COMPOUNDS. Avoiding toxic compounds in plants calls for either *selectively avoiding* such plants or plant parts as one option or having built-in *mechanisms to inactivate* the deleterious materials. An interesting mammalian example is the koala, which has adapted to a diet of plant parts that are rich in *essential oils* and phenols (in the eucalypti). Experience is required! Actually, there are many examples of adaptation of native fauna to local plant species. Presumably, animal species survived or evolved that would either avoid or could detoxify the toxicants.

PHYSIOLOGICAL RESPONSES. In some cases, the gut flora can adapt to some toxicants by metabolizing them to a form less hazardous to the mammalian host. A *period of adaptation* is required. Some animals are wary and cautious of plants with new flavors not experienced previously. Deer, for example, cannot handle Douglas fir because of its toxic ingredients but, after adaptation, can use the plant safely. Saliva is a remarkable protectant for some foregut fermenters. By copious secretion of well-buffered saliva, many ruminant species protect their rumen microbiota against too rapid acid fermentation. There can be a remarkable chemical ability of saliva to neutralize some dietary toxicants to the rumen microflora (e.g., compounds that bind with and inactivate cellulases, thereby limiting fiber digestion). Alternatively and more directly, a block can occur to a host's digestive enzyme secretions (e.g., tannins and other phenols that block the digestive enzymes of the abomasum or intestine). However, these *protective proteins are neither found nor inducible in the saliva of cattle and sheep*. Grazing animals usually encounter low levels of secondary toxicant compounds and are much less well equipped to deal with them than the specialist browsers.

LUPIN TOXIC COMPONENTS. Lupins have been developed for livestock feeds, but they had to be modified genetically to greatly reduce the toxicants they contained in the wild state. Some of these cause hepatotoxicity and anorexia. Several, such as lupinine, are neurotoxic. The neurotoxic syndrome in cattle includes incoordination, staggering, falling, convulsions, dyspnea, and frothing at the mouth. These signs are indicative of antagonism of brain γ-aminobutyric acid (GABA), with which lupinine has structural analogies. *Wild lupins* are recognized as a neurotoxic hazard for sheep. Lupin seed was only safe to feed before the seeds were ripe, but Australian researchers developed a *low-toxicant variety* that is safe. Attractive because of its drought tolerance and high protein content, the safe strains are cultivated there and in Southern Africa. An analogous situation occurred with the "taming" of toxicity in rape varieties with help of toxicologists, plant breeders, and animal physiologists in temperate North America.

PRESYNAPTIC CHOLINERGIC (NICOTINIC) TERMINALS. Presynaptic cholinergic terminals are vulnerable sites to a wide range of toxicants: Biological products of bacteria, poisonous plants, and animal venoms may be involved, along with numerous synthetic chemicals. The affected synapses may be central or peripheral, somatic or autonomic. Some of the targets include

1. Plasmalemmal Na^+-dependent choline transport system: *Hemicholinium* causes neuromuscular blockade by competing with choline for the choline carrier, inhibiting its uptake. *Choline mustard aziridinium* analogs compete with choline for entry into cholinergic neurons.
2. In synthesis of ACh via choline acetylase, *naphtoquinones* and *halogenated cholines* reduce ACh synthesis, though there are also *false cholinergic neurotoxicants.*

PLANT NEUROTOXINS. Synthesis of toxic substances in plants is a widespread phenomenon that is one factor in reducing animal and insect predation of plants. It imparts a survival advantage over competitors that lack them. In a given family or genus, not all species produce such agents, but plants in general have evolved a remarkable library of toxic constituents that impact mammalian systems. It has been estimated that there are *at least 7000 species of plants that are toxic to animals.* Probably about 4% of these can produce toxic effects on the CNS. Not surprisingly, a considerable amount of the terminology of the neurosciences is derived from plant-derived neurotoxins.

Plant Poisoning in Livestock Is Variable. Range-grazing livestock are exposed to the flora of the ecosystem they are living in wherever it may be in the world. However, the plant communities are constantly changing due to climatic changes, introduction of new species or strains, and adventive changes. Some get more aggressive and others less so. Such things are also affected by differences in management practices, including the use of pesticides or changes in other factors, such as stage of growth, grazing species, stocking rate, fencing, and use of land for nonagricultural pur-

poses. An important aspect is palatability. Even if a plant species is perceived to be unpalatably bitter by a herbivore, it often gets down to choices between a lack of nourishing palatable species and availability of unpleasant but available forage on a species at a stage of growth that may contain toxicants.

Behavioral Adaptations. Introduction of domesticated animals to new environments after colonization and settlement proved to be a very hazardous endeavor until the toxic species were recognized and measures were taken either to avoid areas where they were prevalent or to eradicate them. Postsettlement Australasia and the Americas are good examples of this phenomenon. In particular, settlement of areas having a unique and unfamiliar flora, such as Western Australia and Southern Africa, proved to be a formidable challenge to veterinary investigators (e.g., Dunlop 1995)

PLANT NEUROTOXICANTS FOR LIVESTOCK: WITH EXAMPLES FROM WESTERN AUSTRALIA. The goal is to distill some biochemical and pathophysiological insights into serious dysfunctions that can occur following consumption of toxic plants by domestic animals by grazing, browsing, or being fed feeds prepared from parts of them that are poisonous (Dorling et al. 1995).

SWAINSONIA GENUS. This group of plants can produce a trihydroxyindolizine alkaloid that causes a lysosomal storage disease, α-mannosidosis. The toxin acts by inhibiting mannosidases. Sheep, cattle, and horses that graze on such plants develop locomotor and behavioral disorders, followed by a progressive loss of condition and weight. Cellular changes involving abnormal organelles and vacuolar inclusions occur in many tissues. The cells become stuffed initially with gangliosides in lysosomes that give rise to functional changes in targeted populations of neurons. The compound swainsonine has been identified as the cause of toxicity arising from poisonous species of the locoweeds, *Astragalus* and *Oxytropis*. This agent has been found to be an immunomodulator, as well, that can inhibit metastases in certain experimental cancers in mice.

BIRDSVILLE INDIGO: *INDIGOFERRA LIUNAEI*. These plants cause a progressive neural dysfunction affecting hindlimb function in horses (Australia). Incoordination results, and, if the horse is stressed, the outcome can be tetanic spasms and collapse. The plant tissues are rich in β-nitropropionic acid, a member of the family that includes agents that cause lathyrism. Domestic ruminants graze the plant readily but show no signs of the disease, probably because of metabolism by rumen microbiota.

YELLOW STAR THISTLE: *CENTAUREA SOLSTITIALIS*. This plant is toxic to horses. The agents responsible may be sesquiterpene lactones, which are toxic to cultured neuronal cells. Ingestion of the plant results in *chewing disease*, with twitching of the lips, flicking of the tongue, purposeless and chewing movements, along with difficulty in prehension of food and swallowing it. The toxin induces hypotonia of the muscles supplied by cranial nerves 5, 7, and 12. The outcome is bilateral focal symmetrical lesions in the substantia nigra and anterior globus pallidus. There are discrete foci of neuronal necrosis, described as nigropallidal encephalomalacia.

CYCAS AND *MACROZAMIA*. These plants, prevalent in Western Australia, contain the toxicants, cycasin and macrozamin, respectively. These are glycosides of methylazomethanol. When grazed, they can cause hepatic necrosis. Zamia staggers of cattle and sheep results from chronic ingestion of the zamia palm, an African cycad popular there. Clinical signs include posterior ataxia, reflecting a spinal proprioceptive dysfunction that may progress to posterior paralysis with severe hindlimb atrophy. Axonal degeneration in the fasciculus gracilis and the dorsal spinocerebellar tracts are seen on necropsy.

PHALARIS AQUATICA. Present in pastures, this has caused heavy losses of stock in South Australia via the plant's dimethyltryptamine alkaloids that inhibit monoamine oxidase, thereby interfering with the normal role of serotonin and catecholamines, as well as with their metabolism and detoxification. The result of ingestion is convulsive spasms and arrhythmic tachycardia. Head nodding and limb weakness are chronic forms.

GRASS TREES: *XANTHORRHEA* SPECIES. Stock graze the young flower spikes. The affected animals lose their sense of balance and may fall heavily: the *wamps*. The pathophysiology involves areas of demyelination in both the central nervous system and peripheral nerves. Slow recovery can occur once the stock can no longer access the grass trees.

BLINDGRASS: *STYPANDRA IMBRICATA*. This Western Australian plant contains a tetrahydroxybinaphthalene (stypandrol) that causes selective degeneration of the optic nerve and retinal photoreceptors, resulting in blindness. It also causes acute edema of myelin centrally and peripherally. This involves vacuolation and may give rise to cerebral edema. It should be noted that photoreceptors have a system of compacted membranes surrounding them; hence, they are somewhat analogous to myelin structurally. Affected horses, sheep, and goats also develop unexplained posterior paralysis.

STRYCHNOS SPECIES. Poisoning by this species has been common in dogs. These plants contain strychnine or brucine that will interact with γ-aminobutyric acid (GABA) receptors in the brain and glycine receptors in the spinal cord. GABA and glycine are transmitters of inhibitory neurons that modulate skeletal muscle activity. When blocked by these toxicants, opposing muscle groups are overstimulated, leading to tetanic convulsions. Because of their investigative and foraging nature, anything that smells attractive as a potential meal makes dogs susceptible to poisoning in baits.

JAPANESE YEW: *TAXUS* CUSPIDATE. This plant is a not uncommon cause of poisoning in cattle. The animals may be found dead, with their rumen containing twigs and leaves upon necropsy. It is considered the most hazardous of ornamental shrubs and trees. Death can result within hours, often without prodromal signs or with, at most, tremors. The narrow green leaves (and other less palatable parts) contain the cardiotoxic alkaloid taxine, which depresses cardiac conduction and induces cardiac failure.

LUPIN POISONING AND MYCOTOXIC LUPINOSIS: *LUPINUS* SPECIES. Alkaloids present in wild lupins cause a neurological disorder, but the plant is bitter and unpalatable. The alkaloids are in higher concentration in seeds and survive haymaking. The acute syndrome causes dyspnea, hyperexcitability, and struggling that progress to convulsions and respiratory paralysis. There is no icterus, and recovery is likely if the animal survives the crisis. A less visible syndrome is a teratogenic effect in cattle if ingested between days 40 and 70 of gestation (particularly if grazed early in plant growth or during seed formation), leading to calves being born with the skeletal defects of crooked-calf disease. It is attributed to an alkaloid, anagyrine. These calves show arthrogryposis, scoliosis, torticollis and cleft palate. Sweet white and yellow lupins have been developed that are relatively free of most of the poisonous principles found in the wild strains. These new lupins became popular for livestock feeds. However, a new "lupinosis" syndrome appeared in sheep (and seen occasionally in other species) that was manifested by anorexia, lassitude, stupor, icterus, and severe hepatic pathology with ketosis and a high mortality. Ingestion of moldy seed, pods, haulm, and stubble affected by *Phomopsis leptostromiformis*, the black-spot stem blight fungus, was shown to be the cause. Fungus-resistant strains of the lupins are being bred, as the disease has become a major scourge of the sheep industry in South Africa, Australia, and New Zealand.

LOCOWEED: *OXYTROPIS* AND *ASTRAGALUS*. Locoweed poisoning is a result of range livestock (cattle, sheep, and horses) grazing on *Oxytropis* and *Astragalus* plants. The alkaloid indolizidine-1,2,8-triol inhibits α-mannosidase, causing a syndrome resembling genetic mannosidosis in cattle. Neurological signs include emaciation, visual impairment, depression, anorexia, ataxia, hyperexcitability, and violent responses to stimuli (hence the name) especially in horses. There is widespread vacuolation of tissues, particularly the brain and kidneys. Damage to the central nervous system is irreversible. Ingested by ewes or cows, spontaneous abortions may result. As the toxic agent is transferred in the milk, calves and lambs suffer musculoskeletal defects.

RHODODENDRON: *ANDROMEDA* SPECIES. The leaves of this plant tend to be eaten by cattle in spring or winter. The andromedotoxins occur in all parts of the plant.

They affect the medulla, triggering acute hypotension with nausea and attempted vomiting, an abnormal event in ruminants. Anorexia, bloat, convulsions, lacrimation, and paralysis may ensue. Sheep are particularly vulnerable in winter. The toxin appears to act directly on vagal nerve endings in the gastrointestinal tract.

FLUOROACETATE-CONTAINING PLANTS. The genera *Gastrolobium* and *Oxylobium* are a unique group of poisonous plants comprised of numerous toxic species that are mainly components of the native flora of the Southwestern Vegetation Province of Western Australia. Over 30 toxic species have been described and studied in this region. They have caused livestock losses ever since settlers brought horses, cattle, goats, and sheep to the area. The primary toxicant in the plants, which was not identified until 1964, is monofluroroacetic acid (short name *fluoroacetate*). Formulated as the sodium salt, it is now the well-known poison *1080* that has been widely used in Australia to destroy rabbits. It is used in North America for rodent and coyote control. It is a very stable substance that survives for years in preserved specimens and forages. Acid soils enhance the uptake of fluorine by the plants. After ingestion, it is converted to fluorocitrate that blocks the tricarboxylic acid cycle by blocking aconitase. Ingestion of such plants by sheep results in extreme tachycardia, hyperpnea, and nervous agitation. This leads to progressive cardiac failure, ventricular fibrillation, and death. Affected herbivores often die close to their source of drinking water, as drinking accelerates absorption of the poison, which is water soluble. Excretion is slow. A low-protein diet increases the susceptibility of the host. When carnivores such as dogs ingest the agent, typically the clinical signs are neural, with either convulsions or just severe depression leading up to respiratory arrest. Less than half a milligram is sufficient to kill a medium-sized dog, indicating the extreme metabolic blockade of function in the vital organs. Swine and cats experience both cardiovascular and neural pathophysiology.

RECOMMENDED READING

Adams NR. 1995. Detection of the effects of phytoestrogens on sheep and cattle. J Anim Sci 73:1509–1515.

Barnes AL, Croker KP, Allen JG, Costa ND. 1996. Lupinosis of ewes around the time of mating reduces reproductive performance. Aust J Agric Res 47:1305–1314

Burrows GE, Tyrl RJ. 2001. Toxic Plants of North America. Ames: Iowa State University Press.

Curtis SE. 1983. Environmental Management in Agriculture. Ames: Iowa State University Press.

Dejours P, Bolis L, Taylor CR, Weibel ER, eds. 1987. Comparative Physiology: Life in Water and on Land. In: FIDIA Research Series, vol 9. Berlin: Springer-Verlag.

Dorling PR, Colegate SM, Huxtable CR. 1995. Plant neurotoxins. In: Chang LW, Dyer RS, eds. Handbook of Neurotoxicology. New York: Marcel Dekker.

Dunlop RH. 1997. The Hagyard, Davidson and McGee Practice: A cornerstone in the development of Kentucky's racing industry. Vet Heritage 20:1–13.

Majak W, Benn MH. N.d. Glycosides. In: Hui YH, Gorham JR, Murrell KD, Oliver DO, eds. Disease Handbook of Foodborne Diseases Caused by Hazardous Substances, vol 3. New York: Marcel Dekker (reprint undated).

McBarron EJ. 1976. Medical and Veterinary Aspects of Plant Poisons in New South Wales. Department of Agriculture, New South Wales.

McNab BK. 2002. The Physiological Ecology of Vertebrates: A View from Energetics. Ithaca: Cornell University Press.

Poison Plants of Western Australia. N.d. The toxic species of the genera *Gastrolobium* and *Oxylobium*. Bulletin 3772. Perth: Western Australian Department of Agriculture.

Tanner GJ, Moate PJ, Davis LH, et al. 1995. Proanthocyanidins (condensed tannin) destabilise plant protein foams in a dose dependent manner. Aust J Agric Res 46:1101–1109.

PART 3: PATHOPHYSIOLOGY OF SOME NONPLANT TOXICANTS

INORGANIC AND SYNTHETIC ORGANIC TOXIC CHEMICALS, INCLUDING MANY PESTICIDES AND PHARMACEUTICALS. There is a vast range of chemical elements and substances that are not of biological origin that are poisonous to mammals if the amount ingested or otherwise exposed to is sufficiently high, that is, that are not *biotoxins* per se (Murphy 1996). It would be impossible to do justice to this wider spectrum of toxicology in a single chapter of a book on pathophysiology. Therefore, aside from touching on a few examples of unique mechanisms of toxicity, this chapter is restricted to coverage of selected highlights drawn mainly from biotoxins and a few miscellaneous ones with molecular mechanisms of special interest to veterinary medicine. The wider field can be readily addressed by referring to a number of excellent, more encyclopedic, edited books that do cover aspects over a more comprehensive range of chemical toxicants. Examples include Radeleff (1964), Clarke et al. (1981), Osweiler et al. (1985), Rang et al. (1995), Aiello (1998), Hardman and Limberg (2001), Josephy (1997), Voet et al. (1999), Radostits et al. (2000), Spencer and Schaumberg (2000), and Smith (2002).

Mycotoxins and Antinutritional Factors. The major toxicogenic fungi are from the genera *Aspergillus*, *Penicillium*, *Fusarium*, *Acremonium*, *Claviceps*, *Phomopsis*, *Pithomyces*, and *Alternaria* (D'Mello 2000; CAST 2003). Toxigenic strains form metabolites called *mycotoxins*. Fortunately, the synthesis of most mycotoxins is limited to a fairly low number of strains. On the other hand, those few can cause widespread hazards to man and beast. The spotlight became focused on this class of toxicants in 1960 when a major epidemic of *Turkey X disease* in the United Kingdom was shown to be caused by mycotoxins from *Aspergillus flavus*, christened *aflatoxins*. Much later, a second agent, cyclopiazonic acid, was isolated from the old samples, indicating the potential for encountering multiple agents in a given syndrome. A range of aflatoxins has been isolated and studied. One has been isolated from bovine milk from cows consuming contaminated feeds. Aspergilli are storage fungi that thrive on high humidity and temperature; that is, they thrive typically in tropical environments (but also shower rooms and the respiratory tracts of birds). The contaminated feeds were first derived from groundnuts (peanuts) from West Africa. Corn (maize) that is grown in warm humid areas may be infected before harvest. The aflatoxins caused an acute disease, with poults dying in droves having hepatic necrosis and bile duct proliferation. Once its epidemiology and toxicants were understood, precautions were taken that averted a recurrence. Although numerous mycotoxins have been identified subsequently, the majority cause chronic syndromes rather than acute mortalities. Even with the original aflatoxins, the current concern is much more focused on potential carcinogenic effects than on liver damage per se.

ERGOTISM AND FESCUE FOOT MYCOTOXICOSIS. The toxic agents in these conditions are numerous ergot alkaloids that are lysergic acid derivatives and cause severe vasoconstriction of arterioles, particularly in vessels in the extremities (tail and hooves). Their stimulant effect on smooth muscle includes actions on adrenoceptors and 5-HT (5-hydroxytryptamine or serotonin) receptors. The vascular changes may progress to dry gangrene because the vasoconstriction can become arterial spasm with endothelial degeneration and dermal necrosis. Hooves may be sloughed. The feet are tender or painful, and knuckling of the pastern sometimes occurs. There is a neurological form with depression or excitability, loss of appetite, ataxia, weight loss, diarrhea, and clonic convulsions. In ergotism, the source of the toxins is a fungus, *Claviceps purpura*, that grows in the mature seeds of grains such as rye and certain grasses.

In fescue foot, the source is a different endophytic fungus, *Acremonium coenophialum*, which affects the widely grown tall fescue (*Festuca arundinacea* Schreb) at all stages of growth. The ergopeptine alkaloid toxins, and particularly ergovaline, cause vasoconstriction and vascular spasm in the arteries of the feet, and some also antagonize prolactin. The latter effect can cause agalactia in sows, cows, and mares. Mares may develop prolonged gestation and thickened placentas, and may abort. Affected animals are more vulnerable to heat stress, and growth rates are inhibited. It appears to be the cause of "summer slump." Another grass—perennial ryegrass—may be infected by *Acremonium lolii*, which synthesizes lolitrem B, an indole isoprenoid lolitrem alkaloid.

Lupin stubbles used for fodder by sheep in Australia are often infected with the fungus *Phomopsis leptostromiformis*, which forms the mycotoxin phomopsin A, a substituted hexapeptide. This is the cause of lupinosis in sheep that results in ill-thrift, hepatic failure, and death.

Sporidesmin A is a mycotoxin formed by *Pithomyces chartarum*, a widespread pasture saprophyte. The toxin is a diketopiperazine that results in facial eczema in sheep.

The mycotoxins deoxynivalenol (DON) and one of the tricothecenes, known as T-2, give rise to gastric lesions in swine.

Ochratoxin A, which is formed by *Aspergillus ochraceus* in cereal grains grown in temperate climates, is implicated in porcine nephropathy and appears to be a teratogen and a carcinogen.

MYCOTOXICOSES AFFECTING THE CENTRAL NERVOUS SYSTEM. Feeding horses *moldy corn* (maize) can cause an outbreak of *equine leukoencephalomalacia* (ELE). *Fusarium* species form toxins called *fumonisins* (from the Latin *F. moniliforme*). In equidae, ELE causes liquefactive necrosis of the white matter of the brain. This is often unilateral and accompanied by neurological signs that may include apathy, drowsiness, blindness, pharyngeal paralysis, circling, staggering, recumbency, and death. ELE is the result of fumonisin toxicity produced in *F. moniliforme*, which is a fungus growing on corn. *Pigs* are susceptible to fumonisin toxins. They develop anorexia and acute *pulmonary edema* [permeability pulmonary edema (PPE)] with hydrothorax and hepatotoxicosis. This syndrome used to go under the name *moldy-corn poisoning*, which has been replaced by titles for specific mycotoxicoses: aflatoxicosis, estrogenism, ochrotoxicosis, tricothecine (fusariotoxicosis) toxicosis, and leukoencephalomalacia.

Regulatory control programs for mycotoxins have been established in the United States because of human risk. The list of mycotoxins includes aflatoxins, the only group for which specific action levels have been established, DON, fumonisins, and patulins (the latter in apples and apple products). Evaluation is continuous for several others, including ochratoxin A, zearalenone, citrinin, cyclopiazonic acid, and several *Alternaria* toxins.

Essential aspects of protection from mycotoxins entering the mammalian diet include the following: Good agronomic practices and sound storage practices, including protection from the elements and microbial contaminations, as well as insects, mites, rodents, and animal wastes. Since many fungi are slow growing, duration of storage can be important. In particular, temperature and humidity control can be critical. Various physical and dietary stresses and infections can have important effects on host resistance to mycotoxins. The key factor, however, is the nature of the specific toxin or toxins present.

BLUE-GREEN ALGAE TOXINS. Four genera predominate the list of cyanobacteria that have been associated with toxic water blooms on freshwater systems: *Microcystis*, *Nodularia*, *Anabena*, and *Aphanizomenon*. *Microcystis* produces microcystin, an extremely potent hepatotoxin (20 times as toxic as cyanide!) that is a cyclopeptide. The liver damage can result in blood loss and hypovolemic shock with pulmonary embolism. The result can be sudden death. This syndrome tends to occur in late summer in stagnant ponds or small lakes when a wind has blown the algal cover to the shore and then drops again. If cattle drink from the scummy layer, there can be catastrophic losses. *Nodularia* gives rise to nodularin, which is also a cyclic peptide that causes hepatotoxicity. *Anabena* produces anatoxins, one of which causes depolarization of nicotinic ganglia and neuromuscular junctions (NMJs), resulting in paralysis and respiratory failure. Another anatoxin inhibits peripheral cholinesterase after the fashion of organophosphate compounds. *Aphanizomenon* forms alkaloid toxins that are structurally similar to saxitoxin, the notorious agent of shellfish poisoning that kills some sea mammals. Alkaloid toxins are sodium channel blockers.

Exotoxic Endospore-forming Anaerobic Bacteria. The genus *Clostridium* is of enormous importance to farm animal production and veterinary medicine, as well as to the survival of people and companion animals (Schaechter et al. 1998; Madigan et al. 2000; Mims et al. 2001). These pathogenic species are Gram-positive anaerobes that form endospores (sporulate) when their environment is hostile to their survival (such as a lack of accessible nutrients). As only a single spore forms from each parent cell that is in the vegetative state, spore formation is a survival strategy, not a replicative one. When in the active vegetative phase, however, each species of *Clostridium* can form several types of toxin.

Some species can multiply in the gastrointestinal tract and form toxins there that cause severe disease— for example, *C. perfringens* type C in young pigs (up to 3 weeks of age) that penetrates the epithelial barrier of the jejunum, where its β-toxin causes necrosis of the villi, accompanied by hemorrhagic diarrhea. Clostridial enterotoxemia is also an important consequence of clostridial disease (food poisoning) in people and other animal species—type A in dogs (necrotic enteritis), horses (colic), and pigs (diarrhea). Type B in sheep can cause lamb dysentery in neonatals and "struck" (sudden death) in adults; in calves, types B and C can result in acute diarrhea with pain, convulsions, and opisthotonos. In foals, very acute diarrhea and pain followed by dehydration, toxemia, and shock are typical, whereas adults tend to manifest enterocolitis. Newborn or recently weaned lambs are vulnerable to type D, particularly if well fed on milk and/or feed. This causes pulpy kidney and *overeating disease*, named after the rapid postmortem autolysis of the kidneys, sometimes but not always present along with opisthotonos, circling, and head pressing. The rich ingesta favors growth of type D, which forms epsilon toxin that causes vascular damage to capillaries, crucially in the brain. *Clostridium chauvoei* causes blackleg in cattle after spores gain entry before localizing in skeletal muscle, historically causing heavy losses. *Clostridium septicum*, the main cause of malignant edema, and *C. chauvoei* are both soil organisms that enter opportunistically and result in necrotic, gangrenous lesions.

Other histotoxic clostridia gain entry to the body through wounds that are deep enough to create an anaerobic environment. Because of the toxins they produce, such wounds can result in necrosis of all tissue layers where blood supply has been damaged: decubitus ulcers may overlie myonecrosis and even osteonecrosis, requiring complete debridement of the dying anoxic tissues. The classic tetanus toxin arises from closed wounds infected with the spores of *C. tetani* that are widely dispersed in the environment, particularly when accompanied by foreign bodies that foster a hypoxic medium allowing the spores to germinate. The uterus and umbilicus are subject to similar conditions if contaminated around the time of parturition. The large toxin is called *tetanospasmin*, which enters at motor end plates and travels centrally by retrograde axonal transport up α motoneurons and then achieves a crossover to interneurons, its sites of action. The toxin acts as a protease, with zinc at the active site that targets a specific protein, syntaxin, that mediates translocation across the synapse and membrane fusion, blocking the release of inhibitory neurotransmitters such as glycine or GABA. Lacking this constraint, the skeletal musculature contracts excessively, resulting in spastic paralysis, a very pathophysiological tetanus. Tetanus toxin from *C. tetani* also has two polypeptide chains, one of which attaches to the presynaptic nerve membrane, facilitating the entry of the other one into the terminal. The latter is carried retrogradely by fast axonal transport to motoneurons in the spinal cord, where, remarkably, it translocates and binds to the plasmalemma of attached spinal inhibitory neuron terminals. There, the tetanus fragment cleaves two proteins: synaptobrevin and cellubrevin. The effect is blockade of inhibition of motoneurons and sympathetic neurons, resulting in excess motor and sympathetic nerve activity.

Neurotoxicity of Chemicals Used to Kill Pests and Fungi. *Metaldehyde* is a polymer of acetaldehyde used to kill slugs and snails but often unintentionally accessible to domestic stock, particularly dogs and, less commonly, cats, horses, and small ruminants (Clarke et al. 1981:159). Concentrations of GABA, 5-HT, and norepinephrine in the brain are decreased. Metabolized to acetaldehyde polymers that pass the blood-brain barrier, this results in acidosis. Clinical signs include severe tremors, ataxia, hyperesthesia, and hyperpnea. Cats are especially prone to manifest nystagmus. Opisthotonos and continuous tonic convulsions generate acute hyperthermia.

Neurotoxicant Effects Via Neurotransmitter Systems. Neurotoxicants (NTs) may influences the neurotransmitter system in one of three ways:

1. Presynaptic NT release: *increase* or *decrease*
2. Residence time of NT in synaptic cleft: *change*
3. Postsynaptic receptor: *antagonist* or *agonist*

Many NTs act via plasmalemmal receptors, either at ligand-gated ion channels (LGICs) or G proteins that influence intracellular effectors. The LGIC have receptors for inhibitory NTs: GABA$_a$, glycine, and 5-HT, plus most glutamate and nicotinic receptors. The G protein-linked effectors bond to guanine nucleotides while the nongated ion channels (NGICs) influence receptors that respond to glutamate (GLU), GABA$_b$, β-adrenergic, or muscarinic ACh receptors.

Exocytosis of NTs at presynaptic axon terminals involves entry of calcium ions into the cytosol; then synaptic vesicles move to the plasmalemma, where fusion proteins enable release of the NTs. Some biological toxins act as proteases that block transmitter release at these sites.

BOTULINUM TOXIN. Botulinum toxin comes from *Clostridium botulinum* strains that make several serotypes (A–G). These polypeptide toxins consist of two types of chains. The heavier one establishes the bond to the plasmalemma, facilitating the entry of the

lighter one, which is a zinc endopeptidase, into the axon terminal. Once there, it cleaves the synaptic vesicle fusion proteins needed for exocytosis, thereby blocking synaptic transmission. The consequence is blockade of depolarization-induced transmitter release at the NMJ, resulting in flaccid paralysis (Figure 13.4). The syndrome occurs after ingestion of preformed toxin by mammals or birds. Although it is excluded from the brain, it causes descending paralysis via cranial nerve and NMJ involvement. This affects the musculature of the neck, thorax, and extremities while swallowing and voiding may be affected, too. Minute doses of botulinum toxin have been used in therapy of pathophysiologically excess movement of some critical muscles.

α-LATROTOXIN. α-Latrotoxin, from *Latrodectus* spp. (the female black widow spider), is a large peptide that

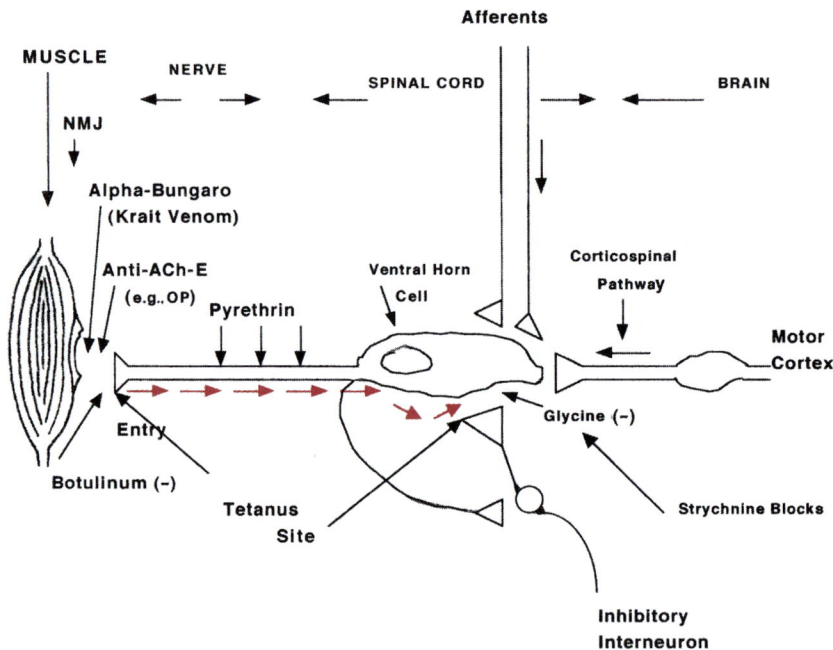

FIG. 13.4—Primary sites of toxic actions in the principal motor pathway from cortex to neuromuscular junction (NMJ). The ventral horn cells of the spinal cord are affected by tetanus toxin that enters the axon at the periphery and is transported retrogradely up to the neuronal soma. It is an endopeptidase that then enters the inhibitory interneuron that synapses with the motoneuron and blocks exocytosis in the interneuron. The unfettered motoneuron then causes tetanic contractions.

Strychnine blocks interneurons at all glycine receptors. Blocking their inhibition, it enhances neuronal activity and leads to exaggerated reflexes. It also blocks inhibition between antagonistic muscle groups (e.g., flexors versus extensors) and recurrent spinal inhibition by intraspinal collaterals of motoneurons mediated by Renshaw cells.

Botulinum toxin is another endopeptidase that lyses proteins in plasma membranes (syntaxin and SNAP-25) and the synaptic vesicle (synaptobrevin, required for exocytosis), where it blocks depolarization induced by acetylcholine (ACh) release at the presynaptic terminal of the neuromuscular junction. This causes flaccid paralysis. The toxin does not cross the blood-brain barrier.

The insecticide pyrethrin causes sodium channels in the axon membrane to stay open for longer than normal after a potential arrives, prolonging the depolarizing afterpotentials. Their toxicity is much greater for insects than for mammals because of their much more rapid biotransformation in the latter, a fine example of selective toxicity. Anti-ACh-E agents have widespread effects on body functions. At the NMJ, the prolonged presence of ACh at the junction causes excessive twitching. Some shellfish and algal toxins act at ganglia and NMJs.

Also, α-latrotoxin in the venom of the black widow spider (*Latrodectus*) is a highly toxic peptide that causes massive ACh release at NMJs.

binds to neurexin 1α and causes massive NT (norepi-nephrine and ACh) release at NMJs with widespread severe muscle cramping. It appears that the mechanism is unusual in that it does not involve calcium ions, bypassing their normal role in NT release. (Aiello 1998:2155) (Figure 13.4).

Axonal Transport in Neurotoxicity. Various axonal metabolic components are transported within nerve fibers: *anterograde* (from neuronal soma to axon ter-minal). Some metabolites are *fast transported* at up to 200 to 400 mm/day, whereas others, notably mitochon-drial components, are transported much more slowly (in the range of 30 to 70 mm/day). Among the fast ones, many go to the end, turn around, and return *ret-rogradely*. These are mainly membrane bound and resemble lysosomes. Of interest to this discussion, they may ferry foreign materials (xenobiotics such as toxi-cants, metals, and toxins). Any chemical-induced pathophysiology is usually observed first at the distal ends of the largest and longest axons. This leads to the "stocking and glove" pattern of distribution of, first, sensory dysfunction, followed by motor weakness in a similar pattern of peripheral nerves and spinal cord tracts. There is also involvement of neural pathways in the brain. Distal nerve fibers subjected to chemically induced degeneration show accumulation of organelles at the periphery that are normally transported *retro-gradely* within the axon.

Progress is being made in identifying cellular effects of some neurotoxicants so that understanding the processes leading to neuronal dysfunction can be advanced. This involves following the time sequence of morphological lesion development and the molecular and pathophysiological dynamics of functional changes. It requires tracking these events in the various classes of neurons, for example, dorsal root and auto-nomic ganglia as well as those within the CNS. Such studies require identification of the individual cells and their types, fiber pathways, synapses, and neurotrans-mitters, along with their insulating cladding and sup-port cells (e.g., myelin, Schwann cells, and glial cells). Changes may be demonstrable in the neuronal soma (cell body), with their setting in a veritable forest of receptors, dendrites, axons, glial cells, interneuronal processes, and synapses.

Neurotoxicants of Some Snake Venoms and Rabies Virus. There is a connection between mad dogs and snake strikes! Rabies has a lethal affinity for the CNS: the virus makes its way via peripheral nerves to the brain, where it infects specific groups of neurons. The glycoprotein that forms spikes on the envelope of the virus enables it to bind to receptors on normal cells. Comparisons were made between the structures of rabies virus and the neurotoxic proteins present in the venom of snakes, such as cobras and sea snakes, that act by blocking Ach receptors. The viral glycoprotein and the venom proteins had identical sequences of amino acids in several regions. This close match makes it very likely that the virus, like the venom, exerts its neurotoxic

effect by binding to the ACh receptors of neurons. Some viruses might possess structures that are very similar to the domains of molecules that normally bind to receptors on cells. If so, such similarity may form the basis of some autoimmune diseases. The immune system may respond to certain viral infections by producing antibod-ies that create havoc by reacting with cellular receptors.

AUTOINTOXICATION AND ALLERGY, CYTO-KINES, AND CHEMOKINES. The thymus is an intriguing organ that emerges early in the development of the mammalian immune system. It screens the mil-lions of antibody specificities for any reactivity to self. Reactive clones of T lymphocytes are eliminated to protect against future self-destruction. Having accom-plished this goal, the thymus sacrifices itself, undergo-ing atrophy.

Cell-mediated immunity arises when maturing T cells differentiate into subsets of cytotoxic T lympho-cytes or T helper cells. This process differs from that of B cells, whose terminally differentiated state is to become an antibody-producing plasma cell.

T cells express T-cell receptors (TCRs) on their sur-face that recognize only antigenic peptides associated with major histocompatibility complex (MHC) mole-cules that are on the surfaces of most cells. These pro-teins allow recognition of an infected cell as an *infected self cell* that should be eliminated. Cytotoxic T lym-phocytes (CTLs) require prior sensitization to respond fully. They then produce perforins (proteases that cre-ate holes in protective cell membranes, allowing entry of granzymes that trigger apoptosis). Macrophages col-laborate with CTLs in producing cytokines (inter-leukins) that help focus on entering antigens.

Natural killer (NK) cells are specialized lympho-cytes that arise from bone marrow precursors that can release granules and kill cells carrying certain antigens that the animal has not encountered before. Peripheral blood lymphocytes are comprised of a majority of T cells, with minorities of NK cells and B cells.

Dendritic cells are remarkable stellate-shaped cells of the monocyte-macrophage series with long dendritic processes extending through the lymphatic and splenic systems that entrap particles traveling in the incoming lymph flow. They occur in all body surface areas and orifices with stratified squamous epithelium, including the epidermis and all penetrating tubular systems lead-ing in via simple surface epithelium that is constantly being replaced, such as the gastrointestinal tract, uro-genital tract, and respiratory tract that drain via inter-stitial fluid and lymphatic channels to their nodal col-lectors. They act as antigen-presenting cells that ensure that any incoming organisms encounter cytotoxic lym-phocytes and immunologic activation.

This system is believed to participate in the initial response to prions entering via the gastrointestinal tract at the level of the ileum. Langerhans' cells in skin and gut are of this type.

Physiological aspects of cellular defense systems must be considered from the perspective of time and cellular differentiation, multiplication, interactions with other cells, and potent chemical factors such as cytokines. Myeloid growth factors stimulate proliferation and differentiation of one or more myeloid cell lines and enhance the function of their mature forms. Myeloid growth factors (GFs) are made by fibroblasts, endothelial cells, macrophages, and T cells.

Pluripotent stem cells of the embryo give rise to a variety of hematopoietic and lymphopoietic cells under the influence of GFs that are glycoproteins. GFs are produced by bone marrow cells and similar cells in peripheral tissues. The hormone controlling erythropoiesis–*erythropoietin*–was isolated in 1977. The GFs for lymphocytes, granulocytes, macrophages, and megakaryocytes followed. Erythropoietin is made in peritubular interstitial cells in the kidney and then moves to the bone marrow. Infection or inflammation suppresses erythropoietin production via inflammatory cytokines. The dynamism of cell turnover in these systems is phenomenal. For example, hematopoiesis generates about 200 billion new red blood cells every day. On top of this, when need arises, this base can be increased severalfold.

Cytokines is a term encompassing a myriad of cellular proteins with proinflammatory and anti-inflammatory effects. Cellular products released from the cytoplasm into the extracellular space that act as the hormones of the immune system is how they have been described. They act at receptor sites in a remarkably diverse way linking neural, endocrine, and immune systems. As such, they have great potential for both beneficial and harmful effects on mammalian systems. With advancing knowledge acquired through recent research, definitions have had to be expanded. *Interleukins* (ILs) for example, were initially referred to as products of leukocytes that acted on leukocytes but now are known to play a much wider spectrum of roles involving many types of cells and a variety of functional outcomes. IL-1 causes fever, induces sleep, and modulates inflammatory and immune responses. The ILs are assigned numbers based on their chronology of discovery, which is not particularly helpful in gaining an understanding of their roles, interactions, and participation in various functions and dysfunctions. *Chemokines* are cytokines that direct chemotaxis (migration) of target cells and affect the function of microbial pathogens.

A major focus of research on the application of cytokines has been their potential use in therapy of infectious diseases, hopefully through amplification of host defenses against pathogens and potentially in minimizing the negative aspects of responses to infection (Holland 2001).

Examples include the deployment of granulocyte colony-stimulating factor (G-CSF) to treat neutropenias. Interferon γ (IFN-γ) shows promise in treating chronic granulomatous diseases. Cytokine immune adjuvants combined with appropriate antimicrobials may bring new life to therapy of chronic intracellular infections. Specific suppression of chronic inflammatory conditions by using anticytokines (e.g., versus tumor-necrosis factor α) may achieve the therapeutic goal without having to resort to chronic glucocorticoid administration with its often undesirable consequences. Anticytokines have considerable potential for dampening uncontrolled responses of the immune system. This is an exciting field of current research in mammalian pathophysiology.

In 1906, von Pirquet coined the term *allergy*. He recognized that antigens induced changed reactivity in both protective immunity and hypersensitivity responses. He proposed that host responses began as uncommitted biologically and able to achieve either beneficial immunity or harmful allergic disease. The latter includes mainly respiratory, dermal, and digestive disorders; that is, surfaces where agents from the outside world interface with the lining tissues after inhalation, contact, or ingestion and evoke reactive responses, including involvement of associated neural and vascular components. *Atopic* (derived from the Greek for "out of place") is a term applied to individual mammals that have a hereditary predisposition to produce immunoglobulin E (IgE) antibodies against certain antigens. Nonallergic individuals produce allergen-specific IgG antibodies and low-grade cellular reactions of the Th-1 type with the cytokines, IFN-γ, and IL-2. Allergic individuals, on the other hand, produce cytokines of the Th-2 type: ILs 4, 5, and 13. This grouping is the immunopathological hallmark of allergic disease (Kay 2000).

Anaphylaxis is a very severe allergic reaction that results from massive release of histamine, kinins, and products of the arachidonic cascade, typically a consequence of IgE-mediated hypersensitivity to an ingested agent, an insect sting, or an injected substance. Histamine induces respiratory difficulty, including bronchoconstriction and laryngeal edema, vasodilation, and hypotension. Its toxic effects can be reversed by prompt administration of epinephrine. More detailed perspectives can be found in Eyre and Burka (1978:100, Fig. 1) and in more recent publications expanding on the roles of various cytokines and mediators.

RECOMMENDED READING

Abramson D. 1997 Toxicants of the genus *Penicillium*. In: D'Mello JPF, ed. Handbook of Plant and Fungal Toxicants. Boca Raton, FL: CRC, pp 303–317.

Aiello SE, ed. 1998. The Merck Veterinary Manual, 8th ed. Whitehouse Station, NJ: Merck.

CAST (Council for Agricultural Science and Technology). 2003. Mycotoxins: Risks in Plant, Animal and Human Systems. Task Force Report no. 139. Ames, IA: CAST.

Cheeke PR. 1998. Natural Toxicants in Feeds, Forages, and Poisonous Plants, 2nd ed. Danville, IL: Interstate.

Cheeke PR. 1998. Natural Toxicants in Feeds, Forages, and Poisonous Plants, 2nd ed. Danville, IL: Interstate.

Clarke ML, Harvey DG, Humphreys DJ. 1981. Veterinary Toxicology, 2nd ed. London: Ballière, Tindall.

D'Mello JPF, ed. 1997. Handbook of Plant and Fungal Toxicants. Boca Raton, FL: CRC.

D'Mello JPF. 2000. Anti-nutritional Factors and Mycotoxins. In: D'Mello JPF, ed. Farm Animal Metabolism and Nutrition. Wallingford, UK: CAB International.

Eyre P, Burka JF. 1978. Hypersensitivity in cattle and sheep: A pharmacological review. J Vet Pharmacol Ther 1:97–109.

Henderson B, Wilson M, McNab R, Lax AJ. 1999. Cellular Microbiology: Bacteria-Host Interactions in Health and Disease. New York: Wiley.

Kay AB 2000. Overview of "Allergy and allergic diseases: with a view to the future." Br Med Bull 56:843–864.

Lock EA, Wilks MF. 2001. Paraquat. In: Handbook of Pesticide Toxicology. New York: Academic.

Mims C, Nash A, Stephen J. 2001. Mims' Pathogenesis of Infectious Disease, 5th ed. San Diego: Academic.

Murphy MJ. 1996. A Field Guide to Common Animal Poisons. Ames: Iowa State University Press.

Pestka JJ, Bondy GS. 1994. Immunotoxic effects of mycotoxins. In: Miller JD, Trenholm HL, eds. Mycotoxins in Grain: Compounds Other than Aflatoxin. St Paul, MN: Eagan, pp 339–358.

Porter JK. 1997. Endophyte alkaloids. In: D'Mello JPF, ed. Handbook of Plant and Fungal Toxicants. Boca Raton, FL: CRC, pp 51–62.

Porter JK, Thompson FN. 1992. Effects of fescue toxicosis on reproduction in livestock. J Anim Sci 70:1594–1603.

Schaechter M, Engleberg NC, Eisenstein BI, Medoff G, eds. 1998. Mechanisms of Microbial Disease, 3rd ed. Baltimore: Williams and Wilkins.

Sevcik C, Brito JC, D'Suze G, et al. 1993. Toxicology of a bovine paraplegic syndrome. Toxicon 12:1581–1594.

Whitten PL, Kudo S, Okubo KK. 1997. Isoflavonoids. In: D'Mello JPF, ed. Handbook of Plant and Fungal Toxicants. Boca Raton, FL: CRC, pp 117–137.

PART 4: PATHOPHYSIOLOGY OF SPONGIFORM ENCEPHALOPATHIES

THOUGHTS ON BOVINE SPONGIFORM ENCEPHALOPATHY, SCRAPIE, AND THE PRION IDEA: TOXICANT EXPOSURE, GENETIC SUSCEPTIBILITY, AND TRANSMISSIBILITY. The prion concept espoused by Prusiner to explain the etiology of the transmissible spongiform encephalopathies (TSEs) is brilliant but seems to have a flaw. The evidence for it being the agent of a truly *infectious* disease is lacking. It is *transmissible*, but is it infectious in situations other than naturally occurring scrapie of sheep and goats and chronic wasting disease (CWD) of cervids such as deer and elk? Perhaps the agent can become infectious when accompanied by other factors or changes, but it does not appear to be an infectious protein per se in all the conditions in which prions have been isolated. Bovine spongiform encephalopathy (BSE) (Figure 13.5) is more like kuru than scrapie, which is a disease that varies greatly in transmissibility with the genetic makeup of the sheep and the agent. Also, BSE and kuru are not shed by affected animals or people but have been amplified by ingestion of processed carcass material (from cattle affected with BSE) or by cannibalism of the brain tissue of the cadavers of affected subjects (kuru). Experimental reproduction of the Creutzfeldt-Jakob disease (CJD) syndrome in primates involved injection directly into the brain. How do we tell a truly infectious condi-

tion from an apparently infectious one? Critical questions are "Is there proof of lateral transmission?" "Does the disease maintain itself in a population?" Epidemiologically, BSE is recognized from Wilesmith's work to be attributable to ingestion of a preformed protein prion agent that can affect virtually every bovine mammal that may consume it at a young age. This concept was based on the data available on experimental reproduction of the disease that followed ingestion of contaminated meat and bone meal (A.R. Austin personal communication). It does not spread from cow to cow like a true infection: if it did, it would not be expected to infect all that consumed the agent. Can we point to a known infection that does that? A strange feature of the BSE epidemic was that most affected dairy herds had only one or a low number of cases.

The concept of a prion protein being the causative agent of transmissible spongiform encephalopathies (TSEs) involves conversion of a normal protein component of CNS tissues, known as the normal cellular isoform of the prion protein or PrP^c to a disease-causing isoform, PrP^{Sc}. PrP^c is rich in alpha-helix and very low in beta-sheet folding form. PrP^{Sc}, on the other hand, is the opposite: high in beta and low in alpha. Thus, a transition from alpha to beta is the fundamental event in creation of a toxic disease-inducing agent. It is unfortunate that modern research on TSEs was so derivative from the British work on scrapie at Compton and Edinburgh that Prusiner used the abbreviation PrP^{Sc}, denoting scrapie form to identify his rogue protein for CJD. The naturally occurring ovine disease, scrapie, has been known for well over 200 years, and no case of a human with CJD has been traced unequivocally to consumption of ovine tissue.

In fact, the claim of infectivity for prions in general seems an overgeneralization. In most cases, they appear to behave more like an intoxication related to genetic susceptibility than to a true infection. Only scrapie of sheep and goats and CWD of cervids seem to be capable of spreading spontaneously in a flock or herd. Kuru in people, TME in mink, and BSE in cattle appeared only after consumption of processed, i.e., rendered, ruminant tissues. When this was recognized, the syndrome was finally eliminated after any further exposure was terminated. Felidae, including captive species in zoos, were found to be susceptible, but no dogs have been reported affected. The latter observation merits investigation. TSEs that have occurred in nondomestic mammals include transmissible mink encephalopathy (TME). However, this was a disease that appeared in captive mink raised for pelt fur production that had been exposed through being fed diets now believed to have contained TSE agent-containing ingredients. TME was the first animal TSE to be recognized after scrapie. It does not occur in mink if they do not consume ruminant-derived animal wastes or meat-and-bone meals. A second TSE to be recognized in nondomestic species appeared in farmed cervids (deer species, mule deer, elk). Several such species are farmed for antler velvet and/or venison production in

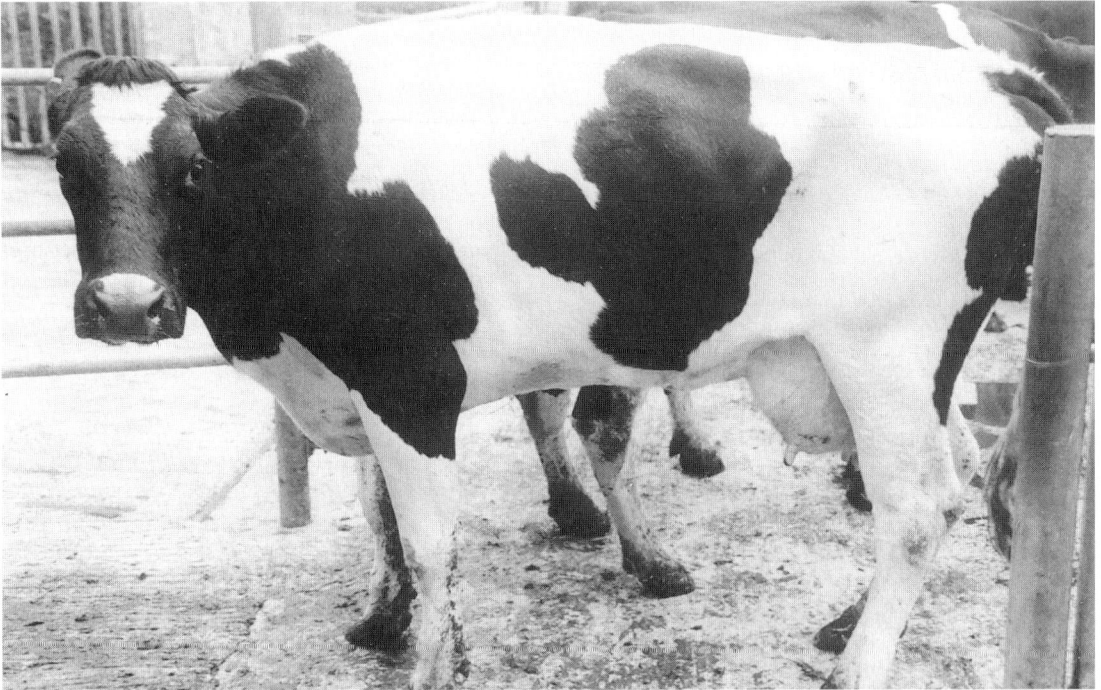

FIG. 13.5—Bovine spongiform encephalopathy (BSE) in a cow during the epidemic in the United Kingdom in 1993 on a Wiltshire farm in Little Langford. Typically cases were over 3 years old because of the long lag period after ingestion prior to clinical signs, even though it is thought that most cases arose from eating rations containing meat and bone meal derived in part from recycled bovine tissues.

Early signs were mild, including unsteadiness especially of the hindfeet and on turning, with stiffness, mild tremors or twitching, and slight arching of the back. The ears have abnormal positions and movements that may be related to hypersensitivity to noise. Touch sensations also show increased sensitivity. Nose licking plus grinding of teeth was commonly seen. Anxiety and mildly aggressive behaviors were common. The aggression was often pseudoaggressive behavior directed at inanimate objects or plants. When animals were subjected to unfamiliar treatments or noises, shipping, and handling, they were more unsettled, uncoordinated, and anxious. This resulted in unpredictable, occasionally aggressive, behavior directed at the persons responsible. The disease was progressive, with weight loss and suppression or cessation of reticuloruminal cyclic contractions suggesting failure of vagal motor control of forestomach motility. On the other hand, cardiac rate was slowed, indicating an increase in vagal tone. The condition worsened, leading to weakness, collapse, and terminal recumbency. The transmissible spongiform encephalopathy agent enters neurons and kills them slowly, leaving a space that is the basis for the term *spongiform encephalopathy*. The rations fed the animals included meat and bone meal that was derived from rendered tissues of BSE-affected cattle, the source of the intoxication. That leaves unanswered the question of where the first contamination of a bovine, or other species, carcass arose to initiate the cascading epidemic. Domestic and exotic Felidae have been affected by ingestion of the bovine agent, but dogs have not. Reproduction of the disease required intracerebral inoculation with brain extracts from affected cattle or oral dosing with meat and bone meal derived from clinical cases. In the latter situation, a prion toxicant analogous to PrP[Sc] was detected in Peyer's patches in the distal ileum, as well as in bone marrow, dorsal root ganglia, spinal cord, and brain. In field cases, however, it was found only in brain and spinal cord 32 to 40 months after oral challenge.

the modern era, often under much closer confinement than would occur in free-ranging animals. After the disease appeared in these confined environments, which included game parks, zoos, and research units, it spread without human laboratory challenge being involved. Is it conceivable that a toxicant that entered via a dietary ingredient could acquire the capacity to spread?

A very important question involves the factors that led to the first occurrence of TSE disease in each species. Could sheep scrapie have occurred as a result of the massive inbreeding techniques employed to fix desired productive traits or appearances in sheep from Bakewell's time? He lived from 1726 to 1795, and early reports of scrapie in Britain date to the middle of the 18th century. His experiments were preceded by Spanish work on Merino sheep to fix the type for very fine wool, and the disease was reported to have arrived in Britain from Southern Europe.

As already noted, the pathophysiology of TSEs is thought to result from the conversion of the normal prion protein into a so-called scrapie form. The latter is thought to trigger an autocatalytic transformation of the normal PrP[c] to its PrP[Sc] three-dimensional structure. This form tends to aggregate spontaneously in such a way that plaques form in the brain. These lead to neuronal destruction and the spongiform state typical of the pathology found after clinical signs appear (Eigen 1996). The disease is unusual because the degenerative process in the brain takes so long to appear. The time scale of the changes requires a clearer molecular explanation, other than the simplistic term *incubation period*.

The prion theory still cannot explain the full picture of the corruption of normal prion proteins to the destructive form. An explanation proposed for the mechanism by some researchers is that an unspecified factor, labeled *protein X*, is required to bind to a normal prion molecule, thereby acting as a "molecular chaperone," a catalyst-like agent to shepherd the PrP^c into proximity with the arriving PrP^{Sc} to achieve the refolding reaction they define as a form of *replication*. At this point, the chaperone dissociates from the original prion, leaving two PrP^{Sc} molecules where one was before (Aunger 2002). So it seems that the PrP^{Sc} molecules, having gained entry to the brain, cannot "go it alone" as infectious parasites but rather depend upon a molecular process that will not be understood until the chaperones are identified. Until then, perhaps, the prion-related diseases seem to be more like intoxications than infections.

It is now clear that TSE diseases require a genetic susceptibility that renders some strains much more susceptible than others. Selection for desired traits may unwittingly have been accompanied by selection for TSE vulnerability.

Ingested neurotoxic prions, after gaining entry to the brain, have the capacity to wreak pathophysiological havoc in consumers that is remarkable in its prolonged slow molecular disruption of the function of the brain. *Incubation*, a term implying infection in common usage, seems inappropriate, although there definitely is a degenerative process going on over a long period after it gains entry. Recording of physiological events in unrestrained cattle throughout a full 24-hour day, in a Ruckebusch-style approach to pathophysiology, Austin and colleagues (1993) showed that the onset of CNS damage to vagus nuclei was manifested by suppression of rumination and altered (a slowed rate) cardiac performance. The toxic prion is nonbiodegradable by the host's tissues, so it just builds up in the brain and damages the tissue progressively. This allows or causes it to acquire its toxicant efficacy via a new form of bioaccumulation not too different from that seen in Alzheimer's disease.

Rather than being a new kind of infectious agent, perhaps a better description would be a new kind of *toxicant*. One should look back to Gajdusek and Hadlow's concept of an infectious cause of kuru after it was shown to be transmissible by intracerebral inoculation of extracts of material from brains of kuru cases to chimpanzees. However, once the etiology of the disease was established to be the consumption of human cadaver tissue from affected cases and con-

trols were instituted to eliminate the practice, it soon disappeared from the tribes that had indulged in the deadly rite. Hadlow noted that the resulting neural lesions bore a striking resemblance on histopathology to those of scrapie, which was then a mysterious but naturally occurring disease that was considered to be infectious but in a controversial and limited way. Parry (1962, 1983a, b) showed that susceptibility of sheep to scrapie depended on genetics, with the Suffolk breed having the highest incidence. His insights were criticized at the time, but the remarkable progress in the molecular biology of susceptibility and resistance to the hazardous prions has led to a plan to exploit the resistance of some ovine strains to scrapie in an eradication strategy involving genetic typing as a basis for selective breeding against susceptible strains.

The difference between scrapie and BSE seems to lie in the fact that BSE can be eradicated by ensuring that the agent does not enter the diet of a susceptible host. Scrapie, however, does spread among *susceptible* sheep. It would be reassuring to farmers, who do not want their products to be a threat to human health, and to consumers who want to avoid risk, if the specter of an enormous potential epidemic of a prion-based disease could be lifted. Obviously, recycling dead tissue back into animal diets after rendering must be avoided worldwide. Just as toxic amines that are present in carcasses of mammals that died can be eaten with apparent impunity by scavengers like vultures, crows, and hyenas, it may be that these types of recycling creatures (including dogs) are also uniquely adapted to processing prions in decaying dead tissue. New ways must be developed to dispose of unwanted animal tissues. CWD is a special risk because it spreads by direct passage once it enters the cervid populations in which it causes progressive emaciation or wasting away. Intensive studies are under way (Spraker et al. 2002). Although the agent has not been shown to spread to noncervid species, hunters are advised to abstain from dining on the fruits of their efforts in the hunt. Mabbott and Bruce (2001) have proposed a new hypothesis for the way in which transmissible spongiform TSE agents like BSE gain entry via the intestinal epithelium's M cells to dendritic cells and ganglion cells of the enteric nervous system that convey it centrally to the brain (Figure 13.6).

Research directed at seeking a therapeutic approach to the syndrome known as variant of CJD (vCJD) thought to be caused by ingestion of preformed BSE prions via an affected dietary component has shown promise in laboratory animal studies. There have been about 100 such human cases so far, and one compound that has shown promise is pentosan phosphate infused directly into the brain. It appears that this type of agent can combine with and perhaps neutralize the toxicants to some extent.

Since the disease is usually, if not always, fatal, this research has become a high priority. Again the "Parry

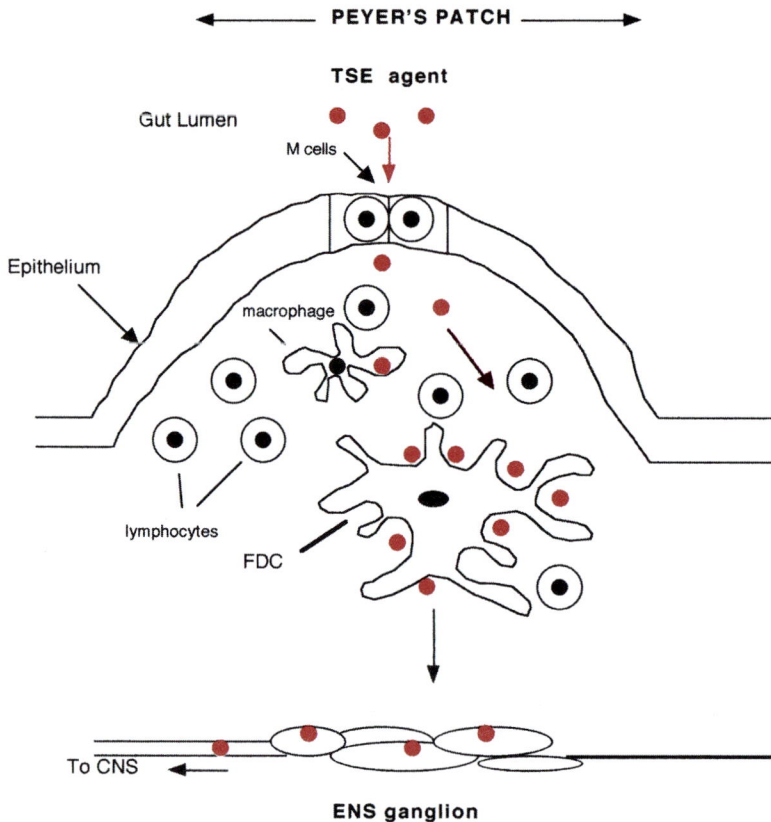

<- — **PEYER'S PATCH** — ->

TSE agent

Gut Lumen

M cells

Epithelium

macrophage

lymphocytes

FDC

To CNS

ENS ganglion

FIG. 13.6—Hypothesis for access of the transmissible spongiform encephalopathy (TSE) agent to the central nervous system (CNS). Following ingestion of recycled ruminant tissues in the form of meat and bone meal derived from affected cows and the passage of the indigestible toxicant to the intestine, it crosses the epithelium. This occurs at specialized membranous cells known as M cells overlying Peyer's patches of lymphoid tissue. Some of the particles may be engulfed by macrophages and interact with lymphocytes. However, the most important element may be the mysterious octopus-like follicular dendritic cells (FDCs) that may act as antigen-processing cells. The TSE agent may be a misfolded prion protein that, after conditioning, enters ganglion cells of the enteric nervous system (ENS) and then travels rostrally up their axons to spinal cord and brain, where it wreaks its destructive effect. The syndrome was not infectious from bovine to bovine, and the epidemic declined as soon as the agent was eliminated from the diet.

initiative," identifying genetically susceptible and resistant subpopulations, has borne fruit. All of the vCJD cases in humans have been methionine 121 homozygous, indicating that genetics is important in susceptibility to the human syndrome of vCJD. Deer and elk species and strains vary in their susceptibility to CWD.

RECOMMENDED READING

Aunger R. 2002. The replication zoo. In: The Electric Meme: A New Theory of How We Think. New York: Free Press, pp 93–101.

Austin AR, Simmons MM. 1993. Reduced rumination in bovine spongiform encephalopathy and scrapie. Vet Rec 132:324–325.

Austin AR, Hawkins SAC, Kelay NS, Simmons MM. 1993. New observations on the clinical signs of BSE and scrapie. In: Bradley R, Marchant B, eds. Transmissible Spongiform Encephalopathies. Proceedings of Consultation on BSE with the Scientific Veterinary Community Of the European Communities, Brussels, 9/14–9/15, 1993.

Badiola JJ, Monleon E, Monzon M, et al. 2002. Description of the first cases of BSE in Spain. Vet Rec 151:509–510.

Eigen M. 1996. Prionics or the kinetic basis of prion diseases. Biophys Chem 63:A1–A18.

Kimberlin RH. 1996. Speculations on the Origin of BSE and the Epidemiology of CJD. In: Gibbs CJ, ed. Bovine Spongiform Encephalopathy. New York: Springer-Verlag.

Lasmézas CI, Adams DB, coordinators. 2003. Risk Analysis of Prion Diseases in Animals. OIE Sci Tech Rev 22(1), 331 pp.

Mabbott NA, Bruce ME. 2001. The immunobiology of TSE diseases. J Gen Virol 82:2307–2318.

Parry HB. 1962. Scrapie: A transmissible and hereditary disease of sheep. Heredity 17:75–105.

Parry HB. 1983a. Recorded occurrences of scrapie from 1750. In: Oppenheimer DR, ed. Scrapie Disease in Sheep. London: Academic, pp 31–59.

Parry HB. 1983b. Scrapie Disease in Sheep. London: Academic.

Spraker TR, Zink RR, Cummings BA, et al. 2002. Distribution of protease-resistant prion protein and spongiform encephalopathy in free-ranging mule deer (*Odocoileus hemionus*) with chronic wasting disease. Vet Pathol 39:546–556.

PART 5: GENERAL READINGS WITH BROAD COVERAGE

Aiello SE, ed. 1998. The Merck Veterinary Manual, 8th ed. Whitehouse Station, NJ: Merck.

Albert A. 1987. Xenobiosis. New York: Chapman and Hall.

Andrews P, Widdicombe J, eds. 1993. Pathophysiology of the Gut and Airways: An Introduction. Chapel Hill, NC: Portland Bar.

Blaxter K. 1989. Energy Metabolism in Animals and Man. New York: Cambridge University Press.

Burrows GE, Tyrl RJ. 2001. Toxic Plants of North America. Ames: Iowa State University Press.

CAST (Council for Agricultural Science and Technology). 2003. Mycotoxins: Risks in Plant, Animal and Human Systems. Task Force Report no. 139. Ames, IA: CAST.

Cheeke PR. 1998. Natural Toxicants in Feeds, Forages, and Poisonous Plants, 2nd ed. Danville, IL: Interstate.

Clarke ML, Harvey DG, Humphreys DJ. 1981. Veterinary Toxicology, 2nd ed. London: Ballière, Tindall.

D'Mello JPF, ed. 1997. Handbook of Plant and Fungal Toxicants. Boca Raton, FL: CRC.

D'Mello JPF. 2000. Anti-nutritional Factors and Mycotoxins. In: D'Mello JPF, ed. Farm Animal Metabolism and Nutrition. Wallingford, UK: CAB International.

Fruton JS. 1992. A Skeptical Biochemist. Cambridge: Harvard University Press.

Garland T, Barr AC. 1998. eds. Toxic Plants and Other Natural Toxicants. New York: AB International.

Greger R, Windhorst U. 1996. Comprehensive Human Physiology, 2 vols. New York: Springer-Verlag.

Hardman JG, Limberg LE. 2001. Goodman and Gilman's The Pharmacological Basis of Therapeutics, 10th ed. New York: McGraw-Hill.

Henderson B, Wilson M, McNab R, Lax AJ. 1999. Cellular Microbiology: Bacteria-Host Interactions in Health and Disease. New York: Wiley.

Holland SM, ed. 2001. Cytokine Therapeutics in Infectious Diseases. Philadelphia: Lippincott Williams and Wilkins.

Josephy PD. 1997. Molecular Toxicology. New York: Oxford University Press.

Lingappa VR, Farey K. 2000. Physiological Medicine: A Clinical Approach to Basic Medical Physiology. New York: McGraw-Hill, Medical Publishing Division, ch 11: Physiology of the hypothalamus and pituitary; ch 13: Adrenal physiology, ch 19: Introduction to host defence.

Mabbott NA, Bruce ME. 2001. The immunobiology of TSE diseases. J Gen Virol 82:2307–2318.

Madigan MT, Martinko JM, Parker J. 2000. Brock: Biology of Microorganisms, 9th ed. Upper Saddle River, NJ: Prentice Hall.

McDowell LR. 2000. Vitamins in Animal and Human Nutrition. Ames: Iowa State University Press.

Osweiler GD, Carson TL, Buck WB, Van Gelder GA. 1985. Clinical and Diagnostic Veterinary Toxicology. Dubuque, IA: Kendall/Hunt.

Panksepp J. 1998. Affective Neuroscience: The Foundations of Human and Animal Emotions. New York: Oxford University Press.

Pough FH, Janis CM, Heison JB. 2002. Vertebrate Life, 6th ed. Upper Saddle River, NJ: Prentice Hall.

Radeleff RD. 1964. Veterinary Toxicology. Philadelphia: Lea and Febiger.

Radostits OM, Gay CC, Blood DC, Hinchcliff KW. 2000. Veterinary Medicine, 9th ed. London: WB Saunders.

Rang HP, Dale MM, Ritter JM, Gardner P. 1995. Pharmacology. New York: Churchill Livingstone.

Ruckebusch Y, Phaneuf L-P, Dunlop RH. 1981. Physiology of Small and Large Animals. Philadelphia: BC Decker.

Ruckebusch Y. 1981. Physiologie, Pharmacologie, Therapeutique Animales. Paris: Maloine.

Schmidt-Nielsen K. 1997. Animal Physiology: Adaptation and Environment, 5th ed. New York: Cambridge University Press.

Shepherd GM. 1994. Neurobiology, 3rd ed. New York: Oxford University Press, Aversion Learning, pp 633–635.

Silbernagl S, Lang F. 2000. Color Atlas of Pathophysiology. New York: Thieme.

Spencer PS, Schaumberg HH, eds. 2000. Experimental and Clinical Toxicology, 2nd ed. Oxford: Oxford University Press.

Underwood EJ, Suttle NF. 2001. The Mineral Nutrition of Livestock, 3rd ed. New York: CAB International.

Voet D, Voet JG, Pratt CW. 1999. Fundamentals of Biochemistry. New York: John Wiley and Sons.

CONCLUSION RELEVANT TO THE ENTIRE TEXT.

Because it states the goal of pathophysiology so appropriately, it seems worth repeating the quote by Greger and Windhorst cited in the Preface:

> The challenge is to cope with the rising flood of outcomes of reductionist research and, at the same time deal with the fundamental question of how the parts and pieces interact. How cells are coordinated to function as an organ, how the organs are coordinated and cooperate in systems, and how the systems' functions are integrated in the somatomotor and neurovegetative behavior of the whole organism when adapting to internal and external needs—a highly dynamic science based on functional thinking and embedded in the fascinating ever-continuing process of learning more about life. [To which I would add, "including its resilience and its frailty."] (Greger and Windhorst 1996)

A hierarchy of biological rhythms superimposed on homeostatic autoregulatory feedback circuits play an important role in the coordination of various body functions. This requires crossing borders to new ways of thinking and other disciplines and concepts—the mathematics of rhythmic self-organizing systems. Note the PNI paradigm: *psychoneuroimmunology*.

Greger and Windhorst also quote W.B. Cannon: "Indeed, regulation in the organism is the central problem in physiology."

INDEX

Page references in *italics* denote figures. References followed by a t denote tables.

Abomasum
  disturbances with parasitic
    infections, 120–121
  mechanisms controlling function,
    120, *121*
  motility and transport, 119–120
ABPE (acute bovine pulmonary
  edema emphysema), 173
Absorption, gastrointestinal tract
  alterations
    enteroinvasive diarrhea, 124
    enterotoxigenic diarrhea,
      123–124
  of calcium, 404
  electrogenic substrate-couple
    sodium absorption in small
    intestine, 121–122
  electroneutral sodium chloride
    adsorption, 122, *122*
  mechanism, basic, 121
ACE (angiotensin-converting
  enzyme), 205
Acetaminophen
  excretion and hepatotoxicity of,
    389
  hepatic necrosis from, 393, *393*
Acetoacetate, 382
Acetylcholine, 304–305
ACh receptors, toxicant effects on,
  502, *503*
Acid-base balance
  clinical assessment, 15
  defenses against acidosis and
    alkalosis, 14
  renal regulation of, 11
  SID (strong ion differences), 15
  treatment of disturbances, 14–15
Acidosis, 14
Acini, liver, 372
Acremonium coenophialum, 500
Acremonium lolii, 500
Acrosome, 226
ACTH (adrenocorticotropic
  hormone), 346, 480–483
Actin, 260–261
Active sodium transport
  inhibitor/endogenous digitalis-
  like inhibitor (ASTI/EDLI), 6,
  12
Acute abdomen. *See* Colic
Acute bovine pulmonary edema
  emphysema (ABPE), 173
Acutely transforming oncoviruses,
  49

Acute-phase proteins, 384–385, 385t
Adaptive cytoprotection, 126
Adaptive immune defenses, 99–108
Adaptive relaxation, stomach, 112
ADCC (antibody-dependent cell-
  mediated cytotoxicity), 65
Adenocarcinoma, hypercalcemia
  and, 437
Adenoma, thyroid, 451
Adenosarcoma, 69
Adenosine triphosphate (ATP)
  muscle use, 262–263
  production of, 480
ADH (antidiuretic hormone), 6,
  10–11
Adhesion, of infectious agents,
  85–86, *86*
Adrenocorticotropic hormone
  (ACTH), 346, 480–483
Adult respiratory distress syndrome
  (ARDS), 168
Aerobes, 84
Aerobic exercise, skeletal muscle
  responses to, 263, 263t
Affective attack, 310
Aflatoxins, 55, 499–500
African trypanosomiasis, 99–101,
  100
Afterload, 188, *188*
Aggression, 310, 358–359
Aging, pathophysiology of, 316
AhR (arylhydrocarbon-activated
  receptor), 389
Airway resistance to airflow, 145
Alanine aminotransferase (ALT),
  396
Albumin, 383–384, 397
Aldosterone, 6, 11, 12
Alkali disease, 328
Alkaline phosphatase, 396
Alkaloids, 308, 496, 498, 500, 501
Alkalosis, 14
Allergic bronchitis, 152
Allergy, 504
Alpha-amino-3-hydroxy-5-methyl-4-
  isoxazole propionic acid
  (AMPA), 306, *307,* 314
α-fetoprotein, 64
1α-hydroxylase, 417, *418,* 424–425,
  438, 452
α-latrotoxin, *502,* 502–503
α-mannosidosis, 497
5α-reductase, 215, 218
ALT (alanine aminotransferase), 396

Alternaria, 500
Alternative pathway, 98
Altrenogest (Regumate), 236
ALV (avian leukosis virus), 51, *51*
Alveolar edema, 163, *164*
Alveolitis, fibrosing, 154–155
Amanita phalloides, 393
Amino acids, liver metabolism of,
  383–385
Ammonia
  as air pollutant, 169
  in hepatic encephalopathy, 392,
    396
  hyperammonemia, 329–330, 332
Ammoniated forage toxicosis, 332
AMPA (alpha-amino-3-hydroxy-5-
  methyl-4-isoxazole propionic
  acid), 306, *307,* 314
Amygdala, 310
Amyloidosis, islet, 471–474
Anabena, 501
Anabolic steroids, 235–236
Anaerobes, 84
Anaerobic bacteria, exotoxic
  endospore-forming, 501
Anaerobic exercise, skeletal muscle
  responses to, 263, 263t
Anaphase, 28, *29*
Anaphylactic shock, 209
Anaphylatoxins, 137, 138, 138t
Anaphylaxis, 504
Androgens
  anabolic steroids, 235–236
  disorders in sexual differentiation,
    218
  metabolic balance and, 480–481
Andromeda, 498–499
Anestrus, pathological, 224
Aneurysm, 201
Angiogenesis, 44–45, 206, *207*
Angiogenic switch, 44
Angiotensin, 12, 17
Angiotensin-converting enzyme
  (ACE), 205
Angiotensin II, 6, 205
Anhydrosis, 487
Anion gap, 15
Anovulatory follicles in mares, 225
ANP. *See* Atrial natriuretic peptide
Antibody
  natural, 95
  structure and function, 101–102
Antibody-dependent cell-mediated
  cytotoxicity (ADCC), 65